# PTEXAM
## The Complete Study Guide

**SCOREBUILDERS** / PTEXAM: The Complete Study Guide

# Copyright ©2013

ISBN 978-1-890989-32-3

The enclosed material is the exclusive property of **Scorebuilders**.
No part of this publication may be reproduced or transmitted,
in any form, without the express written consent of **Scorebuilders**.

For additional information on our review texts, review courses,
and web-based testing programs for physical therapists
and physical therapist assistants, please contact **Scorebuilders**.

# SCOREBUILDERS

P.O. Box 7242
Scarborough, Maine 04070-7242

Toll Free: (866) PTEXAMS
Phone: (207) 885-0304
Fax: (207) 883-8377

## Web Site: www.scorebuilders.com

## Legal Notice

**Scorebuilders** strives to ensure that the information presented in **PTEXAM: The Complete Study Guide** is both accurate and relevant to the NPTE. **Scorebuilders** assumes no responsibility for the accuracy or reliability of the information within the review book. Under no circumstances will **Scorebuilders** be liable for incidental or consequential damage arising from the use of our licensing products. Candidate performance on the sample examinations should be used only as a method to assess strengths and weaknesses and should not be utilized as a predictor of actual examination performance. Any similarity in the questions contained within the sample examinations and the questions on any version of the National Physical Therapy Examination is purely coincidental.

# PT EXAM
## The Complete Study Guide

**Scott M. Giles PT, DPT, MBA**

President, Scorebuilders

Your Ticket to Success

# Acknowledgments

## Dedication

The new edition of ***PTEXAM: The Complete Study Guide*** and every future edition is dedicated to Gwenn Hoyt. Thanks for your years of support, love, and expertise. You are greatly missed for so many reasons.

## Special Thanks

### Therese Giles PT, MS
I would like to thank my wife, Traci, for her substantial contributions to all areas of the project. You are a great teammate and, of course, my best friend.

### Michael Fillyaw PT, MS
I would like to thank Mike for his many contributions to this project.

### Shawn Paquette
I would like to thank Shawn for all of his editing efforts and tremendous attention to detail.

### Jennifer Vance
I would like to thank Jen for her efforts to coordinate the photo shoots and for her involvement in many other important aspects of this project.

### Heather Ganter
I would like to thank Heather for her willingness to share her considerable photography talent. The images are a wonderful addition to the new edition.

### Allyson Harvey
I would like to thank Allyson for her technical and creative skills.

### Erin Giles and Grace Farnkoff
I would like to thank Erin and Grace for their many contributions throughout the creating of the new edition.

## Thank Yous

Thanks to the many student volunteers from academic programs throughout the country that served as reviewers throughout the project.

## Book and Cover Design

### Lucian Burg, LuDesign Studios, Portland, Maine
I would like to thank Lucian for his technical and artistic expertise throughout the creation of the new edition. You did a fantastic job bringing the new edition to life.

## CD Design and Creation

### Jeff Cullaton, Plan C Solutions
I would like to thank Jeff for his technical expertise and willingness to create and adapt the CD to the many nuances associated with the current National Physical Therapy Examination.

# Contributing Authors

## Scott M. Giles P.T., D.P.T., M.B.A.
President, Scorebuilders
Scarborough, Maine

## Therese Giles P.T., M.S.
Vice President, Scorebuilders
Scarborough, Maine

## Michael Fillyaw P.T., M.S.
Clinical Associate Professor
Department of Physical Therapy
University of New England
Portland, Maine

## Danielle Cowan P.T., B.S., CLT-LANA
Developer, Scorebuilders
Scarborough, Maine

## Ryan Bailey P.T., D.P.T.
Holistic Physical Therapy Services
South Portland, Maine

# Introduction

The new edition of **PTEXAM: The Complete Study Guide** is the most comprehensive resource available for the National Physical Therapy Examination and sets a new standard for review book excellence. The resource is a virtual visual delight with full color and hundreds of images. We have significantly expanded the academic review section and have added chapter essentials and proficiency exercises to ensure student mastery of critical National Physical Therapy Examination content.

**PTEXAM: The Complete Study Guide** provides candidates with a number of powerful study tools each designed to prepare candidates for the breadth and depth associated with the current National Physical Therapy Examination. A brief description of each unit in the study guide is listed below.

## Unit 1 - Introduction to the National Physical Therapy Examination

The unit provides candidates with information on the purpose, development, scoring, and administration of the National Physical Therapy Examination. Candidates are introduced to a systematic approach to answering multiple-choice questions and are exposed to recent developments in item construction. The unit also provides a detailed analysis of each of the content outline and system specific areas of the National Physical Therapy Examination. By exploring the categories and subcategories of each of the content outline and system specific areas candidates gain a better understanding of the breadth and depth of the current examination and as a result spend less time covering topics that are not clinically relevant. The unit offers a variety of study concepts that candidates can utilize to increase the effectiveness of study sessions when preparing for the National Physical Therapy Examination.

## Unit 2 - Academic Review

The unit provides candidates with an efficient method to review didactic information from a physical therapy curriculum. The academic review consists of eight distinct chapters of academic information. The first six chapters consist of academic content in specific systems (e.g., musculoskeletal) and non-systems (e.g., equipment and devices) areas. The final chapter in the unit includes a description of the physical therapy management of 60 commonly encountered medical diagnoses on the National Physical Therapy Examination. The academic review avoids attempting to cover every aspect of a physical therapist's academic training and instead focuses on the most essential information necessary to maximize examination performance. Since the examination is designed to assess entry-level practice it is likely that candidates will encounter the information presented in the academic review frequently on the actual examination. Mastery of the information can significantly increase candidates' scores on the National Physical Therapy Examination.

## Unit 3 - Computer-Based Examinations

The unit provides candidates with three, 200 question sample examinations located on a CD. The examinations were developed based on selected specifications from the current content outline and are designed to expose candidates to the nuances of computer based testing. Candidates are able to generate a detailed performance analysis summary that identifies current strengths and weaknesses according to content outline and system specific areas. The examinations provide candidates with the opportunity to refine their test taking skills and to assess their current preparedness for the examination. An answer key includes an explanation specifying why the correct answer is correct and an explanation specifying why each incorrect answer is incorrect. The answer key also includes a cited resource with page number, and the assigned content outline and system specific area.

*Additional resources to assist candidates with their preparation for the National Physical Therapy Examination are located at the conclusion of the text.

# Author's Note

Congratulations on your decision to purchase **PTEXAM: The Complete Study Guide**. I am extremely confident that you will be pleased with your purchase. Leave no stone unturned in your preparation for this important examination and strive to make your examination score reflect your academic knowledge. Candidates that have a firm grasp of didactic information combined with a meaningful study plan emphasizing applied knowledge are often richly rewarded on this challenging examination. We are confident that our text will be a valuable component of your comprehensive study program. Although undoubtedly there will be many magical moments in your life, you will never forget the moment when you become licensed as a physical therapist. **Best of luck on the examination and in your future career endeavors!**

# Table of Contents

| Chapter 1 Unit 1 | 2 | **National Physical Therapy Examination Basics** *Scott Giles* |
|---|---|---|
| Chapter 2 Unit 1 | 14 | **National Physical Therapy Examination Blueprint** *Scott Giles* |
| Chapter 3 Unit 1 | 32 | **Study Concepts** *Scott Giles* |
| Chapter 4 Unit 2 | 44 | **Musculoskeletal System** *Scott Giles* |
| Chapter 5 Unit 2 | 134 | **Neuromuscular and Nervous Systems** *Therese Giles* |
| Chapter 6 Unit 2 | 234 | **Cardiovascular/Pulmonary and Lymphatic Systems** *Michael Fillyaw* |
| Chapter 7 Unit 2 | 312 | **Other Systems** *Therese Giles, Scott Giles, Danielle Cowan, Ryan Bailey* |
| Chapter 8 Unit 2 | 404 | **Equipment and Devices; Therapeutic Modalities** *Scott Giles* |
| Chapter 9 Unit 2 | 484 | **Safety and Protection; Professional Responsibilities; Research** *Scott Giles, Therese Giles, Michael Fillyaw* |
| Chapter 10 Unit 2 | 554 | **Clinical Application Templates** *Scott Giles, Therese Giles* |
| Chapter 11 Unit 3 | 688 | **Exam One** *Scott Giles* |
| Chapter 12 Unit 3 | 792 | **Exam Two** *Scott Giles* |
| Chapter 13 Unit 3 | 894 | **Exam Three** *Scott Giles* |
| | 996 | **Exam References, Exam & Academic Review Indexes, Motivational Moments and Resources** |

# 1

# NATIONAL PHYSICAL THERAPY EXAMINATION BASICS

## Scott Giles

4 Examination Content Outline

4 Examination Scoring

4 Applying for the Examination

6 Examination Administration

7 Test Taking Skills

7 Multiple-Choice Questions

9 Activity One

11 Activity Two

13 Time Constraints

13 Preparing for the Examination

SCOREBUILDERS

The National Physical Therapy Examination (NPTE) is a 250 question (200 scored, 50 pre-test), multiple-choice examination designed to determine if candidates possess the minimal competency necessary to practice as physical therapists.

The examination is created under the auspices of the Federation of State Boards of Physical Therapy (FSBPT). According to the *National Physical Therapy Examination Candidate Handbook*, the examination program serves three important purposes:

1. Provide examination services to regulatory authorities charged with the regulation of physical therapists and physical therapist assistants.

2. Provide a common element in the evaluation of candidates so that standards will be comparable from jurisdiction to jurisdiction.

3. Protect the public interest in having only those persons who have the requisite knowledge of physical therapy be licensed to practice physical therapy.

There are two primary methods to obtain a license to practice as a physical therapist in the United States. They are termed examination and endorsement. Licensure by examination is obtained after a candidate meets or exceeds the minimum scoring requirement on the National Physical Therapy Examination and has satisfied all other state requirements. This form of obtaining licensure is the traditional method for candidates seeking initial licensure.

Licensure by endorsement makes it possible for candidates who have already been licensed in a state by virtue of an examination to potentially gain licensure in another state without retaking the examination. Examination scores can be transferred to any physical therapy state licensing agency via the Federation of State Boards of Physical Therapy Score Transfer Service. The web site address for the Federation of State Boards of Physical Therapy is available in the Appendix.

Although the National Physical Therapy Examination is 250 questions, 50 of the questions serve only as pre-test items and are not officially scored. The pre-test items allow new examination questions to be evaluated throughout the year and eliminate lengthy delays in score reporting when new examinations are introduced. Candidates are unable to differentiate between pre-test and scored items on the examination.

The 250 questions are administered to candidates in five sections consisting of 50 questions each. Each section contains scored items and pre-test items, although the number of pre-test and scored items in each section may vary slightly. Candidates have five hours to complete the five sections at their own pace. Since the sections are not timed individually, it is important for candidates to effectively manage their allotted time as they progress through each of the five sections. Candidates have the opportunity to take one scheduled break at the conclusion of section two, immediately prior to beginning section three. Additional unscheduled breaks can be taken at the conclusion of a given section, however, the elapsed time will not stop. If a candidate does not want to take the break or prefers a shorter break, they can end the break by following the directions displayed on the computer screen. Candidates can leave the examination only when either a scheduled or unscheduled break message is displayed on the computer. Leaving the testing room while not on a designated break will result in an examination irregularity being reported to the FSBPT.

Candidates are unable to return to previously completed sections once a new section is initiated. The academic content is randomized within each section and scoring is based only on the number of questions a candidate answers correctly out of the 200 scored items. As a result, each of the examinations in **PTEXAM: The Complete Study Guide** consists of only 200 questions (four sections, each consisting of 50 questions). Candidates will have four hours to complete each of the 200 question sample examinations.

The FSBPT publishes a content outline which describes the specific categories and subcategories of the examination. The categories and subcategories are based on the tasks and roles that comprise the practice of physical therapy. Once established, the content outline remains active for a period of approximately five years. The most recent version was implemented in January of 2013. The five main categories of the examination are listed here, although the entire content outline will be discussed in detail in **Chapter 2**.

Candidates should attempt to integrate this information in conjunction with the performance analysis summary to accurately identify current strengths and weaknesses and develop appropriate remedial strategies. The computer-based examinations include a number of helpful tools to assist candidates to integrate this information. Candidates should avoid becoming overly excited or depressed based on the results of a given sample examination and use the number of questions answered correctly only as a general indicator of their current level of preparedness. Studying for the examination is much closer to running a marathon than running a sprint. By engaging in meaningful self-assessment activities, candidates can gather valuable information to improve future examination performance.

## Examination Content Outline

**Physical Therapy Examination**

**Foundations for Evaluation, Differential Diagnosis, & Prognosis**

**Interventions**

**Equipment & Devices; Therapeutic Modalities**

**Safety and Protection; Professional Responsibilities; Research and Evidence-Based Practice**

According to the FSBPT, the involvement of a large representative group of practicing physical therapists and other professionals at each stage of examination development ensures that the examinations are relevant to the practice of physical therapy. Individual physical therapists are responsible for writing examination questions. The physical therapists involved are required to attend item-writing workshops that are taught by experienced testing professionals. Questions, once completed, are analyzed independently to make sure they are reflective of the current examination content outline. Examination questions tend to focus on decision making and not purely rote memorization of fact. Successful candidates on the examination must demonstrate the ability to apply knowledge in a safe and effective manner.

## Examination Scoring

The questions on the examination are multiple-choice with four possible answers to each question. Each option is listed as 1, 2, 3, 4. Options such as "none of the above," "all of the above," and "1 and 2 only" are not included on the examination. Candidates are asked to identify the best answer to each of the questions. Each question has only one best answer while the other possible answers serve as distracters. A candidate's score is determined based on the number of scored questions answered correctly. Since there is no penalty for questions answered incorrectly it is imperative that candidates answer all of the available questions. A candidate's cumulative score is termed the total raw score. The maximum total raw score for the National Physical Therapy Examination is 200.

Criterion-referenced scoring is used to determine passing scores on the National Physical Therapy Examination. Passing scores are based on the judgment of selected experts on the minimum number of questions that should be answered correctly by a minimally qualified candidate. Criterion-referenced passing scores are determined independently of candidate performance and are designed to reflect the difficulty level of each examination. For example, if a given examination was judged to be particularly difficult, the criterion-referenced passing score would be lower than the criterion-referenced passing score for another examination that was judged to be less difficult. All state licensing agencies have adopted the FSBPT criterion-referenced passing score and therefore do not individually determine passing scores at the state level. As a result, a passing score for a given examination will always be the same in all jurisdictions.

Since the minimum passing score varies based on the difficulty level of each examination, it is impossible to determine an automatic passing score. Criterion-referenced passing scores often range from 135 - 145. If the criterion-referenced passing score was established as 142 for a given examination, a total raw score of greater than or equal to 142 would be considered a passing score, while a total raw score of less than 142 would be considered a failing score. Within a given examination cycle, criterion-referenced passing scores usually fluctuate in a relatively small range, perhaps by as few as five questions.

An individual examination score is often reported to candidates in the form of a scaled score. Scaled scores range from 200 - 800 with the minimum passing score always being equal to a scaled score of 600. Scaled scores are necessary as a method of equating examinations with different criterion-referenced passing scores. A few state licensing agencies use a slightly different scaled score system where the minimum passing score is equivalent to a scaled score of 75.

## Applying for the Examination

Candidates planning to take the examination should request an application from the state licensing agency in the jurisdiction where they intend to practice as a physical therapist. Candidates are not permitted to apply for the examination in more than one jurisdiction at a time. The address, phone number, and web site for each agency is available at the Federation of State Boards of Physical Therapy (FSBPT) web site, www.fsbpt.org. All state licensing agencies offer online registration for the examination through the FSBPT.

Each state licensing agency can establish its own criteria to be eligible to sit for the National Physical Therapy Examination. A variety of items may be required as part of the application process. These items often include a photograph, a notarized birth certificate, an official transcript from an accredited school, professional reference letters, and a check or money order for the required application, examination, and licensing fees. After the necessary application forms have been completed, the information is returned along with any necessary fees to the state licensing agency or an identified intermediary. Candidates should recognize that even a small departure from the established eligibility criteria can lead to a significant delay in processing a candidate's application. To avoid such delays, it is prudent to read the application carefully and to inquire as to the status of the application approximately two weeks after the completed application has been submitted.

Foreign trained therapists are often subjected to a myriad of requirements before they are eligible to become licensed in the United States. Since the requirements vary significantly by state, it is recommended that candidates contact the state licensing agency within the state they intend to practice. The state licensing agency can provide detailed information on their individual requirements.

There are two general requirements for foreign trained therapists that seem to be consistent in all states:

- Applicants are required to submit their educational credentials for evaluation of their equivalence to the United States trained applicant.
- Applicants must meet or exceed the minimum scoring requirement on the National Physical Therapy Examination.

Other state requirements can include, but are not limited to, the following:

- Demonstrate proficiency in written and spoken English
- Submit letters of reference
- Obtain a valid visa and resident alien card
- Complete an internship or period of supervised practice
- Appear for an interview
- Attain the United States equivalent of a grade of "C" or higher in all professional coursework

Some states offer candidates with verifiable employment the opportunity to practice prior to being licensed by issuing a temporary license. Typically, candidates are required to have a completed application on file and have met all other qualifications for licensure before being considered for the temporary license. In most states temporary licenses are revoked if a candidate receives notification that they were unsuccessful on the National Physical Therapy Examination.

In addition to the National Physical Therapy Examination, a significant number of states require candidates to successfully complete a jurisprudence examination. This type of examination is based on the state rules and regulations governing physical therapy practice. The examination can include multiple-choice items, short-answer questions or fill in the blanks. States can administer the examination using computer-based testing or even as a take-home examination.

The NPTE officially moved from continuous testing to fixed-date testing on July 1, 2011. The change was necessitated by the need to substantially reduce or eliminate candidates' ability to gain a score advantage by having advance access to NPTE questions. The move to fixed-date testing has resulted in the establishment of a number of important dates and deadlines that are critical for all candidates. Candidates taking the NPTE in 2013 must register for one of the four established testing dates.

| Fixed-Date Testing | Registration and Payment Deadline | Jurisdiction Approval Deadline | Seat Reservation Deadline | Scores Reported |
|---|---|---|---|---|
| January 29 | December 22* | December 31* | January 8 | February 5 |
| April 30 | March 23 | April 1 | April 9 | May 7 |
| July 24 | June 17 | June 24 | July 3 | July 31 |
| October 30 | September 23 | September 30 | October 9 | November 6 |

*indicates 2012 date

2014 dates are presently unavailable, however, they will most likely be released in the summer of 2013. Candidates are encouraged to visit the FSBPT web site frequently since established dates and/or registration deadlines are subject to change. A dedicated fixed-date testing page has been integrated into the FSBPT web site: www.fsbpt.org/ForCandidatesAndLicensees/NPTE/FixedDateTestingInfo/

## Examination Administration

The examination is offered on computer at over 300 Prometric Testing Centers within the United States. Candidates are encouraged to make an appointment at a Prometric Testing Center as soon as they receive notification from the FSBPT that they are eligible. The move to fixed-date testing has created shortages at selected Prometric Testing Centers on specific fixed dates. As a result, the FSBPT recommends that candidates wait to make travel arrangements until after they have secured a scheduled test date and location.

Many Prometric Testing Centers will offer both a morning and afternoon appointment. When possible, candidates should schedule their examination at a time consistent with their optimal level of functioning. For example, if a candidate tends to be a "morning person," it would be prudent to schedule the examination in the morning. Candidates with significant anxiety may also want a morning appointment in order to avoid worrying about the examination throughout the day. If candidates are not familiar with the exact location of the examination site, it may be desirable to travel to the site before the actual examination date. The trip will provide candidates with an accurate idea of the time necessary to travel to the site and avoid the possibility of getting lost and subsequently being late for the examination.

Within each Prometric Testing Center, candidates can concentrate on the examination without environmental distracters. Private, modular booths provide adequate work space with proper lighting and ventilation. All Prometric Testing Centers are fully accessible and in compliance with the Americans with Disabilities Act. Candidates requesting accommodation for a documented disability must do so through the state licensing agency. Candidates are not limited to the testing centers within the state they are applying for licensure. For example, a candidate that has recently graduated from a physical therapy program in Maine could apply for licensure in California and take the required examination while still residing in Maine.

Candidates must arrive 30 minutes prior to their scheduled appointment with two forms of acceptable identification which include a government issued photo ID and another piece of identification preprinted with a name and a signature. The first and last names on both forms of ID must match the name on the Authorization to Test letter issued by the FSBPT. Candidates are photographed and a digital image of their fingerprint is taken prior to beginning the examination. Candidates cannot bring any electronic devices (e.g., watches, cell phones) or food and drink into the testing area. A locker will be provided to store personal items. Candidates can request headphones if they want to minimize background noise.

It is important to note that computer skills are not necessary with computer-based testing. Prior to beginning the examination, candidates utilize a tutorial that explains topics such as selecting answers and navigating within the examination. Time spent on the computer tutorial does not count toward the allotted time for the actual examination. The tutorial typically takes candidates less than ten minutes and if necessary, candidates can go through the tutorial a second time.

Candidates have the option of entering their answers using a computer keyboard or mouse. Candidates can go back to previously answered or unanswered questions and make any desired changes within a given section of 50 questions. Once a candidate submits a given section, they are unable to return to the questions within the section. Paper and pencil are not permitted in the Prometric Testing Centers, however, candidates are given an erasable note board or an electronic writing board to utilize during the examination.

The FSBPT is responsible for scoring the examination and reporting results to the individual state licensing agencies. According to the FSBPT, scores will be reported one week after the test date. This time allows the FSBPT to receive, process, and deliver to jurisdictions several thousand exam score files. The state licensing agencies then notify candidates as to their performance on the examination. Formal notification typically occurs through the mail, however, many state licensing agencies have web sites that allow candidates to determine their licensing status online. Some states permit candidates to access their examination status online within one week through the FSBPT.

If a candidate successfully completes the examination, in most cases they have fulfilled the final requirement for licensure. Conversely, if a candidate is unsuccessful on the examination, they are required to reapply to the state licensing agency. With computer-based testing there is no mandatory waiting period before retaking the examination, however, candidates will need to wait until the next fixed date. Some states limit the number of times a candidate can take the examination as well as mandate remedial coursework. In all states, candidates are prohibited from taking the examination more than three times in a 12 month period.

Candidates that were unsuccessful on the National Physical Therapy Examination can receive role feedback from the FSBPT. The role feedback report compares individual examination performance using the content outline and system specific categories with the performance of other candidates exposed to the same examination. Additional information on role feedback is available through the FSBPT.

## Test Taking Skills

Test taking skills are specific skills that allow individuals to utilize the characteristics and format of a selected examination in order to maximize their performance. These skills can be valuable when taking an examination such as the National Physical Therapy Examination. Despite the importance of this topic, very little, if any, academic time is set aside to address test taking skills. The good news is that test taking skills can be learned and that through dedication, desire, and determination, these skills can serve to improve examination performance.

The National Physical Therapy Examination consists of multiple-choice questions with four potentially correct answers to each question. Candidates are instructed to select the "best answer" to complete each question. Before exploring selected test taking strategies, we need to identify the various components of a multiple-choice question. Multiple-choice questions can be dissected into specific identifiable components:

**Item**   An item refers to an individual multiple-choice question and the corresponding potential answers. The National Physical Therapy Examination contains 200 scored items and 50 pre-test items. Each item consists of a stem and four options. Items may vary in content and length, but should utilize a consistent format.

**Stem**   The stem refers to the statement that asks the question. Typically, the stem conveys to the reader the necessary information needed to respond correctly to the question. In addition to the necessary information, extraneous information may be included in the stem. This information, when not recognized by the candidate as unnecessary, often can serve as a significant distracter.

The stem commonly takes on the form of a complete sentence or an incomplete sentence. The stem can be expressed in a positive or negative form. A positive form requires a candidate to identify correct information, while a negative form requires a candidate to identify incorrect information. It is important to scrutinize each stem, since a single key word such as "NOT," "EXCEPT" or "LEAST" can turn a positive stem into a negative stem. Failure to identify this can lead to the identification of an incorrect answer.

**Options**   The options refer to the potential answers to the question asked. One option in each item will be the "best answer," while the others are considered distracters. Options can take on a variety of forms, including a single word, a group of words, an incomplete sentence, a complete sentence or a group of sentences. The method for analyzing each option does not change, regardless of form.

## Approach for Answering Multiple-Choice Questions

On the National Physical Therapy Examination there are 250 items (200 scored, 50 pre-test) that candidates must answer within a five hour time period. Due to the length of the examination and the time constraints associated with it, candidates need to approach the examination in a systematic and organized fashion. Loss of control during the examination will yield poor results that are not reflective of a candidate's actual knowledge. To assist candidates to minimize the impact of this potential pitfall, we will introduce a systematic approach to utilize when answering sample examination items.

The following six-step approach is recommended as a method for answering examination items:

1. Read the stem carefully to become familiar with the item and to determine the command words that indicate the desired action.
2. Read the stem again and identify relevant words or groups of words based on the identified command words.
3. Attempt to generate an answer to the stem.
4. Examine each option completely before moving to the next option.
5. Attempt to identify the best option.
6. Utilize deductive reasoning strategies.

The six-step approach begins with a candidate reading the stem. Candidates should read the stem initially to determine the command words and the associated desired action. Once this has been determined, candidates can reread the stem and attempt to extract the necessary components including relevant words or groups of words.

Perhaps the most important step in the six-step approach is to have candidates attempt to generate an answer to each question based on the identified command words. This is the only opportunity a candidate will have to objectively evaluate the question prior to exposing each of the options. Once a candidate exposes the options, they are no longer able to examine the question in a fully objective manner and instead become more likely to have their interpretation of the question influenced by a presented option. If for some reason a candidate is unable to generate a specific answer, they should attempt to think about the general topic and recall related information. Once a possible answer is generated, candidates should then begin to examine each option one at a time. It is important to read the entire option, since one word can often make a potentially correct answer incorrect. If the generated answer is consistent with one of the available options, the candidate should give the option strong consideration, however, since more than one option can be correct, it is imperative to analyze each presented option.

If candidates finish analyzing an item and are still unable to select one of the available options they should consider using a deductive reasoning strategy. Deductive reasoning strategies allow candidates to improve examination scores without direct knowledge of subject matter. This type of strategy should be applied only when candidates are unable to identify the correct response using academic knowledge. Deductive reasoning strategies often allow candidates to eliminate one or more of the potential answers. Elimination of any option significantly increases the probability of identifying the correct answer. On the National Physical Therapy Examination, eliminating one option increases the chance of selecting a correct answer from 25% to 33%. Eliminating two options increases the chance of selecting a correct answer to 50%. On the surface, this may not seem terribly significant, however, on an examination such as the National Physical Therapy Examination, this can often be the difference between a passing and a failing score. Selected deductive reasoning strategies that can be used effectively on the National Physical Therapy Examination are presented.

### Absurd options

Many times a multiple-choice item will include an option that is not consistent with what the stem is asking or with the other options. In many cases, this option can be eliminated. Rapid elimination of specific options will allow candidates to spend additional time analyzing other more viable options.

### Similar options

When two or more options have a similar meaning or express the same fact, they often imply each other's incorrectness. For this reason, candidates can often eliminate both options.

### Obtainable information

There is a great deal of factual material that candidates must sift through when taking the National Physical Therapy Examination. In some instances, the material can provide candidates with valuable information that can assist them when answering other examination questions.

### Degree of qualification

Particularly in the sciences, there seems to be many exceptions to general rules. Therefore, specific wording such as "always" or "never" often overqualify an option.

# Activity One

In this activity, three sample questions are presented. Candidates should attempt to identify the best answer to each question by utilizing the six-step approach.

An analysis section immediately follows each of the three sample questions. The analysis section begins by showing the sample question with key terms underlined and command words in bold type. A brief narrative follows, which describes how the six-step approach can be applied to the sample question.

An answer key located at the conclusion of the exercise indicates the best answer and an explanation for each question.

## Sample Question One

A physical therapist instructs a patient with a Foley catheter in ambulation activities. During ambulation, the therapist should position the collection bag:

1. above the level of the patient's bladder
2. below the level of the patient's bladder
3. above the level of the patient's heart
4. below the level of the patient's heart

### Analysis

A physical therapist instructs a patient with a <u>Foley catheter in ambulation activities</u>. During ambulation, the therapist should **position the collection bag**:

1. above the level of the patient's bladder
2. below the level of the patient's bladder
3. above the level of the patient's heart
4. below the level of the patient's heart

A candidate should attempt to generate an answer to the question after reading the stem and identifying the pertinent information and command words. The candidate should then begin to reveal each of the available options one at a time. If a generated answer is consistent with one of the available options, there is a high probability that the answer is correct.

If a candidate was not able to generate an answer, they should expose the first option and give it careful consideration before moving on to the next option. They should progress through the remaining options in a similar manner. Candidates should remember it is possible to have more than one option that satisfactorily answers the question. It is then the candidate's responsibility to select the best answer from the viable options.

## Sample Question Two

A group of physical therapists attempts to determine the relationship between two variables on an examination form. Which of the following correlation coefficients would indicate the strongest relationship?

1. +.86
2. +.45
3. -.34
4. -.89

### Analysis

A group of physical therapists attempts to determine <u>the relationship between two variables</u> on an examination form. Which of the following <u>correlation coefficients</u> would indicate the **strongest relationship**?

1. +.86
2. +.45
3. -.34
4. -.89

After reading the stem and identifying the pertinent information and command words, a candidate should recognize that it is virtually impossible to generate an answer prior to viewing the available options. A candidate should, however, begin to think about correlation coefficients and determining the strength of the relationship between variables. The candidate should then expose each of the available options and attempt to identify the correct response.

Although the six-step approach does not directly supply a candidate with the correct response, by carefully reading the stem, a candidate can avoid an unnecessary mistake. In this item, the stem asks the candidate to identify the correlation coefficient that indicates the strongest relationship between the two variables. If a candidate does not read the question carefully, they may make an assumption that the stem is asking for the strongest positive relationship and subsequently answer the question incorrectly.

It is important that a candidate answer each item based only on the given information. By making even small assumptions or by not reading each item carefully, a candidate can make careless mistakes.

## Sample Question Three

A physical therapist completes an isokinetic examination on an 18-year-old male rehabilitating from a medial meniscectomy. The therapist notes that the patient generates 140 ft/lbs of force using the uninvolved quadriceps at 60 degrees per second. Assuming a normal ratio of hamstrings to quadriceps strength, which of the following would be an acceptable hamstrings value at 60 degrees per second?

1. 64 ft/lbs
2. 84 ft/lbs
3. 114 ft/lbs
4. 116 ft/lbs

### Analysis

A physical therapist completes an isokinetic examination on an 18-year-old male rehabilitating from a medial meniscectomy. The therapist notes that the patient generates 140 ft/lbs of force using the uninvolved quadriceps at 60 degrees per second. Assuming a normal ratio of hamstrings to quadriceps strength, which of the following would be **an acceptable hamstrings** value at 60 degrees per second?

1. 64 ft/lbs
2. 84 ft/lbs
3. 114 ft/lbs
4. 116 ft/lbs

For the purpose of discussion, let's assume a candidate has no idea of the normal ratio of quadriceps/hamstrings strength at 60 degrees per second. Lack of specific academic knowledge will result in a candidate not being able to identify the correct answer using the first five steps of the six-step approach. However, by utilizing deductive reasoning strategies, a candidate can significantly increase their chances of identifying the best answer without applying direct academic knowledge.

In this item, the stem asks a candidate to identify a value that would be representative of a normal quadriceps/hamstrings ratio at 60 degrees per second. As with many measurements in physical therapy, precise normal values are difficult to ascertain, and therefore often are expressed in ranges. Since options 3 and 4 are so close in value, they likely imply each other's incorrectness and can therefore be eliminated. Although in this example deductive reasoning strategies were not able to identify the correct answer, they were able to eliminate two of the four possible options. By eliminating two options, a candidate now has a 50% chance of identifying the best answer, even without utilizing any direct academic or clinical knowledge.

# Activity One – Answer Key

### 1. Correct Answer: 2

The effect of gravity necessitates the collection bag being below the level of the patient's bladder.

### 2. Correct Answer: 4

Correlation coefficients range from +1.00 to -1.00. Since the question does not ask for a positive or negative correlation, the strongest relationship is indicated by -.89.

### 3. Correct Answer: 2

A gross estimate of quadriceps:hamstrings ratio is 3:2. Option 2, 84 ft/lbs is therefore the most consistent with the expressed ratio.

## Recent Developments in Item Construction

There have been a number of changes in item construction on the National Physical Therapy Examination within the past few years, most notably the introduction of graphically enhanced items. Although representing a relatively small percentage of the total examination, candidates need to be comfortable answering this type of item. Graphically enhanced items will be incorporated into each of the sample examinations.

**Graphically Enhanced Items**

Graphically enhanced items consist of figures, diagrams, pictures or other static images that are combined with traditional text in an examination item.

## Activity Two

Two graphically enhanced items are presented. Candidates should attempt to identify the best answer to each question. An answer key located at the conclusion of the exercise indicates the best answer and an explanation for each question.

**The following image should be used to answer question 1:**

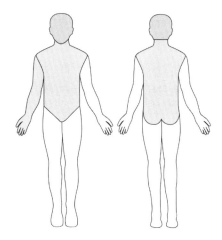

1. A 32-year-old male sustained extensive burns in a house fire. The shaded portion of the body diagrams represents the areas affected by the burns. Using the rule of nines, what percentage of the patient's body was involved?

   1. 40.5%

   2. 44.0%

   3. 49.5%

   4. 54.5%

**The following image should be used to answer question 2:**

2. A physical therapist instructs a patient to complete an exercise activity using a piece of elastic band as pictured. The patient is a 14-year-old female rehabilitating from a lower extremity injury sustained in a soccer contest. The therapist's primary objective for the activity is to:

   1. strengthen the right hip abductor muscles
   2. strengthen the right hip adductor muscles
   3. stretch the right hip abductor muscles
   4. stretch the right hip adductor muscles

# Activity Two – Answer Key

**1. Correct Answer: 3**

The percentage of the body surface burned in an adult can be calculated using the rule of nines: anterior thorax (18%) + posterior thorax (18%) + head (9%) + anterior arm (4.5%) = 49.5%.

**2. Correct Answer: 2**

Successful completion of the activity requires the adductor muscles to exert a force greater than the tension supplied by the elastic band while moving into hip adduction. Muscles acting to adduct the hip include the adductor longus, adductor brevis, adductor magnus, and gracilis.

## Time Constraints

Like many objective examinations, candidates have a specific allotted time to complete the National Physical Therapy Examination. For physical therapists, the available time is five hours. Since the examination consists of 250 questions, candidates will have 72 seconds available to answer each question. This number, although correct when viewing the examination as a whole, can be misleading. There will be many questions that a candidate will be able to answer in much less than 72 seconds, whereas other questions will take somewhat longer. The key to success lies in progressing through the examination in a consistent and predictable manner.

Although 72 seconds per question does not seem like a great deal of time, the majority of candidates will have ample time to complete the examination. Despite this fact, it is important to pay attention to the elapsed time during the examination. It also is important to know your test taking history. Are you typically one of the first, one of the last, or somewhere in the middle of individuals completing an examination? This information is important as you plan your test taking strategy. In order to make sure your pace is appropriate during practice sessions and during the actual examination, it is important to formally check on the elapsed time, at a very minimum, when completing each section of 50 questions. This action will allow candidates to assess their progress and modify their pace, if necessary.

## Preparing for the Examination

The simple thought of preparing for a comprehensive examination such as the National Physical Therapy Examination can be overwhelming. Many candidates ask themselves how it is possible to prepare adequately for an examination that encompasses up to three years of professional coursework. To further complicate matters, the majority of candidates take the National Physical Therapy Examination shortly after graduation. This can be a very anxious and unsettled time. Candidates often are actively seeking employment or are attempting to adjust to a new job. As a result, it is critical that candidates outline a well conceived and deliberate study plan for the examination.

One of the largest advantages of taking an examination such as the National Physical Therapy Examination is that it does not require candidates to demonstrate mastery of new material. On the surface, this may not seem like a significant advantage, but since candidates are, in effect, only reviewing or relearning previously presented information, their level of attainment should be significantly greater. Many candidates fail to utilize this advantage. Candidates who attempt to learn large quantities of new information, instead of focusing on understanding and applying basic concepts, often do themselves a tremendous disservice. It is true that there undoubtedly will be questions that contain information that was not part of a selected curriculum, but to attempt to study this new information in any significant detail would be a large mistake for most candidates. Instead, candidates should focus on reviewing or relearning basic concepts that are an integral component of all accredited physical therapy programs. It is this type of information that will make up the vast majority of the examination. Individuals who take this common sense approach optimize their chances of success.

In physical therapy academic programs, candidates constantly are learning new information on a variety of topics. Although students typically exhibit mastery of selected material during a scheduled examination, they do not always retain the information for later use. Often times, simply reviewing information is enough for candidates to relearn the material, however, in some cases, a more in-depth approach is necessary.

It is recommended that candidates pay particular attention to their practice-oriented professional coursework. Practice-oriented professional coursework includes, but is not limited to, study of the musculoskeletal, neuromuscular, cardiopulmonary, and integumentary systems. The content outline from the FSBPT clearly demonstrates the need for candidates to also review "other systems" (i.e., metabolic and endocrine, gastrointestinal, genitourinary, multi-system). In addition, candidates usually have coursework in patient care skills, physical agents, administration, ethics, research, and education. Each of these topics are important components of the content outline for the National Physical Therapy Examination, although the weighting of each item differs significantly. **Chapter 2** will offer specific information on the relative weighting of each area according to systems and non-systems categories.

Special attention must be taken not to become bogged down in one specific area for any significant amount of time. General concepts that are understood should be scanned quickly, while other concepts that are more difficult for a candidate should be read carefully. Concepts that remain unclear after being reviewed should be written down for future study sessions.

Other foundational coursework encountered earlier in the professional curriculum can be consulted as needed during various study sessions. This type of coursework often includes, but is not limited to anatomy and physiology, neuroanatomy, exercise physiology, and kinesiology. It is important to limit the amount of time spent reviewing this type of foundational coursework. Candidates often can make better use of their allotted time by reviewing coursework encountered later in the curriculum that may be more practice-oriented. By reviewing practice-oriented information, candidates not only keep their studying consistent with the format of the examination, but also at the same time indirectly review much of the information presented in the foundational coursework.

Before beginning to study, develop specific goals for each study session. Ideally, these goals should be established on a weekly basis. Establishing goals will ensure that candidates cover the desired material and will serve as a mechanism to keep them on schedule with their study plan. Candidates should be realistic with the goals they establish and should not attempt to cover more material than is possible in a particular study session.

# 2

# NATIONAL PHYSICAL THERAPY EXAMINATION BLUEPRINT

Scott Giles

15 Content Outline Summary

22 System Specific Summary

SCOREBUILDERS

Perhaps the most valuable piece of information a candidate can utilize when preparing for the National Physical Therapy Examination is the National Physical Therapy Examination Blueprint. The blueprint provides a detailed analysis of each of the content areas of the National Physical Therapy Examination. A thorough understanding of the content outline and system specific weighting will streamline a candidate's preparation. Less time will be spent covering topics that are not clinically relevant to the actual examination and as a result, more time will be available for reviewing and relearning.

This chapter will explore the examination in detail according to the content outline and system specific areas. Each of the sample examinations in **PTEXAM: The Complete Study Guide** offers candidates the opportunity to view their performance according to five system specific and five content outline categories. Candidates must be familiar with the content contained in each system specific and content outline category and use this information to develop remedial plans to improve performance on sample examinations. We will begin with an exploration of the National Physical Therapy Examination Content Outline.

# Content Outline Summary

| Content | Percentage | Questions (Range) |
|---|---|---|
| Physical Therapy Examination | 26.5% | 53 (50-56) |
| Foundations for Evaluation, Differential Diagnosis, & Prognosis | 32.5% | 65 (60-70) |
| Interventions | 28.5% | 57 (56-64) |
| Equipment & Devices; Therapeutic Modalities | 6.0% | 12 (11-14) |
| Safety and Protection; Professional Responsibilities; Research | 6.5% | 13 (11-14) |
| | 100.0% | 200 |

## Content Outline Summary

### NPTE - Content Outline Weighting

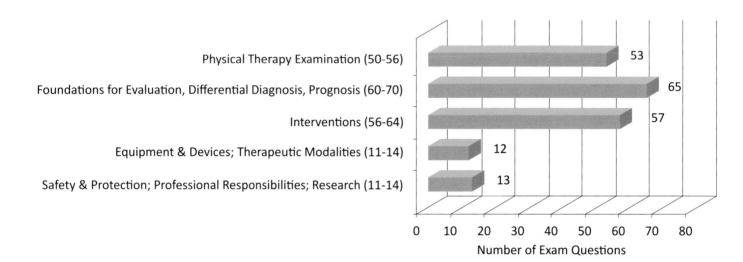

Physical Therapy Examination (50-56) — 53

Foundations for Evaluation, Differential Diagnosis, Prognosis (60-70) — 65

Interventions (56-64) — 57

Equipment & Devices; Therapeutic Modalities (11-14) — 12

Safety & Protection; Professional Responsibilities; Research (11-14) — 13

*Number of Exam Questions*

### NPTE - Content Outline Weighting

Physical Therapy Examination
(50-56 Questions)

Equipment & Devices;
Therapeutic Modalities
(11-14 Questions)

Interventions
(56-64 Questions)

Foundations for Evaluation,
Differential Diagnosis, Prognosis
(60-70 Questions)

Safety & Protection,
Professional Responsibilities,
Research (11-14 Questions)

## Physical Therapy Examination

**Target: 26.5% (53 questions)**

This category refers to knowledge of the types and applications of specific system tests/measures, including outcome measures, according to current best evidence, and their relevance to information collected from the history and systems review. The category includes the reaction of the specific system to tests/measures. Information covered in these areas supports appropriate and effective patient/client management for rehabilitation, health promotion, and performance across the lifespan.

**[Range: 50-56]**

Adapted from the *Physical Therapist NPTE Test Content Outline, Federation of State Boards of Physical Therapy, www.fsbpt.org*

**Physical Therapy Examination**

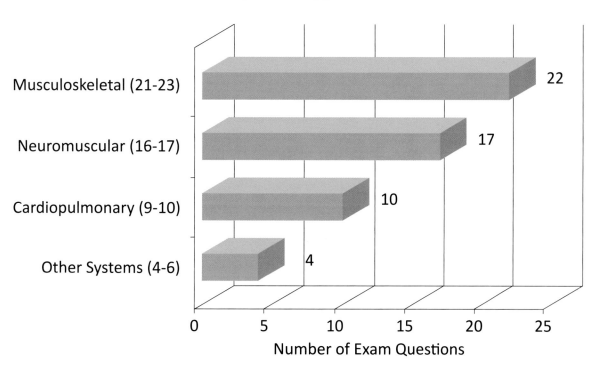

Number of Exam Questions

**Other Systems**

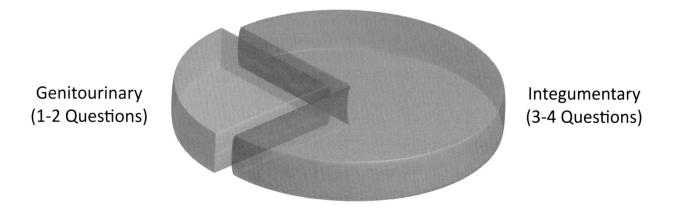

## Foundations for Evaluation, Differential Diagnosis, and Prognosis

**Target: 32.5% (65 questions)**

This category refers to the interpretation of knowledge about diseases/conditions impacting a specific system, according to current best evidence, in order to ensure appropriate and effective patient/client treatment and management decisions for rehabilitation, health promotion, and performance across the lifespan.

**[Range: 60-70]**

Adapted from the *Physical Therapist NPTE Test Content Outline, Federation of State Boards of Physical Therapy, www.fsbpt.org*

**Foundations for Evaluation, Differential Diagnosis, and Prognosis**

**Other Systems**

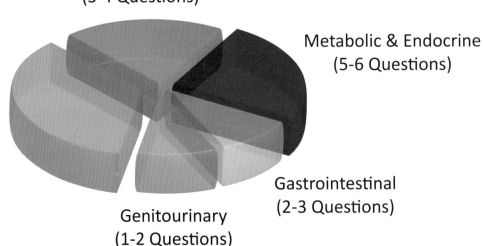

## Interventions

**Target: 28.5% (57 questions)**

This category refers to specific system interventions (including types, applications, responses, and potential complications), according to current best evidence, as well as the impact on the specific system of interventions performed on other systems in order to support patient/client management for rehabilitation, health promotion, and performance across the lifespan.

**[Range: 56-64]**

Adapted from the *Physical Therapist NPTE Test Content Outline, Federation of State Boards of Physical Therapy, www.fsbpt.org*

### Interventions

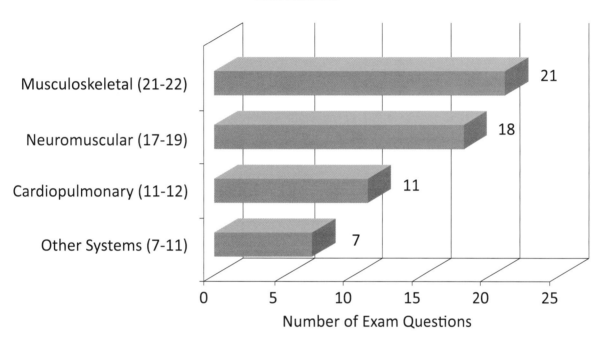

Number of Exam Questions

### Other Systems

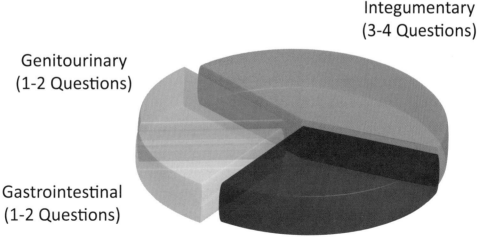

## Equipment and Devices

**Target: 2.5% (5 questions)**

**[Range: 5-6]**

This category refers to the different types of equipment and devices, use requirements, and/or contextual determinants, as well as any other influencing factors involved in the selection and application of equipment and devices, including consideration of current best evidence, in order to support patient/client treatment and management decisions for rehabilitation, health promotion, and performance across the lifespan.

- Assistive and adaptive devices
- Prosthetic devices
- Protective, supportive, and orthotic devices

## Therapeutic Modalities

**Target: 3.5% (7 questions)**

**[Range: 6-8]**

This category refers to the underlying principles for the use of therapeutic modalities as well as the justification for the selection and use of various types of therapeutic modalities, including consideration of current best evidence, in order to support patient/client treatment and management decisions for rehabilitation, health promotion, and performance across the lifespan.

- Thermal modalities
- Iontophoresis
- Electrotherapy modalities, excluding iontophoresis
- Phonophoresis
- Ultrasound modalities, excluding phonophoresis
- Mechanical modalities (e.g., mechanical motion devices, traction devices)
- Biofeedback
- Electromagnetic radiation (e.g., diathermy)
- Pneumatic compression modalities

Adapted from the *Physical Therapist NPTE Test Content Outline, Federation of State Boards of Physical Therapy, www.fsbpt.org*

**Equipment and Devices; Therapeutic Modalities**

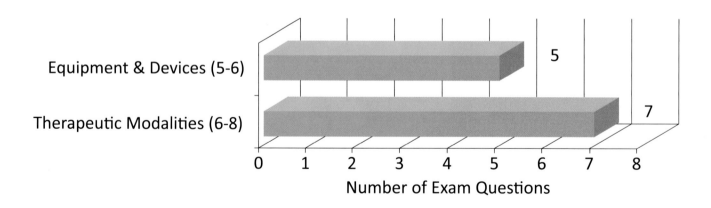

## Safety and Protection

**Target: 2.5% (5 questions)**

[Range: 4-5]

This category refers to the critical issues involved in patient/client safety and protection and the responsibilities of health-care providers to ensure that patient/client management and health-care decisions take place in a secure environment.

- Factors influencing safety and injury prevention
- Function, implications, and precautions related to intravenous lines, tubes, catheters, and monitoring devices
- Emergency preparedness (e.g., CPR, first aid, disaster response)
- Infection control procedures (e.g., standard/universal precautions, isolation techniques, sterile technique)
- Signs/symptoms of physical, sexual, and psychological abuse and neglect

## Professional Responsibilities

**Target: 2.0% (4 questions)**

[Range: 3-4]

This category refers to the responsibilities of health-care providers to ensure that patient/client management and health-care decisions take place in a trustworthy environment.

- Standards of documentation
- Patient/client rights (e.g., ADA, IDEA, HIPAA)
- Human resource legal issues (e.g., OSHA, sexual harassment)
- Roles and responsibilities of physical therapist assistants in relation to physical therapists and other health-care professionals
- Roles and responsibilities of other health-care professionals and support staff

## Research and Evidence-Based Practice

**Target: 2.0% (4 questions)**

[Range: 4-5]

This category refers to the application of measurement principles and research methods to make reasoned and appropriate assessment and to the interpretation of information sources and practice research to support patient/client management decisions fundamental to evidence-based practice.

- Research design and interpretation (e.g., qualitative, quantitative, hierarchy of evidence)
- Measurement science (e.g., reliability, validity)
- Statistics (e.g., t-test, chi-square, correlation coefficient, ANOVA, likelihood ratio)
- Data collection techniques (e.g., surveys, direct observation)

Adapted from the *Physical Therapist NPTE Test Content Outline, Federation of State Boards of Physical Therapy, www.fsbpt.or*g

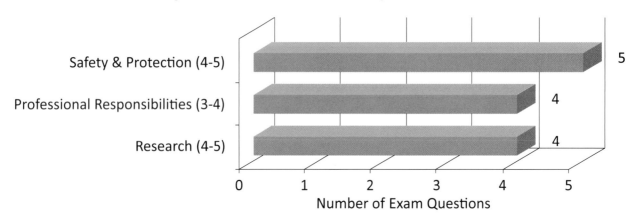

Safety and Protection; Professional Responsibilities; Research

Number of Exam Questions

## System Specific Summary

| Systems (175) | Percentage | Questions (Range) |
|---|---|---|
| Musculoskeletal System | 30.5% | 61 (59-63) |
| Neuromuscular & Nervous Systems | 25.0% | 50 (48-52) |
| Cardiovascular/Pulmonary and Lymphatic Systems | 16.5% | 33 (32-35) |
| Other Systems | | |
| Integumentary System | 5.0% | 10 (9-12) |
| Metabolic and Endocrine Systems | 3.5% | 7 (7-9) |
| Gastrointestinal System | 1.5% | 3 (3-5) |
| Genitourinary System | 2.0% | 4 (3-6) |
| System Interactions | 3.5% | 7 (6-8) |
| Non-Systems (25) | | |
| Equipment & Devices; Therapeutic Modalities | | |
| Equipment & Devices | 2.5% | 5 (5-6) |
| Therapeutic Modalities | 3.5% | 7 (6-8) |
| Safety and Protection; Professional Responsibilities; Research | | |
| Safety and Protection | 2.5% | 5 (4-5) |
| Professional Responsibilities | 2.0% | 4 (3-4) |
| Research & Evidence-Based Practice | 2.0% | 4 (4-5) |
| | 100.0% | 200 |

**NPTE - System Specific Weighting**

Number of Exam Questions

**NPTE - System Specific Weighting**

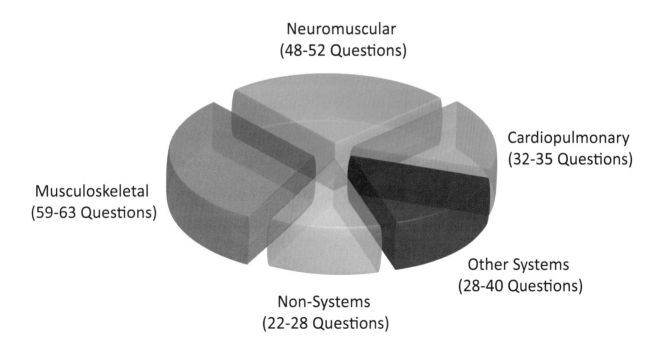

## Musculoskeletal System

**Target: 30.5% (61 questions)**

[Range: 59-63]

**Physical Therapy Examination:** This category refers to knowledge of the types and applications of musculoskeletal system tests/measures, including outcome measures, according to current best evidence, and their relevance to information collected from the history and systems review. The category includes the reaction of the musculoskeletal system to tests/measures and the mechanics of body movement as related to the musculoskeletal system. Information covered in these areas supports appropriate and effective patient/client management for rehabilitation, health promotion, and performance across the lifespan.

- Musculoskeletal system tests/measures, including outcome measures, and their applications according to current best evidence
- Anatomy and physiology of the musculoskeletal system as related to tests/measures
- Movement analysis as related to the musculoskeletal system
- Joint biomechanics and their applications
- Physical therapy ultrasound imaging of the musculoskeletal system

**Foundations for Evaluation, Differential Diagnosis, and Prognosis:** This category refers to the interpretation of knowledge about diseases/conditions of the musculoskeletal system, according to current best evidence, in order to ensure appropriate and effective patient/client treatment and management decisions for rehabilitation, health promotion, and performance across the lifespan.

- Differential diagnoses related to diseases/conditions of the muscular and skeletal systems
- Differential diagnoses related to diseases/conditions of the connective tissue
- Muscular and skeletal diseases/conditions and their pathophysiology to establish and carry out a plan of care, including prognosis
- Connective tissue diseases/conditions and their pathophysiology to establish and carry out a plan of care, including prognosis
- Nonpharmacological medical management of the musculoskeletal system (e.g., diagnostic imaging, laboratory test values, other medical tests, surgical procedures)
- Pharmacological management of the musculoskeletal system

**Interventions:** This category refers to musculoskeletal system interventions (including types, applications, responses, and potential complications), according to current best evidence, as well as the impact on the musculoskeletal system of interventions performed on other systems in order to support patient/client management for rehabilitation, health promotion, and performance across the lifespan.

- Musculoskeletal system physical therapy interventions and their applications for rehabilitation, health promotion, and performance according to current best evidence
- Anatomy and physiology of the musculoskeletal system as related to physical therapy interventions, daily activities, and environmental factors
- Secondary effects or complications from physical therapy and medical interventions on the musculoskeletal system
- Secondary effects or complications on the musculoskeletal system from physical therapy and medical interventions used on other systems

Adapted from the *Physical Therapist NPTE Test Content Outline, Federation of State Boards Physical Therapy, www.fsbpt.org*

## Neuromuscular and Nervous Systems

**Target: 25.0% (50 questions)**

[Range: 48-52]

**Physical Therapy Examination:** This category refers to knowledge of the types and applications of neuromuscular/nervous systems tests/measures, including outcome measures, according to current best evidence, and their relevance to information collected from the history and systems review. The category includes the reaction of the neuromuscular/nervous systems to tests/measures and the mechanics of body movement as related to the neuromuscular/nervous systems. Information covered in these areas supports appropriate and effective patient/client management for rehabilitation, health promotion, and performance across the lifespan.

- Neuromuscular/nervous systems tests/measures, including outcome measures, and their applications according to current best evidence
- Anatomy and physiology of the neuromuscular/nervous systems as related to tests/measures
- Movement analysis as related to the neuromuscular/nervous systems

**Foundations for Evaluation, Differential Diagnosis, and Prognosis:** This category refers to the interpretation of knowledge about diseases/conditions of the neuromuscular/nervous systems, according to current best evidence, in order to ensure appropriate and effective patient/client treatment and management decisions for rehabilitation, health promotion, and performance across the lifespan.

- Differential diagnoses related to diseases/conditions of the neuromuscular/nervous system (CNS, PNS, ANS)
- Neuromuscular/nervous system (CNS, PNS, ANS) diseases/conditions and their pathophysiology to establish and carry out a plan of care, including prognosis
- Nonpharmacological medical management of the neuromuscular/nervous systems (e.g., diagnostic imaging, laboratory test values, other medical tests, surgical procedures)
- Pharmacological management of the neuromuscular/nervous systems

**Interventions:** This category refers to neuromuscular/nervous systems interventions (including types, applications, responses, and potential complications), according to current best evidence, as well as the impact on the neuromuscular/nervous systems of interventions performed on other systems in order to support patient/client management for rehabilitation, health promotion, and performance across the lifespan.

- Neuromuscular/nervous systems physical therapy interventions and their applications for rehabilitation, health promotion, and performance according to current best evidence
- Anatomy and physiology of the neuromuscular/nervous systems as related to physical therapy interventions, daily activities, and environmental factors
- Secondary effects or complications from physical therapy and medical interventions on the neuromuscular/nervous systems
- Secondary effects or complications on the neuromuscular/nervous systems from physical therapy and medical interventions used on other systems
- Motor control as related to neuromuscular/nervous systems physical therapy interventions
- Motor learning as related to neuromuscular/nervous systems physical therapy interventions

Adapted from the *Physical Therapist NPTE Test Content Outline, Federation of State Boards Physical Therapy, www.fsbpt.org*

## Cardiovascular/Pulmonary and Lymphatic Systems

**Target: 16.5% (33 questions)**

**[Range: 32-35]**

**Physical Therapy Examination:** This category refers to knowledge of the types and applications of cardiovascular/pulmonary and lymphatic systems tests/measures, including outcome measures, according to current best evidence, and their relevance to information collected from the history and systems review. The category includes the reaction of the cardiovascular/pulmonary and lymphatic systems to tests/measures and the mechanics of body movement as related to the cardiovascular/pulmonary and lymphatic systems. Information covered in these areas supports appropriate and effective patient/client management for rehabilitation, health promotion, and performance across the lifespan.

- Cardiovascular/pulmonary systems tests/measures, including outcome measures, and their applications according to current best evidence
- Anatomy and physiology of the cardiovascular/pulmonary systems as related to tests/measures
- Movement analysis as related to the cardiovascular/pulmonary systems (e.g., rib cage excursion)

**Foundations for Evaluation, Differential Diagnosis, and Prognosis:** This category refers to the interpretation of knowledge about diseases/conditions of the cardiovascular/pulmonary and lymphatic systems according to current best evidence, in order to ensure appropriate and effective patient/client treatment and management decisions for rehabilitation, health promotion, and performance across the lifespan.

- Differential diagnoses related to diseases/conditions of the cardiovascular/pulmonary systems
- Differential diagnoses related to diseases/conditions of the lymphatic system
- Cardiovascular/pulmonary systems diseases/conditions and their pathophysiology to establish and carry out a plan of care, including prognosis
- Lymphatic system diseases/conditions and their pathophysiology to establish and carry out a plan of care, including prognosis
- Nonpharmacological medical management of the cardiovascular/pulmonary systems (e.g., diagnostic imaging, laboratory test values, other medical tests, surgical procedures)
- Pharmacological management of the cardiovascular/pulmonary systems
- Nonpharmacological medical management of the lymphatic system (e.g., diagnostic imaging, laboratory test values, other medical tests, surgical procedures)

**Interventions:** This category refers to cardiovascular/pulmonary and lymphatic systems interventions (including types, applications, responses, and potential complications) according to current best evidence, as well as the impact on the cardiovascular/pulmonary and lymphatic systems of interventions performed on other systems in order to support patient/client management for rehabilitation, health promotion, and performance across the lifespan.

- Cardiovascular/pulmonary systems physical therapy interventions and their applications for rehabilitation, health promotion, and performance according to current best evidence
- Anatomy and physiology of the cardiovascular/pulmonary systems as related to physical therapy interventions, daily activities, and environmental factors
- Secondary effects or complications from physical therapy and medical interventions on the cardiovascular/pulmonary systems
- Secondary effects or complications on the cardiovascular/pulmonary systems from physical therapy and medical interventions used on other systems
- Lymphatic system physical therapy interventions and their applications for rehabilitation, health promotion, and performance according to current best evidence
- Anatomy and physiology of the lymphatic system as related to physical therapy interventions, daily activities, and environmental factors
- Secondary effects or complications from physical therapy and medical interventions on the lymphatic system
- Secondary effects or complications on the lymphatic system from physical therapy and medical interventions used on other systems

Adapted from the *Physical Therapist NPTE Test Content Outline, Federation of State Boards Physical Therapy, www.fsbpt.org*

# Other Systems (overview)

**Target: 15.5% (31 questions)**

The Other Systems category includes the Integumentary System, Metabolic and Endocrine Systems, Gastrointestinal System, Genitourinary System, and System Interactions.

**[Range: 28-40]**

**Other Systems**

- Integumentary (9-12): 10
- Metabolic & Endocrine (7-9): 7
- Gastrointestinal (3-5): 3
- Genitourinary (3-6): 4
- System Interactions (6-8): 7

Number of Exam Questions

## Integumentary System

**Target: 5.0% (10 questions)**

**Physical Therapy Examination:** This category refers to knowledge of the types and applications of integumentary system tests/measures, including outcome measures, according to current best evidence, and their relevance to information collected from the history and systems review. The category includes the reaction of the integumentary system to tests/measures and the mechanics of body movement as related to the integumentary system. Information covered in these areas supports appropriate and effective patient/ client management for rehabilitation, health promotion, and performance across the lifespan.

**[Range: 9-12]**

- Integumentary system tests/measures, including outcome measures, and their applications according to current best evidence
- Anatomy and physiology of the integumentary system as related to tests/measures
- Movement analysis as related to the integumentary system (e.g., friction, shear, pressure, and scar mobility)

**Foundations for Evaluation, Differential Diagnosis, and Prognosis:** This category refers to the interpretation of knowledge about diseases/conditions of the integumentary system, according to current best evidence, in order to ensure appropriate and effective patient/client treatment and management decisions for rehabilitation, health promotion, and performance across the lifespan.

- Differential diagnoses related to diseases/conditions of the integumentary system
- Integumentary system diseases/conditions and their pathophysiology to establish and carry out a plan of care, including prognosis
- Nonpharmacological medical management of the integumentary system (e.g., diagnostic imaging, laboratory test values, other medical tests, surgical procedures)
- Pharmacological management of the integumentary system

**Interventions:** This category refers to integumentary system interventions (including types, applications, responses, and potential complications), according to current best evidence, as well as the impact on the integumentary system of interventions performed on other systems in order to support patient/client management for rehabilitation, health promotion, and performance across the lifespan.

- Integumentary system physical therapy interventions and their applications for rehabilitation, health promotion, and performance according to current best evidence
- Anatomy and physiology of the integumentary system as related to physical therapy interventions, daily activities, and environmental factors
- Secondary effects or complications from physical therapy and medical interventions on the integumentary system
- Secondary effects or complications on the integumentary system from physical therapy and medical interventions used on other systems

## Metabolic and Endocrine Systems

**Target: 3.5% (7 questions)**

**Foundations for Evaluation, Differential Diagnosis, and Prognosis:** This category refers to the interpretation of knowledge about diseases/conditions of the metabolic and endocrine systems, according to best current evidence, in order to ensure appropriate and effective patient/client treatment and management decisions for rehabilitation, health promotion, and performance across the lifespan.

**[Range: 7-9]**

- Differential diagnoses related to diseases/conditions of the metabolic and endocrine systems
- Metabolic and endocrine systems diseases/conditions and their pathophysiology to establish and carry out a plan of care, including prognosis
- Nonpharmacological medical management of the metabolic and endocrine systems (e.g., diagnostic imaging, laboratory test values, other medical tests, surgical procedures)
- Pharmacological management of the metabolic and endocrine systems

**Interventions:** This category refers to metabolic and endocrine systems interventions (including types, applications, responses, and potential complications), according to current best evidence, as well as the impact on the metabolic and endocrine systems of interventions performed on other systems in order to support patient/client management for rehabilitation, health promotion, and performance across the lifespan.

- Metabolic and endocrine systems physical therapy interventions and their applications for rehabilitation, health promotion, and performance according to current best evidence
- Anatomy and physiology of the metabolic and endocrine systems as related to physical therapy interventions, daily activities, and environmental factors
- Secondary effects or complications from physical therapy and medical interventions on the metabolic and endocrine systems
- Secondary effects or complications on the metabolic and endocrine systems from physical therapy and medical interventions used on other systems

## Gastrointestinal System

**Target: 1.5% (3 questions)**

**Foundations for Evaluation, Differential Diagnosis, and Prognosis:** This category refers to the interpretation of knowledge about diseases/conditions of the gastrointestinal system, according to current best evidence, in order to ensure appropriate and effective patient/client treatment and management decisions for rehabilitation, health promotion, and performance across the lifespan.

**[Range: 3-5]**

- Gastrointestinal system diseases/conditions and their pathophysiology to establish and carry out a plan of care, including prognosis
- Differential diagnoses related to diseases/conditions of the gastrointestinal system
- Nonpharmacological medical management of the gastrointestinal system (e.g., diagnostic imaging, laboratory test values, other medical tests, surgical procedures)
- Pharmacological management of the gastrointestinal system

**Interventions:** This category refers to gastrointestinal system interventions (including types, applications, responses, and potential complications), according to current best evidence, as well as the impact on the gastrointestinal system of interventions performed on other systems in order to support patient/client management for rehabilitation, health promotion, and performance across the lifespan.

- Gastrointestinal system physical therapy interventions and their applications for rehabilitation and health promotion according to current best evidence (e.g., positioning for reflux prevention, bowel programs)

- Anatomy and physiology of the gastrointestinal system as related to physical therapy interventions, daily activities, and environmental factors

- Secondary effects or complications from physical therapy and medical interventions on the gastrointestinal system

- Secondary effects or complications on the gastrointestinal system from physical therapy and medical interventions used on other systems

## Genitourinary System

**Target: 2.0% (4 questions)**

[Range: 3-6]

**Physical Therapy Examination:** This category refers to knowledge of the types and applications of genitourinary system tests/measures, including outcome measures, according to current best evidence, and their relevance to information collected from the history and systems review. The category includes the reaction of the genitourinary system to tests/measures and the mechanics of body movement as related to the genitourinary system. Information covered in these areas supports appropriate and effective patient/client management for rehabilitation, health promotion, and performance across the lifespan.

- Genitourinary system tests/measures, including outcome measures, and their applications according to current best evidence

- Anatomy and physiology of the genitourinary system as related to tests/measures

- Physiological response of the genitourinary system to various types of tests/measures

**Foundations for Evaluation, Differential Diagnosis, and Prognosis:** This category refers to the interpretation of knowledge about diseases/conditions of the genitourinary system, according to current best evidence, in order to ensure appropriate and effective patient/client treatment and management decisions for rehabilitation, health promotion, and performance across the lifespan.

- Differential diagnoses related to diseases/conditions of the genitourinary system

- Genitourinary system diseases/conditions and their pathophysiology to establish and carry out a plan of care, including prognosis

- Nonpharmacological medical management of the genitourinary system (e.g., diagnostic imaging, laboratory test values, other medical tests, surgical procedures)

- Pharmacological management of the genitourinary system

**Interventions:** This category refers to genitourinary system interventions (including types, applications, responses, and potential complications), according to current best evidence, as well as the impact on the genitourinary system of interventions performed on other systems in order to support patient/client management for rehabilitation, health promotion, and performance across the lifespan.

- Genitourinary system physical therapy interventions and their applications for rehabilitation and health promotion according to current best evidence (e.g., bladder programs, biofeedback, pelvic floor retraining)

- Anatomy and physiology of the genitourinary system as related to physical therapy interventions, daily activities, and environmental factors

- Secondary effects or complications from physical therapy and medical interventions on the genitourinary system

- Secondary effects or complications on the genitourinary system from physical therapy and medical interventions used on other systems

## System Interactions

**Target: 3.5% (7 questions)**

[Range: 6-8]

**Foundations for Evaluation, Differential Diagnosis, and Prognosis:** This category refers to the interpretation of knowledge about system interactions, according to current best evidence, in order to ensure appropriate and effective patient/client treatment and management decisions for rehabilitation, health promotion and performance across the lifespan.

- Differential diagnoses related to diseases/conditions where the primary impact is on more than one system
- Diseases/conditions where the primary impact is on more than one system to establish and carry out a plan of care, including prognosis
- Impact of comorbidities/coexisting conditions on patient/client management (e.g., diabetes and hypertension, obesity and arthritis, hip fracture and dementia)
- Psychological and psychiatric conditions that impact patient/client management (e.g., depression, schizophrenia)
- Nonpharmacological medical management of multiple systems (e.g., diagnostic imaging and other medical tests, surgical procedures)
- Pharmacological management of multiple systems, including polypharmacy

Adapted from the *Physical Therapist NPTE Test Content Outline, Federation of State Boards Physical Therapy, www.fsbpt.orgw*

# Non-Systems

## Equipment and Devices

**Target: 2.5% (5 questions)**

[Range: 5-6]

This category refers to the different types of equipment and devices, use requirements, and/or contextual determinants, as well as any other influencing factors involved in the selection and application of equipment and devices, including consideration of current best evidence, in order to support patient/client treatment and management decisions for rehabilitation, health promotion, and performance across the lifespan.

- Assistive and adaptive devices
- Prosthetic devices
- Protective, supportive, and orthotic devices

## Therapeutic Modalities

**Target: 3.5% (7 questions)**

[Range: 6-8]

This category refers to the underlying principles for the use of therapeutic modalities as well as the justification for the selection and use of various types of therapeutic modalities, including consideration of current best evidence, in order to support patient/client treatment and management decisions for rehabilitation, health promotion, and performance across the lifespan.

- Thermal modalities
- Iontophoresis
- Electrotherapy modalities, excluding iontophoresis
- Phonophoresis
- Ultrasound modalities, excluding phonophoresis
- Mechanical modalities (e.g., mechanical motion devices, traction devices)

- Biofeedback
- Electromagnetic radiation (e.g., diathermy)
- Pneumatic compression modalities

Adapted from the *Physical Therapist NPTE Test Content Outline, Federation of State Boards Physical Therapy, www.fsbpt.org*

## Safety and Protection

**Target: 2.5% (5 questions)**

This category refers to the critical issues involved in patient/client safety and protection and the responsibilities of health-care providers to ensure that patient/client management and health-care decisions take place in a secure environment.

**[Range: 4-5]**

- Factors influencing safety and injury prevention
- Function, implications, and precautions related to intravenous lines, tubes, catheters, and monitoring devices
- Emergency preparedness (e.g., CPR, first aid, disaster response)
- Infection control procedures (e.g., standard/universal precautions, isolation techniques, sterile technique)
- Signs/symptoms of physical, sexual, and psychological abuse and neglect

## Professional Responsibilities

**Target: 2.0% (4 questions)**

This category refers to the responsibilities of health-care providers to ensure that patient/client management and health-care decisions take place in a trustworthy environment.

- Standards of documentation

**[Range: 3-4]**

- Patient/client rights (e.g., ADA, IDEA, HIPAA)
- Human resource legal issues (e.g., OSHA, sexual harassment)
- Roles and responsibilities of physical therapist assistants in relation to physical therapists and other health-care professionals
- Roles and responsibilities of other health-care professionals and support staff

## Research and Evidence-Based Practice

**Target: 2.0% (4 questions)**

This category refers to the application of measurement principles and research methods to make reasoned and appropriate assessment and to the interpretation of information sources and practice research to support patient/client management decisions fundamental to evidence-based practice.

**[Range: 4-5]**

- Research design and interpretation (e.g., qualitative, quantitative, hierarchy of evidence)
- Measurement science (e.g., reliability, validity)
- Statistics (e.g., t-test, chi-square, correlation coefficient, ANOVA, likelihood ratio)
- Data collection techniques (e.g., surveys, direct observation)

Adapted from the *Physical Therapist NPTE Test Content Outline, Federation of State Boards Physical Therapy, www.fsbpt.org*

# 3

# STUDY CONCEPTS

**Scott Giles**

34 Learning Styles

35 Time Management

36 Levels of Knowledge and Understanding

37 Golden Rules

38 Automaticity

39 Truths and Myths

40 Blood Pressure

41 Lines, Tubes, and Equipment

42 Emergent Conditions

43 Assessment

SCOREBUILDERS

The inclusion of Study Concepts in **PTEXAM: The Complete Study Guide** serves to remind candidates that preparing for the National Physical Therapy Examination requires more than simply reviewing academic content and taking sample examinations.

Each of the presented Study Concepts provides candidates with an idea or concept to potentially integrate into their comprehensive study plan. For example, perhaps a candidate has a strong learning style preference where they tend to favor active learning over passive learning. To date, their study plan has consisted of purely passive activities such as reading the academic review section of a review book and reviewing class notes. Not surprisingly, the candidate has experienced a great deal of difficulty moving through the academic review and class notes and has serious doubts about how much of the material they have retained. In addition, the candidate finds they are unable to concentrate after approximately 90 minutes of studying and typically discontinues the study session at this point.

The presented Study Concept entitled "Learning Styles" offers a number of practical suggestions to assist candidates to identify their own unique learning style and to design study sessions to incorporate these preferences. Study plans that are designed to address decided learning preferences yield a much greater return on investment than generic study plans.

As a second example, consider the Study Concept entitled "Golden Rules." This item explores whether it is possible to develop specific rules that allow candidates to differentiate between two or more plausible options on multiple-choice questions used on the National Physical Therapy Examination. A potential rule would be something like the following: "When choosing between a number of acceptable interventions, always select the most conservative option in an effort to minimize any potential safety risk to the patient."

Potential rules like this are very tempting since they provide candidates with a means to make questions more objective and therefore less amorphous. The problem, however, is that the National Physical Therapy Examination is designed to assess a candidate's ability to make clinical decisions rather than to rely on memorization or simply apply a set of standardized rules. The Study Concept presents a variety of potential rules and walks candidates through a number of clinical scenarios demonstrating why rules are better used as only loose guidelines to consider when answering multiple-choice questions.

| Study Concepts | |
|---|---|
| Study Concept 1 | **Learning Styles** |
| Study Concept 2 | **Time Management** |
| Study Concept 3 | **Levels of Knowledge and Understanding** |
| Study Concept 4 | **Golden Rules** |
| Study Concept 5 | **Automaticity** |
| Study Concept 6 | **Truths and Myths** |
| Study Concept 7 | **Blood Pressure** |
| Study Concept 8 | **Lines, Tubes, and Equipment** |
| Study Concept 9 | **Emergent Conditions** |
| Study Concept 10 | **Assessment** |

In truth, many questions on the examination require candidates to make unique judgments based on the exact circumstances presented in the two to four sentences that make up the question stem. Candidates who develop the flexibility to apply clinical information in a wide variety of scenarios are well poised to be successful on the National Physical Therapy Examination.

Enjoy each of the presented Study Concepts and use the notes section to make observations of your present performance related to each of these unique topics.

# Study Concept 1: Learning Styles

Studying for a comprehensive examination such as the National Physical Therapy Examination can be a significant challenge for any candidate. Given the volume of information required to be reviewed or relearned, it is critical for candidates to be as efficient as possible as they move through their established study plan. In order to maximize the efficiency of established study sessions, candidates should consider their preferred learning channels.

Perhaps the most critical question to answer relates to your preferred learning style for input and processing. Is your preferred learning style for input and processing more active or passive? Here is a brief description of each style that may assist you to label your individual preference.

**Active learning style** – when exposed to new material, a learner who likes to hear it, see it, say it, question it, interact with it, and then keep on doing this. Learners with this style tend to be multisensoral (visual, auditory, tactile/kinesthetic).

**Passive learning style** – when exposed to new material, a learner who likes to hear it or read it and then keep on doing this. Learners with this style tend to determine the relationship to known material after input and before processing.

It is important to recognize that one learning style is not better than another, but each learning style can come with particular strengths and weaknesses. For example, a candidate who is active for both input and processing may be able to focus intently on the application and utility of ideas, however, may consider details boring and have a short attention span. Conversely, a candidate who is passive for both input and processing may be effective at sequential thinking and focusing on details, but may miss the "big picture."

Please recognize that an individual's learning style varies depending on the situation, however, it is equally important to recognize that most candidates have decided learning style preferences that when harnessed can result in greater efficiency of study sessions.

## General Recommendations for Specific Learning Styles

### Active learning style

Study sessions should consist of 60-90 minute sessions of interactive study. Study sessions should take place as frequently as possible. Group studying is recommended since multisensory stimulation is difficult to achieve alone. Learning tools should include items such as discussions, simulations, hands-on practice, and role playing.

### Passive learning style

Study sessions should be two to three hours in length and focus on large pieces of material. Study sessions should take place three to five times per week. Group studying is recommended periodically with members who are application driven. Learning tools should include items such as lectures, briefings, observations, handouts, texts, and notes.

Awareness of one's learning style will not make an unqualified candidate qualified, however, it can significantly increase the rate of new learning, reviewing, and relearning. A well conceived study plan combined with an awareness of learning style is a powerful one-two combination that can pay significant dividends for candidates on the National Physical Therapy Examination.

Notes:

# Study Concept 2: Time Management

Physical therapy students by definition tend to have strong time management skills, however, these skills are severely tested when preparing for the National Physical Therapy Examination. The majority of students take the National Physical Therapy Examination shortly after graduation, which can be a very anxious and unsettled time. Candidates are often actively seeking employment or are attempting to adjust to a new job. They may have relocated to a different residence or perhaps moved to another part of the country.

The thought of preparing for an examination that represents a minimum of three years of graduate study makes it critical that available study time is spent in areas that will yield the highest return on investment. To illustrate this point, consider the relative systems weighting of the current examination.

| System | Percentage |
|---|---|
| Musculoskeletal System | 30.5% |
| Neuromuscular & Nervous Systems | 25.0% |
| Cardiovascular/Pulmonary and Lymphatic Systems | 16.5% |
| Other Systems | 15.5% |
| Non-Systems | 12.5% |

For example, on a typical examination a candidate will have 61 musculoskeletal system questions and 31 other systems questions. The number of questions is determined by multiplying the percentage of questions specified in each system area by two since the National Physical Therapy Examination consists of a total of 200 scored items. Given the relative weighting of these areas, a typical candidate should spend almost twice as much time studying musculoskeletal content than other systems content. The actual percentage of time spent in each area may vary from candidate to candidate, but the relative weighting of the system on the examination should always remain an important variable to consider when determining the necessary breadth and depth in each area. Fortunately, there are a number of specific strategies candidates can utilize to ensure that they make meaningful progress in their study sessions.

## Strategy: Master Study Schedule

Develop a master schedule for studying which emphasizes the relative weighting of the Systems and Non-Systems areas on the National Physical Therapy Examination.

**Step One** – Create a monthly calendar that identifies specific study days and the anticipated duration of each session.

**Step Two** – Allocate more frequent study sessions and therefore additional study time to systems that are more heavily weighted on the National Physical Therapy Examination.

**Step Three** – Integrate weekly activities that are designed to maintain a balance in life. These areas may address emotional, intellectual, physical, and social needs.

**Step Four** – Reassess your progress on a weekly basis and make any necessary changes to the master schedule.

**PTEXAM: The Complete Study Guide** offers a great deal of additional information on the National Physical Therapy Examination Blueprint. The blueprint specifies the relative weighting of the Systems and Non-Systems areas and introduces the Content Outline.

Notes:

# Study Concept 3: Levels of Knowledge and Understanding

The National Physical Therapy Examination has evolved into an examination that requires candidates to demonstrate their ability to make clinical decisions rather than purely recall factual information. Candidates need to demonstrate solid didactic knowledge of entry-level physical therapy concepts, however, they also need to be able to apply the information in diverse clinical scenarios usually presented in multiple-choice questions of two to four sentences. Candidates who can effectively integrate physical therapy concepts into the various presented scenarios and make informed clinical decisions tend to perform strongly on the examination, while candidates who struggle with this skill tend to perform poorly.

When reviewing academic content, it is important that candidates familiarize themselves with the content at multiple levels of breadth and depth. The following table depicts a hierarchy of knowledge and understanding.

Typically, within a physical therapy academic program, students acquire the information in a hierarchical progression beginning with the lower cognitive levels (i.e., vocabulary level, literal level) and progress over time to higher cognitive levels (i.e., interpretive level and applied level). As candidates begin to prepare for the National Physical Therapy Examination, it is likely that the majority of candidates are comfortable at the vocabulary and literal level, however, there is far greater variability in comfort level at the interpretive and applied levels. Varying levels of comfort may result from exposure or lack thereof to specific subject matter on clinical education experiences or opportunities to develop competence with applied learning activities in the classroom. Regardless of where a candidate is on this spectrum, it is critical that candidates constantly challenge themselves to explore higher level cognitive knowledge as they progress through their academic review.

The presented hierarchy of knowledge and understanding can also be useful for candidates when answering multiple-choice questions. After reading the stem of a given examination question, it may be beneficial for candidates to ask themselves what the question is specifically asking. In this manner, candidates can ensure that their interpretation of the question is consistent with the intended meaning of each question. Failure to interpret the specific meaning of a question often results in a candidate selecting an incorrect response to a multiple-choice item. Test taking mistakes can be extremely harmful on the examination since once this occurs a candidate's examination score is no longer consistent with their true ability. As a candidate's score moves further away from their true ability there is a greater risk of failing the examination.

**Applied Level: (How)**
*Process Analysis, Process Synthesis, Evaluation*

**Interpretive Level: (Why, When, Which)**
*Composition, Classification, Example of Purpose*

**Literal Level: (What, Where)**
*Characteristics, Background, Location, Function*

**Vocabulary Level: (Who, What, When)**
*Names, Definitions*

Notes:

# Study Concept 4: Golden Rules

We have all used certain rules to help us move through our education such as "I before E, except after C." When preparing for the National Physical Therapy Examination, candidates often look for similar rules that can assist them to make important distinctions between two or more plausible options to a given question. Unfortunately, these types of rules do not exist on the National Physical Therapy Examination since every question relies on the nuances of a particular scenario that is typically conveyed in two to four sentences. Perhaps this is best demonstrated by stating a possible rule and then providing several examples to explore the rule in more detail.

**Hypothetical Golden Rule Number One:** When confronted with a situation where patient safety is potentially compromised, always contact the referring physician.

**Rule Buster:** Candidates must be vigilant to identify and act on any potential threat to patient safety, but this does not mean that it is always necessary to contact the referring physician. In some cases, it would be appropriate for a physical therapist to minimize the threat to safety themselves. For example, consider the situation where a patient has a sudden and dramatic drop in their systolic blood pressure while working on vertical positioning. In this case, it may only be necessary for the physical therapist to lower the patient toward the horizontal; in other cases contact with the physician would undoubtedly be necessary.

**New Rule:** It depends.

**Hypothetical Golden Rule Number Two:** When choosing between a number of acceptable interventions, always select the most conservative option in an effort to minimize any potential safety risk to the patient.

**Rule Buster:** Patient safety is a critical component on the National Physical Therapy Examination, but in many cases, it is equally important to weigh the relative benefit of a selected option to achieving a desired patient outcome. How aggressive a therapist should be in a particular situation can only be determined after carefully weighing the relative risk versus the relative reward of each option. It is also important to recognize that all interventions have some degree of risk. If each of the available options to a given question offered no tangible difference in patient outcome, but were considered to be very different in terms of the relative degree of risk, it would then be sensible to select the safest or most conservative option.

**New Rule:** It depends.

**Hypothetical Golden Rule Number Three:** Physical therapist assistants should always contact the supervising physical therapist prior to changing any aspect of a patient's therapy session.

**Rule Buster:** Physical therapist assistants are licensed personnel in the vast majority of states and tend to have a fairly standardized list of acceptable work activities. Communication between a physical therapist and physical therapist assistant is strongly encouraged, however, in some instances, it may not always be necessary. For example, what about the case where a physical therapist assistant wants to change the sequence of resistive exercises or needs to increase or decrease a weight on an existing progressive resistive exercise? In this case, formal communication with the physical therapist would typically not be necessary since physical therapist assistants are able to engage in ongoing assessment. In other instances, formal communication would be necessary. For example, a physical therapist assistant may want to introduce a new intervention that falls outside the current established plan of care or perhaps identifies several findings that indicate a relevant change in a patient's medical status.

**New Rule:** It depends.

As you can see, the only safe rule to rely on is "it depends." Stated differently, the answer to a given question is always dependent on the specific terms and conditions presented in each clinical scenario. Candidates should attempt to inform future clinical decision making based on their experiences with previous sample examination items, but should avoid becoming inflexible or attempting to develop general rules that apply to all situations.

Notes:

# Study Concept 5: Automaticity

On occasion, candidates attempt to complete an academic review by simply taking sample examinations and then reviewing and memorizing the correct answers. This strategy, although potentially helpful, is at best a scattered approach since the scope of the review is dependent solely on the questions asked.

For example, a given series of sample examinations may have a total of eight questions on ultrasound, but it is possible that the questions do not address necessary subject matter such as ultrasound using the underwater technique or explore important concepts such as beam nonuniformity ratio or effective radiating area. This example emphasizes the need for a thorough academic review which allows candidates access to the vast majority of didactic content potentially encountered on the National Physical Therapy Examination.

Consider another example dealing with accessibility standards such as a ramp. Most candidates would quickly recall that the ratio of rise:run is 1:12 or stated differently, each inch of rise requires a minimum of 12 inches of run. Although candidates are likely to be familiar with this concept, they may not be prepared to handle each of the various ways this concept could be tested on the National Physical Therapy Examination.

**An examination item could require a candidate to:**

- Determine the minimum length of a ramp after being given a specific height in inches or feet

- Determine the minimum height of a ramp after being given a specific length in inches or feet

- Determine if a ramp violates the minimum ADA requirements given a height and length in inches or feet

- Determine a given maximum percentage grade for a ramp (using rise:run formula)

- Determine if a ramp violates the maximum percentage grade given a height and length in inches or feet

- Determine the minimum length of a ramp in inches or feet given the need to safely traverse a height the equivalent of a given number of standard size steps

The example illustrates both the need to be familiar with specific didactic content and the need to apply the information in different scenarios. In truth, each of the listed examination items related to ramps relies on the same basic formula (i.e., rise:run), but a candidate's ability to answer the question correctly will depend on their ability to recognize this and in some cases, utilize related information (i.e., the relationship of percentage grade to rise:run and the size of a standard step).

Candidates who have this skill are demonstrating automaticity. Automaticity is a test taking term that describes the ability to quickly recall relevant facts, procedures, and routines and apply this information within the context of a clinically-oriented multiple-choice question. As candidates become increasingly comfortable with the academic knowledge and the ability to apply the information via multiple-choice questions, they tend to score higher on sample examinations.

When reviewing completed sample examination items, candidates greatly benefit from considering other possible scenarios related to the same subject matter or topic being tested. In many cases, the incorrect options for a question are often correct for a variation of the question. For example, a question may ask specifically about the testing procedure for a given cranial nerve. In this case, a candidate may identify option 1 as being correct, but upon reviewing the question later may recognize that options 2, 3, and 4 are also correct for different cranial nerves. Given that there are literally thousands of potential questions that could be asked on the National Physical Therapy Examination, candidates who possess greater flexibility with particular subject matter have a greater probability of answering the item correctly.

**Notes:**

# Study Concept 6: Truths and Myths

There are a variety of popular myths that exist in regard to the National Physical Therapy Examination. Most of the myths are simply misinformation that becomes perpetuated over time. The following section addresses some of the more common myths about the current examination and then sets the record straight.

**Truths and Myths Number One:** The National Physical Therapy Examination has several different forms (i.e., versions), each which has a particular emphasis in terms of systems weighting. For example, a given form may emphasize the musculoskeletal system while another may emphasize the neuromuscular and nervous system.

**Answer:** False
**Explanation:** Each form of the National Physical Therapy Examination is designed based on the same blueprint. The blueprint provides a targeted number of items in each system and content outline area, however, slight variation is permitted in each area within a specified range. The Federation of State Boards of Physical Therapy publicly disseminates the blueprint that provides detailed information on the current examination.

**Truths and Myths Number Two:** When studying for the examination, it is critical to be familiar with multiple academic resources for a selected topic since a given question could require knowledge from a specific resource.

**Answer:** False
**Explanation:** An examination question would not require a candidate to differentiate between multiple academic sources. For example, different academic resources sometimes have subtle differences in select subject matter such as dermatomes or temperature ranges for physical agents. Instead of focusing on this level of detail, a candidate should become comfortable with a given source and have confidence that if this information is encountered on the examination, their answer will be correct.

**Truths and Myths Number Three:** The 50 questions on the National Physical Therapy Examination that are considered pre-test items are clearly identifiable from scored items on the examination.

**Answer:** False
**Explanation:** The 50 pre-test items are intermingled with 200 scored items to make up the 250 question National Physical Therapy Examination. The pre-test items are not distinguishable from scored items and exist in each of the five sections of the examination.

**Truths and Myths Number Four:** Candidates have exactly one hour to complete each of the five sections of the National Physical Therapy Examination.

**Answer:** False
**Explanation:** Candidates have a total of five sections, each with 50 questions, to complete on the National Physical Therapy Examination, however, they are not timed independently. The examination clock will begin at five hours and count down from this value regardless of the rate at which each of the sections is completed. The examination will conclude when the candidate submits their final section or when the five hours has elapsed.

**Truths and Myths Number Five:** A score of 75% correct or 150 of 200 scored items is necessary to pass the National Physical Therapy Examination in most states.

**Answer:** False
**Explanation:** Each form of the examination has an individual criterion-referenced passing score. The passing score may differ by a relatively small amount from form to form. If a particular form was determined to be slightly more difficult than another form, the more difficult form would have a slightly lower criterion-referenced passing score. Individual states do not have the ability to determine passing scores in their respective jurisdictions and instead rely on the established national criterion-referenced passing scores. Recently, criterion-referenced passing scores have been below 150 or 75% of the questions answered correctly.

**Truths and Myths Number Six:** Scores on subsequent attempts of sample examinations are good indicators of success on the National Physical Therapy Examination.

**Answer:** False
**Explanation:** Scores on subsequent attempts of a given sample examination are usually better indicators of memory and less accurate as predictors of future performance. Candidates should always review correct and incorrect answers from a given sample examination, however, they should resist the urge to retake the same examination for the purpose of assessing performance.

**Notes:**

# Study Concept 7: Blood Pressure

Vital signs serve as an important screening tool for physical therapists and should be formally measured for all examinations and then periodically thereafter based on the particular medical diagnosis and specific physical therapy interventions. Given the obvious safety implications associated with measuring and interpreting the results of vital signs, it is critical that candidates have in-depth knowledge of this particular content. This section will present a variety of detailed information related to blood pressure.

- Systolic pressure measures the force exerted against the arteries during the ejection cycle, while diastolic pressure measures the force exerted against the arteries during rest.

- Blood pressure is directly related to cardiac output and peripheral vascular resistance and therefore is an effective non-invasive performance measure of the pumping mechanism of the heart.

- Systolic pressure increases with exertion in a linear progression, often at a rate of 8-12 mm Hg per metabolic equivalent, however, with sustained activity, no further increases typically occur. If systolic pressure does not rise with increasing workload, it may indicate that the functional reserve capacity of the heart has been exceeded.

- Diastolic pressure may increase or decrease a maximum of 10 mm Hg due to adaptive dilation of peripheral vasculature. In a typical clinical setting, the exercise session should be terminated if the systolic pressure exceeds 210 mm Hg or if the diastolic pressure exceeds 110 mm Hg.

- Pulse pressure, which is the difference between systolic and diastolic pressure, generally increases in direct proportion to the intensity of exercise since systolic pressure increases with exercise and diastolic pressure tends to stay the same.

In a healthy adult it is common to see a 40-50 mm Hg change in systolic pressure with intense exercise. Excessive pulse pressure may be indicative of stiffening of the aorta secondary to atherosclerosis.

- Normally, systolic blood pressure in the legs is 10-20% higher than the pressure in the arms (brachial artery). This is why in some cases an ankle-brachial index value of greater than 1.0 is still considered to be normal. Blood pressure readings that are lower in the legs as compared to the arms are abnormal and may be indicative of peripheral vascular disease.

- Blood pressure increases during dynamic resistance exercise, such as free weights, machines or isokinetics, and continues to increase as an exercise set progresses. Blood pressure response is higher during weight training that incorporates a concentric and eccentric phase compared to isokinetic exercise. Blood pressure tends to be higher during the concentric phase of the repetition or when the Valsalva maneuver is used.

- With advancing age, the same amount of blood fills the ventricles, but the pumping mechanism is less effective. As a result, the body compensates by increasing blood pressure in an attempt to maintain homeostasis.

- During exercise testing, a systolic blood pressure that fails to increase or decrease with increasing workloads may signal a plateau or decrease in cardiac output.

- Systolic blood pressure normally decreases promptly with the cessation of exercise. As a general guideline, the three-minute post exercise systolic blood pressure should be less than 90% of the systolic blood pressure at peak exercise.

Notes:

# Study Concept 8: Lines, Tubes, and Equipment

The National Physical Therapy Examination is designed to protect consumers from unqualified practitioners. Given the purpose of the examination, it is inevitable that candidates will encounter a variety of questions that deal with patients with a significantly compromised medical status.

This section presents information on various types of lines, tubes, and equipment. The purpose is to remind physical therapists of some of the more critical elements to consider when treating patients using these devices. Please remember that this is not an all-inclusive list and additional detail will be provided on the vast majority of items throughout **PTEXAM: The Complete Study Guide.**

## Lines

### Arterial Lines (A Line)

- Avoid applying a blood pressure cuff above the infusion site
- Grasp the IV line support pole so the infusion site is at heart level
- Avoid activities that require the infusion site to be above the level of the heart for a prolonged period
- Exercise is possible with the line, but avoid disturbing the apparatus

### Swan-Ganz Catheters (Pulmonary Artery Catheters), Central Venous Pressure Catheters, Indwelling Right Atrial Catheters

- Exercise is possible with the line, but mobility may need to be restricted near the catheter insertion

### Total Parenteral Nutrition, Hyperalimentation Devices (Intravenous Feeding)

- Alarm sound indicates the fluid source is empty or the system has become unbalanced
- Disruption or disconnection may result in an air embolus
- Shoulder motion on the side of the infusion site may be restricted primarily in flexion and abduction
- Exercise is possible with the line, but mobility may need to be restricted near the catheter insertion

### Intracranial Monitoring

- Isometric exercise and the Valsalva maneuver should be avoided since these activities increase intracranial pressure
- Avoid neck flexion, hip flexion greater than 90 degrees, and lying down in a prone position
- Venous drainage is maximal with the head of the bed elevated 30 degrees
- Momentary elevation of intracranial pressure is normal, but sustained increases are not and therefore should be reported

## Tubes

### Nasogastric Tube (NG Tube)

- Patient will not be able to eat food or drink fluids by mouth while the nasogastric tube is in place
- Enteral feedings can be disconnected temporarily for mobility
- Exercise requiring movements of the head and neck should be avoided, especially forward bending

### Gastrostomy Tube (G Tube)

- Distal tubing can inadvertently become caught on items such as furniture and be pulled out
- Enteral feedings should be turned off temporarily prior to and during treatment
- Enteral feedings can be disconnected temporarily for mobility

### Urinary Catheters

- Tubes should be placed below the region being drained since the devices rely on gravity
- The collection bag should not be raised above the level of the bladder for any sustained period
- Avoid disrupting, stretching, disconnecting or occluding the tube during exercise

### Chest Tubes

- When ambulating, collection bottles should be kept below the level of the inserted tube location
- Monitor the patient for changes in breath sounds before and after intervention
- Avoid pressing directly on the chest tube during mobility activities

## Equipment

### Mechanical Ventilation

- Alarm may indicate disconnected tube, coughing or change in respiratory pattern
- Develop nonverbal means of communication with the patient
- Patient is at greater risk for developing contractures, skin ulcers, and deconditioning

### Supplemental Oxygen Delivery System

- Be aware of signs of respiratory distress (i.e., dyspnea, cyanosis, cramping)
- Monitor $SaO_2$, $PaO_2$, and hemodynamics prior to, during, and after physical therapy intervention
- Exercise is possible, but avoid disturbing the tubing

# Study Concept 9: Emergent Conditions

According to the Federation of State Boards of Physical Therapy, the National Physical Therapy Examination is designed to assess basic entry-level competence of the licensure candidate who has graduated from an accredited program. The primary purpose of the examination is therefore to protect the public from unqualified practitioners. Given the purpose of the examination, it is reasonable to expect that a high percentage of examination items will deal with safety-related issues including the identification and management of potentially emergent conditions. When encountering this type of question, it is critical that candidates are armed with the necessary knowledge to make informed clinical decisions.

**The following provides relevant information on three commonly encountered emergent conditions.**

## Pulmonary Embolism

**Description:** A blockage of the pulmonary artery or one of its branches, usually precipitated by a blood clot from a vein (venous thrombus) becoming dislodged from its site of formation. The dislodged blood clot then travels to the arterial blood supply of one of the lungs.

**Clinical presentation:** Difficulty breathing, chest pain that often mimics a heart attack, rapid pulse; in more severe cases circulatory instability and death

**Risk factors:** Surgery, long periods of inactivity, increased levels of clotting factor in the blood, and abnormal factors in the vessel wall

**Diagnosis:** Pulmonary angiography is the most accurate method to diagnose pulmonary embolism, however, because the procedure carries inherent risks to the patient, other diagnostic procedures such as chest x-ray, lung scan, and spiral computerized tomography scan are more commonly utilized.

**Treatment:** Anticoagulant medication such as Heparin and Warfarin

**Notes:** Pulmonary embolism remains the leading cause of hospital death in the United States.

## Hypovolemic Shock

**Description:** A life-threatening condition caused by insufficient circulating blood volume. Primary causes include hemorrhage or severe burns.

**Clinical presentation:** Hypotension due to lack of circulating volume, anxiety, altered mental state, cool and clammy skin, rapid and thready pulse, thirst, and fatigue due to inadequate oxygenation

**Risk factors:** Exposure to severe trauma or burns

**Diagnosis:** Primarily through the identification of the described clinical presentation

**Treatment:** Management of suspected shock includes activating the emergency medical system. Positional management includes lying in supine with the legs elevated approximately 12 inches in situations where it is tolerated. Management of confirmed shock includes controlling bleeding and attempting to restore blood volume by providing infusions of balanced salt solutions or blood in more severe cases.

**Notes:** There are several other common forms of shock including cardiogenic, septic, and anaphylactic. Cardiogenic shock is characterized by failure of the heart to pump effectively. Management includes oxygen therapy and administering cardiac medications. Septic shock is characterized by an overwhelming infection leading to vasodilation. Management includes restoring intravascular volume and identifying and controlling the source of infection. Anaphylactic shock is characterized by a severe and sometimes fatal reaction to an allergen, antigen or drug which causes vasodilation leading to hypotension and increased capillary permeability. Management includes identifying and removing the causative antigen and administering countermediators such as anti-histamine.

## Autonomic Dysreflexia

**Description:** A massive sympathetic discharge that can occur in association with a spinal cord injury or disease. The condition is triggered by a variety of noxious stimuli including bladder distention, urinary tract infection, skin ulcers, and bowel impaction.

**Clinical presentation:** Sweating above the level of the lesion, flushing of the skin above the level of the lesion, elevated blood pressure, and blurred vision

**Risk factors:** Patients with spinal cord injuries at and above the T6 level

**Diagnosis:** Primarily through the identification of the described clinical presentation

**Treatment:** Management of autonomic dysreflexia includes immediate determination and removal of the triggering stimuli. Positional management includes sitting the patient upright to lower the elevated blood pressure below dangerous levels. Tight clothing and stockings should also be removed. If the noxious stimuli cannot be identified, medical management may include vasodilators to assist with symptomatic relief.

**Notes:** Prevalence rates for autonomic dysreflexia have been reported ranging from 48-90% of all individuals with spinal cord injuries at T6 and above. The occurrence of autonomic dysreflexia is increased as an individual moves out of spinal shock.

**Notes:**

# Study Concept 10: Assessment

Candidates must carefully assess their examination performance when taking sample examinations. Each of the sample examinations in *PTEXAM: The Complete Study Guide* offers candidates the opportunity to view their performance according to six system specific and six content outline categories. The shaded areas in the tables below will be used in the performance analysis section to express the number of questions answered correctly in each category, the total number of questions in the category, and the percentage of questions correct.

| System Specific Summary | | |
|---|---|---|
| **Musculoskeletal System** | | |
| **Neuromuscular & Nervous Systems** | | |
| **Cardiovascular/Pulmonary and Lymphatic Systems** | | |
| **Other Systems** | | |
| **Non-Systems** | | |

| Content Outline Summary | | |
|---|---|---|
| **Physical Therapy Examination** | | |
| **Foundations for Evaluation, Differential Diagnosis, & Prognosis** | | |
| **Interventions** | | |
| **Equipment & Devices; Therapeutic Modalities** | | |
| **Safety & Protection; Professional Responsibilities; Research** | | |

Candidates should use this information to develop remedial plans to improve performance on sample examinations. Candidates must be familiar with the content contained in each system specific and content outline category and carefully assess how their performance changes over time.

The academic review section of *PTEXAM: The Complete Study Guide* is arranged according to the exact categories used in the system specific summary and therefore serves as an excellent resource for candidates to utilize when initially remediating deficient areas. In some instances, a candidate may determine that it is necessary to access a more formal academic resource such as a textbook to locate information not covered in the review book. In these situations it is important for candidates to stay focused and avoid purely exploring the textbook since often candidates do not emerge for several hours.

The content outline is less intuitive than the system specific categories since the content outline is not system based, however, it is still very useful given the detailed information available on the National Physical Therapy Examination Blueprint. For example, a candidate may find that they tend to perform very well on questions within the "Physical Therapy Examination" category, but have more difficulty on questions within the "Foundations for Evaluation, Differential Diagnosis, and Prognosis" category. By consulting the National Physical Therapy Examination Blueprint, a candidate will quickly realize that the "Physical Therapy Examination" category deals primarily with tests and measures, anatomy and physiology, and movement analysis, while the "Foundations for Evaluation, Differential Diagnosis, and Prognosis" category deals primarily with diseases/conditions, pathophysiology, and differential diagnosis. The information from the content outline combined with the system specific information allows candidates to gain greater insight toward their current performance and should assist them to be more specific when selecting appropriate remedial activities.

Candidates are encouraged to look for general trends in their scoring when taking sample examinations and avoid making a definitive statement on their level of competence in any given category based on the results of a single sample examination. This is especially true in a category where there is a smaller number of questions such as the integumentary system. As the number of questions in each category diminishes, the category becomes less accurate as a predictor of actual performance. In some instances, candidates will have a few glaring areas of deficiency (e.g., "Musculoskeletal" and "Other Systems"), while in other cases, candidates will demonstrate more consistency. Consistency can be a very good thing if the scores are consistent at a very high level (i.e., a high percentage of questions answered correctly in the majority of areas) or more problematic if the scores are consistent at a very low level (i.e., a low percentage of questions answered correctly in the majority of areas).

In summary, studying for the examination is analogous to developing a plan of care for a patient; the more specific the plan of care is for the particular needs of the patient, the better the patient outcome. In terms of preparing for the examination, the more specific a remedial plan is to the particular needs of a given candidate, the better the candidate's outcome.

# 4

# MUSCULOSKELETAL SYSTEM

## Scott Giles

Musculoskeletal System represents approximately 30.5% (61 questions) of the National Physical Therapy Examination.

The actual number of questions in this category can range from 59 to 63 questions.

45 Exercise Physiology

45 Kinesiology

48 Muscle Action

73 Muscle Testing

77 Gait

82 Range of Motion

90 Special Tests

101 Osteokinematics

104 Pathology

112 Pharmacology

113 Orthotics

114 Amputations and Prosthetics

120 Essentials

122 Proficiencies

SCOREBUILDERS

# Exercise Physiology

## Energy Systems[1]

ATP-PC or Phosphagen System

Anaerobic Glycolysis or Lactic Acid System

Aerobic or Oxygen System

## Anaerobic Metabolism

### ATP-PC System

This energy system is used for ATP production during high intensity, short duration exercise such as sprinting 100 meters. Phosphocreatine decomposes and releases a large amount of energy that is used to construct ATP. There is two to three times more phosphocreatine in cells of muscles than ATP. This process occurs almost instantaneously, allowing for ready and available energy needed by the muscles. The system provides energy for muscle contraction for up to 15 seconds.

The phosphagen system represents the most rapidly available source of ATP for use by the muscle. The energy system is able to function in the described manner since:

- It does not depend on a long series of chemical reactions.
- It does not depend on transporting the oxygen we breathe to the working muscles.
- Both ATP and PC are stored directly within the contractile mechanisms of the muscle.

### Anaerobic Glycolysis

This energy system is a major supplier of ATP during high intensity, short duration activities such as sprinting 400 or 800 meters. Stored glycogen is split into glucose, and through glycolysis, split again into pyruvic acid. The energy released during this process forms ATP. The process does not require oxygen. Anaerobic glycolysis results in the formation of lactic acid, which causes muscular fatigue.

This system is nearly 50% slower than the phosphocreatine system, and can provide a person with 30 to 40 seconds of muscle contraction. The energy system is able to function in the described manner since:

- It does not require the presence of oxygen.
- It only uses carbohydrates (glycogen and glucose).
- It releases enough energy for the resynthesis of only small amounts of ATP.

## Aerobic Metabolism

The aerobic system is used predominantly during low intensity, long duration exercise such as running a marathon. The oxygen system yields by far the most ATP, but it requires several series of complex chemical reactions. This system provides energy through the oxidation of food. The combination of fatty acids, amino acids, and glucose with oxygen releases energy that forms ATP. This system will provide energy as long as there are nutrients to utilize.

# Kinesiology

## Anatomical Position[2,3]

The anatomical position is an erect posture of the body with the face forward, feet pointing forward and slightly apart, arms at the side, and palms forward with fingers and thumbs in extension (Figs. 4-1, 4-2). The position serves as a point of reference for definitions and descriptions of movement including the cardinal planes and associated axes.

## Planes of the Body[3,4]

Motions are described as occurring in three cardinal planes of the body (frontal, sagittal, transverse). Movement in the cardinal planes occurs around three corresponding axes (anterior-posterior, medial-lateral, vertical).

### Frontal plane (coronal)

The frontal (or coronal) plane divides the body into anterior and posterior sections. Motions in the frontal plane, such as abduction and adduction, occur around an anterior-posterior axis.

### Sagittal plane

The sagittal plane divides the body into right and left sections. Motions in the sagittal plane, such as flexion and extension, occur around a medial-lateral axis.

### Transverse plane

The transverse plane divides the body into upper and lower sections. Motions in the transverse plane, such as medial and lateral rotation, occur around a vertical axis.

## Class 2 Lever

A class 2 lever has the resistance (load) between the axis of rotation (fulcrum) and the effort (force). The length of the effort arm is always longer than the resistance arm. In most instances, gravity is the effort and muscle activity is the resistance, however, there are class 2 levers where the muscle is the effort when the distal attachment is on a weight bearing segment. An example of a class 2 lever is a wheelbarrow.

## Class 3 Lever

A class 3 lever has the effort (force) between the axis of rotation (fulcrum) and the resistance (load). The length of the effort arm is always shorter than the length of the resistance arm. Shoulder abduction with weight at the wrist is a class 3 lever. Class 3 levers usually permit large movements at rapid speeds and are the most common type of lever in the body. An example of a class 3 lever is elbow flexion.

**Fig. 4-1 (Left):** Anatomical position - anterior view.

**Fig. 4-2 (Right):** Anatomical position - posterior view.

## Classes of Levers[4]

### Class 1 Lever

A class 1 lever has the axis of rotation (fulcrum) between the effort (force) and resistance (load). There are very few class 1 levers in the body. A class 1 lever is illustrated with the triceps brachii force on the olecranon with an external counterforce pushing on the forearm. Another example of a class 1 lever is a seesaw.

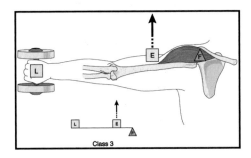

# Joint Classification[4,5,6]

## Fibrous Joints (Synarthroses)

Fibrous joints are composed of bones that are united by fibrous tissue and are nonsynovial. Movement is minimal to none with the amount of movement permitted at the joint dependent on the length of the fibers uniting the bones.

**Suture** – (e.g., sagittal suture of the skull)

- Union of two bones by a ligament or membrane
- Immovable joint
- Eventual fusion is termed synostosis

**Syndesmosis** – (e.g., the tibia and fibula with interosseous membrane)

- Bone connected to bone by a dense fibrous membrane or cord
- Very little motion

**Gomphosis** – (e.g., a tooth in its socket)

- Two bony surfaces connect as a peg in a hole
- The teeth and corresponding sockets in the mandible/maxilla are the only gomphosis joints in the body
- The periodontal membrane is the fibrous component of the joint

## Cartilaginous Joints (Amphiarthroses)

Cartilaginous joints have a hyaline cartilage or fibrocartilage that connects one bone to another. These are slightly moveable joints.

**Synchondrosis** – (e.g., sternum and true rib articulation)

- Hyaline cartilage
- Cartilage adjoins two ossifying centers of bone

- Provides stability during growth
- May ossify to a synostosis once growth is completed
- Slight motion

**Symphysis** – (e.g., pubic symphysis)

- Generally located at the midline of the body
- Two bones covered with hyaline cartilage
- Two bones connected by fibrocartilage
- Slight motion

### Synovial Joints (Diarthroses)

Synovial joints provide free movement between the bones they join. They have five distinguishing characteristics: joint cavity, articular cartilage, synovial membrane, synovial fluid, and fibrous capsule. These joints are the most complex and vulnerable to injury. They are further classified by the type of movement and shape of the articulating bones.

**Uniaxial joint** – one motion around a single axis in one plane of the body

- Hinge (ginglymus) – elbow joint
- Pivot (trochoid) – atlantoaxial joint

**Biaxial joint** – movement occurs in two planes and around two axes through the convex/concave surfaces

- Condyloid – metacarpophalangeal joint of a finger
- Saddle – carpometacarpal joint of the thumb

**Multi-axial joint** – movement occurs in three planes and around three axes

- Plane (gliding) – carpal joints
- Ball and socket – hip joint

# Joint Receptors[1,4]

### Free Nerve Endings

| | |
|---|---|
| Location | Joint capsule, ligaments, synovium, fat pads |
| Sensitivity | One type is sensitive to non-noxious mechanical stress; other type is sensitive to noxious mechanical or biochemical stimuli |
| Primary Distribution | All joints |

### Pacinian Corpuscles

| | |
|---|---|
| Location | Fibrous layer of joint capsule |
| Sensitivity | High frequency vibration, acceleration, and high velocity changes in joint position |
| Primary Distribution | All joints |

### Golgi Ligament Endings

| | |
|---|---|
| Location | Ligaments, adjacent to ligaments' bony attachment |
| Sensitivity | Tension or stretch on ligaments |
| Primary Distribution | Majority of joints |

### Ruffini Endings

| | |
|---|---|
| Location | Fibrous layer of joint capsule |
| Sensitivity | Stretching of joint capsule; amplitude, and velocity of joint position |
| Primary Distribution | Greater density in proximal joints, particularly in capsular regions |

### Golgi-Mazzoni Corpuscles

| | |
|---|---|
| Location | Joint capsule |
| Sensitivity | Compression of joint capsule |
| Primary Distribution | Knee joint, joint capsule |

## Muscle Action

### Head

#### Temporomandibular Joint

**Depress:**
- Lateral pterygoid
- Suprahyoid
- Infrahyoid

**Elevate:**
- Temporalis
- Masseter
- Medial pterygoid

**Protrusion:**
- Masseter
- Lateral pterygoid
- Medial pterygoid

**Retrusion:**
- Temporalis
- Masseter
- Digastric

**Side to Side:**
- Medial pterygoid
- Lateral pterygoid
- Masseter
- Temporalis

### Spine

#### Cervical Intervertebral Joints

**Flexion:**
- Sternocleidomastoid
- Longus colli
- Scalenus muscles

**Extension:**
- Splenius cervicis
- Semispinalis cervicis
- Iliocostalis cervicis
- Longissimus cervicis
- Multifidus
- Trapezius

**Rotation and Lateral Bending:**
- Sternocleidomastoid
- Scalenus muscles
- Splenius cervicis
- Longissimus cervicis
- Iliocostalis cervicis
- Levator scapulae
- Multifidus

#### Thoracic and Lumbar Intervertebral Joints

**Flexion:**
- Rectus abdominis
- Internal oblique
- External oblique

**Extension:**
- Erector spinae
- Quadratus lumborum
- Multifidus

**Rotation and Lateral Bending:**
- Psoas major
- Quadratus lumborum
- External oblique
- Internal oblique
- Multifidus
- Longissimus thoracis
- Iliocostalis thoracis
- Rotatores

### Upper Extremity

#### Scapula

**Elevation:**
- Upper trapezius
- Levator scapulae

**Depression:**
- Latissimus dorsi
- Pectoralis major
- Pectoralis minor
- Lower trapezius

**Protraction:**
- Serratus anterior
- Pectoralis minor

**Retraction:**
- Trapezius
- Rhomboids

**Upward Rotation:**
- Trapezius
- Serratus anterior

**Downward Rotation:**
- Rhomboids
- Levator scapulae
- Pectoralis minor

#### Shoulder Joint

**Flexion:**
- Anterior deltoid
- Coracobrachialis
- Pectoralis major
- Biceps brachii

**Extension:**
- Latissimus dorsi
- Posterior deltoid
- Teres major

**Abduction:**
- Middle deltoid
- Supraspinatus

**Adduction:**
- Pectoralis major
- Latissimus dorsi
- Teres major

**Lateral Rotation:**
- Teres minor
- Infraspinatus
- Posterior deltoid

**Medial Rotation:**
- Subscapularis
- Teres major
- Pectoralis major
- Latissimus dorsi
- Anterior deltoid

# Upper Extremity (continued)

## Elbow Joint

**Flexion:**
- Biceps brachii
- Brachialis
- Brachioradialis

**Extension:**
- Triceps brachii
- Anconeus

## Radioulnar Joint

**Supination:**
- Biceps brachii
- Supinator

**Pronation:**
- Pronator teres
- Pronator quadratus

## Wrist Joint

**Flexion:**
- Flexor carpi radialis
- Flexor carpi ulnaris
- Palmaris longus

**Extension:**
- Extensor carpi radialis longus
- Extensor carpi radialis brevis
- Extensor carpi ulnaris

**Radial Deviation:**
- Extensor carpi radialis
- Flexor carpi radialis
- Extensor pollicis longus and brevis

**Ulnar Deviation:**
- Extensor carpi ulnaris
- Flexor carpi ulnaris

# Lower Extremity

## Hip Joint

**Flexion:**
- Iliopsoas
- Sartorius
- Rectus femoris
- Pectineus

**Extension:**
- Gluteus maximus and medius
- Semitendinosus
- Semimembranosus
- Biceps femoris

**Abduction:**
- Gluteus medius
- Gluteus minimus
- Piriformis
- Obturator internus
- Tensor fasciae latae

**Adduction:**
- Adductor magnus
- Adductor longus
- Adductor brevis
- Gracilis

**Medial Rotation:**
- Tensor fasciae latae
- Gluteus medius
- Gluteus minimus
- Pectineus
- Adductor longus

**Lateral Rotation:**
- Gluteus maximus
- Obturator externus
- Obturator internus
- Piriformis
- Gemelli
- Sartorius

## Knee Joint

**Flexion:**
- Biceps femoris
- Semitendinosus
- Semimembranosus
- Sartorius

**Extension:**
- Rectus femoris
- Vastus lateralis
- Vastus intermedius
- Vastus medialis

## Ankle Joint

**Plantar Flexion:**
- Tibialis posterior
- Gastrocnemius
- Soleus
- Peroneus longus
- Peroneus brevis
- Plantaris
- Flexor hallucis

**Dorsiflexion:**
- Tibialis anterior
- Extensor hallucis longus
- Extensor digitorum longus
- Peroneus tertius

**Inversion:**
- Tibialis posterior
- Tibialis anterior
- Flexor digitorum longus

**Eversion:**
- Peroneus longus
- Peroneus brevis
- Peroneus tertius

# Specific Joints - Upper Extremity

## Shoulder[5,7-11]

The shoulder complex is formed by a series of unique articulations including the glenohumeral joint, sternoclavicular joint, acromioclavicular joint, and scapulothoracic articulation.

## Articulations

### Glenohumeral joint

The glenohumeral joint is formed by the convex head of the humerus and the concave glenoid fossa of the scapula. The glenohumeral joint is a ball and socket synovial joint with three degrees of freedom. The relatively small articular surface of the glenoid fossa in relation to the size of the humeral head, makes the glenohumeral joint inherently unstable.

### Glenohumeral Snapshot

**Osteokinematic motions:** flexion, extension, abduction, adduction, medial rotation, lateral rotation

**Loose packed position:** 55 degrees abduction, 30 degrees horizontal adduction

**Close packed position:** abduction and lateral rotation

**Capsular pattern:** lateral rotation, abduction, medial rotation

### Sternoclavicular joint

The sternoclavicular joint is formed by the medial end of the clavicle and the manubrium of the sternum. The joint is a saddle-shaped synovial joint with three degrees of freedom. A fibrocartilaginous disc between the manubrium and clavicle enhances the stability of the joint. The disc acts as a shock absorber and serves as the axis for clavicular rotation.

### Sternoclavicular Snapshot

**Osteokinematic motions:** elevation, depression, protraction, retraction, medial rotation, lateral rotation

**Loose packed position:** arm resting by the side

**Close packed position:** maximum shoulder elevation

**Capsular pattern:** pain at extremes of range of movement

### Acromioclavicular joint

The acromioclavicular joint is formed by the acromion process of the scapula and the lateral end of the clavicle. The joint is a plane synovial joint with three degrees of freedom. The acromioclavicular joint functions to maintain the relationship between the scapula and clavicle during glenohumeral range of motion.

### Acromioclavicular Snapshot

**Osteokinematic motions:** anterior tilting, posterior tilting, upward rotation, downward rotation, protraction, retraction

**Loose packed position:** arm resting by the side

**Close packed position:** arm abducted to 90 degrees

**Capsular pattern:** pain at extremes of range of movement

### Scapulothoracic articulation

The scapulothoracic articulation is formed by the body of the scapula and the muscles covering the posterior chest wall. Motion consists of sliding of the scapula on the thorax. The articulation is not a true anatomical joint because it lacks the necessary synovial joint characteristics.

## Muscle Action

**Shoulder flexion:** anterior deltoid, coracobrachialis, pectoralis major, biceps brachii

**Shoulder extension:** latissimus dorsi, posterior deltoid, teres major

**Shoulder abduction:** middle deltoid, supraspinatus

**Shoulder adduction:** pectoralis major, latissimus dorsi, teres major

**Shoulder lateral rotation:** teres minor, infraspinatus, posterior deltoid

**Shoulder medial rotation:** subscapularis, teres major, pectoralis major, latissimus dorsi, anterior deltoid

**Scapula elevation:** upper trapezius, levator scapulae

**Scapula depression:** latissimus dorsi, pectoralis major, pectoralis minor, lower trapezius

**Scapula protraction:** serratus anterior, pectoralis minor

**Scapula retraction:** trapezius, rhomboids

**Scapula upward rotation:** trapezius, serratus anterior

**Scapula downward rotation:** rhomboids, levator scapulae, pectoralis minor

## Primary Structures

### Glenoid labrum

The glenoid labrum is a fibrocartilaginous structure that serves to deepen the glenoid fossa and increases the size of the articular surface. The glenoid labrum consists of a dense fibrous connective tissue that is often damaged with recurrent shoulder instability.

### Joint capsule

The joint capsule arises from the glenoid fossa and the glenoid labrum to blend with the muscles of the rotator cuff. The volume of the joint capsule is twice as large as the size of the humeral head. The capsule is reinforced by the glenohumeral ligaments and the coracohumeral ligament.

### Subacromial bursa

The subacromial bursa extends over the supraspinatus tendon and distal muscle belly, beneath the acromion and deltoid muscle. The bursa facilitates movement of the deltoid muscle over the fibrous capsule of the shoulder joint and supraspinatus tendon. The bursa is often involved with impingement beneath the acromial arch.

### Subscapular bursa

The subscapular bursa overlies the anterior joint capsule and lies beneath the subscapularis muscle. Anterior shoulder fullness may indicate articular effusion secondary to distention of the bursa.

### Elbow[5,8-10]

The elbow joint is a synovial joint consisting of three bones (i.e., humerus, radius, ulna) and three primary articulations (i.e., radiohumeral, ulnohumeral, proximal radioulnar) enclosed within a single joint capsule. The elbow is classified as a hinge joint formed by the articulation of the ulna with the humerus.

## Articulations

### Radiohumeral joint

The proximal joint surface of the radiohumeral joint is the ball-shaped capitulum of the distal humerus. The distal joint surface is the concave head of the radius.

### Radiohumeral Snapshot

**Osteokinematic motions:** flexion, extension, pronation, supination

**Loose packed position:** full extension, supination

**Close packed position:** 90 degrees flexion, 5 degrees supination

**Capsular pattern:** flexion, extension, supination, pronation

### Ulnohumeral joint

The ulnohumeral joint is formed by the hourglass-shaped trochlea of the humerus and the trochlear notch of the ulna.

### Ulnohumeral Snapshot

**Osteokinematic motions:** flexion, extension

**Loose packed position:** 70 degrees of elbow flexion, 10 degrees supination

**Close packed position:** extension

**Capsular pattern:** flexion, extension

### Proximal radioulnar joint

The proximal radioulnar joint consists of the concave radial notch of the ulna and the convex rim of the radial head.

### Proximal Radioulnar Snapshot

**Osteokinematic motions:** pronation, supination

**Loose packed position:** 70 degrees elbow flexion, 35 degrees supination

**Close packed position:** 5 degrees supination

**Capsular pattern:** supination, pronation

## Muscle Action

**Elbow flexion:** biceps brachii, brachialis, brachioradialis

**Elbow extension:** triceps brachii, anconeus

**Forearm supination:** biceps brachii, supinator

**Forearm pronation:** pronator teres, pronator quadratus

## Primary Structures

### Radial collateral ligament (i.e., lateral collateral ligament)

The radial collateral ligament extends from the lateral epicondyle of the humerus to the lateral border and olecranon process of the ulna and to the annular ligament. It is a fan-shaped ligament that prevents adduction of the elbow joint, and provides reinforcement for the radiohumeral articulation.

### Ulnar collateral ligament (i.e., medial collateral ligament)

The ulnar collateral ligament runs from the medial epicondyle of the humerus to the proximal portion of the ulna. The ligament prevents excessive abduction of the elbow joint.

## Consider This
### Mechanisms of Injury for Elbow Ligaments

The ulnar and radial collateral ligaments can become stretched, frayed or torn through the stress of repetitive throwing motions. If the force on the soft tissues is greater than the tensile strength of the structure, tiny tears of the ligaments can develop. Months (and even years) of throwing can cause microtears, degeneration, and finally, rupture of the ligaments. Baseball pitchers are the athletes treated most often for this problem. Tennis, track and field, football, ice hockey, and water polo participants have also been reported to injure the collateral ligaments. A fall on an outstretched arm can lead to collateral ligament rupture, often with associated elbow dislocation.

### Annular ligament

The annular ligament consists of a band of fibers that surrounds the head of the radius. It allows the head of the radius to rotate and retain contact with the radial notch of the ulna.

### Anterior ligament

The anterior ligament is capsular in nature and function. It stretches from the radial collateral ligament and attaches above the upper edge of the coronoid fossa, extending to just below the coronoid process.

### Posterior ligament

The posterior ligament resembles the anterior ligament. It blends on each side with the collateral ligaments and is attached to the upper portion of the olecranon fossa, and to just below the olecranon process.

### Wrist[5,8,9,10,12]

The wrist complex is formed by the radiocarpal and midcarpal joints. The radiocarpal joint attaches the hand to the forearm. The midcarpal joint is formed by the articulations of the proximal and distal row of carpals.

### Articulations

#### Radiocarpal joint

The proximal joint surface of the radiocarpal joint is formed by the distal radius and the radioulnar articular disc, which connects the medial aspect of the distal radius to the distal ulna. The distal joint surface is formed by the scaphoid, lunate, and triquetrum. The radiocarpal joint has two degrees of freedom. It is encased in a strong capsule reinforced by numerous ligaments shared with the midcarpal joint.

#### Radiocarpal Snapshot

**Osteokinematic motions:** flexion, extension, radial deviation, ulnar deviation

**Loose packed position:** neutral with slight ulnar deviation

**Close packed position:** extension with radial deviation

**Capsular pattern:** flexion and extension equally limited

### Midcarpal joint

Motion of the wrist results in complex motion between the proximal and distal row of carpals with the exception of the pisiform. The joint surfaces are reciprocally convex and concave.

### Muscle Action

**Wrist flexion:** flexor carpi radialis, flexor carpi ulnaris, palmaris longus

**Wrist extension:** extensor carpi radialis longus, extensor carpi radialis brevis, extensor carpi ulnaris

**Radial deviation:** extensor carpi radialis, flexor carpi radialis, extensor pollicis longus, extensor pollicis brevis

**Ulnar deviation:** extensor carpi ulnaris, flexor carpi ulnaris

### Primary Structures

#### Dorsal radiocarpal ligament

The dorsal radiocarpal ligament is the only major ligament on the dorsal surface of the wrist. The ligament originates on the posterior surface of the distal radius and styloid process of the radius and attaches to the lunate and triquetrum. The ligament serves to limit wrist flexion.

#### Palmar radiocarpal ligament

The palmar radiocarpal ligament maintains the alignment of the associated joint structures and limits hyperextension of the wrist. The ligament originates from the anterior surface of the distal radius and attaches to the capitate, triquetrum, and scaphoid.

#### Radial collateral ligament

The radial collateral ligament serves to limit ulnar deviation and becomes taut when the wrist is in extremes of extension and flexion. The ligament originates from the styloid process of the radius and inserts on the scaphoid and trapezium.

#### Carpal tunnel

The carpal tunnel is located close to the deep surface of the flexor retinaculum. The median nerve enters the palm through the carpal tunnel. Any condition that significantly reduces the size of the carpal tunnel (e.g., tenosynovitis, inflammation of the flexor retinaculum) may result in compression of the median nerve.

#### Interosseous membrane

The interosseous membrane consists of a dense band of fibrous connective tissue that runs obliquely from the radius to the ulna. The structure spans from the proximal radioulnar joint to the distal radioulnar joint and serves as a stabilizer against axial forces applied to the wrist.

**Fig. 4-3:** Muscles of the anterior upper limb.

**Fig. 4-4:** Muscles of the posterior upper limb.

**Fig. 4-5:** Muscles of the volar surface of the forearm.

Extensor carpi ulnaris

Extensor digitorum

Abductor pollicis longus
Extensor pollicis brevis
Extensor pollicis longus

**Fig. 4-6:** Muscles of the dorsal surface of the forearm.

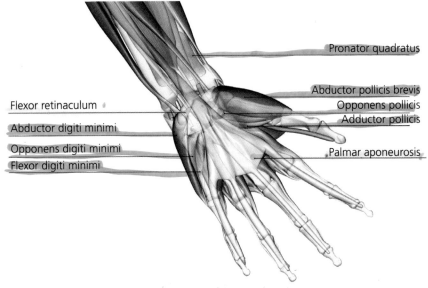

Pronator quadratus

Abductor pollicis brevis
Opponens pollicis
Adductor pollicis

Flexor retinaculum

Abductor digiti minimi

Opponens digiti minimi
Flexor digiti minimi

Palmar aponeurosis

**Fig. 4-7:** Muscles of the volar surface of the wrist and hand.

Abductor pollicis

Extensor retinaculum

Dorsal interosseus

Abductor digiti minimi

Extensor digitorum tendons

Extensor digiti minimi tendon

**Fig. 4-8:** Muscles of the dorsal surface of the wrist and hand.

# Specific Joints - Lower Extremity

## Hip[5,8-10]

The hip (iliofemoral) joint is a synovial joint formed by the head of the femur and the acetabulum. The hip is classified as a ball and socket joint with three degrees of freedom.

## Articulations

### Iliofemoral joint

The proximal joint surface of the iliofemoral joint consists of the acetabulum which is oriented laterally, inferiorly, and anteriorly. The distal joint surface consists of the convex head of the femur.

### Iliofemoral Snapshot

**Osteokinematic motions:** flexion, extension, abduction, adduction, medial rotation, lateral rotation

**Loose packed position:** 30 degrees flexion, 30 degrees abduction, slight lateral rotation

**Close packed position:** full extension, medial rotation

**Capsular pattern:** flexion, abduction, medial rotation (sometimes medial rotation is most limited)

## Muscle Action

**Hip flexion:** iliopsoas, sartorius, rectus femoris, pectineus

**Hip extension:** gluteus maximus, gluteus medius, semitendinosus, semimembranosus, biceps femoris

**Hip abduction:** gluteus medius, gluteus minimus, piriformis, obturator internus, tensor fasciae latae

**Hip adduction:** adductor magnus, adductor longus, adductor brevis, gracilis

**Hip medial rotation:** tensor fasciae latae, gluteus medius, gluteus minimus, pectineus, adductor longus

**Hip lateral rotation:** gluteus maximus, obturator externus, obturator internus, piriformis, gemelli, sartorius

## Primary Structures

### Articular capsule

A strong articular capsule extends from the rim of the acetabulum to the neck of the femur. The capsule is reinforced by the iliofemoral, pubofemoral, and ischiofemoral ligaments.

### Iliofemoral ligament

The iliofemoral ligament consists of a thickened portion of the articular capsule that extends from the anterior inferior iliac spine of the pelvis to the intertrochanteric line of the femur. The structure is considered to be the strongest ligament in the body and serves to prevent excessive hip extension and assists to maintain upright posture.

### Pubofemoral ligament

The pubofemoral ligament consists of a thickened portion of the articular capsule that extends from the pubic portion of the rim of the acetabulum to the neck of the femur. The structure serves to prevent excessive abduction of the femur and limits hip extension.

### Ischiofemoral ligament

The ischiofemoral ligament consists of a thickened portion of the articular capsule that extends from the ischial wall of the acetabulum to the neck of the femur. The structure is the weakest of the three ligaments, however, it serves to reinforce the articular capsule.

### Acetabular labrum

The acetabular labrum consists of a fibrocartilaginous rim attached to the margin of the acetabulum. The structure enhances the depth of the acetabulum.

## Knee[8-12]

The knee joint is a synovial joint consisting of three bones (i.e., femur, tibia, patella) and two primary articulations (i.e., tibiofemoral, patellofemoral) enclosed within a single joint capsule. The knee is classified as a hinge joint, formed by the articulation of the tibia with the femur, with two degrees of freedom.

## Articulations

### Tibiofemoral joint

The proximal joint surface of the tibiofemoral joint is formed by the convex medial and lateral condyles of the distal femur. The distal joint surface is formed by the concave medial and lateral condyles of the proximal tibia.

### Tibiofemoral Snapshot

**Osteokinematic motions:** flexion, extension, medial rotation, lateral rotation

**Loose packed position:** 25 degrees flexion

**Close packed position:** full extension, lateral rotation of tibia

**Capsular pattern:** flexion, extension

## Consider This

### Common Mechanisms of Injury for Knee Ligaments

Stability of the knee is enhanced by the role of four primary ligaments. The ligaments are capable of functioning in isolation or collectively. Due to the unique function of each ligament, it is possible to identify specific mechanisms of injury often associated with a particular ligamentous injury.

**Anterior cruciate ligament (ACL)**

The ACL may be injured through a noncontact twisting injury associated with hyperextension and varus or valgus stress to the knee. Other mechanisms for ACL damage include the tibia being driven anteriorly on the femur, the femur being driven posteriorly on the tibia or severe knee hyperextension. Special tests designed to assess the integrity of the ACL include the anterior drawer test, Lachman test, lateral pivot shift test, and Slocum test.

**Posterior cruciate ligament (PCL)**

The PCL may be injured when the superior portion of the tibia is struck while the knee is flexed. A common example of this occurs in a motor vehicle accident when a passenger's leg collides against the dashboard. Other mechanisms for PCL damage include the tibia being driven posteriorly on the femur, the femur being driven anteriorly on the tibia or severe knee hyperflexion. Special tests designed to assess the integrity of the PCL include the posterior drawer test and posterior sag sign.

**Medial collateral ligament (MCL)**

The MCL may be injured with a pure valgus load at the knee without rotation. This type of injury is often sustained with contact activities such as a lateral blow to the knee during a football game. Injury to the MCL often involves injury to other knee structures such as the ACL or medial meniscus. A valgus stress test can assess the integrity of the MCL.

**Lateral collateral ligament (LCL)**

The LCL may be injured with a pure varus load at the knee without rotation. This type of injury is often sustained with contact activities such as a medial blow to the knee. The LCL is rarely completely torn without a concurrent injury to the ACL or PCL. A varus stress test can assess the integrity of the LCL.

### Patellofemoral joint

The patellofemoral joint is formed by the convex patella and the concave trochlear groove of the femur. The patella slides superiorly in knee extension and inferiorly in knee flexion. Patella rotation and tilting also occur during knee extension and flexion.

## Muscle Action

**Knee flexion:** biceps femoris, semitendinosus, sartorius, semimembranosus

**Knee extension:** rectus femoris, vastus lateralis, vastus intermedius, vastus medialis

## Primary Structures

### Bursae

The knee has several important bursae including the prepatellar bursa, superficial infrapatellar bursa, and deep infrapatellar bursa. The prepatellar bursa lies over the patella and allows for greater freedom of movement of the skin covering the anterior aspect of the patella. The superficial infrapatellar bursa lies between the patellar tendon and skin, while the deep infrapatellar bursa lies between the patellar tendon and the tibia.

### Anterior cruciate ligament

The ACL runs from the anterior intercondylar area of the tibia to the medial aspect of the lateral femoral condyle in the intercondylar notch. The ACL prevents anterior displacement of the tibia on the femur.

### Posterior cruciate ligament

The PCL runs from the posterior intercondylar area of the tibia to the lateral aspect of the medial femoral condyle in the intercondylar notch. The PCL prevents posterior displacement of the tibia on the femur.

### Medial collateral ligament

The MCL runs from slightly above the medial femoral epicondyle to the medial aspect of the shaft of the tibia. The deep capsular fibers are attached to the medial meniscus. The MCL prevents excessive valgus displacement of the tibia relative to the femur.

### Lateral collateral ligament

The LCL runs from the lateral femoral epicondyle to the fibular head. The LCL prevents excessive varus displacement of the tibia relative to the femur.

## Arcuate ligament complex

The arcuate ligament complex consists of the arcuate ligament, oblique popliteal ligament, lateral collateral ligament, popliteus tendon, and lateral head of the gastrocnemius. The complex assists the cruciate ligaments in controlling posterolateral rotatory instability of the knee and provides support to the posterolateral joint capsule.

## Menisci

The medial and lateral menisci are firmly attached to the proximal surface of the tibia. The menisci are thick at the periphery and thinner at their internal unattached edges. Menisci function to deepen the articular surfaces of the tibia where they articulate with the femoral condyles. The menisci function as shock absorbers and contribute to lubrication and nutrition of the joint.

## Ankle and Foot[8-12]

The ankle and foot are formed by a series of unique articulations including the distal tibiofibular joint, talocrural joint, subtalar joint, midtarsal joint, and forefoot.

## Articulations

### Distal tibiofibular joint

The distal tibiofibular joint is formed by a fibrous union between the lateral aspect of the distal tibia and the distal fibula.

### Talocrural joint

The talocrural joint is formed by the articulations of the distal tibia, talus, and fibula. The joint is a synovial hinge joint with one degree of freedom. The talocrural joint offers significant stability in dorsiflexion, however, it becomes much more mobile with plantar flexion.

### Talocrural Snapshot

**Osteokinematic motions:** dorsiflexion, plantar flexion

**Loose packed position:** 10 degrees plantar flexion, midway between maximum inversion and eversion

**Close packed position:** maximum dorsiflexion

**Capsular pattern:** plantar flexion, dorsiflexion

### Subtalar joint

The subtalar joint is formed by three articulations (anterior, middle, posterior) between the talus and calcaneus. The joint has one degree of freedom. The anterior and middle articulations are formed by two convex facets on the talus and two concave facets on the calcaneus. The posterior articulation is formed by a concave facet on the inferior surface of the talus and a convex facet on the body of the calcaneus.

### Subtalar Snapshot

**Osteokinematic motions:** inversion, eversion

**Loose packed position:** midway between extremes of range of movement

**Close packed position:** supination

**Capsular pattern:** limitation of varus range of movement

### Midtarsal joint

The midtarsal (transverse tarsal) joint is formed by the talocalcaneonavicular joint and the calcaneocuboid joint. The joint is considered to have two axes, one longitudinal and one oblique. Motions around both axes are triplanar.

### Midtarsal Snapshot

**Osteokinematic motions:** inversion, eversion

**Loose packed position:** midway between extremes of range of movement

**Close packed position:** supination

**Capsular pattern:** dorsiflexion, plantar flexion, adduction, medial rotation

### Forefoot

The forefoot consists of the tarsometatarsal joints, metatarsophalangeal joints, and interphalangeal joints.

## Muscle Action

**Plantar flexion:** tibialis posterior, gastrocnemius, soleus, peroneus longus, peroneus brevis, plantaris, flexor hallucis

**Dorsiflexion:** tibialis anterior, extensor hallucis longus, extensor digitorum longus, peroneus tertius

**Inversion:** tibialis posterior, tibialis anterior, flexor digitorum longus

**Eversion:** peroneus longus, peroneus brevis, peroneus tertius

## Primary Structures

### Ligaments

The majority of the ligaments in the ankle are areas of increased density within the joint capsule. As a result, damage to the ankle ligaments typically produces damage to the joint capsule and irritation of the synovial lining.

## Anterior talofibular ligament

The anterior talofibular ligament is taut during plantar flexion and resists inversion of the talus and calcaneus. The ligament also resists anterior translation of the talus on the tibia.

## Calcaneofibular ligament

The calcaneofibular ligament is an extracapsular ligament that resists inversion of the talus within the midrange of talocrural motion.

## Posterior talofibular ligament

The ligament resists posterior displacement of the talus on the tibia.

## Deltoid ligament

The deltoid ligament is formed by the anterior tibiotalar ligament, tibiocalcaneal ligament, posterior tibiotalar ligament, and tibionavicular ligament. The ligament provides medial ligamentous support by resisting eversion of the talus.

## Interosseous membrane

The interosseous membrane consists of a strong fibrous tissue that serves to fixate the fibula to the tibia. Distally, the structure blends into the anterior and posterior tibiofibular ligaments and provides additional support at the distal tibiofibular syndesmosis joint.

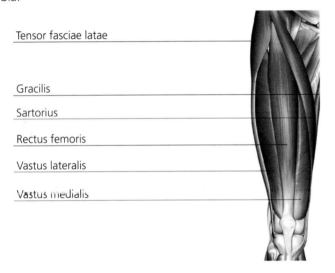

**Fig. 4-9:** Muscles of the anterior upper leg.

**Fig. 4-10:** Muscles of the posterior upper leg.

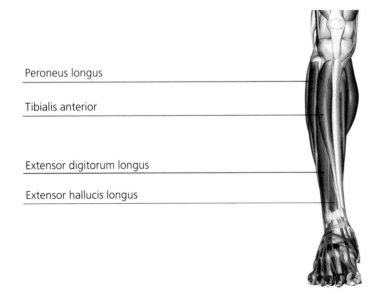

**Fig. 4-11:** Muscles of the anterior lower leg.

**Fig. 4-12:** Muscles of the posterior lower leg.

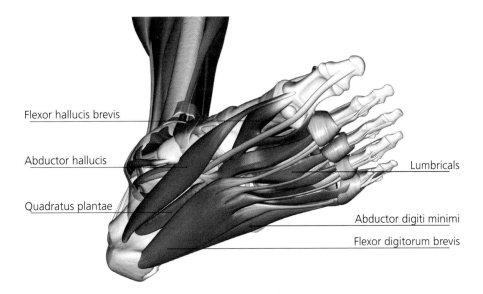

Flexor hallucis brevis

Abductor hallucis

Quadratus plantae

Lumbricals

Abductor digiti minimi

Flexor digitorum brevis

**Fig. 4-13:** Muscles of the volar surface of the foot.

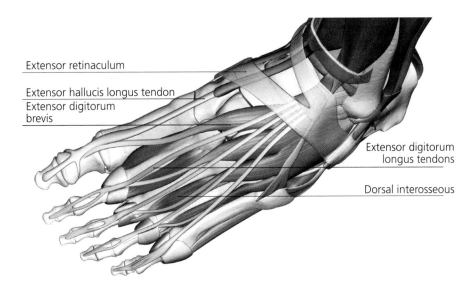

Extensor retinaculum

Extensor hallucis longus tendon

Extensor digitorum brevis

Extensor digitorum longus tendons

Dorsal interosseous

**Fig. 4-14:** Muscles of the dorsal surface of the foot.

# Spine

## Cervical Spine[3,10,13,14]

The cervical spine consists of seven cervical vertebrae. The first two, the atlas and axis, are unique. The atlas (C1) supports the weight of the head through two facet joints which form the atlanto-occipital joint. The axis (C2) has a superior projection called the dens. The articulation between the dens and the anterior arch of the atlas forms the atlantoaxial joint.

## Articulations

### Atlanto-occipital joint

The atlanto-occipital joint is a condylar synovial joint that permits flexion and extension of the cranium. This motion is often noted when nodding the head to say "yes."

### Atlantoaxial joints

The atlantoaxial joints are plane synovial joints that permit flexion, extension, lateral flexion, and rotation of the cervical spine. The majority of rotation of the skull on the spinal column occurs at the atlantoaxial joints.

### Intervertebral joints

The intervertebral joints are formed by the superior and inferior surfaces of the vertebral bodies and the associated intervertebral disks.

### Zygapophyseal joints

The zygapophyseal joints are formed by the right and left superior articular facets of one vertebra and the right and left inferior articular facets of an adjacent superior vertebra.

## Muscle Action

**Cervical flexion:** sternocleidomastoid, longus colli, scalenus muscles

**Cervical extension:** splenius cervicis, semispinalis cervicis, iliocostalis cervicis, longissimus cervicis, multifidus, trapezius

**Cervical rotation and lateral bending:** sternocleidomastoid, scalenus muscles, splenius cervicis, longissimus cervicis, iliocostalis cervicis, levator scapulae, multifidus

## Primary Structures

### Anterior longitudinal ligament

The anterior longitudinal ligament limits extension of the spine and reinforces the anterior portion of the intervertebral disks and vertebrae.

### Posterior longitudinal ligament

The posterior longitudinal ligament limits flexion of the spine and reinforces the posterior aspect of the intervertebral disks.

### Ligamentum nuchae

The ligamentum nuchae restricts flexion in the cervical spine.

### Interspinous ligaments

The interspinous ligaments are located between the spinous processes and serve to limit flexion and rotation of the spine.

### Ligamentum flavum

The ligamentum flavum connects the lamina of one vertebra to the lamina of the vertebra above it. The structure serves to limit flexion and rotation of the spine.

### Intervertebral disks

Intervertebral disks are formed by a dense layer of collagen fibers and fibrocartilage called the annulus fibrosus as well as a flexible inner layer called the nucleus pulposus. The annulus fibrosus is firmly attached to the adjacent vertebrae and provides tensile strength to the disk during spinal movement. The nucleus pulposus is a gelatinous mass located centrally in the disk. Flexion of a vertebral segment causes the anterior portion of the disk to be compressed and the posterior portion of the disk to be distracted.

### Intervertebral foramina

The intervertebral foramina are located in the posterior pillar of each vertebral segment. Spinal nerves and blood vessels exit the spinal canal via the foramina. The size of the intervertebral foramen increases with flexion and contralateral sidebending and decreases with extension and ipsilateral sidebending. Nerve root entrapment can result from closure or narrowing of the intervertebral foramen due to arthritic changes, spurring or narrowing of the intervertebral disks.

### Cervical Spine Snapshot

**Osteokinematic motions:** flexion, extension, lateral flexion, rotation

**Loose packed position:** midway between flexion and extension

**Close packed position:** extension

**Capsular pattern:** lateral flexion and rotation equally limited, extension

## Thoracolumbar Spine[3,9,10,14-16]

The thoracic spine consists of 12 vertebrae with long prominent spinous processes. The first ten thoracic vertebrae have articular facets on each transverse process where the ribs articulate. The lumbar spine consists of five vertebrae that provide the primary stability for the low back.

## Articulations

### Intervertebral joints

The intervertebral joints are formed by the superior and inferior surfaces of the vertebral bodies and the associated intervertebral disks.

### Zygapophyseal joints

The zygapophyseal joints are formed by the right and left superior articular facets of one vertebra and the right and left inferior articular facets of an adjacent superior vertebra.

## Muscle Action

**Thoracic and lumbar flexion:** rectus abdominis, internal oblique, external oblique

**Thoracic and lumbar extension:** erector spinae, quadratus lumborum, multifidus

**Thoracic and lumbar rotation and lateral bending:** psoas major, quadratus lumborum, external oblique, internal oblique, multifidus, longissimus thoracis, iliocostalis thoracis, rotatores

## Primary Structures

### Ribs

Ribs 1-10 articulate with the thoracic vertebrae through the costovertebral joints and the costotransverse joints. Ribs 1-7 are attached to the sternum through costal cartilage and ribs 8-10 join with the costal cartilage of ribs 1-7. Ribs 11-12 articulate only with the vertebral bodies of T11-T12, but not the transverse process of the same vertebrae. Ribs 11-12 are classified as floating because they do not attach to the sternum or the costal cartilage at their distal end.

### Anterior longitudinal ligament

The anterior longitudinal ligament limits extension of the spine and reinforces the anterior portion of the intervertebral disks and vertebrae.

### Posterior longitudinal ligament

The posterior longitudinal ligament limits flexion of the spine and reinforces the posterior aspect of the intervertebral disks.

### Supraspinous ligament

The supraspinous ligament restricts flexion in the thoracic and lumbar spine.

### Thoracic and Lumbar Spine Snapshot

**Osteokinematic motions:** flexion, extension, lateral flexion, rotation

**Loose packed position:** midway between flexion and extension

**Close packed position:** extension

**Capsular pattern:** lateral flexion and rotation equally limited, extension

### Interspinous ligaments

The interspinous ligaments are located between the spinous processes and serve to limit flexion and rotation of the spine.

### Ligamentum flavum

The ligamentum flavum connects the lamina of one vertebra to the lamina of the vertebra above it. The structure serves to limit flexion and rotation of the spine.

### Intervertebral disks

Intervertebral disks are formed by a dense layer of collagen fibers and fibrocartilage called the annulus fibrosus as well as a flexible inner layer called the nucleus pulposus. The annulus fibrosus is firmly attached to the adjacent vertebrae and provides tensile strength to the disk during spinal movement. The nucleus pulposus is a gelatinous mass located slightly posterior to the center of the disk in the lumbar spine. Flexion of a vertebral segment causes the anterior portion of the disk to be compressed and the posterior portion of the disk to be distracted.

### Intervertebral foramina

The intervertebral foramina are located in the posterior pillar of each vertebral segment. Spinal nerves and blood vessels exit the spinal canal via the foramina. The size of the intervertebral foramen increases with flexion and contralateral sidebending and decreases with extension and ipsilateral sidebending. Nerve root entrapment can result from closure or narrowing of the intervertebral foramen due to arthritic changes, spurring or narrowing of the intervertebral disks.

### Lumbar plexus

The lumbar plexus is formed by the nerve roots of T12 and L1-L4. The plexus innervates the anterior and medial muscles of the thigh and the dermatomes of the medial leg and foot. The largest and most important branches of the plexus are the obturator and femoral nerves.

### Sacral plexus

The sacral plexus is formed by the lumbosacral trunk, the ventral rami of S1-S3, and the descending portion of S4. The plexus supplies the muscles of the buttocks, and through the sciatic nerve, innervates the muscles of the posterior thigh and lower leg.

**Sacrum**

The sacrum is a broad, thick bone consisting of five fused vertebrae that fixate the spinal column to the pelvis. The main functions of the sacrum are to provide an attachment for the iliac bones and to protect the pelvic organs. The sacrum is attached to the pelvis by strong ligaments forming the sacroiliac joint.

**Coccyx**

The coccyx articulates with the sacrum and most often consists of four small, fused vertebral bodies. The coccyx does not have a specific purpose and is most often considered an embryological remnant.

# Muscle Physiology

| Classification of Muscle Fibers | |
| --- | --- |
| Type I | Type II |
| Aerobic | Anaerobic |
| Red | White |
| Tonic | Phasic |
| Slow twitch | Fast twitch |
| Slow-oxidative | Fast glycolytic |

| Functional Characteristics of Muscle Fibers | |
| --- | --- |
| Type I | Type II |
| Low fatigability | High fatigability |
| High capillary density | Low capillary density |
| High myoglobin content | Low myoglobin content |
| Smaller fibers | Larger fibers |
| Extensive blood supply | Less blood supply |
| Large amount of mitochondria | Fewer mitochondria |
| Examples: marathon, swimming | Examples: high jump, sprinting |

# Muscle Receptors

## Muscle Spindle

Muscle spindles are distributed throughout the belly of the muscle. They function to send information to the nervous system about muscle length and/or the rate of change of its length. The muscle spindle is important in the control of posture, and with the help of the gamma system, involuntary movements.

## Golgi Tendon Organ

Golgi tendon organs are encapsulated sensory receptors through which the muscle tendons pass immediately beyond their attachment to the muscle fibers. They are very sensitive to tension, especially when produced from an active muscle contraction. They function to transmit information about tension or the rate of change of tension within the muscle.

An average of 10-15 muscle fibers are usually connected in series with each Golgi tendon organ. The Golgi tendon organ is stimulated through the tension produced by muscle fibers. Golgi tendon organs provide the nervous system with instantaneous information on the degree of tension in each small muscle segment.

# Types of Muscular Contraction

**Concentric:** A concentric contraction occurs when the muscle shortens while developing tension.

**Eccentric:** An eccentric contraction occurs when the muscle lengthens while developing tension.

**Isometric:** An isometric contraction occurs when tension develops, but there is no change in the length of the muscle.

**Isotonic:** An isotonic contraction occurs when the muscle shortens or lengthens while resisting a constant load.

**Isokinetic:** An isokinetic contraction occurs when the tension developed by the muscle, while shortening or lengthening at a constant speed, is maximal over the full range of motion.

# Open-Chain versus Closed-Chain Activities

**Open-Chain:** Open-chain activities involve the distal segment, usually the hand or foot, moving freely in space. An example of an open-chain activity is kicking a ball with the lower extremity (Fig. 4-15).

**Closed-Chain:** Closed-chain activities involve the body moving over a fixed distal segment. An example of a closed-chain activity is a squat lift (Fig. 4-16).

**Fig. 4-15:** An example of an open-chain exercise.

**Fig. 4-16:** An example of a closed-chain exercise.

## Resistive and Overload Training

**Isometric Exercise:** Muscular force is generated without a change in muscle length. Isometric exercises are often performed against an immovable object. Submaximal isometric exercises are traditionally used in rehabilitation programs.

**Isotonic Exercise:** Muscular contraction is generated with the muscle exerting a constant tension. This can also be thought of as muscle movement with a constant load. Isotonic exercises are performed against resistance, often employing equipment such as handheld weights.

**Isokinetic Exercise:** Muscular contraction is generated with a constant maximal speed and variable load. In isokinetic exercise, the reaction force is identical to the force applied to the equipment. Cybex, Biodex, and Lido are a few of the companies making isokinetic exercise equipment.

## Pain

### McGill Pain Questionnaire

A pain assessment tool that is divided into four parts with a total of 70 questions.

**Part 1** Patient marks on a drawing of the body to indicate area and type of pain (internal or external)

**Part 2** Patient chooses one word that best describes the pain from each of the twenty categories

**Part 3** Patient describes pattern of pain, factors that increase and relieve pain

**Part 4** Patient rates the intensity of pain on a scale of zero to five

This tool can be used to establish a baseline, evaluate particular treatment regimens, and monitor progress. It is valid, reliable, and the most widely used pain assessment scale.

### Numerical Rating Scale

A tool used to assess pain intensity by rating pain on a scale of 0-10 or 0-100. The 0 represents no discernable pain and the 10 or 100 represent the worst pain ever. The information is used as a baseline and should be reassessed at regular intervals in order to monitor progress. This scale is easy to administer, assess, and monitor.

### Visual Analogue Scale

A tool used to assess pain intensity using a 10-15 cm line with the left anchor indicating "no pain" and the right anchor indicating "the worst pain you can have." The level of perceived pain is indicated on the line and is reassessed frequently over the course of physical therapy to record changes and progress, and to predict patient outcome. This scale can be highly sensitive if small increments such as millimeters are used to measure the patient's point of pain on the scale. The visual analogue scale is a valid tool if measurements are taken accurately.

# Exercise Programs

| DeLorme | Protocol |
|---|---|
| First Set | 10 repetitions x 50% of 10 repetition maximum |
| Second Set | 10 repetitions x 75% of 10 repetition maximum |
| Third Set | 10 repetitions x 100% of 10 repetition maximum |

| Oxford Technique | Protocol |
|---|---|
| First Set | 10 repetitions x 100% of 10 repetition maximum |
| Second Set | 10 repetitions x 75% of 10 repetition maximum |
| Third Set | 10 repetitions x 50% of 10 repetition maximum |

# Musculoskeletal System Examination

## Upper Quarter Screening [10,13,17-18]

The upper quarter screen provides a rapid assessment of mobility and neurologic function of the cervical spine and upper extremities. The screen is traditionally performed with the patient in sitting.

The following are components of an upper extremity screening:

### Posture

- Postural assessment

## Range of Motion

- Active range of motion of the cervical spine
- Active range of motion of the upper extremities
- Passive overpressure of the cervical spine and upper extremities, if the patient does not exhibit signs and symptoms of pathology

| Resistive Testing (C1 – T1) | |
|---|---|
| **Resistive Test** | **Innervation Level** |
| Cervical rotation | C1 |
| Shoulder elevation | C2 – C4 |
| Shoulder abduction | C5 |
| Elbow flexion | C5 – C6 |
| Wrist extension | C6 |
| Elbow extension | C7 |
| Wrist flexion | C7 |
| Thumb extension | C8 |
| Finger adduction | T1 |

| Reflex Testing (C5 – C7) | |
|---|---|
| **Reflex Test** | **Innervation Level** |
| Biceps | C5 |
| Brachioradialis | C6 |
| Triceps | C7 |

### Dermatome Testing (C2 – T1)

| Area of Skin | Innervation Level |
|---|---|
| Posterior head | C2 |
| Posterior-lateral neck | C3 |
| Acromioclavicular joint | C4 |
| Lateral arm | C5 |
| Lateral forearm and thumb | C6 |
| Palmar distal phalanx – middle finger | C7 |
| Little finger and ulnar border of the hand | C8 |
| Medial forearm | T1 |

### Resistive Testing (L1 – S1)

| Resistive Test | Innervation Level |
|---|---|
| Hip flexion | L1 – L2 |
| Knee extension | L3 – L4 |
| Ankle dorsiflexion | L4 – L5 |
| Great toe extension | L5 |
| Ankle plantar flexion | S1 |

### Reflex Testing (L4 – S1)

| Reflex Test | Innervation Level |
|---|---|
| Patella | L4 |
| Achilles | S1 |

## Lower Quarter Screening [10,13,18]

The lower quarter screen provides a rapid assessment of mobility and neurologic function of the lumbosacral spine and lower extremities. The screen is traditionally performed with the patient in standing or sitting.

The following are components of a lower extremity screening:

**Posture**

- Postural assessment

**Range of Motion**

- Active range of motion of the lumbosacral spine
- Active range of motion of the lower extremities
- Passive overpressure of the lumbosacral spine and lower extremities, if the patient does not exhibit signs and symptoms of pathology

### Functional Testing (L4 – S1)

| Functional Test | Innervation Level |
|---|---|
| Heel walking | L4 – L5 |
| Toe walking | S1 |
| Straight leg raise | L4 – S1 |

### Dermatome Testing (L2 – S5)

| Area of Skin | Innervation Level |
|---|---|
| Anterior thigh | L2 |
| Middle third of anterior thigh | L3 |
| Patella and medial malleolus | L4 |
| Fibular head and dorsum of foot | L5 |
| Lateral and plantar aspect of foot | S1 |
| Medial aspect of posterior thigh | S2 |
| Perianal area | S3 – S5 |

## Scanning Examination to Rule Out Referral of Symptoms from Other Tissues

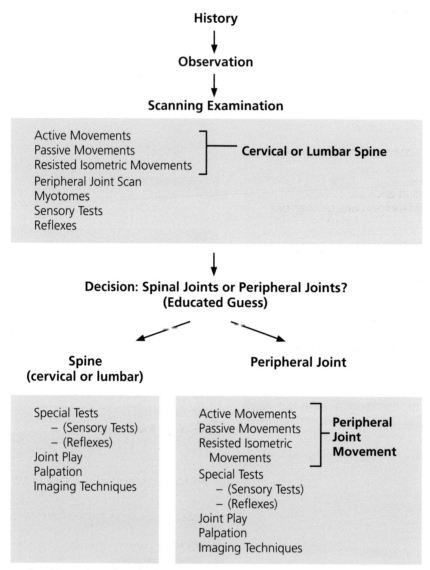

From Magee, DJ: Orthopedic Physical Assessment. W.B. Saunders Company, Philadelphia 2002, p.15, with permission.

# Body Composition[19]

Body composition is defined as the relative percentage of body weight that is comprised of fat and fat-free tissue. There are multiple methods for testing the percentage of body fat including hydrostatic weighing, skinfold measurements, plethysmography, body mass index, and bioelectrical impedance analysis. A healthy range of body fat is 12-18% for males and 18-23% for females.

### Densitometry

**Hydrostatic Weighing:** This method calculates the density of the body by immersing a person in water and measuring the amount of water that becomes displaced. The percentage of body fat is then determined by calculating the measured amount of water displaced in an equation based on Archimedes' principle. This method is the most widely used laboratory procedure to determine body density. Limitations of this method include the need to account for residual lung volume during submersion and evaluating patients that must tolerate water submersion during the testing. The standard error for this method is estimated at 2 to 2.5%.

**Plethysmography:** This method calculates the density of the body utilizing the amount of air displacement during testing within a specialized closed chamber. The change in pressure within the chamber is measured and converted to the percentage of body fat using a standardized equation.

## Anthropometry

**Skinfold Measurement:** This method determines the overall percentage of body fat through the measurement of nine standardized sites. The correlation relies on the theory that the amount of subcutaneous fat is proportional to the total fat in the body. Limitations of this method include the requisite of an experienced examiner as well as variance from the standards based on gender, age, and ethnicity. Accuracy of measurement is within +/-3% with appropriate technique and equipment.

### Skinfold Measurement Procedure

- All measurements should be taken on the right side of the body

- Take multiple measurements at each site to ensure accuracy and retest if the difference is greater than one to two millimeters

- Skinfold calipers should be positioned one centimeter away from the examiner's fingers when pinching the side, positioned perpendicular to the skinfold, and centered between the base and top of the fold (Fig. 4-17)

- Wait one to two seconds before reading the caliper

- Maintain pinching of the site during the reading of the caliper

**Fig. 4-17:** A therapist measuring a skinfold with skinfold calipers at the triceps site.

### Standard Skinfold Sites

| | |
|---|---|
| Abdominal | Midaxillary |
| Triceps * | Subscapular * |
| Biceps | Suprailiac |
| Chest/pectoral | Thigh |
| Medial calf | |

There are seven-site and three-site formulas to calculate the percentage of body fat using particular sites. There are also specific formulas for gender, sport, ethnicity, and age.

* Indicates the most commonly utilized sites

### Other Techniques

**Body Mass Index (BMI)**

**(See Cardiovascular and Pulmonary Systems Unit)**

**Bioelectrical Impedance Analysis (BIA)**

This method of assessing body composition uses a small electrical current and measures the resistance or opposition to the current flow. This technique is based on the principle that resistance to electrical current is inversely related to the composition of water within the body. The formula of height$^2$/resistance is used for the general population while population-specific equations are also available. The standard error compares to the accuracy of skinfold measurements at approximately +/-3%. Limitations include the requisite for the subjects to be properly hydrated as well as following all guidelines for the BIA protocol.

### BIA Protocol

- Abstain from eating or drinking within four hours prior to testing

- Abstain from vigorous physical activity within 12 hours prior to testing

- Urinate within 30 minutes prior to testing

- Avoid alcohol consumption for 48 hours prior to testing

- Avoid excessive water intake prior to testing

# Posture

## Good and Faulty Posture: Summary Chart

| Good Posture | Part | Faulty Posture |
|---|---|---|
| Toes should be straight, that is, neither curled downward nor bent upward.<br>They should extend forward in line with the foot and should not be squeezed together or overlap. | **Toes** | Toes bend up at the first joint and down at middle joints so that the weight rests on the tips of the toes (hammer toes). This fault is often associated with wearing shoes that are too short.<br>Big toe slants inward toward the midline of the foot (hallux valgus). "Bunion." This fault is often associated with wearing shoes that are too narrow and pointed at the toes. |
| In standing, the longitudinal arch has the shape of a half dome.<br>Barefoot or in shoes without heels, the feet toe-out slightly.<br>In shoes with heels, the feet are parallel.<br>In walking with or without shoes, the feet are parallel and the weight is transferred from the heel along the outer border to the ball of the foot.<br>In sprinting, the feet are parallel or toe-in slightly. The weight is on the balls of the feet and toes because the heels do not come in contact with the ground. | **Foot** | Low longitudinal arch or flat foot.<br>Low metatarsal arch, usually indicated by calluses under the ball of the foot.<br>Weight borne on the inner side of the foot (pronation). "Ankle rolls in."<br>Weight borne on the outer border of the foot (supination). "Ankle rolls out."<br>Toeing-out while walking, or while standing in shoes with heels ("slue-footed").<br>Toeing-in while walking or standing ("pigeon-toed"). |
| Legs are straight up and down. Kneecaps face straight ahead when feet are in good position. Looking at the knees from the side, the knees are straight (i.e., neither flexed or hyperextended). | **Knees and Legs** | Knees touch when feet are apart (knock-knees).<br>Knees are apart when feet touch (bowlegs).<br>Knee curves slightly backward (hyperextended knee). "Back-knee."<br>Knee bends slightly forward, that is, it is not as straight as it should be (flexed knee).<br>Kneecaps face slightly toward each other (medially rotated femurs).<br>Kneecaps face slightly outward (laterally rotated femurs). |
| Ideally, the body weight is borne evenly on both feet and the hips are level. One side should not be more prominent than the other as seen from front or back, nor is one hip more forward or backward than the other as seen from the side. The spine does not curve to the left or the right side. (A slight deviation to the left in right-handed individuals and to the right in left-handed individuals is not uncommon. Also, a tendency toward a slightly low right shoulder and slightly high right hip is frequently found in right-handed people, and vice versa for left-handed people.) | **Hips, Pelvis, and Spine Back View** | One hip is higher than the other (lateral pelvic tilt). Sometimes it is not really higher but appears so because a sideways sway of the body has made it more prominent. (Tailors and dressmakers often notice a lateral tilt because the hemline of skirts or length of trousers must be adjusted to the difference.)<br>The hips are rotated so that one is farther forward than the other (clockwise or counterclockwise rotation). |

# Good and Faulty Posture: Summary Chart

| Good Posture | Part | Faulty Posture |
|---|---|---|
| The front of the pelvis and the thighs are in a straight line. The buttocks are not prominent in back but slope slightly downward.<br><br>The spine has four natural curves. In the neck and lower back the curve is forward; in the upper back and lowest part of the spine (sacral region) it is backward. The sacral curve is a fixed curve while the other three are flexible. | **Spine and Pelvis Side View** | The low back arches forward too much (lordosis). The pelvis tilts forward too much. The front of the thigh forms an angle with the pelvis when this tilt is present.<br><br>The normal forward curve in the low back has straightened. The pelvis tips backward as in swayback and flat-back postures.<br><br>Increased backward curve in the upper back (kyphosis or round upper back).<br><br>Increased forward curve in the neck. Almost always accompanied by round upper back and seen as a forward head.<br><br>Lateral curve of the spine (scoliosis); toward one side (C-curve), toward both sides (S-curve). |
| In young children, up to about the age of 10, the abdomen normally protrudes somewhat. In older children and adults it should be flat. | **Abdomen** | Entire abdomen protrudes.<br><br>Lower part of the abdomen protrudes while the upper part is pulled in. |
| A good position of the chest is one in which it is slightly up and slightly forward (while the back remains in good alignment).<br><br>The chest appears to be in a position about halfway between that of a full inspiration and a forced expiration. | **Chest** | Depressed or "hollow-chest" position.<br><br>Lifted and held up too high, brought about by arching the back.<br><br>Ribs more prominent on one side than on the other.<br><br>Lower ribs flaring out or protruding. |
| Arms hang relaxed at the sides with palms of the hands facing toward the body. Elbows are slightly bent, so forearms hang slightly forward.<br><br>Shoulders are level and neither one is more forward or backward than the other when seen from the side.<br><br>Shoulder blades lie flat against the rib cage. They are neither too close together or too wide apart. In adults, a separation of about 4 inches is average. | **Arms and Shoulders** | Arms held stiffly in any position forward, backward, or out from the body. Arms turned so that palms of hands face backward.<br><br>One shoulder higher than the other. Both shoulders hiked-up. One or both shoulders drooping forward or sloping. Shoulders rotated either clockwise or counterclockwise.<br><br>Shoulder blades pulled back too hard. Shoulder blades too far apart. Shoulder blades too prominent, standing out from the rib cage (winged scapulae). |
| Head is held erect in a position of good balance. | **Head** | Chin up too high.<br><br>Head protruding forward. Head tilted or rotated to one side. |

From Kendall F, McCreary E, Provance P: Muscle Testing and Function. Lippencott, William & Wilkins, Baltimore 1993, p.115-116, with permission.

## Consider This

### Ideal Plumb Line Alignment[10,18]

A plumb line is a tool that consists of a weight suspended at the end of a string to determine verticality. Ideal positioning of selected body parts in relation to the plumb line is described below.

- Slightly posterior to coronal suture
- Through the external auditory meatus
- Through the axis of the odontoid process
- Midway through the tip of the shoulder
- Through the bodies of the lumbar vertebrae
- Slightly posterior to the hip joint
- Slightly anterior to the axis of the knee joint
- Slightly anterior to the lateral malleolus
- Through the calcaneocuboid joint

Although desirable, rarely will a given patient demonstrate ideal alignment with all of the anatomical landmarks listed above. The following pictures provide an example of a patient with "good posture" and a patient with "faulty posture" (Figs. 4-18, 4-19).

**Fig. 4-18:** An example of a patient with relatively "good posture" using a plumb line. The image demonstrates several anatomical landmarks in ideal alignment and others that are in close proximity.

**Fig. 4-19:** An example of a patient with relatively "faulty posture" using a plumb line.

# Positioning of a Joint[10]

## Loose Packed Position of Joints

| Joint | Position |
|---|---|
| Facet (spine) | Midway between flexion and extension |
| Temporomandibular | Mouth slightly open (freeway space) |
| Glenohumeral | 55° abduction, 30° horizontal adduction |
| Acromioclavicular | Arm resting by side in normal physiological position |
| Sternoclavicular | Arm resting by side in normal physiological postion |
| Ulnohumeral (elbow) | 70° flexion, 10° supination |
| Radiohumeral | Full extension, full supination |
| Proximal radioulnar | 70° flexion, 35° supination |
| Distal radioulnar | 10° supination |
| Radiocarpal (wrist) | Neutral with slight ulnar deviation |
| Carpometacarpal | Midway between abduction - adduction and flexion - extension |
| Metacarpophalangeal | Slight flexion |
| Interphalangeal | Slight flexion |
| Hip | 30° flexion, 30° abduction, slight lateral rotation |
| Knee | 25° flexion |
| Talocrural (ankle) | 10° plantar flexion, midway between maximum inversion and eversion |
| Subtalar | Midway between extremes of range of movement |
| Midtarsal | Midway between extremes of range of movement |
| Tarsometatarsal | Midway between extremes of range of movement |
| Metatarsophalangeal | Neutral |
| Interphalangeal | Slight flexion |

From Magee, DJ: Orthopedic Physical Assessment. W.B. Saunders Company, Philadelphia 2002, p.50, with permission.

## Close Packed Position of Joints

| Joint | Position |
|---|---|
| Facet (spine) | Extension |
| Temporomandibular | Clenched teeth |
| Glenohumeral | Abduction and lateral rotation |
| Acromioclavicular | Arm abducted to 90° |
| Sternoclavicular | Maximum shoulder elevation |
| Ulnohumeral (elbow) | Extension |
| Radiohumeral | Elbow flexed 90°, forearm supinated 5° |
| Proximal radioulnar | 5° supination |
| Distal radioulnar | 5° supination |
| Radiocarpal (wrist) | Extension with radial deviation |
| Metacarpophalangeal (fingers) | Full flexion |
| Metacarpophalangeal (thumb) | Full opposition |
| Interphalangeal | Full extension |
| Hip | Full extension, medial rotation |
| Knee | Full extension, lateral rotation of tibia |
| Talocrural (ankle) | Maximum dorsiflexion |
| Subtalar | Supination |
| Midtarsal | Supination |
| Tarsometatarsal | Supination |
| Metatarsophalangeal | Full extension |
| Interphalangeal | Full extension |

From Magee, DJ: Orthopedic Physical Assessment. W.B. Saunders Company, Philadelphia 2002, p.50, with permission.

## Descriptions of Specific Positions

| | Loose Packed | Close Packed |
|---|---|---|
| **Stress on joint** | Minimal | Maximal |
| **Congruency of joint** | Minimal | Full |
| **Ligament position** | Great laxity | Full tightness |
| **Joint surface** | No volitional separation | Compressed |

## Common Capsular Patterns of Joints[10]

| Joint | Restriction* |
|---|---|
| Temporomandibular | Limitation of mouth opening |
| Atlanto-occipital | Extension, side flexion equally limited |
| Cervical spine | Lateral flexion and rotation equally limited, extension |
| Glenohumeral | Lateral rotation, abduction, medial rotation |
| Sternoclavicular | Pain at extremes of range of movement |
| Acromioclavicular | Pain at extremes of range of movement |
| Ulnohumeral | Flexion, extension |
| Radiohumeral | Flexion, extension, supination, pronation |
| Proximal radioulnar | Supination, pronation |
| Distal radioulnar | Full range of movement, pain at extremes of rotation |
| Radiocarpal (wrist) | Flexion and extension equally limited |
| Trapeziometacarpal | Abduction, extension |
| Metacarpophalangeal and interphalangeal | Flexion, extension |

| Joint | Restriction* |
|---|---|
| Thoracic spine | Lateral flexion and rotation equally limited, extension |
| Lumbar spine | Lateral flexion and rotation equally limited, extension |
| Sacroiliac, symphysis pubis, and sacrococcygeal | Pain when joints are stressed |
| Hip** | Flexion, abduction, medial rotation (sometimes medial rotation is most limited) |
| Knee | Flexion, extension |
| Tibiofibular | Pain when joint stressed |
| Talocrural | Plantar flexion, dorsiflexion |
| Talocalcaneal (subtalar) | Limitation of varus range of movement |
| Midtarsal | Dorsiflexion, plantar flexion, adduction, medial rotation |
| First metatarsophalangeal | Extension, flexion |
| Second to fifth metatarsophalangeal | Variable |
| Interphalangeal | Flexion, extension |

* Movements are listed in order of restriction.**For the hip: flexion, abduction, and medial rotation are the movements most limited in a capsular pattern.
From Magee, DJ: Orthopedic Physical Assessment. W.B. Saunders Company, Philadelphia 2002, p.28, with permission.

# End-Feel[3,20]

## Normal End-Feel

End-feel is the type of resistance that is felt when passively moving a joint through the end range of motion. Certain tissues and joints have a consistent end-feel and are described as firm, hard or soft. Pathology can be identified through noting the type of abnormal end-feel within a particular joint.

### Firm (stretch)

Examples: Ankle dorsiflexion
Finger extension
Hip medial rotation
Forearm supination

### Hard (bone to bone)

Example: Elbow extension

### Soft (soft tissue approximation)

Examples: Elbow flexion
Knee flexion

## Abnormal End-Feel

Abnormal end-feel consists of any end-feel that is felt at an abnormal or inconsistent point in the range of motion or in a joint that normally presents with a different end-feel.

### Empty (cannot reach end-feel, usually due to pain)

Examples: Joint inflammation
Fracture
Bursitis

### Firm

Examples: Increased tone
Tightening of the capsule
Ligament shortening

### Hard

Examples: Fracture
Osteoarthritis
Osteophyte formation

### Soft

Examples: Edema
Synovitis
Ligament instability/tear

# Muscle Testing

## Manual Muscle Testing Grades[2,21]

| | |
|---|---|
| **Zero** (0/5) | The subject demonstrates no palpable muscle contraction. |
| **Trace** (1/5) | The subject's muscle contraction can be palpated, but there is no joint movement. |
| **Poor Minus** (2-/5) | The subject does not complete range of motion in a gravity-eliminated position. |
| **Poor** (2/5) | The subject completes range of motion in a gravity-eliminated position. |
| **Poor Plus** (2+/5) | The subject is able to initiate movement against gravity. |
| **Fair Minus** (3-/5) | The subject does not complete the range of motion against gravity, but does complete more than half of the range. |
| **Fair** (3/5) | The subject completes range of motion against gravity without manual resistance. |
| **Fair Plus** (3+/5) | The subject completes range of motion against gravity with only minimal resistance. |
| **Good Minus** (4-/5) | The subject completes range of motion against gravity with minimal-moderate resistance. |
| **Good** (4/5) | The subject completes range of motion against gravity with moderate resistance. |
| **Good Plus** (4+/5) | The subject completes range of motion against gravity with moderate-maximal resistance. |
| **Normal** (5/5) | The subject completes range of motion against gravity with maximal resistance. |

## Positioning for Muscle Testing[2,21]

### Supine

| | |
|---|---|
| Abdominals | Anterior deltoid* |
| Biceps | Brachioradialis |
| Finger flexors | Finger extensors |
| Iliopsoas | Infraspinatus |
| Lateral rotators of shoulder* | Medial rotators of shoulder* |
| Neck flexors | Pectoralis major |
| Pectoralis minor | Peroneals |
| Pronators | Sartorius |
| Serratus anterior | Supinators |
| Tensor fasciae latae | Teres minor |
| Thumb muscles | Tibialis anterior |
| Tibialis posterior | Toe extensors |
| Toe flexors | Triceps* |
| Wrist extensors | Wrist flexors |

### Sidelying

| | |
|---|---|
| Gluteus medius | Gluteus minimus |
| Hip adductors | Lateral abdominals |

### Prone

| | |
|---|---|
| Back extensors | Gastrocnemius |
| Gluteus maximus | Hamstrings* |
| Lateral rotators of the shoulder* | Latissimus dorsi |
| Lower trapezius | Medial rotators of the shoulder* |
| Middle trapezius | Neck extensors |
| Posterior deltoid* | Quadratus lumborum |
| Rhomboids | Soleus |
| Teres major | Triceps* |

### Sitting

| | |
|---|---|
| Coracobrachialis | Deltoid* |
| Hip flexors* | Lateral rotators of hip |
| Medial rotators of hip | Quadriceps |
| Upper trapezius | Serratus anterior* |

### Standing

| | |
|---|---|
| Ankle plantar flexors | Serratus anterior* |

*Indicates multiple acceptable positions for muscle testing

# Manual Muscle Testing

**Fig. 4-20:** Manual muscle testing of the anterior deltoid.

**Fig. 4-21:** Manual muscle testing of the posterior deltoid.

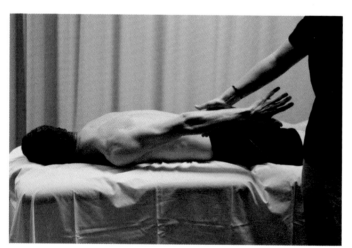

**Fig. 4-22:** Manual muscle testing of the latissimus dorsi.

**Fig. 4-23:** Manual muscle testing of the hip flexors.

**Fig. 4-24:** Manual muscle testing of the gluteus medius.

**Fig. 4-25:** Manual muscle testing of the hip adductors.

**Fig. 4-26:** Manual muscle testing of the hip lateral rotators.

**Fig. 4-27:** Manual muscle testing of the quadriceps femoris.

## Muscle Insufficiency[2,16]

A muscle contraction that is less than optimal due to an extremely lengthened or shortened position of the muscle. There are two types of insufficiency:

**Active:** when a two-joint muscle contracts across both joints simultaneously

**Passive:** when a two-joint muscle is lengthened over both joints simultaneously

## Dynamometry[10]

Dynamometry is the process of measuring forces that are doing work. A dynamometer is a device that measures strength through the use of a load cell or spring-loaded gauge. There are various kinds of dynamometers that are used based on treatment objectives. Three types of dynamometry that will be discussed here include the handheld dynamometer that measures grip strength, the handheld dynamometer used to measure strength of the extremities through isometric contraction, and the dynamometer used to measure strength through isokinetic contraction. Handheld dynamometry demonstrates intrarater reliability of > .94. The same dynamometer should be used each session and the same tester should consistently measure the patient.

- **A handheld dynamometer** can be used to assess the grip strength of a patient (Fig. 4-28). Normally, a patient's dominant grip strength is five to ten pounds greater than the non-dominant grip strength. Handheld dynamometry is also used to measure muscle group strength by having the patient exert maximal force against the dynamometer. Portable, non-electric units include a hydraulic or spring-load system and display the force on a gauge. Electrical units use load cells or strain gauges and display force digitally. Grip strength is usually recorded in pounds or kilograms.

**Fig. 4-28:** A handheld dynamometer. Courtesy Chattanooga, a DJO Global Company.

- **Isometric dynamometry** measures the static strength of a muscle group without any movement. The extremity is restrained by stabilization straps or stabilized with only verbal instruction (Fig. 4-29).

    **Benefits** include attaining peak and average force data, reaction time data, rate of motor recruitment, and maximal exertion data. This method is relatively safe, simple to use, easy to interpret data, and cost effective.

    **Disadvantages** include the inability to convert data to functional activities, as well as the need for caution with patients with acute orthopedic injury, osteoporosis or hernia. This method is contraindicated for patients with fractures and significant hypertension.

**Fig. 4-29:** A patient using a pinch grip dynamometer.

- **Isokinetic dynamometry** measures the strength of a muscle group during a movement with constant, predetermined speed. This device will alter the resistance to accommodate for the change in the length-tension ratio and lever arm throughout the entire arc of motion. The muscle group will therefore maximally contract throughout the motion. Common speeds of motion include 60, 120, and 180 degrees per second.

    **Benefits** include the ability to test the muscle strength at various speeds, the ability to measure the patient's power, and that the patient will never have more resistance than they can handle during the isokinetic testing.

    **Disadvantages** include the high cost of operation for the device, limitations in patterns of movement, a higher level of understanding required by the patient, and that this method does not truly correlate to function since people do not perform at a constant velocity during daily activities.

### Make Test:

A make test is an evaluation procedure where a patient is asked to apply a force against the dynamometer.

### Break Test:

A break test is an evaluation procedure where a patient is asked to hold a contraction against pressure that is applied in the opposite direction to the contraction.

# Gait

| | Standard Terminology | Rancho Los Amigos Terminology |
|---|---|---|
| **Stance Phase (60% of gait cycle)** | Heel strike<br>Foot flat<br>Midstance<br>Heel off<br>Toe off | Initial contact<br>Loading response<br>Midstance<br>Terminal stance<br>Pre-swing |
| **Swing Phase (40% of gait cycle)** | Acceleration<br>Midswing<br>Deceleration | Initial swing<br>Midswing<br>Terminal swing |

## Standard Terminology[4,23]

### Stance Phase

**Heel strike:** Heel strike is the instant that the heel touches the ground to begin stance phase.

**Foot flat:** Foot flat is the point in which the entire foot makes contact with the ground and should occur directly after heel strike.

**Midstance:** Midstance is the point during the stance phase when the entire body weight is directly over the stance limb.

**Heel off:** Heel off is the point in which the heel of the stance limb leaves the ground.

**Toe off:** Toe off is the point in which only the toe of the stance limb remains on the ground.

### Swing Phase

**Acceleration:** Acceleration begins when toe off is complete and the reference limb swings until positioned directly under the body.

**Midswing:** Midswing is the point when the swing limb is directly under the body.

**Deceleration:** Deceleration begins directly after midswing, as the swing limb begins to extend, and ends just prior to heel strike.

## Rancho Los Amigos Terminology[4,22,23]

### Stance Phase

**Initial contact:** Initial contact is the beginning of the stance phase that occurs when the foot touches the ground (Fig. 4-30).

**Loading response:** Loading response corresponds to the amount of time between initial contact and the beginning of the swing phase for the other leg (Fig. 4-31).

**Midstance:** Midstance corresponds to the point in stance phase when the other foot is off the floor until the body is directly over the stance limb (Fig. 4-32).

**Terminal stance:** Terminal stance begins when the heel of the stance limb rises and ends when the other foot touches the ground (Fig. 4-33).

**Pre-swing:** Pre-swing begins when the other foot touches the ground and ends when the stance foot reaches toe off (Fig. 4-34).

### Swing Phase

**Initial swing:** Initial swing begins when the stance foot lifts from the floor and ends with maximal knee flexion during swing (Fig. 4-35).

**Midswing:** Midswing begins with maximal knee flexion during swing and ends when the tibia is perpendicular with the ground (Fig. 4-36).

**Terminal swing:** Terminal swing begins when the tibia is perpendicular to the floor and ends when the foot touches the ground (Fig. 4-37).

**Fig. 4-30:** Initial contact   **Fig. 4-31:** Loading response   **Fig. 4-32:** Midstance   **Fig. 4-33:** Terminal stance

## Normal Gait

| | SWING PHASE 40% | | | STANCE PHASE 60% | | | | |
|---|---|---|---|---|---|---|---|---|
| | **Initial Swing** | **Midswing** | **Terminal Swing** | **Initial Contact** | **Loading Response** | **Midstance** | **Terminal Stance** | **Pre-Swing** |
| **Trunk** | Erect Neutral | Erect Neutral | Erect Neutral | Erect Neutral | Erect Neutral | Erect Neutral | Erect Neutral | Erect Neutral |
| **Pelvis** | Level: Backward Rotation 4-5° | Level: Neutral Rotation | Level: Forward Rotation 4-5° | Level: Maintains Forward Rotation | Level: Less Forward Rotation | Level: Neutral Rotation | Level: Backward Rotation 4-5° | Level: Backward Rotation 4-5° |
| **Hip** | Flexion 20° | Flexion 20° - 30° | Flexion 30° | Flexion 30° | Flexion 30° | Extending to Neutral | Apparent Hyperextension 10° | Neutral Extension |
| | Neutral: Rotation Abduction Adduction | Neutral: Rotation Abduction Adduction | Neutral: Rotation Abduction Adduction | Neutral: Rotation Abduction Adduction | Neutral: Rotation Abduction Adduction | Neutral: Rotation Abduction Adduction | Neutral: Rotation Abduction Adduction | Neutral: Rotation Abduction Adduction |
| **Knee** | Flexion 60° | From 60° to 30° Flexion | Extension to 0° | Full Extension | Flexion 15° | Extending to Neutral | Full Extension | Flexion 35° |
| **Ankle** | Plantar Flexion 10° | Neutral | Neutral | Neutral Heel First | Plantar Flexion 15° | From Plantar Flexion to 10° Dorsiflexion | Neutral with Tibia Stable and Heel Off Prior to Initial Contact Opposite Foot | Plantar Flexion 20° |
| **Toes** | Neutral | Neutral | Neutral | Neutral | Neutral | Neutral | Neutral IP Extended MP | Neutral IP Extended MP |

From Rancho Los Amigos National Rehabilitation Center: Normal and Pathological Gait Syllabus, p. 11, Downey, California, with permission.

**Fig. 4-34:** Pre-swing     **Fig. 4-35:** Initial swing     **Fig. 4-36:** Midswing     **Fig. 4-37:** Terminal swing

| | Double Support | Right Single Support | Double Support | Left Single Support |
|---|---|---|---|---|

Right Heel Initial Contact — Left Pre-Swing — Left Heel Initial Contact — Right Pre-Swing — Right Heel Initial Contact

0%     10%     50%     60%     100%

| Right Stance Phase (60%) | Right Swing Phase (40%) |
|---|---|

**Fig. 4-38:** Timing and sequence of the gait cycle.

## Peak Muscle Activity During the Gait Cycle[4,24]

**Tibialis anterior:** Peak activity is just after heel strike. Responsible for eccentric lowering of the foot into plantar flexion.

**Gastroc-soleus group:** Peak activity is during late stance phase. Responsible for concentric raising of the heel during toe off.

**Quadriceps group:** Two periods of peak activity. In periods of single support during early stance phase and just before toe off to initiate swing phase.

**Hamstrings group:** Peak activity is during late swing phase. Responsible for decelerating the unsupported limb.

## Range of Motion Requirements for Normal Gait

| | |
|---|---|
| **Hip flexion:** | **0 – 30 degrees** |
| **Hip extension:** | **0 – 10 degrees** |
| **Knee flexion:** | **0 – 60 degrees** |
| **Knee extension:** | **0 degrees** |
| **Ankle dorsiflexion:** | **0 – 10 degrees** |
| **Ankle plantar flexion:** | **0 – 20 degrees** |

**SCORE**BUILDERS

## Gait Terminology[4,10]

**Base of support:** The distance measured between the left and right foot during progression of gait. The distance decreases as cadence increases. The average base of support for an adult is two to four inches.

**Cadence:** The number of steps an individual will walk over a period of time. The average value for an adult is 110–120 steps per minute.

**Degree of toe-out:** The angle formed by each foot's line of progression and a line intersecting the center of the heel and second toe. The average degree of toe-out for an adult is seven degrees.

**Double support phase:** The double support phase refers to the two times during a gait cycle where both feet are on the ground. The time of double support increases as the speed of gait decreases. This phase does not exist with running.

**Gait cycle:** The gait cycle refers to the sequence of motions that occur from initial contact of the heel to the next consecutive initial contact of the same heel.

**Pelvic rotation:** Rotation of the pelvis occurs opposite the thorax in order to maintain balance and regulate speed. The average pelvic rotation during gait for an adult is a total of 8 degrees (4 degrees forward with the swing leg and 4 degrees backward with the stance leg).

**Single support phase:** The single support phase occurs when only one foot is on the ground and occurs twice during a single gait cycle.

**Step length:** The distance measured between right heel strike and left heel strike. The average step length for an adult is 28 inches. (Fig. 4-39)

**Stride length:** The distance measured between right heel strike and the following right heel strike. The average stride length for an adult is 56 inches. (Fig. 4-39)

## Abnormal Gait Patterns[10,23]

**Antalgic:** A protective gait pattern where the involved step length is decreased in order to avoid weight bearing on the involved side, usually secondary to pain.

**Ataxic:** A gait pattern characterized by staggering and unsteadiness. There is usually a wide base of support and movements are exaggerated.

**Cerebellar:** A staggering gait pattern seen in cerebellar disease.

**Circumduction:** A gait pattern characterized by a circular motion to advance the leg during swing phase; this may be used to compensate for insufficient hip or knee flexion or dorsiflexion.

**Double step:** A gait pattern in which alternate steps are of a different length or at a different rate.

**Equine:** A gait pattern characterized by high steps; usually involves excessive activity of the gastrocnemius.

**Festinating:** A gait pattern where a patient walks on toes as though pushed. It starts slowly, increases, and may continue until the patient grasps an object in order to stop.

**Hemiplegic:** A gait pattern in which patients abduct the paralyzed limb, swing it around, and bring it forward so the foot comes to the ground in front of them.

**Parkinsonian:** A gait pattern marked by increased forward flexion of the trunk and knees; gait is shuffling with quick and small steps; festinating may occur.

**Scissor:** A gait pattern in which the legs cross midline upon advancement.

**Spastic:** A gait pattern with stiff movement, toes seeming to catch and drag, legs held together, and hip and knee joints slightly flexed. Commonly seen in spastic paraplegia.

**Steppage:** A gait pattern in which the feet and toes are lifted through hip and knee flexion to excessive heights; usually secondary to dorsiflexor weakness. The foot will slap at initial contact with the ground secondary to the decreased control.

**Tabetic:** A high stepping ataxic gait pattern in which the feet slap the ground.

**Trendelenburg:** A gait pattern that denotes gluteus medius weakness; excessive lateral trunk flexion and weight shifting over the stance leg.

**Vaulting:** A gait pattern where the swing leg advances by compensating through the combination of elevation of the pelvis and plantar flexion of the stance leg.

**Fig. 4-39:** Step and stride length.

# Gait Deviations

| | Foot slap | Toe down instead of heel strike | Clawing of toes | Heel lift during midstance | No toe off |
|---|---|---|---|---|---|
| **Ankle and Foot** | • Weak dorsiflexors<br>• Dorsiflexor paralysis | • Plantar flexor spasticity<br>• Plantar flexor contracture<br>• Weak dorsiflexors<br>• Dorsiflexor paralysis<br>• Leg length discrepancy<br>• Hindfoot pain | • Toe flexor spasticity<br>• Positive support reflex | • Insufficient dorsiflexion range<br>• Plantar flexor spasticity | • Forefoot/toe pain<br>• Weak plantar flexors<br>• Weak toe flexors<br>• Insufficient plantar flexion range of motion |
| | **Exaggerated knee flexion at contact** | **Hyperextension in stance** | **Exaggerated knee flexion at terminal stance** | **Insufficient flexion with swing** | **Excessive flexion with swing** |
| **Knee** | • Weak quadriceps<br>• Quadriceps paralysis<br>• Hamstrings spasticity<br>• Insufficient extension range of motion | • Compensation for weak quadriceps<br>• Plantar flexor contracture | • Knee flexion contracture<br>• Hip flexion contracture | • Knee effusion<br>• Quadriceps extension spasticity<br>• Plantar flexor spasticity<br>• Insufficient flexion range of motion | • Flexor withdrawal reflex<br>• Lower extremity flexor synergy |
| | **Insufficient hip flexion at initial contact** | **Insufficient hip extension at stance** | **Circumduction during swing** | **Hip hiking during swing** | **Exaggerated hip flexion during swing** |
| **Hip** | • Weak hip flexors<br>• Hip flexor paralysis<br>• Hip extensor spasticity<br>• Insufficient hip flexion range of motion | • Insufficient hip extension range of motion<br>• Hip flexion contracture<br>• Lower extremity flexor synergy | • Compensation for weak hip flexors<br>• Compensation for weak dorsiflexors<br>• Compensation for weak hamstrings | • Compensation for weak dorsiflexors<br>• Compensation for weak knee flexors<br>• Compensation for extensor synergy pattern | • Lower extremity flexor synergy<br>• Compensation for insufficient ankle dorsiflexion |

# Range of Motion

## Average Adult Range of Motion - Upper and Lower Extremities; Spine[3]

| Upper Extremity | |
|---|---|
| **Shoulder** | |
| Flexion | 0-180 |
| Extension | 0-60 |
| Abduction | 0-180 |
| Medial rotation | 0-70 |
| Lateral rotation | 0-90 |
| **Elbow** | |
| Extension | 0 |
| Flexion | 0-150 |
| **Forearm** | |
| Pronation | 0-80 |
| Supination | 0-80 |
| **Wrist** | |
| Flexion | 0-80 |
| Extension | 0-70 |
| Radial deviation | 0-20 |
| Ulnar deviation | 0-30 |
| **Thumb** | |
| **Carpometacarpal** | |
| Abduction | 0-70 |
| Flexion | 0-15 |
| Extension | 0-20 |
| Opposition | Tip of thumb to base of fifth digit |
| **Metacarpophalangeal** | |
| Flexion | 0-50 |
| **Interphalangeal** | |
| Flexion | 0-80 |
| **Digits – Second to Fifth** | |
| **Metacarpophalangeal** | |
| Flexion | 0-90 |
| Hyperextension | 0-45 |
| **Proximal interphalangeal** | |
| Flexion | 0-100 |
| **Distal interphalangeal** | |
| Flexion | 0-90 |
| Hyperextension | 0-10 |

| Lower Extremity | |
|---|---|
| **Hip** | |
| Flexion | 0-120 |
| Extension | 0-30 |
| Abduction | 0-45 |
| Adduction | 0-30 |
| Medial rotation | 0-45 |
| Lateral rotation | 0-45 |
| **Knee** | |
| Flexion | 0-135 |
| **Ankle** | |
| Dorsiflexion | 0-20 |
| Plantar flexion | 0-50 |
| Inversion | 0-35 |
| Eversion | 0-15 |
| **Subtalar** | |
| Inversion | 0-5 |
| Eversion | 0-5 |

| Spine | |
|---|---|
| **Cervical Spine** | |
| Flexion | 0-45 |
| Extension | 0-45 |
| Lateral flexion | 0-45 |
| Rotation | 0-60 |
| **Thoracic and Lumbar Spine** | |
| Flexion | 0-80 |
| Extension | 0-25 |
| Lateral flexion | 0-35 |
| Rotation | 0-45 |

## Consider This

### Process for Conducting Goniometric Measurement

Goniometric measurement can be reliable (i.e., possessing repeatability of measures) and valid (i.e., meaningful interpretation can be inferred through the measure) when performed by a trained individual following the recommended procedure. The following 12-step process outlines the recommended procedure for conducting goniometric measurement.

1. Place the subject in the recommended testing position.
2. Stabilize the proximal joint segment.
3. Move the distal joint segment through the available range of motion. Make sure that the passive range of motion is performed slowly, the end of the range is attained, and the end-feel is determined.
4. Make a clinical estimate of the range of motion.
5. Return the distal joint segment to the starting position.
6. Palpate bony anatomical landmarks.
7. Align the goniometer.
8. Read and record the starting position. Remove the goniometer.
9. Stabilize the proximal joint segment.
10. Move the distal segment through the full range of motion.
11. Replace and realign the goniometer. Palpate the anatomical landmarks again if necessary.
12. Read and record the range of motion.

Adapted from Norkin and White: Measurement of Joint Motion: A Guide to Goniometry. F.A. Davis Company, Philadelphia, 2003, p.35, with permission.

## Goniometric Technique[3,20]

### Upper Extremity

#### Shoulder*

**Flexion**

Patient position: supine

Stabilization: thorax to prevent extension of the spine

End-feel: firm

Axis: acromial process

Stationary arm: midaxillary line of the thorax

Moveable arm: lateral midline of the humerus using the lateral epicondyle of the humerus for reference

**Extension**

Patient position: prone

Stabilization: thorax to prevent flexion of the spine

End-feel: firm

Axis: acromial process

Stationary arm: midaxillary line of the thorax

Moveable arm: lateral midline of the humerus using the lateral epicondyle of the humerus for reference

**Abduction**

Patient position: supine

Stabilization: thorax to prevent lateral flexion of the spine

End-feel: firm

Axis: anterior aspect of the acromial process

Stationary arm: parallel to the midline of the anterior aspect of the sternum

Moveable arm: medial midline of the humerus

**Adduction**

Patient position: supine

Stabilization: thorax to prevent lateral flexion of the spine

End-feel: firm

Axis: anterior aspect of the acromial process

Stationary arm: parallel to the midline of the anterior aspect of the sternum

Moveable arm: medial midline of the humerus

**Medial rotation**

Patient position: supine with shoulder abducted to 90 degrees and elbow flexed to 90 degrees

Stabilization: distal end of the humerus to maintain the shoulder in 90 degrees of abduction

**End-feel:** firm

**Axis:** olecranon process

**Stationary arm:** parallel or perpendicular to the floor

**Moveable arm:** ulna using the olecranon process and ulnar styloid process for reference

### Lateral rotation

**Patient position:** supine with shoulder abducted to 90 degrees and elbow flexed to 90 degrees

**Stabilization:** distal end of the humerus to maintain the shoulder in 90 degrees of abduction

**End-feel:** firm

**Axis:** olecranon process

**Stationary arm:** parallel or perpendicular to the floor

**Moveable arm:** ulna using the olecranon process and ulnar styloid process for reference

*The supplied stabilization descriptions are for shoulder complex motion. The required stabilization may vary for glenohumeral motions.

## Elbow

### Flexion (Fig. 4-40)

**Patient position:** supine

**Stabilization:** humerus to prevent flexion of the shoulder

**End-feel:** soft

**Axis:** lateral epicondyle of the humerus

**Stationary arm:** lateral midline of the humerus using the center of the acromial process for reference

**Moveable arm:** lateral midline of the radius using the radial head and radial styloid process for reference

**Fig. 4-40:** A therapist measuring elbow flexion with a goniometer.

### Extension

**Patient position:** supine

**Stabilization:** humerus to prevent flexion of the shoulder

**End-feel:** hard

**Axis:** lateral epicondyle of the humerus

**Stationary arm:** lateral midline of the humerus using the center of the acromial process for reference

**Moveable arm:** lateral midline of the radius using the radial head and radial styloid process for reference

## Forearm

### Pronation

**Patient position:** sitting with the elbow flexed to 90 degrees

**Stabilization:** distal end of the humerus to prevent medial rotation and abduction of the humerus

**End-feel:** firm or hard

**Axis:** lateral to the ulnar styloid process

**Stationary arm:** parallel to the anterior midline of the humerus

**Moveable arm:** dorsal aspect of the forearm, just proximal to the styloid process of the radius and ulna

### Supination

**Patient position:** sitting with the elbow flexed to 90 degrees

**Stabilization:** distal end of the humerus to prevent lateral rotation and adduction of the humerus

**End-feel:** firm

**Axis:** medial to the ulnar styloid process

**Stationary arm:** parallel to the anterior midline of the humerus

**Moveable arm:** ventral aspect of the forearm, just proximal to the styloid process of the radius and ulna

## Wrist

### Flexion

**Patient position:** sitting next to a supporting surface with the shoulder abducted to 90 degrees and the elbow flexed to 90 degrees

**Stabilization:** radius and ulna to prevent supination or pronation

**End-feel:** firm

**Axis:** lateral aspect of the wrist over the triquetrum

**Stationary arm:** lateral midline of the ulna using the olecranon and ulnar styloid process for reference

**Moveable arm:** lateral midline of the fifth metacarpal

### Extension

**Patient position:** sitting next to a supporting surface with the shoulder abducted to 90 degrees and the elbow flexed to 90 degrees

**Stabilization:** radius and ulna to prevent supination or pronation

**End-feel:** firm

**Axis:** lateral aspect of the wrist over the triquetrum

**Stationary arm:** lateral midline of the ulna using the olecranon and ulnar styloid process for reference

**Moveable arm:** lateral midline of the fifth metacarpal

### Radial deviation

**Patient position:** sitting next to a supporting surface with the shoulder abducted to 90 degrees and the elbow flexed to 90 degrees

**Stabilization:** radius and ulna to prevent supination or pronation

**End-feel:** firm or hard

**Axis:** over the middle of the dorsal aspect of the wrist over the capitate

**Stationary arm:** dorsal midline of the forearm using the lateral epicondyle of the humerus for reference

**Moveable arm:** dorsal midline of the third metacarpal

### Ulnar deviation

**Patient position:** sitting next to a supporting surface with the shoulder abducted to 90 degrees and the elbow flexed to 90 degrees

**Stabilization:** radius and ulna to prevent supination or pronation

**End-feel:** firm

**Axis:** over the middle of the dorsal aspect of the wrist over the capitate

**Stationary arm:** dorsal midline of the forearm using the lateral epicondyle of the humerus for reference

**Moveable arm:** dorsal midline of the third metacarpal

## Thumb

### Carpometacarpal flexion

**Patient position:** sitting with the forearm and hand on a supporting surface

**Stabilization:** carpals, radius, and ulna to prevent wrist motion

**End-feel:** firm

**Axis:** over the palmar aspect of the first carpometacarpal joint

**Stationary arm:** ventral midline of the radius using the ventral surface of the radial head and radial styloid process for reference

**Moveable arm:** ventral midline of the first metacarpal

### Carpometacarpal extension

**Patient position:** sitting with the forearm and hand on a supporting surface

**Stabilization:** carpals, radius, and ulna to prevent wrist motion

**End-feel:** firm

**Axis:** over the palmar aspect of the first carpometacarpal joint

**Stationary arm:** ventral midline of the radius using the ventral surface of the radial head and radial styloid process for reference

**Moveable arm:** ventral midline of the first metacarpal

### Carpometacarpal abduction

**Patient position:** sitting with the forearm and hand on a supporting surface

**Stabilization:** carpals and second metacarpal to prevent wrist motion

**End-feel:** firm

**Axis:** over the lateral aspect of the radial styloid process

**Stationary arm:** lateral midline of the second metacarpal using the center of the second metacarpophalangeal joint for reference

**Moveable arm:** lateral midline of the first metacarpal using the center of the first metacarpophalangeal joint for reference

### Carpometacarpal adduction

**Patient position:** sitting with the forearm and hand on a supporting surface

**Stabilization:** carpals and second metacarpal to prevent wrist motion

**End-feel:** firm

**Axis:** over the lateral aspect of the radial styloid process

**Stationary arm:** lateral midline of the second metacarpal using the center of the second metacarpophalangeal joint for reference

**Moveable arm:** lateral midline of the first metacarpal using the center of the first metacarpophalangeal joint for reference

## Fingers

### Metacarpophalangeal flexion

**Patient position:** sitting with the forearm and hand on a supporting surface

**Stabilization:** metacarpal to prevent wrist motion

**End-feel:** firm or hard

**Axis:** over the dorsal aspect of the metacarpophalangeal joint

**Stationary arm:** over the dorsal midline of the metacarpal

**Moveable arm:** over the dorsal midline of the proximal phalanx

### Metacarpophalangeal extension

**Patient position:** sitting with the forearm and hand on a supporting surface

**Stabilization:** metacarpal to prevent wrist motion

**End-feel:** firm

**Axis:** over the dorsal aspect of the metacarpophalangeal joint

**Stationary arm:** over the dorsal midline of the metacarpal

**Moveable arm:** over the dorsal midline of the proximal phalanx

### Metacarpophalangeal abduction

**Patient position:** sitting with the forearm and hand on a supporting surface

**Stabilization:** metacarpal to prevent wrist motion

**End-feel:** firm

**Axis:** over the dorsal aspect of the metacarpophalangeal joint

**Stationary arm:** over the dorsal midline of the metacarpal

**Moveable arm:** dorsal midline of the proximal phalanx

### Metacarpophalangeal adduction

**Patient position:** sitting with the forearm and hand on a supporting surface

**Stabilization:** metacarpal to prevent wrist motion

**End-feel:** firm

**Axis:** over the dorsal aspect of the metacarpophalangeal joint

**Stationary arm:** over the dorsal midline of the metacarpal

**Moveable arm:** dorsal midline of the proximal phalanx

### Proximal interphalangeal flexion

**Patient position:** sitting with the forearm and hand on a supporting surface

**Stabilization:** proximal phalanx to prevent motion at the metacarpophalangeal joint

**End-feel:** soft, firm or hard

**Axis:** over the dorsal aspect of the proximal interphalangeal joint

**Stationary arm:** over the dorsal midline of the proximal phalanx

**Moveable arm:** over the dorsal midline of the middle phalanx

### Proximal interphalangeal extension

**Patient position:** sitting with the forearm and hand on a supporting surface

**Stabilization:** proximal phalanx to prevent motion at the metacarpophalangeal joint

**End-feel:** firm

**Axis:** over the dorsal aspect of the proximal interphalangeal joint

**Stationary arm:** over the dorsal midline of the proximal phalanx

**Moveable arm:** over the dorsal midline of the middle phalanx

### Distal interphalangeal flexion

**Patient position:** sitting with the forearm and hand on a supporting surface

**Stabilization:** middle and proximal phalanx to prevent motion at the proximal interphalangeal joint

**End-feel:** firm

**Axis:** over the dorsal aspect of the distal interphalangeal joint

**Stationary arm:** over the dorsal midline of the middle phalanx

**Moveable arm:** over the dorsal midline of the distal phalanx

### Distal interphalangeal extension

**Patient position:** sitting with the forearm and hand on a supporting surface

**Stabilization:** middle and proximal phalanx to prevent motion at the proximal interphalangeal joint

**End-feel:** firm

**Axis:** over the dorsal aspect of the distal interphalangeal joint

**Stationary arm:** over the dorsal midline of the middle phalanx

**Moveable arm:** over the dorsal midline of the distal phalanx

## Lower Extremity

### Hip

#### Flexion (Fig. 4-41)

**Patient position:** supine

**Stabilization:** pelvis to prevent posterior tilting

**End-feel:** soft or firm

**Axis:** over the lateral aspect of the hip joint using the greater trochanter of the femur for reference

**Stationary arm:** lateral midline of the pelvis

**Moveable arm:** lateral midline of the femur using the lateral epicondyle for reference

#### Extension

**Patient position:** prone

**Stabilization:** pelvis to prevent anterior tilting

**End-feel:** firm

**Axis:** over the lateral aspect of the hip joint using the greater trochanter of the femur for reference

**Stationary arm:** lateral midline of the pelvis

**Moveable arm:** lateral midline of the femur using the lateral epicondyle for reference

#### Abduction

**Patient position:** supine

**Stabilization:** pelvis to prevent lateral tilting and rotation; trunk to prevent lateral flexion

**End-feel:** firm

**Axis:** over the anterior superior iliac spine (ASIS) of the extremity being measured

**Stationary arm:** align with imaginary horizontal line extending from one ASIS to the other ASIS

**Moveable arm:** anterior midline of the femur using the midline of the patella for reference

**Fig. 4-41:** A therapist measuring hip flexion with a goniometer.

## Adduction

**Patient position:** supine

**Stabilization:** pelvis to prevent lateral tilting

**End-feel:** firm

**Axis:** over the anterior superior iliac spine (ASIS) of the extremity being measured

**Stationary arm:** align with imaginary horizontal line extending from one ASIS to the other ASIS

**Moveable arm:** anterior midline of the femur using the midline of the patella for reference

## Medial rotation

**Patient position:** sitting

**Stabilization:** distal end of the femur

**End-feel:** firm

**Axis:** anterior aspect of the patella

**Stationary arm:** perpendicular to the floor or parallel to the supporting surface

**Moveable arm:** anterior midline of the lower leg using the crest of the tibia and a point midway between the two malleoli for reference

## Lateral rotation

**Patient position:** sitting

**Stabilization:** distal end of the femur

**End-feel:** firm

**Axis:** anterior aspect of the patella

**Stationary arm:** perpendicular to the floor or parallel to the supporting surface

**Moveable arm:** anterior midline of the lower leg using the crest of the tibia and a point midway between the two malleoli for reference

## Knee

### Flexion

**Patient position:** supine

**Stabilization:** femur to prevent rotation, abduction, and adduction of the hip

**End-feel:** soft or firm

**Axis:** lateral epicondyle of the femur

**Stationary arm:** lateral midline of the femur using the greater trochanter for reference

**Moveable arm:** lateral midline of the fibula using the lateral malleolus and fibular head for reference

### Extension

**Patient position:** supine

**Stabilization:** femur to prevent rotation, abduction, and adduction of the hip

**End-feel:** firm

**Axis:** lateral epicondyle of the femur

**Stationary arm:** lateral midline of the femur using the greater trochanter for reference

**Moveable arm:** lateral midline of the fibula using the lateral malleolus and fibular head for reference

## Ankle

### Dorsiflexion

**Patient position:** sitting with the knee flexed to 90 degrees

**Stabilization:** tibia and fibula to prevent knee and hip motion

**End-feel:** firm

**Axis:** lateral aspect of the lateral malleolus

**Stationary arm:** lateral midline of the fibula using the head of the fibula for reference

**Moveable arm:** parallel to the lateral aspect of the fifth metatarsal

### Plantar flexion

**Patient position:** sitting with the knee flexed to 90 degrees

**Stabilization:** tibia and fibula to prevent knee and hip motion

**End-feel:** firm or hard

**Axis:** lateral aspect of the lateral malleolus

**Stationary arm:** lateral midline of the fibula using the head of the fibula for reference

**Moveable arm:** parallel to the lateral aspect of the fifth metatarsal

### Inversion (Fig. 4-42)

**Patient position:** sitting with the knee flexed to 90 degrees

**Stabilization:** tibia and fibula to prevent knee and hip motion

**End-feel:** firm

**Axis:** anterior aspect of the ankle midway between the malleoli

**Stationary arm:** anterior midline of the lower leg using the tibial tuberosity for reference

**Moveable arm:** anterior midline of the second metatarsal

Fig. 4-42: A therapist measuring ankle complex inversion.

### Eversion

**Patient position:** sitting with the knee flexed to 90 degrees

**Stabilization:** tibia and fibula to prevent knee and hip motion

**End-feel:** firm or hard

**Axis:** anterior aspect of the ankle midway between the malleoli

**Stationary arm:** anterior midline of the lower leg using the tibial tuberosity for reference

**Moveable arm:** anterior midline of the second metatarsal

## Subtalar

### Inversion

**Patient position:** prone with the foot extended over a supporting surface

**Stabilization:** tibia and fibula to prevent knee and hip motion

**End-feel:** firm

**Axis:** posterior aspect of the ankle midway between the malleoli

**Stationary arm:** posterior midline of the lower leg

**Moveable arm:** posterior midline of the calcaneus

### Eversion

**Patient position:** prone with the foot extended over a supporting surface

**Stabilization:** tibia and fibula to prevent knee and hip motion

**End-feel:** firm or hard

**Axis:** posterior aspect of the ankle midway between the malleoli

**Stationary arm:** posterior midline of the lower leg

**Moveable arm:** posterior midline of the calcaneus

## Spine

### Cervical Spine

#### Flexion

**Patient position:** sitting with the thoracic and lumbar spine supported

**Stabilization:** shoulder girdle and chest; the patient's hands should be placed on their knees

**End-feel:** firm

**Axis:** over the external auditory meatus

**Stationary arm:** perpendicular or parallel to the ground

**Moveable arm:** along the base of the nares or if using a tongue depressor, align the goniometer parallel with the tongue depressor

#### Extension

**Patient position:** sitting with the thoracic and lumbar spine supported

**Stabilization:** shoulder girdle and chest to prevent extension of the thoracic and lumbar spine

**End-feel:** firm

**Axis:** over the external auditory meatus

**Stationary arm:** perpendicular or parallel to the ground

**Moveable arm:** along the base of the nares, or if using a tongue depressor, align the goniometer parallel with the tongue depressor

Fig. 4-43: A therapist preparing to measure cervical lateral flexion with a cervical range of motion (CROM) device.

### Lateral flexion (Fig. 4-43)

**Patient position:** sitting

**Stabilization:** shoulder girdle and chest to prevent lateral flexion of the thoracic and lumbar spines

**End-feel:** firm

**Axis:** over the spinous process of the C7 vertebra

**Stationary arm:** with the spinous processes of the thoracic vertebrae so that the arm is perpendicular to the ground

**Moveable arm:** along the dorsal midline of the head using the occipital protuberance for reference

### Rotation (Fig. 4-44)

**Patient position:** sitting with the thoracic and lumbar spine supported

**Stabilization:** shoulder girdle and chest to prevent rotation of the thoracic and lumbar spines

**End-feel:** firm

**Axis:** over the center of the cranial aspect of the head

**Stationary arm:** parallel to an imaginary line between the two acromial processes

**Moveable arm:** with the tip of the nose or if using a tongue depressor, align the goniometer parallel with the tongue depressor

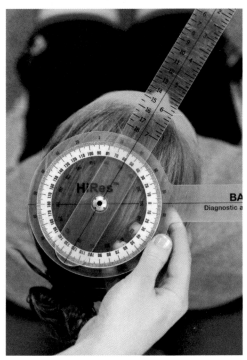

**Fig. 4-44:** A therapist measuring cervical rotation with a goniometer.

## Thoracic and Lumbar Spines

### Flexion and extension (Fig. 4-45)

Flexion of the thoracic and lumbar spines is most commonly measured with a tape measure instead of a goniometer.

The therapist aligns a tape measure between the spinous processes of C7 and S1. The distance is recorded. The patient is then asked to bend forward gradually while the therapist allows the tape measure to unwind. The second distance is recorded. The amount of thoracic and lumbar flexion is determined by calculating the difference between the first and the second measurements. Extension of the thoracic and lumbar spine is measured in a similar manner.

**Fig. 4-45:** A therapist measuring thoracic and lumbar flexion with a double inclinometer.

**Fig. 4-46:** A therapist measuring thoracic and lumbar lateral flexion with a goniometer.

**Lateral flexion (Fig. 4-46)**

**Patient position:** standing with the feet shoulder width apart

**Stabilization:** pelvis to prevent lateral tilting

**End-feel:** firm

**Axis:** over the posterior aspect of the spinous process of S1

**Stationary arm:** perpendicular to the ground

**Moveable arm:** along the posterior aspect of the spinous process of C7

**Rotation**

**Patient position:** sitting on a chair without a back with the feet positioned on the floor for pelvic stabilization

**Stabilization:** pelvis to prevent rotation

**End-feel:** firm

**Axis:** over the center of the cranial aspect of the head

**Stationary arm:** parallel to an imaginary line between the two prominent tubercles on the iliac crests

**Moveable arm:** along an imaginary line between the two acromial processes

## Consider This

### Documentation of Recorded Measures

Health care providers work in an integrated fashion to deliver patient care. The patient medical record is one of the primary ways that health care providers keep each other informed of current patient status and other relevant information. As a result, it is critical that health care providers document relevant information in the medical record in a timely and accurate manner. Failure to meet this standard potentially results in ineffective medical care and may jeopardize patient safety.

The results of goniometric measurements can be used to illustrate this point. Let's assume that a therapist reviews the medical record of a patient recovering from a motor vehicle accident, in which the patient sustained multiple lower extremity injuries. Upon reviewing the medical record, the therapist determines that in successive notes the patient's right knee range of motion was described as 10-105 degrees and 10-0-105 degrees.

Although the recorded measurements appear extremely similar, they are in fact very different. 10-105 degrees indicates that the patient's range of motion begins at 10 degrees of knee flexion and ends at 105 degrees of knee flexion (95 degrees of total available movement). Conversely, the use of "0" between the starting and ending values indicates the patient has 10 degrees of knee hyperextension and 105 degrees of knee flexion (115 degrees of total available movement).

This type of inaccuracy could cause a variety of potential problems including selecting inappropriate parameters for a device such as a continuous passive motion machine, selecting an inappropriate therapeutic exercise activity based on the patient's available range of motion, and potential reimbursement-related questions concerning the extreme variability in recorded measures.

# Special Tests

## Special Tests Outline

## Upper Extremity

### Shoulder

**Dislocation**

Apprehension test for anterior shoulder dislocation

Apprehension test for posterior shoulder dislocation

**Biceps Tendon Pathology**

Ludington's test

Speed's test

Yergason's test

**Rotator Cuff Pathology/Impingement**

Drop arm test

Hawkins-Kennedy impingement test

Neer impingement test

Supraspinatus test

**Thoracic Outlet Syndrome**

Adson maneuver

Allen test

Costoclavicular syndrome test

Roos test

Wright test (hyperabduction test)

**Miscellaneous**

Glenoid labrum tear test

Upper limb tension tests

## Elbow

**Ligamentous Instability**

Varus stress test

Valgus stress test

**Epicondylitis**

Cozen's test

Lateral epicondylitis test

Medial epicondylitis test

Mill's test

**Neurological Dysfunction**

Tinel's sign

## Wrist/Hand

**Ligamentous Instability**

Ulnar collateral ligament instability test

**Vascular Insufficiency**

Allen test

Capillary refill test

   **(See Cardiovascular and Pulmonary Systems Unit)**

**Contracture/Tightness**

Bunnel-Littler test

Tight retinacular ligament test

**Neurological Dysfunction**

Froment's sign

Phalen's test

Tinel's sign

**Miscellaneous**

Finkelstein test

Grind test

Murphy sign

# Lower Extremity

## Hip

**Contracture/Tightness**

Ely's test

Ober's test

Piriformis test

Thomas test

Tripod sign

90-90 straight leg raise test

**Pediatric Tests**

Barlow's test

Ortolani's test

**Miscellaneous**

Craig's test

Patrick's test (Faber test)

Quadrant scouring test

Trendelenburg test

## Knee

**Ligamentous Instability**

Anterior drawer test

Lachman test

Lateral pivot shift test

Posterior drawer test

Posterior sag sign

Slocum test

Valgus stress test

Varus stress test

**Meniscal Pathology**

Apley's compression test

Bounce home test

McMurray test

**Swelling**

Brush test

Patellar tap test

**Miscellaneous**

Clarke's sign

Hughston's plica test

Noble compression test

Patellar apprehension test

## Ankle

**Ligamentous Instability**

Anterior drawer test

Talar tilt

**Miscellaneous**

Homans' sign

   **(See Cardiovascular and Pulmonary Systems Unit)**

Thompson test

Tibial torsion test

True leg length discrepancy test

## Spine

### Cervical Region

Foraminal compression test

Vertebral artery test

### Lumbar/Sacroiliac Region

Sacroiliac joint stress test

Sitting flexion test

Standing flexion test

## Descriptions of Special Tests

## Shoulder

### Dislocation

**Apprehension test for anterior shoulder dislocation[10,26]**

The patient is positioned in supine with the arm in 90 degrees of abduction. The therapist laterally rotates the patient's shoulder. A positive test is indicated by a look of apprehension or a facial grimace prior to reaching an end point (Fig. 4-47).

**Apprehension test for posterior shoulder dislocation[8,10]**

The patient is positioned in supine with the arm in 90 degrees of flexion and medial rotation. The therapist applies a posterior force through the long axis of the humerus. A positive test is indicated by a look of apprehension or a facial grimace prior to reaching an end point.

Fig. 4-47: A therapist observing a patient while administering an apprehension test for anterior shoulder dislocation.

### Biceps Tendon Pathology

**Ludington's test[10,13]**

The patient is positioned in sitting and is asked to clasp both hands behind the head with the fingers interlocked. The patient is then asked to alternately contract and relax the biceps muscles. A positive test is indicated by absence of movement in the biceps tendon and may be indicative of a rupture of the long head of the biceps.

**Speed's test[10,26]**

The patient is positioned in sitting or standing with the elbow extended and the forearm supinated. The therapist places one hand over the bicipital groove and the other hand on the volar surface of the forearm. The therapist resists active shoulder flexion. A positive test is indicated by pain or tenderness in the bicipital groove region and may be indicative of bicipital tendonitis (Fig. 4-48).

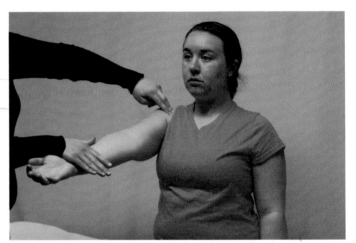

Fig. 4-48: A therapist administering Speed's test. The therapist resists shoulder flexion while palpating the bicipital groove.

**Yergason's test[10,13]**

The patient is positioned in sitting with 90 degrees of elbow flexion and the forearm pronated. The humerus is stabilized against the patient's thorax. The therapist places one hand on the patient's forearm and the other hand over the bicipital groove. The patient is directed to actively supinate and laterally rotate against resistance. A positive test is indicated by pain or tenderness in the bicipital groove and may be indicative of bicipital tendonitis.

### Rotator Cuff Pathology/Impingement

**Drop arm test[10,26]**

The patient is positioned in sitting or standing with the arm in 90 degrees of abduction. The patient is asked to slowly lower the arm to their side. A positive test is indicated by the patient failing to slowly lower the arm to their side or by the presence of severe pain and may be indicative of a tear in the rotator cuff.

## Hawkins-Kennedy impingement test[10]

The patient is positioned in sitting or standing. The therapist flexes the patient's shoulder to 90 degrees and then medially rotates the arm. A positive test is indicated by pain and may be indicative of shoulder impingement involving the supraspinatus tendon (Fig. 4-49).

**Fig. 4-49:** A positive Hawkins-Kennedy impingement test is indicated by the presence of pain.

## Neer impingement test[10,26]

The patient is positioned in sitting or standing. The therapist positions one hand on the posterior aspect of the patient's scapula and the other hand stabilizing the elbow. The therapist elevates the patient's arm through flexion. A positive test is indicated by a facial grimace or pain and may be indicative of shoulder impingement involving the supraspinatus tendon.

## Supraspinatus test[10,13]

The patient is positioned with the arm in 90 degrees of abduction followed by 30 degrees of horizontal adduction with the thumb pointing downward. The therapist resists the patient's attempt to abduct the arm. A positive test is indicated by weakness or pain and may be indicative of a tear of the supraspinatus tendon, impingement or suprascapular nerve involvement.

## Thoracic Outlet Syndrome

### Adson maneuver[10,26]

The patient is positioned in sitting or standing. The therapist monitors the radial pulse and asks the patient to rotate his/her head to face the test shoulder. The patient is then asked to extend his/her head while the therapist laterally rotates and extends the patient's shoulder. A positive test is indicated by an absent or diminished radial pulse and may be indicative of thoracic outlet syndrome.

## Allen test[10,26]

The patient is positioned in sitting or standing with the test arm in 90 degrees of abduction, lateral rotation, and elbow flexion. The patient is asked to rotate the head away from the test shoulder while the therapist monitors the radial pulse. A positive test is indicated by an absent or diminished pulse when the head is rotated away from the test shoulder. A positive test may be indicative of thoracic outlet syndrome.

## Costoclavicular syndrome test[10,18]

The patient is positioned in sitting. The therapist monitors the patient's radial pulse and assists the patient to assume a military posture. A positive test is indicated by an absent or diminished radial pulse and may be indicative of thoracic outlet syndrome caused by compression of the subclavian artery between the first rib and the clavicle.

## Roos test[10,18]

The patient is positioned in sitting or standing with the arms positioned in 90 degrees of abduction, lateral rotation, and elbow flexion. The patient is asked to open and close their hands for three minutes. A positive test is indicated by the inability to maintain the test position, weakness of the arms, sensory loss or ischemic pain. A positive test may be indicative of thoracic outlet syndrome.

## Wright test (hyperabduction test)[10]

The patient is positioned in sitting or supine. The therapist moves the patient's arm overhead in the frontal plane while monitoring the patient's radial pulse. A positive test is indicated by an absent or diminished radial pulse and may be indicative of compression in the costoclavicular space.

## Miscellaneous

### Glenoid labrum tear test[10]

The patient is positioned in supine. The therapist places one hand on the posterior aspect of the patient's humeral head while the other hand stabilizes the humerus proximal to the elbow. The therapist passively abducts and laterally rotates the arm over the patient's head and then proceeds to apply an anterior directed force to the humerus. A positive test is indicated by a clunk or grinding sound and may be indicative of a glenoid labrum tear.

### Upper limb tension tests[10]

Upper limb tension tests are types of neural provocation maneuvers. The tests require an ordered sequence of movements occurring at the shoulder, arm, elbow, forearm, wrist, and hand. Symptoms and relevant changes in symptoms should be identified after each step. A sensitization test is often employed if symptoms are minimal or absent after the identified sequence. Upper limb tension tests are recommended for patients with symptoms in the arm, head, neck, and thoracic spine. Each test begins with the noninvolved side being tested first.

## Upper Limb Tension Tests

| | Upper Limb Tension Test 1 | Upper Limb Tension Test 2 | Upper Limb Tension Test 3 | Upper Limb Tension Test 4 |
|---|---|---|---|---|
| **Joint Positioning Sequence** | shoulder depression with 110 degrees abduction, elbow extension, forearm supination, wrist extension, finger and thumb extension | shoulder depression with 10 degrees abduction, elbow extension, forearm supination, wrist extension, finger and thumb extension, shoulder lateral rotation | shoulder depression with 10 degrees abduction, elbow extension, forearm pronation, wrist flexion ulnar deviation, finger and thumb flexion, shoulder medial rotation | shoulder depression with 10-90 degrees abduction, elbow flexion, forearm supination, wrist extension radial deviation, finger and thumb extension, shoulder lateral rotation |
| **Sensitization Test** | contralateral cervical lateral flexion | contralateral cervical lateral flexion | contralateral cervical lateral flexion | contralateral cervical lateral flexion |
| **Nerve Bias** | median nerve, anterior interosseous nerve | median nerve, musculocutaneous nerve, axillary nerve | radial nerve | ulnar nerve |

## Elbow

### Ligamentous Instability

#### Varus stress test[8,10]

The patient is positioned in sitting with the elbow in 20 to 30 degrees of flexion. The therapist places one hand on the elbow and the other hand proximal to the patient's wrist. The therapist applies a varus force to test the lateral collateral ligament while palpating the lateral joint line. A positive test is indicated by increased laxity in the lateral collateral ligament when compared to the contralateral limb, apprehension or pain. A positive test may be indicative of a lateral collateral ligament sprain.

#### Valgus stress test[8,10]

The patient is positioned in sitting with the elbow in 20 to 30 degrees of flexion. The therapist places one hand on the elbow and the other hand proximal to the patient's wrist. The therapist applies a valgus force to test the medial collateral ligament while palpating the medial joint line. A positive test is indicated by increased laxity in the medial collateral ligament when compared to the contralateral limb, apprehension or pain. A positive test may be indicative of a medial collateral ligament sprain.

### Epicondylitis

#### Cozen's test[10,18]

The patient is positioned in sitting with the elbow in slight flexion. The therapist places his/her thumb on the patient's lateral epicondyle while stabilizing the elbow joint. The patient is asked to make a fist, pronate the forearm, radially deviate, and extend the wrist against resistance. A positive test is indicated by pain in the lateral epicondyle region or muscle weakness and may be indicative of lateral epicondylitis.

#### Lateral epicondylitis test[8,10]

The patient is positioned in sitting. The therapist stabilizes the elbow with one hand and places the other hand on the dorsal aspect of the patient's hand distal to the proximal interphalangeal joint. The patient is asked to extend the third digit against resistance. A positive test is indicated by pain in the lateral epicondyle region or muscle weakness and may be indicative of lateral epicondylitis.

#### Medial epicondylitis test[8,10]

The patient is positioned in sitting. The therapist palpates the medial epicondyle and supinates the patient's forearm, extends the wrist, and extends the elbow. A positive test is indicated by pain in the medial epicondyle region and may be indicative of medial epicondylitis.

### Mill's test[10]

The patient is positioned in sitting. The therapist palpates the lateral epicondyle, pronates the patient's forearm, flexes the wrist, and extends the elbow. A positive test is indicated by pain in the lateral epicondyle region and may be indicative of lateral epicondylitis.

## Neurological Dysfunction

### Tinel's sign[10,13]

The patient is positioned in sitting with the elbow in slight flexion. The therapist taps with the index finger between the olecranon process and the medial epicondyle. A positive test is indicated by a tingling sensation in the ulnar nerve distribution of the forearm, hand, and fingers. A positive test may be indicative of ulnar nerve compression or compromise.

## Wrist/Hand

## Ligamentous Instability

### Ulnar collateral ligament instability test[10]

The patient is positioned in sitting. The therapist holds the patient's thumb in extension and applies a valgus force to the metacarpophalangeal joint of the thumb. A positive test is indicated by excessive valgus movement and may be indicative of a tear of the ulnar collateral and accessory collateral ligaments. This type of injury is referred to as gamekeeper's or skier's thumb.

## Vascular Insufficiency

### Allen test[8,10]

The patient is positioned in sitting or standing. The patient is asked to open and close the hand several times in succession and then maintain the hand in a closed position. The therapist compresses the radial and ulnar arteries. The patient is then asked to relax the hand and the therapist releases the pressure on one of the arteries while observing the color of the hand and fingers. A positive test is indicated by delayed or absent flushing of the radial or ulnar half of the hand and may be indicative of an occlusion in the radial or ulnar artery (Figs. 4-50, 4-51).

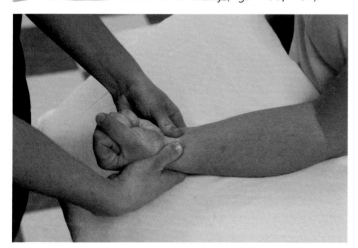

**Fig. 4-50:** A therapist compresses the radial and ulnar arteries while administering the Allen test.

**Fig. 4-51:** The therapist releases the radial artery and observes the color of the hand and fingers.

## Contracture/Tightness

### Bunnel-Littler test[10,26]

The patient is positioned in sitting with the metacarpophalangeal joint held in slight extension. The therapist attempts to move the proximal interphalangeal joint into flexion. If the proximal interphalangeal joint does not flex with the metacarpophalangeal joint extended, there may be a tight intrinsic muscle or capsular tightness. If the proximal interphalangeal joint fully flexes with the metacarpophalangeal joint in slight flexion, there may be intrinsic muscle tightness without capsular tightness.

### Tight retinacular ligament test[10]

The proximal interphalangeal joint is held in a neutral position while the therapist attempts to flex the distal interphalangeal joint. If the therapist is unable to flex the distal interphalangeal joint, the retinacular ligaments or capsule may be tight. If the therapist is able to flex the distal interphalangeal joint with the proximal interphalangeal joint in flexion, the retinacular ligaments may be tight and the capsule may be normal.

## Neurological Dysfunction

### Froment's sign[10,26]

The patient is positioned in sitting or standing and is asked to hold a piece of paper between the thumb and index finger. The therapist attempts to pull the paper away from the patient. A positive test is indicated by the patient flexing the distal phalanx of the thumb due to adductor pollicis muscle paralysis. If at the same time, the patient hyperextends the metacarpophalangeal joint of the thumb, it is termed Jeanne's sign. Both objective findings may be indicative of ulnar nerve compromise or paralysis (Fig. 4-52).

**Fig. 4-52:** A positive Froment's sign is indicated by the patient flexing the distal phalanx of the thumb due to adductor pollicis muscle paralysis.

### Phalen's test[8,10]

The patient is positioned in sitting or standing. The therapist flexes the patient's wrists maximally and asks the patient to hold the position for 60 seconds. A positive test is indicated by tingling in the thumb, index finger, middle finger, and lateral half of the ring finger and may be indicative of carpal tunnel syndrome due to median nerve compression (Fig. 4-53).

**Fig. 4-53:** A patient maintains the test position for Phalen's test.

### Tinel's sign[10,13]

The patient is positioned in sitting or standing. The therapist taps over the volar aspect of the patient's wrist. A positive test is indicated by tingling in the thumb, index finger, middle finger, and lateral half of the ring finger distal to the contact site at the wrist. A positive test may be indicative of carpal tunnel syndrome due to median nerve compression.

## Miscellaneous

### Finkelstein test[10,26]

The patient is positioned in sitting or standing and is asked to make a fist with the thumb tucked inside the fingers. The therapist stabilizes the patient's forearm and ulnarly deviates the wrist. A positive test is indicated by pain over the abductor pollicis longus and extensor pollicis brevis tendons at the wrist and may be indicative of tenosynovitis in the thumb (de Quervain's disease) (Fig. 4-54).

**Fig. 4-54:** A therapist administers the Finkelstein test to a patient in sitting.

### Grind test[10]

The patient is positioned in sitting or standing. The therapist stabilizes the patient's hand and grasps the patient's thumb on the metacarpal. The therapist applies compression and rotation through the metacarpal. A positive test is indicated by pain and may be indicative of degenerative joint disease in the carpometacarpal joint.

### Murphy sign[10,18]

The patient is positioned in sitting or standing and is asked to make a fist. A positive test is indicated by the patient's third metacarpal remaining level with the second and fourth metacarpals. A positive test may be indicative of a dislocated lunate.

## Hip

### Contracture/Tightness

### Ely's test[10,13]

The patient is positioned in prone while the therapist passively flexes the patient's knee. A positive test is indicated by spontaneous hip flexion occurring simultaneously with knee flexion and may be indicative of a rectus femoris contracture (Fig. 4-55).

### Ober's test[10,26]

The patient is positioned in sidelying with the lower leg flexed at the hip and the knee. The therapist moves the test leg into hip extension and abduction and then attempts to slowly lower the test leg. A positive test is indicated by an inability of the test leg to adduct and touch the table and may be indicative of a tensor fasciae latae contracture (Fig. 4-56).

**Fig. 4-55:** A positive Ely's test is indicated by active hip flexion occurring simultaneously with passive knee flexion.

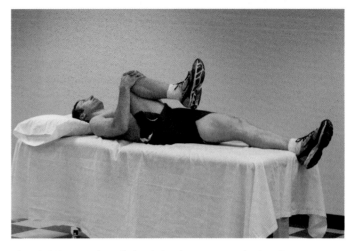

**Fig. 4-57:** A patient brings the knee towards the chest as part of the Thomas test. A positive test is indicated by the straight leg rising from the table.

### Tripod sign[10]

The patient is positioned in sitting with the knees flexed to 90 degrees over the edge of a table. The therapist passively extends one knee. A positive test is indicated by tightness in the hamstrings or extension of the trunk in order to limit the effect of the tight hamstrings.

### 90-90 straight leg raise test[8,10]

The patient is positioned in supine and is asked to stabilize the hips in 90 degrees of flexion with the knees relaxed. The therapist instructs the patient to alternately extend each knee as much as possible while maintaining the hips in 90 degrees of flexion. A positive test is indicated by the knee remaining in 20 degrees or more of flexion and is indicative of hamstrings tightness.

**Fig. 4-56:** A therapist administers Ober's test by moving the patient's leg into hip extension and abduction, and then attempts to lower the leg towards the table.

### Piriformis test[10,13]

The patient is positioned in sidelying with the test leg positioned toward the ceiling and the hip flexed to 60 degrees. The therapist places one hand on the patient's pelvis and the other hand on the patient's knee. While stabilizing the pelvis, the therapist applies a downward (adduction) force on the knee. A positive test is indicated by pain or tightness, and may be indicative of piriformis tightness or compression on the sciatic nerve caused by the piriformis.

### Thomas test[10,26]

The patient is positioned in supine with the legs fully extended. The patient is asked to bring one of his/her knees to the chest in order to flatten the lumbar spine. The therapist observes the position of the contralateral hip while the patient holds the flexed hip. A positive test is indicated by the straight leg rising from the table and may be indicative of a hip flexion contracture (Fig. 4-57).

Pediatric Tests

### Barlow's test[10,27]

The patient is positioned in supine with the hips flexed to 90 degrees and the knees flexed. The therapist tests each hip individually by stabilizing the femur and pelvis with one hand while the other hand moves the test leg into abduction while applying forward pressure posterior to the greater trochanter. A positive test is indicated by a click or a clunk and may be indicative of a hip dislocation being reduced. The test is considered to be a variation of Ortolani's test.

*[handwritten margin note: Adduction]*

### Ortolani's test[10,27]

The patient is positioned in supine with the hips flexed to 90 degrees and the knees flexed. The therapist grasps the legs so that their thumbs are placed along the patient's medial thighs and the fingers are placed on the lateral thighs toward the buttocks. The therapist abducts the patient's hips and gentle pressure is applied to the greater trochanters until resistance is felt at approximately 30 degrees. A positive test is indicated by a click or a clunk and may be indicative of a dislocation being reduced.

## Miscellaneous

### Craig's test[10,18]

The patient is positioned in prone with the test knee flexed to 90 degrees. The therapist palpates the posterior aspect of the greater trochanter and medially and laterally rotates the hip until the greater trochanter is parallel with the table. The degree of femoral anteversion corresponds to the angle formed by the lower leg with the perpendicular axis of the table. Normal anteversion for an adult is 8-15 degrees (Fig. 4-58).

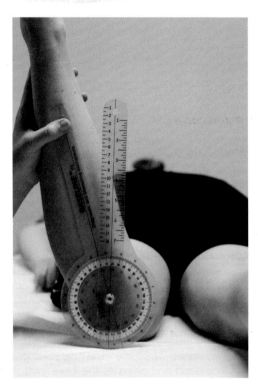

**Fig. 4-58:** A therapist attempts to quantify the amount of femoral anteversion with a goniometer after administering Craig's test.

### Patrick's test (Faber test)[8,10]

The patient is positioned in supine with the test leg flexed, abducted, and laterally rotated at the hip onto the opposite leg. The therapist slowly lowers the test leg through abduction toward the table. A positive test is indicated by failure of the test leg to abduct below the level of the opposite leg and may be indicative of iliopsoas, sacroiliac or hip joint abnormalities.

### Quadrant scouring test[10,13]

The patient is positioned in supine. The therapist passively flexes and adducts the hip with the knee in maximal flexion. The therapist applies a compressive force through the shaft of the femur while continuing to passively move the patient's hip. A positive test is indicated by grinding, catching or crepitation in the hip and may be indicative of pathologies such as arthritis, avascular necrosis or an osteochondral defect.

### Trendelenburg test[8,10]

The patient is positioned in standing and is asked to stand on one leg for approximately ten seconds. A positive test is indicated by a drop of the pelvis on the unsupported side and may be indicative of weakness of the gluteus medius muscle on the supported side.

# Knee

## Ligamentous Instability

### Anterior drawer test[8,10]

The patient is positioned in supine with the knee flexed to 90 degrees and the hip flexed to 45 degrees. The therapist stabilizes the lower leg by sitting on the forefoot. The therapist grasps the patient's proximal tibia with two hands, places their thumbs on the tibial plateau, and administers an anterior directed force to the tibia on the femur. A positive test is indicated by excessive anterior translation of the tibia on the femur with a diminished or absent end-point and may be indicative of an anterior cruciate ligament injury (Fig. 4-59).

**Fig. 4-59:** A therapist administers the anterior drawer test to a patient positioned in supine with the hip in 45 degrees of flexion and the knee in 90 degrees of flexion.

### Lachman test[10,26]

The patient is positioned in supine with the knee flexed to 20-30 degrees. The therapist stabilizes the distal femur with one hand and places the other hand on the proximal tibia. The therapist applies an anterior directed force to the tibia on the femur. A positive test is indicated by excessive anterior translation of the tibia on the femur with a diminished or absent end-point and may be indicative of an anterior cruciate ligament injury (Fig. 4-60).

### Lateral pivot shift test[8,10]

The patient is positioned in supine with the hip flexed and abducted to 30 degrees with slight medial rotation. The therapist grasps the leg with one hand and places the other hand over the lateral surface of the proximal tibia. The therapist medially rotates the tibia and applies a valgus force to the knee while the knee is slowly flexed. A positive test is indicated by a palpable shift or clunk occurring between 20 and 40 degrees of flexion and is indicative of anterolateral rotatory instability. The shift or clunk results from the reduction of the tibia on the femur.

**Fig. 4-60:** A therapist administers the Lachman test by applying an anterior directed force to the tibia on the femur while stabilizing the distal femur.

### Posterior drawer test[8,10]

The patient is positioned in supine with the knee flexed to 90 degrees and the hip flexed to 45 degrees. The therapist stabilizes the lower leg by sitting on the forefoot. The therapist grasps the patient's proximal tibia with two hands, places their thumbs on the tibial plateau, and administers a posterior directed force to the tibia on the femur. A positive test is indicated by excessive posterior translation of the tibia on the femur with a diminished or absent end-point and may be indicative of a posterior cruciate ligament injury.

### Posterior sag sign[8,10]

The patient is positioned in supine with the knee flexed to 90 degrees and the hip flexed to 45 degrees. A positive test is indicated by the tibia sagging back on the femur and may be indicative of a posterior cruciate ligament injury.

### Slocum test[10,13]

The patient is positioned in supine with the knee flexed to 90 degrees and the hip flexed to 45 degrees. The therapist rotates the patient's foot 30 degrees medially to test anterolateral instability. The therapist stabilizes the lower leg by sitting on the forefoot. The therapist grasps the patient's proximal tibia with two hands, places their thumbs on the tibial plateau, and administers an anterior directed force to the tibia on the femur. A positive test is indicated by movement of the tibia occurring primarily on the lateral side and may be indicative of anterolateral instability. The test can also be performed to assess anteromedial instability by rotating the patient's foot 15 degrees laterally.

### Valgus stress test[10,13]

The patient is positioned in supine with the knee flexed to 20-30 degrees. The therapist positions one hand on the medial surface of the patient's ankle and the other hand on the lateral surface of the knee. The therapist applies a valgus force to the knee with the distal hand. A positive test is indicated by excessive valgus movement and may be indicative of a medial collateral ligament sprain. A positive test with the knee in full extension may be indicative of damage to the medial collateral ligament, posterior cruciate ligament, posterior oblique ligament, and posteromedial capsule.

### Varus stress test[10,13]

The patient is positioned in supine with the knee flexed to 20-30 degrees. The therapist positions one hand on the lateral surface of the patient's ankle and the other hand on the medial surface of the knee. The therapist applies a varus force to the knee with the distal hand. A positive test is indicated by excessive varus movement and may be indicative of a lateral collateral ligament sprain. A positive test with the knee in full extension may be indicative of damage to the lateral collateral ligament, posterior cruciate ligament, arcuate complex, and posterolateral capsule.

## Meniscal Pathology

### Apley's compression test[10,18]

The patient is positioned in prone with the knee flexed to 90 degrees. The therapist stabilizes the patient's femur using one hand and places the other hand on the patient's heel. The therapist medially and laterally rotates the tibia while applying a compressive force through the tibia. A positive test is indicated by pain or clicking and may be indicative of a meniscal lesion.

### Bounce home test[8,10]

The patient is positioned in supine. The therapist grasps the patient's heel and maximally flexes the knee. The patient's knee is extended passively. A positive test is indicated by incomplete extension or a rubbery end-feel and may be indicative of a meniscal lesion.

### McMurray test[8,10]

The patient is positioned in supine. The therapist grasps the distal leg with one hand and palpates the knee joint line with the other. With the knee fully flexed, the therapist medially rotates the tibia and extends the knee. The therapist repeats the same procedure while laterally rotating the tibia. A positive test is indicated by a click or pronounced crepitation felt over the joint line and may be indicative of a posterior meniscal lesion.

## Swelling

### Brush test[10,22]

The patient is positioned in supine. The therapist places one hand below the joint line on the medial surface of the patella and strokes proximally with the palm and fingers as far as the suprapatellar pouch. The other hand then strokes down the lateral surface of the patella. A positive test is indicated by a wave of fluid just below the medial distal border of the patella and is indicative of effusion in the knee.

### Patellar tap test[10,22]

The patient is positioned in supine with the knee flexed or extended to a point of discomfort. The therapist applies a slight tap over the patella. A positive test is indicated if the patella appears to be floating and may be indicative of joint effusion.

## Miscellaneous

### Clarke's sign[8,10]

The patient is positioned in supine with the knees extended. The therapist applies slight pressure distally with the web space of their hand over the superior pole of the patella. The therapist then asks the patient to contract the quadriceps muscle while maintaining pressure on the patella. A positive test is indicated by failure to complete the contraction without pain and may be indicative of patellofemoral dysfunction.

### Hughston's plica test[10,22]

The patient is positioned in supine. The therapist flexes the knee and medially rotates the tibia with one hand while the other hand attempts to move the patella medially and palpate the medial femoral condyle. A positive test is indicated by a popping sound over the medial plica while the knee is passively flexed and extended.

### Noble compression test[8,10]

The patient is positioned in supine with the hip slightly flexed and the knee in 90 degrees of flexion. The therapist places the thumb of one hand over the lateral epicondyle of the femur and the other hand around the patient's ankle. The therapist maintains pressure over the lateral epicondyle while the patient is asked to slowly extend the knee. A positive test is indicated by pain over the lateral femoral epicondyle at approximately 30 degrees of knee flexion and may be indicative of iliotibial band friction syndrome.

### Patellar apprehension test[8,10]

The patient is positioned in supine with the knees extended. The therapist places both thumbs on the medial border of the patella and applies a laterally directed force. A positive test is indicated by a look of apprehension or an attempt to contract the quadriceps, in an effort to avoid subluxation and may be indicative of patella subluxation or dislocation.

## Ankle

## Ligamentous Instability

### Anterior drawer test[8,10]

The patient is positioned in supine. The therapist stabilizes the distal tibia and fibula with one hand, while the other hand holds the foot in 20 degrees of plantar flexion and draws the talus forward in the ankle mortise. A positive test is indicated by excessive anterior translation of the talus away from the ankle mortise and may be indicative of an anterior talofibular ligament sprain.

### Talar tilt[10,22]

The patient is positioned in sidelying with the knee flexed to 90 degrees. The therapist stabilizes the distal tibia with one hand while grasping the talus with the other hand. The foot is maintained in a neutral position. The therapist tilts the talus into abduction and adduction. A positive test is indicated by excessive adduction and may be indicative of a calcaneofibular ligament sprain.

## Miscellaneous

### Thompson test[8,10]

The patient is positioned in prone with the feet extended over the edge of a table. The therapist asks the patient to relax and proceeds to squeeze the muscle belly of the gastrocnemius and soleus muscles. A positive test is indicated by the absence of plantar flexion and may be indicative of a ruptured Achilles tendon (Fig. 4-61).

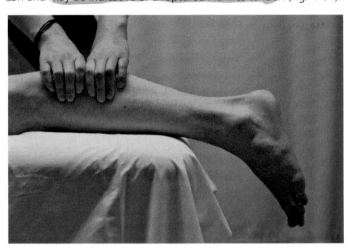

**Fig. 4-61·** A therapist administers the Thompson test by squeezing the muscle belly of the gastrocnemius and soleus muscles.

### Tibial torsion test[10]

The patient is positioned in sitting with the knees over the edge of a table. The therapist places the thumb and index finger of one hand over the medial and lateral malleolus. The therapist then measures the acute angle formed by the axes of the knee and ankle. Normal lateral rotation of the tibia is considered to be 12-18 degrees in an adult.

### True leg length discrepancy test[10]

The patient is positioned in supine with the hips and knees extended, the legs 15 to 20 cm apart, and the pelvis in balance with the legs. Using a tape measure, the therapist measures from the distal point of the anterior superior iliac spines to the distal point of the medial malleoli. A positive test is indicated by a bilateral variation of greater than one centimeter and may be indicative of a true leg length discrepancy.

## Spine

## Cervical Region

### Foraminal compression test[10,22]

The patient is positioned in sitting with the head laterally flexed. The therapist places both hands on top of the subject's head and exerts a downward force. A positive test is indicated by pain radiating into the arm toward the flexed side and may be indicative of nerve root compression.

### Vertebral artery test[10,22]

The patient is positioned in supine. The therapist places the patient's head into extension, lateral flexion, and rotation to the ipsilateral side. A positive test is indicated by dizziness, nystagmus, slurred speech or loss of consciousness and may be indicative of compression of the vertebral artery.

## Lumbar/Sacroiliac Region

### Sacroiliac joint stress test[10]

The patient is positioned in supine. The therapist crosses their arms, placing the palms of the hands on the patient's anterior superior iliac spines. The therapist applies a downward and lateral force to the pelvis. A positive test is indicated by unilateral pain in the sacroiliac joint or gluteal area and may be indicative of sacroiliac joint dysfunction.

### Sitting flexion test[10,22]

The patient is positioned in sitting with the knees flexed to 90 degrees and the feet on the floor. The patient's hips should be abducted to allow the patient to bend forward. The therapist places his/her thumbs on the inferior margin of the posterior superior iliac spines and monitors the movement of the bony structures as the patient bends forward and reaches toward the floor. A positive test is indicated by one posterior superior iliac spine moving farther in a cranial direction and may be indicative of an articular restriction.

### Standing flexion test[10,22]

The patient is positioned in standing with the feet 12 inches apart. The therapist places his/her thumbs on the inferior margin of the posterior superior iliac spines and monitors the movement of the bony structures as the patient bends forward with the knees extended. A positive test is indicated by one posterior superior iliac spine moving farther in a cranial direction and may be indicative of an articular restriction.

# Osteokinematic and Arthrokinematic Motions

## Upper Extremity Joints - Osteokinematic and Arthrokinematic Motion[10,14]

| Joint | Resting Position | Convex/Concave | Osteokinematic/Arthrokinematic Motion |
|---|---|---|---|
| Sternoclavicular | Anatomical position | *Elevation/depression* Convex: clavicle Concave: sternum *Protraction/retraction* Convex: sternum Concave: clavicle | Opposite direction Same direction |
| Acromioclavicular | Anatomical position | Convex: clavicle Concave: acromion | Opposite direction |
| Glenohumeral | 55 degrees abduction, 30 degrees horizontal adduction | Convex: humerus Concave: glenoid | Opposite direction |
| Ulnohumeral | 70 degrees flexion, 10 degrees supination | Convex: humerus Concave: ulna | Same direction |
| Radiohumeral | Full extension, full supination | Convex: humerus Concave: radius | Same direction |
| Proximal radioulnar | 70 degrees flexion, 35 degrees supination | Convex: radius Concave: ulna | Opposite direction |

## Upper Extremity Joints - Osteokinematic and Arthrokinematic Motion (continued)

| Joint | Resting Position | Convex/Concave | Osteokinematic/Arthrokinematic Motion |
|---|---|---|---|
| Distal radioulnar | 10 degrees supination | Convex: ulna<br>Concave: radius | Same direction |
| Radiocarpal | Neutral with slight ulnar deviation | Convex: carpals<br>Concave: radius | Opposite direction |
| Metacarpophalangeal joints of digits 2-5 | Slight flexion | Convex: metacarpals<br>Concave: phalanges | Same direction |
| Proximal and distal interphalangeal joints of digits 2-5 | Slight flexion | Convex: proximal phalanges<br>Concave: distal phalanges | Same direction |

## Lower Extremity Joints - Osteokinematic and Arthrokinematic Motion[10,14]

| Joint | Resting Position | Convex/Concave | Osteokinematic/Arthrokinematic Motion |
|---|---|---|---|
| Hip | 30 degrees flexion, 30 degrees abduction, slight lateral rotation | Convex: femur<br>Concave: acetabulum | Opposite direction |
| Tibiofemoral | 25 degrees flexion | Convex: femur<br>Concave: tibia | Same direction |
| Patellofemoral | 25 degrees flexion | Convex: patella<br>Concave: femur | Opposite direction |
| Proximal tibiofibular | 0 degrees plantar flexion | Convex: tibia<br>Concave: fibula | Same direction |
| Distal tibiofibular | 0 degrees plantar flexion | Convex: fibula<br>Concave: tibia | Opposite direction |
| Talocrural | 10 degrees plantar flexion, midway between maximum inversion and eversion | Convex: talus<br>Concave: tibia and fibula | Opposite direction |
| Subtalar | Midway between extremes of range of movement | Convex: anterior and middle talus<br>Concave: anterior and middle calcaneus<br>Convex: posterior calcaneus<br>Concave: posterior talus | Same direction<br><br>Opposite direction |
| Intermetatarsal | Midway between extremes of range of movement | Convex: more medial metatarsals<br>Concave: more lateral metatarsals | Same direction |
| Metatarsophalangeal | Neutral | Convex: metatarsals<br>Concave: phalanges | Same direction |
| Interphalangeal joints of the toes | Slight flexion | Convex: proximal phalanges<br>Concave: distal phalanges | Same direction |

# Miscellaneous Joints - Osteokinematic and Arthrokinematic Motion[10,14]

| Joint | Resting Position | Convex/Concave | Osteokinematic/ Arthrokinematic Motion |
|---|---|---|---|
| Temporomandibular | Mouth slightly open (freeway space) | Convex: mandible Concave: temporal bone | Opposite direction |

# Mobilization[14,16]

Mobilization is a passive movement technique designed to improve joint function.

**Indications:** restricted joint mobility, restricted accessory motion, desired neurophysiological effects

**Contraindications:** active disease, infection, advanced osteoporosis, articular hypermobility, fracture, acute inflammation, muscle guarding, joint replacement

## Grades of Movement

| | |
|---|---|
| **Grade I** | Small amplitude movement performed at the beginning of range. |
| **Grade II** | Large amplitude movement performed within the range, but not reaching the limit of the range and not returning to the beginning of range. |
| **Grade III** | Large amplitude movement performed up to the limit of range. |
| **Grade IV** | Small amplitude movement performed at the limit of range. |
| **Grade V** | Small amplitude, high velocity thrust technique performed to snap adhesions at the limit of range. |

## Convex-Concave Rule

Determines the direction of decreased joint gliding and the appropriate direction for the mobilizing force.

**Convex surface moving on a concave surface:**

- Roll and slide occur in the opposite direction

- Mobilizing force should be applied in the opposite direction of the bone movement

**Concave surface moving on a convex surface:**

- Roll and slide occur in the same direction

- Mobilizing force should be applied in the same direction as the bone movement

## Mobilization Technique

- The patient should have a general understanding of the purpose of mobilization.

- The patient should be completely relaxed during treatment.

- The therapist should be in a comfortable position while performing mobilization activities.

- The therapist's position should allow for optimal control of movement. Explain specific mobilization techniques to the patient prior to beginning treatment. Complete a general examination of each patient prior to beginning mobilization activities.

- Use gravity to assist with mobilization whenever possible.

- Mobilization activities are usually performed initially with the joint in a loose packed position.

- Maintain contact with the mobilizing hand as close to the joint space as possible.

- Allow one digit to palpate the joint line when possible.

- Mobilize one joint in one direction at a time.

- Use a mobilization belt or wedge to assist with stabilization when necessary.

- Constantly modify mobilization techniques based on individual patient response.

- Compare the quality and quantity of joint play bilaterally.

- Reassess each patient prior to every treatment session.

**Fig. 4-62:** A therapist administers a posterior glide of the humerus on the glenoid. This type of intervention would be most effective to increase glenohumeral flexion, medial rotation, and horizontal adduction range of motion.

**Fig. 4-63:** A therapist administers an anterior glide of the femur on the acetabulum. This type of intervention would be most effective to increase hip extension and lateral rotation.

**Fig. 4-64:** A therapist administers an inferior glide of the femur on the acetabulum. This type of intervention would be most effective to increase hip abduction.

**Fig. 4-65:** A therapist administers a medial glide of the patella. This type of intervention would be most effective to increase accessory motion of the patellofemoral joint.

# Pathology of the Musculoskeletal System

## Achilles Tendonitis[18,28,29]

Achilles tendonitis is a repetitive overuse disorder resulting in microscopic tears of collagen fibers on the surface or in the substance of the Achilles tendon. The tendon is most often impacted in an avascular zone located two to six centimeters above the insertion of the tendon.

**Etiology** - Repetitive overload of the Achilles tendon often caused by changes in training intensity or faulty technique. Patients with limited flexibility and strength in the gastrocnemius and soleus complex and patients with a pronated or cavus foot are at increased risk. Activities frequently associated with Achilles tendonitis include running, basketball, gymnastics, and dancing. A history of Achilles tendonitis increases the likelihood of an Achilles tendon rupture later in life.

**Signs and Symptoms** - aching or burning in the posterior heel, tenderness of the Achilles tendon, pain with increased activity, swelling and thickening in the tendon area, muscle weakness due to pain, morning stiffness

**Treatment** - Initially RICE (Rest, Ice, Compression, Elevation), nonsteroidal anti-inflammatory medications (NSAIDs), and anal-gesics as needed. A heel lift and cross training may be used to limit the amount of tensile loading through the tendon. Prevention includes heel cord stretching exercises, use of appropriate soft-soled footwear, eccentric strengthening of the gastrocnemius and soleus complex, and avoiding sudden changes in intensity of training programs.

## Adhesive Capsulitis[13,28,29]

Adhesive capsulitis results in a loss of range of motion in active and passive shoulder motion due to soft tissue contracture. The condition is caused by adhesive fibrosis and scarring between the capsule, rotator cuff, subacromial bursa, and deltoid.

**Etiology** - The onset may be related to a direct injury to the shoulder or may begin insidiously. Peak incidence occurs in individuals between 40 and 60 years of age with females being affected more than males. Patients with diabetes have an increased incidence of adhesive capsulitis. The condition is self-limiting and typically resolves in one to two years, although some individuals have residual loss of motion.

**Signs and Symptoms** - insidious onset of localized pain often extending down the arm, subjective reports of stiffness, night pain, restricted range of motion in a capsular pattern

**Treatment** - The focus of treatment is on increasing range of motion with glenohumeral mobilization, range of motion exercises, and palliative modalities. The therapist and patient should avoid overstretching and elevating pain since this can result in further loss of motion. Surgical options include suprascapular nerve block and closed manipulation under anesthesia.

## Anterior Cruciate Ligament Sprain[8,13,28]

The anterior cruciate ligament (ACL) runs from the anterior intercondylar area of the tibia to the medial aspect of the lateral femoral condyle in the intercondylar notch. The ligament prevents anterior displacement of the tibia in relation to the femur. The extent of the sprain is classified according to the extent of ligament damage. A grade I sprain involves microscopic tears of the ligament, while a grade III sprain indicates a completely torn ligament.

**Etiology** - Noncontact twisting injury associated with hyperextension, varus or valgus stress to the knee. An ACL sprain often involves injury to other knee structures such as the medial capsule, medial collateral ligament, and menisci.

**Signs and Symptoms** - The patient may report a loud pop or feeling the knee "giving way" or "buckling" followed by dizziness, sweating, and swelling. Special tests to identify the presence of an ACL tear include the anterior drawer test, Lachman test, and lateral pivot shift test.

**Treatment** - Initially RICE, NSAIDs, and analgesics as needed. Conservative treatment includes lower extremity strengthening exercises emphasizing the quadriceps and the hamstrings. Surgery is often warranted for a complete ACL tear (grade III). Surgery most often consists of intra-articular reconstruction using the patellar tendon, iliotibial band or hamstrings tendon. A derotation brace may be beneficial for a patient with an ACL deficient knee, however, it has limited benefit for a patient following surgical reconstruction.

## Congenital Hip Dysplasia[27,30]

Congenital hip dysplasia, also known as developmental dysplasia, is a condition characterized by malalignment of the femoral head within the acetabulum. The condition develops during the last trimester in utero.

**Etiology** - cultural predisposition, malposition in utero, environmental and genetic influences

**Signs and Symptoms** - Clinical presentation includes asymmetrical hip abduction with tightness and apparent femoral shortening of the involved side. Testing for this condition may include the Ortolani's test, Barlow's test, and diagnostic ultrasound.

**Treatment** - The focus of treatment is dependent on age, severity, and initial attempts to reposition the femoral head within the acetabulum through the constant use of a harness, bracing, splinting or traction. Open reduction with subsequent application of a hip spica cast may be required if conservative treatment fails. Physical therapy may be indicated after cast removal for stretching, strengthening, and caregiver education.

## Congenital Limb Deficiencies[27-30]

A congenital limb deficiency is a malformation that occurs in utero, secondary to an altered developmental course. Congenital limb deficiencies are classified as longitudinal or transverse. A longitudinal limb deficiency refers to a reduction or absence of an element or elements within the long axis of the bone. A transverse limb deficiency refers to a limb that has developed to a particular level beyond which no skeletal elements exist.

**Etiology** - The majority of congenital limb deficiencies are idiopathic or are genetic in origin. Other possible etiologies include poor blood supply, constricting amniotic bands, infection, and maternal drug exposure.

**Signs and Symptoms** - structural or acquired abnormality of a limb, phantom limb pain

**Treatment** - The focus of treatment is on symmetrical movements, strengthening, range of motion, weight bearing activities, and prosthetic training when appropriate.

## Congenital Torticollis[30-31]

Congenital torticollis, also known as wry neck, is characterized by a unilateral contracture of the sternocleidomastoid muscle. The condition is most often identified in the first two months of life.

**Etiology** - The cause is unknown, however, it may be associated with malpositioning in utero (e.g., breech) and birth trauma.

**Signs and Symptoms** - Clinical presentation includes lateral cervical flexion to the same side as the contracture, rotation toward the opposite side, and facial asymmetries.

**Treatment** - Initially, treatment is conservative with emphasis on stretching, active range of motion, positioning, and caregiver education. Surgical management is indicated when conservative options have failed and the child is over one year of age. A surgical release followed by physical therapy may be indicated for range of motion and proper alignment.

## Glenohumeral Instability[8,13,18,28]

Glenohumeral instability refers to excessive translation of the humeral head on the glenoid during active rotation. Instability involves varying degrees of injuries to dynamic and static structures that function to contain the humeral head in the glenoid. Subluxation refers to joint laxity, allowing for more than 50% of the humeral head to passively translate over the glenoid rim without dislocation. Dislocation is the complete separation of the articular surfaces of the glenoid and the humeral head. Approximately 85% of dislocations detach the glenoid labrum (i.e., Bankart lesion).

**Etiology** - A combination of forces stress the anterior capsule, glenohumeral ligament, and rotator cuff, causing the humerus to move anteriorly out of the glenoid fossa. An anterior dislocation is the most common and is usually associated with shoulder abduction and lateral rotation.

**Signs and Symptoms** - Subluxation: feeling the shoulder "popping" out and back into place, pain, paresthesias, sensation of the arm feeling "dead," positive apprehension test, capsular tenderness, swelling; Dislocation: severe pain, paresthesias, limited range of motion, weakness, visible shoulder fullness, arm supported by contralateral limb.

**Treatment** - Initial immobilization with a sling for three to six weeks. RICE and NSAIDs are often utilized in the early phase. Following immobilization, range of motion, and isometric strengthening should be initiated followed by progressive resistive exercises emphasizing the internal and external rotators, as well as the large scapular muscles.

## Impingement Syndrome[8,13,18,28]

Impingement syndrome is one of the most common injuries of the shoulder. It is often caused by repetitive microtrauma from upper extremity activity performed above the horizontal plane. Individuals participating in throwing activities, swimming, and racquet sports are particularly susceptible to impingement syndrome.

**Etiology** - Impingement syndrome is caused by the humeral head and the associated rotator cuff attachments migrating proximally and becoming impinged on the undersurface of the acromion and the coracoacromial ligament.

**Signs and Symptoms** - discomfort or mild pain deep within the shoulder, pain with overhead activities, painful arc of motion (i.e., 70-120 degrees abduction), positive impingement sign, tenderness over the greater tuberosity and the bicipital groove

**Treatment** - Initially RICE, NSAIDs, and activity modification. Once tolerated, treatment includes rotator cuff strengthening and scapular stability exercises. Long-term prevention includes continued strengthening of the rotator cuff and scapula stabilizers, along with improved biomechanics related to sport-specific or relevant work activities.

## Juvenile Rheumatoid Arthritis[30,31]

Juvenile rheumatoid arthritis (JRA) is the most common chronic rheumatic disease in children and presents with inflammation of the joints and connective tissues. Classification of JRA includes systemic, polyarticular, and oligoarticular.

**Etiology** - The exact etiology is unknown, however, it is theorized that an external source such as a virus, infection or trauma may trigger an autoimmune response producing JRA in a child with a genetic predisposition.

**Signs and Symptoms** - The clinical presentation is based on the classification of JRA. Systemic JRA occurs in 10-20% of cases and presents with acute onset, high fevers, rash, enlargement of the spleen and liver, and inflammation of the lungs and heart. Polyarticular JRA accounts for 30-40% of cases and presents with high female incidence, significant rheumatoid factor, and arthritis in more than four joints with symmetrical joint involvement. Oligoarticular (pauciarticular) JRA accounts for 40-60% of cases and affects less than five joints with asymmetrical joint involvement.

**Treatment** - Pharmacological management to relieve inflammation and pain through NSAIDs, corticosteroids, antirheumatics, and immunosuppressive agents. Physical therapy management includes passive and active range of motion, positioning, splinting, strengthening, endurance training, weight bearing activities, postural training, and functional mobility. Pain management includes the use of modalities such as paraffin, ultrasound, warm water, and cryotherapy. Surgical intervention may be indicated secondary to pain, contractures or irreversible joint destruction.

## Lateral Epicondylitis[8,28,29]

Lateral epicondylitis refers to an irritation or inflammation of the common extensor muscles at their origin on the lateral epicondyle of the humerus. Individuals who take part in racquet sports or activities requiring throwing are at the greatest risk for developing lateral epicondylitis.

**Etiology** - The condition is caused by eccentric loading of the wrist extensor muscles, usually the extensor carpi radialis brevis, resulting in microtrauma. Lateral epicondylitis can be precipitated by poor mechanics or faulty equipment such as a tennis racquet with a handle that is too small or with strings that possess too much tension. The condition is most common in individuals between 30 and 50 years of age.

**Signs and Symptoms** - Pain is present immediately anterior or distal to the lateral epicondyle of the humerus. Pain typically worsens with repetition and resisted wrist extension.

**Treatment** - Initially RICE, NSAIDs, and activity modification. Physical therapy should attempt to increase strength, flexibility, and endurance of the wrist extensors. A strap placed two to three inches distal to the elbow joint can reduce muscular tension placed on the epicondyle and may diminish or eliminate patient symptoms.

## Legg-Calve-Perthes Disease[30,31]

Legg-Calve-Perthes disease is characterized by degeneration of the femoral head due to a disturbance in the blood supply (i.e., avascular necrosis). The disease is self-limiting and has four distinct stages: condensation, fragmentation, re-ossification, and remodeling.

**Etiology** - trauma, genetic predisposition, synovitis, vascular abnormalities, infection

**Signs and Symptoms** - pain, decreased range of motion, antalgic gait, positive Trendelenburg sign

**Treatment** - Activities are variable based on the clinical presentation, but the primary focus is to relieve pain, maintain the femoral head in the proper position, and improve range of motion. Physical therapy may be required intermittently for stretching, splinting, crutch training, aquatic therapy, traction, and exercise. Orthotic devices and surgical intervention may be indicated depending on classification and severity of the condition.

## Medial Collateral Ligament Sprain[8,13,28]

The medial collateral ligament (MCL) runs from slightly above the medial femoral epicondyle to the medial aspect of the shaft of the tibia. A MCL sprain often involves injury to other knee structures such as the ACL or medial meniscus.

**Etiology** - A contact or noncontact, fixed foot, tibial rotational injury associated with valgus force and external tibia rotation can damage the MCL. This injury is often associated with activities such as football, skiing, and soccer.

**Signs and Symptoms** - Clinical presentation includes knee pain, swelling, antalgic gait, decreased range of motion, and a feeling of instability. A valgus stress test can be used to assess the integrity of the MCL.

**Treatment** - Initially RICE, NSAIDs, and analgesics as needed. Conservative treatment includes decreasing inflammation, protecting the knee joint and ligament, range of motion, and strengthening exercises as tolerated. Strengthening exercises gradually become more aggressive and functional activities are introduced. Surgery is rarely required since the MCL is well vascularized.

## Meniscus Tear[8,13,18,28]

The medial and lateral menisci are firmly attached to the proximal surface of the tibia. The menisci are thick at the periphery and thinner at their internal unattached edges. The medial meniscus is more commonly injured than the lateral meniscus because it is less mobile due to its attachment to the joint capsule. The incidence of medial meniscal tears increases significantly over time with ACL deficiency. Meniscal injuries are definitively diagnosed by arthroscopy or magnetic resonance imaging.

**Etiology** - Meniscal injuries are usually associated with fixed foot rotation while weight bearing on a flexed knee. This action produces compression and rotational forces on the meniscus.

**Signs and Symptoms** - The clinical presentation includes joint line pain, swelling, catching or a locking sensation. Special tests to identify the presence of a meniscus tear include Apley's compression test, bounce home test, and McMurray test.

**Treatment** - Initially RICE, NSAIDs, and analgesics as needed. Conservative treatment consists of palliative modalities and strengthening exercises. Surgery ranging from a partial meniscectomy to a meniscal repair is often warranted for active individuals. Meniscal repairs are typically performed on tears located on the outer edges of the meniscus due to the increased vascularity. Recent advances in technology have increased the incidence of meniscal transplantation.

## Osgood-Schlatter Disease[8,13,29]

Osgood-Schlatter disease, also known as traction apophysitis, is a self-limiting condition that results from repetitive traction on the tibial tuberosity apophysis.

**Etiology** - The condition is caused by repetitive tension to the patellar tendon over the tibial tuberosity in young athletes. This can result in a small avulsion of the tuberosity and subsequent swelling.

**Signs and Symptoms** - point tenderness over the patella tendon at the insertion on the tibial tubercle, antalgic gait, pain with increasing activity

**Treatment** - Conservative treatment focuses on education, icing, flexibility exercises, and eliminating activities that place strain on the patella tendon such as squatting, running or jumping.

## Osteoarthritis[29,31]

Osteoarthritis is a chronic disease that causes degeneration of articular cartilage, primarily in weight bearing joints. Subsequent deformity and thickening of subchondral bone occurs resulting in impaired functional status. Any joint may be involved, however, the most commonly affected sites include the hands and weight bearing joints such as the hips and knees.

**Etiology** - The cause of osteoarthritis is unknown. The condition typically appears during middle age and affects nearly all individuals to some extent by age 70. Osteoarthritis occurs more commonly in men than women up to age 55, however, it is more common in women later in life. Risk factors include being overweight, fractures or other joint injuries, and occupational or athletic overuse.

**Signs and Symptoms** - Clinical presentation includes gradual onset of pain present at the affected joint, increased pain after exercise, increased pain with weather changes, enlarged joints, crepitus, stiffness, limited joint range of motion, Heberden's nodes, and Bouchard's nodes. Blood tests are not helpful in diagnosing osteoarthritis, although radiographs may show diminished joint space or a bone spur.

**Treatment** - The goal of treatment is to reduce pain, promote joint function, and protect the joint. Pharmacological management may include acetaminophen, NSAIDs, and corticosteroids. Some patients benefit from viscosupplementation which is administered through a series of injections of hyaluronic acid into the knee. The goal is to improve lubrication of the knee, reduce pain, and improve range of motion. Physical therapy interventions include passive and active range of motion, heating and cooling agents, patient education, strengthening exercises, transcutaneous electrical nerve stimulation, energy conservation, weight loss, body mechanics, joint protection techniques, and bracing. Surgical intervention can range from arthroscopic surgery to total joint arthroplasty.

## Osteogenesis Imperfecta[30,31]

Osteogenesis imperfecta is a connective tissue disorder that affects the formation of collagen during bone development. There are four classifications of osteogenesis imperfecta that vary in level of severity.

**Etiology** - The cause of osteogenesis imperfecta is genetic inheritance with types I and IV considered autosomal dominant traits and types II and III considered autosomal recessive traits.

**Signs and Symptoms** - pathological fractures, osteoporosis (i.e., brittle bones), hypermobile joints, bowing of the long bones, weakness, scoliosis, impaired respiratory function

**Treatment** - Management begins at birth with caregiver education on proper handling and facilitation of movement. Physical therapy will focus on active range of motion emphasizing symmetrical movements, positioning, functional mobility, fracture management, and the use of orthotics. In severe cases where ambulation is not realistic, wheelchair prescription and training is indicated.

## Patellofemoral Syndrome[8,13,28,29]

Patellofemoral syndrome is a general term describing pain or discomfort in the anterior knee. The condition is often termed chondromalacia patella, which refers to softening of the articular cartilage of the patella.

**Etiology** - Patellofemoral syndrome is a repetitive overuse disorder resulting from increased force at the patellofemoral joint. Factors associated with increased patellofemoral forces include decreased quadriceps strength, decreased lower extremity flexibility, patellar instability, increased tibial torsion or femoral anteversion. Patients at increased risk for developing patello-femoral syndrome include females, individuals experiencing a growth spurt, runners who have recently increased mileage, and overweight individuals.

**Signs and Symptoms** - anterior knee pain, pain with prolonged sitting, swelling, crepitus, pain when ascending and descending stairs

**Treatment** - The focus of treatment is dependent on the contributing factors associated with the abnormal patellar tracking. Possible treatment options include palliative modalities to decrease inflammation and pain, lower extremity flexibility exercises, medial patella glides, biofeedback, and patella taping. Lower extremity strengthening should emphasize the quadriceps and in particular, the vastus medialis oblique, while minimizing patellofemoral compressive forces.

## Plantar Fasciitis[13,28,29]

Plantar fasciitis refers to inflammation of the plantar fascia at the proximal insertion on the medial tubercle of the calcaneus. The plantar fascia is a broad structure comprised of connective tissue which spans from the calcaneus to the metatarsal heads. The structure is designed to provide support to the arch of the foot. Excessive tension over time creates chronic inflammation and microtears at the proximal insertion of the plantar fascia.

**Etiology** - Plantar fasciitis is often associated with an acute injury from excessive loading of the foot or chronic irritation from an excessive amount of pronation or prolonged duration of pronation. The condition is most common in patients between 40 and 60 years of age.

**Signs and Symptoms** - Clinical presentation includes tenderness at the insertion of the plantar fascia, presence of a heel spur, pain that is worse in the morning or after periods of prolonged inactivity, difficulty with prolonged standing, and pain when walking in bare feet.

**Treatment** - Initially RICE, NSAIDs, and analgesics as needed. A heel cup, massage using a tennis ball or rolling pin, medial longitudinal arch taping, and joint mobilization may be helpful. Prevention includes heel cord stretching exercises, use of appropriate soft-soled footwear, and avoiding sudden changes in the intensity of training programs. Orthotics may be used to minimize hyperpronation.

## Posterior Cruciate Ligament Sprain[8,13,28]

The posterior cruciate ligament (PCL) runs from the posterior intercondylar area of the tibia to the lateral aspect of the medial femoral condyle in the intercondylar notch. The ligament prevents posterior displacement of the tibia in relation to the femur.

**Etiology** - The most common causes of a PCL injury are landing on the tibia with a flexed knee or hitting a dashboard in a motor vehicle accident with a flexed knee. Isolated PCL tears are not common and often involve other knee structures such as the ACL, MCL, LCL, and menisci.

**Signs and Symptoms** - The patient may report feeling as if the femur is sliding off the tibia. Swelling and mild pain may be present, but often the patient is asymptomatic. Special tests to identify the presence of a PCL tear include the posterior drawer test and posterior sag sign.

**Treatment** - Initially RICE, NSAIDs, and analgesics as needed. Physical therapy treatment includes lower extremity strengthening exercises and functional progression. Surgical treatment can occur, however, the procedure is not as evolved as the procedure for the ACL. If surgery is performed, isolated hamstrings exercises are often avoided for a minimum of six weeks.

## Rheumatoid Arthritis[31,34,35]

Rheumatoid arthritis is a systemic autoimmune disorder of unknown etiology. The disease presents with a chronic inflammatory reaction in the synovial tissues of a joint that results in erosion of cartilage and supporting structures within the capsule. Onset of rheumatoid arthritis may initially occur at any joint, but it is common in the small joints of the hand, foot, wrist, and ankle. This disease has periods of exacerbation and remission. Rheumatoid arthritis is diagnosed based on the clinical presentation of involved joints, the presence of blood rheumatoid factor, and radiographic changes.

**Etiology** - The cause of rheumatoid arthritis is unknown. One to two percent of the American population is affected. Women are affected three times more than men and the most common age of onset falls between 40 and 60 years of age.

**Signs and Symptoms** - onset may be gradual or immediate, symmetrical involvement, pain and tenderness of affected joints, morning stiffness, warm joints, decrease in appetite, malaise, increased fatigue, swan neck deformity (i.e., DIP flexion, PIP hyperextension), boutonniere deformity (i.e., DIP extension, PIP flexion), low grade fever

**Treatment** - The goal of treatment is to reduce inflammation and pain, promote joint function, and prevent joint destruction and deformity. Pharmacological management includes NSAIDs to reduce inflammation and pain. Corticosteroid medications may be desirable during severe flare-ups or when the patient's condition is not responding to NSAIDs. Disease-modifying antirheumatic medications are slow-acting and take weeks or months to become effective, however, they have the ability to slow the progression of joint destruction and deformity. Physical therapy interventions include passive and active range of motion, heating and cooling agents, splinting, patient education, energy conservation, body mechanics, and joint protection techniques.

## Rotator Cuff Tear[16,29,32,33]

The rotator cuff can be torn due to an acute traumatic incident or as a result of a chronic degenerative pathology. Patients 50 years of age and older are particularly susceptible to tears due to chronic degenerative pathology. Rotator cuff tears are classified as partial-thickness or full-thickness. A partial-thickness tear extends through only a portion of the tendon. A full-thickness tear is a complete tear of the tendon. The size of a tear can range from small (1 centimeter or less) to large (more than 5 centimeters).

**Etiology** - Intrinsic factors associated with rotator cuff tears include impaired blood supply to the tendon, resulting in degeneration. Extrinsic factors include trauma, repetitive microtrauma, and postural abnormalities.

**Signs and Symptoms** - arm positioned in internal rotation and adduction, point tenderness at the greater tubercle and acromion, marked limitation in shoulder flexion and abduction with upper trapezius recruitment evident, increased tone in anterior shoulder structures

**Treatment** - Conservative management includes RICE, NSAIDs, and analgesics as needed. The primary focus of therapy is to prevent adhesive capsulitis and strengthen upper extremity musculature. Surgical management to repair the tendon can be arthroscopic, mini-open with arthroscopic assist or a traditional open approach. Following surgery, the patient will be immobilized in a sling. The amount of immobilization time will vary depending on surgeon preference, surgical procedure, and the size of the tear. A large tear may require four to six weeks of immobilization. Physical therapy begins with passive range of motion and gradually moves to active-assistive motion. Active motion and isometric exercises begin once approved by the surgeon. The patient will gradually become functional with activities of daily living and progress to more aggressive strengthening activities. Return to functional activities requiring dynamic overhead motion occurs in 9-12 months.

## Scoliosis[13,28,29]

Scoliosis refers to a lateral curvature of the spine. The condition is most often quantified using the Cobb method with a standing radiograph. Scoliosis is often classified as functional, neuromuscular or degenerative. Functional scoliosis results from abnormalities in the body that indirectly impact the spine (e.g., leg length discrepancy, muscle imbalance, poor posture). This type of scoliosis is often referred to as nonstructural scoliosis since the curves are flexible and can be corrected with lateral bending. Neuromuscular scoliosis results from developmental pathology resulting in alterations within the structure of the spine. This type of scoliosis is often observed in patients with cerebral palsy or Marfan syndrome. Degenerative scoliosis occurs due to the normal aging process and is facilitated by changes such as osteophyte formation, bone demineralization, and disk herniation. Neuromuscular and degenerative scoliosis are considered to be forms of structural scoliosis since the curves are inflexible and do not reduce with lateral bending.

**Etiology** - The development of scoliosis is typically idiopathic. Idiopathic scoliosis is most commonly diagnosed between 10 and 13 years of age. Girls and boys have a similar risk of developing a mild curve (e.g., 10 degrees or less), however, girls have a significantly greater risk of acquiring a curve greater than 30 degrees.

**Signs and Symptoms** - Shoulder level asymmetry with or without the presence of a rib hump. Pain is not typically associated with the spinal curvature, rather it is a result of the abnormal forces placed on other tissues of the body due to the curvature.

**Treatment** - The focus of treatment is determined based on the magnitude of the curve and the degree of progression. If the curve is not progressing, generally no formal action is taken. Physical therapy treatment includes muscle strengthening and flexibility exercises, shoe lifts, and bracing. A spinal orthosis is often warranted with a curve that ranges between 25 and 40 degrees. Surgical intervention may be required with curves greater than 40 degrees.

## Talipes Equinovarus[30,31]

Talipes equinovarus, also known as "clubfoot," is a deformity characterized by the heel pointing downward and the forefoot turning inward.

**Etiology** - The cause is unknown, however, theories postulate familial tendency, positioning in utero or a defect in the ovum. This condition accompanies other neuromuscular abnormalities including spina bifida and arthrogryposis, and may result from the lack of movement in utero.

**Signs and Symptoms** - The clinical presentation includes adduction of the forefoot, varus positioning of the hindfoot, and equinus at the ankle.

**Treatment** - Medical management begins shortly after birth and includes splinting and serial casting. The goal of intervention is to restore proper positioning of the foot and ankle. Failed management or severe involvement may require surgical intervention and subsequent casting.

## Total Hip Arthroplasty[16,18,29,32,36]

Total hip arthroplasty refers to the removal of the proximal and distal joint surfaces of the hip with subsequent replacement by an acetabular component and a femoral implant. The acetabular component is most often press fit into place, although it is occasionally held in place by screws. Bone is removed from the femur with subsequent shaping to accept the femoral stem with the attached prosthetic femoral head. The surgical procedure can utilize an anterolateral, direct lateral or posterolateral approach. The type of approach selected determines the necessary hip precautions post-operatively.

Fixation can be cemented or cementless. Cemented fixation allows weight bearing as tolerated on the involved lower extremity, often immediately, since the cement achieves maximum fixation in approximately 15 minutes. Cementless and hybrid fixation rely on bone growth and may dictate partial weight bearing or non-weight bearing initially. The level of weight bearing is determined by the surgeon, typically based on the mechanical fixation of the prosthesis within the acetabulum and femur. There are advantages and disadvantages of each type of fixation, however, the primary indication for cementless fixation is a young, active individual (e.g., less than 65 years of age). Minimally invasive surgical techniques require one or two incisions, usually less than 10 centimeters in length. The benefit of minimally invasive procedures is less soft tissue trauma and an accelerated post-operative recovery. The average lifespan for a total hip arthroplasty is 15 to 20 years, and as a result, younger individuals may need one or more revision procedures in their lifetime. Complications for total hip arthroplasty include deep vein thrombosis, infection, pulmonary embolus, heterotopic ossification, femoral fractures, dislocation, and neurovascular injury.

**Etiology** - Total hip arthroplasty is an elective surgical procedure. Medical conditions often associated with the need for total hip arthroplasty include osteoarthritis, rheumatoid arthritis, osteomyelitis, and avascular necrosis.

**Signs and Symptoms** - Prior to surgery, there is severe pain with weight bearing, loss of mobility, gross instability or limitation in range of motion, failure of non-operative management or a previous surgical procedure.

**Treatment** - Initially physical therapy management focuses on decreasing inflammation and allowing tissues to heal, emphasizing adherence to hip precautions, minimizing muscle atrophy, and regaining full passive range of motion. Treatment may include ankle pumps, quadriceps and gluteal sets, active hip flexion within available range of motion, assistive device training, and progressive ambulation. As the patient progresses, treatment moves toward regaining full strength and endurance and attaining independence in the home setting.

## Total Knee Arthroplasty[16,18,29,32,33,36]

Total knee arthroplasty refers to the removal of the proximal and distal joint surfaces of the knee and replacing them with an implant. The procedure is the most commonly performed surgery for advanced arthritis of the knee. Total knee arthroplasty can be classified several different ways. The first classification is based on the number of compartments replaced. Unicompartmental indicates that only the medial or lateral joint surface was replaced. Bicompartmental indicates that the entire surface of the femur and tibia were replaced, while a tricompartmental procedure includes replacement of the femur and tibia along with the patella. The implant design can be classified by the degree of constraint. An unconstrained design offers no inherent stability and relies on soft tissue integrity for stability. This type of design is used primarily with unicompartmental arthroplasty. A semiconstrained design offers some degree of stability without compromising mobility. This is the most common classification of total knee arthroplasty. A fully constrained design offers the most stability by restricting one or more planes of motion. This results in greater implant stress with a higher likelihood of implant problems (e.g., wear, failure, loosening). The average lifespan for a total knee arthroplasty is 15-20 years, and as a result, younger individuals may need one or more revision procedures in their lifetime.

Minimally invasive surgical techniques are becoming more common with total knee arthroplasty. The procedure requires only a 3-5 inch incision instead of the 8-12 inches typically required with a traditional procedure. As a result, there is less soft tissue trauma and minimal damage to the quadriceps muscle, which allows the muscle to initially produce a stronger contraction. This is extremely relevant since quadriceps weakness is correlated with an increased risk of falling. There remains a paucity of research available to determine long-term outcomes associated with the minimally invasive surgical procedure, however, preliminary data suggests positive outcomes including decreased hospital stays, improved range of motion, and improved strength.

Fixation methods include cemented, uncemented (i.e., bone ingrowth), and hybrid. The type of fixation selected is influenced by a variety of factors including patient activity level, comorbidities, life expectancy, and tightness of fit of the femoral component achieved during surgery. Cemented remains the most common method of fixation. Potential complications of total knee arthroplasty include deep vein thrombosis, infection, pulmonary embolus, peroneal nerve palsy, restricted range of motion, periprosthetic fractures, and chronic joint effusion.

**Etiology** - Total knee arthroplasty is an elective surgical procedure. Medical conditions often associated with the need for total knee arthroplasty include osteoarthritis and osteomyelitis.

# Spotlight on Safety
## Total Hip Arthroplasty Precautions[16,18,32,36]

The specific surgical approach utilized for total hip arthroplasty is determined based on a variety of factors including patient activity level, co-morbidities, life expectancy, anticipated compliance, and surgeon familiarity. Physical therapists must have an awareness of each type of approach including the structures impacted and the associated hip precautions.

### Surgical approaches and associated hip precautions:

**Anterolateral approach** - Access to the hip occurs through the interval between the tensor fasciae latae and the gluteus medius muscle. Some portion of the hip abductors are released from the greater trochanter and the hip is dislocated anteriorly.

**Hip precautions:** Avoid flexion of the hip beyond 90 degrees, extension of the hip, lateral rotation, and adduction.

**Direct lateral approach** - This approach leaves the posterior portion of the gluteus medius attached to the greater trochanter. It requires longitudinal division of the tensor fasciae latae and vastus lateralis, along with a release of the anterior portion of the gluteus medius. Since the posterior soft tissues and capsule are left intact, the approach minimizes the probability of dislocation and may be ideal for noncompliant patients.

**Hip precautions:** Avoid flexion of the hip beyond 90 degrees, extension of the hip, lateral rotation, and adduction.

**Posterolateral approach** - Access to the hip occurs by splitting the gluteus maximus muscle in line with the muscle fibers. The short external rotators are then released and the hip abductors are retracted anteriorly. This approach maintains the integrity of the gluteus medius and vastus lateralis muscles. The femur is then dislocated posteriorly. Although it is the most commonly used approach for total hip arthroplasty, the procedure results in a high post-surgical dislocation rate.

**Hip precautions:** Avoid flexion of the hip beyond 90 degrees, adduction, and medial rotation.

**Signs and Symptoms** - Prior to surgery there is severe pain with weight bearing, loss of mobility, gross instability or limitation in range of motion, marked deformity of the knee, failure of non-operative management or a previous surgical procedure.

**Treatment** - Initially, physical therapy treatment focuses on decreasing inflammation and allowing tissues to heal, emphasizing adherence to knee precautions, minimizing muscle atrophy, and regaining full passive range of motion. Knee flexion requires a minimum of 90 degrees for activities of daily living and 105 degrees to rise comfortably from sitting. Therapeutic activities include ankle pumps, quadriceps and gluteal sets, active range of motion within available range, use of a continuous passive motion machine, assistive device training, and progressive ambulation. As the patient progresses, treatment moves toward regaining full strength, endurance, and independence in the home setting. Advanced therapeutic activities include wall slides, controlled lunges, stationary cycling, and step ups.

## Consider This

### Discharge Guidelines Following Total Hip Arthroplasty[16,18,32,36]

Patients may need to remain compliant with a strict set of discharge guidelines, typically for up to three months following total hip arthroplasty. Failure to follow the guidelines potentially jeopardizes the integrity of the surgical procedure and creates an unnecessary safety risk. The specific guidelines that are most critical for a patient upon discharge will be heavily influenced by the surgical approach and the type of fixation utilized.

**General guidelines include:**

- Avoid crossing the legs when in a sitting position.

- Sit in firm chairs and avoid sitting in low or soft furniture. Limit forward bending when sitting or standing up.

- Stand with the feet in a neutral position (avoid turning the toes inward).

- Use a pillow or splint between the legs when in bed.

- Avoid pulling blankets up in bed with forward bending.

- Place a nightstand on the same side of the bed as the uninvolved side.

- Use a raised toilet seat or portable commode for toileting activities.

- Use a rubber, non-skid bath mat in the shower.

- Use a long handled brush to avoid leaning forward when bathing.

- Remove all throw rugs and always walk with appropriate footwear.

- When walking, turn to the uninvolved side to avoid pivoting on the involved side.

- Walk for short periods and gradually increase the time period to improve endurance.

- When ascending stairs, step up with the uninvolved leg.

- When descending stairs, step down with the involved leg.

*These guidelines apply to traditional total hip arthroplasty and may not be necessary with minimally invasive procedures.

# Types of Fractures[31]

**Avulsion fracture:** A portion of a bone becomes fragmented at the site of tendon attachment due to a traumatic and sudden stretch of the tendon.

**Closed fracture:** A break in a bone where the skin over the site remains intact.

**Comminuted fracture:** A bone that breaks into fragments at the site of injury.

**Compound fracture:** A break in a bone that protrudes through the skin.

**Greenstick fracture:** A break on one side of a bone that does not damage the periosteum on the opposite side. This type of fracture is often seen in children.

**Nonunion fracture:** A break in a bone that has failed to unite and heal after nine to twelve months.

**Stress fracture:** A break in a bone due to repeated forces to a particular portion of the bone.

**Spiral fracture:** A break in a bone shaped like an "S" due to torsion and twisting.

# Pharmacological Management of the Musculoskeletal System[37,38,39]

## Nonopioid Agents

**Action:** Nonopioid agents provide analgesia and pain relief, produce anti-inflammatory effects, and initiate anti-pyretic (reduces fever) properties. These drugs promote a reduction of prostaglandin formation that decreases the inflammatory process, decreases uterine contractions, lowers fever, and minimizes impulse formation of pain fibers.

**Indications:** mild to moderate pain of various origins, fever, headache, muscle ache, inflammation (except acetaminophen), primary dysmenorrhea, reduction of risk of myocardial infarction (aspirin only)

**Side effects:** nausea, vomiting, vertigo, abdominal pain, gastrointestinal distress or bleeding, ulcer formation, potential for Reye syndrome in children (aspirin only)

**Implications for PT:** Patients are at increased risk for masked pain that would allow for movement beyond limitation or false understanding of their level of mobility. Complaints of stomach pain should be taken seriously with a subsequent referral to a physician

**Examples:** Tylenol (acetaminophen); Nonsteroidal anti-inflammatories (NSAIDs): Aspirin (acetylsalicylic acid), Aleve (naproxen), Advil (ibuprofen), Celebrex (celecoxib)

## Opioid Agents (Narcotics)

**Action:** Opioid agents provide analgesia for acute severe pain management. The medication stimulates opioid receptors within the CNS to prevent pain impulses from reaching their destination. Certain drugs are also used to assist with dependency and withdrawal symptoms.

**Indications:** moderate to severe pain of various origins, induction of conscious sedation prior to a diagnostic procedure, management of opioid dependence, relief of severe and persistent cough (codeine)

**Side effects:** mood swings, sedation, confusion, vertigo, dulled cognitive function, orthostatic hypotension, constipation, incoordination, physical dependence, tolerance

**Implications for PT:** A therapist must monitor the patient for potential side effects, especially signs of respiratory depression. Treatment that is otherwise painful should be scheduled approximately two hours after administration to maximize the analgesic benefit. A patient may not accurately report if a particular technique is painful.

**Examples:** Roxanol (morphine), Demerol (meperidine), Oxy-Contin (oxycodone), Sublimaze (fentanyl), Paveral (codeine)

## Glucocorticoid Agents (Corticosteroids)

**Action:** Glucocorticoids provide hormonal, anti-inflammatory, and metabolic effects including suppression of articular and systemic diseases. These agents reduce inflammation in chronic conditions that can damage healthy tissue through a series of reactions. Vasoconstriction results from stabilizing lysosomal membranes and enhancing the effects of catecholamines.

**Indications:** replacement therapy for endocrine dysfunction, anti-inflammatory and immunosuppressive effects; treatment of rheumatic, respiratory, and various other disorders

**Side effects:** muscle atrophy, gastrointestinal distress, glaucoma, adrenocortical suppression, drug-induced Cushing syndrome, weakening with breakdown of supporting tissues (bone, ligament, tendon, skin), mood changes, hypertension

**Implications for PT:** A therapist must wear a mask when working with patients on glucocorticoid therapy since their immune system is weakened. A therapist must be aware of signs of toxicity including moon face, buffalo hump, and personality changes. Patients are at risk for osteoporosis and muscle wasting. Treatment of an injected joint will require special care due to ligament and tendon laxity or weakening.

**Examples:** Dermacort (hydrocortisone or cortisol), Cordrol (prednisone), Pediapred (prednisolone), Medrol (methylprednisolone), Decadrol (dexamethasone), Nasonex (mometasone)

## Disease-modifying Antirheumatic Agents

**Action:** Disease-modifying antirheumatic drugs (DMARD) slow or halt the progression of rheumatic disease. They are used early during the disease process to slow the progression prior to widespread damage of the affected joints. They act to induce remission by modifying the pathology and inhibiting the immune response responsible for rheumatic disease.

**Indications:** rheumatic disease, preferably during early treatment

**Side effects:** (depending on classification of DMARD) nausea, headache, joint pain and swelling, toxicity, gastrointestinal distress, sore throat, fever, liver dysfunction, hair loss, potential for sepsis, retinal damage

**Implications for PT:** Therapists should recognize that many of the agents have a high incidence of toxicity.

**Examples:** Rheumatrex (methotrexate), Arava (leflunomide), Antimalarial: Aralen (chloroquine), Plaquenil (hydroxychloroquine); Gold compounds: Ridaura (auranofin), Solganal (aurothioglucose); Tumor necrosis factor inhibitors: Humira (adalimumab), Enbrel (etanercept).

# Musculoskeletal System Terminology[2,10,16]

**Bursitis:** A condition caused by acute or chronic inflammation of the bursae. Symptoms may include a limitation in active range of motion secondary to pain and swelling.

**Contusion:** A sudden blow to a part of the body that can result in mild to severe damage to superficial and deep structures. Treatment includes active range of motion, ice, and compression.

**Edema:** An increased volume of fluid in the soft tissue outside of a joint capsule.

**Effusion:** An increased volume of fluid within a joint capsule.

**Genu valgum:** A condition where the knees touch while standing with the feet separated. Genu valgum will increase compression of the lateral tibial condyle and increase stress to the medial structures. Genu valgum is also termed knock-knee.

**Genu varum:** A condition where there is bowing of the legs with added space between the knees while standing with the feet together. Genu varum will increase compression of the medial tibial condyle and increase stress to the lateral structures. Genu varum is also termed bowleg.

**Kyphosis:** An excessive curvature of the spine in a posterior direction, usually identified in the thoracic spine. Common causes include osteoporosis, compression fractures, and poor posture secondary to paralysis.

**Lordosis:** An excessive curvature of the spine in an anterior direction, usually identified in the cervical or lumbar spine. Common causes include weak abdominal muscles, pregnancy, excessive weight in the abdominal area, and hip flexion contractures.

**Q angle:** The degree of angulation present when measuring from the midpatella to the anterior superior iliac spine and to the tibial tubercle. A normal Q angle measured in supine with the knee straight is 13 degrees for a male and 18 degrees for a female. An excessive Q angle can lead to pathology and abnormal tracking.

**Sprain:** An acute injury involving a ligament.

- **Grade I** – mild pain and swelling, little to no tear of the ligament

- **Grade II** – moderate pain and swelling, minimal instability of the joint, minimal to moderate tearing of the ligament, decreased range of motion

- **Grade III** – severe pain and swelling, substantial joint instability, total tear of the ligament, substantial decrease in range of motion

**Strain:** An injury involving the musculotendinous unit that involves a muscle, tendon or their attachments to bone.

- **Grade I** – localized pain, minimal swelling, and tenderness

- **Grade II** – localized pain, moderate swelling, tenderness, and impaired motor function

- **Grade III** – a palpable defect of the muscle, severe pain, and poor motor function

**Tendonitis:** A condition caused by acute or chronic inflammation of a tendon. Symptoms may include gradual onset, tenderness, swelling, and pain.

# Orthotics

An orthotic is an external device that provides support or stabilization, improves function, corrects deformities, and distributes pressure from one area to another. Orthotics are made from a variety of materials including plastic, metal, leather, fabric, elastic or hybrid materials. They can be custom made or over-the-counter and are available in various prefabricated sizes. Orthotics should be lightweight, adjustable, and easy to don and doff.

Functions of orthotics include preventing deformity, maintaining proper alignment, inhibiting tone, assisting weak limbs, protecting against injury, and facilitating motion.

Factors to consider when prescribing an orthotic include static versus dynamic, temporary versus permanent, level of support required, energy efficiency, cosmesis, and cost.

## Lower Extremity[36, 40-42]

### Foot Orthotics

A semirigid or rigid insert worn inside a shoe that corrects foot alignment and improves function. May also be used to relieve pain. Foot orthotics are custom molded and are often designed for a specific level of functioning.

### Ankle-foot Orthosis (AFO)

A metal ankle-foot orthosis consists of two metal uprights connected proximally to a calf band and distally to a mechanical ankle joint and shoe. The ankle joint may have the ability to be locked and not allow any motion, or set to have limited anterior/posterior capability depending on the patient's need. A plastic ankle-foot orthosis is fabricated by a cast mold of the patient's lower extremity. The use of plastic is more cosmetic, lighter, and requires that if a patient presents with edema it does not significantly fluctuate. Proper fit of a plastic ankle-foot orthosis requires that a patient be casted in a subtalar neutral position. A footplate can be incorporated into the ankle-foot orthosis to assist with tone reduction. Solid ankle-foot orthoses control dorsiflexion/plantar flexion and also inversion/eversion with a trim line anterior to the malleoli. They can be fabricated to keep the ankle positioned at 90 degrees or can be fabricated with an articulating ankle joint. This articulation allows the tibia to advance over the foot during the mid to late stance phase of gait. A posterior leaf spring is a plastic AFO with a trim line posterior to the malleoli. Its primary purpose is to assist with dorsiflexion and prevent foot drop. It requires adequate medial/lateral control by the patient. Ankle-foot orthoses can also influence knee control. A floor reaction AFO assists with knee extension during stance through positioning of a calf band and/or positioning at the ankle. Ankle-foot orthoses are commonly prescribed for patients with peripheral neuropathy, nerve lesions or hemiplegia.

### Knee-ankle-foot Orthosis (KAFO)

A knee-ankle-foot orthosis provides support and stability to the knee and ankle. The orthosis can be fabricated using two metal uprights extending from the foot/shoe to the thigh with calf and thigh bands. Plastic knee-ankle-foot orthoses are fabricated by a cast mold of the patient's lower extremity. A plastic thigh shell is connected to a plastic ankle-foot orthosis through metal uprights lateral and medial to the knee joint. Both types allow for a lock mechanism at the knee that provides stability. The ankle is also held in proper alignment.

### Craig-Scott knee-ankle-foot Orthosis

A knee-ankle-foot orthosis designed specifically for persons with paraplegia. This design allows a person to stand with a posterior lean of the trunk.

### Hip-knee-ankle-foot Orthosis (HKAFO)

A hip-knee-ankle-foot orthosis is indicated for patients with hip, foot, knee, and ankle weakness. It consists of bilateral knee-ankle-foot orthoses with an extension to the hip joints and a pelvic band. The orthosis can control rotation at the hip and abduction/adduction. The orthosis is heavy and restricts patients to a swing-to or swing-through gait pattern.

### Reciprocating Gait Orthosis (RGO)

Reciprocating gait orthoses are a derivative of the HKAFO and incorporate a cable system to assist with advancement of the lower extremities during gait. When the patient shifts weight onto a selected lower extremity, the cable system advances the opposite lower extremity. The orthoses are used primarily for patients with paraplegia.

### Parapodiums

A parapodium is a standing frame designed to allow a patient to sit when necessary. It is a prefabricated frame and ambulation is achieved by shifting weight and rocking the base across the floor. It is primarily used by the pediatric population.

---

**Spine[36, 40, 41]**

### Corset

A corset is constructed of fabric and may have metal uprights within the material to provide abdominal compression and support. Corsets are utilized to provide pressure and relieve pain associated with mid and low back pathologies.

### Halo Vest Orthosis

The halo vest is an invasive cervical thoracic orthosis that provides full restriction of all cervical motion. A metal ring with four posts that attach to a vest is placed on a patient and secured by inserting four pins through the ring into the skull. This orthosis is commonly used with cervical spinal cord injuries to prevent further damage or dislocation during the recovery period. A patient will wear a halo vest until the spine becomes stable.

### Milwaukee Orthosis

The Milwaukee orthosis is designed to promote realignment of the spine due to scoliotic curvature. The orthosis is custom made and extends from the pelvis to the upper chest. Corrective padding is applied to the areas of severity of the curve.

### Taylor Brace

The Taylor brace is a thoracolumbosacral orthosis that limits trunk flexion and extension through a three-point control design.

### Thoracolumbosacral Orthosis (TLSO)

A custom molded TLSO is utilized to prevent all trunk motions and is commonly utilized as a means of post-surgical stabilization. The rigid shell is fabricated from plastics in a bivalve style using straps/Velcro to secure the orthosis.

# Amputation and Prosthetics

Amputation is the surgical removal of a body part, partial or full extremity, due to disease, trauma or injury. Lower extremity amputations are significantly more common than upper extremity amputations, with peripheral vascular disease serving as the primary etiology. Amputation is considered the last course of action, but for many patients with various pathologies, it may become the only viable treatment option.

Prosthetics attempt to replace the missing body part to allow a patient improved function and cosmesis. A patient will be evaluated by a team of health care professionals to ensure that they meet specific criteria to be a candidate for a prosthesis. Prosthetic prescription provides the patient with an appropriate prosthesis that best meets their stated needs and goals. Physical and occupational therapy are usually indicated for functional retraining with the prosthesis.

## Types of Upper Extremity Amputations

**Forequarter (scapulothoracic):** surgical removal of the upper extremity including the shoulder girdle

**Shoulder disarticulation:** surgical removal of the upper extremity through the shoulder

**Transhumeral:** surgical removal of the upper extremity proximal to the elbow joint

**Elbow disarticulation:** surgical removal of the lower arm and hand through the elbow joint

**Transradial:** surgical removal of the upper extremity distal to the elbow joint

**Wrist disarticulation:** surgical removal of the hand through the wrist joint

**Partial hand:** surgical removal of a portion of the hand and/or digits at either the transcarpal, transmetacarpal or transphalangeal level

**Digit amputation:** surgical removal of a digit at either the metacarpophalangeal, proximal interphalangeal or distal interphalangeal level

## Types of Lower Extremity Amputations

**Hemicorporectomy:** surgical removal of the pelvis and both lower extremities

**Hemipelvectomy:** surgical removal of one half of the pelvis and the lower extremity

**Hip disarticulation:** surgical removal of the lower extremity from the pelvis

**Transfemoral:** surgical removal of the lower extremity above the knee joint

**Knee disarticulation:** surgical removal of the lower extremity through the knee joint

**Transtibial:** surgical removal of the lower extremity below the knee joint

**Syme's:** surgical removal of the foot at the ankle joint with removal of the malleoli

**Chopart's:** disarticulation at the midtarsal joint

**Transmetatarsal:** surgical removal of the midsection of the metatarsals

### Components of an Upper Extremity Prosthesis

| | Transradial | Transhumeral |
|---|---|---|
| **Socket** | • Standard socket covers two-thirds of forearm <br> • Standard socket may be shortened to allow for increased pronation/supination ability <br> • Supracondylar sockets are self-suspending and require no additional harness apparatus | • Standard socket extends to acromion level <br> • Modified design allows for more stability with rotational movements <br> • Lightweight friction units may be used with passive prosthetic arms |
| **Suspension** | • Triceps cuff <br> • Harness <br> • Cable system | • Harness <br> • Cable system <br> • Suction |
| **Elbow unit** | • Attaches to either triceps cuff or upper arm pad <br> • Flexible or rigid hinge connects socket to proximal component | • Internal or external locking elbow unit |
| **Wrist unit** | • Quick change unit <br> • Wrist flexion unit <br> • Ball and socket <br> • Constant friction | • Same as transradial |
| **Terminal device** | • Voluntary opening or closing <br> • Body-powered, externally powered, myoelectric or hybrid <br> • Hook, mechanical hand, cosmetic glove | • Same as transradial |

## Types of Post-Operative Dressings[40,43,44]

| Rigid (Plaster of Paris) | |
|---|---|
| **Advantages** | **Disadvantages** |
| • Allows early ambulation with pylon<br>• Promotes circulation and healing<br>• Stimulates proprioception<br>• Provides protection<br>• Provides soft tissue support<br>• Limits edema | • Immediate wound inspection is not possible<br>• Does not allow for daily dressing change<br>• Requires professional application |

| Semi-rigid (Una paste, air splint) | |
|---|---|
| **Advantages** | **Disadvantages** |
| • Reduces post-operative edema<br>• Provides soft tissue support<br>• Allows for earlier ambulation<br>• Provides protection<br>• Easily changeable | • Does not protect as well as the rigid dressing<br>• Requires more changing than rigid dressing<br>• May loosen and allow for development of edema |

| Soft (Ace wrap, shrinker) | |
|---|---|
| **Advantages** | **Disadvantages** |
| • Reduces post-operative edema<br>• Provides some protection<br>• Relatively inexpensive<br>• Easily removed for wound inspection<br>• Allows for active joint range of motion | • Tissue healing is interrupted by frequent dressing changes<br>• Joint range of motion may delay the healing of the incision<br>• Increased risk of joint contractures<br>• Less control of residual limb pain<br>• Cannot control the amount of tension in the bandage<br>• Risk of a tourniquet effect |

## Components of a Lower Extremity Prosthesis[40,45]

| | Transfemoral | Transtibial |
|---|---|---|
| **Socket** | • Quadrilateral socket<br>• Ischial containment socket | • Patella tendon bearing socket (PTB)<br>• Supracondylar patella tendon socket (PTS)<br>• Supracondylar – suprapatellar socket (SC-SP) |
| **Suspension** | • Complete suction<br>• Partial suction<br>  – Silesian bandage<br>  – Pelvic belt/band | • Supracondylar cuff<br>• Thigh corset<br>• Supracondylar brim<br>• Rubber sleeve suspension<br>• Waist belt with fork strap |
| **Knee** | • Single axis knee<br>• Polycentric knee<br><br>**Friction mechanisms:**<br>  – Constant friction<br>  – Variable friction<br>  – Sliding friction<br>  – Hydraulic friction<br>  – Pneumatic friction | • Not needed |
| **Shank** | • Exoskeleton – rigid exterior<br>• Endoskeleton – pylon covered with foam | • Same as transfemoral shank |
| **Foot** | • Solid ankle cushion heel (SACH)<br>• Stationary attachment flexible endoskeleton (SAFE)<br>• Single axis foot<br>• Multi-axis foot | • Same as transfemoral foot |

## Considerations for Prosthetic Training[40,43]

### Forequarter (scapulothoracic)
- Loss of all shoulder, elbow, and hand function
- Most common cause is malignancy
- Functional prosthesis use is uncommon
- A lightweight cosmetic prosthetic is typically well-tolerated

### Shoulder disarticulation
- Loss of all shoulder, elbow, and hand function
- Most commonly the result of malignancy or severe electrical injuries
- Functional prosthetic use is possible
- An external prosthetic shoulder joint is typically required

### Transhumeral amputation
- Loss of all elbow and hand function
- Most commonly due to trauma
- Typically 7-10 centimeters proximal to the distal humeral condyles
- Trauma associated fracture, dislocation or peripheral nerve injury may delay prosthetic interventions
- Second most common level of upper extremity amputation

### Elbow disarticulation
- Loss of all elbow and hand function
- Most commonly due to trauma
- Allows for self-suspending socket
- An external prosthetic elbow joint is typically required

### Transradial amputation
- Loss of all hand function
- Must be a minimum of five centimeters proximal to the distal radius
- Typically the result of trauma
- Trauma associated fracture, dislocation or peripheral nerve injury may delay prosthetic interventions
- Functionally preferred over wrist disarticulation or selected partial hand amputations
- Most common level of upper extremity amputation

### Wrist disarticulation
- Loss of all hand function
- Relatively uncommon level of amputation
- Cosmetic and functional prosthetic disadvantages

### Partial hand amputation
- Loss of a portion of digit/hand function
- Limb sparing technique utilized when functional pinch can be preserved
- Toe transfer to replace a thumb may be considered if prosthesis fails

### Digit amputation
- Preserved function is highly variable depending on number of digits involved and level of amputation
- Prostheses are not typically utilized

- A long transradial amputation may be more functional if multiple digits are involved at proximal levels

### Hemipelvectomy and hip disarticulation
- All functions of the hip, knee, ankle, and foot are absent
- Most common cause is malignancy
- Does not allow for activation of the prosthesis through a residual limb
- Prosthetic motion must be initiated through weight bearing

### Transfemoral amputation
- Length of the residual limb with regard to leverage and energy expenditure
- No ability to weight bear through the end of the residual limb
- Susceptible to hip flexion contracture
- Adaptation required for balance, weight of prosthesis, and energy expenditure

### Knee disarticulation
- Loss of all knee, ankle, and foot function
- The residual limb can weight bear through its end
- Susceptible to hip flexion contracture
- Knee axis of the prosthesis is below the natural axis of the knee
- Gait deviations can occur secondary to the malalignment of the knee axis

### Transtibial amputation
- Loss of ankle and foot functions
- Residual limb does not allow for weight bearing at its end
- Weight bearing in the prosthesis should be distributed over the total residual limb
- Patellar tendon should be the area of primary weight bearing
- Adaptations required for balance
- Susceptible to knee flexion contracture

### Syme's amputation
- Loss of all foot functions
- Residual limb can weight bear through its end
- Residual limb is bulbous with a non-cosmetic appearance
- Dog ears must be reduced for proper prosthetic fit
- Adaptation required for the increased weight of the prosthesis
- Adaptation required due to diminished toe off during gait

### Transmetatarsal and Chopart's amputation
- Loss of forefoot leverage
- Loss of balance
- Loss of weight bearing surface
- Loss of proprioception
- Tendency to develop equinus deformity

## Wrapping Guidelines[40,43]

- Elastic wrap should not have any wrinkles
- Diagonal and angular patterns should be used
- Do not wrap in circular patterns
- Provide pressure distally to enhance shaping
- Anchor wrap above the knee for transtibial amputations
- Anchor wrap around pelvis for transfemoral amputations

- Promote full elbow extension for transradial amputations
- Promote full knee extension for transtibial amputations
- Promote full hip extension for transfemoral amputations
- Secure the wrap with tape; do not use clips
- Use 2-4 inch wrap for upper extremity amputations
- Use 3-4 inch wrap for transtibial amputations
- Use 6 inch wrap for transfemoral amputations
- Rewrap frequently to maintain adequate pressure

# Spotlight on Safety

## Complications Following Amputation[40,43]

There are a multitude of potential complications patients may experience following amputation. Therapists should be aware of the potential signs and symptoms associated with these complications and, when warranted, be prepared to take immediate action.

Several of the more common complications following amputation are discussed.

### Contractures
Failure to initiate full range of motion early in the post-operative phase and poor positioning of the residual limb significantly increase the likelihood of a contracture. The joint immediately proximal to the amputation site is the most susceptible. The most likely contractures based on level of amputation are: transmetatarsal and Syme's - equinus deformity; transtibial - knee flexion; transfemoral - hip flexion and abduction.

### Deep Vein Thrombosis
A deep vein thrombosis is a blood clot that forms in a vein with the potential to dislodge as an embolism and travel until it blocks an artery. This is a serious medical condition since the embolus may obstruct a selected artery. Heparin is an anticoagulant commonly used to reduce the risk of deep vein thrombosis following surgery.

### Hypersensitivity
Hypersensitivity of the residual limb can significantly impede or even prevent the appropriate fit and functional use of a prosthesis. Specific desensitization techniques and early fitting of a temporary prosthesis are key components in post-amputation rehabilitation. Weight bearing, massage, tapping, and residual limb wrapping are all commonly utilized interventions that facilitate desensitization.

### Neuroma
A neuroma is a bundle of nerve endings that group together and can produce pain due to scar tissue, pressure from the prosthesis or tension on the residual limb.

### Phantom Limb
Phantom limb refers to a painless sensation where the patient feels that the limb is still present. This is common immediately after amputation and will usually subside with desensitization and prosthetic use, however, it may continue for extended periods of time for some patients.

### Phantom Pain
Phantom pain refers to the patient's perception of some form of painful stimuli as it relates to the residual limb. The pain can be continuous or intermittent, local or general, and short-term or permanent. This type of pain can disable the patient and interfere with successful rehabilitation. Treatment options include TENS, ultrasound, icing, relaxation techniques, desensitization techniques, and prosthetic use.

### Psychological Impact
It is extremely common for patients to experience a variety of negative thoughts and emotions following amputation. This can include denial, grief, anxiety, depression or suicidal feelings. The intensity of the thoughts and emotions may be elevated in patients following emergency amputation since the patient had insufficient time to mentally prepare for the loss.

### Wound Infections
The residual limb can become infected following the surgical procedure. Antibiotics are administered at the time of surgery to reduce the risk of infection.

# Gait Deviations[22,40]

| Prosthetic Causes | Amputee Causes |
|---|---|
| **Lateral Bending** | |
| Prosthesis may be too short<br><br>Improperly shaped lateral wall<br><br>High medial wall<br><br>Prosthesis aligned in abduction | Poor balance<br><br>Abduction contracture<br><br>Improper training<br><br>Short residual limb<br><br>Weak hip abductors on prosthetic side<br><br>Hypersensitive and painful residual limb |
| **Abducted Gait** | |
| Prosthesis may be too long<br><br>High medial wall<br><br>Poorly shaped lateral wall<br><br>Prosthesis positioned in abduction<br><br>Inadequate suspension<br><br>Excessive knee friction | Abduction contracture<br><br>Improper training<br><br>Adductor roll<br><br>Weak hip flexors and adductors<br><br>Pain over lateral residual limb |
| **Circumducted Gait** | |
| Prosthesis may be too long<br><br>Too much friction in the knee<br><br>Socket is too small<br><br>Excessive plantar flexion of prosthetic foot | Abduction contracture<br><br>Improper training<br><br>Weak hip flexors<br><br>Lacks confidence to flex the knee<br><br>Painful anterior distal residual limb<br><br>Inability to initiate prosthetic knee flexion |
| **Excessive Knee Flexion During Stance** | |
| Socket set forward in relation to foot<br><br>Foot set in excessive dorsiflexion<br><br>Stiff heel<br><br>Prosthesis too long | Knee flexion contracture<br><br>Hip flexion contracture<br><br>Pain anteriorly in residual limb<br><br>Decrease in quadriceps strength<br><br>Poor balance |

| Prosthetic Causes | Amputee Causes |
|---|---|
| **Vaulting** | |
| Prosthesis may be too long<br><br>Inadequate socket suspension<br><br>Excessive alignment stability<br><br>Foot in excessive plantar flexion | Residual limb discomfort<br><br>Improper training<br><br>Fear of stubbing toe<br><br>Short residual limb<br><br>Painful hip/residual limb |
| **Rotation of Forefoot at Heel Strike** | |
| Excessive toe-out built in<br>Loose fitting socket<br>Inadequate suspension<br>Rigid SACH heel cushion | Poor muscle control<br>Improper training<br>Weak medial rotators<br>Short residual limb |
| **Forward Trunk Flexion** | |
| Socket too big<br><br>Poor suspension<br><br>Knee instability | Hip flexion contracture<br><br>Weak hip extensors<br><br>Pain with ischial weight bearing<br><br>Inability to initiate prosthetic knee flexion |
| **Medial or Lateral Whip** | |
| Excessive rotation of the knee<br><br>Tight socket fit<br><br>Valgus in the prosthetic knee<br><br>Improper alignment of toe break | Improper training<br><br>Weak hip rotators<br><br>Knee instability |

# Musculoskeletal System Essentials

1. The body's three sources of adenosine triphosphate (ATP) include the ATP-PC (Phosphagen) System, Anaerobic Glycolysis (Lactic Acid) System, and Aerobic (Oxygen) System.

2. The ATP-PC (Phosphagen) System is used for ATP production during high intensity, short duration exercise, such as sprinting 100 meters. The system provides energy for muscle contraction for up to 15 seconds.

3. The anaerobic glycolysis system supplies ATP during high intensity, short duration exercise, such as sprinting 400 or 800 meters. The system provides energy for muscle contraction for 30-40 seconds.

4. The aerobic system supplies ATP during low intensity, long duration activities, such as running a marathon. The amount of ATP production is far greater, but requires a complicated series of chemical reactions.

5. Motion occurs in three cardinal planes of the body (frontal, sagittal, transverse) around three corresponding axes (anterior-posterior, medial-lateral, vertical).

6. Common joint receptors include free nerve endings, Golgi ligament endings, Golgi-Mazzoni corpuscles, Pacinian corpuscles, and Ruffini endings.

7. The upper extremity consists of the shoulder, elbow, and wrist. The shoulder complex is formed by the glenohumeral joint, sternoclavicular joint, acromioclavicular joint, and scapulothoracic articulations. The elbow joint is formed by the radiohumeral joint, ulnohumeral joint, and proximal radioulnar joint. The wrist complex is formed by the radiocarpal and midcarpal joints.

8. The lower extremity consists of the hip, knee, ankle, and foot. The hip joint is a synovial joint formed by the head of the femur and the acetabulum. The knee joint is formed by the tibiofemoral joint and patellofemoral joint. The ankle and foot are formed by the distal tibiofibular joint, talocrural joint, subtalar joint, midtarsal joint, and forefoot.

9. The cervical spine consists of 7 vertebrae. The thoracic spine consists of 12 vertebrae, and the lumbar spine consists of 5 vertebrae.

10. Type I muscle fibers are described as aerobic, red, tonic, slow twitch, and slow-oxidative. Type II muscle fibers are described as anaerobic, white, phasic, fast twitch, and fast-glycolytic.

11. Muscle spindles are distributed throughout the belly of the muscle and function to send information to the nervous system about muscle length and/or the rate of change of its length.

12. Resistive training programs often employ isometric, isotonic, and isokinetic exercise.

13. Golgi tendon organs are encapsulated sensory receptors that are sensitive to tension, especially when produced by active muscle contraction. They function to transmit information about tension or the rate of change of tension within the muscle.

14. Open-chain activities involve the distal segment moving freely in space, while closed-chain activities involve the body moving over a fixed distal segment.

15. An upper and lower quarter screen should, at a minimum, consist of an assessment of posture, range of motion, resistive testing, reflex testing, and dermatome testing.

16. Body composition refers to the relative percentage of body weight that is comprised of fat and fat-free tissue. A healthy range of body fat is 12-18% for males and 18-23% for females.

17. Common methods to assess body composition include hydrostatic weighing, plethysmography, skinfold measurement, body mass index, and bioelectrical impedance.

18. The loose packed position of a joint is characterized by minimal stress on the joint, minimal joint congruency, and maximum ligament laxity. The close packed position of a joint is characterized by maximal stress on the joint, full joint congruency, and maximum ligament tightness.

19. End-feel refers to the type of resistance felt when passively moving a joint through the end range of motion. An end-feel classified as firm, hard or soft can be normal or abnormal depending on the joint, while an end-feel classified as empty is always abnormal.

20. Manual muscle testing grades range from zero (0/5) to normal (5/5) based on the ability to move a body segment through range with and without varying levels of resistance.

21. Active muscle insufficiency occurs when a two-joint muscle contracts across both joints simultaneously. Passive insufficiency occurs when a two-joint muscle is lengthened over both joints simultaneously.

22. Standard gait terminology includes heel strike, foot flat, midstance, heel off, toe off, acceleration, midswing, and deceleration.

23. Rancho Los Amigos gait terminology includes initial contact, loading response, midstance, terminal stance, pre-swing, initial swing, midswing, and terminal swing.

# Musculoskeletal System Essentials

24. The stance phase represents approximately 60% of the gait cycle and the swing phase represents 40% of the gait cycle.

25. Step length refers to the distance measured between right heel strike and left heel strike. Stride length refers to the distance measured between right heel strike and the following right heel strike.

26. Biceps tendon pathology can be identified through Ludington's test, Speed's test, and Yergason's test.

27. Rotator cuff pathology/impairment can be identified through the drop arm test, Hawkins-Kennedy impingement test, Neer impingement test, and supraspinatus test.

28. Contractures, or tightness of the hip, can be identified through Ely's test, Ober's test, piriformis test, Thomas test, tripod sign, and 90-90 straight leg raise test.

29. An anterior cruciate ligament sprain can be identified through the anterior drawer test, Lachman test, and lateral pivot shift test.

30. Meniscal pathology of the knee can be identified through Apley's compression test, bounce home test, and McMurray test.

31. Grades I and IV mobilizations are considered small amplitude movement, while grades II and III are considered large amplitude movements.

32. Grade V manipulation is defined as small amplitude, high velocity thrust technique performed to snap adhesions at the limit of range of motion.

33. The convex/concave rule specifies that when a convex surface is moving on a concave surface, roll and slide occur in the opposite direction. When a concave surface is moving on a convex surface, roll and slide occur in the same direction.

34. Adhesive capsulitis results in a loss of range of motion in active and passive shoulder motion caused by adhesive fibrosis and scarring between the capsule, rotator cuff, subacromial bursa, and deltoid.

35. Impingement syndrome is often caused by repetitive microtrauma from upper extremity activity performed above the horizontal plane.

36. Osteoarthritis is a chronic disease that causes degeneration of articular cartilage primarily in weight bearing joints.

37. Rheumatoid arthritis is a systemic autoimmune disorder caused by a chronic inflammatory reaction in the synovial tissues of a joint that results in erosion of cartilage and supporting structures within the capsule.

38. Hip precautions following total hip arthroplasty using a posterolateral surgical approach include avoiding hip flexion beyond 90 degrees, adduction, and hip medial rotation.

39. Common pharmacological agents used in the treatment of musculoskeletal disorders include opioid agents, nonopioid agents, glucocorticoid agents, and disease-modifying antirheumatic agents.

40. Common types of fractures include avulsion, closed, comminuted, compound, greenstick, nonunion, stress, and spiral.

41. Kyphosis refers to an excessive curvature of the spine in a posterior direction usually identified in the thoracic spine. Lordosis refers to an excessive curvature of the spine in an anterior direction usually in the cervical or lumbar spine.

42. An orthotic is an external device that provides support or stabilization, improves function, corrects deformities, and distributes pressure from one area to another.

43. Lower extremity amputations are significantly more common than upper extremity amputations with peripheral vascular disease serving as the primary etiology.

44. Components of an upper extremity prosthesis include the socket, suspension, elbow unit, wrist unit, and terminal device.

45. Components of a lower extremity prosthesis include socket, suspension, knee, shank, and foot.

46. Potential complications following amputation include contractures, deep vein thrombosis, hypersensitivity, neuroma, phantom limb, phantom pain, psychological impact, and wound infections.

47. Common gait deviations with a prosthesis include lateral bending, vaulting, forward trunk flexion, medial or lateral whip, abducted gait, circumducted gait, excessive knee flexion during stance, and rotation of the forefoot at heel strike.

**Musculoskeletal System Proficiencies**

## 1. Musculoskeletal Upper Extremity Anatomy

Identify the appropriate term for each of the specified locations. Answers must be selected from the Word Bank and can be used only once.

**Word Bank:** brachioradialis, flexor carpi radialis, flexor carpi ulnaris, flexor digitorum superficialis, palmaris longus, pronator quadratus, pronator teres

Biceps aponeurosis

g

f

a

b

e

c

d

## 2. Musculoskeletal Lower Extremity Anatomy I

Identify the appropriate term for each of the specified locations. Answers must be selected from the Word Bank and can be used only once.

**Word Bank:** gracilis, rectus femoris, sartorius, tensor fasciae latae, vastus lateralis, vastus medialis

a

b

c

d

e

f

QUIZ **Musculoskeletal System Proficiencies**

## 3. Musculoskeletal Lower Extremity Anatomy II

Identify the appropriate term for each of the specified locations. Answers must be selected from the Word Bank and can be used only once.

**Word Bank:** abductor digiti minimi, abductor hallucis, flexor digitorum brevis, flexor hallucis brevis, lumbricals, quadratus plantae

a

b

c

f

e

d

## 4. Muscle Function - Upper Extremity

Identify the muscle that contributes to performing each of the listed motions. Each muscle in the Word Bank must be used only once. Since a given muscle may contribute to multiple motions, it is essential for answers to be selected in a manner that allows for all muscles to be utilized.

**Word Bank:** anconeus, brachioradialis, coracobrachialis, extensor carpi ulnaris, flexor carpi radialis, latissimus dorsi, palmaris longus, teres major, teres minor

| Shoulder | Muscle |
|---|---|
| flexion | a |
| extension | b |
| lateral rotation | c |
| medial rotation | d |
| **Elbow** | **Muscle** |
| flexion | e |
| extension | f |
| **Wrist** | **Muscle** |
| flexion | g |
| extension | h |
| radial deviation | i |

**SCORE**BUILDERS

## 5. Muscle Function - Lower Extremity

Identify the muscle that contributes to performing each of the listed motions. Each muscle in the Word Bank must be used only once. Since a given muscle may contribute to multiple motions, it is essential for answers to be selected in a manner that allows for all muscles to be utilized.

**Word Bank:** biceps femoris, extensor hallucis longus, gluteus medius, gracilis, iliopsoas, peroneus longus, piriformis, tibialis posterior, vastus medialis

| Hip | Muscle |
|---|---|
| flexion | a |
| adduction | b |
| lateral rotation | c |
| medial rotation | d |
| **Knee** | **Muscle** |
| flexion | e |
| extension | f |
| **Ankle** | **Muscle** |
| dorsiflexion | g |
| inversion | h |
| eversion | i |

## 6. Muscle Fibers

Identify the type of muscle fiber most closely associated with each described characteristic. Answers must be selected from the Word Bank.

**Word Bank:** Type I, Type II

| Characteristic | Type |
|---|---|
| low capillary density | a |
| aerobic | b |
| large amount of mitochondria | c |
| white | d |
| fast-glycolytic | e |
| low myoglobin content | f |
| extensive blood supply | g |
| slow twitch | h |

# QUIZ Musculoskeletal System Proficiencies

## 7. Manual Muscle Testing

Identify the manual muscle testing grade most closely associated with the supplied description. Answers must be selected from the Word Bank and can be used only once.

**Word Bank:** zero, trace, poor minus, poor, poor plus, fair minus, fair, fair plus, good minus, good, good plus, normal

| Grade | Description |
|---|---|
| a | The subject does not complete range of motion in a gravity-eliminated position. |
| b | The subject's muscle contraction can be palpated, but there is no joint movement. |
| c | The subject does not complete the range of motion against gravity, but does complete more than half of the range. |
| d | The subject completes range of motion against gravity with maximal resistance. |
| e | The subject completes range of motion against gravity with minimal-moderate resistance. |
| f | The subject completes range of motion with gravity eliminated. |
| g | The subject completes range of motion against gravity with only minimal resistance. |
| h | The subject completes range of motion against gravity with moderate resistance. |

## 8. Gait - Standard Terminology

Identify the sequence and phase of the gait cycle starting with heel strike and ending with deceleration. Answers must be selected from the Word Bank and can be used only once.

**Word Bank:** **Sequence** - 2nd, 3rd, 4th, 5th, 6th, 7th

**Phase** - acceleration, foot flat, heel off, midstance, midswing, toe off

| Sequence | Phase | Description |
|---|---|---|
| 1st | heel strike | The instant the heel touches the ground to begin stance phase. |
| a | b | The point in which only the toe of the stance limb remains on the ground. |
| c | d | The point when the swing limb is directly under the body. |
| e | f | The point in which the entire foot makes contact with the ground. |
| g | h | Begins when toe off is complete and the reference limb swings until positioned directly under the body. |
| i | j | The point in which the heel of the stance limb leaves the ground. |
| k | l | The point during the stance phase when the entire body weight is directly over the stance limb. |
| 8th | deceleration | Begins directly after midswing as the swing limb begins to extend and ends just prior to heel strike. |

# Musculoskeletal System Proficiencies

## 9. Abnormal Gait

Identify the abnormal gait pattern most closely associated with the supplied description. Answers must be selected from the Word Bank and can be used only once.

**Word Bank:** antalgic, circumduction, parkinsonian, scissor, steppage, tabetic, Trendelenburg, vaulting

| Gait Pattern | Description |
|---|---|
| a | A gait pattern in which the feet and toes are lifted through hip and knee flexion to excessive heights. |
| b | A gait pattern characterized by the legs crossing midline upon advancement. |
| c | A gait pattern characterized by a circular motion to advance the leg during swing phase. |
| d | A protective gait pattern where the involved step length is decreased in order to avoid weight bearing on the involved side. |
| e | A gait pattern where the swing leg advances through a combination of elevation of the pelvis and plantar flexion of the stance leg. |
| f | A gait pattern characterized by excessive lateral trunk flexion and weight shifting over the stance leg due to gluteus medius weakness. |
| g | A gait pattern marked by quick and small steps with increased forward flexion of the trunk and knees. |
| h | A high stepping ataxic gait pattern in which the feet slap the ground. |

## 10. Goniometry

Complete the blank cells with the appropriate information based on the supplied information. The number of desired responses for each cell is identified in parentheses.

| Joint | | Motion | | Axis | |
|---|---|---|---|---|---|
| shoulder | | flexion | | a | (1) |
| shoulder | | b | (2) | olecranon process | |
| c | (1) | pronation | | lateral to the ulnar styloid process | |
| wrist | | radial deviation | | d | (1) |
| hip | | e | (2) | anterior aspect of the patella | |
| ankle | | f | (2) | lateral aspect of the lateral malleolus | |
| g | (1) | h | (2) | posterior aspect of the ankle midway between the malleoli | |

# Musculoskeletal System Proficiencies

## 11. Special Tests

Complete the blank cells with the appropriate information based on the supplied information.

| Special Test | Patient Position | Positive Sign |
|---|---|---|
| Vertebral artery test | a | b |
| Speed's test | sitting or standing | c |
| d | e | failing to slowly lower the arm to their side or by the presence of severe pain |
| Allen test (thoracic outlet) | f | g |
| h | i | pain in the lateral epicondyle region or muscle weakness |
| j | supine | straight leg rising from the table |
| Ober's test | sidelying | k |
| Patrick's test | l | m |
| Anterior drawer test (knee) | supine | n |
| Apley's compression test | o | pain or clicking |
| p | q | absence of plantar flexion |
| Homan's sign | r | s |

# Musculoskeletal System Proficiencies

## 12. Osteokinematic and Arthrokinematic Motions

Identify the concave and convex joint surface associated with the listed joints. Answers must be selected from the Word Bank and can be used more than once.

**Word Bank:** acetabulum, carpals, femur, fibula, glenoid, humerus, radius, talus, tibia

| Joint | Concave | | Convex | |
|---|---|---|---|---|
| glenohumeral | a | (1) | b | (1) |
| radiohumeral | c | (1) | d | (1) |
| radiocarpal | e | (1) | f | (1) |
| hip | g | (1) | h | (1) |
| tibiofemoral | i | (1) | j | (1) |
| talocrural | k | (2) | l | (1) |

## 13. Musculoskeletal System Basics

Mark each statement as True or False. If the statement is False correct the statement in the space provided.

| True/False | Statement |
|---|---|
| a | An end-feel classified as empty can be classified as normal or abnormal depending on the joint. |
| Correction | |
| b | The loose packed position of the hip is 30 degrees flexion, 30 degrees abduction, and slight medial rotation. |
| Correction | |
| c | Stride length refers to the distance measured between right heel strike and left heel strike. |
| Correction | |

# Musculoskeletal System Proficiencies

| True/False | Statement |
|---|---|
| d | The capsular pattern of the glenohumeral joint is lateral rotation, abduction, and medial rotation. |
| **Correction** | |
| e | According to Rancho Los Amigos gait terminology, pre-swing, midswing, and terminal swing are components of swing phase. |
| **Correction** | |
| f | Peak activity of the tibialis anterior occurs during the gait cycle just after heel strike. |
| **Correction** | |
| g | Normal elbow flexion is 0-135 degrees. |
| **Correction** | |
| h | The tensor fasciae latae, gluteus medius, and piriformis function as medial rotators of the hip. |
| **Correction** | |
| i | Muscle testing of the lower trapezius, rhomboids, and latissimus dorsi occurs with the patient positioned in prone. |
| **Correction** | |
| j | Sixty percent of the gait cycle occurs in the stance phase. |
| **Correction** | |

# Musculoskeletal System Answer Key

**1. Musculoskeletal Upper Extremity Anatomy**
a.   palmaris longus
b.   flexor carpi radialis
c.   flexor carpi ulnaris
d.   pronator quadratus
e.   flexor digitorum superficialis
f.   brachioradialis
g.   pronator teres

**2. Musculoskeletal Lower Extremity Anatomy I**
a.   tensor fasciae latae
b.   gracilis
c.   sartorius
d.   rectus femoris
e.   vastus lateralis
f.   vastus medialis

**3. Musculoskeletal Lower Extremity Anatomy II**
a.   flexor hallucis brevis
b.   abductor hallucis
c.   quadratus plantae
d.   flexor digitorum brevis
e.   abductor digiti minimi
f.   lumbricals

**4. Muscle Function - Upper Extremity**
a.   coracobrachialis
b.   latissimus dorsi
c.   teres minor
d.   teres major
e.   brachioradialis
f.   anconeus
g.   palmaris longus
h.   extensor carpi ulnaris
i.   flexor carpi radialis

**5. Muscle Function - Lower Extremity**
a.   iliopsoas
b.   gracilis
c.   piriformis
d.   gluteus medius
e.   biceps femoris
f.   vastus medialis
g.   extensor hallucis longus
h.   tibialis posterior
i.   peroneus longus

**6. Muscle Fibers**
a.   Type II
b.   Type I
c.   Type I
d.   Type II
e.   Type II
f.   Type II
g.   Type I
h.   Type I

**7. Manual Muscle Testing**
a.   poor minus
b.   trace
c.   fair minus
d.   normal
e.   good minus
f.   poor
g.   fair plus
h.   good

**8. Gait - Standard Terminology**
a.   5th
b.   toe off
c.   7th
d.   midswing
e.   2nd
f.   foot flat
g.   6th
h.   acceleration
i.   4th
j.   heel off
k.   3rd
l.   midstance

**9. Abnormal Gait**
a.   steppage
b.   scissor
c.   circumduction
d.   antalgic
e.   vaulting
f.   Trendelenburg
g.   parkinsonian
h.   tabetic

# Musculoskeletal System Answer Key

## 10. Goniometry

a. acromial process

b. lateral rotation and medial rotation

c. forearm

d. over the middle of the dorsal aspect of the wrist over the capitate

e. lateral rotation and medial rotation

f. dorsiflexion and plantar flexion

g. subtalar

h. inversion and eversion

## 11. Special Tests

a. supine

b. dizziness, nystagmus, slurred speech or loss of consciousness

c. pain or tenderness in the bicipital groove region

d. drop arm test

e. sitting or standing

f. sitting or standing

g. absent or diminished radial pulse

h. lateral epicondylitis test

i. sitting

j. Thomas test

k. inability of the test leg to adduct and touch the table

l. supine

m. failure of the test leg to abduct below the level of the opposite leg

n. excessive anterior translation of the tibia on the femur with a diminished or absent end-point

o. prone

p. Thompson test

q. prone

r. supine

s. pain in the calf

## 12. Osteokinematic and Arthrokinematic Motions

a. glenoid

b. humerus

c. radius

d. humerus

e. radius

f. carpals

g. acetabulum

h. femur

i. tibia

j. femur

k. tibia and fibula

l. talus

## 13. Musculoskeletal System Basics*

a. FALSE: Correction - An end-feel classified as empty is always considered abnormal due to the presence of pain.

b. FALSE: Correction - The loose packed position of the hip is 30 degrees flexion, 30 degrees abduction, and slight lateral rotation.

c. FALSE: Correction - Step length refers to the distance measured between right heel strike and left heel strike.

d. TRUE

e. FALSE: Correction - Pre-swing is a component of stance phase. Initial swing, midswing, and terminal swing are components of swing phase.

f. TRUE

g. FALSE: Correction - Normal elbow flexion is 0-150 degrees.

h. FALSE: Correction - The tensor fasciae latae and gluteus medius function as medial rotators of the hip. The piriformis functions as a lateral rotator of the hip.

i. TRUE

j. TRUE

*The correction presented for each false statement is an example of several possible corrections.

# Musculoskeletal System References

1. Guyton A. *Textbook of Medical Physiology.* W.B. Saunders Company, 1986.

2. Kendall F, McCreary E, Provance P. *Muscle Testing and Function*. Fifth Edition. Williams & Wilkins, 2005.

3. Norkin C, White D. *Measurement of Joint Motion: A Guide to Goniometry*. Third Edition. F.A. Davis Company, 2003.

4. Levangie P, Norkin C. *Joint Structure and Function: A Comprehensive Analysis*. Fourth Edition. FA Davis Company, 2005.

5. Tortora G, Derrickson B. *Principles of Anatomy and Physiology*. Twelfth Edition. John Wiley & Sons Inc., 2009.

6. Moore K. *Clinically Oriented Anatomy*. Second Edition. Williams & Wilkins, 1985.

7. Patton K, Thibodeau G. *Anatomy and Physiology*. Seventh Edition. Elsevier Inc., 2010.

8. Anderson MK., Hall SJ, Martin M. *Fundamentals of Sports Injury Management*. Fourth Edition. Lippincott Williams & Wilkins, 2009.

9. Bickley L, Szilagyi P. *Bates' Guide to Physical Examination and History Taking*. Tenth Edition. Lippincott Williams & Wilkins, 2009.

10. Magee D. *Orthopedic Physical Assessment*. Fifth Edition. W.B. Saunders Company, 2007.

11. Starkey C, Ryan J. *Evaluation of Orthopedic and Athletic Injuries*. F.A. Davis Company, 2002.

12. Hoppenfeld S. *Physical Examination of the Spine and Extremities*. Appleton-Century-Crofts, 1982.

13. Hertling D, Kessler R. *Management of Common Musculoskeletal Disorders*. Fourth Edition. Lippincott Williams & Wilkins, 2005.

14. Edmond S. *Joint Mobilization/Manipulation: Extremity and Spinal Techniques*. Second Edition. Mosby Inc., 2006.

15. Hall C, Brody L. *Therapeutic Exercise: Moving Toward Function*. Second Edition. Lippincott Williams & Wilkins, 2004.

16. Kisner C, Colby L. *Therapeutic Exercise Foundations and Techniques*. Fifth Edition. F.A. Davis Company, 2007.

17. Prentice W, Voight M. *Techniques in Musculoskeletal Rehabilitation*. McGraw-Hill Inc., 2001.

18. Dutton M. *Orthopaedic Examination, Evaluation, and Intervention*. Second Edition. McGraw-Hill Inc., 2008.

19. *American College of Sports Medicine: ACSM's Resource Manual for Guidelines for Exercise Testing and Prescription*. Sixth Edition. Lippincott Williams & Wilkins, 2010.

20. Reese N, Bandy WD. *Joint Range of Motion and Muscle Length Testing*. Second Edition. W.B. Saunders Company, 2009.

21. Hislop HJ, Montgomery J. *Daniels and Worthingham's Muscle Testing: Techniques of Manual Examination*. Eighth Edition, W.B. Saunders Company, 2007.

22. Rothstein J, Roy S, Wolf S. *The Rehabilitation Specialist's Handbook*. Third Edition. F.A. Davis Company, 2005.

23. Perry J, Burnfield J. *Gait Analysis: Normal and Pathological Function*. Second Edition. Slack Incorporated, 2010.

24. Hamill J, Knutzen K. *Biomechanical Basis of Human Movement*. Third Edition. Lippincott Williams & Wilkins, 2008.

25. Oatis C. *Kinesiology: The Mechanics and Pathomechanics of Human Movement*. Second Edition. Lippincott Williams & Wilkins, 2009.

26. Reider B. *The Orthopaedic Physical Examination*. W.B. Saunders Company, 1999.

27. Tecklin J. *Pediatric Physical Therapy*. Fourth Edition. Lippincott Williams & Wilkins, 2007.

28. Birrer R, O'Connor F. *Sports Medicine for the Primary Care Physician*. Third Edition. CRC Press, 2004.

29. Sueki D, Brechter J. *Orthopedic Rehabilitation Clinical Advisor*. Mosby Inc., 2010.

30. Campbell S. *Physical Therapy for Children*. Third Edition. W.B. Saunders Company, 2006.

31. Goodman C, Boissonnault W, Fuller K. *Pathology: Implications for the Physical Therapist*. Third Edition. W.B. Saunders Company, 2008.

32. Brotzman SB, Wilk KE. *Clinical Orthopedic Rehabilitation*. Mosby Inc., 2003.

33. Maxey L, Magnusson J. *Rehabilitation for the Postsurgical Orthopedic Patient*. Mosby Inc., 2001.

34. *Nurse's 3-Minute Clinical Reference*. Second Edition. Lippincott Williams & Wilkins, 2007.

35. Goodman C, Snyder T. *Differential Diagnosis in Physical Therapy*. Fourth Edition. W.B. Saunders Company, 2007.

## Musculoskeletal System References

36. Cameron M, Monroe L. *Physical Rehabilitation: Evidence-Based Examination, Evaluation, and Intervention*. Saunders, 2007.

37. Roach S. *Pharmacology for Health Professionals*. Lippincott Williams & Wilkins, 2005.

38. Gladson B. *Pharmacology for Physical Therapists*. Saunders, 2006.

39. Ciccone C. *Pharmacology for Rehabilitation*. Fourth Edition. F.A. Davis Company, 2007.

40. Seymour R. *Prosthetics and Orthotics: Lower Limb and Spinal*. Lippincott Williams & Wilkins, 2002.

41. Palmer L, Toms J. *Manual for Functional Training*. Third Edition. F.A. Davis Company, 1992.

42. Radomski MV, Latham CAT. *Occupational Therapy for Physical Dysfunction*. Sixth Edition. Lippincott, Williams & Wilkins, 2008.

43. Braddom RL. *Physical Medicine and Rehabilitation*. Third Edition. Saunders, Elsevier, 2007.

44. Tan JC. *Practical Manual of Physical Medicine and Rehabilitation*. Second Edition. Mosby Inc., 2005.

45. DeRuyter O. *Clinician's Guide to Assistive Technology*. Mosby Inc., 2002.

# 5

# Neuromuscular and Nervous Systems

## Therese Giles

Neuromuscular and Nervous Systems represents approximately 25% (50 questions) of the National Physical Therapy Examination.

The actual number of questions in this category can range from 48 to 52 questions.

135 Neuroanatomy

149 Cranial Nerves

154 Reflexes

158 Sensation

166 Balance

172 Communication Disorders

175 Pharmacology

176 Pathology

181 Cerebrovascular Accident

184 Neurological Rehabilitation

197 Spinal Cord Injury

205 Traumatic Brain Injury

208 Pediatrics and Development

217 Essentials

220 Proficiencies

SCOREBUILDERS

# Neuroanatomy: Anatomical Divisions of the Nervous System[1,2,3]

## Central Nervous System (CNS)

### Brain

**forebrain (prosencephalon)**
- **telencephalon:** cerebrum, hippocampus, basal ganglia, amygdala
- **diencephalon:** thalamus, hypothalamus, subthalamus, epithalamus

**midbrain (mesencephalon)**
- **tectum:** superior and inferior colliculi
- **tegmentum:** cerebral aqueduct, periaqueductal gray, reticular formation, substantia nigra, red nucleus

**hindbrain (rhombencephalon)**
- **metencephalon:** cerebellum, pons
- **myelencephalon:** medulla oblongata

### Brainstem

**midbrain, pons, medulla oblongata**
- Brainstem is noted separately to acknowledge its components since it incorporates the midbrain with specific sections of the hindbrain.

### Spinal Cord
- cervical, thoracic, lumbar, sacral, and coccygeal levels
- afferent and efferent tracts
- inner core of gray matter and superficial white matter

## Characteristics

- main centers where integration and coordination of nervous system information occurs
- covered in a system of meninges and suspended in cerebrospinal fluid for protection
- surrounded by skull and vertebral column for protection
- gray matter - consists of unmyelinated neurons and contains capillaries, glial cells, cell bodies, and dendrites
- white matter - consists of myelinated axons and contains nerve fibers without dendrites
- white matter of the spinal cord is divided into three funiculi: anterior, lateral, and dorsal columns
- brain is divided into left and right cerebral hemispheres
- each hemisphere of the brain contains a frontal lobe, temporal lobe, parietal lobe, and occipital lobe

## Peripheral Nervous System (PNS)

**Cranial Nerves and Ganglia**
- 12 pairs of cranial nerves exit the skull through the foramina

**Spinal Nerves and Ganglia/Plexuses**
- 31 pairs of spinal nerves exit the vertebral column through the intervertebral foramina
  - 8 cervical, 12 thoracic, 5 lumbar, 5 sacral, 1 coccygeal

### Characteristics

- bundles of nerve fibers and axons are supported by connective tissue and conduct information to the CNS
- encased in fibrous sheaths, however, relatively unprotected
- spinal nerves each have an anterior root carrying motor information away from the CNS (efferent fibers)
- spinal nerves each have a posterior root carrying information regarding sensation to the CNS (afferent fibers)
- ganglia are clusters or swellings of cells that give rise to the peripheral and central nerve fibers
- ganglia are divided into sensory ganglia and autonomic ganglia

## Autonomic Nervous System (ANS)

**Sympathetic Division**
- prepares the body for emergency response; norepinephrine neurotransmitter; generally a stimulating response    *Fight or Flight*

**Parasympathetic Division**
- conserving and restoring energy; acetylcholine neurotransmitter; generally an inhibitory response    *Rest + Digest*

### Characteristics

- anatomically contains portions of the CNS and PNS
- concerned with innervation for involuntary processes, glands, internal organs, and smooth muscle
- emphasis on homeostasis and a person's response to stress
- impulses often do not reach our consciousness
- impulses produce largely automatic responses

## Somatic Nervous System (SNS)

* peripheral and motor nerve fibers

### Characteristics

* peripheral nerve fibers send sensory information to the CNS
* motor nerve fibers send information to skeletal muscles
* somatic motor neurons travel directly to skeletal muscle without intervening synapses
* all nerve fibers are myelinated
* controls voluntary movements and provides the ability to sense touch, smell, sight, taste and sound
* all five senses are influenced by the SNS

## Limbic System[4]

* corpus callosum, olfactory tract, mammillary bodies, fornix, thalamic nuclei, amygdala, hippocampus, parahippocampal gyrus, cingulate gyrus, hypothalamic nuclei

### Characteristics

* involved in the control and expression of mood and emotion, processing and storage of recent memory, olfaction, control of appetite, and emotional responses to food
* lesions to the limbic system can also result in a variety of behaviors including aggression, extreme fearfulness, altered sexual behavior, and changes in motivation.

## Consider This

### Autonomic Nervous System Disorders[5]

* The autonomic nervous system (ANS) influences all internal organs, blood vessels, pupils and muscles of the eye, as well as sweat, salivary, and digestive glands as it relates to homeostasis. The ANS controls blood pressure, heart and breathing rates, body temperature, digestion, metabolism, electrolyte balance, production of saliva, sweat and tears, urination, defecation, sexual response, and other bodily processes.
* Disorders of the ANS can affect any body part or process. Autonomic disorders may result from outside pathology that damages autonomic nerves, such as diabetes or alcoholism, or there may be primary damage to the system. Autonomic disorders may be reversible or progressive in nature.
* Examples of ANS disorders include constipation, erectile dysfunction, Horner's syndrome, vasovagal syncope, orthostatic hypotension, and postural tachycardia syndrome.
* ANS disorders are typically treated with pharmacological intervention. These disorders may or may not have an impact on the physical therapy plan of care. Therapists need to possess an understanding of the impact of a patient's disorder and modify treatment based on their findings.

# Central Nervous System

## Brain

### Forebrain (Prosencephalon)[1,2,6]

#### Telencephalon

The telencephalon is the largest division of the human brain and consists of the cerebrum (cerebral cortex), hippocampus, basal ganglia, and amygdala (Fig. 5-1).

#### Cerebrum

The cerebrum, which encompasses the major portion of the brain, is divided into the right and left cerebral hemispheres (Fig. 5-2). The two hemispheres are joined at the bottom by white matter, termed corpus callosum, which relays information from one side of the brain to the other. The surface of the cerebrum contains billions of neurons and glia that form the cerebral cortex. The outer surface of the cerebrum is termed gray matter and the interior is termed white matter. Sulci and fissures demark the specific lobes of the brain. Each lobe is responsible for different functions.

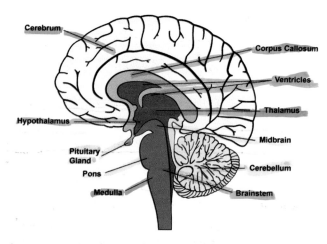

**Fig. 5-1:** A sagittal view of the human brain.

#### Fissures

- interhemispheric fissure (medial longitudinal): separates the two cerebral hemispheres
- Sylvian fissure (lateral): anterior portion separates the temporal and frontal lobes; posterior portion separates the temporal and parietal lobes

#### Sulci

- central sulcus (sulcus of Rolando): separates frontal and parietal lobes laterally
- parieto-occipital sulcus: separates the parietal and occipital lobes medially
- calcarine sulcus: separates the occipital lobe into superior and inferior halves

## Hemisphere Specialization/Dominance[6,7]

### Left

- Language
- Sequence and perform movements
- Understand language
- Produce written and spoken language
- Analytical
- Controlled
- Logical
- Rational
- Mathematical calculations
- Express positive emotions such as love and happiness
- Process verbally coded information in an organized, logical, and sequential manner

### Right

- Nonverbal processing
- Process information in a holistic manner
- Artistic abilities
- General concept comprehension
- Hand-eye coordination
- Spatial relationships
- Kinesthetic awareness
- Understand music
- Understand nonverbal communication
- Mathematical reasoning
- Express negative emotions
- Body image awareness

**Fig. 5-2:** The two hemispheres of the brain and the corresponding characteristics of each.

## Lobes of the Cerebrum[2,7,8]

| Lobe | Function | Impairment |
|------|----------|------------|
| Frontal | • voluntary movement (primary motor cortex/ precentral gyrus), intellect, orientation<br>• Broca's area (typically located in the left hemisphere): speech, concentration<br>• personality, temper, judgment, reasoning, behavior, self-awareness, executive functions | • contralateral weakness<br>• perseveration, inattention<br>• personality changes, antisocial behavior<br>• impaired concentration, apathy<br>• Broca's aphasia (expressive deficits)<br>• delayed or poor initiation<br>• emotional lability |
| Parietal | • associated with sensation of touch, kinesthesia, perception of vibration, and temperature<br>• receives information from other areas of the brain regarding hearing, vision, motor, sensory, and memory<br>• provides meaning for objects<br>• interprets language and words<br>• spatial and visual perception | • dominant hemisphere (typically located in the left hemisphere): agraphia, alexia, agnosia<br>• non-dominant hemisphere (typically located in the right hemisphere): dressing apraxia, constructional apraxia, anosognosia<br>• contralateral sensory deficits<br>• impaired language comprehension<br>• impaired taste |
| Temporal | • primary auditory processing and olfaction<br>• Wernicke's area (typically located in the left hemisphere): ability to understand and produce meaningful speech, verbal and general memory, assists with understanding language<br>• the rear of the temporal lobe enables humans to interpret other peoples' emotions and reactions | • learning deficits<br>• Wernicke's aphasia (receptive deficits)<br>• antisocial, aggressive behaviors<br>• difficulty with facial recognition<br>• difficulty with memory, memory loss<br>• inability to categorize objects |
| Occipital | • main processing center for visual information<br>• processes visual information regarding colors, light, and shapes<br>• judgment of distance, seeing in three dimensions | • homonymous hemianopsia *– visual field loss on same side of both eyes*<br>• impaired extraocular muscle movement and visual deficits<br>• impaired color recognition<br>• reading and writing impairment<br>• cortical blindness with bilateral lobe involvement |

### Hippocampus

The hippocampus is deeply embedded within the lower temporal lobe. It is responsible for the process of forming and storing new memories of one's personal history and other declarative memory. It also possesses great importance in learning language. This "memory indexer" sends memories to appropriate areas of the cerebral hemispheres for long-term storage and retrieves memories when needed.

### Basal ganglia

The basal ganglia are gray matter masses located deep within the white matter of the cerebrum and include the caudate, putamen, globus pallidus, substantia nigra, and subthalamic nuclei. The basal ganglia are collectively responsible for voluntary movement, regulation of autonomic movement, posture, muscle tone, and control of motor responses. Basal ganglia dysfunction has been associated with conditions including Parkinson's disease, Huntington's disease, Tourette's syndrome, attention-deficit disorder, obsessive-compulsive disorder, and many addictions.

### Amygdala

The amygdala is a small, almond-shaped nuclei located within the temporal lobes of each hemisphere of the brain. It lies adjacent to the hippocampus and just beneath the surface of the front, medial portion of the temporal lobe. This positioning results in the bulge on the surface called the uncus. The main function of amygdala is emotional and social processing. It is involved with fear and pleasure responses, arousal, processing of memory, and the formation of emotional memories.

### Diencephalon[9]

The diencephalon is located beneath the cerebral hemispheres and contains the thalamus, hypothalamus, subthalamus, and epithalamus. The diencephalon is the area of the brain where the major motor and sensory tracts synapse. It acts as an interactive site between the central nervous system and the endocrine system, as well as complementing the limbic system.

## Consider This

### Treatment Challenges That Result from Specific Lobe Damage[2,4]

When treating a patient with brain damage, there are predictable patterns of deficits based on the area of the brain that sustained injury. A therapist must recognize the particular concerns as it relates to the affected area(s) of the brain and integrate this into the plan of care.

- Frontal lobe lesions will produce deficits that range from paralysis and apraxia to loss of executive functions and goal-directed behaviors. Modifications to therapy may include response to perseveration, apraxia, and impaired executive functions. Patients with a frontal lobe lesion may present with apathy or may be uninhibited, distractible, and lack judgment.

- Parietal lobe lesions affect sensory awareness, interpretation, and perception. Somatosensory deficits elicit abnormal movement patterns for patients. Deficits in directional concepts hinder movement planning and require modification of therapy.

- Temporal lobe lesions will affect short and long-term memory. Damage to Wernicke's area (left hemisphere) impairs the comprehension of spoken language. Modification to therapy would include a more kinesthetic approach, relying on demonstration. New learning is available, but patients are usually unable to recall the steps that surround the new skill.

- Occipital lobe lesions produce various visual deficits that can hinder therapy. Cortical blindness occurs with damage to the occipital cortex and affects a patient's ability to receive, but not to perceive visual information. Therapy should avoid the use of diagrams, written materials, and reading. Environmental modification is required secondary to visual deficits, field cuts, and potential for visual agnosia.

### Thalamus

The thalamus is a relay or processing station for the majority of information that goes to the cerebral cortex. It coordinates sensory perception and movement with other parts of the brain and spinal cord that also have a role in sensation and movement. It receives information from the cerebellum, basal ganglia, and all sensory pathways except for the olfactory tract. The thalamus then relays the information to the appropriate association cortex. Damage to the thalamus can produce thalamic pain syndrome where there is spontaneous pain on the contralateral side of the body to the thalamic lesion.

### Hypothalamus

The hypothalamus receives and integrates information from the autonomic nervous system and assists in regulating hormones. The structure also controls functions such as hunger, thirst, sexual behavior, and sleeping. It regulates body temperature, the adrenal glands, the pituitary gland, and many other vital activities. It is located below the thalamus at the base of the diencephalon. Lesions can produce a variety of impairments based on the area of damage including obesity, sexual disinterest, poor temperature control, and diabetes insipidus.

### Subthalamus

The subthalamus is located between the thalamus and the hypothalamus and is primarily represented by the subthalamic nucleus. It is important for regulating movements produced by skeletal muscles. It has association with the basal ganglia and substantia nigra.

### Epithalamus

The epithalamus is primarily represented by the pineal gland. This gland secretes melatonin and is involved in circadian rhythms, the internal clock, selected regulation of motor pathways, and emotions. It is associated with the limbic system and basal ganglia.

## Midbrain (Mesencephalon)[9]

The midbrain is one of the three components of the brainstem and is located at the base of the brain above the spinal cord. The midbrain connects the forebrain to the hindbrain and functions as a large relay area for information passing from the cerebrum, cerebellum, and spinal cord. It is also a reflex center for visual, auditory, and tactile responses. Two key areas of the midbrain include:

- **tectum:** superior and inferior colliculi
- **tegmentum:** cerebral aqueduct, periaqueductal gray, reticular formation, substantia nigra, red nucleus

## Hindbrain (Rhombencephalon)[2,3]

The hindbrain consists of the cerebellum, pons, and medulla oblongata. The pons and medulla oblongata are components of the brainstem and control the body's vital functions. The cerebellum coordinates movement and assists with maintaining balance.

### Cerebellum

The cerebellum (metencephalon) is located at the posterior of the brain below the occipital lobes and is separated from the cerebrum by the tentorium. The cerebellum is responsible for fine tuning of movement and assists with maintaining posture and balance by controlling muscle tone and positioning of the extremities in space. The cerebellum controls the ability to perform rapid alternating movements. The cerebellum consists of two hemispheres of gray matter, and is divided into three lobes: the anterior, posterior, and flocculonodular lobes, with the fourth ventricle lying anterior to the lobes. Damage to one side of the cerebellum will produce ipsilateral impairment to the body. Cerebellar lesions may produce ataxia, nystagmus, tremor, hypermetria, poor coordination, and deficits in postural reflexes, balance, and equilibrium depending on the area of cerebellar lesion.

## Pons

The pons (also metencephalon) is located below the midbrain and superior to the medulla oblongata. It assists with regulation of respiration rate and is associated with the orientation of the head in relation to visual and auditory stimuli. Cranial nerves V through VIII originate from the pons.

## Medulla oblongata

The medulla oblongata (myelencephalon) is cone-shaped, connects to the pons superiorly, and to the spinal cord inferiorly. It's composed of white matter on the surface and gray matter within the interior. The medulla influences autonomic nervous activity and the regulation of respiration and heart rate. Reflex centers for vomiting, coughing, and sneezing are found within the medulla. Damage to motor tracts crossing within the medulla produces

contralateral impairment. The medulla is also responsible for relaying somatic sensory information from internal organs and for the control of arousal and sleep. Cranial nerves IX, X, XI, and XII originate from the medulla oblongata.

## Brainstem

The brainstem is a separate classification within the brain and is located in front of the cerebellum with connection to the spinal cord. It consists of three structures: the midbrain, pons, and medulla oblongata. These structures are found both within the midbrain and hindbrain. The brainstem works as a relay station, sending messages between various parts of the body and the cerebral cortex. Many of the primitive functions that are essential for survival, such as regulation of heart rate and respiratory rate, are located within the brainstem. The reticular activating system is found within the midbrain, pons, medulla, and a portion of the thalamus. Severe damage to the brainstem will often result in "brain death" secondary to the key functions that are controlled within this area. The majority of cranial nerves originate within the brainstem.

## Blood Supply[2,6]

The brain's blood supply consists of the two internal carotid arteries and the two vertebral arteries. The branches of these main arteries form the Circle of Willis (Fig. 5-3).

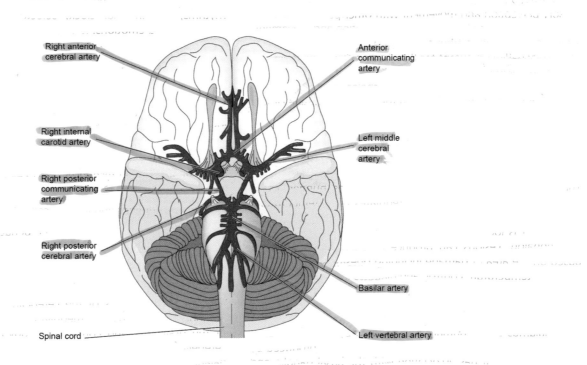

**Fig. 5-3:** The vascular supply to the brain; Circle of Willis.

## Blood Supply to the Brain

| Blood Supply to the Brain | Expected Possible Impairment Based on Extent of Vascular Involvement |
|---|---|
| **Anterior cerebral artery (ACA)[10]** | |
| • Anterior frontal lobe<br>• Medial surface of frontal and parietal lobes | • Contralateral lower extremity motor and sensory involvement<br>• Loss of bowel and bladder control<br>• Loss of behavioral inhibition<br>• Significant mental changes<br>• Neglect<br>• Aphasia<br>• Apraxia and agraphia<br>• Perseveration<br>• Akinetic mutism with significant bilateral involvement |
| **Middle cerebral artery (MCA)[11,12]** | |
| • Most of outer cerebrum<br>• Basal ganglia<br>• Posterior and anterior internal capsule<br>• Putamen<br>• Pallidum<br>• Lentiform nucleus | • Most common site of a CVA<br>• Wernicke's aphasia in dominant hemisphere<br>• Homonymous hemianopsia<br>• Apraxia<br>• Flat affect with right hemisphere damage<br>• Contralateral weakness and sensory loss of face and upper extremity with lesser involvement in the lower extremity<br>• Impaired spatial relations<br>• Anosognosia in non-dominant hemisphere<br>• Impaired body schema |
| **Posterior cerebral artery (PCA)[2,6]** | |
| • Portion of midbrain<br>• Subthalamic nucleus<br>• Basal nucleus<br>• Thalamus<br>• Inferior temporal lobe<br>• Occipital and occipitoparietal cortices | • Contralateral pain and temperature sensory loss<br>• Contralateral hemiplegia (central area), mild hemiparesis<br>• Ataxia, athetosis or choreiform movement<br>• Quality of movement is impaired<br>• Thalamic pain syndrome<br>• Anomia — *type of aphasia*<br>• Prosopagnosia with occipital infarct *(face blindness)*<br>• Hemiballismus<br>• Visual agnosia<br>• Homonymous hemianopsia<br>• Memory impairment<br>• Alexia, dyslexia<br>• Cortical blindness from bilateral involvement |
| **Vertebral-basilar artery[9]** | |
| • Lateral aspect of pons and midbrain together with superior surface of cerebellum<br>• Cerebellum - branches from the basilar artery (posterior inferior cerebellar, anterior inferior cerebellar, and superior cerebellar arteries)<br>• Medulla - posterior inferior cerebellar artery, smaller branches from the vertebral arteries<br>• Pons - branches from the basilar artery<br>• Midbrain and thalamus - posterior cerebral arteries<br>• Occipital cortex - posterior cerebral artery, basilar artery | • Loss of consciousness<br>• Hemiplegia or tetraplegia<br>• Comatose or vegetative state<br>• Inability to speak<br>• Locked-in syndrome<br>• Vertigo<br>• Nystagmus<br>• Dysphagia<br>• Dysarthria<br>• Syncope<br>• Ataxia |

# Consider This

## Occlusion to a Specific Artery will Produce Predictable Patterns of Impairment[2,10,11]

Blood supply is specific to particular areas within the brain. When a particular artery sustains damage via occlusion or hemorrhage, there is a specific pattern of disability that will occur. The extent of disability is determined by the extent of occlusion, the area of the brain involved, availability of collateral circulation to the affected area of the brain, and if the involved artery produces unilateral or bilateral damage. Bilateral arterial involvement will typically produce the most significant impairments.

### Anterior cerebral artery

Bilateral occlusion of the anterior cerebral artery will typically produce paraplegia. Other findings include incontinence, abulic aphasia, frontal lobe symptoms such as personality changes, and potential akinetic mutism (i.e., conscious unresponsiveness).

### Middle cerebral artery

Bilateral occlusion of the middle cerebral artery at the stem will produce contralateral hemiplegia and sensory impairment. Dominant hemisphere impairment includes global, Wernicke's or Broca's aphasia. Since the middle cerebral artery supplies the larger portion of the cortex, other impairments are lobe dependent.

### Posterior cerebral artery

Two of the most significant impairments with posterior cerebral artery occlusion are thalamic pain syndrome and cortical blindness. Thalamic pain presents with abnormal sensation of pain, temperature, touch, and proprioception. The perceived sensation of pain can become debilitating. Cortical blindness is the loss of vision due to damage to the visual portion of the occipital cortex. Although the affected eye is physically normal, there is full or partial vision loss. The pupil continues to dilate and constrict in response to light since this occurs without influence of the brain.

### Vertebral-basilar artery

There is a wide variety of clinical symptoms and syndromes based on the complex vascularity of the vertebral-basilar artery system. Severe impairment can cause locked-in syndrome, coma or vegetative state. Wallenberg syndrome secondary to lateral medullary infarct presents with ipsilateral facial pain, ipsilateral ataxia, vertigo, contralateral pain, and thermal impairment.

## Supporting Systems of the Brain and Spinal Cord[2,7]

### Meninges

Meninges consist of three layers of connective tissue covering the brain and spinal cord. The meninges provide protection from contusion and infection. There are blood vessels and cerebrospinal fluid (CSF) within the meninges.

- **dura mater:** outer most meninge; has four folds; lines the periosteum of the skull and protects the brain; subdural space separates this from the arachnoid matter
- **arachnoid:** the middle meninge; the arachnoid is impermeable; surrounds the brain in a loose manner; subarachnoid space separates this from the pia mater
- **pia mater:** inner most meninge; covers the contours of the brain; forms the choroid plexus in the ventricular system

dura mater ← epidural space
← subdural space
arachnoid
← subarachnoid space
pia mater

# Spotlight on Safety

## Meningitis[1,13]

Meningitis is the inflammation of the meninges of the brain and spinal cord. There are various forms of meningitis with bacterial meningitis being potentially fatal within hours of onset. Acute meningitis is considered to be a medical emergency. A therapist must be aware of the signs and symptoms of meningitis including:

- fever, headache, vomiting
- complaints of a stiff and painful neck, nuchal rigidity
- pain in the lumbar area and posterior thigh
- Brudzinski's sign (flexion of the neck facilitates flexion of the hips and knees)
- Kernig's sign (pain with hip flexion combined with knee extension)
- sensitivity to light

A lumbar puncture is the gold standard for diagnosis. Early diagnosis is essential to avoid permanent neurological damage. Treatment includes antibiotic, antimicrobial, and steroid pharmacological intervention.

### Dural Spaces[5,9]

- **epidural space:** an area between the skull and outer dura mater that can be abnormally occupied; also the area in the spinal cord between the dura mater and the periosteum of the vertebrae

- **subdural space:** the area between the dura and arachnoid meninges

- **subarachnoid space:** the area between the arachnoid and pia mater that contains CSF and the circulatory system for the cerebral cortex

### Ventricular System[5,9]

The ventricular system is designed to protect and nourish the brain. It is comprised of four fluid-filled cavities called ventricles and multiple foramina that allow the passage of cerebrospinal fluid (CSF). Each ventricle contains specialized tissue called choroid plexus that makes CSF. An excess of CSF in the brain can cause an enlargement in the ventricles causing hydrocephalus; excess fluid within the spinal cord is termed syringomyelia.

#### Cerebrospinal fluid

Cerebrospinal fluid (CSF) is a clear, fluid-like substance that cushions the brain and spinal cord from injury and provides mechanical buoyancy and support. CSF is produced constantly with a yield of 500-700 ml/day. CSF provides nutrition to the central nervous system, serves as a conduit for removal of metabolites, and is constantly being absorbed and replenished within the brain and spinal cord.

### Blood-brain Barrier[5,9]

The blood-brain barrier consists of the meninges, protective glial cells, and capillary beds of the brain. It is responsible for exchange of nutrients between the central nervous system and the vascular system. The blood-brain barrier provides protection for the central nervous system by restricting certain molecules from crossing the barrier while others are able to do so freely.

## Spotlight on Safety
### Hydrocephalus[1,14,15]

Hydrocephalus is an increase of CSF within the ventricles of the brain typically due to poor resorption, obstruction of flow or excessive production of CSF. It can be classified as congenital, acquired or idiopathic as well as communicating or non-communicating. Associated conditions and causative factors vary but may include spina bifida, choroid plexus neoplasm, cerebral palsy, tumor, meningitis or encephalocele. Successful treatment includes surgical placement of a shunt or performing an endoscopic third ventriculostomy (ETV). Often repeated neurosurgical procedures are necessary to treat hydrocephalus. Long-term health outcomes for patients with hydrocephalus remain unpredictable.

Signs of hydrocephalus or a blocked shunt include:

- enlarged head or bulging fontanelles in infants
- headache
- changes in vision
- large veins noted on scalp
- behavioral changes
- seizures
- alteration in appetite, vomiting
- "sun setting" sign or downward deviation of the eyes
- incontinence

Physical therapists working with patients with hydrocephalus or at risk for hydrocephalus must be aware of signs and symptoms of the condition as well as shunt malfunction, and when necessary, immediately notify appropriate medical personnel. There must be immediate medical intervention to alleviate the excessive fluid within the brain. Failure to act in a timely manner can result in coma and/or death.

## Spinal Cord[6,9]

The spinal cord is a component of the central nervous system and a direct continuation of the brainstem. The spinal cord functions as a relay for information between peripheral structures and the brain in order to process information. The cord is surrounded by meninges and contained within the vertebral canal of the vertebral column (Fig. 5-4). The spinal cord contains both white and gray matter with the largest amount of gray matter found in the lumbar region. The vertebral artery forms the anterior spinal artery and two posterior spinal arteries that all surround the spinal cord. The spinal cord runs from the foramen magnum to the conus medullaris (between the 1st and 2nd lumbar vertebrae). There are 31 segments with a pair of spinal nerves arising from each segment and these nerves are components of the peripheral nervous system. Each spinal nerve contains a dorsal root (sensory) with afferent fibers and a ventral root (motor) with efferent fibers (Fig. 5-5).

Cervical spine

Thoracic spine

Lumbar spine

Sacrum

Coccyx

**Fig. 5-4:** A sagittal view of the spine.

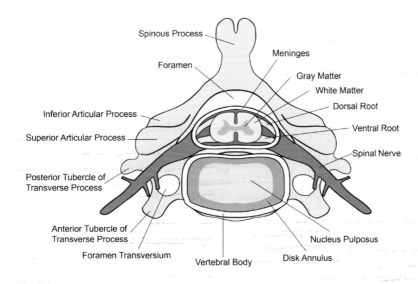

**Fig. 5-5:** A cross section of a vertebral segment.

## Ascending Tracts[7,16,17]

Sensory tracts ascending in the white matter of the spinal cord arise either from cells of spinal ganglia or from intrinsic neurons within the gray matter that receive primary sensory input. Ascending tracts relay sensory feedback to the cerebrum and cerebellum. The primary afferent tracts include:

**Fasciculus cuneatus (posterior or dorsal column):** sensory tract for trunk, neck, and upper extremity proprioception, vibration, two-point discrimination, and graphesthesia

**Fasciculus gracilis (posterior or dorsal column):** sensory tract for trunk and lower extremity proprioception, two-point discrimination, vibration, and graphesthesia

**Spinocerebellar tract (dorsal):** sensory tract that ascends to the cerebellum for ipsilateral subconscious proprioception, tension in muscles, joint sense, and posture of the trunk and lower extremities

**Spinocerebellar tract (ventral):** sensory tract that ascends to the cerebellum, some fibers crossing with subsequent recrossing at the level of the pons for ipsilateral subconscious proprioception, tension in muscles, joint sense, and posture of the trunk, upper extremities, and lower extremities

**Spino-olivary tract:** ascends to the cerebellum and relays information from cutaneous and proprioceptive organs

**Spinoreticular tract:** the afferent pathway for the reticular formation that influences levels of consciousness

**Spinotectal tract:** sensory tract providing afferent information for spinovisual reflexes and assists with movement of eyes and head towards a stimulus

**Spinothalamic tract (anterior):** sensory tract for light touch and pressure

**Spinothalamic tract (lateral):** sensory tract for pain and temperature sensation

## Descending Tracts[7,16,17]

Tracts descending to the spinal cord are involved with voluntary motor function, muscle tone, reflexes and equilibrium, visceral innervation, and modulation of ascending sensory signals. The largest, the corticospinal tract, originates in the cerebral cortex. Smaller descending tracts originate in nuclei in the midbrain, pons, and medulla oblongata. The primary efferent tracts include:

**Corticospinal tract (anterior):** pyramidal motor tract responsible for ipsilateral voluntary, discrete, and skilled movements

**Corticospinal tract (lateral):** pyramidal motor tract responsible for contralateral voluntary fine movement

- Damage to the corticospinal (pyramidal) tracts results in a positive Babinski sign, absent superficial abdominal reflexes and cremasteric reflex, and the loss of fine motor or skilled voluntary movement.

**Reticulospinal tract:** extrapyramidal motor tract responsible for facilitation or inhibition of voluntary and reflex activity through the influence on alpha and gamma motor neurons

**Rubrospinal tract:** extrapyramidal motor tract responsible for motor input of gross postural tone, facilitating activity of flexor muscles, and inhibiting the activity of extensor muscles

**Tectospinal tract:** extrapyramidal motor tract responsible for contralateral postural muscle tone associated with auditory/visual stimuli

**Vestibulospinal tract:** extrapyramidal motor tract responsible for ipsilateral gross postural adjustments subsequent to head movements; facilitating activity of the extensor muscles and inhibiting activity of the flexor muscles

- Damage to the extrapyramidal tracts results in significant paralysis, hypertonicity, exaggerated deep tendon reflexes, and clasp-knife reaction.

## Consider This

### Brown-Sequard's Syndrome[18,19]

Afferent and efferent pathways provide consistent and predictable deficits with injury. Depending on the location of a lesion and whether or not a pathway crossed or remained on the originating side, symptoms will be noted ipsilaterally or contralaterally to the lesion. Thorough examination of a patient will allow a therapist to potentially target particular pathways that may be damaged.

As an example, Brown-Sequard's syndrome is an incomplete lesion typically caused by a stab wound, which produces hemisection of the spinal cord. There is paralysis and loss of vibratory sense and position sense on the same side as the lesion due to the damage to the corticospinal tracts and dorsal columns. There is a loss of pain and temperature sense on the opposite side of the lesion from damage to the lateral spinothalamic tract.

# Peripheral Nervous System

The peripheral nervous system (PNS) contains nerves that originate within the brain and spinal cord, but end peripherally. The PNS consists of motor, sensory, and autonomic neurons that innervate end-organs that include sensory receptors, muscles, and glands. The PNS consists of 12 pairs of cranial nerves, 31 pairs of spinal nerves, and all associated ganglia and sensory receptors. Most peripheral nerves contain motor (efferent) and sensory (afferent) components (Fig. 5-6). Sensory nerves originate in the dorsal root ganglia while motor nerves originate in the anterior horn of the spinal cord. The autonomic neurons are divided into the sympathetic and parasympathetic nerves. The sympathetic nerves originate in the lateral horn of the thoracic spinal cord and the parasympathetic nerves originate from the lateral gray matter of the sacral level of the spinal cord and from the brain itself. Peripheral nerves are typically classified by axon diameter or speed of conduction.

## Cutaneous Sensory End-organ Receptors[20]

- Thermoreceptors
- Nociceptors
- Mechanoreceptors
  - Merkel's disc
  - Ruffini's corpuscle
  - Pacinian corpuscle
  - Meissner's corpuscle
  - muscle spindle
  - free nerve ending
  - Golgi tendon organ
- Chemoreceptors
- Photoreceptors

## Peripheral Nervous System Terminology[2,3,20]

**Axon:** a projection of a nerve away from the cell body that conducts impulses

**Dendrite:** an extension of the cell body that receives signals from other neurons

**Endoneurium:** the inner most covering of a peripheral nerve that surrounds each individual axon

**Epineurium:** the outer most covering of a peripheral nerve that surrounds the entire nerve and provides a buffer for the peripheral nerve

**Motor unit:** a single motor neuron and all of the muscle fibers that it innervates

**Myelin:** proteins and lipids that form to create a sheath around particular nerves; increases conductivity of the nerve impulse

**Nerve conduction velocity:** measures the speed of a nerve impulse along the axon of a nerve

**Neurons:** nerve cells that receive and send signals to other nerve cells; comprised of a cell body, axon, and dendrites

**Nodes of Ranvier:** brief gaps in myelination of an axon; serves to facilitate rapid conduction of a nerve impulse via jumping from gap node to gap node

Fig. 5-6: A cross section of the spinal cord noting the spinal nerves.

**Perineurium:** the middle layer of covering surrounding the peripheral nerve that envelopes fascicles or groups of axons and maintains the blood-nerve barrier

**Saltatory conduction:** an action potential moving along an axon in a jumping fashion from node to node; decreases the use of sodium-potassium pumps and increases speed of conduction

**Schwann cell:** cells that cover the nerve fibers within the peripheral nervous system and form the myelin sheath

## Classification of Peripheral Nerves[20]

**A Fibers**

- Large fibers
- Myelinated
- High conduction rate
- Alpha, beta, gamma, delta subsets
  - **Alpha:** alpha motor neurons, muscle spindle primary endings, Golgi tendon organs, touch
  - **Beta:** touch, kinesthesia, muscle spindle secondary endings
  - **Gamma:** touch, pressure, gamma motor neurons
  - **Delta:** pain, touch, pressure, temperature

- Sensory components include:
  - **Muscle spindle (primary afferent endings):** primary for low-threshold stretch
  - **Muscle spindle (secondary afferent endings):** receptors that respond to changes in length
  - **Golgi tendon organ:** responds to tension/stretch of a tendon

**B Fibers**

- Medium fibers
- Myelinated
- Reasonably fast conduction rate
- Pre-ganglionic fibers of the autonomic system

**C Fibers**

- Small fibers
- Poorly myelinated or unmyelinated
- Slowed conduction rate
- Post-ganglionic fibers of the sympathetic system
- Exteroceptors for pain, temperature, and touch

# Nerve Root Dermatomes, Myotomes, Reflexes, and Paresthetic Areas[21]

| Nerve Root | Dermatome* | Muscle Weakness (Myotome) | Reflexes Affected | Paresthesias |
|---|---|---|---|---|
| C1 | Vertex of skull | None | None | None |
| C2 | Temple, forehead, occiput | Longus colli, sternocleidomastoid, rectus capitis | None | None |
| C3 | Entire neck, posterior cheek, temporal area, prolongation forward under mandible | Trapezius, splenius capitis | None | Cheek, side of neck |
| C4 | Shoulder area, clavicular area, upper scapular area | Trapezius, levator scapulae | None | Horizontal band along clavicle and upper scapula |
| C5 | Deltoid area, anterior aspect of entire arm to base of thumb | Supraspinatus, infraspinatus, deltoid, biceps | Biceps, brachioradialis | None |
| C6 | Anterior arm, radial side of hand to thumb and index finger | Biceps, supinator, wrist extensors | Biceps, brachioradialis | Thumb and index finger |
| C7 | Lateral arm and forearm to index, long, and ring fingers | Triceps, wrist flexors (rarely, wrist extensors) | Triceps | Index, long, and ring fingers |
| C8 | Medial arm and forearm to long, ring, and little fingers | Ulnar deviators, thumb extensors, thumb adductors (rarely, triceps) | None | Little finger alone or with two adjacent fingers; not ring or long fingers, alone or together (C7) |

# Nerve Root Dermatomes, Myotomes, Reflexes, and Paresthetic Areas[21]

| Nerve Root | Dermatome* | Muscle Weakness (Myotome) | Reflexes Affected | Paresthesias |
|---|---|---|---|---|
| T1 | Medial side of forearm to base of little finger | | | |
| T2 | Medial side of upper arm to medial elbow, pectoral and midscapular areas | Disk lesions at upper two thoracic levels do not appear to give rise to root weakness. Weakness of intrinsic muscles of the hand is due to other pathology (e.g., thoracic outlet pressure, neoplasm of lung, and ulnar nerve lesion). | | |
| T3 – T12 | T3-T6, upper thorax; T5-T7, costal margin; T8-T12, abdomen and lumbar region | Articular and dural signs and root pain are common. Root signs (cutaneous analgesia) are rare and have such indefinite area that they have little localizing value. Weakness is not detectable. | | |
| L1 | Back, over trochanter and groin | None | None | Groin; after holding posture, which causes pain |
| L2 | Back, front of thigh to knee | Psoas, hip adductors | None | Occasionally anterior thigh |
| L3 | Back, upper buttock, anterior thigh and knee, medial lower leg | Psoas, quadriceps, thigh atrophy | Knee jerk sluggish, PKB positive, pain on full SLR | Medial knee, anterior lower leg |
| L4 | Medial buttock, lateral thigh, medial leg, dorsum of foot, big toe | Tibialis anterior, extensor hallucis | SLR limited, neck flexion pain, weak or absent knee jerk, side flexion limited | Medial aspect of calf and ankle |
| L5 | Buttock, posterior and lateral thigh, lateral aspect of leg, dorsum of foot, medial half of sole, first, second, and third toes | Extensor hallucis, peroneals, gluteus medius, dorsiflexors, hamstrings and calf atrophy | SLR limited one side, neck flexion painful, ankle decreased, crossed-leg raising pain | Lateral aspect of leg, medial three toes |
| S1 | Lateral and plantar aspect of foot | Calf and hamstrings, wasting of gluteals, peroneals, plantar flexors | SLR limited, Achilles reflex weak or absent | Lateral two toes, lateral foot, lateral leg to knee, plantar aspect of foot |
| S2 | Buttock, thigh, and leg posterior | Same as S1 except peroneals | Same as S1 | Lateral leg, knee, and heel |
| S3 | Groin, medial thigh to knee | None | None | None |
| S4 | Perineum, genitals, lower sacrum | Bladder, rectum | None | Saddle area, genitals, anus, impotence, massive posterior herniation |

*In any part of which pain may be felt. PKB = prone knee bending; SLR = straight leg raising.

Adapted from Magee, DJ: Orthopedic Physical Assessment. W.B. Saunders Company, Philadelphia 2002, p.16, with permission.

## Cranial Nerves and Methods of Testing[21]

| Nerve | Afferent (Sensory) | Efferent (Motor) | Test |
|---|---|---|---|
| Olfactory | Smell: Nose | | Identify familiar odors (e.g., chocolate, coffee) |
| Optic | Sight: Eye | | Test visual fields |
| Oculomotor | | Voluntary motor: Levator of eyelid; superior, medial, and inferior recti; inferior oblique muscle of eyeball<br>Autonomic: Smooth muscle of eyeball | Upward, downward, and medial gaze<br>Reaction to light |
| Trochlear | | Voluntary motor: Superior oblique muscle of eyeball | Downward and lateral gaze |
| Trigeminal | Touch, pain: Skin of face, mucous membranes of nose, sinuses, mouth, anterior tongue | Voluntary motor: Muscles of mastication | Corneal reflex<br>Face sensation<br>Clench teeth; push down on chin to separate jaws |
| Abducens | | Voluntary motor: Lateral rectus muscle of eyeball | Lateral gaze |
| Facial | Taste: Anterior tongue | Voluntary motor: Facial muscles<br>Autonomic: Lacrimal, submandibular, and sublingual glands | Close eyes tight<br>Smile and show teeth<br>Whistle and puff cheeks<br>Identify familiar tastes (e.g., sweet, sour) |
| Vestibulocochlear (acoustic nerve) | Hearing: Ear<br>Balance: Ear | | Hear watch ticking<br>Hearing tests<br>Balance and coordination tests |
| Glossopharyngeal | Touch, pain: Posterior tongue, pharynx<br>Taste: Posterior tongue | Voluntary motor: Select muscle of pharynx<br>Autonomic: Parotid gland | Gag reflex<br>Ability to swallow |
| Vagus | Touch, pain: Pharynx, larynx, bronchi<br>Taste: Tongue, epiglottis | Voluntary motor: Muscles of palate, pharynx, and larynx<br>Autonomic: Thoracic and abdominal viscera | Gag reflex<br>Ability to swallow<br>Say "Ahhh" |
| Accessory | | Voluntary motor: Sternocleidomastoid and trapezius muscle | Resisted shoulder shrug |
| Hypoglossal | | Voluntary motor: Muscles of tongue | Tongue protrusion (if injured, tongue deviates toward injured side) |

From Magee, DJ: Orthopedic Physical Assessment. W.B. Saunders Company, Philadelphia 2002, p.69, with permission.

## Cranial Nerve Testing Procedures[21,22]

The cranial nerves refer to twelve pairs of nerves that have their origin in the brain. Certain cranial nerves contain both sensory and motor fibers, however, many possess either sensory or motor fibers. Since lesions affecting the cranial nerves produce specific and predictable alterations, it is often prudent to perform cranial nerve testing as part of a neurological examination. The following information is a summary of some of the more common methods of testing selected cranial nerves.

### Cranial Nerve I - Olfactory

The patient is positioned in sitting with the eyes closed or blindfolded. The therapist places an item with a familiar odor under the patient's nostril and the patient is asked to identify the odor. A positive test may be indicated by an inability to identify familiar odors.

### Cranial Nerve II - Optic

The patient is positioned in standing a selected distance from a chart or diagram. The therapist asks the patient to identify objects or read selected items from the chart or diagram. A positive test may be indicated by an inability to identify objects at a reasonable distance.

### Cranial Nerve III - Oculomotor

The patient is positioned in sitting and is asked to follow an object such as a writing utensil with their eyes as it is moved vertically, horizontally, and diagonally. The therapist should make sure the patient does not rotate their head during the testing and should inspect the patient's eyes for asymmetry or ptosis. A positive test is indicated by an identified tracking deficit, asymmetry or ptosis.

### Cranial Nerve IV - Trochlear (Fig. 5-7)

The patient is positioned in sitting and asked to follow an object such as a writing utensil with their eyes as it is moved in an inferior direction. The therapist should make sure the patient does not move his head downward. A positive test is indicated by an inability to depress the eyes and/or complaints of diplopia.

**Fig. 5-7:** Examination of the trochlear nerve. The patient should be able to follow the tongue depressor as it is moved in an inferior direction without moving the head.

### Cranial Nerve V - Trigeminal

The patient is positioned in sitting and is asked to close their eyes. The therapist uses a piece of cotton and a safety pin to alternately touch the patient's face. The patient is asked to classify each contact with the face as "sharp" or "dull." A positive test for the sensory component may be identified by impaired or absent sensation or the inability to differentiate between "sharp" or "dull." The motor component is tested by asking the patient to perform mandibular protrusion, retrusion, and lateral deviation. A positive test may be indicated by an impaired ability to move the mandible through the specified motions.

### Cranial Nerve VI - Abducens (Fig. 5-8)

The patient is positioned in sitting. The therapist asks the patient to abduct their eyes without rotating the head. A positive test is indicated by an inability to abduct the eyes.

**Fig. 5-8:** Examination of the abducens nerve. The patient should be able to abduct the eyes without moving the head.

### Cranial Nerve VII - Facial (Fig. 5-9)

The patient is positioned in sitting and is asked to distinguish between sweet and salty substances placed on the anterior portion of the tongue. A positive test for the sensory component may be identified by an inability to accurately identify sweet and salty substances. The motor component is tested by performing a manual muscle test of selected muscles involved in facial expression. A positive test for the motor component may be indicated by an inability to mimic selected facial expressions due to muscle impairment.

**Fig. 5-9:** Examination of the facial nerve. The patient should be able to mimic facial expressions. The sensory component of the nerve distinguishes between sweet and salty taste over the anterior tongue.

## Cranial Nerve VIII - Vestibulocochlear

The patient is positioned in sitting in a quiet location. The therapist, positioned behind the patient and to one side, slowly brings a ticking watch toward the patient's ear. The therapist records the distance from the ear when the patient is able to identify the ticking sound. The therapist repeats the procedure on the contralateral ear and compares the measurements. A positive test is indicated by an inability to hear the ticking sound at 18-24 inches or a significant bilateral difference. Alternate tests include the Weber and Rinne tests which require a 512 Hz tuning fork.

## Cranial Nerve IX - Glossopharyngeal (Fig. 5-10)

The patient is positioned in sitting. The therapist touches the pharynx with a tongue depressor. A positive test may be indicated by lack of gagging or an inability to feel the tongue depressor touch the back of the throat. The sensory component is tested by assessing the patient's ability to distinguish objects by taste after they are placed on the posterior portion of the tongue. A positive test for the sensory component may be identified by an inability to accurately identify tasted substances, especially sour and bitter substances, placed on the posterior third of the tongue.

**Fig. 5-10:** Examination of the glossopharyngeal and vagus nerves. The tongue depressor on the tongue should produce a gag response.

## Cranial Nerve X - Vagus (Fig. 5-10)

The patient is positioned in sitting. The therapist touches the pharynx with a tongue depressor. A positive test may be indicated by a lack of gagging or an inability to feel the tongue depressor touch the back of the throat (same description for Cranial Nerve IX - Glossopharyngeal). If the gag reflex is absent the therapist should carefully assess the movement of the soft palate and uvula.

## Cranial Nerve XI - Accessory (Fig. 5-11)

The patient is positioned in sitting with the arms at the side. The therapist asks the patient to shrug their shoulders and maintain the position while the therapist applies resistance through the shoulders in the direction of shoulder depression. A positive test may be indicated by an inability to maintain the test position against resistance.

**Fig. 5-11:** Examination of the accessory nerve. The patient should be able to maintain a shoulder shrug against resistance.

## Cranial Nerve XII - Hypoglossal (Fig. 5-12)

The patient is positioned in sitting. The therapist asks the patient to protrude the tongue. A positive test may be indicated by an inability to fully protrude the tongue or the tongue deviating to one side during protrusion.

**Fig. 5-12:** Examination of the hypoglossal nerve. The patient should be able to protrude the tongue in a symmetrical fashion.

# Nerves of the Brachial Plexus[23]

| Origin | Nerves | Muscles |
|---|---|---|
| From the rami of the plexus | Dorsal scapular | Rhomboids<br>Levator scapulae |
| | Long thoracic | Serratus anterior |
| From the trunks of the plexus | Nerve to subclavius | Subclavius |
| | Suprascapular | Infraspinatus<br>Supraspinatus |
| From the lateral cord of the plexus | Lateral pectoral | Pectoralis major - clavicular head |
| | Musculocutaneous | Coracobrachialis<br>Biceps brachii<br>Brachialis |
| | Lateral root of the median | Flexor muscles in the forearm, except flexor carpi ulnaris, and five muscles in the hand |
| From the medial cord of the plexus | Medial pectoral | Pectoralis major<br>Pectoralis minor |
| | Ulnar | Flexor carpi ulnaris<br>Flexor digitorum profundus<br>Most small muscles of the hand |
| | Medial root of the median | Flexor muscles in the forearm, except flexor carpi ulnaris, and five muscles of the hand |
| From the posterior cord of the plexus | Upper subscapular | Subscapularis |
| | Thoracodorsal | Latissimus dorsi |
| | Lower subscapular | Subscapularis<br>Teres major |
| | Axillary | Deltoid<br>Teres minor |
| | Radial | Brachioradialis<br>Triceps<br>Supinator<br>Wrist extensors<br>Anconeus |

# Lower Extremity Innervation[23]

| Lumbar Plexus | Sciatic Nerve - Tibial Division |
|---|---|
| Psoas major<br>Psoas minor<br>Quadratus lumborum | Semitendinosus<br>Semimembranosus<br>Biceps femoris (long head) |

| Sacral Plexus | Sciatic Nerve - Common Peroneal Division |
|---|---|
| Piriformis<br>Superior gemelli<br>Inferior gemelli<br>Obturator internus<br>Quadratus femoris | Biceps femoris (short head) |

| Inferior Gluteal Nerve | Deep Peroneal Nerve |
|---|---|
| Gluteus maximus | Tibialis anterior<br>Extensor digitorum longus<br>Extensor hallucis longus<br>Peroneus tertius<br>Extensor digitorum brevis |

| Superior Gluteal Nerve | Superficial Peroneal Nerve |
|---|---|
| Gluteus medius<br>Gluteus minimus<br>Tensor fasciae latae | Peroneus longus<br>Peroneus brevis |

| Femoral Nerve | Medial Plantar Nerve |
|---|---|
| Vastus lateralis<br>Rectus femoris<br>Vastus medialis<br>Vastus intermedius<br>Iliacus<br>Sartorius<br>Pectineus | Abductor hallucis<br>Lumbrical I<br>Flexor digitorum brevis<br>Flexor hallucis brevis |

| Obturator Nerve | Lateral Plantar Nerve |
|---|---|
| Adductor longus<br>Adductor brevis<br>Adductor magnus<br>Obturator externus<br>Gracilis | Abductor digiti minimi<br>Flexor digiti minimi<br>Opponens digiti minimi<br>Dorsal interossei<br>Quadratus plantae<br>Adductor hallucis<br>Lumbrical II, III, IV<br>Plantar interossei |

| Tibial Nerve | |
|---|---|
| Soleus<br>Popliteus<br>Plantaris<br>Tibialis posterior<br>Gastrocnemius<br>Flexor hallucis longus<br>Flexor digitorum longus | |

## Superficial Reflexes[6,22]

A reflex is a motor response to a sensory stimulation that is used to examine the integrity of the nervous system. Superficial reflexes are a response to stimulation of the receptors within the skin. Superficial reflexes are quite different from the muscle stretch (or deep tendon) reflexes since the sensory signal must reach the spinal cord, and must ascend the cord to reach the brain. The motor component also must descend the spinal cord to reach the motor neurons making this a polysynaptic reflex.

## Procedure Guidelines for Superficial Reflex Testing[6,22]

- The patient should be relaxed and understand the testing procedure.
- Position the patient properly.
- Reflexes are typically graded as present or absent, although a large difference between left and right will also indicate an abnormal response.
- The examination should provide a comparison of both sides of the body.
- Examination results should assist the therapist to recognize a deficit within the nervous system.

| | Superficial Reflex Testing[22] | | |
|---|---|---|---|
| **Common Superficial Reflexes** | **Spinal Level** | **Procedure** | **Normal Response** |
| **Abdominal reflex** | T8-L1 | stroke briskly and lightly with a blunt object (tongue depressor) from each quadrant of the abdomen in a diagonal manner towards the umbilicus | contraction of the abdominals and deviation of the umbilicus in the direction of stimulus |
| **Corneal "blink" reflex** | trigeminal and facial nerves | ask the patient to look up and away from you; stroke the cornea using a piece of cotton | both eyes will blink with contact to one eye |
| **Cremasteric reflex** | L1-L2 | scratch the skin of the upper medial thigh | a brisk and brief elevation of the testicle on the ipsilateral side |
| **Gag reflex** | glossopharyngeal and vagus nerves | the therapist lightly stimulates each side of the back of the throat and notes the reaction | a gag will occur post stimulation; may be absent in some percentage of the normal population |
| **Plantar reflex** (Fig. 5-13) | L5-S1 | stroke the lateral aspect of the sole of the foot with the blunt end of a reflex hammer from the heel to the ball of the foot and medially to the base of the great toe | flexion of the toes *Babinski reflex is the abnormal response that indicates CNS lesion (Fig. 5-14) |

**Fig. 5-13:** A normal plantar reflex response.

**Fig. 5-14:** A positive Babinski reflex response.

- Avoid "pecking" at the tendon with the hammer as this will not produce valid results.
- Reflexes can be graded as depressed (hypo), normal or exaggerated (hyper) on a scale of 0-4.
- If the therapist has difficulty eliciting a reflex, the Jendrassik maneuver should be employed to distract the patient, increase reflex activity, and decrease guarding. The patient can be directed to perform the Jendrassik maneuver by locking the fingers together and directly pulling against each other immediately prior to the reflex stimulus.
- The examination should provide a comparison of both sides of the body and should include all deep tendon reflexes.
- The examination should provide a comparison of "normal" areas to suspected areas of impairment.
- Examination results should assist the therapist to identify deficits within the nervous system.

## Deep Tendon Reflexes[6,22,24]

Deep tendon reflexes (DTR) elicit a muscle contraction when the muscle's tendon is stimulated due to the reflex arc involving the spinal or brainstem segment that innervates the specific muscle. Hyperreflexia refers to hyperactivity or clonic reflexes. This can be indicative of a suprasegmental lesion (a lesion above the level of the spinal reflex pathways). Hyporeflexia refers to a diminished or absent response to tapping of the tendon. This can be indicative of disease that involves one or multiple components of the reflex arc itself.

### Procedure Guidelines for Deep Tendon Reflex Testing[6,22]

- The patient should be relaxed and understand the testing procedure.
- Position the patient properly and symmetrically with the muscle placed on a slight stretch.
- A reflex hammer should be utilized to deliver a direct strike on the tendon with an anticipated immediate response (Fig. 5-15).

**Fig. 5-15:** A standard reflex hammer used to assess deep tendon reflexes.

| Reflex Grading Scale[25] | |
| --- | --- |
| **Reflex Grading** | **Interpretation** |
| 0 = no response | always abnormal |
| 1+ = diminished/depressed response | may or may not be normal |
| 2+ = active normal response | normal |
| 3+ = brisk/exaggerated response | may or may not be normal |
| 4+ = very brisk/hyperactive; abnormal response | always abnormal |

## Deep Tendon Reflex Testing[6,22,25]

### Biceps tendon (Fig. 5-16)

**Spinal Level:** C5-C6
**Procedure:** support the elbow in partial flexion in sitting or supine; place the thumb firmly over the biceps tendon at the elbow and strike the hammer through the thumb
**Normal Response:** Contraction of the biceps muscle; flexion of the elbow

Fig. 5-16: Examination of the biceps deep tendon reflex.

### Brachioradialis tendon (Fig. 5-17)

**Spinal Level:** C5-C6
**Procedure:** rest the hand on the lap in sitting with the forearm supported and in neutral; strike the radius one to two inches superior to the wrist
**Normal Response:** Contraction of the brachioradialis muscle; elbow flexion and/or forearm supination

Fig. 5-17: Examination of the brachioradialis deep tendon reflex.

### Triceps tendon (Fig. 5-18)

**Spinal Level:** C6-C7
**Procedure:** support the upper extremity through the humerus and allow the lower portion to hang with elbow flexion; strike the triceps tendon directly above the elbow
**Normal Response:** Contraction of the triceps muscle; elbow extension

Fig. 5-18: Examination of the triceps deep tendon reflex.

### Patellar tendon (Fig. 5-19)

**Spinal Level:** L3-L4
**Procedure:** supported knee flexion with the patient in sitting or supine; strike the tendon directly inferior to the patella
**Normal Response:** Contraction of the quadriceps; knee extension

**Fig. 5-19:** Examination of the patellar deep tendon reflex.

### Achilles tendon (Fig. 5-20)

**Spinal Level:** S1-S2
**Procedure:** in sitting, flex the foot at the ankle putting the Achilles on stretch; strike the Achilles tendon above the foot
**Normal Response:** Plantar flexion of the foot

**Fig. 5-20:** Examination of the Achilles deep tendon reflex.

# Spotlight on Safety
## Clinical Relevance of Reflex Testing[25]

**Deep tendon reflex (DTR)** testing can assist the therapist in determining the type of pathology that exists. Absent DTRs will indicate a lesion in the reflex arc itself. If absent reflexes accompany sensory loss in the distribution of the nerve that is supplying a particular reflex, the lesion is found within the afferent arc of the reflex and is located in either the nerve or dorsal horn. If an absent DTR accompanies paralysis, fasciculations or atrophy, the lesion is found within the efferent arc of the reflex and may include the efferent nerve, anterior horn cells or both.

**Peripheral neuropathy** is the most common etiology surrounding absent reflexes. Associated conditions can include diabetes, alcoholism, vitamin deficiencies such as pernicious anemia, certain cancers, and certain toxins (lead, arsenic, vincristine). Neuropathies will typically present with sensory, motor or mixed impairments and may affect all components of the reflex arc.

**Hyperactive DTRs** are found when there is interruption of the cortical supply to the lower motor neuron (secondary to upper motor neuron lesion). The interruption exists above the segment of the reflex arc, with other findings determining localization of the exact lesion. Assessment of the DTRs can provide information as to the level of lesion that exists within the central nervous system.

## Sensation

There are several types of sensation that a physical therapist will evaluate including superficial, deep (proprioceptive), and cortical (combined) sensations. A therapist should examine superficial and deep sensations first, followed by cortical sensations.

- **Superficial:** temperature, light touch, pain
- **Deep:** proprioception, kinesthesia, vibration
- **Cortical:** bilateral simultaneous stimulation, stereognosis, two-point discrimination, barognosis, localization of touch

### Procedure Guidelines for Sensory Testing[6,22]

- The patient should be relaxed and understand the expectations of the required response.
- The examination should be conducted in an efficient manner so that the sensory system does not fatigue and allow for unreliable responses.
- The patient's vision should be obscured or the patient blindfolded so that their vision does not influence the perceived sensation.
- The pace of the examination should vary so that the patient does not expect a stimulus or respond merely to the rhythm of the test.
- The therapist should have a complete understanding of areas of the skin that have heightened or decreased sensitivity based on the type of sensation that is tested (i.e., temperature versus light touch).
- The examination should provide a comparison of both sides of the body and should include all extremities and the trunk.
- The examination should provide a comparison of "normal" areas to suspected areas of impairment.
- The examination should provide a comparison of distal versus proximal response for each tested area.
- The therapist may examine dermatomes and peripheral nerve distribution or patterns of sensation such as:
  - bilateral shoulders - C4
  - medial and lateral aspects of bilateral forearms - C6 to T1
  - thumbs and little fingers - C6 and C8
  - bilateral anterior thighs - L2 and L3
  - medial and lateral aspects of bilateral lower legs (calf)- L4 and L5
  - bilateral little toes - S1
  - saddle area - S4
- Examination results should assist the therapist to recognize the deficit as CNS, plexus or peripheral nerve pattern damage.
- Patients with sensory deficits or who are at risk for sensory impairments should be tested using Semmes Weinstein monofilaments for objective data collection regarding protective sensation (Figs. 5-21, 5-22, 5-23).

**Fig. 5-21:** Semmes Weinstein monofilaments.

**Fig. 5-22:** Testing protocol requires the monofilament to be held perpendicular to the surface tested.

**Fig. 5-23:** Proper pressure has been applied when the monofilament deforms.

## Consider This

### Screening of Superficial, Deep, and Cortical Sensations[6,26]

When screening a patient's sensation, there are typical stimuli that produce an expected response that measures a patient's sensation as normal or impaired.

- **Barognosis:** perceive the weight of different objects in the hand
- **Deep pain:** squeeze the forearm or calf muscle
- **Graphesthesia:** identify a number or letter drawn on the skin without visual input
- **Kinesthesia:** identify direction and extent of movement of a joint or body part
- **Light touch:** perceive touch through light pressure or use of a cotton ball
- **Localization:** ability to identify the exact location of light touch on the body using a verbal response or gesturing
- **Proprioception:** identify a static position of an extremity or body part
- **Stereognosis:** identify an object without sight (Fig. 5-24)
- **Superficial pain:** perceive noxious stimulus using a pen cap, paper clip end or pin
- **Temperature:** perceive warm and cold test tubes
- **Two-point discrimination:** using a two-point caliper on the skin, identify one or two points without visual input (Fig. 5-25)
- **Vibration:** tuning fork

Impairment found with any of the above sensations may designate lesion or pathology to a particular pathway or region of the brain. The therapist can utilize this information to enhance understanding of the neurological impairment as well as to customize the plan of care.

Fig. 5-24: The patient is trying to identify the paper clip without visual feedback and using only the sense of touch. This is an examination of stereognosis.

Fig. 5-25: Examination of two-point discrimination.

## Sensory Testing[6,22,25]

### Light touch (Fig. 5-26)

- instruct and demonstrate the testing procedure to the patient and ask for a response
- attempt to initiate the testing in a normal area so the patient can anticipate what to expect
- performed through touching the skin lightly or using cotton
- with eyes closed, ask patient to identify when they feel a touch
- compare sides of the body, proximal versus distal areas, and identify patterns or innervation level of impairment

**Fig. 5-26:** Examination of light touch sensation using a cotton ball.

### Pain (Fig. 5-27)

- instruct and demonstrate the testing procedure to the patient and have them note the sharp versus dull side of a pin or appropriate instrument such as a Wartenberg pinwheel (Fig. 5-28)
- performed through touching the skin while alternating in a random fashion between the sharp and dull ends of the pin
- attempt to initiate the testing in an intact area so the patient can anticipate what to expect
- with eyes closed, ask the patient to identify if they feel a sharp or dull sensation
- allow the patient to make comparisons by asking if the stimulus is the same or different when testing different areas
- compare sides of the body, proximal versus distal areas, identify patterns or innervation level of impairment

**Fig. 5-27 (Left):** Examination of sharp versus dull sensation using a Wartenberg pinwheel.

**Fig. 5-28 (Right):** Wartenberg pinwheels.

### Temperature

- temperature discrimination should utilize test tubes, warm water in one and cold water in the other
- avoid extreme temperatures as this is a test of discrimination, not of a patient's tolerance to extreme temperatures
- instruct and demonstrate the testing procedure to the patient with the expectation of a response of "hot" or "cold" for each stimulus
- attempt to initiate the testing in an intact area so the patient can anticipate what to expect
- touch the skin while alternating in a random fashion between the warm and cold test tubes

- with eyes closed, ask the patient to identify if they sense a warm or cold temperature
- allow the patient to make comparisons by asking if the stimulus is the same temperature or a different temperature when testing different areas
- compare sides of the body, proximal versus distal areas, identify patterns or distribution levels of impairment
- testing for temperature discrimination will also predict pain sensation since there are sensory receptors with each modality that overlap

## Sensory Testing[6,22,25]

### Vibration (Fig. 5-29)

- instruct and demonstrate the testing procedure to the patient
- preferably performed using a 128 Hz tuning fork and alternating the testing with vibration and without vibration (Fig. 5-30)
- initiate the test by tapping the tuning fork to produce vibration and placing it over the interphalangeal joint of a patient's finger or the interphalangeal joint of the great toe
- with eyes closed, ask patient to identify what they feel
- strike the tuning fork tines with each attempt, but stop the vibration on intermittent trials to ensure that the patient will recognize vibration versus touch or pressure
- if there is impairment, test bony prominences proximally including the wrist, elbow, spinous processes, clavicles, medial malleolus, patella, ASIS, etc.
- allow the patient to make comparisons by asking if the stimulus is the same or different when testing the different bony areas of a limb or right versus left sides of the body

**Fig. 5-29 (Above):** Examination of vibration using a tuning fork.

**Fig. 5-30 (Below):** A tuning fork.

### Pressure

- instruct and demonstrate the testing procedure to the patient and ask for a response
- attempt to initiate the testing in an intact area so the patient can anticipate what to expect
- touch the skin with a fingertip using direct pressure firm enough to stimulate the deep receptors
- with eyes closed, ask patient to identify when they feel anything

- alternate light touch and deep pressure with the patient responding "light" or "deep"
- compare sides of the body, proximal versus distal areas, identify patterns or distribution level of impairment

## Consider This

### Abnormalities in Sensory Perception[2,17,20]

When treating a patient with peripheral nerve damage, all areas of the face, trunk, and extremities should be assessed for each modality of sensation and documented. Sensation should be tested without the influence of visual feedback to the patient so that the results are not influenced by what a patient anticipates as the response to the stimuli that the therapist provides. Sensory testing requires patience and practice in order to generate the most accurate results.

- **Allodynia:** the sensation of pain in response to a stimulus that would not typically produce pain
- **Analgesia:** the absence of pain while remaining conscious
- **Anesthesia:** the absence of touch sensation
- **Causalgia:** constant, relentless, burning hyperesthesia and hyperalgesia that develops after a peripheral nerve injury
- **Dysesthesia:** distortion of any of the senses, especially the sense of touch
- **Hyperesthesia:** heightened sensation
- **Hyperpathia:** an extreme exaggerated response to pain
- **Hypesthesia:** a diminished sensation of touch
- **Neuralgia:** severe and multiple shock-like pains that radiate from a specific nerve distribution
- **Pallanesthesia:** loss of vibration sensation
- **Paresthesia:** abnormal sensations such as tingling, pins and needles or burning sensations

## Peripheral Nerve Lesions[20]

A lesion of the nerve can occur through many mechanisms of injury. Possible etiologies include mechanical (compression injury), crush and percussion (fracture, compartment syndrome), laceration, penetrating trauma (stab wound), stretch (traction injury), high velocity trauma (motor vehicle accident), and cold (frostbite). When there is peripheral nerve degeneration, the voluntary muscles first exhibit an altered response to acetylcholine, with wasting of the sarcoplasm and loss of fibrils. This results in total loss of muscle over time with replacement by fibrous tissues.

**Double crush syndrome:** existence of two separate lesions along the same nerve that create more severe symptoms than if only one lesion existed

**Mononeuropathy:** an isolated nerve lesion; associated conditions include trauma and entrapment

**Neuroma:** abnormal growth of nerve cells; associated conditions include vasculitis, AIDS, and amyloidosis

**Peripheral neuropathy:** impairment or dysfunction of the peripheral nerves; associated conditions include diabetic peripheral neuropathy, trauma, alcoholism

**Polyneuropathy:** diffuse nerve dysfunction that is symmetrical and typically secondary to pathology and not trauma; associated conditions include Guillain-Barre syndrome, peripheral neuropathy, use of neurotoxic drugs, and HIV

**Wallerian degeneration:** degeneration that occurs distally, specifically to the myelin sheath and axon

### Classification of Acute Nerve Injuries[9,27]

**Neurapraxia**

- Mildest form of injury
- Conduction block usually due to myelin dysfunction
- Axonal continuity preserved
- Axons, epineurium, perineurium, and endoneurium intact
- Nerve conduction is preserved proximal and distal to the lesion
- Nerve fibers are not damaged, no evidence of nerve degeneration is noted
- Symptoms include pain, minimal muscle atrophy, numbness or greater loss of motor and sensory function, diminished proprioception
- Recovery is rapid and complete and will occur within 4-6 weeks
- Pressure injuries are the most common

## Consider This

### Peripheral Nerve Injury: Typical Etiologies[2,13,20]

Both upper and lower extremity nerves have typical etiologies that subsequently produce specific patterns of impingement or compression injuries.

In the upper extremity, brachial plexus injuries can result from trauma, penetration, traction or compression. The following lists common etiologies associated with specific nerve injuries.

**Axillary:** fracture of the neck of the humerus, anterior dislocation of the shoulder

**Musculocutaneous:** fracture of the clavicle

**Radial:** compression of the nerve in the radial tunnel, fracture of the humerus

**Median:** compression in the carpal tunnel, pronator teres entrapment

**Ulnar:** compression in the cubital tunnel, entrapment in Guyon's canal

In the lower extremity, many nerve injuries for women are secondary to labor, delivery or surgical procedures around the pelvis. The following lists common etiologies associated with specific nerve injuries.

**Femoral:** total hip arthroplasty, displaced acetabular fracture, anterior dislocation of the femur, hysterectomy, appendectomy

**Sciatic:** blunt force trauma to the buttocks, total hip arthroplasty, accidental injection to the nerve

**Obturator:** fixation of a femur fracture, total hip arthroplasty

**Peroneal:** femur, tibia or fibula fracture, positioning during surgical procedures

**Tibial:** tarsal tunnel entrapment, popliteal fossa compression

**Sural:** fracture of the calcaneus or lateral malleolus

Recovery is based on the degree of injury and potential for regeneration of the nerve. The majority of research indicates that children tend to have better outcomes after peripheral nerve damage than adults, although some research sees no difference between the populations. The earlier repair of a nerve yields a better outcome; the more distal the lesion, the better the outcome secondary to the nerve length that requires recovery.

## Axonotmesis

- A more severe grade of injury to a peripheral nerve

- Reversible injury to damaged fibers since they maintain an anatomical relationship to each other

- Damage occurs to the axons with preservation of the endoneurium (neural connective tissue sheath), epineurium, Schwann cells, and supporting structures

- Distal Wallerian degeneration can occur

- The nerve can regenerate distal to the site of the lesion at a rate of one millimeter per day

- Recovery is spontaneous and varies from spotty to no recovery; surgery may be required for repair

- Traction, compression, and crush injuries are the most common

## Neurotmesis

- The most severe grade of injury to a peripheral nerve

- Axon, myelin, connective tissue components are all damaged or transected

- Irreversible injury; no possibility of regeneration

- Flaccid paralysis and wasting of muscles occur; total loss of sensation to area supplied by the nerve

- All motor and sensory loss distal to the lesion becomes permanently impaired

- No spontaneous recovery; with surgical reattachment, potential regenerating axons may grow at one millimeter per day with proximal recovery first; sensory recovery occurs sooner than motor fibers

- Complete transection of the nerve trunk

## Peripheral Nervous System Pathology[2,3,9]

### Anterior Horn Cell

- Sensory component intact
- Motor weakness and atrophy
- Fasciculations
- Decreased deep tendon reflexes
- **Example:** amyotrophic lateral sclerosis (ALS), poliomyelitis

### Muscle

- Sensory component intact
- Motor weakness; fasciculations are rare
- Normal or decreased deep tendon reflexes
- **Example:** muscular dystrophy

### Neuromuscular Junction

- Sensory component intact
- Motor fatigue is greater than actual weakness
- Normal deep tendon reflexes
- **Example:** myasthenia gravis

### Peripheral Nerve (Mononeuropathy)

- Sensory loss along the nerve route
- Motor weakness and atrophy in a peripheral distribution; may have fasciculations
- **Example:** trauma

### Peripheral Polyneuropathy

- Sensory impairments; "stocking glove" distribution
- Motor weakness and atrophy; weaker distally than proximally; may have fasciculations
- Decreased deep tendon reflexes
- **Example:** diabetic peripheral polyneuropathy

### Spinal Roots and Nerves

- Sensory component will have corresponding dermatomal deficits
- Motor weakness in an innervated pattern; may have fasciculations
- Decreased deep tendon reflexes
- **Example:** herniated disk

## Upper Motor Neuron Disease

An upper motor neuron disease is characterized by a lesion found in descending motor tracts within the cerebral motor cortex, internal capsule, brainstem, or spinal cord. Symptoms include weakness of involved muscles, hypertonicity, hyperreflexia, mild disuse atrophy, and abnormal reflexes. Damaged tracts are in the lateral white column of the spinal cord.

**Examples of upper motor neuron lesions include:**

- cerebral palsy
- hydrocephalus
- ALS (both upper and lower)
- CVA
- birth injuries
- multiple sclerosis
- Huntington's chorea
- traumatic brain injury
- pseudobulbar palsy
- brain tumors

## Lower Motor Neuron Disease

A lower motor neuron disease is characterized by a lesion that affects nerves or their axons at or below the level of the brainstem, usually within the "final common pathway." The ventral gray column of the spinal cord may also be affected. Symptoms include flaccidity or weakness of the involved muscles, decreased tone, fasciculations, muscle atrophy, and decreased or absent reflexes.

**Examples of lower motor neuron lesions include:**

- poliomyelitis
- ALS (both upper and lower)
- Guillain-Barre syndrome
- tumors involving the spinal cord
- trauma
- progressive muscular atrophy
- infection
- Bell's palsy
- carpal tunnel syndrome
- muscular dystrophy
- spinal muscular atrophy

## Upper versus Lower Motor Neuron Disease[1,2,3]

|  | UMND | LMND |
|---|---|---|
| **Reflexes** | Hyperactive | Diminished or absent |
| **Atrophy** | Mild from disuse | Present |
| **Fasciculations** | Absent | Present |
| **Tone** | Hypertonic | Hypotonic to flaccid |

## Involuntary Movement/Movement Disorders[1,6,22]

An involuntary movement is defined as a movement that the person does not start or stop at the person's own command or with an observer's command. Muscle fiber contractions of either central or peripheral origin can create small or large scale patterns. Common forms of hypokinesia include apraxia, rigidity, and bradykinesia. Common forms of hyperkinesia include ataxia, athetosis, chorea, tics, tremors, dysmetria, and dystonia. Select movement disorders are highlighted below.

### Tremors

Tremors are involuntary, rhythmic, oscillatory movements that are typically classified into three groupings:

- **Resting:** Tremors are observable at rest and may or may not disappear with movement; may increase with mental stress. An example is the pill-rolling tremor associated with Parkinson's disease.
- **Postural:** Tremors are observable during a voluntary contraction to maintain a posture. Examples include the rapid tremor associated with hyperthyroidism, fatigue or anxiety, and benign essential tremor.
- **Intention (kinetic):** Tremors are absent at rest, but observable with activity and typically increase as the target approaches. These tremors likely indicate a lesion of the cerebellum or its efferent pathways and are typically seen with multiple sclerosis.

### Tics

Tics are sudden, brief, repetitive coordinated movements that will usually occur at irregular intervals. There are simple and complex tics that vary from myoclonic jerks to jumping movements that may include vocalization and repetition of other sounds. Tourette syndrome is an example of a pathology that presents with tics.

### Chorea

Chorea is a form of hyperkinesia that presents with brief, irregular contractions that are rapid, but not to the degree of myoclonic jerks. Chorea is typically secondary to damage of the caudate nucleus. Chorea is often equated to "fidgeting." Ballism is a form of chorea that includes choreic jerks of large amplitude. Ballism produces flailing movements of the limbs and is typically secondary to damage of the subthalamic nucleus. Huntington's disease is an example of a pathology that presents with chorea.

### Dystonia

Dystonia is a syndrome of sustained muscle contractions that frequently causes twisting, abnormal postures, and repetitive movements. All muscles can be affected and the involuntary movements are often accentuated during volitional movement and with progression, can produce overflow. Presentation varies as there are multiple types and etiologies surrounding dystonia. Etiologies range from genetic or acquired to environmental or a secondary effect from medications. Presentations can include sustained contractions of agonist and antagonist muscles; repeatedly persisting within the same muscle group; voluntary movements that create involuntary movement secondary to overflow; torsion spasms that are continual, patterned and twisting; as well as other presentations based on etiology. Common diagnoses that may include dystonia are Parkinson's disease, cerebral palsy, and encephalitis.[13]

### Athetosis

Athetosis is a movement disorder that presents with slow, twisting, and writhing movements that are large in amplitude. Athetoid movement is primarily seen in the face, tongue, trunk, and extremities. When the movements are brief, they merge with chorea (choreoathetosis), and when sustained, they merge with dystonia, and it is typically associated with spasticity. Athetosis is a common finding in several forms of cerebral palsy secondary to basal ganglia pathology.

## Muscle/Movement Impairment Terminology[1,13,24]

**Akinesia:** The inability to initiate movement; commonly seen in patients with Parkinson's disease.

**Asthenia:** Generalized weakness, typically secondary to cerebellar pathology.

**Ataxia:** The inability to perform coordinated movements.

**Athetosis:** A condition that presents with involuntary movements combined with instability of posture. Peripheral movements occur without central stability.

**Bradykinesia:** Movement that is very slow.

**Chorea:** Movements that are sudden, random, and involuntary.

**Clasp-knife response:** A form of resistance seen during range of motion of a hypertonic joint where there is greatest resistance at the initiation of range that lessens with movement through the range of motion.

**Clonus:** A characteristic of an upper motor neuron lesion; involuntary alternating spasmodic contraction of a muscle precipitated by a quick stretch reflex.

**Cogwheel rigidity:** A form of rigidity where resistance to movement has a phasic quality to it; often seen with Parkinson's disease.

**Dysdiadochokinesia:** The inability to perform rapidly alternating movements.

**Dysmetria:** The inability to control the range of a movement and the force of muscular activity.

**Dystonia:** Closely related to athetosis, however, there is larger axial muscle involvement rather than appendicular muscles.

**Fasciculation:** A muscular twitch that is caused by random discharge of a lower motor neuron and its muscle fibers; suggests lower motor neuron disease, however, can be benign.

**Hemiballism:** An involuntary and violent movement of a large body part.

**Kinesthesia:** The ability to perceive the direction and extent of movement of a joint or body part.

**Lead pipe rigidity:** A form of rigidity where there is uniform and constant resistance to range of motion; often associated with lesions of the basal ganglia.

**Rigidity:** A state of severe hypertonicity where a sustained muscle contraction does not allow for any movement at a specified joint.

**Tremor:** Involuntary, rhythmic, oscillatory movements secondary to a basal ganglia lesion. There are various classifications secondary to specific etiology.

## Consider This

### Modified Ashworth Scale for Grading Spasticity[20]

The Modified Ashworth Scale is a widely used qualitative scale for the assessment of spasticity; it measures the amount of resistance to passive stretch. Clinical assessment of spasticity may also include muscle grading, deep tendon reflexes (DTRs), and range of motion (ROM) evaluation.

Spasticity is a component of an upper motor neuron lesion, which is also characterized by exaggerated phasic (tendon jerks) and tonic (spastic) stretch reflexes that can occur after injury to the CNS. Spasticity is not a primary condition, but a secondary effect from CNS damage also allowing for a loss of movement dexterity.

#### Modified Ashworth Scale for Grading Spasticity

| Grade | Description |
|---|---|
| 0 | no increase in muscle tone |
| 1 | slight increase in muscle tone, manifested by a catch and release or by minimal resistance at the end of the range of motion when the affected part(s) is moved in flexion or extension |
| 1+ | slight increase in muscle tone, manifested by a catch, followed by minimal resistance throughout the remainder (less than half) of the ROM |
| 2 | more marked increase in muscle tone through most of the ROM, but affected part(s) easily moved |
| 3 | considerable increase in muscle tone, passive movement difficult |
| 4 | affected part(s) rigid in flexion or extension |

Other methods for evaluating spasticity include the Bilateral Adductor Tone Score, the Spasm Frequency Score, and electrophysiologic studies, however, most of these methods are time consuming, expensive, and require specialized equipment.

## Balance[23,26,28]

Balance can be defined as:

- a state of physical equilibrium
- maintenance and control of the center of gravity
- achieving and maintaining an upright posture

All definitions assume integrated somatosensory, visual, and vestibular information within the central nervous system. Balance is best assessed through investigation of all three components of balance.

### Somatosensory Input

Somatosensory receptors are located in the joints, muscles, ligaments, and skin to provide proprioceptive information regarding length, tension, pressure, pain, and joint position. Proprioceptive and tactile input from the ankles, knees, hips, and neck provide balance information to the brain.

- **Challenging the somatosensory system:** examination of pressure and vibration; observation of a patient when changing the surface they are standing on. Examples would be slopes, uneven surfaces, standing on foam. (Figs. 5-31, 5-32)

Fig. 5-31: Examination of balance while stressing the somatosensory system by using an altered surface.

**Fig. 5-32:** Examination of balance by stressing the somatosensory system by using an altered surface and closing the patient's eyes. This does not allow for visual feedback regarding balance.

## Visual Input

Visual receptors allow for perceptual acuity regarding verticality, motion of objects and self, environmental orientation, postural sway, and movements of the head/neck. Children rely heavily on this system for maintenance of balance.

- **Challenging the visual system:** examination of quiet standing with eyes open; observing balance strategies to maintain center of gravity with and without visual input. Assessment of potential visual field cuts, hemianopsia, pursuits, saccades, double vision, gaze control, and acuity is necessary. (Fig. 5-33)

## Vestibular Input

The vestibular system provides the central nervous system with feedback regarding the position and movement of the head with relation to gravity. The labyrinth consists of three semicircular canals filled with endolymph and two otolith organs. Semicircular canals respond to the movement of fluid with head motion. Otoliths measure the effects of gravity and movement with regard to acceleration/deceleration.

- **Challenging the vestibular system:** examination of balance with movement of the head; testing such as Dix-Hallpike maneuver, bithermal caloric testing, assessment for nystagmus, head thrust sign; testing of the vestibuloocular reflex.

### Balance Reflexes

**Vestibuloocular reflex (VOR):** VOR allows for head/eye movement coordination. This reflex supports gaze stabilization through eye movement that counters movements of the head. This maintains a stable image on the retina during movement.

**Vestibulospinal reflex (VSR):** VSR attempts to stabilize the body and control movement. The reflex assists with stability while the head is moving as well as coordination of the trunk during upright postures.

### Automatic Postural Strategies

Automatic postural strategies are automatic motor responses that are used to maintain the center of gravity over the base of support. These responses always react or respond to a particular stimulus.

**Ankle strategy:** The ankle strategy is the first strategy to be elicited by a small range and slow velocity perturbation when the feet are on the ground. Muscle groups contract in a distal to proximal fashion to control postural sway from the ankle joint.

**Hip strategy:** The hip strategy is elicited by a greater force, challenge or perturbation through the pelvis and hips. The hips will move (in the opposite direction from the head) in order to maintain balance. Muscle groups contract in a proximal to distal fashion in order to counteract the loss of balance.

**Fig. 5-33:** Examination of balance with a decrease in the base of support.

**Suspensory strategy:** The suspensory strategy is used to lower the center of gravity during standing or ambulation in order to better control the center of gravity. Examples of this strategy include knee flexion, crouching or squatting. This strategy is often used when both mobility and stability are required during a task (such as surfing).

**Stepping strategy:** The stepping strategy is elicited through unexpected challenges or perturbations during static standing or when the perturbation produces such a movement that the center of gravity is beyond the base of support. The lower extremities step and/or upper extremities reach to regain a new base of support.

Vertigo is used to describe a sense of movement and rotation of oneself or the surrounding environment. It typically is a sensation of spinning, but can also present as linear motion or falling. Vertigo may have a peripheral or central origin.

## Characteristics of Central Versus Peripheral Vertigo[1]

| Peripheral vertigo | Central vertigo |
| --- | --- |
| • episodic and short duration<br>• autonomic symptoms present<br>• precipitating factor<br>• pallor, sweating<br>• nausea and vomiting<br>• auditory fullness (fullness within the ears)<br>• tinnitus | • autonomic symptoms less severe<br>• loss of consciousness can occur<br>• neurological symptoms present including:<br>  – diplopia<br>  – hemianopsia<br>  – weakness<br>  – numbness<br>  – ataxia<br>  – dysarthria |

## Etiology of Central Versus Peripheral Vertigo[1]

| Peripheral | Central |
| --- | --- |
| Benign paroxysmal positional vertigo (BPPV) | Meningitis |
| Meniere's disease | Migraine headache |
| Infection | Complications of neurologic origin post ear infections |
| Trauma/tumor | Trauma/tumor |
| Metabolic disorders (i.e., diabetes mellitus) | Cerebellar degeneration disorders (i.e., alcoholism) |
| Acute alcohol intoxication | Multiple sclerosis |

**Benign paroxysmal positional vertigo (BPPV):** This condition is comprised of repeated episodes of vertigo that occur subsequent to changes in head position. BPPV only lasts a few seconds and is typically first noted while in a recumbent position since it most commonly affects the posterior semicircular canal. The etiology is usually otoconia (canalith) that loosens and travels into the posterior semicircular canal, causing vertigo. Nystagmus is present and can be noted when assessing a patient using the Dix-Hallpike test. Patients with BPPV typically find it self-limiting and can be successfully treated with canalith repositioning maneuvers which are passive movements used to remove the otoconia from the canals, thus remediating the vertigo.

**Dix-Hallpike test:** This maneuver is a vertiginous position test used in assessment and treatment. The test stimulates the posterior semicircular canal and attempts to determine if otoconia exist within the canal. If the patient experiences nystagmus and vertigo, the test is performed to determine if a patient presents with BPPV or a central lesion. (Figs. 5-34, 5-35, 5-36)

**Fig. 5-34:** The initial positioning for the Dix-Hallpike test where the patient starts in sitting with the legs extended on the table and head rotated 45 degrees to one side.

**Fig. 5-35:** The patient is rapidly moved to a supine position with the head (still in 45 degrees rotation) extended 30 degrees beyond horizontal off the end of the table.

**Fig. 5-36:** The therapist continues to hold the patient's head in this position for 20-30 seconds observing the potential for nystagmus. If nystagmus exists, the direction of the eyes and appearance of the nystagmus can determine inner ear versus CNS lesion.

# Consider This
## Nystagmus[24]

Nystagmus is abnormal eye movement that entails nonvolitional, rhythmic oscillation of the eyes. The speed of movement is faster in one direction than the other direction. A patient with nystagmus will also commonly complain of vertigo, nausea, and oscillopsia (movement of objects viewed).

### Observation

**Eye movement:** Horizontal, vertical, rotatory or mixed movements

**Type of eye movement:** Pendular or jerk

**Direction:** Bidirectional or unidirectional

**Nystagmus movement:** Binocular or monocular with symmetrical or dissociated movement. Effects of change of position of the head or posture on nystagmus

### Congenital Nystagmus

This form of nystagmus is typically mild and does not change in severity over the person's lifetime. It is not usually associated with other pathology.

### Acquired Nystagmus

**Spontaneous nystagmus:** Nystagmus caused by an imbalance of vestibular signals to the oculomotor neurons that causes a constant drift in one direction that is countered by a quick movement in the opposite direction. This typically occurs after an acute vestibular lesion and will last approximately 24 hours.

**Peripheral nystagmus:** Nystagmus that occurs with a peripheral vestibular lesion and is inhibited when the patient fixates their vision on an object.

**Central nystagmus:** Nystagmus that occurs with a central lesion of the brainstem/cerebellum and is not inhibited by visual fixation on an object.

**Positional nystagmus:** Nystagmus that is induced by a change in head position. The semicircular canals stimulate the nystagmus that typically lasts only a few seconds.

**Gaze-evoked nystagmus:** Nystagmus that occurs when the eyes shift from a primary position to an alternate position. The nystagmus is caused by the patient's inability to maintain the stable gaze position. This is typically indicative of CNS pathology and is associated with brain injury and multiple sclerosis.

| Characteristics of Central Versus Peripheral Nystagmus[24] | | |
|---|---|---|
| **Symptoms of Nystagmus** | **Central Lesion** | **Peripheral Lesion** |
| **Direction** | Either bidirectional or unidirectional | Unidirectional with the fast segment of movement indicating the opposite direction of lesion |
| **Visual fixation** | No inhibition with fixation | Will inhibit nystagmus and vertigo |
| **Vertigo** | Mild | Significant |
| **Length of symptoms** | May be chronic | Minutes, days, weeks, but finite period of time; recurrent |
| **Etiology** | Demyelination of nerves, vascular lesion, cancer/tumor | Meniere's disease, vascular disorders, trauma, toxicity, infection of inner ear |

## Balance Tests and Measures[24,29,30]

There are various tests and measures to assess the different facets of balance. Selection of the most appropriate instrument is determined based on clinical diagnosis and patient presentation. Common balance tests and measures are discussed below.

### Berg Balance Scale

This is a tool designed to assess a patient's risk for falling. There are fourteen tasks, each scored on an ordinal scale from 0-4. These tasks include static activities, transitional movements, and dynamic activities in sitting and standing positions. The maximum score is a 56 with a score less than 45 indicating an increased risk for falling. This tool can be used as a one-time examination or as an ongoing tool to monitor a patient who may be at risk for falls.

<45
↑ risk of falls

### Fregley-Graybiel Ataxia Test Battery

A tool that consists of eight test conditions used in the battery with each leg measured on two accounts, the time spent in each test position and the number of steps that a patient takes without falling. Five trials of each condition are performed. The test conditions include:

- stand on beam with eyes open
- stand on beam with eyes closed
- walk on beam with eyes open
- sharpened Romberg (heel-toe static positioning)
- standing with eyes open
- standing with eyes closed
- standing on one leg with eyes closed
- walking on the floor with eyes closed

The therapist scores each condition on a pass/fail basis with normative data for comparison. This tool is best suited for patients with high level motor skills since each condition is challenging. Therapists use this tool to assess and treat balance dysfunction, however, patient performance does not assist the therapist to diagnose the cause of balance dysfunction.

### Fugl-Meyer Sensorimotor Assessment of Balance Performance Battery

This tool is designed as a subset of the Fugl-Meyer Physical Performance Battery and is designed to assess balance specifically for patients with hemiplegia. Each of the seven items assessed is scored from 0-2, specific to each item with the maximum score being 14. Even though a 14 is the best score that a person can receive, the patient still may not have normal balance.

### Functional Reach Test (Figs. 5-37, 5-38)

A single task screening tool used to assess standing balance and risk of falling. A person is required to stand upright with a static base of support. A yardstick is positioned to measure the forward distance that a patient can reach without moving the feet. Three trials are performed and averaged together.

The following are age-related standard measurements for functional reach:

20 - 40 years: 14.5 - 17 inches

41 - 69 years: 13.5 - 15 inches

70 - 87 years: 10.5 - 13.5 inches

A patient that falls below the age appropriate range for functional reach has an increased risk for falling. The outcome measure demonstrates high test-retest correlation and intrarater reliability.

**Fig. 5-37:** Initial positioning for the Functional Reach Test.

**Fig. 5-38:** Reaching forward during the Functional Reach Test.

**Fig. 5-39:** Romberg testing for postural sway with eyes closed.

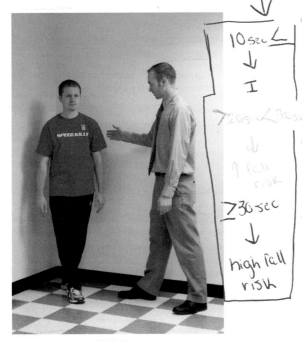

10 sec
↓
I

≥20s < 30s
↓
↑ fall risk

≥30 sec
↓
high fall risk

**Fig. 5-40:** Testing using the sharpened Romberg for postural sway with eyes open.

### Romberg Test

This is an assessment tool of balance and ataxia that initially positions the patient in unsupported standing, feet together, upper extremities folded, looking at a fixed point straight ahead with eyes open. With the eyes open, three sensory systems (visual, vestibular, somatosensory) provide input to the cerebellum to maintain standing stability. If there is a mild lesion in the vestibular or somatosensory systems, the patient will typically compensate through the visual sense.

Next the patient maintains the same standing posture, but closes the eyes (Fig. 5-39). A patient receives a grade of "normal" if they are able to maintain the position for 30 seconds. An abnormal response occurs with the inability to maintain balance when standing erect with the feet together and the eyes closed. Patients may exhibit excessive sway or begin to fall. When the visual input is removed, instability will be present if there is a larger somatosensory or vestibular deficit producing the instability. If a patient demonstrates ataxia and has a positive Romberg test, this indicates sensory ataxia and not cerebellar ataxia.

There is also a Sharpened Romberg test where the patient's balance is further assessed by performing in the same manner but with a heel-to-toe stance, typically with the non-dominant foot in front. The patient would first be tested with eyes open (Fig. 5-40) and then with eyes closed. This modification increases the challenge to the vestibular and somatosensory systems.

### Timed Get Up and Go Test

This is a functional performance screening tool used to assess a person's level of mobility and balance. The person initially sits in a supported chair with a firm surface, transfers to a standing position, and walks approximately 10 feet. The patient must then turn around without external support, walk back towards the chair, and return to a sitting position. The patient is scored based on amount of postural sway, excessive movements, reaching for support, side stepping or other signs of loss of balance. The 5-point ordinal rating scale designates a score of one as normal and a score of five as severely abnormal. In an attempt to increase overall reliability the use of time was implemented. Patients who are independent can complete the multi-task process in 10 seconds or less. Patients that require over 20 seconds to complete the process are at the limit for functional independence and may be at an increased risk for falling. Patients that require 30 seconds are at a high risk for a fall.

### Tinetti Performance Oriented Mobility Assessment

A tool used to screen patients and identify if there is an increased risk for falling. The first section assesses balance through sit to stand and stand to sit from an armless chair, immediate standing balance with eyes open and closed, tolerating a slight push in the standing position, and turning 360 degrees. A patient is scored from 0-2 in most categories with a maximum score of 16. The second section assesses gait at normal speed and at a rapid, but safe speed. Items scored in this section include initiation of gait, step length and height, step asymmetry and continuity, path, stance during gait, and trunk motion. A patient is scored 0-2 for each with a maximum score of 12. The tool has a combined maximum total of 28 with the risk of falling increasing as the total score decreases. A total score less than 19 indicates a high risk for a fall.

< 19 = high risk for a fall

### Vestibular Rehabilitation

Vestibular rehabilitation is a therapeutic intervention that can be highly successful for patients with vestibular or central balance system disorders. Exercise protocols for vestibular retraining utilize compensation, adaptation, and plasticity to increase the brain's sensitivity, restore symmetry, improve vestibuloocular control, and subsequently increase motor control and movement.

### Goals for Vestibular Rehabilitation

- Improve balance
- Improve trunk stability
- Increase strength and range of motion in order to improve musculoskeletal balance responses and strategies
- Decrease the rate and risk of falls
- Minimize dizziness

### Vestibuloocular Retraining Therapeutic Guidelines

- Vestibuloocular reflex (VOR) and vestibulospinal reflex (VSR) stimulation exercises
- Ocular motor exercises
- Balance exercises
- Gait exercises
- Combination exercises (obstacle courses, functioning in a public place)
- Habituation training exercises (use only with appropriate patients)

- Individualize each program based on the patient's specific impairments (rehabilitation versus compensation training)
- Use of practice, feedback, and repetition are vital for skill refinement
- Use of gravity, varying surface conditions, visual conditions, and environmental cues should be included in therapeutic planning
- The center of gravity must be controlled at each stage of treatment
- Strategy (hip, ankle, stepping, suspense) training should be implemented during treatment so that strategies become automatic responses
- Force plate systems, electromyographic biofeedback, optokinetic visual stimulation, and videography are all technical systems that can provide feedback to motor learning during vestibular rehabilitation
- Foam, mirrors, rocker boards, BAPS boards, Swiss balls, foam rollers, trampolines, and wedges are lower "tech" treatment tools that are successfully used for vestibular rehabilitation

# Communication Disorders

## Aphasia[1]

Aphasia is an acquired neurological impairment of processing for receptive and/or expressive language. Aphasia is the result of brain injury, head trauma, CVA, tumor or infection. Diagnosis is based on the site of lesion in the brain and the blood vessels involved. Patients with aphasia are classified based on observation of fluent or non-fluent aphasia. Approximately 95% of right-handed persons and 66% of left-handed persons are left hemisphere dominant for language.

Prognosis is dependent on the individual patient, location, and extent of the lesion. Typically, the more sudden the onset of damage, as in the case of an acute CVA, the higher extent of aphasia can be expected. The following characteristics associated with aphasia are often associated with a poor prognosis: perseveration of speech, severe auditory comprehension impairments, unreliable yes/no answers, and the use of empty speech without recognition of impairments.

### Fluent Aphasia[5,9,31]

- Lesion varies based on the type of fluent aphasia but frequently involves the temporal lobe, Wernicke's area or regions of the parietal lobe
- Word output and speech production are functional
- Prosody is acceptable, but empty speech/jargon
- Speech lacks any substance, use of paraphasias
- Use of neologisms (substitution within a word that is so severe it makes the word unrecognizable)

### Non-fluent Aphasia[5,9,31]

- Lesion varies based on the type of non-fluent aphasia, but frequently the frontal lobe (anterior speech center) of the dominant hemisphere is affected
- Poor word output and dysprosodic speech (impairment in the rhythm and inflection of speech)
- Poor articulation and increased effort for speech
- Content is present, but impaired syntactical words

## Types of Fluent Aphasia[5,9,31]

### Wernicke's Aphasia

- Lesion: posterior region of superior temporal gyrus
- Also known as "receptive aphasia"
- Comprehension (reading/auditory) impaired
- Good articulation, use of paraphasias
- Impaired writing
- Poor naming ability
- Motor impairment not typical due to the distance from Wernicke's area to the motor cortex

### Conduction Aphasia

- Lesion: supramarginal gyrus, arcuate fasciculus
- Severe impairment with repetition
- Intact fluency, good comprehension
- Speech interrupted by word-finding difficulties
- Reading intact, writing impaired

## Types of Non-fluent Aphasia[5,9,31]

### Broca's Aphasia

- Lesion: 3rd convolution of frontal lobe
- Also known as "expressive aphasia"
- Most common form of aphasia
- Intact auditory and reading comprehension
- Impaired repetition and naming skills
- Frustration with language skill errors
- Paraphasias are common
- Motor impairment typical due to proximity of Broca's area to the motor cortex

### Global Aphasia

- Lesion: frontal, temporal, parietal lobes
- Comprehension (reading/auditory) is severely impaired
- Impaired naming, writing, repetition skills
- May involuntarily verbalize, usually without correct context
- May use nonverbal skills for communication

### Verbal Apraxia[1]

Apraxia is a non-dysarthric and non-aphasic impairment of prosody and articulation of speech. Verbal expression is impaired secondary to deficits in motor planning. A patient is unable to initiate learned movement (articulation of speech) even though they understand the task. Lesions are usually found in the left frontal lobe adjacent to Broca's area.

### Dysarthria[1]

Dysarthria is a motor disorder of speech that is caused by an upper motor neuron lesion that affects the muscles that are used to articulate words and sounds. Speech is often noted as "slurred" and there may also be an effect on respiratory or phonatory systems due to the weakness.

## Spotlight on Safety

### Treating Aphasia[8]

Treating a patient with aphasia typically requires a physical therapist to alter the traditional methods of treatment in order to enhance communication and provide a safe and comfortable environment for the patient. The physical therapist may want to co-treat or consult with the speech pathologist to establish the best means of communication with the patient. The following may be considered when treating a patient that presents with aphasia:

- Cueing strategies must avoid verbal input and use tactile and visual cues.
- Attempt to have only one person speak to the patient at a time. Extra noise and multiple voices will only confuse the patient.
- Use concise sentences and yes/no questioning for ease of understanding and response.
- Allow the patient adequate time to process and respond before progressing with treatment.
- Allow for ample time for communication during treatment. If communication is rushed, this can decrease the effectiveness of the therapy session. The patient may also become frustrated with feeling pressure to respond.
- Attempt to allow the patient to perform an activity or segment of therapy without repetitive feedback.

# Medical Procedures/Testing for Neurological Dysfunction[32]

| Procedure/Test | Rationale |
|---|---|
| Cerebral angiography | A cerebral angiogram is an invasive procedure that can determine the narrowing or blockage of an artery within the brain. This can be used when diagnosing a potential CVA, brain tumor, aneurysm or vascular malformation. The catheter is threaded up through the body into an artery within the neck and contrast dye is released into the bloodstream. A series of x-rays is then taken. |
| Computed tomography (CT scan) | Brain scan imaging is typically non-invasive and provides cross sections of the area tested, with precise two dimensional views of bones, tissues, and organs. Dyes or contrast are occasionally used to provide the best view of any pathology that may exist within the tissues. A CT scan of the brain or spinal cord is required to rule out vascular malformations, tumors, cysts, herniated disks, hemorrhage, epilepsy, encephalitis, spinal stenosis, intracranial bleeding, and head injury. |

| Procedure/Test | Rationale |
|---|---|
| Discography | Invasive procedure to evaluate the integrity and pathology of a spinal disk. Contrast dye is injected and CT scanning is performed in order to better assess suspected damaged areas of intervertebral disks. |
| Electroencephalography (EEG) | Non-invasive procedure that can continuously measure electrical activity of the brain using multiple electrodes attached to the skull. Baseline electrical activity is determined, and then various stimuli are presented and brain waves are analyzed. An EEG is used to rule out seizure disorders, brain death, brain tumors, brain damage, inflammation, alcoholism, select psychiatric disorders, and degenerative disorders that affect the brain. |
| Electromyography (EMG) | Invasive procedure that is used to assess nerve and muscle dysfunction or spinal cord disease. EMG records the electrical activity from the brain or spinal cord to the peripheral nerve root being tested. An EMG is used to rule out muscle pathology, nerve pathology, spinal cord disease, denervated muscle, and lower motor neuron injury. |
| Evoked potentials | Non-invasive procedure using two sets of electrodes that records the time it takes for an impulse to reach the brain. External stimuli (auditory, visual, proprioceptive) are used to evoke electrical potentials within the brain. This is used to rule out multiple sclerosis, brain tumor, acoustic neuroma (small tumors of the inner ear), and spinal cord injury. |
| Magnetic resonance imaging (MRI) | Brain scan imaging that is typically non-invasive and provides detailed images including tissues, organs, bones, and nerves. A contrast dye may be used to enhance imaging of certain tissues. The MRI is used to rule out tumors of the brain or spinal cord, multiple sclerosis, and head trauma. |
| Myelography | Invasive procedure of the spinal canal using contrast dye and x-ray imaging. The procedure has a high risk for headache following the spinal tap, but is used to rule out potential abnormalities surrounding the subarachnoid space, spinal nerve injury, herniated disks, fractures, back or leg pathology, and spinal tumors. |
| Nerve conduction velocity (NCV) | Non-invasive stimulation of a peripheral nerve to determine the nerve action potentials and the nerve's ability to send a signal. NCV rules out peripheral neuropathies, carpal tunnel syndrome, demyelination pathology, and peripheral nerve compression. |
| Positron emission tomography (PET) | Brain scan imaging that provides two and three-dimensional pictures of brain activity and is used to rule out cerebral circulatory pathology, metabolism dysfunction, tumors, blood flow, and brain changes following injury or drug abuse. |
| Spinal puncture (lumbar) | Invasive procedure that inserts a needle through lumbar puncture below the level of L1-L2 for cerebral spinal fluid sample. A spinal puncture primarily rules out hemorrhage, inflammation, infection, meningitis, and tumor. |

# Pharmacology - Neuromuscular Management[13,33]

## Antiepileptic Agents

**Action:** Antiepileptic agents reduce or eliminate seizure activity within the brain. These agents attempt to inhibit the firing of certain cerebral neurons through various effects on the CNS. Chemical classifications include barbiturates, benzodiazepines, carboxylic acids, hydantoins, iminostilbenes, succinimides, and second generation drugs.

**Indications:** seizure activity (partial seizures, generalized seizures, unclassified seizures)

**Side effects:** (agent dependent) ataxia, skin issues, behavioral changes, gastrointestinal distress, headache, blurred vision, weight gain

**Implications for PT:** Therapists must have adequate knowledge of established protocols for responding to a seizure as well as potential side effects of antiepileptic medications. Patients with epilepsy may show greater sensitivity to environmental surroundings such as light or noise level.

**Examples:** Seconal (secobarbital), Klonopin (clonazepam), Depakote (valproic acid), Dilantin (phenytoin), Tegretol (carbamazepine), Celontin (methsuximide), Neurontin (gabapentin).

## Antispasticity Agents

**Action:** Antispasticity agents promote relaxation in a spastic muscle. Spasticity is an exaggerated stretch reflex of the muscle that can occur after injury to the CNS. Spasticity is not a primary condition, but a secondary effect from CNS damage. Agents bind selectively within the CNS or within the skeletal muscle cells to reduce spasticity.

**Indications:** increased tone, spasticity, spinal cord injury, CVA, multiple sclerosis

**Side effects:** drowsiness, confusion, headache, dizziness, generalized muscle weakness, hepatotoxicity potential with Dantrium, tolerance, dependence

**Implications for PT:** Therapists must balance the need to decrease spastic muscles with the loss of function that a patient may experience with the reduction of hypertonicity. Once spasticity is reduced, therapists should focus on therapeutic handling techniques, facilitation, and strengthening to promote overall mobility. Sedation may also alter the scheduling of therapy to allow for maximal participation.

**Examples:** Lioresal (baclofen), Valium (diazepam), Dantrium (dantrolene), Zanaflex (tizanidine)

## Cholinergic Agents

**Action:** Cholinergic direct stimulant agents mimic acetylcholine and bind directly to the cholinergic receptor to activate and create a response at the cellular level. Indirect acting cholinergic stimulants increase cholinergic synapse activity through the inhibition of acetylcholinesterase (which normally destroys acetylcholine). The increase of acetylcholine at the synapse increases cholinergic synaptic transmission.

**Indications:** glaucoma, dementia due to Alzheimer's disease, postoperative decrease in gastrointestinal motility, myasthenia gravis, reversal of anticholinergic toxicity

**Side effects:** gastrointestinal distress, impaired visual accommodation, bronchoconstriction, bradycardia, flushing, other parasympathetic effects

**Implications for PT:** Patients may experience a decrease in heart rate and dizziness. Therapists should be aware of characteristics of both sympathetic and parasympathetic systems and notify the physician if a patient begins to exhibit unexpected side effects. Patients with Alzheimer's disease and myasthenia gravis may be better able to participate in therapeutic activities when taking cholinergic agents.

**Examples:** Direct: Duvoid (bethanechol), Pilocar (pilocarpine); Indirect: Aricept (donepezil), Tensilon (edrophonium), Prostigmin (neostigmine), Cognex (tacrine)

## Dopamine Replacement Agents

**Action:** Dopamine replacement agents assist to relieve the symptoms of Parkinson's disease secondary to the decrease in endogenous dopamine. These agents are able to cross the blood-brain barrier through active transport and transform to dopamine within the brain.

**Indications:** Parkinson's disease, Parkinsonism

**Side effects:** arrhythmias (levodopa), gastrointestinal distress, orthostatic hypotension, dyskinesias, mood and behavioral changes, tolerance

**Implications for PT:** Therapists and patients attain maximal benefit from scheduling therapy one hour after administration of levadopa. Therapists must understand the debilitating effects of drug holidays and should monitor the patient's blood pressure frequently due to the potential for orthostatic hypotension.

**Examples:** Sinemet or Madopar (levodopa), Symmetrel (amantadine)

## Muscle Relaxant Agents

**Action:** Muscle relaxant agents promote relaxation in muscles that typically present with spasm that is a continuous, tonic contraction. Spasms typically occur secondary to a musculoskeletal or peripheral nerve injury rather than CNS injury.

**Indications:** muscle spasm

**Side effects:** (agent dependent) sedation, drowsiness, dizziness, nausea, vomiting, headache, tolerance, dependence

**Implications for PT:** Therapists must be aware of potential side effects, however, maximize the potential for relaxation through therapeutic techniques and the use of modalities during treatment. Prevention of reinjury through stretching, posture retraining, and education should assist the patient to achieve desired outcomes.

**Examples:** Valium (diazepam), Flexeril (cyclobenzaprine), Paraflex (chlorzoxazone)

# Neuromuscular and Nervous Systems Pathology

## Alzheimer's Disease[1,6,24]

Alzheimer's disease is a progressive neurodegenerative disorder that results in deterioration and irreversible damage within the cerebral cortex and subcortical areas of the brain. Neurons that are normally involved with acetylcholine transmission deteriorate within the cerebral cortex. Development of amyloid plaques and neurofibrillary tangles result in further damage to the nervous system.

**Etiology** – The exact etiology of Alzheimer's disease is unknown, however, hypothesized causes include lower levels of neurotransmitters, higher levels of aluminum within brain tissue, genetic inheritance, autoimmune disease, abnormal processing of the substance amyloid, and virus. The risk of developing Alzheimer's disease increases with age and there is a higher incidence in women.

**Signs and symptoms** – Alzheimer's disease is initially noted by a change in higher cortical functions such as difficulty with new learning and subtle changes in memory and concentration. Progression includes a loss of orientation, word finding difficulties, depression, poor judgment, rigidity, bradykinesia, shuffling gait, and impaired ability to perform self-care skills. End-stage disease includes severe intellectual and physical destruction, incontinence, functional dependence, and an inability to speak.

**Treatment** – There is no curative treatment for the disease process. Medications are administered to inhibit acetylcholinesterase, alleviate cognitive symptoms, and control behavioral changes. Tacrine (Cognex), donepezil (Aricept), and rivastigmine (Exelon) are common pharmacological agents, however, the side effects can be substantial. Physical therapy management should focus on maximizing the patient's remaining function and providing family and caregiver education. Many patients require a long-term Alzheimer's care facility secondary to personality changes, aggressive behavior, and end-stage complications.

## Amyotrophic Lateral Sclerosis[1,13]

Amyotrophic lateral sclerosis (ALS) is a chronic degenerative disease that produces both upper and lower motor neuron impairments. Significant loss of anterior horn cells in the spinal cord and the motor cranial nerve nuclei in lower brainstem produces weakness and muscle atrophy. Demyelination of corticospinal and corticobulbar tracts produce the upper motor neuron symptoms. The rapid degeneration causes denervation of muscle fibers, muscle atrophy, and weakness.

**Etiology** – The exact etiology of ALS is unknown (90% of all cases), however, theories include genetic inheritance, virus, metabolic disturbances, and toxicity of lead and aluminum. There is a higher incidence in men and the disease typically begins between 40 to 70 years of age.

**Signs and symptoms** – Early clinical presentation of ALS may include both upper and lower motor neuron involvement. Lower motor neuron signs include asymmetric muscle weakness, fasciculations, cramping, and atrophy within the hands. Weakness spreads in a distal to proximal path. Upper motor neuron symptoms can include incoordination of movement, spasticity, clonus, and a positive Babinski reflex. A patient with ALS will exhibit fatigue, oral motor impairment, motor paralysis, and eventual respiratory paralysis.

**Treatment** – Effective management of ALS is based on supportive care and symptomatic therapy. Pharmacological intervention may include riluzole (Rilutek). Physical, occupational, speech, respiratory, and nutritional therapies may be warranted with the focus on quality of life and caregiver training.

## Spotlight on Safety

### Irreversible Dementia[13,20,24]

A therapist must be aware of each patient's medical history and level of orientation prior to treatment. This is achieved through screening of cognition, memory, and judgment irregardless of the primary diagnosis. Certain pathologies can cause irreversible dementia including:

**Degenerative pathology:** Alzheimer's disease, Huntington's disease, multiple sclerosis

**Infectious pathology:** tuberculosis, AIDS

**Vascular pathology:** CVA, anoxia, arteriovenous malformation, multi-infarct dementia

**Miscellaneous conditions at risk for dementia:** head injury, hydrocephalus, toxins, alcoholism

A therapist should modify the plan of care in order to ensure that the therapeutic goals are achieved and the patient remains safe. In early stages of dementia, patients will typically attempt to conceal their shortcomings and this can significantly compromise patient safety. Thorough assessment for at-risk patients will minimize safety risks.

## Bell's Palsy[13]

Bell's palsy is a temporary unilateral facial paralysis secondary to trauma with demyelination and/or axonal degeneration of the facial nerve. This is a common clinical condition with the highest incidence in individuals between 15 and 45 years of age.

**Etiology** – The exact etiology of Bell's palsy is unclear, however, the condition may be secondary to a viral infection, specifically the herpes simplex/herpes zoster virus. Inflammation and subsequent pressure injure the nerve with varying degrees of damage. The inflammation within the auditory canal produces subsequent demyelination of the nerve and if ischemia occurs, there is axonal degeneration of the nerve.

**Signs and symptoms** – A patient with Bell's palsy will present with an asymmetrical facial appearance with "drooping" of the eyelid and mouth, potential for drooling, dryness of the eye, and inability to close the eyelid due to weakness.

**Treatment** – The sooner the person is diagnosed and treated, the better the outcome. Some patients have very mild involvement and their symptoms typically resolve within two weeks time without formal medical intervention. In cases with greater severity, the patient may be treated with anti-viral medications along with high-dose corticosteroids. Physical therapy may be indicated for stimulation of the facial nerve, facial massage and/or exercise, depending on the degree of injury.

## Carpal Tunnel Syndrome[13,20]

Carpal tunnel syndrome (CTS) is a peripheral nerve entrapment injury that occurs as a result of compression of the median nerve where it passes through the carpal tunnel. Normal tissue pressure within the tunnel is approximately 3 to 7 mm Hg, but CTS can result in pressure greater than 30 mm Hg with the wrist at rest which produces ischemia within the nerve. This results in sensory and motor disturbances in the median nerve distribution of the hand.

**Etiology** – The exact etiology of CTS is unclear, however, associated conditions that contribute to CTS include repetitive use, rheumatoid arthritis, pregnancy, diabetes, cumulative trauma disorders, tumor, hypothyroidism, and wrist sprain or fracture.

**Signs and symptoms** – A patient with CTS will initially present with sensory changes and paresthesia along the median nerve distribution in the hand. It may also radiate into the upper extremity, shoulder, and neck. Symptoms include night pain, weakness of the hand, muscle atrophy, decreased grip strength, clumsiness, and decreased wrist mobility.

**Treatment** – There is no universally accepted treatment of CTS, however, typically a patient with CTS will initially receive conservative management including splinting, ergonomic measures, local corticosteroid injections, and physical therapy management. Severe cases may require surgical release of the carpal tunnel.

## Cerebellar Disorders[1,13,24]

Cerebellar disorders have numerous etiologies and present differently based on etiology and location of the lesion within the cerebellum.

**Etiology** – Etiologies vary and include congenital malformations, hereditary ataxias, and genetic and acquired conditions.

- **Congenital malformations** manifest early in life and are non-progressive. Manifestations vary depending on the structures involved; ataxia is usually present.

- **Hereditary ataxias** may be autosomal recessive or autosomal dominant. The most common autosomal recessive ataxia is Friedreich's ataxia. Friedreich's ataxia results from a gene mutation causing abnormal repetition of the DNA sequence and ultimately, impaired mitochondrial function. Gait unsteadiness begins early in life and it is followed by upper extremity ataxia, dysarthria, and paresis. Mental function declines and slight tremors may be seen. Reflexes, vibration, and position senses are impaired.

- **Spinocerebellar ataxias** are the main autosomal dominant ataxias. Manifestations vary with many forms affecting multiple areas in the central and peripheral nervous systems. They commonly present with neuropathy, pyramidal signs, ataxia, and restless leg syndrome.

- **Acquired ataxias** may result from nonhereditary neurodegenerative systemic disorders, toxin exposure or can be idiopathic. Systemic disorders include alcoholism, hypothyroidism, and vitamin E deficiency. Toxins include carbon monoxide, heavy metals, and lithium.

**Signs and symptoms** – Signs and symptoms vary based on etiology, but typically include ataxia.

**Treatment** – Treatment is diagnosis dependent and typically supportive unless it is acquired and/or reversible. Some systemic disorders such as hypothyroidism and toxin exposure can be treated; surgical intervention may be appropriate for structural lesions (tumor, hydrocephalus), however, the majority of treatment is typically supportive.

## Diabetic Neuropathy[13,34]

Diabetic neuropathy is a complication and direct effect of diabetes mellitus. Nerve ischemia results from microvascular disease combined with the direct effects of hyperglycemia on neurons resulting in the impairment of nerve function. There are many forms including cranial neuropathies, radiculopathies, and mononeuropathies. The most common include symmetric polyneuropathy and autonomic neuropathy.

**Etiology** – The primary etiology is the diagnosis of diabetes mellitus. Continued research attempts to understand the cause and effect of prolonged exposure to high blood glucose and its exact impact on nerve function. There are multiple factors that lead to all forms of diabetic neuropathy including metabolic factors, high blood glucose, duration of diabetes, neurovascular factors, impairment with transport of oxygen and nutrients to the nerves, autoimmune factors, inflammation in nerves, inherited traits, and the impact of environmental and lifestyle choices such as alcohol and smoking.

**Signs and symptoms** – Symptoms vary depending on the form of diabetic neuropathy, but typically weakness and sensory disturbances occur distally in a symmetrical pattern. Initial symptoms typically include tingling, numbness or pain, especially in the feet. Symptoms can involve the sensory, motor or autonomic systems. Additional symptoms may include wasting of muscles in the feet or hands, "stocking glove" sensory distribution impairments, orthostatic hypotension, weakness, urinary impairments, and significant pain.

**Treatment** – Patients require strict monitoring of blood glucose levels to prevent further nerve pathology. Physical therapy is typically indicated to address the various symptoms including pain management, foot care, and overall fitness. Pharmacological intervention may also be warranted.

## Epilepsy[13,27,34]

Epilepsy is a chronic condition where there is temporary dysfunction of the brain that results in hypersynchronous electrical discharge of cortical neurons and seizure activity that is typically unprovoked and unpredictable. A seizure is a transient event that is a symptom of interrupted brain functioning. A seizure is the hallmark sign of epilepsy, however, one seizure does not signal epilepsy.

**Etiology** – There are various classifications of seizures, however, many cases are idiopathic. Other associated conditions that increase risk of epilepsy include genetic influence, head trauma, dementia, CVA, cerebral palsy, Down syndrome, and autism.

**Signs and symptoms** – Seizure symptoms vary, depending on type and extent of the seizure. Loss of awareness or consciousness and disturbances of movement, sensation, mood or mental function may occur.

**Treatment** – Many patients require antiepileptic medication to manage seizures, however, there is no current medical treatment to "cure" epilepsy. Initiating antiepileptic medication is a serious decision since side effects can produce a variety of adverse effects. Surgical intervention is sometimes warranted when pharmacological management has failed and there is a high disruption of the quality of the person's life.

## Guillain-Barre Syndrome[13,24]

Guillain-Barre syndrome (GBS), or acute polyneuropathy, is a temporary inflammation and demyelination of the peripheral nerves' myelin sheaths, potentially resulting in axonal degeneration. The autoantibodies of GBS attack segments of the myelin sheath of the peripheral nerves. GBS can occur at any age, however, there is a peak in frequency in the young adult population and again in adults that are between their fifth and eighth decades.

**Etiology** – The exact etiology of GBS is unknown, however, it is hypothesized to be an autoimmune response to a previous respiratory infection, influenza, immunization or surgery. Viral infections, Epstein-Barr syndrome, cytomegalovirus, bacterial infections, surgery, and vaccinations have been associated with the development of GBS.

**Signs and symptoms** – GBS results in motor weakness in a distal to proximal progression, sensory impairment, and possible respiratory paralysis. A patient with GBS will initially present with distal symmetrical motor weakness, mild distal sensory impairments, and transient paresthesias that progress towards the upper extremities and head. The level of disability usually peaks within two to four weeks after onset. Muscle and respiratory paralysis, absence of deep tendon reflexes, and the inability to speak or swallow may also occur. GBS can be life-threatening with respiratory involvement.

**Treatment** – Medical management of a patient with GBS typically requires hospitalization for treatment of symptoms. Pharmacological intervention often includes immunosuppressive and analgesic/narcotic medications. Cardiac monitoring, plasmapheresis, and mechanical ventilation may be required. Physical, occupational, and speech therapies are typically indicated. Physical therapy may include pulmonary rehabilitation, strengthening, mobility training, wheelchair and orthotic prescription and/or assistive device training. Intervention and rate of progression are dependent on the ultimate level of disability from GBS.

# Spotlight on Safety
### Seizures: Before, During, and After[13,27]

Epilepsy is responsible for the majority of seizures. There are various classifications of seizures including partial, generalized, and unclassified; seizures that can be simple or complex (unimpaired versus impaired consciousness), and convulsive versus nonconvulsive. Regardless of the form of seizure, a therapist should be aware of the potential course of the seizure in order to provide safe emergency treatment.

A prodromal period is rare, but can occur days or hours prior to a seizure and may include mood changes, lightheadedness, sleep disturbances, irritability, and difficulty concentrating. An aura will briefly occur within minutes before a complex partial or generalized tonic-clonic seizure. The aura is actually a simple partial seizure and produces symptoms that alert the person that something is about to happen. Symptoms vary but can include restlessness, nervousness, anxiety, heaviness, and a general feeling that something within the body is not quite right.

The therapist should consider the following when attempting to manage a person that is having a seizure:

- Stay calm and prevent injury
- Remove all objects surrounding the person to ensure that there is nothing that could harm the person during the seizure
- Maintain awareness of the length of time of the seizure
- Ensure that the person is as comfortable as possible
- Do not allow other people near the person in an effort to keep the individual isolated
- Consider your safety and do not hold the person down; there is no need for restraint if the person is thrashing during the seizure
- Avoid placing anything into the person's mouth (the person is not capable of swallowing their tongue)
- Avoid providing any water, food or medicine until the person is fully alert
- Be prepared to call 911 if the seizure lasts longer than five minutes

After the seizure is over, place the person on their left side to avoid choking in case the person vomits. The person should remain in this position until they are fully alert. The therapist should stay with the person until they have recovered which typically takes five to twenty minutes. Therapists should be aware of patients that are at-risk for seizure activity in order to avoid any unnecessary safety risks.

## Huntington's Disease[13,20]

Huntington's disease (HD), also known as Huntington's chorea, is a neurological disorder of the CNS and is characterized by degeneration and atrophy of the basal ganglia and cerebral cortex within the brain. The neurotransmitters become deficient and are unable to modulate movement.

**Etiology** – HD is genetically transmitted as an autosomal dominant trait with the defect linked to chromosome four and to the gene identified as IT-15. The disease is usually perpetuated by a person that has children prior to diagnosis. The average age for developing symptoms is between 35 and 55 years, however, symptoms can develop at any age.

**Signs and symptoms** – HD is a movement disorder that includes affective dysfunction and cognitive impairment. The patient may present with involuntary choreic movements, mild alteration in personality, grimacing, protrusion of the tongue, and ataxia with choreoathetoid movements. Late stage HD includes mental deterioration, decrease in IQ, depression, dysphagia, incontinence, immobility, and rigidity.

**Treatment** – Medical management of HD requires genetic, psychological, and social counseling for the patient and family. Pharmacological management is initiated once choreiform movement impairs a patient's functional capacity. Physical therapy should maximize endurance, strength, balance, postural control, and functional mobility.

## Multiple Sclerosis[13,20,24]

Multiple sclerosis (MS) produces patches of demyelination of the myelin sheaths that surround nerves within the brain and spinal cord. This decreases the efficiency of nerve impulse transmission and symptoms will vary based on the location and the extent of demyelination. There is subsequent plaque development and eventual failure of impulse transmission.

**Etiology** – The exact etiology of MS is unknown. Genetics, viral infections, and environment all have a role in the development of MS. It is theorized that a slow-acting virus initiates the autoimmune response in individuals that have environmental and genetic factors associated with the disease. MS can occur at any age with the highest incidence between 20-35 years of age.

**Signs and symptoms** – Symptoms vary based on the type of disease, location, extent of demyelination, and degree of sclerosis. Initial symptoms include visual problems, paresthesias and sensory changes, clumsiness, weakness, ataxia, balance dysfunction, and fatigue. The clinical course usually consists of periods of exacerbations and remissions, with the degree of neurologic dysfunction and subsequent recovery following typical patterns related to the specific type of MS. The frequency and intensity of exacerbations may indicate the speed/course of the disease process.

**Treatment** – Management of MS includes pharmacological, medical, and therapeutic interventions. The goal is to lessen the length of exacerbations and maximize the health of the patient. Pharmacological intervention is indicated along with physical, occupational, and speech therapies throughout the disease process. Nutritional and psychological counseling are also important components of medical management. Physical therapy intervention includes regulation of activity level, relaxation and energy conservation techniques, normalization of tone, balance and gait training, core stabilization, and adaptive/assistive device training.

## Myasthenia Gravis[13,20,24]

Myasthenia gravis is an autoimmune disease resulting in neuromuscular junction pathology. There is a defect specifically in the transmission of nerve impulses to the muscles at the neuromuscular junction. Antibodies block or destroy the receptors that are needed for acetylcholine uptake and this prevents muscle contraction.

**Etiology** – This is an autoimmune disease process that also has an association with an enlarged thymus. There is also an association with diabetes, rheumatoid arthritis, lupus, and other immune disorders. There are multiple forms of myasthenia gravis that range from mild to severe involvement.

**Signs and symptoms** – The cardinal signs of myasthenia gravis include extreme fatiguability and skeletal muscle weakness that can fluctuate within minutes or over an extended period. The ocular muscles are typically affected first and approximately half of the patients experience ptosis and diplopia. Dysphagia, dysarthria, and cranial nerve weakness are also common findings.

**Treatment** – The disease process of myasthenia gravis will fluctuate and a patient will experience remissions and exacerbations. A myasthenia gravis "crisis" is a medical emergency where there is an exacerbation that includes the respiratory muscles and requires a ventilator. Anticholinesterase drug therapy, plasmapheresis, and immunosuppressive therapy may be utilized. Physical and occupational therapies are also indicated intermittently with supportive goals. Physical therapy will typically focus on obtaining a respiratory baseline and pulmonary intervention as needed. Energy conservation techniques and strengthening using isometric contractions are appropriate for most patients. Since patients typically require long-term corticosteroids, physical therapy may also focus on secondary osteoporosis.

## Parkinson's Disease[13,20,24]

Parkinson's disease is a primary degenerative disorder and is characterized by a decrease in production of dopamine (neurotransmitter) within the corpus striatum of the basal ganglia. The basal ganglia stores the majority of dopamine and is responsible for modulation and control of voluntary movement.

**Etiology** – Primary Parkinson's disease has an unknown etiology and accounts for the majority of patients with Parkinsonism. Contributing factors that can produce symptoms of Parkinson's disease include genetic defect, toxicity from carbon monoxide, excessive manganese or copper, carbon disulfide, vascular impairment of the striatum, encephalitis, and other neurodegenerative diseases such as Huntington's disease or Alzheimer's disease. The majority of patients are between 50 and 79 years of age and approximately 10% are diagnosed before 40 years.

## Consider This

### Facts and Physical Therapy Guidelines for Treating Myasthenia Gravis[13]

Treating a patient with myasthenia gravis requires an understanding of the disease process, precautions, and contraindications to treatment. Common facts associated with myasthenia gravis include:

- myasthenia gravis encompasses mild to severe symptoms and can fluctuate in severity from hour to hour at times
- proximal muscle groups are typically more affected than distal muscle groups
- difficulty with speech, swallowing, and chewing may persist due to weakness of the pharyngeal muscles and muscles of mastication
- involvement of the cranial nerves may result in eyelid weakness, diplopia, and ptosis
- typified by exacerbations, remissions, and atypically, "crisis" which is life-threatening
- remissions are not typically complete or permanent

**Physical therapy guidelines in the treatment of myasthenia gravis should include:**

- acquire a baseline for respiratory and neurological status
- monitor respiratory function on a regular basis to ensure that the muscles of respiration are not weakening
- review proper techniques for positioning during meals to prevent aspiration
- observe for signs of a myasthenia "crisis" (e.g., respiratory difficulty, swallowing issues, labored talking or chewing)
- review signs of toxicity and side effects of pharmacological intervention
- educate the patient to plan activity around periods of increased energy
- instruct and review energy conservation techniques
- avoid strenuous exercise and stress
- avoid excessive heat or cold as it exacerbates symptoms
- educate regarding signs of osteoporosis for patients that are using long-term corticosteroids
- initiate strengthening for patients with mild to moderate symptoms using moderate to maximal isometric contractions, while avoiding muscle fatigue
- treatment should always be based on the patient's current symptoms, strength, and level of fatigue

**Signs and symptoms** – The majority of patients with Parkinson's disease will initially notice a resting tremor in the hands (sometimes called a pill-rolling tremor) or feet that increases with stress and disappears with movement or sleep. Early symptoms can include balance disturbances, difficulty rolling over and rising from bed, and impairment with fine manipulative movements seen in writing, bathing, and dressing. Progression of the disease process includes hypokinesia, sluggish movement, difficulty with initiating (akinesia) and stopping movement, festinating and shuffling gait, bradykinesia, poor posture, dysphagia, and "cogwheel" or "lead pipe" rigidity of skeletal muscles. Patients may also experience "freezing" during ambulation, speech, blinking, and movements of the arms. A patient with Parkinson's disease may also have a mask-like appearance with no facial expression.

**Treatment** – The medical management of Parkinson's disease relies heavily on pharmacological intervention. Dopamine replacement therapy is most effective in reducing movement disorders, bradykinesia, rigidity, and tremor. Physical, occupational, and speech therapies may be warranted intermittently throughout the course of the disease. Physical therapy intervention should include maximizing endurance, strength, and functional mobility. Verbal cueing and visual feedback are also effective tools to use with this population.

### Post-polio Syndrome (PPS)[13]

Poliomyelitis is a viral infection resulting in neuropathy that includes focal and asymmetrical motor impairments. In the United States, this virus was all but eradicated in the 1960s with the development of a vaccine. Post-polio syndrome is a lower motor neuron pathology that affects the anterior horn cells of those previously affected with polio. Surviving axons were originally able to increase the size of their innervation ratio to assist denervated muscle. PPS occurs when the compensated reinnervation fails and results in ongoing muscle denervation.

**Etiology** – A previous diagnosis of polio is essential to diagnose PPS. Approximately 25-50% of persons with polio experience PPS decades after their initial recovery (average interval is approximately 25 years).

**Signs and symptoms** – Symptoms vary, however, commonly there is slow and progressive weakness, fatigue, muscle atrophy, pain, and swallowing issues.

**Treatment** – There is no pharmacological intervention to alter the progression of PPS. Emphasis of treatment surrounds lifestyle modification and symptomatic intervention. Physical therapy should emphasize supervised exercise, functional independence, adaptive equipment, and education to assist patients to maintain as much independence as possible.

# Cerebrovascular Accident

A cerebrovascular accident is a specific event that results in a lack of oxygen supply to a specific area of the brain secondary to either ischemia or hemorrhage. The outcome of a CVA greatly varies and is based on etiology, extent of the CVA, the area of the brain that is affected, subsequent collateral damage, and the patient's co-morbidities and overall health status.

## Spotlight on Safety
### Risk Factors for Cerebrovascular Accident[13,20,24]

There are a number of primary and secondary risk factors that can lead to the development of a CVA. Patient education regarding risk factors and impairments secondary to CVA should be included in all treatment plans for patients that are at increased risk. Many risk factors are modifiable and can be altered to improve a patient's risk profile and overall health.

| Primary | Secondary |
|---|---|
| Hypertension | Obesity |
| Cardiac disease or arrhythmias | High cholesterol |
| Diabetes mellitus | Behaviors related to hypertension (i.e., stress, excessive salt intake) |
| Cigarette smoking | Physical inactivity |
| Transient ischemic attacks | Increased alcohol consumption |

## Types of Cerebrovascular Accidents[13,20,24]

### Transient Ischemic Attack (TIA)

A transient ischemic attack is usually linked to an atherosclerotic thrombosis which causes a temporary interruption of blood supply to an area of the brain. The effects may be similar to a CVA, but symptoms resolve quickly, typically within 24 to 48 hours. A TIA most often occurs in the carotid and vertebrobasilar arteries and may indicate future CVA.

### Completed Stroke

A CVA that presents with total neurological deficits at the onset.

### Stroke in Evolution

A CVA, usually caused by a thrombus that gradually progresses. Total neurological deficits are not seen for one to two days after onset.

### Ischemic Stroke

Once there is a loss of perfusion to a portion of the brain (within just seconds), there is a central area of irreversible infarction surrounded by an area of potential ischemia.

- **Embolus (20% of ischemic CVAs)**

  Associated with cardiovascular disease, an embolus may be a solid, liquid or gas, and can originate in any part of the body. The embolus travels through the bloodstream to the cerebral arteries causing occlusion of a blood vessel and a resultant infarct. The middle cerebral artery is most commonly affected by an embolus from the internal carotid arteries. Due to the sudden onset of occlusion, tissues distal to the infarct can sustain higher permanent damage than those of thrombotic infarcts. An embolic CVA occurs rapidly with no warning, and often presents with a headache. Common cardiac disorders that can lead to embolism include valvular disease (i.e., rheumatic mitral stenosis), ischemic heart disease, acute myocardial infarction, arrhythmias (i.e., atrial fibrillation), patent foramen ovale, cardiac tumors, and post cardiac catheterization.

- **Thrombus**

An atherosclerotic plaque develops in an artery and eventually occludes the artery or a branching artery causing an infarct. This type of CVA is extremely variable in onset where symptoms can appear in minutes or over several days. A thrombotic CVA usually occurs during sleep or upon awakening after a myocardial infarction or post-surgical procedure.

## Hemorrhage (10 - 15% of CVAs)

Hemorrhage is an abnormal bleeding in the brain due to a rupture in blood supply. The infarct is due to disruption of oxygen to an area of the brain and compression from the accumulation of blood. Hypertension is usually a precipitating factor causing rupture of an aneurysm or arteriovenous malformation. Trauma can also precipitate hemorrhage and subsequent CVA. Characteristics include severe headache, vomiting, high blood pressure, and an abrupt onset of symptoms. Hemorrhage usually occurs during the day with symptoms evolving in relation to the speed of the bleed. Approximately 50% of deaths from hemorrhagic stroke occur within the first 48 hours.

## Characteristics of a Cerebrovascular Accident[1,2,30]

| Left Hemisphere | Right Hemisphere | Brainstem | Cerebellum |
|---|---|---|---|
| Weakness, paralysis of the right side | Weakness, paralysis of the left side | Unstable vital signs | Decreased balance |
| Increased frustration | Decreased attention span | Decreased consciousness | Ataxia |
| Decreased processing | Left hemianopsia | Decreased ability to swallow | Decreased coordination |
| Possible aphasia (expressive, receptive, global) | Decreased awareness and judgment | Weakness on both sides of the body | Nausea |
| Possible dysphagia | Memory deficits | Paralysis on both sides of the body | Decreased ability for postural adjustment |
| Possible motor apraxia (ideomotor and ideational) | Left inattention | | Nystagmus |
| Decreased discrimination between left and right | Decreased abstract reasoning | | |
| Right hemianopsia | Emotional lability | | |
| | Impulsive behaviors | | |
| | Decreased spatial orientation | | |

## Synergy Patterns[35]

When the central nervous system is damaged as with a CVA, the higher centers of the brain are also damaged. The higher centers are responsible for both complex motor patterns and the inhibition of massive gross motor patterns. Synergy patterns result when the higher centers of the brain lose control and the uncontrolled or partially controlled stereotyped patterns of the middle and lower centers emerge.

### Upper Limb

|  | Flexor Synergy | Extensor Synergy |
|---|---|---|
| Scapula | Elevation and retraction | Depression and protraction |
| Shoulder | Abduction and lateral rotation | Medial rotation and adduction |
| Elbow | Flexion | Extension |
| Forearm | Supination | Pronation |
| Wrist | Flexion | Extension |
| Fingers | Flexion with adduction | Flexion with adduction |
| Thumb | Flexion and adduction | Adduction and flexion |

- The flexor synergy is seen when the patient attempts to lift up their arm or reach for an object.

### Lower Limb

|  | Flexor Synergy | Extensor Synergy |
|---|---|---|
| Hip | Abduction and lateral rotation | Extension, medial rotation and adduction |
| Knee | Flexion | Extension |
| Ankle | Dorsiflexion with supination | Plantar flexion with inversion |
| Toes | Extension | Flexion and adduction |

- The flexor synergy is characterized by great toe extension and flexion of the remaining toes secondary to spasticity.

## CVA Tests and Measures[20,24,29]

There are various tests and measures to assess the different impairments secondary to CVA. Patients are administered specific tests based on clinical diagnosis and patient presentation.

- **National Institute of Health (NIH) Stroke Scale:** assessment of an acute CVA relative to impairment

- **Functional Independence Measure (FIM):** provides a level of burden through assessment of mobility and ADL management

- **Stroke Impact Scale:** assessment of physical and social disability or level of impairment secondary to CVA

- **Fugl-Meyer Assessment of Physical Performance:** motor, sensory, and balance impairment; also assesses pain and range of motion

# Neurological Rehabilitation

Neurological rehabilitation may incorporate a variety of treatments based on the patient's pathology, problem list, and deficits. There are many forms of neurological rehabilitation based on each construct's beliefs regarding motor control and motor learning. A therapist must use therapeutic techniques that meet the individual patient's therapeutic objectives and goals. The following are various theories of neurological rehabilitation based on each theory's interpretation of motor control and motor learning.

## Motor Control[28,30]

Motor control is the study of the nature of movement; or the ability to regulate or direct essential movement. Historically, control was thought to arise from reflex or hierarchical models where the cortex was perceived as the highest functioning component of the system and spinal level reflexes were the lowest functioning components. New models of motor control challenge these theories and believe that there is a greater distribution of control and that the cortex is not solely at the top of the hierarchy.

Theories in general should provide a framework to interpret the issue or behavior, guide clinical action and treatment, provide new ideas, and utilize working hypotheses for examination and intervention. There are multiple theories of motor control that each embrace abstract ideas regarding the actual control of movement and are based on a specific interpretation of how the brain functions and interacts with other body systems. Some of the motor control theories include the Reflex theory, Hierarchical theory, Motor programming theory, Task-oriented theory, and Ecological theory.

### Motor Learning[28,36]

Motor learning is the study of the acquisition or modification of movement. Motor learning differentiates learning versus performance, provides guidelines for appropriate use of feedback, prioritizes the impact of practice as it relates to skill and movement, and also focuses on the transfer of learning across tasks and environments of practice. Two of the initial theories of motor learning include:

- **Adam's closed loop theory:** The first attempt at the creation of a comprehensive motor learning theory with the premise of sensory feedback as an ongoing process for the nervous system to compare current movement with stored information on memory of past movement; high emphasis on the concept of practice.

- **Schmidt's schema theory:** This theory was created in response to the limitations of the closed loop theory. Its main construct relies on open loop control processes and a motor program concept; promotes clinical value of feedback and importance of variation with practice.

## Three Stage Model of Motor Learning[7,26,36]

**Cognitive Stage:** This is the initial stage of learning where there is a high concentration of conscious processing of information. The person will acquire information regarding the goal of the activity and begin to problem solve as to how to attain the goal. A controlled environment is ideal for learning during this stage and participation is a must for the person to progress.

### Characterized by:

- large amount of errors
- inconsistent attempts
- repetition of effort allows for improvement in strategies
- inconsistent performance
- high degree of cognitive work: listening, observing, and processing feedback

**Associative Stage:** This is the intermediate stage of learning where a person is able to more independently distinguish correct versus incorrect performance. The person is linking the feedback that has been received with the movement that has been performed and the ultimate goal. A controlled environment is helpful but at this stage, the person can progress to a less structured or more open environment. Avoid excessive external feedback as the person should have improved internal or proprioceptive feedback for the task at hand.

### Characterized by:

- decreased errors with new skill performance
- decreased need for concentration and cognition regarding the activity
- skill refinement
- increased coordination of movement
- large amount of practice yields refinement of the motor program surrounding the activity

**Autonomous Stage:** This is the final stage of learning or skilled learning where a person improves the efficiency of the activity without a great need for cognitive control. The person can also perform the task with interference from a variable environment.

### Characterized by:

- automatic response
- mainly error-free regardless of environment
- patterns of movement are non-cognitive and automatic
- distraction does not impact the activity
- the person can simultaneously perform more than one task if needed
- extrinsic feedback should be very limited or should not be provided
- internal feedback or self-assessment should be dominant

## Feedback[36]

Feedback is imperative for the progression of motor learning. A patient will rely on both intrinsic and extrinsic feedback as it relates to movement. Feedback allows for correction and adaptation within the environment. Current research supports reducing the extrinsic feedback (fading of feedback) in order to ultimately enhance learning.

**Intrinsic (inherent) feedback:** represents all feedback that comes to the person through sensory systems as a result of the movement including visual, vestibular, proprioceptive, and somatosensory inputs.

**Extrinsic (augmented) feedback:** represents the information that can be provided while a task or movement is in progress or subsequent to the movement. This is typically in the form of verbal feedback or manual contacts.

**Knowledge of results:** is an important form of extrinsic feedback and includes terminal feedback regarding the outcome of a movement that has been performed in relation to the movement's goals.

**Knowledge of performance:** is extrinsic feedback that relates to the actual movement pattern that someone used to achieve their goal of movement.

## Practice[36]

Practice refers to repeated performance of an activity in order to learn or perfect a skill. Physical practice allows for direct physical experience and kinesthetic stimulation to assist with acquisition of the skill. Mental practice is the cognitive rehearsal of a task or experience without any physical movement.

There are several commonly used terms that describe various types of practice:

**Massed practice:** The practice time in a trial is greater than the amount of rest between trials. *practice > rest*

**Distributed practice:** The amount of rest time between trials is equal to or is greater than the amount of practice time for each trial. *rest ≥ practice*

**Constant practice:** Practice of a given task under a uniform condition.

**Variable practice:** Practice of a given task under differing conditions.

**Random practice:** Varying practice amongst different tasks.

**Blocked practice:** Consistent practice of a single task.

**Whole training:** Practice of an entire task.

**Part training:** Practice of an individual component or selected components of a task.

## Key Terminology[28,36]

**Closed system model:** This is characterized by transfer of information that incorporates multiple feedback loops and larger distribution of control. In this model, the nervous system is seen as an active "participant" with the ability to enable the initiation of movement as opposed to solely "reacting" to stimuli.

**Compensation:** The ability to utilize alternate motor and sensory strategies due to an impairment that limits the normal completion of a task.

**Habituation:** The decrease in response that will occur as a result of consistent exposure to non-painful stimuli.

**Learning:** The process of acquiring knowledge about the world that leads to a relatively permanent change in a person's capability to perform a skilled action.

- **Non-associative:** a single repeated stimulus (habituation, sensitization)
- **Associative:** gaining understanding of the relationship between two stimuli, causal relationships or stimulus and consequence (classical conditioning, operant conditioning)
- **Procedural:** learning tasks that can be performed without attention or concentration to the task; a task is learned by forming movement habits (developing a habit through repetitive practice)
- **Declarative:** requires attention, awareness, and reflection in order to attain knowledge that can be consciously recalled (mental practice)

**Motor learning:** The ability to perform a movement as a result of internal processes that interact with the environment and produce a consistent strategy to generate the correct movement. It is the acquisition of, or modification of movement.

**Motor program:** A concept of a central motor pattern that can be activated by sensory stimuli or central processes. Motor programs are seen as containing the rules for creating spatial and temporal patterns of motor activity needed to carry out a given motor task.

**Open system model:** This is characterized by a single transfer of information without any feedback loop (reflexive hierarchical theory). In this theory, the nervous system is seen as awaiting stimuli in order to react.

**Performance:** A temporary change in motor behavior seen during a particular session of practice that is a result of many variables, however, only one variable is focusing on the act of learning. Performance is not an absolute measure of learning since there are multiple variables that potentially affect performance.

**Plasticity:** The ability to modify or change at the synapse level either temporarily or permanently in order to perform a particular function.

**Postural control:** The ability of the motor and sensory systems to stabilize position and control movement.

**Recovery:** The ability to utilize previous strategies to return to the same level of functioning.

**Sensitization:** The increase in response that will occur as a result of a noxious stimuli.

**Strategy:** A plan used to produce a specific result or outcome that will influence the structure or system.

## Consider This

### Motor Learning Intervention Constructs[28,30,36]

The following are general concepts of motor learning that should be considered when evaluating, developing a plan of care, and treating patients. Many therapists will utilize therapeutic interventions from various theories of neurological rehabilitation based on the individual patient.

- Models of motor control vary based on the interpretation of brain function
- Examination determines the degree of impairment
- Intervention is designed at the level of impairment
- It is essential for a patient to relearn how to perform a functional task in order to maximize recovery and independence
- Sensory, motor, and cognitive strategies should be used to acquire postural control
- Focus is both on recovery and compensatory techniques
- Belief that sensory, motor, and perceptual input contribute to motor control
- Movement is based around a behavioral goal
- Type and amount of feedback (visual, verbal, tactile) should be determined for each individual patient
- Emphasis on postural control, alignment, and sequencing of movements is essential
- Intervention should create multiple ways to solve a movement disorder
- Belief that performance is observed, the act of learning is not
- Environmental factors must be considered with intervention, planning, and implementation

### Carr and Shepherd: Motor Relearning Approach[28,37,38]

An approach developed by Janet Carr and Roberta Shepherd in the 1970's that targets normal movement and how it is relearned after neurological insult. Carr and Shepherd's construct is that factors that are involved with learning are also involved with relearning and should include:[28]

- identification of a goal

- inhibition of any unnecessary activity that does not relate to normal movement

- the ability to adjust during activity to the effects of gravity and balance

- proper body alignment

- proper motivation

- incorporate internal or mental practice as well as external or physical practice

- feedback

- knowledge of results

A significant construct of this approach is centered around a therapist's observation of the patient during examination in order to identify the variations in normal movement. Through critical assessment, the therapist is able to identify components of movement that are missing or abnormal and the corresponding interventions. Treatment relies on techniques inherent to this approach as well as other various approaches to neurological rehabilitation. Intrinsic feedback through sensory, visual, proprioceptive or tactile channels as well as external feedback through an observer is necessary for the patient to influence their progress towards their goals.

### Key Terminology[30,37,38]

**Closed motor skill:** A skill that is performed under a stable and unchanging environment.

**Knowledge of results:** Providing the patient with external feedback regarding a patient's performance of a task. This can include observations as well as objective data and can be positive or negative in nature with the goal of influencing the learner.

**Open motor skill:** A skill that is performed under a consistently changing environment.

**Transfer of learning:** An action cannot be separated from the environment that it is performed in. A patient must be able to transfer the skill or motor task into different environments.

## Consider This

### Motor Relearning Intervention Constructs[37,38]

The following are general concepts of motor relearning that should be considered when evaluating, developing a plan of care, and treating patients. Many therapists will utilize therapeutic interventions from various theories of neurological rehabilitation based on the individual patient.

- Utilizes various techniques from other treatment approaches

- Belief that treatment cannot be routine or based on diagnosis, must be individual to the patient

- Developmental sequence may not be necessary in treatment when treating adults

- Practice may include breaking the task into discrete components, followed by practice of the task as a whole

- Use of Bobath techniques for handling, facilitation, inhibitive casting, use of therapeutic ball (Figs. 5-41, 5-42)

- Use of Rood techniques of application of ice, brushing, tapping for facilitation

- Biofeedback should be utilized for decreasing hypertonicity with movement or for targeting facilitation of a muscle group

- Self-correction and self-awareness should be incorporated into treatment through the use of a mirror, verbal feedback, and biofeedback

- Intrinsic and extrinsic (augmented) feedback are important during treatment

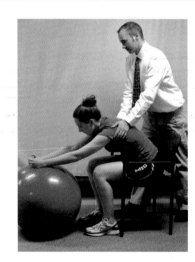

**Fig. 5-41:** Facilitation of movement patterns using a therapeutic ball.

**Fig. 5-42:** Therapist uses handling techniques and facilitation to assist with functional activities.

### Bobath: Neuromuscular Developmental Treatment (NDT)[30,39]

An approach developed by Karl and Berta Bobath based on the hierarchical model of neurophysiologic function. Abnormal postural reflex activity and abnormal muscle tone are caused by the loss of central nervous system control at the brainstem and spinal cord levels. The concept recognizes that interference of normal function within the brain caused by central nervous system dysfunction leads to a slowing down or cessation of motor de-

velopment and the inhibition of righting reactions, equilibrium reactions, and automatic movements. The patient should learn to control movement through activities that promote normal movement patterns that integrate function.

New assumptions that have been incorporated into NDT resulting from current motor control research include:[28]

- Postural control can be learned and modified through experience

- Postural control uses both feedback and feed-forward mechanisms for execution of tasks

**SCORE**BUILDERS

- Postural control is initiated from a patient's base of support
- Postural control is required for skill development
- Postural control develops by assuming progressive positions in which there is an increase in the distance between the center of gravity and base of support; the base of support should also decrease

### Key Terminology

**Facilitation:** A technique utilized to elicit voluntary muscular contraction.

**Inhibition:** A technique utilized to decrease excessive tone or movement.

**Key points of control:** Specific handling of designated areas of the body (shoulder, pelvis, hand, and foot) will influence and facilitate posture, alignment, and control (Fig. 5-43).

**Placing:** The act of moving an extremity into a position that the patient must hold against gravity.

**Reflex inhibiting posture:** Designated static positions that Bobath found to inhibit abnormal tonal influences and reflexes.

**Fig. 5-43:** Facilitation using key points of control.

## Consider This

### NDT Intervention Constructs[30,39]

The following are general concepts of NDT that should be considered when evaluating, developing a plan of care, and treating patients. Many therapists will utilize therapeutic interventions from various theories of neurological rehabilitation based on the individual patient.

- Inhibition of abnormal patterns of movement with simultaneous facilitation of normal patterns

- Alteration of abnormal tone and influencing isolated active movement

- Avoid utilization of abnormal reflexes or associated reactions during treatment

- Utilize manual contact and handling through key points of control for facilitation and inhibition (Fig. 5-44)

- Achieve a balance between muscle groups during therapeutic interventions

- Utilize the developmental sequence, dynamic reflex inhibiting patterns, and functional activities with varying levels of difficulty during therapeutic intervention

- Emphasize the use of rotation during treatment activities (Fig. 5-45)

- Provide the patient with the sensation of normal movement by inhibiting abnormal postural reflex activity

- Treatment should be active and dynamic, incorporating function

- Provide orientation to midline control by moving in and out of midline with dynamic activity (Fig. 5-46)

- Belief that compensation techniques are unnecessary and should be avoided

**Fig. 5-44:** The therapist uses a NDT technique of manual contacts and therapeutic handling to decrease tonal influence during motor output and functional activity. Key points of control can facilitate or inhibit tone based on the therapeutic goals.

**Fig. 5-45:** NDT encourages the use of rotation during therapeutic activities.

**Fig. 5-46:** Using developmental sequence to gain midline control. The therapist can facilitate the patient to move in and out of midline to improve dynamic mobility and control.

## Brunnstrom: Movement Therapy in Hemiplegia[24,40,41]

Movement therapy in hemiplegia developed by Signe Brunnstrom is based on the hierarchical model by Hughlings Jackson. This approach created and defined the term synergy and initially encouraged the use of synergy patterns during rehabilitation. The belief was to immediately practice synergy patterns and subsequently develop combinations of movement patterns outside of the synergy. Synergies are considered primitive patterns that occur at the spinal cord level as a result of the hierarchical organization of the central nervous system. Reinforcing synergy patterns is rarely utilized now as research has indicated that reinforced synergy patterns are very difficult to change. Brunnstrom developed the seven stages of recovery, which are used for evaluation and documentation of patient progress.

### Key Terminology

**Associated reaction:** An involuntary and automatic movement of a body part as a result of an intentional active or resistive movement in another body part.

**Homolateral synkinesis:** A flexion pattern of the involved upper extremity facilitates flexion of the involved lower extremity.

**Limb synergies:** A group of muscles that produce a predictable pattern of movement in flexion or extension patterns.

**Raimiste's phenomenon:** The involved lower extremity will abduct or adduct with applied resistance to the uninvolved lower extremity in the same direction.

**Souques' phenomenon:** Raising the involved upper extremity above 100 degrees with elbow extension will produce extension and abduction of the fingers.

**Stages of recovery:** Brunnstrom separates neurological recovery into seven separate stages based on progression through abnormal tone and spasticity. These seven stages of recovery describe tone, reflex activity, and volitional movement.

### Seven Stages of Recovery[28]

**Stage 1:** No volitional movement initiated.

**Stage 2:** The appearance of basic limb synergies. The beginning of spasticity.

**Stage 3:** The synergies are performed voluntarily; spasticity increases.

**Stage 4:** Spasticity begins to decrease. Movement patterns are not dictated solely by limb synergies.

**Stage 5:** A further decrease in spasticity is noted with independence from limb synergy patterns.

**Stage 6:** Isolated joint movements are performed with coordination.

**Stage 7:** Normal motor function is restored.

## Consider This
### Movement Therapy in Hemiplegia Intervention Constructs[28,41]

The following are general concepts of movement therapy in hemiplegia that should be considered when evaluating, developing a plan of care, and treating patients. Many therapists will utilize therapeutic interventions from various theories of neurological rehabilitation based on the individual patient.

- Evaluation of strength focuses on patterns of movement rather than straight plane motion at a joint

- Sensory examination is required to assist with treating motor deficits

- Initially limb synergies are encouraged as a necessary milestone for recovery

- Encourage overflow to recruit active movement of the weak side

- Repetition of task and positive reinforcement should be emphasized during treatment activities

- A patient will follow the stages of recovery, but may experience a plateau at any point so that full recovery may not be achieved

- Movement combinations that deviate from the basic limb synergies should be introduced in stage 4 of recovery

- Treatment should incorporate only tasks that the patient can master or almost master

### Kabat, Knott, and Voss: Proprioceptive Neuromuscular Facilitation (PNF)[30,40]

PNF was introduced in the early 1950's using the hierarchical model as its framework. The original goal of treatment was to establish gross motor patterns within the central nervous system. This approach is based on the premise that stronger parts of the body are utilized to stimulate and strengthen the weaker parts. Normal movement and posture is based on a balance between control of antagonist and agonist muscle groups. Development will follow the normal sequence through a component of motor learning. This theory places great emphasis on manual contacts and correct handling. Short and concise verbal commands are used along with resistance throughout the full movement pattern. The PNF approach utilizes methods that promote or hasten the response of the neuromuscular mechanism through stimulation of the proprioceptors. Movement patterns follow diagonals or spirals that each possess a flexion, extension, and rotatory component and are directed toward or away from midline.

### Key Terminology

**Chopping:** A combination of bilateral upper extremity asymmetrical patterns performed as a closed-chain activity (Fig. 5-47).

**Developmental sequence:** A progression of motor skill acquisition. The stages of motor control include mobility, stability, controlled mobility, and skill.

**Mass movement patterns:** The hip, knee, and ankle move into flexion or extension simultaneously.

**Overflow:** Muscle activation of an involved extremity due to intense action of an uninvolved muscle or group of muscles.

**Fig. 5-47:** Chopping is a PNF technique using bilateral upper extremity patterns of movement to improve strength, stability, and control.

## Consider This

### PNF Intervention Constructs (Kabat, Knott, Voss)[30,40]

The following are general concepts of PNF that should be considered when evaluating, developing a plan of care, and treating patients. Many therapists will utilize therapeutic interventions from various theories of neurological rehabilitation based on the individual patient.

- A patient learns diagonal patterns of movement
- Techniques must have accurate timing, specific commands, and correct hand placement
- Verbal commands must be short and concise
- Repetition of task or activity is important in motor learning
- Resistance given during the movement pattern is greater if the objective is stability (Fig. 5-48), less if the objective is mobility (Fig. 5-49)
- Techniques should utilize isometric and isotonic muscle contractions
- Treatment objectives will dictate the use of techniques through either full movement or at points within the range
- Developmental sequence is used in conjunction with PNF techniques in order to increase the balance between agonists and antagonists
- PNF techniques are implemented to progress a patient through the stages of motor control
- Functional patterns of movement are used to increase control
- Techniques should be utilized that increase strength or improve relaxation by enhancing overflow from the stronger to the weaker muscles

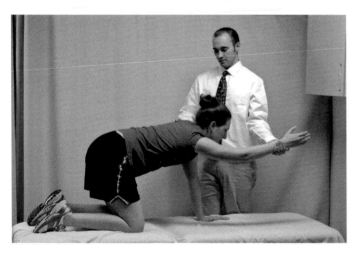

**Fig. 5-48:** A therapist can provide a graded amount of resistance based on therapeutic goals. This patient is working through the developmental sequence and the therapist is providing a larger amount of resistance to improve stability with a varying base of support.

**Fig. 5-49:** The therapist is using minimal resistance during a lower extremity PNF pattern to improve mobility and active movement.

## PNF Diagonal Patterns – Upper Extremity Responses

|  | **D1 Flexion Pattern** (Fig. 5-50) | **D1 Extension Pattern** | **D2 Flexion Pattern** | **D2 Extension Pattern** |
|---|---|---|---|---|
| **Scapula** | Elevation<br>Abduction<br>Upward rotation | Depression<br>Adduction<br>Downward rotation | Elevation<br>Adduction<br>Upward rotation | Depression<br>Abduction<br>Downward rotation |
| **Shoulder** | Flexion<br>Adduction<br>Lateral rotation | Extension<br>Abduction<br>Medial rotation | Flexion<br>Abduction<br>Lateral rotation | Extension<br>Adduction<br>Medial rotation |
| **Elbow** | Flexion or extension | Flexion or extension | Flexion or extension | Flexion or extension |
| **Radioulnar** | Supination | Pronation | Supination | Pronation |
| **Wrist** | Flexion<br>Radial deviation | Extension<br>Ulnar deviation | Extension<br>Radial deviation | Flexion<br>Ulnar deviation |
| **Thumb** | Adduction | Abduction | Extension | Opposition |

## PNF Diagonal Patterns – Lower Extremity Responses

|  | **D1 Flexion Pattern** | **D1 Extension Pattern** | **D2 Flexion Pattern** (Fig. 5-51) | **D2 Extension Pattern** |
|---|---|---|---|---|
| **Pelvis** | Protraction | Retraction | Elevation | Depression |
| **Hip** | Flexion<br>Adduction<br>Lateral rotation | Extension<br>Abduction<br>Medial rotation | Flexion<br>Abduction<br>Medial rotation | Extension<br>Adduction<br>Lateral rotation |
| **Knee** | Flexion or extension | Flexion or extension | Flexion or extension | Flexion or extension |
| **Ankle and Toes** | Dorsiflexion<br>Inversion | Plantar flexion<br>Eversion | Dorsiflexion<br>Eversion | Plantar flexion<br>Inversion |

**Fig. 5-50:** D1F pattern of the upper extremity.

**Fig. 5-51:** D2F pattern of the lower extremity.

## Levels of Motor Control[40]

### Mobility

The ability to initiate movement through a functional range of motion.

### Stability

The ability to maintain a position or posture through cocontraction and tonic holding around a joint. Unsupported sitting with midline control is an example of stability.

### Controlled Mobility

The ability to move within a weight bearing position or rotate around a long axis. Activities in prone on elbows or weight shifting in quadruped are examples of controlled mobility. (Fig. 5-52).

### Skill

The ability to consistently perform functional tasks and manipulate the environment with normal postural reflex mechanisms and balance reactions. Skill activities include ADLs and community locomotion.

**Fig. 5-52:** The patient working in modified plantigrade is an example of controlled mobility.

## PNF Therapeutic Exercises

| Technique | Mobility | | Stability | Controlled Mobility | Skill | | Strength |
|---|---|---|---|---|---|---|---|
| | Increased ROM | Initiate Movement | | | Distal Functional Movement | Proximal Dynamic Stability | |
| Agonistic Reversals | | | | X | | X | |
| Alternating Isometrics | | | X | | | | X |
| Contract-Relax | X | | | | | | |
| Hold-Relax | X | | | | | | |
| Hold-Relax Active Movement | | X | | | | | |
| Joint Distraction | X | X | | | | | |
| Normal Timing | | | | | X | | |
| Repeated Contractions | | X | | | | | X |
| Resisted Progression | | | | | | X | X |
| Rhythmic Initiation | | X | | | | | |
| Rhythmical Rotation | X | X | | | | | |
| Rhythmic Stabilization | X | | X | | | | |
| Slow Reversal | | | X | X | X | | |
| Slow Reversal Hold | | | X | X | X | | |
| Timing for Emphasis | | | | | X | | X |

## PNF Therapeutic Exercise Descriptions

*Red colored terms indicate the level of developmental sequence.

### Agonistic Reversals (AR)

**Controlled mobility, skill:** An isotonic concentric contraction performed against resistance followed by alternating concentric and eccentric contractions with resistance. AR requires use in a slow and sequential manner, and may be used in increments throughout the range to attain maximum control.

### Alternating Isometrics (AI)

**Stability:** Isometric contractions are performed alternating from muscles on one side of the joint to the other side without rest. AI emphasizes endurance or strengthening.

### Contract-Relax (CR)

**Mobility:** A technique used to increase range of motion. As the extremity reaches the point of limitation, the patient performs a maximal contraction of the antagonistic muscle group. The therapist resists movement for eight to ten seconds with relaxation to follow. The technique is repeated until no further gains in range of motion are noted during the session.

### Hold-Relax (HR)

**Mobility:** An isometric contraction used to increase range of motion. The contraction is facilitated for all muscle groups at the limiting point in the range of motion. Relaxation occurs and the extremity moves through the newly acquired range to the next point of limitation until no further increases in range of motion occur. The technique is often used for patients that present with pain.

### Hold-Relax Active Movement (HRAM)

**Mobility:** A technique to improve initiation of movement to muscle groups tested at 1/5 or less. An isometric contraction is performed once the extremity is passively placed into a shortened range within the pattern. Overflow and facilitation may be used to assist with the contraction. Upon relaxation, the extremity is immediately moved into a lengthened position of the pattern with a quick stretch. The patient is asked to return the extremity to the shortened position through an isotonic contraction.

### Joint Distraction

**Mobility:** A proprioceptive component used to increase range of motion around a joint. Consistent manual traction is provided slowly and usually in combination with mobilization techniques. It can also be used in combination with quick stretch to initiate movement.

### Normal Timing (NT)

**Skill:** A technique used to improve coordination of all components of a task. NT is performed in a distal to proximal sequence. Proximal components are restricted until the distal components are activated and initiate movement. Repetition of the pattern produces a coordinated movement of all components.

### Repeated Contractions (RC)

**Mobility:** A technique used to initiate movement and sustain a contraction through the range of motion. RC is used to initiate a movement pattern, throughout a weak movement pattern or at a point of weakness within a movement pattern. The therapist provides a quick stretch followed by isometric or isotonic contractions.

### Resisted Progression (RP)

**Skill:** A technique used to emphasize coordination of proximal components during gait. Resistance is applied to an area such as the pelvis, hips or extremity during the gait cycle in order to enhance coordination, strength or endurance.

### Rhythmic Initiation (RI)

**Mobility:** A technique used to assist in initiating movement when hypertonia exists. Movement progresses from passive ("let me move you"), to active assistive ("help me move you"), to slightly resistive ("move against the resistance"). Movements must be slow and rhythmical to reduce the hypertonia and allow for full range of motion.

### Rhythmical Rotation (RR)

**Mobility:** A passive technique used to decrease hypertonia by slowly rotating an extremity around the longitudinal axis. Relaxation of the extremity will increase range of motion.

### Rhythmic Stabilization (RS)

**Mobility, stability:** A technique used to increase range of motion and coordinate isometric contractions. The technique requires isometric contractions of all muscles around a joint against progressive resistance. The patient should relax and move into the newly acquired range and repeat the technique. If stability is the goal, RS should be applied as a progression from AI in order to stabilize all muscle groups simultaneously around the specific body part.

### Slow Reversal (SR)

**Stability, controlled mobility, skill:** A technique of slow and resisted concentric contractions of agonists and antagonists around a joint without rest between reversals. This technique is used to improve control of movement and posture.

### Slow Reversal Hold (SRH)

**Stability, controlled mobility, skill:** Using slow reversal with the addition of an isometric contraction that is performed at the end of each movement in order to gain stability.

### Timing for Emphasis (TE)

**Skill:** Used to strengthen the weak component of a motor pattern. Isotonic and isometric contractions produce overflow to weak muscles.

## Rood[28,30]

This theory is based on Sherrington and the reflex stimulus model. Rood believed that all motor output was the result of both past and present sensory input. Treatment is based on sensorimotor learning. It takes into account the autonomic nervous system and emotional factors as well as motor ability. Rood used a developmental sequence, which was seen as "key patterns" in the enhancement of motor control. A goal of this approach is to obtain homeostasis in motor output and to activate muscles to perform a task independent of a stimulus. Exercise is seen as a treatment technique only if the response is correct and if it provides sensory feedback that enhances the motor learning of that response. Once a response is obtained during treatment, the stimulus should be withdrawn. Rood introduced the use of sensory stimulation to facilitate or inhibit responses such as icing and brushing in order to elicit desired reflex motor responses.

### Sensory Stimulation Techniques

| Facilitation | Inhibition |
| --- | --- |
| • Approximation (Fig. 5-53) | • Deep pressure |
| • Joint compression | • Prolonged stretch |
| • Icing | • Warmth |
| • Light touch | • Prolonged cold |
| • Quick stretch | |
| • Resistance | |
| • Tapping | |
| • Traction | |

**Fig. 5-53:** The therapist is providing approximation to the hips while the patient is in standing in order to improve cocontraction around the joint and subsequent stability.

### Key Terminology

**Heavy work:** A method used to develop stability by performing an activity (work) against gravity or resistance. Heavy work focuses on the strengthening of postural muscles.

**Light work:** A method used to develop controlled movement and skilled function by performing an activity (work) without resistance. Light work focuses on the extremities.

**Key patterns:** A developmental sequence designed by Rood that directs patients' mobility recovery from synergy patterns through controlled motion.

## Consider This

### Rood Sensory Intervention Constructs[28,30]

The following are general concepts of Rood that should be considered when evaluating, developing a plan of care, and treating patients. Many therapists will utilize therapeutic interventions from various theories of neurological rehabilitation based on the individual patient.

- Utilization of sensory stimulation to achieve motor output during treatment
- Movement is considered autonomic and noncognitive
- Homeostasis of all systems is essential
- Techniques such as neutral warmth, maintained pressure, and slow rhythmical stroking can be used to calm a patient
- Tactile stimulation is used to facilitate normal movement
- The environment can influence the effects of therapeutic intervention
- Exercise must provide proper sensory feedback in order to be therapeutic
- Belief in techniques used to stimulate the proprioceptive, exteroceptive, and vestibular channels of the central nervous system

# Neuromuscular and Nervous Systems Terminology[1,2,3,27]

**Agnosia:** The inability to interpret information.

**Agraphesthesia:** The inability to recognize symbols, letters or numbers traced on the skin.

**Agraphia:** The inability to write due to a lesion within the brain and is typically found in combination with aphasia.

**Alexia:** The inability to read or comprehend written language secondary to a lesion within the dominant lobe of the brain.

**Anosognosia:** The denial or unawareness of one's illness; often associated with unilateral neglect.

**Aphasia:** The inability to communicate or comprehend due to damage to specific areas of the brain.

**Apraxia:** The inability to perform purposeful learned movements or activities even though there is no sensory or motor impairment that would hinder completion of the task.

**Astereognosis:** The inability to recognize objects by sense of touch.

**Body schema:** Having an understanding of the body as a whole and the relationship of its parts to the whole.

**Constructional apraxia:** The inability to reproduce geometric figures and designs. A person is often unable to visually analyze how to perform a task.

**Decerebrate rigidity:** A characteristic of a corticospinal lesion at the level of the brainstem that results in extension of the trunk and all extremities (Fig. 5-54).

**Decorticate rigidity:** A characteristic of a corticospinal lesion at the level of the diencephalon where the trunk and lower extremities are positioned in extension and the upper extremities are positioned in flexion (Fig. 5-55).

**Diplopia:** Double vision

**Dysarthria:** Slurred and impaired speech due to a motor deficit of the tongue or other muscles essential for speech.

**Dysphagia:** The inability to properly swallow.

**Dysprosody:** Impairment in the rhythm and inflection of speech.

**Emotional lability:** A characteristic of a right hemisphere infarct where there is an inability to control emotions and outbursts of laughing or crying that are inconsistent with the situation.

**Fluent aphasia:** Characteristic of receptive aphasia where speech produces functional output regarding articulation, but lacks content and is typically dysprosodic using neologistic jargon.

**Hemiparesis:** A condition of weakness on one side of the body.

**Hemiplegia:** A condition of paralysis on one side of the body.

**Homonymous hemianopsia:** The loss of the right or left half of the field of vision in both eyes.

**Ideational apraxia:** The inability to formulate an initial motor plan and sequence tasks where the proprioceptive input necessary for movement is impaired.

**Ideomotor apraxia:** A condition where a person plans a movement or task, but cannot volitionally perform it. Automatic movement may occur, however, a person cannot impose additional movement on command.

**Neologism:** Substitution within a word that is so severe that it makes the word unrecognizable.

**Non-fluent aphasia:** Characteristic of expressive aphasia where speech is non-functional, effortful, and contains paraphasias. Writing is also impaired.

**Perseveration:** The state of repeatedly performing the same segment of a task or repeatedly saying the same word/phrase without purpose.

**Synergy:** Mass movement patterns that are primitive in nature and coupled with spasticity due to brain damage.

**Unilateral neglect:** The inability to interpret stimuli and events on the contralateral side of a hemispheric lesion. Left-sided neglect is most common with a lesion to the right inferior parietal or superior temporal lobes.

Fig. 5-54: Decerebrate positioning.

Fig. 5-55: Decorticate positioning.

# Spinal Cord Injury (SCI)

When there is sufficient force exerted on the spinal cord, there can be permanent damage with extensive neurological deficits. There are approximately 250,000 people in the United States today with traumatic spinal cord injuries. Motor vehicle accidents are the largest cause of traumatic SCI. Other etiologies include stabbing, falls, sports injuries, and high-risk behaviors. The mechanism of injury often dictates the predicted pattern of deficits. Flexion injuries occur most often at the C5-C6 level of the spine while extension injuries occur most at the C4-C5 level. Axial loading and rotatory injuries are other mechanisms for spinal cord damage. A spinal cord injury will have an area of primary damage followed by an area of secondary damage that can extend multiple spinal segments beyond the initial segment of injury.

## Types of Spinal Cord Injury[18,19,24]

**Complete lesion:** A lesion to the spinal cord where there is no preserved motor or sensory function below the level of the lesion.

**Incomplete lesion:** A lesion to the spinal cord with incomplete damage to the cord. There may be scattered motor function, sensory function or both below the level of the lesion.

## Specific Incomplete Lesions[18,19,24]

### Anterior Cord Syndrome

An incomplete lesion that results from compression and damage to the anterior part of the spinal cord or anterior spinal artery. The mechanism of injury is usually cervical flexion. There is loss of motor function and pain and temperature sense below the lesion due to damage of the corticospinal and spinothalamic tracts.

### Brown-Sequard's Syndrome

An incomplete lesion usually caused by a stab wound, which produces hemisection of the spinal cord. There is paralysis and loss of vibratory and position sense on the same side as the lesion due to the damage to the corticospinal tract and dorsal columns. There is a loss of pain and temperature sense on the opposite side of the lesion from damage to the lateral spinothalamic tract. Pure Brown-Sequard's syndrome is rare since most spinal cord lesions are atypical.

### Cauda Equina Injuries

An injury that occurs below the L1 spinal level where the long nerve roots transcend. Cauda equina injuries can be complete, however, they are frequently incomplete due to the large number of nerve roots in the area. A cauda equina injury is considered a peripheral nerve injury. Characteristics include flaccidity, areflexia, and impairment of bowel and bladder function. Full recovery is not typical due to the distance needed for axonal regeneration.

### Central Cord Syndrome

An incomplete lesion that results from compression and damage to the central portion of the spinal cord. The mechanism of injury is usually cervical hyperextension that damages the spinothalamic tract, corticospinal tract, and dorsal columns. The upper extremities present with greater involvement than the lower extremities and greater motor deficits exist as compared to sensory deficits.

### Posterior Cord Syndrome

A relatively rare syndrome that is caused by compression of the posterior spinal artery and is characterized by loss of pain perception, proprioception, two-point discrimination, and stereognosis. Motor function is preserved.

## Spinal Cord Injury Tests and Measures

### ASIA Impairment Scale
### (American Spinal Injury Association)[42]

| | |
|---|---|
| **A =** | **Complete:** No sensory or motor function is preserved in sacral segments S4-S5. |
| **B =** | **Sensory Incomplete:** Sensory but not motor function is preserved below the neurologic level and extends through sacral segments S4-S5. |
| **C =** | **Motor Incomplete:** Motor function is preserved below the neurologic level, and most key muscles below the neurologic level have a muscle grade less than 3. |
| **D =** | **Motor Incomplete:** Motor function is preserved below the neurologic level, and most key muscles below the neurologic level have a muscle grade greater than or equal to 3. |
| **E =** | **Normal:** Sensory and motor functions are normal. |

## Classification of Level of Injury

**Motor level:** The motor level is determined by the most caudal key muscles that have muscle strength of 3 or greater with the superior segment tested as normal or 5.

**Motor index scoring:** Testing each key muscle using the 0-5 scoring, with total points of 25 per extremity for the total possible score of 100.

**Sensory level:** The sensory level is determined by the most caudal dermatome with a normal score of 2/2 for pinprick and light touch.

## Key Muscles Tested

| | |
|---|---|
| C5 | Elbow flexors (biceps, brachialis) |
| C6 | Wrist extensors (extensor carpi radialis longus and brevis) |
| C7 | Elbow extensors (triceps) |
| C8 | Finger flexors (flexor digitorum profundus) to the middle finger |
| T1 | Small finger abductors (abductor digiti minimi) |
| L2 | Hip flexors (iliopsoas) |
| L3 | Knee extensors (quadriceps) |
| L4 | Ankle dorsiflexors (tibialis anterior) |
| L5 | Long toe extensors (extensor hallucis longus) |
| S1 | Ankle plantar flexors (gastrocnemius, soleus) |

## Potential Complications of Spinal Cord Injury[18,19,24]

### Deep Vein Thrombosis (DVT)

Deep vein thrombosis results from the formation of a blood clot that becomes dislodged and is termed an embolus. This is considered a serious medical condition since the embolus may obstruct a selected artery. A patient with a spinal cord injury has a greater risk of developing a DVT due to the absence or decrease in the normal pumping action by active contractions of muscles in the lower extremities. Homans' sign is a special test designed to confirm the presence of a DVT. Prevention of a DVT should include prophylactic anticoagulant therapy, maintaining a positioning schedule, range of motion, proper positioning to avoid excessive venous stasis, and use of elastic stockings.

**Symptoms:** Swelling of the lower extremity, pain, sensitivity over the area of the clot, and warmth in the area are cardinal symptoms of DVT.

**Treatment:** Once a DVT is suspected, there should be no active or passive movement performed to the involved lower extremity. Bed rest and anticoagulant pharmacological intervention are usually indicated. Surgical procedures can be performed if necessary.

## Sensory Testing for Light Touch and Pinprick

0=Absent, 1=Impaired/hyperesthesia, 2=Intact

| Level | Site for Sensory Testing |
|---|---|
| C2 | Occipital protuberance |
| C3 | Supraclavicular fossa |
| C4 | Top of the acromioclavicular joint |
| C5 | Lateral side of antecubital fossa |
| C6 | Thumb |
| C7 | Middle finger |
| C8 | Little finger |
| T1 | Medial side of antecubital fossa |
| T2 | Apex of axilla |
| T3 | Third intercostal space (IS) |
| T4 | Fourth IS at the nipple line |
| T5 | Fifth IS (midway between T4 and T6) |
| T6 | Sixth IS at the level of the xiphisternum |
| T7 | Seventh IS (midway between T6 and T8) |
| T8 | Eighth IS (midway between T6 and T10) |
| T9 | Ninth IS (midway between T8 and T10) |
| T10 | 10th IS or umbilicus |
| T11 | 11th IS (midway between T10 and T12) |
| T12 | Midpoint of inguinal ligament |
| L1 | Half the distance between T12 and L2 |
| L2 | Midanterior thigh |
| L3 | Medial femoral condyle |
| L4 | Medial malleolus |
| L5 | Dorsum of the foot at third metatarsophalangeal joint |
| S1 | Lateral heel |
| S2 | Popliteal fossa in the midline |
| S3 | Ischial tuberosity |
| S4-5 | Perianal area (taken as 1 level) |

# Spotlight on Safety

## Autonomic Dysreflexia: A Medical Emergency[18,43]

Autonomic dysreflexia is perhaps the most dangerous complication of spinal cord injury and can occur in patients with lesions at or above T6. A noxious stimulus below the level of the lesion triggers the autonomic nervous system causing a sudden elevation in blood pressure. Common causes include distended or full bladder, kink or blockage in the catheter, bladder infections, pressure ulcers, extreme temperature changes, tight clothing or even an ingrown toenail. If not treated, this condition can lead to convulsions, hemorrhage, and death.

**Symptoms:** High blood pressure, severe headache, blurred vision, stuffy nose, profuse sweating, goose bumps below the level of the lesion, and vasodilation (flushing) above the level of injury.

**Treatment:** The therapist should immediately check the catheter for blockage while having the patient assume or remain in a sitting position. Lying a patient down is contraindicated and will only assist to further elevate blood pressure. The patient should be examined for any other irritating stimuli and potentially checked for bowel impaction. If the cause remains unknown, the patient should receive immediate medical intervention.

## Ectopic Bone

Ectopic bone or heterotopic ossification refers to the spontaneous formation of bone in the soft tissue. It typically occurs adjacent to larger joints such as the knees or the hips. Theories regarding etiology range from tissue hypoxia to abnormal calcium metabolism.

**Symptoms:** Early symptoms include edema, decreased range of motion, and increased temperature of the involved joint.

**Treatment:** Pharmacological intervention usually involves diphosphates that inhibit ectopic bone formation. Physical therapy and surgery are often incorporated into treatment. Physical therapy should focus on maintaining functional range of motion and allowing the patient the most independent functional outcome possible.

## Orthostatic Hypotension

Orthostatic hypotension or postural hypotension occurs due to a loss of sympathetic control of vasoconstriction in combination with absent or severely reduced muscle tone. Venous pooling is fairly common during the early stages of rehabilitation. A decrease in systolic blood pressure greater than 20 mm Hg after moving from a supine position to a sitting position is typically indicative of orthostatic hypotension.

**Symptoms:** Complaints of dizziness, lightheadedness, nausea, and "blacking out" when going from a horizontal to a vertical position are primary symptoms of this condition.

**Treatment:** Monitoring vital signs assists with minimizing the effects of orthostatic hypotension. The use of elastic stockings, ace wraps to the lower extremities, and abdominal binders are common. Gradual progression to a vertical position using a tilt table is often indicated. Pharmacological intervention may be indicated in order to increase blood pressure.

## Pressure Ulcers

A pressure ulcer is caused by sustained pressure, friction, and/or shearing to a surface. The most common areas susceptible to pressure ulcers are the coccyx, sacrum, ischium, trochanters, elbows, buttocks, malleoli, scapulae, and prominent vertebrae. Pressure ulcers require immediate medical intervention and often can significantly delay the rehabilitation process.

# Spotlight on Safety

## SCI: Prevention of Pressure Ulcers[13,18,19]

Recent data shows that between 60-80% of people with SCI develop a pressure ulcer within their lifetime. Patients with spinal cord injury potentially experience many of the risk factors associated with the development of a pressure ulcer including:

- immobility
- decreased or absent sensation
- prolonged pressure to an area
- shearing forces
- poor positioning
- poor nutrition

**Prevention should include:**

**Proper positioning while sitting and in bed:** protecting all bony prominences, equal distribution of weight, use of equipment such as specialized cushions, mattress pads, and other pressure relief devices

**Proper skin care:** full cleansing and drying of skin, consistently inspect all skin and monitor any red areas closely; use of skin care products that are recommended by health care professionals

**Proper changing of position:** consistently change position every two hours; need to weight shift in sitting at a minimum of every 15-20 minutes

**Proper nutrition:** attain adequate nutrition and calories each day, drink the recommended amount of water, limit empty calories and alcohol intake

**Clothing:** wear clothing that is not high risk for skin breakdown (e.g., zippers), avoid tight clothing; clothing should be breathable with a comfortable fit

**Mobility:** daily activity is recommended and should include a cardiovascular component; however, avoid activities with a high shear or drag component

**Symptoms:** Primarily there is a reddened area that persists or an open area of the skin.

**Treatment:** Prevention is of greatest importance. A patient should change position frequently, maintain proper skin care, sit on an appropriate cushion, consistently weight shift, and maintain proper nutrition and hydration. Surgical intervention is often necessary with advanced pressure ulcers.

### Spasticity

Spasticity can occasionally be useful to a patient with a spinal cord injury, however, more often serves to interfere with functional activities. Spasticity can be enhanced by both internal and external sources such as stress, decubiti, urinary tract infections, bowel or bladder obstruction, temperature changes or touch.

**Symptoms:** Increased involuntary contraction of muscle groups, increased tonic stretch reflexes, and exaggerated DTRs.

**Treatment:** Medications are usually administered in an attempt to reduce the degree of spasticity (Dantrium, Baclofen, Lioresal). Aggressive treatment includes phenol blocks, rhizotomies, myelotomies, and other surgical interventions. Physical therapy intervention includes positioning, aquatic therapy, weight bearing, functional electrical stimulation, range of motion, resting splints, and inhibitive casting.

## Functional Outcomes for Complete Lesions[24]

| Functional Skills | Level of Assistance Required (by SCI level groups) | | | |
|---|---|---|---|---|
| | High Tetraplegia (C1-C5) | Mid-level Tetraplegia (C6) | Low Tetraplegia (C7-C8) | Paraplegia |
| **Bed Mobility**<br>• Rolling side to side<br>• Rolling supine/prone<br>• Supine/sitting<br>• Scooting all directions | – Dependent (C1-C4)<br>– Moderate to maximal assistance (C5)<br>– Verbally direct | – Minimal assistance to modified independent with equipment<br>– Verbally direct | – Independent with all | – Independent |
| **Transfers**<br>• Bed<br>• Car<br>• Toilet<br>• Bath equipment<br>• Floor<br>• Upright wheelchair | – Dependent (C1-C4)<br>– Maximal assistance with level sliding board transfers (C5)<br>– Verbally direct | – Minimal assistance to modified independent for sliding board transfers<br>– Dependent with wheelchair loading in car<br>– Dependent with floor transfers and uprighting wheelchair<br>– Verbally direct | – Modified independent to independent with level surface transfer (sliding board)<br>– Moderate assistance to modified independent with car transfer<br>– Maximal to moderate assistance with floor transfers and uprighting wheelchair<br>– Verbally direct | – Independent with level surface and car transfers (depression)<br>– Minimal assistance to independent with floor transfers and uprighting wheelchair<br>– Verbally direct |
| **Weight Shifts**<br>• Pressure relief<br>• Repositioning in wheelchair | – Setup to modified independent with power recline/tilt weight shift<br>– Dependent with manual recline/tilt/lean weight shift<br>– Verbally direct | – Modified independent with power recline/tilt weight shift<br>– Minimal assistance to modified independent with side to side/forward lean weight shift<br>– Verbally direct | – Modified independent with side to side/forward lean, or depression weight shift | – Modified independent with depression weight shift |
| **Wheelchair Management**<br>• Wheel locks<br>• Armrests<br>• Footrests/legrests<br>• Safety strap(s)<br>• Cushion adjustment<br>• Anti-tip levers<br>• Wheelchair maintenance | – Dependent with all<br>– Able to verbally direct | – Some assistance required<br>– Able to verbally direct | – May require assistance with cushion adjustment, anti-tip levers, and wheelchair maintenance<br>– Able to verbally direct | – Independent with all |

# Functional Outcomes for Complete Lesions[24]

| Functional Skills | Level of Assistance Required (by SCI level groups) | | | |
|---|---|---|---|---|
| | High Tetraplegia (C1-C5) | Mid-level Tetraplegia (C6) | Low Tetraplegia (C7-C8) | Paraplegia |
| **Wheelchair Mobility**<br>• Smooth surfaces<br>• Up/down ramps<br>• Up/down curbs<br>• Rough terrain<br>• Up/down steps (manual wheelchair only) | – Supervision/ setup to modified independent on smooth, ramp, and rough terrain with power wheelchair<br>– Modified independent with manual wheelchair on smooth surface in forward direction (C5)<br>– Maximal assistance to dependent with manual wheelchair in all other situations (C5)<br>– Able to verbally direct | – Modified independent in smooth, ramp, and rough terrain with power wheelchair<br>– Dependent to maximal assistance up/down curb with power wheelchair<br>– Modified independent on smooth surfaces with manual wheelchair<br>– Moderate to minimal assistance on ramps and rough terrain with manual wheelchair<br>– Maximal to moderate assistance up/down curbs with manual wheelchair<br>– Able to verbally direct | – Modified independent on smooth, ramp, and rough terrain with power wheelchair<br>– Dependent to maximal assistance up/down curb with power wheelchair<br>– Modified independent on smooth surfaces and up/ down ramps with manual wheelchair<br>– Minimal assistance to modified independent on rough terrain<br>– Moderate to minimal assistance up/down curbs with manual wheelchair<br>– Dependent to maximal assistance up/down steps with manual wheelchair<br>– Can verbally direct | – Minimal assistance to modified independent up/ down 6" curbs with manual wheelchair<br>– Modified independent with descending steps with manual wheelchair<br>– Maximal to minimal assistance to ascend steps with manual wheelchair<br>– Able to verbally direct |
| **Gait**<br>• Don/doff orthoses<br>• Sit/stand<br>• Smooth surfaces<br>• Up/down ramps<br>• Up/down curbs<br>• Up/down steps<br>• Rough terrain<br>• Safe falling | – Not applicable | – Not applicable | – Not applicable | – Abilities range from:<br>– exercise only with KAFOs*<br>– household gait with KAFOs<br>– limited community gait with KAFOs or AFOs*<br>– functional community ambulation with or without orthoses |
| **ROM/Positioning**<br>• PROM to trunk, legs, and arms<br>• Pad/position in bed | – Dependent<br>– Able to verbally direct | – Moderate assistance to modified independent with all<br>– Able to verbally direct | – Minimal assistance to modified independent with all<br>– Able to verbally direct | – Independent |
| **Feeding**<br>• Drinking<br>• Finger feeding<br>• Utensil feeding | – Dependent (C1-C4)<br>– Minimal assistance with adaptive equipment (C5)<br>– Able to verbally direct | – Modified independent with adaptive equipment | – Modified independent with adaptive equipment (C7) | – Independent |

# Functional Outcomes for Complete Lesions[24]

| Functional Skills | Level of Assistance Required (by SCI level groups) | | | |
|---|---|---|---|---|
| | High Tetraplegia (C1-C5) | Mid-level Tetraplegia (C6) | Low Tetraplegia (C7-C8) | Paraplegia |
| **Grooming**<br>• Face<br>• Teeth<br>• Hair<br>• Makeup<br>• Shaving face | – Dependent (C1-C4)<br>– Minimal assistance with adaptive equipment for face, teeth, makeup/shaving (C5)<br>– Maximal/moderate assistance for hair grooming (C5)<br>– Able to verbally direct | – Modified independent with adaptive equipment | – Modified independent | – Independent |
| **Dressing**<br>• Dressing and undressing (in bed or wheelchair)<br>• Upper body/lower body (in bed or wheelchair) | – Dependent<br>– Able to verbally direct | – Modified independent for upper body in bed or wheelchair<br>– Minimal assistance with lower body dressing in bed<br>– Moderate assistance with lower body undressing in bed<br>– Able to verbally direct | – Modified independent for upper/lower body dressing in bed<br>– Minimal assistance with lower body dressing/undressing in wheelchair (C7)<br>– Modified independent for upper/lower body dressing/undressing in wheelchair (C8)<br>– Able to verbally direct | – Modified independent |
| **Bathing**<br>• Bathing and drying off<br>• Upper body and lower body | – Dependent<br>– Able to verbally direct | – Minimal assistance for upper body bathing and drying<br>– Moderate assistance for lower body bathing and drying<br>– Use of shower or tub chair<br>– Able to verbally direct | – Modified independent with all using shower or tub chair | – Modified independent with all on tub bench or tub bottom cushion |
| **Bowel/Bladder Problems**<br>• Intermittent catheterization<br>• Leg bag care<br>• Condom application<br>• Clean up<br>• In bed/wheelchair (bladder)<br>• Feminine hygiene<br>• Bowel program | – Dependent<br>– Able to verbally direct | **Bladder:**<br>– Minimal assistance for male in bed or wheelchair<br>– Moderate assistance for female in bed<br>**Bowel:**<br>– Moderate assistance with use of equipment<br>– Able to verbally direct | **Bladder:**<br>– Modified independent for male in bed or wheelchair<br>– Modified independent for female in bed; moderate assistance for female in wheelchair<br>**Bowel:**<br>– Minimal assistance to modified independent with use of equipment<br>– Able to verbally direct | **Bladder:**<br>– Modified independent for male and female<br>**Bowel:**<br>– Modified independent for male and female |

*KAFO = knee-ankle-foot orthosis; AFO = ankle-foot orthosis

From Umphred DA: Neurological Rehabilitation. Mosby-Year Book, Inc. 1995, p. 502-505, with permission.

## Spinal Cord Injury Terminology[18,19,24]

**Cauda equina injury:** A term used to describe injuries that occur below the L1 level of the spine. A cauda equina injury is considered to be a lower motor neuron lesion.

**Dermatome:** Designated sensory areas based on spinal segment innervation.

**Head-hips relationship:** A principle of mechanics used during mobility training with upper extremity weight bearing used as a fulcrum for activity. This technique requires the head to move in the opposite direction from the hips.

**Myelotomy:** A surgical procedure that severs certain tracts within the spinal cord in order to decrease spasticity and improve function.

**Myotome:** Designated motor areas based on spinal segment innervation.

**Neurectomy:** A surgical removal of a segment of a nerve in order to decrease spasticity and improve function.

**Neurogenic bladder:** The bladder empties reflexively for a patient with an injury above the level of S2. The sacral reflex arc remains intact.

**Neurologic level:** The lowest segment (most caudal) of the spinal cord with intact strength and sensation. Muscle groups at this level must receive a grade of fair.

**Nonreflexive bladder:** The bladder is flaccid as a result of a cauda equina or conus medullaris lesion. The sacral reflex arc is damaged.

**Paradoxical breathing:** A form of abnormal breathing that is common in tetraplegia where the abdomen rises and the chest is pulled inward during inspiration. On expiration the abdomen falls and the chest expands.

**Paraplegia:** A term used to describe injuries that occur at the level of the thoracic, lumbar or sacral spine.

**Rhizotomy:** A surgical resection of the sensory component of a spinal nerve in order to decrease spasticity and improve function.

**Sacral sparing:** An incomplete lesion where some of the innermost tracts remain innervated. Characteristics include sensation of the saddle area, movement of the toe flexors, and rectal sphincter contraction.

**Spinal shock:** A physiologic response that occurs between 30 and 60 minutes after trauma to the spinal cord and can last up to several weeks. Spinal shock presents with total flaccid paralysis and loss of all reflexes below the level of injury.

**Tenodesis:** Patients with tetraplegia that do not possess motor control for grasp can utilize the tight finger flexors in combination with wrist extension to produce a form of grasp.

**Tenotomy:** A surgical release of a tendon in order to decrease spasticity and improve function.

**Tetraplegia (quadriplegia):** A term adopted by the American Spinal Cord Injury Association to describe injuries that occur at the level of the cervical spine.

**Zone of preservation:** A term used to describe poor or trace motor or sensory function for up to three levels below the neurologic level of injury.

# Consider This

## Spinal Cord Injury Intervention Constructs[13,20,24]

Patients with spinal cord injury will likely have a unique course of rehabilitation based on their primary diagnosis, secondary complications, co-morbidities, and level of impairment. The following guidelines, however, reflect areas that should be incorporated into the plan of care for patients with spinal cord injury.

- Positioning
- Prevention of pressure ulcers
- Pressure relief techniques and equipment
- Range of motion
- Family/caregiver teaching
- Bowel and bladder programming
- Respiratory training/airway clearance
  - Assisted cough and secretion clearance
  - Breathing exercises
  - Abdominal binders
  - Mechanical ventilation
  - Glossopharyngeal breathing (GPB)

- Wheelchair, cushion (Figs. 5-56, 5-57), and orthotic prescriptions
- Wheelchair mobility
- Balance and center of gravity retraining
- Motor function retraining (transitioning between positions, seated scooting) (Figs. 5-58, 5-59)
- Mobility training including floor transfers if appropriate (Figs. 5-60, 5-61, 5-62)
- Pain management
- Use of FES, biofeedback, TENS if appropriate
- Self-care skills
- Gait training (T9 or lower)

**Fig. 5-56:** Roho high profile specialized cushion with cover.

**Fig. 5-57:** Roho high profile specialized cushion for wheelchair seating.

**Fig. 5-58:** Functional retraining of a patient with spinal cord injury, specifically transfers from the wheelchair to the mat surface.

**Fig. 5-59:** The patient must compensate by looping the upper extremity under the lower extremity in combination with momentum in order to swing the lower extremity onto the mat surface.

**Fig. 5-60:** The patient initiates the roll by manually crossing legs, using the upper extremities to create movement and momentum.

**Fig. 5-61:** The patient begins to roll using momentum and gravity.

**Fig. 5-62:** The patient ends in prone position as anticipated.

# Traumatic Brain Injury

According to the Centers for Disease Control and Prevention, more than 1.7 million people annually sustain a traumatic brain injury. Approximately 52,000 die from the trauma and an additional 80,000 experience long-term impairment and disability on an annual basis. The leading risk factor for TBI is a motor vehicle accident, followed by falls, high risk behaviors, and gunshot wounds. Brain injury is classified as open versus closed with primary and secondary brain damage. Secondary damage within the brain can be significant due to the widespread areas that are affected.

## Types of Brain Injury[20,44]

### Open Injury

An injury of direct penetration through the skull to the brain. Location, depth of penetration, and pathway determine the extent of brain damage. Examples include gunshot wound, knife or sharp object penetration, skull fragments, and direct trauma.

### Closed Injury

An injury to the brain without penetration through the skull. Examples include concussion, contusion, hematoma, injury to extracranial blood vessels, hypoxia, drug overdose, near drowning, and acceleration or deceleration injuries.

### Primary Injury

Initial injury to the brain sustained by impact. Examples include skull penetration, skull fractures, and contusions to gray and white matter.

**Coup lesion:** A direct lesion of the brain under the point of impact. Local brain damage is sustained.

**Contrecoup lesion:** An injury that results on the opposite side of the brain. The lesion is due to the rebound effect of the brain after impact.

### Secondary Injury

Brain damage that occurs as a response to the initial injury. Examples include hematoma, hypoxia, ischemia, increased intracranial pressure, and post-traumatic epilepsy.

**Epidural hematoma:** A hemorrhage that forms between the skull and dura mater.

**Subdural hematoma:** A hemorrhage that forms due to venous rupture between the dura and arachnoid.

### Levels of Consciousness[20,44]

**Coma:** A state of unconsciousness and a level of unresponsiveness to all internal and external stimuli.

**Stupor:** A state of general unresponsiveness with arousal occurring from repeated stimuli.

**Obtundity:** A state of consciousness that is characterized by a state of sleep, reduced alertness to arousal, and delayed responses to stimuli.

**Delirium:** A state of consciousness that is characterized by disorientation, confusion, agitation, and loudness.

**Clouding of consciousness:** A state of consciousness that is characterized by quiet behavior, confusion, poor attention, and delayed responses.

**Consciousness:** A state of alertness, awareness, orientation, and memory.

## Spotlight on Safety
### Concussions[13,43]

A concussion can occur as a result of injury, specifically a blow to the head. This may or may not produce a temporary loss of consciousness. There is damage to the reticular activating system that allows for immediate changes in vital signs. Concussions occur frequently secondary to acute trauma such as motor vehicle accidents or through athletics.

**The American Academy of Neurology classifies concussions as:**

**Grade 1** – A concussion that results from head injury where there was no loss of consciousness but typically some transient confusion by the patient. Symptoms will typically resolve within 15 minutes of the event. The patient may exhibit full memory of the event. An athlete should be removed from the competition and return only if symptom free after one week of rest.

**Grade 2** – A concussion that results from a moderate head injury with transient confusion that will last longer than 15 minutes. The patient may exhibit poor concentration, retrograde and antegrade amnesia. An athlete should be removed immediately from the competition and receive a medical evaluation. CT scan is indicated if symptoms worsen and return to play should be deferred until the athlete is asymptomatic for two weeks at rest and with exertion.

**Grade 3** – A concussion that results from head injury with any form of loss of consciousness. A patient should require transport to the emergency room for full neurological evaluation. Hospitalization is warranted if altered consciousness or mental status persists. An athlete should be withheld from competition after a grade 3 concussion once symptom free for a minimum of one month. This form of concussion is secondary to diffuse axonal injury and, if severe, can result in coma.

## Traumatic Brain Injury Tests and Measures

**Rancho Los Amigos Levels of Cognitive Functioning[24]**

### I. NO RESPONSE

Patient appears to be in a deep sleep and is completely unresponsive to any stimuli.

### II. GENERALIZED RESPONSE

Patient reacts inconsistently and non-purposefully to stimuli in a nonspecific manner. Responses are limited and often the same regardless of stimulus presented. Responses may be physiological changes, gross body movements, and/or vocalization.

## III. LOCALIZED RESPONSE

Patient reacts specifically, but inconsistently to stimuli. Responses are directly related to the type of stimulus presented. May follow simple commands such as closing the eyes or squeezing the hand in an inconsistent, delayed manner.

## IV. CONFUSED-AGITATED

Patient is in a heightened state of activity. Behavior is bizarre and non-purposeful relative to the immediate environment. Does not discriminate among persons or objects; is unable to cooperate directly with treatment efforts. Verbalizations frequently are incoherent and/or inappropriate to the environment; confabulation may be present. Gross attention to environment is very brief; selective attention is often nonexistent. Patient lacks short and long-term recall.

## V. CONFUSED-INAPPROPRIATE

Patient is able to respond to simple commands fairly consistently. However, with increased complexity of commands or lack of any external structure, responses are non-purposeful, random, or fragmented. Demonstrates gross attention to the environment, but is highly distractible and lacks the ability to focus attention on a specific task. With structure, may be able to converse on a social automatic level for short periods of time. Verbalization is often inappropriate and confabulatory. Memory is severely impaired; often shows inappropriate use of objects; may perform previously learned tasks with structure, but is unable to learn new information.

## VI. CONFUSED-APPROPRIATE

Patient shows goal-directed behavior, but is dependent on external input or direction. Follows simple directions consistently and shows carryover for relearned tasks such as self-care. Responses may be incorrect due to memory problems, but they are appropriate to the situation. Past memories show more depth and detail than recent memory.

## VII. AUTOMATIC-APPROPRIATE

Patient appears appropriate and oriented within the hospital and home setting. Goes through daily routine automatically, but frequently robot-like. Patient shows minimal to no confusion and has shallow recall of activities. Shows carryover for new learning, but at a decreased rate. With structure is able to initiate social or recreational activities; judgment remains impaired.

## VIII. PURPOSEFUL-APPROPRIATE

Patient is able to recall and integrate past and recent events and is aware of and responsive to environment. Shows carryover for new learning and needs no supervision once activities are learned. May continue to show a decreased ability relative to premorbid abilities, abstract reasoning, tolerance for stress, and judgment in emergencies or unusual circumstances.

From Professional Staff Association, Rancho Los Amigos Hospital, p.87-88, with permission

## Glasgow Coma Scale[24]

A neurological assessment tool used initially after injury to determine arousal and cerebral cortex function. A total score of eight or less correlates to severe brain injury and coma in 90% of patients. Scores of 9 to 12 indicate moderate brain injuries and scores from 13 to 15 indicate mild brain injuries.

### Glasgow Coma Scale

| Eye Opening | E |
|---|---|
| Spontaneous | 4 |
| To speech | 3 |
| To pain | 2 |
| Nil | 1 |
| **Best Motor Response** | **M** |
| Obeys commands | 6 |
| Localizes pain | 5 |
| Withdraws | 4 |
| Abnormal flexion | 3 |
| Extensor response | 2 |
| Nil | 1 |
| **Verbal Response** | **V** |
| Oriented | 5 |
| Confused conversation | 4 |
| Inappropriate words | 3 |
| Incomprehensible sounds | 2 |
| Nil | 1 |
| **Coma Score (E+M+V) = 3 to 15** | |

From Management of Head Injuries by Bryan Jennett and Graham Teasdale, Copyright-1981 by Oxford University Press, Inc. Used by permission of Oxford University Press, Inc.

## Memory Impairments

**Anterograde memory:** The inability to create new memory. Anterograde memory is usually the last to recover after a comatose state. Contributing factors include poor attention, distractibility, and impaired perception of stimuli.

**Post-traumatic amnesia:** The time between the injury and when the patient is able to recall recent events. The patient does not recall the injury or events up until this point of recovery. Post-traumatic amnesia is used as an indicator of the extent of damage.

**Retrograde amnesia:** An inability to remember events prior to the injury. Retrograde amnesia may progressively decrease with recovery.

# Consider This

## Traumatic Brain Injury Intervention Constructs[20,24,44]

Patients with brain injury will likely have a unique course of rehabilitation based on their primary diagnosis, secondary complications, co-morbidities, and level of impairment. The following guidelines, however, reflect areas that should be incorporated into the plan of care for patients with a brain injury.

- Emphasis on motivation

- Promote independence

- Therapy should be goal-directed, functional, and recreational

- Focus on orientation

- Focus on behavior modification activities

- Repetition is typically helpful

- Educate patient in compensatory strategies for success

- Structure is essential depending on the level of the patient

- Avoid overstimulation during therapy

- A calm voice and simple commands are desirable when interacting with the patient

- Perform activities that are both familiar and enjoyable for the patient

- Family education and support can enhance and assist the rehabilitation process

- Allow patient to choose activities on occasion

- Flexibility in treatment is needed based on patient's immediate needs and state of mind

- Intervention should include:

  - Cognitive and orientation training

  - Therapeutic exercise

  - Positioning

  - Sensory integration

  - Balance and vestibular training

  - Range of motion

  - Motor function training

  - Wheelchair and adaptive equipment prescription

  - Splinting and serial casting

  - Mobility training

# Pediatrics and Development

## Concepts of Development[45,46]

**Cephalic to Caudal:** A person develops head and upper extremity control prior to trunk and lower extremity control. There is a general skill acquisition from the direction of head to toe.

**Gross to Fine:** A general trend for large muscle movement acquisition with progression to small muscle skill acquisition.

**Mass to Specific:** A general trend for a person to acquire simple movements and progress towards complex movements.

**Proximal to Distal:** A concept that uses the midline of the body as the reference point. Trunk control (midline stability) is acquired first with subsequent gain in distal control (extremities).

## Infant Reflexes and Possible Effects if Reflex Persists Abnormally[47]

| Primitive Reflex | Possible Negative Effect on Movement with Abnormal Persistence of Reflex |
|---|---|

### Asymmetrical Tonic Neck Reflex (ATNR)

**Stimulus:** Head position, turned to one side
**Response:** Arm and leg on face side are extended, arm and leg on scalp side are flexed, spine curved with convexity toward face side
**Normal age of response:** Birth to 6 months

**Interferes with:**
- Feeding
- Visual tracking
- Midline use of hands
- Bilateral hand use
- Rolling
- Development of crawling
- Can lead to skeletal deformities (e.g., scoliosis, hip subluxation, hip dislocation)

### Symmetrical Tonic Neck Reflex (STNR)

**Stimulus:** Head position, flexion or extension
**Response:** When head is in flexion, arms are flexed, legs extended. When head is in extension, arms are extended, legs are flexed
**Normal age of response:** 6 to 8 months

**Interferes with:**
- Ability to prop on arms in prone position
- Attaining and maintaining hands-and-knees position
- Crawling reciprocally
- Sitting balance when looking around
- Use of hands when looking at object in hands in sitting position

### Tonic Labyrinthine Reflex (TLR)

**Stimulus:** Position of labyrinth in inner ear - reflected in head position
**Response:** In the supine position, body and extremities are held in extension; in the prone position, body and extremities are held in flexion
**Normal age of response:** Birth to 6 months

**Interferes with:**
- Ability to initiate rolling
- Ability to prop on elbows with extended hips when prone
- Ability to flex trunk and hips to come to sitting position from supine position
- Often causes full body extension, which interferes with balance in sitting or standing

### Galant Reflex

**Stimulus:** Touch to skin along spine from shoulder to hip
**Response:** Lateral flexion of trunk to side of stimulus
**Normal age of response:** 30 weeks of gestation to 2 months

**Interferes with:**
- Development of sitting balance
- Can lead to scoliosis

# Infant Reflexes and Possible Effects if Reflex Persists Abnormally[47]

| Primitive Reflex | Possible Negative Effect on Movement with Abnormal Persistence of Reflex |
|---|---|

### Palmar Grasp Reflex

**Stimulus:** Pressure in palm on ulnar side of hand
**Response:** Flexion of fingers causing strong grip
**Normal age of response:** Birth to 4 months

**Interferes with:**
- Ability to grasp and release objects voluntarily
- Weight bearing on open hand for propping, crawling, protective responses

### Plantar Grasp Reflex

**Stimulus:** Pressure to base of toes
**Response:** Toe flexion
**Normal age of response:** 28 weeks of gestation to 9 months

**Interferes with:**
- Ability to stand with feet flat on surface
- Balance reactions and weight shifting in standing

### Rooting Reflex

**Stimulus:** Touch on cheek
**Response:** Turning head to same side with mouth open
**Normal age of response:** 28 weeks of gestation to 3 months

**Interferes with:**
- Oral-motor development
- Development of midline control of head
- Optical righting, visual tracking, and social interaction

### Moro Reflex

**Stimulus:** Head dropping into extension suddenly for a few inches
**Response:** Arms abduct with fingers open, then cross trunk into adduction; cry
**Normal age of response:** 28 weeks of gestation to 5 months

**Interferes with:**
- Balance reactions in sitting
- Protective responses in sitting
- Eye-hand coordination, visual tracking

### Startle Reflex

**Stimulus:** Loud, sudden noise
**Response:** Similar to Moro response, but elbows remain flexed and hands closed
**Normal age of response:** 28 weeks of gestation to 5 months

**Interferes with:**
- Sitting balance
- Protective responses in sitting
- Eye-hand coordination, visual tracking
- Social interaction, attention

### Positive Support Reflex

**Stimulus:** Weight placed on balls of feet when upright
**Response:** Stiffening of legs and trunk into extension
**Normal age of response:** 35 weeks of gestation to 2 months

**Interferes with:**
- Standing and walking
- Balance reactions and weight shift in standing
- Can lead to contractures of ankles into plantar flexion

### Walking (Stepping) Reflex

**Stimulus:** Supported upright position with soles of feet on firm surface
**Response:** Reciprocal flexion/extension of legs
**Normal age of response:** 38 weeks of gestation to 2 months

**Interferes with:**
- Standing and walking
- Balance reactions and weight shifting in standing
- Development of smooth, coordinated reciprocal movements of lower extremities

From Ratliffe KT: Clinical Pediatric Physical Therapy: A Guide for the Physical Therapy Team. Mosby Inc., Philadelphia 1998, p.266, with permission.

# Developmental Gross and Fine Motor Skills[47]

| Gross Motor Skills | Fine Motor Skills |
|---|---|
| **Newborn to 1 Month** | |

**Prone**
Physiological flexion
Lifts head briefly
Head to side

**Supine**
Physiological flexion
Rolls partly to side

**Sitting**
Head lag in pull to sit

**Standing**
Reflex standing and walking

Regards objects in direct line of sight
Follows moving object to midline
Hands fisted
Arm movements jerky
Movements may be purposeful or random

| Gross Motor Skills | Fine Motor Skills |
|---|---|
| **2 to 3 Months** | |

**Prone**
Lifts head 90 degrees briefly
Chest up in prone position with some weight through forearms
Rolls prone to supine

**Supine**
Asymmetrical tonic neck reflex (ATNR) influence is strong
Legs kick reciprocally
Prefers head to side

**Sitting**
Head upright, but bobbing
Variable head lag in pull to sitting position
Needs full support to sit

**Standing**
Poor weight bearing
Hips in flexion, behind shoulders

Can see farther distances
Hands open more
Visually follows through 180 degrees
Grasp is reflexive
Uses palmar grasp

| Gross Motor Skills | Fine Motor Skills |
|---|---|
| **4 to 5 Months** | |

**Prone**
Bears weight on extended arms
Pivots in prone to reach toys

**Supine**
Rolls from supine to side position
Plays with feet to mouth

**Sitting**
Head steady in supported sitting position
Turns head in sitting position
Sits alone for brief periods

**Standing**
Bears all weight through legs in supported standing

Grasps and releases toys
Uses ulnar-palmar grasp

| Gross Motor Skills | Fine Motor Skills |
|---|---|
| **6 to 7 Months** | |

**Prone**
Rolls from supine to prone position
Holds weight on one hand to reach for toy

**Supine**
Lifts head

**Sitting**
Lifts head and helps when pulled to sitting position
Gets to sitting position without assistance
Sits independently

**Mobility**
May crawl backward

Approaches objects with one hand
Arm in neutral when approaching toy
Radial-palmar grasp
"Rakes" with fingers to pick up small objects
Voluntary release to transfer objects between hands

# Developmental Gross and Fine Motor Skills[47]

| Gross Motor Skills | Fine Motor Skills |
|---|---|
| **8 to 9 Months** | |

**Prone**
Gets into hands-knees position

**Supine**
Does not tolerate supine position

**Sitting**
Moves from sitting to prone position
Sits without hand support for longer periods
Pivots in sitting position

**Standing**
Stands at furniture
Pulls to stand at furniture
Lowers to sitting position from supported stand

**Mobility**
Crawls forward
Walks along furniture (cruising)

Develops active supination
Radial-digital grasp develops
Uses inferior pincer grasp
Extends wrist actively
Points with index finger
Pokes with index finger
Release of objects is more refined
Takes objects out of container

| Gross Motor Skills | Fine Motor Skills |
|---|---|
| **10 to 11 Months** | |

**Standing**
Stands without support briefly
Pulls to stand using half-kneel intermediate position
Picks up object from floor from standing with support

**Mobility**
Walks with both hands held
Walks with one hand held
Creeps on hands and feet (bear walk)

Fine pincer grasp developed
Puts objects into container
Grasps crayon adaptively

| Gross Motor Skills | Fine Motor Skills |
|---|---|
| **12 to 15 Months** | |

Walks without support
Fast walking
Walks backward
Walks sideways
Bends over to look between legs
Creeps or hitches upstairs
Throws ball in sitting

Marks paper with crayon
Builds tower using two cubes
Turns over small container to obtain contents

| Gross Motor Skills | Fine Motor Skills |
|---|---|
| **16 to 24 Months** | |

Squats in play
Walking upstairs and downstairs with one hand held using both feet on step
Propels ride-on toys
Kicks ball
Throws ball
Throws ball forward
Picks up toy from floor without falling

Folds paper
Strings beads
Stacks six cubes
Imitates vertical and horizontal strokes with crayon on paper
Holds crayon with thumb and fingers

| Gross Motor Skills | Fine Motor Skills |
|---|---|
| **2 Years** | |

Rides tricycle
Walks backward
Walks on tiptoe
Runs on toes
Walks downstairs alternating feet
Catches large ball
Hops on one foot

Turns knob
Opens and closes jar
Able to button large buttons
Uses child-size scissors with help
Does 12 to 15 piece puzzles
Folds paper or clothes

# Developmental Gross and Fine Motor Skills[47]

| Gross Motor Skills | Fine Motor Skills |
|---|---|
| **Preschool Age (3 to 4 Years)** | |
| Throws ball 10 feet | Controls crayons more effectively |
| Walks on a line 10 feet | Copies a circle or cross |
| Hops 2-10 times on one foot | Matches colors |
| Jumps distances of up to two feet | Cuts with scissors |
| Jumps over obstacles up to 12 inches | Draws recognizable human figures with head and two extremities |
| Throws and catches small ball | Draws squares |
| Runs fast and avoids obstacles | May demonstrate hand preference |
| **Early School Age (5 to 8 Years)** | |
| Skips on alternate feet | Hand preference is evident |
| Gallops | Prints well, starting to learn cursive writing |
| Can play hopscotch, balance on one foot, controlled hopping, and squatting on one leg | Able to button small buttons |
| Jumps with rhythm, control (jump rope) | |
| Bounces large ball | |
| Kicks ball with greater control | |
| Limbs growing faster than trunk allowing greater speed, leverage | |

| Gross Motor Skills | Fine Motor Skills |
|---|---|
| **Later School Age (9 to 12 Years)** | |
| Mature patterns of movement in throwing, jumping, running | Develops greater control in hand usage |
| Competition increases, enjoys competitive games | Learns to draw |
| Improved balance, coordination, endurance, attention span | Handwriting is developed |
| Boys may develop preadolescent fat spurt | |
| Girls may develop prepubescent and pubescent changes in body shape (hips, breasts) | |
| **Adolescence (13 Years+)** | |
| Rapid growth in size and strength, boys more than girls | Develops greater dexterity in fingers for fine tasks (knitting, sewing, art, crafts) |
| Puberty leads to changes in body proportions, center of gravity rises toward shoulders for boys, lowers to hips for girls | |
| Balance and coordination skills, eye-hand coordination, endurance may plateau during growth spurt | |

From Ratliffe KT: Clinical Pediatric Physical Therapy: A Guide for the Physical Therapy Team. Mosby Company Inc., Philadelphia 1998, p.45-47, with permission.

## Pediatric Therapeutic Positioning

Proper positioning is essential to obtain maximum function for the pediatric population. Positioning is used for many purposes including facilitation of desired patterns of movement, inhibition of abnormal reflexes, normalization of tone, midline orientation, enhancement of respiratory capacity, pulmonary hygiene, maintaining skin integrity, and prevention of contractures.

## Ideal Positioning[47]

| | Supine | Prone | Sidelying | Sitting |
|---|---|---|---|---|
| **Pelvis and Hips** | Pelvis in line with trunk. Hips in 30 to 90 degrees of flexion. Neutral rotation of pelvis. Hips symmetrically abducted 10 to 20 degrees. | Pelvis in line with trunk. Hips in extension. Neutral rotation of pelvis. Hips symmetrically abducted 10 to 20 degrees. | Pelvis in line with trunk. Hips in flexion. Neutral rotation. Hips in 10 to 20 degrees abduction. | Pelvis in line with trunk. Hips at 90 degrees flexion. Neutral rotation of pelvis. Hips symmetrically abducted 10 to 20 degrees. |
| **Trunk** | Straight. Shoulders in line with hips. Neutral rotation of trunk. | Straight. Shoulders in line with hips. Neutral rotation. | Straight. Shoulders in line with hips. Slight sidebending okay. | Straight. Shoulders over hips. Not rotated. |
| **Head and Neck** | Head in neutral position. Facing forward. Slight cervical flexion. | Head in neutral position. Facing to one side. Slight cervical flexion. | Head in neutral position. Facing forward. Slight cervical flexion. | Head in neutral position. Facing forward. Head evenly on shoulders. |
| **Shoulders and Arms** | Arms fully supported. Arms forward of trunk. Forearms rest on trunk or pillow. | Arms fully supported. Arms forward of trunk. Flexion at shoulders. Flexion at elbows. | Both arms supported. Lower arm forward, not lying on point of shoulders. Lower arm neutral rotation. Upper arm may have 0 to 40 degrees medial rotation. | Arms fully supported. Elbows in flexion. 0 to 45 degrees internally rotated shoulders. |
| **Legs and Feet** | Knees supported in flexion. Feet positioned at 90 degrees. | Knees extended. Feet positioned at 90 degrees. | Knees in flexion. Feet positioned at 90 degrees. Pillow between knees. | Knees at 90 degrees. Ankles at 90 degrees. Feet fully supported. Thighs fully supported. |

From Ratliffe KT: Clinical Pediatric Physical Therapy: A Guide for the Physical Therapy Team. Mosby Inc., Philadelphia 1998, p.266, with permission.

# Neuromuscular and Nervous Systems Pediatric Pathology

## Arthrogryposis Multiplex Congenita (AMC)[45,46,47]

Arthrogryposis multiplex congenita is a non-progressive neuromuscular disorder that is estimated to occur during the first trimester in utero. The restriction in utero allows for fibrosis of muscles and structures within the joints.

**Etiology** – An exact etiology of AMC is unknown, however, causative factors include poor movement during early development due to myopathic, neuropathic or joint abnormalities. The causative factor for a small percentage of children with this condition is genetic inheritance as an autosomal dominant trait.

**Signs and symptoms** – AMC characteristics include cylinder-like extremities with minimal definition, significant and multiple contractures, dislocation of joints, and muscle atrophy.

**Treatment** – The goal of treatment is to attain the maximum level of developmental skills through positioning, stretching, strengthening, splinting, and use of adaptive equipment. Significant family involvement is required for the home program. Surgical intervention may be indicated.

## Cerebral Palsy (CP)[13,45,46,47]

Cerebral palsy is an umbrella term used to describe movement disorders due to brain damage that are non-progressive and are acquired in utero, during birth or infancy. The brain damage decreases the brain's ability to monitor and control nerve and voluntary muscle activity.

**Etiology** – CP can occur before or during birth secondary to a lack of oxygen, maternal infections, drug or alcohol abuse, placental abnormalities, toxemia, prolonged labor, prematurity, and Rh incompatibility. The etiology of acquired cerebral palsy includes meningitis, CVA, seizures, and brain injury.

**Signs and symptoms** – Characteristics vary from mild and undetectable to severe loss of control accompanied by profound mental retardation. All types of cerebral palsy demonstrate abnormal muscle tone, impaired modulation of movement, presence of abnormal reflexes, and impaired mobility.

### Cerebral Palsy Primary Motor Patterns (mixed motor patterns exist)

- **Spastic** - indicating a lesion in the motor cortex of the cerebrum; upper motor neuron damage
- **Athetoid** - indicating a lesion involving the basal ganglia; cerebellum and cerebellar pathways

### Distribution of Involvement

- **Monoplegia** - one extremity
- **Diplegia** - bilateral lower extremity involvement, however, upper extremities may be affected
- **Hemiplegia** - unilateral involvement of the upper and lower extremities
- **Quadriplegia** - involvement of the entire body

**Treatment** – Treatment of cerebral palsy is a lifelong process. Intervention includes ongoing family and caregiver education, normalization of tone, stretching, strengthening, motor learning and developmental milestones, positioning, weight bearing activities, and mobility skills. Splinting, assistive devices, and specialized seating may be indicated. Surgical intervention may be required for orthopedic management or reduction of spasticity.

## Down Syndrome[45,46,47]

Down syndrome is a genetic abnormality consisting of an extra twenty-first chromosome, termed trisomy 21.

**Etiology** – The etiology of Down syndrome includes incomplete cell division of the 21st pair of chromosomes due to nondisjunction, translocation or mosaic classification. Advanced maternal age increases the risk of genetic imbalance.

**Signs and symptoms** – Signs and symptoms of this syndrome include mental retardation, hypotonia, joint hypermobility, flattened nasal bridge, narrow eyelids with epicanthal folds, small mouth, feeding impairments, flat feet, scoliosis, congenital heart disease, and visual and hearing loss.

**Treatment** – Treatment should emphasize exercise and fitness, stability, maximizing respiratory function, and education for caregivers. Surgical intervention may be indicated for cardiac abnormalities.

## Duchenne Muscular Dystrophy[13,45,46,47]

Duchenne muscular dystrophy is a progressive disorder caused by the absence of the gene required to produce the muscle proteins dystrophin and nebulin. Without dystrophin and nebulin, cell membranes weaken, myofibrils are destroyed, and muscle contractility is lost. Fat and connective tissue eventually replace muscle, and death usually occurs from cardiopulmonary failure prior to age 25, usually in the teenage years.

**Etiology** – The causative factor is inheritance as an X-linked recessive trait. The child's mother is a silent carrier and only male offspring will manifest the disease.

**Signs and symptoms** – Characteristics usually manifest between two and five years of age. Progressive weakness, disinterest in running, falling, toe walking, excessive lordosis, and pseudohypertrophy of muscle groups are common symptoms. Progressive impairment with ADLs and mobility begins around age five and the inability to ambulate follows.

**Treatment** – Intervention focuses on family and caregiver education, respiratory function, submaximal exercise, mobility skills, splinting, orthotics, and adaptive equipment. Medical management includes the use of immunosuppressants, steroids, and surgical intervention for orthopedic impairments.

## Prader-Willi Syndrome[45,46,47]

Prader-Willi syndrome is a genetic condition that is diagnosed by physical attributes and patterns of behavior rather than genetic testing.

**Etiology** – The causative factor is a partial deletion of chromosome 15.

**Signs and symptoms** – Characteristics include physical and behavioral attributes such as small hands, feet, and sex organs, hypotonia, almond-shaped eyes, obesity, and a constant desire for food. This child will present with coordination impairments and mental retardation.

**Treatment** – Physical therapy includes postural control, exercise and fitness, and gross and fine motor skills training.

## Spina Bifida[13,45,46,47]

Spina bifida is a developmental abnormality due to insufficient closure of the neural tube by the 28th day of gestation. This defect usually occurs in the low thoracic, lumbar or sacral regions and affects the central nervous, musculoskeletal, and urinary systems.

**Etiology** – A single etiology has not been identified, however, causative factors include genetic predisposition, environmental influence, low levels of maternal folic acid, maternal hyperthermia, and certain classifications of drugs. Classifications of spina bifida include:

**Spina Bifida Occulta** - An impairment and non-fusion of the spinous processes of a vertebrae, however, the spinal cord and meninges remain intact. There is usually no associated disability.

**Spina Bifida Cystica** - Presents with a cyst-like protrusion through the non-fused vertebrae, which results in impairment.

### Forms of Spina Bifida Cystica

- **Meningocele** - Herniation of meninges and cerebrospinal fluid into a sac that protrudes through the vertebral defect. The spinal cord remains within the canal.

- **Myelomeningocele** - A severe form characterized by herniation of meninges, cerebrospinal fluid, and the spinal cord extending through the defect in the vertebrae. The cyst may or may not be covered by skin.

**Signs and symptoms** – Characteristics and associated impairments of myelomeningocele include motor loss below the level of the defect in the spinal cord, sensory deficits, hydrocephalus, Arnold-Chiari Type II malformation, osteoporosis, clubfoot, scoliosis, tethered cord syndrome, latex allergy, bowel and bladder dysfunction, and learning disabilities.

**Treatment** – Physical therapy treatment emphasizes significant family teaching regarding positioning, handling, range of motion, and therapeutic exercise. Additional therapeutic activities include facilitation of developmental milestones, skin care, strengthening, balance and mobility training, adaptive equipment, splinting, orthotic prescription, and wheelchair prescription. Physical therapy is ongoing through adolescence and is based on the severity of impairments and needs of the child.

## Spinal Muscular Atrophy (SMA)[13,45,46,47]

Spinal muscular atrophy is characterized by progressive degeneration of the anterior horn cell.

**Etiology** – The causative factor of spinal muscular atrophy is an autosomal recessive genetic inheritance. Certain types of this disease involve a mutation on chromosome 5. Categories of spinal muscular atrophy include:

**Acute Infantile SMA (Type 1-Werdnig-Hoffmann disease)** - Occurs between birth and two months of age. Motor degeneration progresses quickly and life expectancy is less than one year.

**Chronic Childhood SMA (Type 2-Chronic Werdnig-Hoffmann disease)** - Presents after six months to one year and has slower progression than infantile SMA. Impairment is steady, however, a child can survive into adulthood.

**Juvenile SMA (Type 3-Kugelberg-Welander SMA)** - Occurs later in childhood from 4-17 years of age. Children with juvenile SMA typically survive into adulthood.

**Signs and symptoms** – Characteristics for all categories of the disease are the same, and vary in onset and speed of progression. Characteristics include progressive muscle weakness and atrophy, diminished or absent deep tendon reflexes, normal intelligence, intact sensation, and end-stage respiratory compromise.

**Treatment** – Treatment includes positioning, vestibular and visual stimulation, and access to play. Treatment for the slower progressing categories is primarily supportive including educating caregivers, mobility training, and use of assistive devices and adaptive equipment.

# Legislation Acts and Amendments for the Education of Children with Disabilities[48]

Over the last 25 years, there have been various forms of legislation that were enacted in order to improve health care, medical benefits, and education specifically for children. The largest reforms are listed below.

### Education for All Handicapped Children Act (enacted 1975)

The groundbreaking law was intended to support states and localities in protecting the rights of, meeting the individual needs of, and improving the results for infants, toddlers, children, and youths with disabilities and their families. This is the origin of the Individuals with Disabilities Education Improvement Act (IDEA).

### Carl D. Perkins Vocational Education Act of 1984

Each state was required to meet the special needs of individuals with handicaps or adults that are disadvantaged, adults in need of training and retraining, single parents or homemakers, programs designed to eliminate sex bias/stereotyping, and criminal offenders.

### Perkins Vocational and Applied Technology Act (enacted 1990)

Reauthorization and modification of the Education for All Handicapped Children Act (EHA). Provides free, appropriate education in the least restrictive environment for individuals with disabilities from age 3-21.

### IDEA (Individuals with Disabilities Education Improvement Act) Amendments (enacted 1991)

Reauthorized early intervention; established Federal Interagency Coordination Council.

### Rehabilitation Act Amendments (enacted 1992)

Transition planning at high school graduation includes coordination of assistive technology services and the rehabilitation system.

### IDEA Amendments (enacted 1997)

Restructuring of IDEA into four distinct and individual parts. It defines the responsibilities of school districts in providing services to ensure that children with certain specified disabilities receive free, appropriate education. School districts must prepare an Individualized Education Program (IEP) for each eligible child. Related services most commonly include speech, physical, and occupational therapies, and child counseling.

### No Child Left Behind Act (enacted 2002)

The most sweeping reform of the Elementary and Secondary Education Act since its enactment in 1965. This act redefines the federal role in K-12 education. It requires accountability for all children, including student groups based on poverty, race and ethnicity, disability, and limited English proficiency (LEP). Its goal is to close the achievement gap between disadvantaged, disabled, and minority students and their peers.

### Before the IDEA

- One in five children with disabilities was educated.
- Over 1 million children with disabilities were excluded from the education system.
- 3.5 million children with disabilities did not receive appropriate services.

### Impact of the IDEA

- Currently 6.5 million children with disabilities are served.
- 96% of students with disabilities are now served in a regular school setting.
- There is an increase in the number of children from birth to three that receive services.

NEXT EXIT

MOTIVATIONAL MOMENT

See Page 1024

# Neuromuscular and Nervous Systems Essentials

1. The nervous system is composed of specialized cells that function to receive, integrate, control, and transmit information throughout the body. Components of the nervous system include the central nervous system (CNS), peripheral nervous system (PNS), autonomic nervous system (ANS), somatic nervous system (SNS), and limbic system.

2. The central nervous system anatomically consists of the brain and the spinal cord. There are two hemispheres of the brain and each hemisphere includes a frontal, temporal, parietal, and occipital lobe. The brain can also be divided into the forebrain, midbrain, and hindbrain. Each area is responsible for interpretation and control of certain biological processes and movement.

3. The peripheral nervous system consists of 12 pairs of cranial nerves and 31 pairs of spinal nerves. These nerves all have afferent and efferent fibers for communication between the body and the central nervous system.

4. The autonomic nervous system (ANS) consists of two divisions: the sympathetic division (generally a stimulating response) and the parasympathetic division (generally an inhibitory response). Anatomically, the ANS contains portions of the CNS and PNS. Impulses to the ANS typically do not reach the level of consciousness and instead produce automatic responses.

5. The somatic nervous system (SNS) regulates body movement through sensory and motor neurons that transmit information from the brain to muscle fibers throughout the body. The SNS controls voluntary movement, influences the five senses, and is responsible for reflex arcs such as deep tendon reflexes.

6. The limbic system is found within the brain and is involved with control and expression of mood, processing, memory, appetite, and olfaction. Lesions to this area can produce aggression, fearlessness, alterations in motivation, and other behaviors.

7. The forebrain consists of the telencephalon (cerebral cortex, hippocampus, basal ganglia, amygdala) and the diencephalon (thalamus, hypothalamus, subthalamus, epithalamus).

8. The cerebrum consists of gray matter on the surface and white matter interiorly, while sulci and fissures demark the specific lobes.

9. The left hemisphere has specific responsibilities including the ability to understand language, sequencing of movements, producing written and spoken language, expression of positive emotions, and the ability to be analytical, controlled, and logical. The right hemisphere has specific responsibilities including nonverbal processing, artistic expression, comprehension of general concepts, spatial relationships, kinesthetic awareness, mathematical reasoning, and body image awareness.

10. Each lobe of the brain has specific responsibilities: **Frontal:** intellect, orientation, voluntary movement, Broca's area, executive functions; **Parietal:** receives information associated with touch, kinesthesia, vibration; **Temporal:** auditory processing, Wernicke's area, production of meaningful speech; **Occipital:** visual processing, judgment of distance, vision in three dimensions.

11. The midbrain is located at the base of the brain above the spinal cord. It consists of the tectum and tegmentum and serves as a relay area, connecting the forebrain to the hindbrain. It is also a reflex center for visual, auditory, and tactile responses.

12. The hindbrain consists of the cerebellum, pons, and medulla oblongata. The cerebellum coordinates movement and assists with maintenance of balance. The pons and medulla assist with control of the body's vital functions.

13. From the Circle of Willis, the anterior cerebral artery, middle cerebral artery, posterior cerebral artery, and vertebral-basilar artery perfuse different regions of the brain and will produce impairments with vascular pathology specific to each artery.

14. The meninges are three layers of connective tissue that provide covering and protection for the brain and spinal cord. The dura mater is the outermost layer, followed by the arachnoid, and the pia mater (innermost layer). Dural spaces are areas normally surrounding meninges that may contain cerebrospinal fluid.

15. Cerebrospinal fluid is a clear fluid-like substance that cushions the brain and spinal cord and provides nutrition to the CNS. The ventricular system assists to produce and circulate CSF.

16. The spinal cord is a component of the CNS and a direct continuation of the brainstem. It serves as a relay for information between the brain and peripheral structures. Spinal nerves each possess afferent and efferent fibers for transmission of information through ascending and descending tracts of the spinal cord.

17. The peripheral nervous system contains nerves that have sensory, motor, and autonomic responsibilities. Cutaneous sensory end organs include thermoreceptors, nociceptors, mechanoreceptors, chemoreceptors, and photoreceptors that provide feedback through different channels of stimulation.

18. Peripheral nerve fibers may be classified as A, B or C fibers. A fibers are large and myelinated with a high conduction speed. B fibers are medium and myelinated with a moderate speed. C fibers are small and unmyelinated or poorly myelinated with a slow speed.

# Neuromuscular and Nervous Systems Essentials

19. Nerve roots from C1 through S4 each innervate a particular region for sensation (dermatome), and for motor innervation (myotome), and provide a pattern of anticipated weakness with impairment.

20. The cranial nerves include olfactory, optic, oculomotor, trochlear, trigeminal, abducens, facial, vestibulocochlear, glossopharyngeal, vagus, accessory, and hypoglossal nerves. Each has a specific testing protocol to ensure accuracy of results.

21. The brachial plexus innervates the muscles of the upper extremity while the lower extremity is innervated by the lumbar plexus and sacral plexus.

22. Superficial reflexes are a response to stimulation of the receptors within the skin. The sensory signal must reach the spinal cord and ascend to the brain for processing. Common superficial reflexes include the abdominal, corneal, cremasteric, gag, and plantar reflexes. The Babinski reflex is an abnormal plantar reflex.

23. Deep tendon reflexes (DTR) elicit a muscle contraction through stimulation of the muscle's tendon through a reflex arc. DTRs are graded from 0 to 4+ and results of testing may be indicative of a lesion to the reflex arc or a suprasegmental lesion.

24. Superficial sensations include light touch, temperature, and pain. Deep sensations include kinesthesia, proprioception, and vibration. Cortical sensations include localization of touch, bilateral simultaneous stimulation, two-point discrimination, stereognosis, and barognosis.

25. Acute injury to a peripheral nerve will produce neurapraxia (the mildest form of injury with axons preserved and recovery rapid and complete), axonotmesis (more severe injury with reversible damage, potential for spontaneous recovery), and neurotmesis (most severe damage, axon and myelin are damaged, irreversible injury, no spontaneous recovery, surgery may allow for some recovery).

26. Upper motor neuron lesions are found within the motor cortex, internal capsule, brainstem or spinal cord. Hyperactive reflexes, mild atrophy, and increased tone are characteristic findings with this form of pathology.

27. Lower motor neuron lesions are found in nerves or their axons at or below the level of the brainstem. Hypoactive or absent reflexes, atrophy, fasciculations, and decreased tone are characteristic findings with this form of pathology.

28. Tremors, tics, chorea, dystonia, and athetosis are all forms of movement disorders that present with involuntary movements.

29. Balance is the state of physical equilibrium with maintenance and control of the center of gravity. There are somatosensory, visual, and vestibular systems that provide feedback to the CNS regarding balance.

30. The vestibuloocular reflex (VOR) supports gaze stabilization through eye movement that counters movements of the head. The vestibulospinal reflex (VSR) attempts to stabilize the body while the head is moving in order to manage upright posture.

31. Vestibular rehabilitation is targeted for patients with central or peripheral balance disorders and can include VOR and VSR exercises, ocular motor exercises, habituation training, balance training, center of gravity control, varying environments, visual conditions, and use of gravity to challenge the balance system.

32. Communication disorders can include all forms of aphasia, verbal apraxia, and dysarthria. Aphasia is typically classified as receptive, expressive or global. Treatment will be modified based on the patient's ability to communicate or understand alternative forms of communication.

33. Common pharmacological agents used in the treatment of neurological disorders include antiepileptic agents, antispasticity agents, cholinergic agents, dopamine replacement agents, and muscle relaxant agents.

34. A cerebrovascular accident (CVA) is a specific event that results in a lack of oxygen to a specific area of the brain secondary to ischemia or hemorrhage. CVAs are typically termed a completed stroke, stroke in evolution, transient ischemic attack, ischemic stroke or hemorrhage.

35. A patient presents with predictable patterns of impairment when ischemia occurs secondary to a CVA in the left hemisphere, right hemisphere, brainstem or cerebellum.

36. The flexor synergy for the upper extremity includes scapular elevation and retraction; shoulder abduction and lateral rotation; elbow flexion; forearm supination; wrist flexion; and finger and thumb flexion with adduction. The extensor synergy for the upper extremity includes scapular depression and protraction; shoulder adduction and medial rotation; elbow extension; forearm pronation; wrist extension; and finger and thumb flexion with adduction.

37. The flexor synergy for the lower extremity includes hip abduction and lateral rotation; knee flexion; ankle dorsiflexion with supination; and toe extension. The extensor synergy for the lower extremity includes hip extension, medial rotation, and adduction; knee extension; ankle plantar flexion with inversion; and toe flexion and adduction.

38. Neurological rehabilitation may incorporate a variety of treatments based on the patient's pathology and goals. The variety of constructs base each of the theories of rehabilitation on their particular interpretation of motor control and motor learning.

# Neuromuscular and Nervous Systems Essentials

39. Motor control is the study of the nature of movement and the ability to direct essential movement. Motor learning is the study of the acquisition or modification of movement. Stages of motor learning include the cognitive stage, associative stage, and autonomous stage. Feedback is imperative for the progression of motor learning.

40. Practice is integral to motor learning. Various types of practice include massed and distributed practice; constant and variable practice; random and blocked practice; and whole training and part training.

41. Bobath developed Neuromuscular Developmental Treatment based on the hierarchical model of neurophysiologic function. This approach includes facilitation and inhibition of tone, reflex inhibiting postures, key points of control, proximal control, and the use of rotation during treatment.

42. Brunnstrom's Movement Therapy in Hemiplegia utilizes synergy patterns to assist with developing movement combinations outside of synergy patterns. Raimiste's phenomenon and Souques' phenomenon are used in treatment along with associated reactions, stages of recovery, overflow, and limb synergies.

43. Proprioceptive Neuromuscular Facilitation (PNF) is based on establishing gross motor patterns within the CNS, allowing for stronger parts to stimulate and strengthen the weaker parts. Treatment emphasizes developmental sequence, mass movement patterns, and diagonal patterns.

44. Rood's theory of neurological rehabilitation is based on the reflex stimulus model where motor output is the result of past and present sensory input. The goal of homeostasis is achieved using key patterns to enhance motor control. Treatment includes sensory stimulation to facilitate or inhibit a response.

45. Spinal cord injury (SCI) refers to permanent damage that can occur to the spinal cord after a sufficient force has been exerted on the spinal cord itself. Motor vehicle accidents have the highest incidence for SCI. There are complete and incomplete lesions with regard to motor and sensory function.

46. Incomplete lesions can include anterior cord syndrome, Brown-Sequard's syndrome, central cord syndrome, posterior cord syndrome, and cauda equina injuries.

47. The ASIA Impairment Scale is widely used for assessment of a patient with a SCI. This tool classifies complete versus incomplete lesions along with key muscles to test.

48. Autonomic dysreflexia is a common complication of a SCI and is considered a medical emergency. An excessive and uncontrolled increase in blood pressure places the patient at risk. A kinked catheter is the most typical stimulus for this condition.

49. Functional outcomes are anticipated for each level of spinal cord injury. A physical therapist must be able to recognize a patient's potential based on expected functional outcomes.

50. Traumatic brain injury is classified as either open or closed with primary and secondary brain damage. Primary injuries typically consist of coup and contrecoup lesions with secondary injury typically due to an epidural or subdural hematoma.

51. The Glasgow Coma Scale is used to assess patients with suspected head injury in order to classify the injury from mild to severe.

52. Rancho Los Amigos Levels of Cognitive Functioning Scale will also assist to classify the level of injury based on where the patient best meets the criteria of each level. The levels include: no response; generalized response; localized response; confused-agitated; confused-inappropriate; confused-appropriate; automatic-appropriate; and purposeful-appropriate.

53. The concepts of development include cephalic to caudal; gross to fine; mass to specific; and proximal to distal.

54. Primitive reflexes are elicited with a predictable stimulus that causes a predictable response until the time when the primitive reflex is integrated. When reflexes do not integrate, there is typically interference with progressing through the developmental milestones.

55. Developmental milestones for gross and fine motor skills follow a tentative schedule that children will follow through the teenage years. Developmental delay and other pediatric pathology may cause the child to experience difficulty progressing through the milestones.

56. Therapeutic positioning is essential to obtain maximum function for the pediatric population and is used to facilitate desired movement, inhibit unwanted tonal influences, normalize tone, prevent contractures, enhance midline orientation, and improve respiratory capacity.

57. Legislation such as the Individuals with Disabilities Education Improvement Act (IDEA), Rehabilitation Act, and No Child Left Behind Act have provided improved services and benefits for children with disabilities. These laws have been updated and amended to improve services for children with disabilities.

## QUIZ Neuromuscular and Nervous Systems Proficiencies

### 1. Brain Anatomy

Identify the appropriate term for each of the specified locations. Answers must be selected from the Word Bank and can be used only once.

**Word Bank:** fornix, hypothalamus, medulla oblongata, midbrain, olfactory bulb, pineal gland, pituitary gland

### 2. Circle of Willis

Identify the appropriate term for each of the specified locations. Answers must be selected from the Word Bank and can be used only once.

**Word Bank:** anterior communicating artery, arterial circle, basilar artery, left middle cerebral artery, left vertebral artery, right anterior cerebral artery, right internal carotid artery, right posterior cerebral artery, right posterior communicating artery

# QUIZ　Neuromuscular and Nervous Systems Proficiencies

## 3. Cranial Nerve Function

Indicate "yes" or "no" in each cell based on the presence or absence of a sensory (afferent) and/or motor (efferent) component for each cranial nerve.

| Cranial Nerve | Sensory | Motor |
|---|---|---|
| Olfactory | a | b |
| Optic | c | d |
| Oculomotor | e | f |
| Trochlear | g | h |
| Trigeminal | i | j |
| Abducens | k | l |
| Facial | m | n |
| Vestibulocochlear | o | p |
| Glossopharyngeal | q | r |
| Vagus | s | t |
| Accessory | u | v |
| Hypoglossal | w | x |

## 4. Cranial Nerve Testing

Identify the most appropriate method of testing for each of the cranial nerves. Answers must be selected from the Word Bank and can be used more than once if indicated.

**Word Bank:** downward and lateral gaze; face sensation; familiar odors; familiar tastes; gag reflex (2); hearing test; lateral gaze; resisted shoulder shrug; tongue protrusion; upward, downward, and medial gaze; visual fields

| Cranial Nerve | Cranial Nerve Test |
|---|---|
| Olfactory | a |
| Optic | b |
| Oculomotor | c |
| Trochlear | d |
| Trigeminal | e |
| Abducens | f |
| Facial | g |
| Vestibulocochlear | h |
| Glossopharyngeal | i |
| Vagus | j |
| Accessory | k |
| Hypoglossal | l |

# QUIZ Neuromuscular and Nervous Systems Proficiencies

## 5. Hemispheric Specialization

Identify the specific hemisphere most closely associated with each described function. Answers must be selected from the Word Bank and can be used more than once.

**Word Bank:** left, right

| Hemisphere | Function |
|---|---|
| a | logical and rational |
| b | understand nonverbal communication |
| c | understand and express language |
| d | spatial relationships |
| e | artistic abilities |
| f | mathematical calculations |
| g | body image awareness |
| h | express positive emotions |
| i | express negative emotions |

## 6. Innervation Levels

Identify the primary innervation level most closely associated with the described myotome, dermatome or reflex. Answers must be selected from the Word Bank and can be used more than once.

**Word Bank:** C4, C5, C6, C7, C8, L4, L5, S1, S3

| Myotome | Innervation Level |
|---|---|
| trapezius | a |
| triceps | b |
| extensor hallucis longus | c |
| gastrocnemius-soleus | d |
| **Dermatome** | **Innervation Level** |
| deltoid area | e |
| radial side of hand to thumb and index finger | f |
| medial arm and forearm to long, ring, and little fingers | g |
| groin, medial thigh to knee | h |
| **Reflex** | **Innervation Level** |
| biceps | i |
| triceps | j |
| patellar | k |
| Achilles | l |

# QUIZ  Neuromuscular and Nervous Systems Proficiencies

## 7. Sensory Testing

Identify the type of sensory testing most closely associated with the supplied description. Answers must be selected from the Word Bank and can be used only once.

**Word Bank:** deep pain, graphesthesia, kinesthesia, light touch, proprioception, temperature, two-point discrimination, stereognosis, superficial pain, vibration

| Sensation | Description |
|---|---|
| a | squeeze the forearm or calf muscle |
| b | use a tuning fork |
| c | identify a static position of an extremity |
| d | use a cotton ball applied to the skin |
| e | identify direction and extent of movement of a body part |
| f | use hot and cold test tubes |
| g | draw a letter on the skin with a finger |
| h | identify one or two points without sight |
| i | identify an object without sight |
| j | use a paper clip end or a pen cap |

## 8. Upper versus Lower Motor Neuron Lesions

Indicate whether each pathology is an upper motor neuron or lower motor neuron lesion. Answers must be selected from the Word Bank and can be used more than once.

**Word Bank:** upper motor neuron, lower motor neuron

| Pathology | Type of Lesion |
|---|---|
| multiple sclerosis | a |
| traumatic brain injury | b |
| Bell's palsy | c |
| Guillain-Barre syndrome | d |
| Huntington's chorea | e |
| muscular dystrophy | f |
| poliomyelitis | g |
| cerebral palsy | h |
| CVA | i |

**SCORE**BUILDERS

# QUIZ   Neuromuscular and Nervous Systems Proficiencies

## 9. Brunnstrom's Stages of Recovery

Identify the appropriate sequence of Brunnstrom's Stages of Recovery based on the supplied description. Answers must be selected from the Word Bank and can be used only once.

**Word Bank:** Sequence - 1, 2, 3, 4, 5, 6, 7

| Sequence | Description |
|----------|-------------|
| a | The synergies are performed voluntarily; spasticity increases. |
| b | Normal motor function is restored. |
| c | The appearance of basic limb synergies. The beginning of spasticity. |
| d | Spasticity begins to decrease. Movement patterns are not dictated solely by limb synergies. |
| e | No volitional movement initiated. |
| f | A further decrease in spasticity is noted with independence from limb synergy patterns. |
| g | Isolated joint movements are performed with coordination. |

## 10. Sensory Stimulation Techniques

Identify whether the sensory stimulation technique is used for facilitation or inhibition. Answers must be selected from the Word Bank and can be used more than once.

**Word Bank:** facilitation, inhibition

| Technique | Use |
|-----------|-----|
| icing | a |
| deep pressure | b |
| warmth | c |
| joint compression | d |
| prolonged stretch | e |
| quick stretch | f |
| tapping | g |
| light touch | h |

# Neuromuscular and Nervous Systems Proficiencies

## 11. Pediatric Reflexes I

Identify the type of pediatric reflex associated with the supplied stimulus. Answers must be selected from the Word Bank and can be used only once.

**Word Bank:** asymmetrical tonic neck reflex, Galant reflex, Moro reflex, palmar grasp reflex, plantar grasp reflex, positive support reflex, rooting reflex, startle reflex, symmetrical tonic neck reflex, walking (stepping) reflex

| Reflex | Stimulus |
|---|---|
| a | touch on the cheek |
| b | head position, turned to one side |
| c | loud, sudden noise |
| d | head position, flexion or extension |
| e | head dropping into extension suddenly for a few inches |
| f | touch to the skin along the spine from the shoulder to the hip |
| g | weight placed on the balls of the feet when upright |
| h | pressure to the base of the toes |
| i | pressure in the palm on the ulnar side of the hand |
| j | supported upright position with the soles of the feet on a firm surface |

## 12. Pediatric Reflexes II

Identify the type of pediatric reflex associated with the described response. Answers must be selected from the Word Bank and can be used only once.

**Word Bank:** asymmetrical tonic neck reflex, Galant reflex, Moro reflex, palmar grasp reflex, plantar grasp reflex, positive support reflex, rooting reflex, symmetrical tonic neck reflex, tonic labyrinthine reflex, walking (stepping) reflex

| Reflex | Response |
|---|---|
| a | arms abduct with fingers open, then cross trunk into adduction; cry |
| b | arm and leg on the face side are extended; arm and leg on the scalp side are flexed |
| c | when the head is in flexion, the arms are flexed and the legs are extended |
| d | when in a supine position, the body and the extremities are held in extension |
| e | flexion of the fingers causing a strong grip |
| f | lateral flexion of the trunk to the side of the stimulus |
| g | toe flexion |
| h | reciprocal flexion and extension of the legs |
| i | turning the head to the same side with the mouth open |
| j | stiffening of the legs and the trunk into extension |

# Neuromuscular and Nervous Systems Proficiencies

## 13. Neuromuscular and Nervous Systems Terminology

Identify the neuromuscular term most closely associated with the supplied description. Answers must be selected from the Word Bank and can be used only once.

**Word Bank:** agraphia, alexia, aphasia, constructional apraxia, dysprosody, emotional lability, hemiparesis, homonymous hemianopsia, ideomotor apraxia, neologism, perseveration, unilateral neglect

| Terminology | Description |
|---|---|
| a | Substitution within a word that is so severe that it makes the word unrecognizable. |
| b | The state of repeatedly performing the same segment of a task or repeatedly saying the same word/phrase without purpose. |
| c | The inability to write due to a lesion within the brain. |
| d | The inability to control emotion with outbursts of laughing or crying that are inconsistent with the situation. |
| e | The loss of the right or left half of the field of vision in both eyes. |
| f | The inability to interpret stimuli and events on the contralateral side of a hemispheric lesion. |
| g | Impairment in the rhythm and inflection of speech. |
| h | A condition where a person plans a movement or task, but cannot volitionally perform it. |
| i | The inability to communicate or comprehend due to damage to specific areas of the brain. |
| j | A condition of weakness on one side of the body. |
| k | The inability to reproduce geometric figures and designs. |
| l | The inability to read or comprehend written language. |

## 14. Neuromuscular and Nervous Systems Basics

Mark each statement as True or False. If the statement is False, correct the statement in the space provided.

| True/False | Statement |
|---|---|
| a | The occipital lobe of the cerebrum contains the primary motor cortex and Broca's area. |
| Correction | |
| b | The meninges consist of three distinct layers termed the dura mater, arachnoid, and pia mater. |

# QUIZ  Neuromuscular and Nervous Systems Proficiencies

| True/False | Statement |
|---|---|
| Correction | |
| c | The fasciculus gracilis is a motor tract responsible for voluntary, discrete, and skilled movement. |
| Correction | |
| d | The axillary and radial nerves originate from the posterior cord of the brachial plexus. |
| Correction | |
| e | The plantar reflex is assessed by stroking the lateral aspect of the sole of the foot to the ball of the foot toward the base of the great toe. |
| Correction | |
| f | A reflex grade of 1+ is indicative of a brisk or exaggerated response. |
| Correction | |
| g | Elbow flexion and/or forearm supination is a normal response when eliciting the brachioradialis deep tendon reflex. |
| Correction | |
| h | Graphesthesia refers to the ability to perceive the weight of different objects placed in the hand. |
| Correction | |
| i | A grade of 0 on the Modified Ashworth Scale is indicative of no increase in muscle tone. |
| Correction | |
| j | Slopes, uneven surfaces, and standing on foam could be used to challenge the somatosensory system during a balance assessment. |

# Neuromuscular and Nervous Systems Proficiencies

| True/False | Statement |
|---|---|
| **Correction** | |
| k | Crouching or squatting is an example of the suspensory postural strategy. |
| **Correction** | |
| l | The Berg Balance Scale consists of fourteen tasks, each scored on an ordinal five point scale. |
| **Correction** | |
| m | Patients with Brown-Sequard's syndrome present with a loss of pain and temperature sense on the ipsilateral side of the lesion. |
| **Correction** | |
| n | Guillain-Barre syndrome results in motor weakness in a proximal to distal progression. |
| **Correction** | |
| o | The Glasgow Coma Scale has a minimum score of 0 and a maximum score of 15. |
| **Correction** | |

# Neuromuscular and Nervous Systems Answer Key

## 1. Brain Anatomy
a. olfactory bulb
b. fornix
c. pituitary gland
d. midbrain
e. medulla oblongata
f. pineal gland
g. hypothalamus

## 2. Circle of Willis
a. right anterior cerebral artery
b. right internal carotid artery
c. right posterior communicating artery
d. right posterior cerebral artery
e. left vertebral artery
f. basilar artery
g. arterial circle
h. left middle cerebral artery
i. anterior communicating artery

## 3. Cranial Nerve Function
a. yes
b. no
c. yes
d. no
e. no
f. yes
g. no
h. yes
i. yes
j. yes
k. no
l. yes
m. yes
n. yes
o. yes
p. no
q. yes
r. yes
s. yes
t. yes
u. no
v. yes
w. no
x. yes

## 4. Cranial Nerve Testing
a. familiar odors
b. visual fields
c. upward, downward, and medial gaze
d. downward and lateral gaze
e. face sensation
f. lateral gaze
g. familiar tastes
h. hearing test
i. gag reflex
j. gag reflex
k. resisted shoulder shrug
l. tongue protrusion

## 5. Hemispheric Specialization
a. left
b. right
c. left
d. right
e. right
f. left
g. right
h. left
i. right

## 6. Innervation Levels
a. C4
b. C7
c. L5
d. S1
e. C5
f. C6
g. C8
h. S3
i. C5
j. C7
k. L4
l. S1

## 7. Sensory Testing
a. deep pain
b. vibration
c. proprioception
d. light touch
e. kinesthesia
f. temperature

# Neuromuscular and Nervous Systems Answer Key

g.  graphesthesia

h.  two-point discrimination

i.  stereognosis

j.  superficial pain

## 8. Upper versus Lower Motor Neuron Lesions

a.  upper motor neuron

b.  upper motor neuron

c.  lower motor neuron

d.  lower motor neuron

e.  upper motor neuron

f.  lower motor neuron

g.  lower motor neuron

h.  upper motor neuron

i.  upper motor neuron

## 9. Brunnstrom's Stages of Recovery

a.  3

b.  7

c.  2

d.  4

e.  1

f.  5

g.  6

## 10. Sensory Stimulation Techniques

a.  facilitation

b.  inhibition

c.  inhibition

d.  facilitation

e.  inhibition

f.  facilitation

g.  facilitation

h.  facilitation

## 11. Pediatric Reflexes I

a.  rooting reflex

b.  asymmetrical tonic neck reflex

c.  startle reflex

d.  symmetrical tonic neck reflex

e.  Moro reflex

f.  Galant reflex

g.  positive support reflex

h.  plantar grasp reflex

i.  palmar grasp reflex

j.  walking (stepping) reflex

## 12. Pediatric Reflexes II

a.  Moro reflex

b.  asymmetrical tonic neck reflex

c.  symmetrical tonic neck reflex

d.  tonic labyrinthine reflex

e.  palmar grasp reflex

f.  Galant reflex

g.  plantar grasp reflex

h.  walking (stepping) reflex

i.  rooting reflex

j.  positive support reflex

## 13. Neuromuscular and Nervous Systems Terminology

a.  neologism

b.  perseveration

c.  agraphia

d.  emotional lability

e.  homonymous hemianopsia

f.  unilateral neglect

g.  dysprosody

h.  ideomotor apraxia

i.  aphasia

j.  hemiparesis

k.  constructional apraxia

l.  alexia

## 14. Neuromuscular and Nervous Systems Basics*

a.  FALSE: Correction - The frontal lobe of the cerebrum contains the primary motor cortex and Broca's area.

b.  TRUE

c.  FALSE: Correction - The corticospinal tract is a motor tract responsible for voluntary, discrete, and skilled movement.

d.  TRUE

e.  TRUE

f.  FALSE: Correction - A reflex grade of 1+ is indicative of a diminished or depressed response.

g.  TRUE

h.  FALSE: Correction - Barognosis refers to the ability to perceive the weight of different objects placed in the hand.

i.  TRUE

j.  TRUE

k.  TRUE

l.  TRUE

# Neuromuscular and Nervous Systems Answer Key

m.  FALSE: Correction - Patients with Brown-Sequard's syndrome present with a loss of pain and temperature sense on the contralateral side of the lesion.

n.  FALSE: Correction - Guillain-Barre syndrome results in motor weakness in a distal to proximal progression.

o.  FALSE: Correction - The Glasgow Coma Scale has a minimum score of 3 and a maximum score of 15.

   *The correction presented for each false statement is an example of several possible corrections.

## Neuromuscular and Nervous Systems References

1. Rowland LP, Pedley TA. *Merritt's Neurology*. 12th Edition. Lippincott Williams & Wilkins, 2009.

2. Snell RS. *Clinical Neuroanatomy*. 7th Edition. Philadelphia, PA: Lippincott Williams & Wilkins, 2009.

3. Lundy-Ekman L. *Neuroscience Fundamentals for Rehabilitation*. Third Edition. WB Saunders Company, 2007.

4. McCaffrey P. The Corpus Striatum, Rhinencephalon, Connecting Fibers, and Diencephalon. www.csuchico.edu/~pmccaffrey/syllabi/CMSD%20320/362unit5.html Neuroscience on the Web Series. November, 2010. Accessed March, 2011.

5. Cohen H. *Neuroscience for Rehabilitation*. JB Lippincott Company, 1999.

6. DeMyer W. *Technique of the Neurologic Examination*. McGraw-Hill Companies, 2004.

7. Bertoti, DB. *Functional Neurorehabilitation Through the Life Span*. FA Davis, 2004.

8. Gillen G, Burtkhardt A. *Stroke Rehabilitation: A Functional Approach*. Mosby, 1998.

9. Conn PM. *Neuroscience in Medicine*. JB Lippincott Company, 2008.

10. Freemon FR. Akinetic Mutism and Bilateral Anterior Cerebral Artery Occlusion. http://www.ncbi.nlm.nih.gov/pmc/articles/PMC1083504/ Journal of Neurology, Neurosurgery, and Psychiatry. Accessed March, 2011.

11. Dawson VL, Hsu CY, Liu TH, Dawson TM, Wamsley JK. Receptor alterations in subcortical structures after bilateral middle cerebral artery infarction of the cerebral cortex. http://www.ncbi.nlm.nih.gov/pubmed/8070526. Accessed April, 2011.

12. Slater D, Curtin S, Johns J. Middle cerebral artery stroke. http://emedicine.medscape.com/article/323120-overview. Accessed March 2011.

13. Goodman C, Boissonnault W, Fuller K. *Pathology: Implications for the Physical Therapist*. Third Edition. WB Saunders Company, 2008.

14. Campbell S. *Physical Therapy for Children*. Third Edition. WB Saunders Company, 2006.

15. Campbell S. *Decision Making in Pediatric Neurologic Physical Therapy*. Churchill Livingstone, 1999.

16. Human Nervous System. Encyclopedia Britannica Online, http://www.britannica.com/EBchecked/topic/409709/human-nervous-system. Updated 2010. Retrieved November 29, 2010.

17. Gutman S. *Quick Reference Neuroscience for Rehabilitation Professionals*. Slack Inc, 2001.

18. Field-Fote E. *Spinal Cord Injury Rehabilitation*. FA Davis Company, 2009.

19. Sisto SA, Druin E, Macht-Sliwinski M. *Spinal Cord Injuries Management and Rehabilitation*. Mosby Elsevier, 2009.

20. Cameron M, Monroe L. *Physical Information-Evidence-Based Examination: Evaluation, and Intervention*. Saunders Elsevier, 2007.

21. Magee DJ. *Orthopedic Physical Assessment*. WB Sanders, 2008.

22. Bickley L, Szilagyi P. *Bates' Guide to Physical Examination and History Taking*. Tenth Edition. Lippincott Williams & Wilkins, 2009.

23. Kendall F. *Muscles Testing and Function with Posture and Pain*. Lippincott Williams & Wilkins, 2005.

24. Umphred D. *Neurological Rehabilitation*. Fifth Edition. Mosby, 2006.

25. Walker HK, Hall WD, Hurst JW. *Clinical Methods: The History, Physical, and Laboratory Examinations*. Third Edition. Butterworths, 1990.

## Neuromuscular and Nervous Systems References

26. O'Sullivan S, Schmitz T. *Physical Rehabilitation: Assessment and Treatment*. Fifth Edition. FA Davis Company, 2007.

27. Rothstein J, Roy S, Wolf S. *The Rehabilitation Specialist's Handbook*. Third Edition. FA Davis Company, 2005.

28. Montgomery PC, Connolly BH. *Clinical Applications for Motor Control*. Slack, Incorporated, 2003.

29. *Physical Therapist's Clinical Companion*, Springhouse Corporation, 2000.

30. Bennett S, Karnes J. *Neurological Disabilities: Assessment and Treatment*. Lippincott-Raven Publishers, 1998.

31. Barnes M, Dobkin B, Bogousslavsky J. *Recovery after Stroke*. Cambridge University Press, 2005.

32. Neurological Diagnostic Tests and Procedures. National Institute of Neurological Disorders and Stroke, National Institutes of Health. http://www.ninds.nih.gov/disorders/misc/diagnostic_tests.htm. Accessed June 2011.

33. Ciccone C. *Pharmacology in Rehabilitation*. Fourth Edition. FA Davis Company, 2007.

34. *Miller-Keane: Encyclopedia and Dictionary of Medicine, Nursing, and Allied Health*. Seventh Edition. WB Saunders Company, 2003.

35. Davies PM. *Steps to Follow: The Comprehensive Treatment of Patients with Hemiplegia*. Sprzinger-Verlag, 2004.

36. Shumway-Cook A, Woollacott M. *Motor Control: Translating Research into Clinical Practice*. Third Edition. Lippincott Williams & Wilkins, 2007.

37. Carr J, Shepard R. *Neurological Rehabilitation: Optimizing Motor Performance*. Butterworth-Heinemann, 1998.

38. Carr J, Shepard R. *Stroke Rehabilitation: Guidelines for Exercise and Training to Optimize Motor Skill*. Elsevier Science Limited, 2003.

39. Bobath B. *Adult Hemiplegia: Evaluation and Treatment*. Third Edition. Butterworth-Heinemann, 1990.

40. Sullivan P, Markos P. *Clinical Decision Making in Therapeutic Exercise*. Appleton & Lange, 1995.

41. Brunnstrom S. *Movement Therapy in Hemiplegia*. Harper and Row Publishers Inc., 1992.

42. Mesulam MM. Motor Exam Guide and Key Sensory Points. National Institute of Health http://www.asia-spinalinjury.org/# American Spinal Injury Association (ASIA). Accessed June 2011.

43. Goodman C, Snyder T. *Differential Diagnosis in Physical Therapy*. Fourth Edition. WB Saunders Company, 2007.

44. Campbell M. *Rehabilitation for Traumatic Brain Injury: Physical Therapy Practice in Context*. Churchill Livingstone, 2000.

45. Long T, Toscano K. *Handbook of Pediatric Physical Therapy*. Second Edition. Lippincott Williams & Wilkins, 2002.

46. Tecklin J. *Pediatric Physical Therapy*. Fourth Edition. Lippincott Williams & Wilkins, 2007.

47. Ratliffe KT. *Clinical Pediatric Physical Therapy: A Guide for the Physical Therapy Team*. Mosby Inc., 1998.

48. Special Education and Rehabilitative Services. ehttp://www2.ed.gov/policy/speced/leg/edpicks.jhtml?src=ln. The US Department of Education. Accessed June 2011.

# 6

# CARDIOVASCULAR/ PULMONARY AND LYMPHATIC SYSTEMS

## Michael Fillyaw

Cardiovascular/Pulmonary and Lymphatic Systems represents approximately 16.5% (33 questions) of the National Physical Therapy Examination.

The actual number of questions in this category can range from 32 to 35 questions.

235 Anatomy and Physiology

242 Lung Volumes and Capacities

243 Pathology

253 Laboratory Tests

256 Diagnostic Procedures

258 Pharmacology

260 Medical Procedures

279 Aerobic Exercise Prescription

280 Airway Clearance Techniques

295 Cardiopulmonary Resuscitation

296 Essentials

298 Proficiencies

SCOREBUILDERS

# Anatomy and Physiology of the Cardiovascular System

## Heart

### Topology of the Heart

**Apex:** The lowest part of the heart formed by the inferolateral part of the left ventricle. It projects anteriorly and to the left at the level of the 5th intercostal space and the left midclavicular line.

**Base:** The upper border of the heart involving the left atrium, part of the right atrium, and the proximal portions of the great vessels. It lies approximately below the second rib at the level of the second intercostal space.

**Endocardium:** The endothelial tissue that lines the interior of the heart chambers and valves.

**Epicardium:** The serous layer of the pericardium. The epicardium contains the epicardial coronary arteries and veins, autonomic nerves, and lymphatics.

**Myocardium:** The thick contractile middle layer of muscle cells that forms the bulk of the heart wall.

**Pericardium:** A double-walled connective tissue sac that surrounds the outside of the heart and great vessels.

### Great Vessels of the Heart

**Aorta:** The body's largest artery and the central conduit of blood from the heart to the body. The aorta begins at the upper part of the left ventricle, and after ascending for a short distance arches backward and to the left (arch of the aorta). It then descends within the thorax (thoracic aorta) and passes into the abdominal cavity (abdominal aorta).

**Superior vena cava:** The vein that returns venous blood from the head, neck, and arms to the right atrium.

**Inferior vena cava:** The vein that returns venous blood from the lower body and viscera to the right atrium.

**Pulmonary arteries:** The arteries that carry deoxygenated blood from the right ventricle to the left and right lungs.

**Pulmonary veins:** The veins that carry oxygenated blood from the right and left lungs to the left atrium.

### Heart Chambers and Valves

The superior chambers of the heart are the right atrium (RA) and left atrium (LA). The wall between the atria is the atrial septum. The two inferior chambers of the heart are the right ventricle (RV) and left ventricle (LV). The wall between the ventricles is the ventricular septum. The right chambers collect blood from the body and pump it to the lungs. The left chambers collect blood from the lungs and pump it to the rest of the body.

The heart has four valves that function to maintain unidirectional blood flow (Fig. 6.1). The atrioventricular valves (AV) are between the atria and ventricles and are named by the number of leaflets or cusps. The right AV valve, or tricuspid valve, has three leaflets. It controls blood flow between the RA and RV. The left AV valve, or mitral valve, has two leaflets. It controls blood flow between the LA and LV. The aortic valve is between the LV and aorta; the pulmonary valve is between the RV and pulmonary artery.

Venous blood from the superior and inferior vena cava enters the RA and is pumped through the tricuspid valve into the RV. The tricuspid valve closes while the RV contracts to pump blood through the pulmonary valve and into the pulmonary trunk, which divides into right and left pulmonary arteries serving the right and left lungs, respectively. After picking up oxygen and releasing carbon dioxide in the pulmonary capillaries, oxygenated blood returns via the pulmonary veins to the LA. Contraction of the LA forces blood through the mitral valve into the LV. The mitral valve closes when the LV contracts to pump blood through the aortic valve into the aorta where it is distributed into the coronary circulation and systemic circulation (Fig. 6-1).

### Coronary Arteries

The coronary arteries are a network of progressively smaller vessels that carry oxygenated blood to the myocardium. The right and left coronary arteries arise from the ascending aorta just beyond where the aorta leaves the left ventricle. These arteries and their branches supply all parts of the myocardium (Fig. 6-2).

# HEART
## Chambers of the Heart

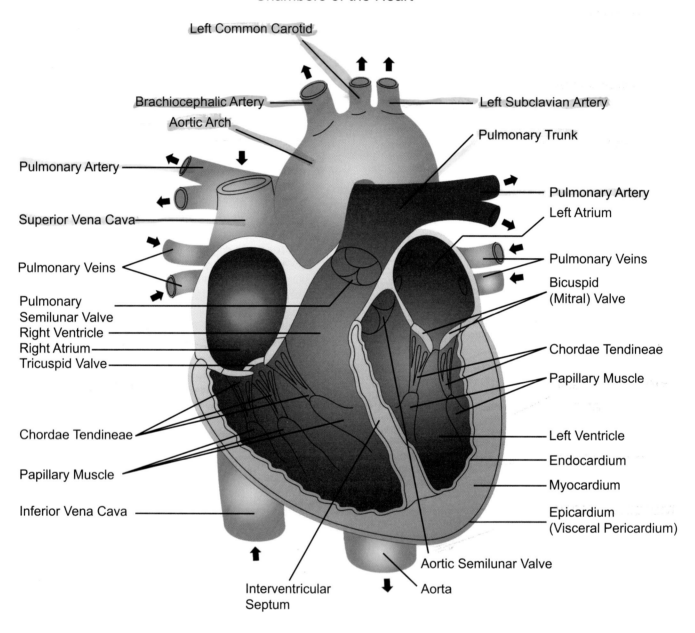

Left Common Carotid

Brachiocephalic Artery

Aortic Arch

Left Subclavian Artery

Pulmonary Trunk

Pulmonary Artery

Superior Vena Cava

Pulmonary Artery

Left Atrium

Pulmonary Veins

Pulmonary Veins

Pulmonary Semilunar Valve

Bicuspid (Mitral) Valve

Right Ventricle

Right Atrium

Tricuspid Valve

Chordae Tendineae

Papillary Muscle

Chordae Tendineae

Left Ventricle

Papillary Muscle

Endocardium

Myocardium

Inferior Vena Cava

Epicardium (Visceral Pericardium)

Aortic Semilunar Valve

Interventricular Septum

Aorta

Anterior View

**Fig. 6-1:** Cross section of the anterior of the heart showing the chambers and valves.

| Coronary Artery and Main Branches | Areas Supplied |
|---|---|
| **Right coronary artery** | |
| Sinus node artery | Right atrium |
| Right marginal artery | Right ventricle |
| Posterior descending artery | Inferior walls of both ventricles<br>Inferior portion of the interventricular septum |
| **Left coronary artery** | |
| Circumflex artery | Left atrium<br>Posterior and lateral walls of the left ventricle<br>Anterior and inferior walls of the left ventricle |
| Left anterior descending artery | Anterior portion of the interventricular septum |

**Fig. 6-2:** Anterior surface of the heart showing the great vessels and coronary arteries.

## Coronary Veins

The coronary venous circulation includes the coronary sinus, cardiac veins, and thebesian veins. The great cardiac vein, along with the small and middle cardiac veins, drain into the coronary sinus, emptying into the right atrium. The thebesian veins arise in the myocardium and drain into all chambers of the heart, but primarily into the right atrium and right ventricle.

## Cardiac Conduction System

The components of the cardiac conduction system include the sinoatrial (SA) node, internodal tracts, atrioventricular (AV) node, common AV bundle or bundle of His, right and left bundle branches, and Purkinje fibers. Each cardiac myocyte has an intrinsic ability to depolarize and propagate electrical impulses from cell to cell without nerve stimulation.

The SA node is the normal pacemaker of the heart. Specialized conduction tracts conduct the cardiac impulse between the SA node and AV node and to the atrial musculature. The Bachmann bundle appears to conduct the cardiac impulse preferentially from the right to the left atrium. At the lower end of the AV node, the nodal fibers form the common bundle of His which passes to the interventricular septum and divides into right and left bundle branches. The branches divide into the Purkinje fibers that extend into both ventricular walls.

## Innervation of the Heart

Although cardiac automaticity is intrinsic to the SA node; heart rate, rhythm, and contractility are also influenced by the autonomic nervous system. The vagus and sympathetic cardiac nerves converge to form the cardiac plexus at the base of the heart.

- The sympathetic influence is achieved by release of epinephrine and norepinephrine. Sympathetic nerves stimulate the chambers to beat faster (chronotropic effect) and with greater force of contraction (inotropic effect).

- The parasympathetic influence is achieved via acetylcholine release from the vagus nerve. Parasympathetic nerves slow the heart rate (chronotropic effect) primarily through their influence on the SA node.

## Neural Reflexes and Circulatory Control

The balance between the sympathetic and parasympathetic components of the autonomic nervous system determines cardiovascular responses.

**Baroreceptor reflex:** Baroreceptors are mechanoreceptors that detect changes in pressure. The reflexes by which blood pressure is maintained are collectively known as the baroreflex, which includes arterial baroreceptors (high pressure receptors located in the carotid sinus, aortic arch, and origin of the right subclavian artery) and cardiopulmonary receptors (low pressure receptors). Sympathetic activation leads to increased cardiac contractility, increased heart rate, venoconstriction, and arterial vasoconstriction, ultimately leading to increased blood pressure via elevation of total peripheral resistance and cardiac output. Parasympathetic

activation leads to a decrease in heart rate and a small decrease in contractility, resulting in a decrease in blood pressure.

**Bainbridge reflex:** An increase in venous return stretches receptors in the wall of the right atrium which sends vagal afferent signals to the cardiovascular center within the medulla. The signals inhibit parasympathetic activity, resulting in an increased heart rate.

**Chemoreceptor reflex:** Chemosensitive cells located in the carotid bodies and the aortic body respond to changes in pH status and blood oxygen tension. At an arterial partial oxygen pressure of less than 50 mm Hg or in conditions of acidosis, the chemoreceptors stimulate the respiratory centers and increase the depth and rate of ventilation. In addition, the ensuing activation of the parasympathetic system reduces heart rate and myocardial contractility. In the case of persistent hypoxia, the CNS will be directly stimulated with a resultant increase in sympathetic activity.

**Valsalva maneuver:** Forced expiration against a closed glottis produces increased intrathoracic pressure, increased central venous pressure, and decreased venous return. The resultant decrease in cardiac output and blood pressure is sensed by baroreceptors, which reflexively increase heart rate and myocardial contractility through sympathetic stimulation. When the glottis opens, venous return increases and blood pressure and heart contractility increase. The increase in blood pressure is sensed by baroreceptors, which reflexively decrease the heart rate through the parasympathetic efferent pathways.

## Cardiac Cycle

The cardiac cycle refers to the sequence of events that occur when the heart beats.

**Atrial systole:** The contraction of the right and left atria pushing blood into the ventricles.

**Atrial diastole:** The period between atrial contractions when the atria are repolarizing.

**Ventricular systole:** Contraction of the right and left ventricles pushing blood into the pulmonary arteries and aorta.

**Ventricular diastole:** The period between ventricular contractions when the ventricles are repolarizing.

**Preload:** Refers to the tension in the ventricular wall at the end of diastole. It reflects the venous filling pressure that fills the left ventricle during diastole.

**Afterload:** Refers to the forces that impede the flow of blood out of the heart, primarily the pressure in the peripheral vasculature, the compliance of the aorta, and the mass and viscosity of blood.

**Stroke volume (SV):** Refers to the volume of blood ejected by each contraction of the left ventricle. Normal SV ranges from 60 to 80 ml depending on age, sex, and activity.

**Cardiac output (CO):** The amount of blood pumped from the left or right ventricle per minute. It is equal to the product of stroke volume and heart rate. Normal CO for an adult male at rest is 4.5 to 5.0 L/min with women producing slightly less. CO can increase up to 25 L/min during exercise.

**Venous return:** The amount of blood that returns to the right atrium each minute. This is similar in volume to the CO. Because the cardiovascular system is a closed loop, venous return must equal CO when averaged over time.

## Systemic Circulation

The systemic arterial circulation carries oxygenated blood from the left ventricle through the aorta, arteries, and arterioles to the capillaries in the tissues of the body. From the capillaries, deoxygenated blood returns through a series of venules and veins. The veins of the upper and lower extremities are subdivided into superficial and deep. The superficial veins are beneath the skin between the two layers of superficial fascia; the deep veins accompany the arteries. Both types of veins have valves, but they are more numerous in the deep veins than in the superficial veins and in lower extremity veins more than upper extremity veins.

## Blood and Components of Blood[1]

Blood transports oxygen and nutrients to the cells of the body and returns waste products from these cells. Normal blood volume of an adult is between 4.5 and 5.0 L, with women's volume being slightly less than men. Hypovolemia refers to decreased blood volume, specifically the volume of plasma. Causes of hypovolemia include bleeding, dehydration from vomiting, diarrhea, sweating, severe burns, and diuretic medications used to treat hypertension. Signs and symptoms of hypovolemia include orthostatic hypotension, tachycardia, and elevated body temperature. Hypervolemia, or fluid overload, refers to increased blood plasma. Causes of hypervolemia include excess intake of fluids (e.g., IV or blood transfusion) and sodium or fluid retention (e.g., heart failure, kidney disease). Signs and symptoms of hypervolemia include swelling in the legs, ascites (fluid in the abdomen), and fluid in the lungs.

### Plasma

Plasma is the liquid component of blood, in which the blood cells and platelets are suspended. Plasma consists of water, electrolytes, and proteins, and accounts for more than half of the total blood volume. Plasma is important in regulating blood pressure and temperature.

### Red blood cells

Red blood cells (i.e., erythrocytes) make up approximately 40% of blood volume. Red blood cells contain hemoglobin, a protein that gives blood its red color and enables it to bind with oxygen. When the number of red blood cells is too low (anemia), the blood carries less oxygen, resulting in fatigue and weakness. If the number of red blood cells is too high (polycythemia), the blood is too thick, increasing the risk of stroke or heart attack.

### Blood platelets

Blood platelets (i.e., thrombocytes) assist in blood clotting by clumping together at a bleeding site and forming a plug that helps to seal the blood vessel. A low number of platelets (thrombocytopenia) increases the risk for bruising and abnormal bleeding. A high number of platelets (thrombocythemia) increases the risk of thrombosis, which may result in a stroke or heart attack.

### White blood cells

White blood cells (i.e., leukocytes) protect against infection. A low number of white blood cells (leukopenia) increases the risk of infection. An abnormally high number of white blood cells (leukocytosis) can indicate an infection or leukemia. There are five main types of white blood cells (Fig. 6-3):

**Neutrophils:** help protect the body against infections by ingesting bacteria and debris.

**Lymphocytes:** consist of three main types - T lymphocytes and natural killer cells, which help protect against viral infections and can detect and destroy some cancer cells, and B lymphocytes, which develop into cells that produce antibodies.

**Monocytes:** ingest dead or damaged cells and help defend against infectious organisms.

**Eosinophils:** kill parasites, destroy cancer cells, and are involved in allergic responses.

**Basophils:** participate in allergic responses.

Erythrocytes    Thrombocytes

Fig. 6-3: Blood cells. Left to right: top row - erythrocytes and thrombocytes; bottom row – monocyte, basophil, eosinophil, neutrophil, lymphocyte.

# Anatomy and Physiology of the Respiratory System

## Thorax

The bony thorax encloses and protects the heart, lungs and other organs and provides attachment sites for ventilatory muscles and other muscles. The thorax is bounded posteriorly by the 12 thoracic vertebrae, intervertebral disks, and ribs; anteriorly by the sternum, costal cartilages, and ribs; and laterally by the ribs. Although not considered part of the thorax, the clavicles and scapulae provide attachment sites for the accessory muscles of inspiration.

### Sternum

The sternum consists of three parts – manubrium, body, and xiphoid process. The manubrium, the superior portion, articulates with the right and left clavicles at the clavicular notch. The manubrium articulates with the body of the sternum forming the sternal angle (angle of Louis). A notch at the junction of the manubrium and body provides for the articulation of the second rib. The xiphoid process is the inferior portion of the sternum.

### Ribs

Most of the bony thorax is formed by the 12 pairs of ribs. Anteriorly, ribs 1 through 7 (true ribs) attach to the sternum by costal cartilage. The costal cartilages of ribs 8 through 10 (false ribs) attach to the cartilage of the rib above and do not reach the sternum. The ventral ends of ribs 11 and 12 (floating ribs) have no skeletal attachment.

### Thoracic vertebrae

Except for ribs 1, 10, 11, and 12, which articulate only with one vertebra, the head of each rib has both a superior and inferior facet for articulation with the bodies of two adjacent thoracic vertebrae. The inferior facet articulates with the superior costal facet of the vertebra of the same number. The superior facet articulates with the inferior costal facet of the vertebra numbered one lower. The transverse process of each vertebra has a transverse costal facet that articulates with the facet on the tubercle of the rib forming the costotransverse joints.

## Muscles of Inspiration

The diaphragm, external intercostals, and internal intercostals are considered principal muscles of inspiration.

The diaphragm is the primary muscle of inspiration. It is a dome-shaped muscle that separates the thoracic cavity from the abdominal cavity. Contraction of the diaphragm causes the chest to expand longitudinally and the lower ribs to elevate to allow for inspiration.

The intercostal muscles occupy the spaces between the ribs. External intercostal muscles are oriented obliquely upward and backward from the upper border of one rib to the lower border of the rib above. Internal intercostal muscles are oriented obliquely upward and forward from the upper border of one rib to the lower border of the rib above. Contraction of the external and internal intercostal muscles elevates the ribs. Upward

movement of the upper ribs increases the anterior-posterior (A-P) diameter of the chest; elevation of the lower ribs increases the transverse diameter.

Other muscles that attach to the sternum and ribs and ordinarily contribute to movement of the chest wall only during high levels of ventilation are considered accessory muscles of inspiration. These include the sternocleidomastoid, scalenes, pectoralis major (sternocostal portion), pectoralis minor, and serratus anterior.

## Muscles of Exhalation

During quiet breathing, exhalation results from passive recoil of the lungs and rib cage. During forceful breathing, the rectus abdominus, external oblique, internal oblique, and transverse abdominus depress the lower ribs and compress the abdominal contents, thus pushing up the diaphragm and assisting with active exhalation.

## Upper Respiratory Tract

The upper respiratory tract includes the nasal cavity, pharynx (nasopharynx, oropharynx, laryngopharynx), and larynx. In addition to serving as gas conduits, these passages humidify, cool or warm inspired air, and filter foreign matter before it can reach the alveoli. The hairs in the nostrils filter out many particles while the remaining particles settle on mucous membranes in the nose or near the tonsils and adenoids.

## Lower Respiratory Tract

The lower respiratory tract extends from the larynx to the alveoli in the lungs and consists of the conducting airways and the terminal respiratory units. Between the trachea and the alveoli, the airways divide approximately 23 times.

### Trachea

Beginning at the larynx (approximately at the base of the neck) and ending at the carina (at the level of the fourth thoracic vertebra and the sternal angle) the trachea consists of a series of horseshoe-shaped rings of cartilage which support the anterior and lateral walls. Posteriorly, the trachea is composed of longitudinal bundles of smooth muscle, fibrous and elastic tissues, and numerous mucous glands. The trachea divides at the carina into the right and left main bronchi.

## Lung Lobes and Segments

The lungs are located on either side of the mediastinum, each within its own pleural cavity. The right lung has three lobes (upper, middle, and lower) and the left lung has two lobes (upper and lower). The lingula of the left upper lobe is analogous to the right middle lobe (Fig. 6-4).

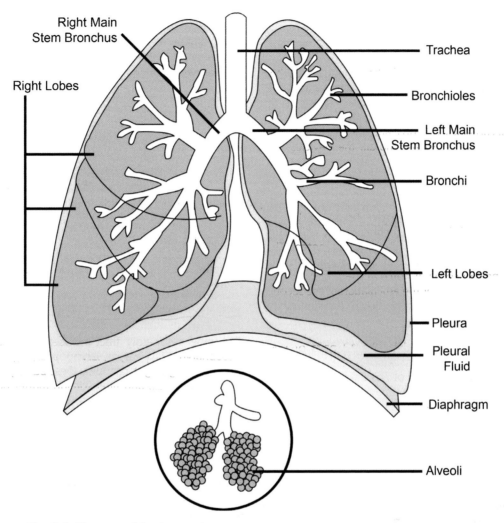

**Fig. 6-4:** Diagram of the human lungs.

## Bronchopulmonary segments

The bronchopulmonary segments are the topographic units of the lungs. There are 10 bronchopulmonary segments in the right lung and eight bronchopulmonary segments in the left lung. The right and left main bronchi branch into lobar bronchi. Each lobar bronchus branches into segmental bronchi, corresponding to the bronchopulmonary segments of the right and left lungs, which branch into bronchioles and end in terminal bronchioles.

### Right lung

The right main bronchus gives rise to the superior, middle, and inferior lobar bronchi. The right superior lobar bronchus divides into three segmental bronchi: apical, anterior, and posterior. The right middle lobar bronchus divides into two segmental bronchi: medial and lateral. The right inferior lobar bronchus divides into five segmental bronchi: superior, medial basal, anterior basal, lateral basal, and posterior basal.

### Left lung

The left main bronchus divides into the superior and inferior lobar bronchi, which correspond to the upper and lower lobes,

respectively. The left superior lobar bronchus subdivides into a superior division and an inferior (lingular) division. The superior division divides into the anterior segmental bronchus and the apicoposterior segmental bronchus (corresponding to the apical and posterior segmental bronchi of the right upper lobe). The inferior or lingular division subdivides into the superior segmental bronchus and inferior segmental bronchus. The left inferior lobar bronchus divides into the superior, lateral basal, posterior basal, and anteromedial basal segmental bronchi (corresponding to the anterior and medial segmental bronchi of the right lower lobe).

### Alveolar–capillary units

The bronchi branch many times before terminating in the acinus or respiratory unit of the lung. Oxygen diffuses across the alveolar-capillary septum into the red blood cells in the lung capillaries where it combines with hemoglobin to be transported back to the heart. Carbon dioxide diffuses in the opposite direction.

## Pleurae

A membranous serous sac called visceral pleura covers each lung. The pleura covering the surface of the lungs is called the visceral pleura. The pleural tissue covering the inner surfaces of the chest wall, ribs, vertebrae, diaphragm, and mediastinum is called parietal pleura. Normally, the two pleurae remain in contact throughout the respiratory cycle, separated only by serous fluid. Under abnormal circumstances, the pleural space may contain air (pneumothorax), blood (hemothorax), pus or increased amounts of serous fluid, which compress the lung and cause respiratory distress.

## Pulmonary Circulation

The portion of the circulatory system that carries deoxygenated blood from the heart to the lungs via the pulmonary arterial trunk, right and left pulmonary arteries, lobar arteries, arterioles, and capillaries. The pulmonary circulation returns oxygenated blood from the lungs to the left atrium via the pulmonary veins.

## Bronchial Circulation

The portion of the circulatory system that supplies oxygenated blood to the bronchi and connective tissue of the lungs via the bronchial arteries, which drain directly into the bronchial veins.

## Innervation of the Lungs

The lungs, trachea, and bronchi are innervated by both sympathetic and parasympathetic nerves containing efferent and afferent fibers. Postganglionic sympathetic fibers innervate the smooth muscles of the bronchi and pulmonary blood vessels. Parasympathetic innervation of these structures is via the vagus nerve. The nerves to the lungs reach the pulmonary vessels and lung tissue through the anterior and posterior pulmonary plexuses.

## Control of Breathing[2]

Although spontaneous breathing is largely an involuntary process, also it is under voluntary control. Breathing control is achieved by integrated activity of the central respiratory center in the brainstem and peripheral receptors in the lungs, airways, chest wall, and blood vessels. The respiratory center integrates the information transmitted from the central and peripheral chemoreceptors and mechanoreceptors in the chest wall to stimulate motor neurons that innervate the respiratory muscles.

The central chemoreceptors in the medulla respond to increases in the partial pressure of $CO_2$ and hydrogen ion by increasing ventilation. In addition to sensing changes in the partial pressure of $CO_2$ and hydrogen ion concentration, the peripheral chemoreceptors in the carotid bodies also respond to hypoxemia by increasing ventilation. Mechanoreceptors inhibit muscle activity when the force of contraction reaches potentially injurious levels.

## Lung Volumes and Capacities

| | |
|---|---|
| Anatomic dead space volume (VD) | The volume of air that occupies the non-respiratory conducting airways. |
| Expiratory reserve volume (ERV) | The maximal volume of air that can be exhaled after a normal tidal exhalation. ERV is approximately 15% of total lung volume. |
| Forced expiratory volume (FEV) | The maximal volume of air exhaled in a specified period of time: usually the 1st, 2nd, and 3rd second of a forced vital capacity maneuver. |
| Forced vital capacity (FVC) | The volume of air expired during a forced maximal expiration after a forced maximal inspiration. |
| Functional residual capacity (FRC) | The volume of air in the lungs after normal exhalation. FRC = ERV + RV. FRC is approximately 40% of total lung volume. |
| Inspiratory capacity (IC) | The maximal volume of air that can be inspired after a normal tidal exhalation. IC = TV + IRV. IC is approximately 60% of total lung volume. |
| Inspiratory reserve volume (IRV) | The maximal volume of air that can be inspired after normal tidal volume inspiration. IRV is approximately 50% of total lung volume. |
| Minute volume ventilation (VE) | The volume of air expired in one minute. VE = TV x respiratory rate. |
| Peak expiratory flow (PEF) | The maximum flow of air during the beginning of a forced expiratory maneuver. |
| Residual volume (RV) | The volume of gas remaining in the lungs at the end of a maximal expiration. RV is approximately 25% of total lung volume. |
| Tidal volume (TV) | Total volume inspired and expired with each breath during quiet breathing. TV is approximately 10% of total lung volume. |
| Total lung capacity (TLC) | The volume of air in the lungs after a maximal inspiration; the sum of all lung volumes. TLC = RV + VC or TLC = FRC + IC. |
| Vital capacity (VC) | The volume change that occurs between maximal inspiration and maximal expiration. VC = TV + IRV + ERV. VC is approximately 75% of total lung volume. |

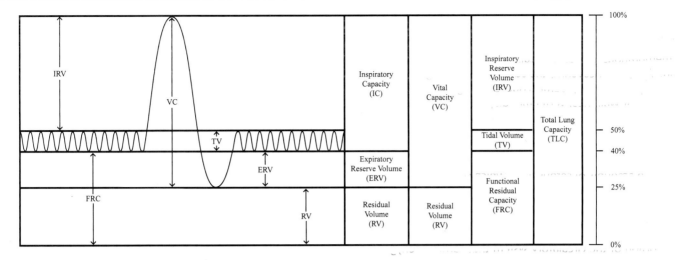

ERV = ~15% total volume
IRV = ~50% total volume
FRC = ~40% total volume
VC = ~75% total volume

RV = ~25% total volume
IC = ~60% total volume
TV = ~10% total volume
TLC = 100% volume

**Fig. 6-5:** Spirogram showing lung volumes and capacities.

## Oxygen and Carbon Dioxide Transport

Oxygen is physically dissolved in the blood plasma and chemically combined with hemoglobin in red blood cells. Much more oxygen is combined with hemoglobin than is dissolved in the plasma. Only about 0.3 mL $O_2$ is dissolved in 100 mL of arterial blood. However, the physically dissolved oxygen contributes to the $PaO_2$, which determines how much oxygen combines chemically with hemoglobin.

Carbon dioxide is physically dissolved in the blood, chemically combined with the amino acids of hemoglobin as carbamino compounds, and as bicarbonate ions. About 5-10% of the total carbon dioxide transported by the blood is dissolved in physical solution. A similar percentage is in the form of carbamino compounds. The remaining 80-90% of the carbon dioxide is transported by the blood as bicarbonate ions.

# Pathology of the Heart and Blood Vessels

## Aneurysm[3]

A localized abnormal dilation of a blood vessel, usually an artery. Common sites include the thoracic and abdominal aorta and vessels within the brain.

**Etiology** – Congenital defect; weakness in the wall of the vessel often due to chronic hypertension; connective tissue disease (e.g., Marfan Syndrome); trauma; infection.

**Signs and symptoms** – Variable based on the site. Aortic aneurysms are usually asymptomatic, but may include generalized abdominal or low back pain. Abdominal aortic aneurysms may cause pulsations near the navel. A cerebral aneurysm can cause a sudden and severe headache, nausea and vomiting, stiff neck, seizure, loss of consciousness, and double vision.

**Treatment** – Antihypertensive medications may be recommended for hypertension. Surgery is recommended to repair large aortic aneurysms and consists of replacing the aneurysm with a synthetic fabric graft. Two surgical options for ruptured brain aneurysms are surgical clipping and endovascular coiling.

## Angina Pectoris[3]

A transient precordial sensation of pressure or discomfort resulting from myocardial ischemia. Common types of angina pectoris are:

- **Stable angina** - Occurs at a predictable level of exertion, exercise or stress and responds to rest or nitroglycerin.

- **Unstable angina** - Usually is more intense, lasts longer, is precipitated by less exertion, occurs spontaneously at rest, is progressive, or any combination of these features.

- **Prinzmetal (variant) angina** - Occurs due to coronary artery spasm most often associated with coronary artery disease.

**Etiology** – Inadequate blood flow and oxygenation of the heart muscle mostly due to coronary artery disease.

**Signs and symptoms** – Usually described as pressure, heaviness, fullness, squeezing, burning or aching behind the sternum, but may also be felt in the neck and back, jaw, shoulders, and arms. The sensation may be associated with difficulty breathing, nausea or vomiting, sweating, anxiety or fear (anginal equivalents). It is typically triggered by exertion or strong emotion and subsides with rest.

**Treatment** – Treatments for acute angina include supplemental oxygen, nitroglycerin, and rest. Chronic or recurring angina pectoris is treated with long-acting nitrates, beta blockers, and calcium channel blockers. Angioplasty with stenting of the coronary arteries or coronary artery bypass surgery may be performed when medications are not effective.

## Atherosclerosis[3]

A slow progressive accumulation of fatty plaques on the inner walls of arteries. Over time the plaque can restrict blood flow, causing a blood clot.

**Etiology** – Although the exact cause is unknown, the process may begin with damage or injury to the inner wall of the artery from hypertension, high cholesterol, smoking or diabetes. Over time, fatty plaques made of cholesterol and other cellular waste products build up at the site of the injury and harden, narrowing the artery and impeding blood flow (Fig. 6-6).

**Signs and symptoms** – Varies based on the severity of disease and the artery affected. When the coronary arteries are affected, angina pectoris may result. When cerebral arteries are affected, numbness or weakness of the arms or legs, difficulty speaking or slurred speech, or drooping face muscles may result. When peripheral arteries are affected, intermittent claudication may result.

**Treatment** – Lifestyle changes, medications, and surgery may be recommended. Lifestyle changes include smoking cessation, regular exercise, healthy diet, and stress management. Medications may include antihypertensive, antiplatelet, and antilipidemic agents. Surgical procedures may include: angioplasty, endarterectomy, and bypass surgery.

Normal cross section of artery

Cholesterol particles

A plaque forms in the artery

Artery becomes narrowed

Narrowed artery becomes blocked by a blood clot

**Fig. 6-6:** Changes in an artery due to atherosclerosis.

## Cardiomyopathy[3]

Cardiomyopathy refers to a group of conditions that affect the myocardium, impairing the ability of the heart to contract and relax. Three types of cardiomyopathy are dilated, hypertrophic, and restrictive.

**Etiology** – There are many causes of cardiomyopathy, including coronary artery disease and valvular heart disease.

**Signs and symptoms** – None during the early stages. As the condition progresses, signs and symptoms include breathlessness with exertion or even at rest; swelling of the legs, ankles and feet; bloating of the abdomen due to fluid buildup; fatigue; irregular heartbeat; dizziness, lightheadedness and fainting.

**Treatment** – Variable depending on type of cardiomyopathy.

- **Dilated cardiomyopathy** – Common medications include ACE inhibitors, beta blockers, digoxin, and diuretics. Surgical intervention may include a biventricular pacemaker or an implantable cardioverter-defibrillator for patients at risk for serious arrhythmias.

- **Hypertrophic cardiomyopathy** – Medications to slow the heart rate and stabilize its rhythm. Common medications include Lopressor and calcium channel blockers. If medications are unsuccessful, surgical interventions may include septal myectomy (removal of the thickened interventricular septum); septal alcohol ablation (destruction of the interventricular septum by alcohol injection); pacemaker implantation; and implantable cardioverter-defibrillator.

- **Restrictive cardiomyopathy** – Medications focus on improving symptoms and may include diuretics, antihypertensives, and antiarrhythmics. In severe cases, surgical options include a ventricular assist device or a heart transplant.

## Chronic Venous Insufficiency (CVI)[3]

A condition in which the veins and valves in the lower extremity are damaged and cannot keep blood flowing toward the heart. This causes the veins to remain filled with blood.

**Etiology** – Weak or damaged valves inside the veins. Risk factors include age, female gender, obesity, pregnancy, and prolonged sitting or standing.

**Signs and symptoms** – Leg swelling, varicose veins, aching, heaviness or cramping, itching, redness or skin ulcers of the legs and ankles.

**Treatment** – Compression stockings and elevation of the legs help decrease chronic swelling. Varicose vein stripping may be performed for cases with persistent leg pain or skin ulcers due to poor circulation.

## Congenital Heart Defects[3]

A malformation of the interior walls or valves of the heart or the major arteries and veins near the heart that are present at birth. Blood flow through the heart may be slowed, blocked or misdirected. Congenital heart defects are the most common type of major birth defect.

## Atrial septal defect (ASD)

A hole in the wall of the heart separating the right and left atria. In fetal circulation, there is normally an opening between the two atria to allow blood to bypass the lungs. This opening is termed foramen ovale and usually closes at birth. If the ASD persists, blood continues to flow from the left to the right atria and is called a shunt. In severe cases, blood may flow from the right to the left atria.

**Etiology** – Congenital heart defects arise from errors early in the heart's development. Genetics and environmental factors may play a role.

**Signs and symptoms** – Small to moderate sized defects may produce no symptoms or symptoms that appear after 30 years of age. Large or long-standing atrial septal defects may cause:

- Heart murmur
- Shortness of breath, especially when exercising
- Fatigue
- Swelling of the legs, feet or abdomen
- Heart palpitations
- Frequent lung infections
- Stroke
- Cyanosis of the skin

**Treatment** – Surgical closure is recommended if the defect is large, the heart is swollen or symptoms occur. A non-surgical procedure involves placing a closure device into the heart and across the ASD using a catheter.

## Coarctation of the aorta

A congenital heart defect in which the aorta is narrowed near the ductus arteriosus. The coarctation may range from mild to severe and may not be detected until adulthood, depending on the amount of narrowing. It usually occurs along with other congenital defects including patent ductus arteriosus, ventricular septal defect, and bicuspid aortic valve.

**Etiology** – Congenital heart defects arise from errors early in the heart's development, but there is often no clear cause. Genetics and environmental factors may play a role. Rarely, it may develop later in life due to atherosclerosis or inflammation of the aorta.

**Signs and symptoms** – Depend on the severity of the narrowing. In infants with severe narrowing, pale skin, sweating, and shortness of breath are noted soon after birth. In older children and adults, the most common sign is high blood pressure in the arms, but low blood pressure in the legs. Other signs and symptoms may include shortness of breath on exercise, intermittent claudication, weakness, and headache.

**Treatment** – Depends on age when diagnosed and the degree of narrowing of the aorta, but usually consists of surgical repair (resection, patch, bypass), or balloon angioplasty.

## Patent ductus arteriosus (PDA)

A congenital heart defect in which the ductus arteriosus, which normally shunts blood from the pulmonary artery directly to the descending aorta in utero, does not close after birth.

**Etiology** – Congenital heart defects arise from errors early in the heart's development, but there is often no clear cause. Genetics and environmental factors may play a role. Risk factors include premature birth, other heart defects, family history, rubella infection or diabetes during pregnancy, and exposure to alcohol, drugs, chemicals or radiation during pregnancy.

**Signs and symptoms** – A small ductus may be asymptomatic, whereas a large ductus may present with tachycardia, respiratory distress, poor eating, weight loss, and congestive heart failure.

**Treatment** – Non-surgical treatments to reduce the size of the ductus include diuretics and indomethacin. Surgical repair may be necessary for a large ductus or when initial management fails. Left untreated, a PDA can cause pulmonary hypertension, heart failure, and other complications.

## Ventricular septal defect (VSD)

A hole in the septum separating the right and left ventricles. If the hole is large, too much blood will be pumped to the lungs, leading to heart failure.

**Etiology** – Congenital heart defects arise from errors early in the heart's development, but there is often no clear cause. Genetics and environmental factors may play a role. Risk factors include rubella or diabetes during pregnancy, exposure to alcohol, drugs, chemicals, and radiation during pregnancy.

**Signs and symptoms** – A small defect may have no symptoms and the hole may eventually close as the interventricular wall continues to grow after birth. A large defect may cause:

- Cyanosis of the skin, lips, and fingernails
- Poor eating, failure to thrive
- Fast breathing or breathlessness
- Fatigue
- Swelling of the legs, feet or abdomen
- Rapid heart rate (i.e., tachycardia)

**Treatment** – A common approach involves surgical patching or stitching to close the hole.

## Tetralogy of Fallot

A combination of four heart defects including: (1) ventricular septal defect (VSD); (2) pulmonary stenosis; (3) right ventricular hypertrophy; (4) aorta overriding the ventricular septal defect. It is often diagnosed during infancy, but may not be detected until later in life, depending on the severity of the defects and symptoms.

**Etiology** – In most cases the cause is unknown. Risk factors include poor maternal nutrition, viral illness or genetic disorders.

**Signs and symptoms** – Depend on the obstruction of blood flow from the right ventricle, but may include:

- Cyanosis of the skin
- Shortness of breath and rapid breathing, especially during feeding
- Fainting
- Clubbing of fingers and toes

- Poor weight gain
- Tiring easily during play
- Irritability and prolonged crying
- Heart murmur

**Treatment** – Surgery is the only effective treatment. Usually, cardiac surgery involves placing a patch over the VSD and widening the pulmonary valve and pulmonary arteries. Untreated cases usually develop severe complications including infective endocarditis, which may result in death or disability by early adulthood.

## Cor Pulmonale[4]

Cor pulmonale, also known as pulmonary heart disease, refers to hypertrophy of the right ventricle caused by altered structure or function of the lungs.

**Etiology** – Pulmonary hypertension from chronically increased resistance in the pulmonary circulation.

**Signs and symptoms** – The cardinal symptom is progressive shortness of breath, especially with exertion. Other signs and symptoms are fatigue, palpitations, atypical chest pain, swelling of the lower extremities, dizziness, and syncope.

**Treatment** – Supplemental oxygen sufficient to maintain $SaO_2$ > 90% and/or $PaO_2$ > 60 mm Hg. General measures include diuretics and anticoagulation.

## Coronary Artery Disease (CAD)[3]

CAD is the narrowing or blockage of the coronary arteries due to atheromatous plaques resulting in diminished blood flow.

**Etiology** – CAD is thought to begin with damage or injury to the inner layer of a coronary artery. Once the inner wall is damaged, fatty plaques made of cholesterol and other cellular waste products tend to accumulate at the site of injury. If a plaque ruptures, platelets will clump at the site to try to repair the artery. This clump can block the artery, leading to a heart attack. Risk factors for CAD are the same as those for atherosclerosis: high blood levels of LDL cholesterol, low blood levels of HDL cholesterol, type 2 diabetes mellitus, smoking, obesity, and physical inactivity. Genetic factors, hypertension, and hypothyroidism also contribute to risk.

**Signs and symptoms** – The degree of stenosis required to produce signs and symptoms varies with the oxygen demand. The diminished blood flow may cause angina, shortness of breath or other symptoms, which may not be felt until >70% of the lumen is occluded. A complete blockage can cause a heart attack.

**Treatment** – Aggressive modification of atherosclerosis risk factors to slow progression and induce regression of existing plaques and restore or improve coronary blood flow. This includes smoking cessation; weight loss; a heart-healthy diet low in saturated fat, cholesterol and sodium; regular exercise; modification of serum lipids; and control of hypertension and diabetes. Drug therapy includes: antiplatelet agents (e.g., aspirin, Clopidogrel), ACE inhibitors, angiotensin II receptor blockers, and statins. Percutaneous angioplasty and coronary artery bypass graft surgery are considered for patients at high risk of mortality.

## Deep Vein Thrombosis (DVT)[3]

A condition in which a blood clot forms in one or more of the deep veins, usually in the lower extremities. DVT is a serious condition because the clot can break loose and travel to the lungs, resulting in a pulmonary embolism.

**Etiology** – Any condition that impairs normal circulation or normal blood clotting. Many factors increase the risk of a DVT including prolonged sitting or bed rest, inherited blood clotting disorders, injury or surgery of the veins, pregnancy, cancer, birth control or hormone replacement therapy, being overweight, obesity, and smoking.

**Signs and symptoms** – About 50% of DVT cases are asymptomatic. When signs and symptoms occur they can include swelling, pain, redness, and warmth in the affected leg.

**Treatment** – The goal of treatment is to prevent the blood clot from getting bigger and to prevent it from breaking loose and causing a pulmonary embolism. Medications include anticoagulant and thrombolytic agents. "Filters" may be surgically inserted into the vena cava to prevent clots from reaching the lungs. Compression stockings may be recommended to reduce blood pooling.

## Endocarditis[3]

Endocarditis is inflammation of the endothelium that lines the heart and cardiac valves. If left untreated, endocarditis can damage or destroy heart valves and become life-threatening.

**Etiology** – Caused by bacteria that may enter the blood from catheters or needles, dental procedures, gum disease, sexually transmitted disease or inflammatory bowel disease. Individuals with a damaged heart valve, an artificial heart valve or other heart defects are at the greatest risk.

**Signs and symptoms** – May develop slowly, depending on the cause of the infection and if the heart is affected, but can include fever, chills, heart murmur, fatigue, shortness of breath, weight loss, blood in urine, and skin petechiae.

**Treatment** – Antibiotics are the first line of treatment. Surgery may be needed to treat persistent infections or replace a damaged heart valve.

## Heart Failure[5]

Also known as congestive heart failure, heart failure is a progressive condition in which the heart cannot maintain a normal cardiac output to meet the body's demands for blood and oxygen. Heart failure often develops after other conditions have damaged or weakened the heart. The ventricles weaken and dilate to the point that the heart can't pump efficiently. It can affect the right side, left side or both sides of the heart, but typically begins with the left ventricle. The term "congestive heart failure" comes from blood backing up into the liver, abdomen, lower extremities, and lungs. The condition can be acute or chronic.

**Etiology** – Coronary artery disease, hypertension, diabetes mellitus, myocardial infarction, abnormal heart valves, and cardiomyopathy.

**Signs and symptoms** – Shortness of breath; fatigue and weakness; swelling in the legs, feet and abdomen; rapid or irregular heartbeat with S3 or S4 heart sound; persistent cough or wheezing; and weight gain from fluid retention.

**Treatment** – Sometimes treating the underlying cause can correct heart failure (e.g., repairing a damaged heart valve or controlling an abnormal heart rhythm). In most cases, treatment is a balance of medications, devices, and lifestyle changes to help the heart contract normally. Medications include anticoagulants, antihypertensives, and digitalis to increase the strength of contraction. In severe cases, surgery and medical devices may be needed to correct the underlying cause of the heart failure. These include coronary artery bypass graft, heart valve repair, implantable cardioverter-defibrillators (ICD), biventricular pacemakers, left ventricular assist device, and heart transplant. Lifestyle changes include smoking cessation, restricting sodium intake, maintaining healthy weight, limiting alcohol and fluids, stress reduction, and moderate exercise.

## Heart Murmur[3]

An abnormal swishing or whooshing sound heard by auscultation sometime during the cardiac cycle.

**Etiology** – Innocent heart murmurs occur when blood flows rapidly through the heart due to activity, pregnancy, fever, and anemia. Abnormal heart murmurs may be caused by turbulent blood flow through a damaged or narrowed heart valve or a hole in one of the heart's walls. Other causes include rheumatic fever, endocarditis, calcified valves, and mitral valve prolapse.

**Signs and symptoms** – Innocent murmurs are not usually associated with other signs or symptoms. Abnormal murmurs may be associated with cyanosis, limb edema, shortness of breath, enlarged neck veins, weight gain, chest pain, dizziness, and fainting.

**Treatment** – Innocent murmurs usually do not require treatment. Treatment for abnormal heart murmurs depends on the underlying cause and can include medications or surgery. Common medications are: digoxin, anticoagulants, diuretics, and other antihypertensive agents. Surgical procedures include valve replacement or patching atrial or ventricular septal defects.

## Hypertension[6]

Arterial hypertension in adults is a sustained elevation of systolic pressure ≥ 140 mm Hg or diastolic pressure ≥ 90 mm Hg. Hypertension in children and adolescents is defined as systolic and/or diastolic blood pressure that is consistently equal to or greater than the 95th percentile of the blood pressure distribution.

**Etiology** – Primary or essential hypertension has no known cause. Hypertension with an identified cause (usually renal disease) is called secondary hypertension.

**Signs and symptoms** – Hypertension is often asymptomatic until complications develop in the organs. An S4 heart sound is an early sign. Severe hypertension (DBP > 120 mm Hg) can cause significant CNS symptoms (e.g., confusion, cortical blindness, hemiparesis, seizures), cardiovascular symptoms (e.g., chest pain, dyspnea), and renal involvement.

**Treatment** – Recommendations include lifestyle modifications (aerobic physical activity at least 30 min/day most days of the week; weight loss to a body mass index of 18.5 to 24.9; smoking cessation; reduced intake of dietary sodium and alcohol; increased consumption of fruits, vegetables, and low-fat dairy products with reduced saturated and total fat content); and medications. Classes of medications for hypertension include diuretics, beta blockers, calcium channel blockers, ACE inhibitors, angiotensin II receptor blockers, and direct vasodilators.

### Classification of Hypertension in Adults[7]

| BP Classification | SBP mm Hg* | DBP mm Hg* |
|---|---|---|
| Normal | <120 | <80 |
| Prehypertensive | 120–139 | 80–89 |
| Stage 1 hypertension | 140–159 | 90–99 |
| Stage 2 hypertension | ≥160 | ≥100 |

*Classification determined by higher BP category

## Lymphedema

Edema, or swelling, due to an accumulation of lymph in the extremities.

**Etiology** – Primary lymphedema is a rare, inherited condition caused by problems with the development of lymph vessels. Causes of secondary lymphedema include any condition or procedure that damages or obstructs lymph nodes or vessels.

**Signs and symptoms** – Swelling with restricted motion of the upper or lower extremity; aching and heaviness or a feeling of fullness; brawny, fibrous, non pitting edema in one or more limbs.

**Treatment** – There is no cure, but treatments focused on reducing swelling and controlling pain may lessen symptoms and slow or halt progression. Treatments include: gentle active exercise, pressure gradient bandages, massage, pneumatic compression, and compression garments. Surgery to remove excess tissue in the affected extremity may be considered.

## Myocardial Infarction (MI)[8]

Also known as a heart attack, a MI occurs when the blood flow through one or more of the coronary arteries is severely reduced or cut off completely. This causes irreversible necrosis to the portion of myocardium supplied by the blocked artery.

**Etiology** – Most heart attacks occur when a ruptured atherosclerotic plaque or blood clot blocks the flow of blood through a coronary artery. An uncommon cause is a spasm of a coronary artery.

**Signs and symptoms** – Chest discomfort with pressure, squeezing or pain; shortness of breath; discomfort in the upper body including the arms, shoulder, neck or back; nausea, vomiting, dizziness, sweating, and palpitations.

**Treatment** – Treatment of a MI varies from medication to surgery, or both, depending on the severity and the amount of heart damage. Medications used to treat the acute MI include anticoagulants and thrombolytic agents, pain relievers, antihypertensives, and cholesterol-lowering medications. Surgical procedures may include coronary angioplasty with stenting or coronary artery bypass surgery. Recommended lifestyle changes include smoking cessation, moderate exercise, maintaining a healthy diet and weight, stress reduction, and consuming alcohol only in moderation.

## Spotlight on Safety
### Warning Signs of a Heart Attack[8]

Heart attack symptoms vary. Not all people who have heart attacks experience the same symptoms or experience them to the same degree. Some heart attacks are sudden and intense, but most start slowly, with mild pain or discomfort. Signs that can indicate a heart attack include:

- Discomfort in the center of the chest that lasts more than a few minutes, or that goes away and comes back. It can feel like uncomfortable pressure, squeezing, fullness or pain.

- Pain or discomfort in one or both upper extremities, the back, neck, jaw or stomach.

- Shortness of breath with or without chest discomfort.

- Breaking out in a cold sweat, nausea or lightheadedness.

The most common heart attack symptom is chest pain or discomfort in both men and women. Women are somewhat more likely than men to experience shortness of breath, nausea/vomiting, and back or jaw pain.

Often people affected aren't sure what's wrong and wait too long before getting help. Even if a patient or therapist is not sure it's a heart attack, they should have it checked by a doctor. Patients should not wait more than five minutes to call 911 or an emergency response number. It is best to call Emergency Medical Services (EMS) for rapid transport to an emergency room. EMS staff can begin treatment when they arrive and can revive someone whose heart has stopped.

## Myocarditis

Myocarditis refers to inflammation and weakness of the myocardium. Myocarditis can cause the myocardium to become thick and swollen, which can lead to symptoms of heart failure.

**Etiology** – Usually caused by a viral (e.g., influenza, coxsackie virus, adenovirus) or bacterial (e.g., polio, rubella, Lyme disease) infection.

**Signs and symptoms** – Depend on the cause and severity of the disease. Common symptoms include arrhythmias, chest pain, shortness of breath, fatigue, and signs of fever (headache, muscle aches, sore throat, diarrhea or rashes).

**Treatment** – Treatment focuses on the underlying cause and may include antibiotics, anti-inflammatory agents, diuretics, beta blockers, and calcium channel blockers to reduce the workload of the heart. Severe cases may require surgical implantation of a ventricular assist device or intra-aortic balloon pump.

## Pericarditis[3]

Pericarditis refers to an inflammation of the pericardium of the heart. The pericardium has an inner and outer layer with a small amount of lubricating fluid between them. When the pericardium becomes inflamed, the amount of fluid between the two layers increases (pericardial effusion). This condition may be acute or chronic, both of which can disrupt the heart's normal rhythm and/or function and possibly, although rarely, lead to death.

**Etiology** – Usually a complication of viral infections (e.g., coxsackie, influenza, HIV), but it can also result from bacterial and fungal infections. Other causes include heart attack, chest trauma, surgery, immunosuppressive medications, and radiation to the chest.

**Signs and Symptoms** – Chest pain, shortness of breath, dry cough, anxiety, fatigue, and fever.

**Treatment** – Analgesics or anti-inflammatory medications are given to relieve pain; antibiotics are prescribed if the pericarditis is due to a bacterial infection. Most cases are mild and clear up on their own or with rest and simple treatment. More intense treatment may be needed to prevent complications like cardiac tamponade. Cardiac tamponade occurs when fluid in the pericardium creates pressure on the heart preventing the heart from properly filling with blood. As a result, less blood leaves the heart, which causes a sharp drop in blood pressure. If left untreated, cardiac tamponade can be fatal. Treatment consists of pericardiocentesis, in which a needle or catheter is inserted to remove excess fluid in the pericardium.

## Peripheral Arterial Disease[9]

Stenotic, occlusive, and aneurysmal diseases of the aorta and peripheral arteries.

**Etiology** – Caused primarily by atherosclerosis and thromboembolic processes that alter the structure and function of the aorta and its branches.

**Signs and symptoms** – Fatigue, aching, numbness, or pain primarily in the buttock, thigh, calf, or foot at rest or when walking; poorly healing wounds of the legs or feet; distal hair loss, trophic skin changes, and hypertrophic nails.

**Treatment** – For patients with asymptomatic disease, treatment consists of smoking cessation, lipid lowering medications, and control of diabetes and hypertension (with beta blockers). For patients with disabling intermittent claudication, treatment consists of revascularization procedures (e.g., angioplasty, stent, lasers, atherectomy devices) and surgery (e.g., aortobifemoral bypass, aortoiliac bypass, aortofemoral bypass, iliofemoral bypass) may be recommended. Supervised exercise training should be performed for a minimum of 30 to 45 minutes, at least three times per week, for a minimum of 12 weeks.

## Rheumatic Fever[3]

An inflammatory disease that can develop as a complication of untreated or poorly treated strep throat from group A streptococcus bacteria. Rheumatic fever can damage the heart valves and cause heart failure.

**Etiology** – Streptococcus pyogenes or group A streptococcus that cause strep throat or scarlet fever.

**Signs and symptoms** – Result from the inflammation of the heart, joints, skin or central nervous system and may include red, swollen, fever, and painful joints, heart palpitations, chest pain, shortness of breath, and skin rash.

**Treatment** – The goals of treatment are to destroy group A streptococcal bacteria, relieve symptoms, and control inflammation. Medications include antibiotics and anti-inflammatory agents.

## Valvular Heart Disease[10]

Damage to one or more of the heart's valves results in regurgitation or stenosis of blood flow. In regurgitation, also known as insufficiency or incompetence, the blood leaks backward through the damaged valve. Stenosis happens when the leaflets thicken, stiffen or fuse together and do not open wide enough to allow adequate blood flow through the valve.

**Etiology** – Congenital defects, calcific degeneration, infective endocarditis, coronary artery disease, myocardial infarction, and rheumatic fever.

**Signs and symptoms** – Varies based on the type and severity of valve disease, but may include heart palpitations, shortness of breath, chest pain, coughing, ankle swelling, and fatigue.

**Treatment** – Patients with minimal symptoms may not require treatment. Treatment for moderate cases includes medications to reduce the workload of the heart, regulate the heart rhythm, and prevent clotting. These medications may include digitalis, diuretics, antiplatelet and anticoagulant agents, beta blockers, and calcium channel blockers. Severe cases may require balloon valvuloplasty or surgery to repair or replace the affected valve.

# Pathology of the Airways and Lungs

## Acute Respiratory Distress Syndrome (ARDS)[3]

ARDS is sudden respiratory failure due to fluid accumulation in the alveoli. ARDS usually occurs in people who are already critically ill or who have significant injuries. Severe shortness of breath develops within a few hours to a few days after the original disease or trauma. ARDS is fatal in 25 to 40 percent of the people who develop it. Survivors of ARDS may not regain full lung function for a year or more.

**Etiology** – The mechanical cause of ARDS is fluid leaking from the smallest blood vessels in the lungs into the alveoli. Normally, a protective membrane keeps this fluid in the vessels, however, inflammation undermines the membrane's integrity, leading to the fluid leakage. A number of conditions can injure the lungs and lead to inflammation including:

- Severe viral or bacterial pneumonia
- Infection spreading through the blood (sepsis)
- Heart failure
- Multiple or massive blood transfusions
- A serious head or chest injury
- Fractures of long bones, which cause a fat embolism
- Prolonged use of large volumes of supplemental oxygen
- Accidental inhalation of vomit or chemicals, such as ammonia or chlorine
- Smoke inhalation
- Near drowning
- An adverse reaction to cancer drugs or other medications
- Drug overdose, most commonly with heroin
- Shock from any cause

**Signs and symptoms** – Varies based on the cause and severity of ARDS. They include severe shortness of breath, labored and unusually rapid breathing, hypotension, confusion, extreme fatigue, cough, and fever.

**Treatment** – It is important to determine the cause of ARDS because it can determine treatment and predict the chances for survival. The first goal of treatment is to get oxygen to the lungs and organs. Most people will be treated with supplemental oxygen and mechanical ventilation. Treating the underlying condition then becomes equally important. Medications are given to prevent and treat infection, relieve pain, provide sedation, and prevent blood clot formation.

## Asthma[11]

Asthma is a chronic inflammation of the airways caused by an increased airway hypersensitivity to various stimuli.

**Etiology** – Factors that trigger asthma include respiratory infections; allergens such as pollen, mold, animal dander, feathers, dust, food, and cockroaches; exposure to cold air or sudden temperature change; cigarette smoke; excitement/stress; and exercise.

**Signs and symptoms** – Range from mild to severe depending on the level of airway restriction. A mild attack presents with wheezing, chest tightness, and slight shortness of breath. A severe attack presents with dyspnea, flaring nostrils, diminished wheezing, anxiety, cyanosis, and the inability to speak. A severe attack can result in respiratory failure if left untreated.

**Treatment** – Reducing exposure to known triggers is a critical step toward controlling asthma. Two classes of medications are used to treat asthma: anti-inflammatory agents and bronchodilators. Anti-inflammatory agents interrupt bronchial inflammation and have a preventive action. These agents include inhaled corticosteroids, cromolyn sodium, and leukotriene modifiers. Bronchodilators dilate the airways by relaxing bronchial smooth muscle. They include beta-adrenergic agonists, methylxanthines, and anticholinergics. Physical therapy management includes caregiver education, airway clearance, breathing exercises, relaxation, and endurance and strength training.

## Atelectasis[12]

A condition in which one or more areas of the lungs collapse or do not inflate properly.

**Etiology** – Conditions and factors that prevent deep breathing and coughing can cause atelectasis. These include postoperative pain, pleural effusion, tumor, ARDS, asthma, COPD, and cystic fibrosis.

**Signs and symptoms** – If a small area of the lung is affected, there may be no signs or symptoms. If a large area is affected, there may be cyanosis, shortness of breath, increased breathing rate, and increased heart rate.

**Treatment** – Treatments vary based on the underlying cause of the atelectasis. Deep breathing, changing positions, and airway clearance techniques assist to fully expand the lungs. Positive end-expiratory pressure or continuous positive airway pressure devices use mild air pressure to help keep the airways and alveoli open. Medications include supplemental oxygen, nebulized bronchodilators, and mucolytic agents. Bronchoscopy may be used to remove foreign objects or mucous plugs blocking the airways.

## Bronchial Carcinoma[3]

Bronchial carcinoma or lung cancer refers to any epithelial carcinoma occurring in the bronchopulmonary tree. Cancers are broadly divided into two main groups: small cell lung carcinomas and non-small cell lung carcinomas, including squamous cell carcinoma, adenocarcinoma, and large cell carcinoma.

**Etiology** – Smoking is the primary cause of the majority of lung cancers, but it can occur in people who have never smoked or had prolonged exposure to secondhand smoke. In these cases, the exact etiology may be unknown.

**Signs and symptoms** – A new cough or changes in a chronic cough, coughing up blood, shortness of breath, wheezing, weight loss, and bone pain. Typically, signs and symptoms are not present until the disease is advanced.

**Treatment** – Surgery (wedge resection, segmental resection, lobectomy, pneumonectomy), chemotherapy, and radiation therapy.

## Bronchiectasis[12]

A progressive obstructive lung disease that produces abnormal dilation of a bronchus. This is an irreversible condition usually associated with chronic infections, aspiration, cystic fibrosis or immune system impairment. The bronchial walls weaken over time due to infection and allow for permanent dilation of bronchi and bronchioles.

**Etiology** – Injury to the airways or lung infection (pneumonia, whooping cough, measles, tuberculosis, fungal infections).

**Signs and symptoms** – Consistent productive cough, hemoptysis, weight loss, anemia, crackles, wheezes, and loud breath sounds.

**Treatment** – Medications include antibiotics, bronchodilators, expectorants, and mucolytics.

## Bronchitis[3]

Bronchitis is an inflammation of the bronchi characterized by hypertrophy of the mucus secreting glands, increased mucus secretions, and insufficient oxygenation due to mucus blockage. Chronic bronchitis is characterized by a productive cough for three months over the course of two consecutive years.

**Etiology** – Acute bronchitis may be caused by cold viruses and exposure to smoke and other air pollutants. Cigarette smoking is the primary cause of chronic bronchitis, but exposure to air pollutants, dust, or toxic gases in the environment or workplace can also contribute.

**Signs and symptoms** – Persistent cough with production of thick sputum, increased use of accessory muscles of breathing, wheezing, dyspnea, cyanosis, and increased pulmonary artery pressure. Patients with chronic bronchitis present with a cough that is worse in the morning and in damp weather and may experience frequent respiratory infections.

**Treatment** – Focuses on relieving symptoms and improving breathing. For acute bronchitis, treatment includes rest, fluids, breathing warm and moist air, cough suppressants, and acetaminophen or aspirin. For chronic bronchitis, treatments include antibiotics, anti-inflammatory agents, and bronchodilators. Recommended lifestyle changes include smoking cessation, avoiding respiratory irritants, using an air humidifier, using a cold-air face mask if cold air aggravates cough and promotes shortness of breath, and pulmonary rehabilitation (airway clearance, breathing exercises, and endurance and strength training).

## Chronic Obstructive Pulmonary Disease (COPD)[3]

COPD refers to a group of lung diseases that block airflow due to narrowing of the bronchial tree. Emphysema and chronic bronchitis are the two main conditions that make up COPD. COPD can also refer to damage caused by chronic asthmatic bronchitis. Progression of the disease includes alveolar destruction and subsequent air trapping. Patients have an increased total lung capacity with a significant increase in residual volume.

**Etiology** – In the majority of cases, COPD is caused by long-term smoking or exposure to secondhand smoke. Other irritants can cause COPD, including air pollution and certain occupational fumes. In rare cases, COPD results from a genetic disorder that causes low levels of the protein alpha-1-antitrypsin.

**Signs and symptoms** – Excessive mucus production, chronic productive cough, wheezing, shortness of breath, fatigue, and reduced exercise capacity.

**Treatment** – Medications include bronchodilators, inhaled steroids, supplemental oxygen, and antibiotics (if a bacterial infection is present). Surgery may include lung volume reduction surgery, bullectomy, and lung transplantation. Lifestyle modifications include smoking cessation, influenza shots, avoiding respiratory irritants, maintaining good nutrition, and pulmonary rehabilitation (airway clearance, breathing exercises, and endurance and strength training).

## Cystic Fibrosis (CF)[13]

CF is an autosomal recessive genetic disease of the exocrine glands that primarily affects the lungs, pancreas, liver, intestines, sinuses, and sex organs. People who have CF inherit two faulty CF genes, one from each parent.

**Etiology** – The causative factor is a mutation of the cystic fibrosis transmembrane conductance regulator on chromosome 7. A defective gene and its protein product cause the body to produce unusually thick, sticky mucus that leads to life-threatening lung infections, obstructs the pancreas, and inhibits normal digestion and absorption of food.

**Signs and symptoms** – Symptoms vary with the progression of the disease and may include salty tasting skin, persistent and productive coughing, frequent lung infections, wheezing, shortness of breath, poor growth/weight gain in spite of a good appetite, and frequent greasy, bulky stools.

**Treatment** – Medications include antibiotics, nutritional supplements, pancreatic enzyme replacements, mucolytics, and bronchodilators. Physical therapy includes airway clearance, breathing techniques, assisted cough, and ventilatory muscle training. General exercise is indicated to improve overall strength and endurance, except with severe lung disease.

## Emphysema[3]

In emphysema, the alveolar walls are gradually destroyed and the alveoli are turned into large, irregular pockets with gaping holes in the walls. In addition, the elastic fibers that hold open the bronchioles are destroyed, so that they collapse during exhalation, not letting air escape from the lungs. The alveoli are permanently overinflated and dead space increases within the lungs.

**Etiology** – Smoking is the leading cause of emphysema. One to two percent of individuals with emphysema have a genetic disorder that causes low levels of the protein alpha-1-antitrypsin, which protects the elastic structures in the lungs. Without this protein, enzymes can cause progressive lung damage, eventually resulting in emphysema.

**Signs and symptoms** – Shortness of breath, wheezing, chronic coughing, orthopnea, barrel chest, increased use of accessory muscles, increased respiration rate, fatigue, and reduced exercise capacity.

**Treatment** – Medications include bronchodilators, inhaled steroids, supplemental oxygen, and antibiotics (if a bacterial infection is present). Surgery may include lung volume reduction surgery, bullectomy, and lung transplantation. Lifestyle modifications include smoking cessation, annual influenza inoculation, avoiding respiratory irritants, maintaining good nutrition, and pulmonary rehabilitation (airway clearance, breathing exercises, and endurance and strength training).

## Pleural Effusion[3]

A pleural effusion is a buildup of fluid in the pleural space between the lungs and chest cavity. The excess fluid can push the pleura against the lung making it hard to breathe and, in some cases, causing an atelectasis. If the fluid gets infected and turns into an abscess, the condition is called empyema.

**Etiology** – Pleuritis, or inflammation of the visceral and parietal pleura. Pleuritis can be caused by a viral infection, pneumonia, pulmonary embolism, and autoimmune diseases such as lupus and rheumatoid arthritis.

**Signs and symptoms** – Shortness of breath. If the fluid becomes infected, dry cough, fever, and chills may appear.

**Treatment** – Treatment is directed at the underlying condition causing the signs and symptoms. For example, if the pleuritis is caused by a bacterial pneumonia, an antibiotic will be used to treat the infection. Most viral infections run their course without requiring treatment. Nonsteroidal anti-inflammatory drugs may help relieve some of the signs and symptoms. If the fluid buildup is large, a chest tube may be inserted to drain the fluid.

## Pneumonia[3]

Pneumonia refers to inflammation of the lungs (Fig. 6-7).

**Etiology** – Usually caused by bacterial, viral, fungal, or parasitic infection.

**Signs and symptoms** – Symptoms are variable depending on the cause of the infection. Common signs and symptoms include fever, cough, shortness of breath, sweating, shaking chills, chest pain that fluctuates with breathing, headache, muscle pain, and fatigue.

**Treatment** – Variable depending on the severity of the symptoms and the type of pneumonia. Antibiotics are used for bacterial and mycoplasma pneumonias. Antiviral agents are used to treat a few forms of viral pneumonia. Antifungal agents are used to treat fungal pneumonia. Lifestyle remedies include rest and drinking plenty of liquids.

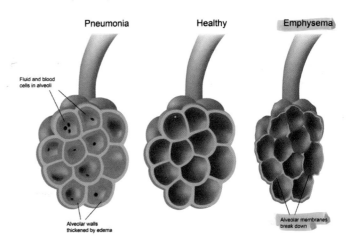

**Fig. 6-7:** Changes in alveoli with pneumonia and emphysema.

## Pulmonary Edema[3]

Pulmonary edema occurs when fluid collects in the alveoli within the lungs, making it difficult to breathe. Acute pulmonary edema is a medical emergency.

**Etiology** – In most cases, pulmonary edema occurs when the left ventricle is unable to pump blood adequately (e.g., left-sided heart failure). As a result, pressure increases inside the left atrium and then in the pulmonary veins and capillaries, causing fluid to be pushed through the capillary walls into the alveoli. In noncardiac pulmonary edema, fluid leaks from the capillaries within the alveoli since the capillaries themselves become more permeable. This may result from pneumonia, exposure to certain toxins and medications, smoke inhalation, respiratory distress syndrome, and living at high elevations.

**Signs and symptoms** – Depending on the cause, symptoms can develop suddenly or slowly. Signs and symptoms that come on suddenly may include extreme shortness of breath and difficulty breathing; a feeling of suffocating or drowning; wheezing or gasping for breath; anxiety; restlessness; a sense of apprehension; coughing; frothy, blood-tinged sputum; chest pain (if a cardiac cause); and a rapid, irregular pulse.

**Treatment** – Variable depending on the underlying cause, but often includes supplemental oxygen and medications.

## Spotlight on Safety

### Signs and Symptoms of Acute Pulmonary Edema[3]

Acute pulmonary edema is life-threatening. Call 911 or emergency medical services immediately if any of the following signs or symptoms develop:

- Extreme shortness of breath or difficulty breathing with profuse sweating
- A bubbly, wheezing or gasping sound during breathing
- A cough that produces frothy sputum that may be tinged with blood
- Cyanotic skin color
- A rapid, irregular pulse
- A severe drop in blood pressure

## Pulmonary Embolism (PE)[3]

PE is a condition where one or more arteries in the lungs become blocked. PE can be life-threatening, but prompt treatment with anti-clotting medications can greatly reduce the risk of death.

**Etiology** – In most cases, PE is caused by blood clots from the lower extremities.

**Signs and Symptoms** – Symptoms can vary greatly, depending on how much of the lung is involved, the size of the clot, and overall health of the patient (especially the presence or absence of underlying lung disease or heart disease). Common signs and symptoms include sudden onset of shortness of breath; chest pain that becomes worse with deep breathing, coughing, eating or bending; and coughing up bloody or blood-streaked sputum. Other signs and symptoms include wheezing, lower extremity swelling, excessive sweating, rapid or irregular pulse, and lightheadedness or fainting.

**Treatment** – Pulmonary embolism can be life-threatening, but prompt treatment with anticoagulants and thrombolytic agents greatly reduces the risk of death. Surgery may be done to remove the clot or insert a filter into the inferior vena cava. Preventing clot formation in the deep leg veins reduces the risk of PE. Prevention includes compression stockings, pneumatic compression, physical activity, and drinking fluids.

## Pulmonary Fibrosis[3]

A condition in which microscopic damage to the alveoli causes irreversible scarring of the interstitial tissue. Normally, the tissue is highly elastic, expanding and contracting with each breath. Scarring makes the interstitial tissue stiff and thick and the alveoli less flexible, making breathing more difficult.

**Etiology** – In most cases, the cause is unknown (idiopathic pulmonary fibrosis). Chronic exposure to silica dust (silicosis), asbestos fibers (asbestosis), grain dust, sugar cane, and bird and animal droppings can cause pulmonary fibrosis. Radiation for lung or breast cancer, chemotherapy drugs (methotrexate, cyclophosphamide), certain antiarrhythmic medications (amiodarone, propranolol), and some antibiotics (nitrofurantoin, sulfasalazine) can also cause fibrosis.

**Signs and Symptoms** – The most common symptoms are shortness of breath, especially during or after physical activity, and a dry cough, which usually does not appear until the disease is advanced and irreversible lung damage has already occurred. Other symptoms include fatigue, unexplained weight loss, and aching muscles and joints.

**Treatment** – Although the lung scarring is irreversible and no current treatment has proven effective in stopping the progression of the disease, some treatments may improve symptoms temporarily and improve quality of life. A combination of corticosteroids and immunosuppressive agents are often prescribed initially. Lung transplantation may be used in cases of advanced disease. Other treatments to reduce symptoms and improve quality of life include supplemental oxygen and pulmonary rehabilitation (breathing exercises, nutrition counseling, emotional support).

## Restrictive Lung Dysfunction (RLD)[14]

RLD is an abnormal reduction in lung expansion and pulmonary ventilation.

**Etiology** - RLD is caused by abnormal lung parenchyma (e.g., atelectasis, pneumonia, pulmonary fibrosis, pulmonary edema, acute respiratory distress syndrome), abnormal pleura (e.g., pleural effusion, pleural fibrosis, pneumothorax, hemothorax), and disorders affecting ventilatory pump function (e.g., decrease in respiratory drive, neurologic and neuromuscular diseases, muscle disease or weakness, thoracic deformity or trauma, connective tissue disorders affecting the thoracic joints, pregnancy, obesity, and ascites).

**Signs and Symptoms** – Dyspnea on exertion, a persistent non-productive cough, increased respiratory rate, hypoxemia, decreased vital capacity, abnormal breath sounds, and reduced exercise tolerance.

**Treatment** – Variable depending on the etiology (e.g., antibiotics for pneumonia, treatment of edema, reversal of CNS depression). Additional supportive measures include mechanical ventilation, supplemental oxygen, nutrition support, and pulmonary rehabilitation (airway clearance, breathing exercise, respiratory muscle training, endurance and strength training).

# Common Laboratory Tests

## Arterial Blood Gas (ABG)

Arterial blood gases are collected to evaluate acid–base status (pH), ventilation ($PaCO_2$), and oxygenation of arterial blood ($PaO_2$). The partial pressure of oxygen in arterial blood ($PaO_2$) and the percent oxygen saturation of hemoglobin ($SaO_2$) provide information about how well the lungs are functioning to oxygenate the blood. The partial pressure of carbon dioxide in arterial blood ($PaCO_2$) provides information on how well the lungs are able to remove carbon dioxide. Changes in $PaCO_2$ directly affect the balance of pH in the body. Blood pH is tightly regulated, as an imbalance in either direction can affect the nervous system and can cause convulsions or coma. Bicarbonate ($HCO_3$-) is an important component of the chemical buffering system that keeps the blood from becoming too acidic or basic and is often part of an ABG test.

**Mean (range) of adult normal ABG values:**

**pH:** 7.4 (7.35 - 7.45)

**$PaCO_2$:** 40 mm Hg at sea level breathing ambient air (35 - 45 mm Hg)

**$PaO_2$:** 97 mm Hg at sea level breathing ambient air (80 - 100 mm Hg)

**$HCO_3$-:** 24 mEq/L (22 – 26 mEq/L)

**$SaO_2$:** 95 - 98%

**By convention, ABG results are written or spoken in the following order:** pH→$PaCO_2$→$PaO_2$→$HCO_3$- (e.g., 7.4/40/97/24)

**Acidemia:** elevated acidity of blood (pH < 7.35)

**Alkalemia:** decreased acidity of blood (pH > 7.45)

**Eucapnia:** normal level of $CO_2$ in arterial blood ($PaCO_2$ 35 - 45 mm Hg)

**Hypercapnia:** elevated level of $CO_2$ in arterial blood ($PaCO_2$ > 45 mm Hg)

**Hypocapnia:** low level of $CO_2$ in arterial blood ($PaCO_2$ < 35 mm Hg)

**Hypoxemia:** low level of $O_2$ in arterial blood ($PaO_2$ < 80 mm Hg)

**Mild hypoxemia:** $PaO_2$ 60 - 79 mm Hg

**Moderate hypoxemia:** $PaO_2$ 40 - 59 mm Hg

**Severe hypoxemia:** $PaO_2$ < 40 mm Hg

**Hypoxia:** low level of $O_2$ in the tissue despite adequate perfusion of the tissue

## Cardiac Biomarkers[15]

Certain enzymes leak out of the heart cells and into the blood after a myocardial infarction. Cardiac enzyme studies measure the levels of creatine phosphokinase (CK) and the protein troponin in the blood. CK-MB is a relatively specific test for myocardial infarction. It appears in blood approximately four hours after infarction, peaks at 12–24 hours, and declines over 48–72 hours. Cardiac troponin-I is also a specific marker for infarction, and unlike CK-MB levels, it remains elevated for 5-7 days.

## Cholesterol Test[15]

Also called a lipid panel or lipid profile, a cholesterol test measures the amount of cholesterol and triglycerides in the blood in order to determine the risk of atherosclerosis. Cholesterol is carried in the circulation in association with lipoproteins. A complete lipid profile includes the measurement of four types of lipids in the blood: total cholesterol, high-density lipoprotein (HDL) cholesterol, low-density lipoprotein (LDL) cholesterol, and triglycerides. HDL cholesterol is referred to as the "good" cholesterol because it helps carry away LDL cholesterol and is protective against atherogenesis. LDL cholesterol is referred to as the "bad" cholesterol since it is associated with the buildup of fatty plaques within the arteries which reduce blood flow. The body converts any calories it does not need to use right away into triglycerides, which are stored in adipose tissue. High levels of triglycerides are seen in overweight people, in those consuming too many sweets or too much alcohol, and in people with diabetes who have elevated blood sugar levels.

## Complete Blood Count (CBC)[15]

A CBC measures red blood cell count, total white blood cell count, white blood cell differential, platelets, hemoglobin, and hematocrit. A CBC is performed to assess health, to diagnose and monitor a medical condition, and to monitor the effects of medical treatment.

## Hematocrit (Hct)[15]

Hematocrit is the percentage of red blood cells in total blood volume. A low hematocrit may indicate anemia, blood loss, and vitamin or mineral deficiencies. A high hematocrit may indicate dehydration or polycythemia vera, a condition that causes an overproduction of red blood cells.

# Consider This

## Systematic Analysis of Arterial Blood Gas

Using a standard approach to interpreting arterial blood gas values improves the therapist's understanding of the patient's acid-base, ventilation, and oxygenation status.

### STEP 1
### Examine pH to assess acid-base balance

pH < 7.40 indicates acidosis

pH > 7.40 indicates alkalosis

### STEP 2
### Examine the $PaCO_2$ as an indicator of ventilatory status

$PaCO_2$ = 35 – 45 mm Hg indicates adequate ventilation; no respiratory problem and no respiratory compensation for metabolic problem

$PaCO_2$ < 30 mm Hg indicates alveolar hyperventilation

$PaCO_2$ > 50 mm Hg indicates alveolar hypoventilation, ventilatory failure

### STEP 3
### Interpret $PaCO_2$ in relation to pH

$PaCO_2$ > 45 mm Hg and pH < 7.40 indicate respiratory acidosis

$PaCO_2$ > 45 mm Hg and pH > 7.40 indicate retention of $CO_2$ to compensate for metabolic alkalosis

$PaCO_2$ < 35 mm Hg and pH > 7.40 indicate respiratory alkalosis

$PaCO_2$ < 35 mm Hg and pH < 7.40 indicate elimination of $CO_2$ to compensate for metabolic acidosis

### STEP 4
### Interpret the $HCO_3$- in relation to pH

$HCO_3$- = 22 – 26 mEq/L indicates no primary metabolic problem and no metabolic compensation for a respiratory problem

$HCO_3$- < 22 mEq/L and pH < 7.40 indicate metabolic acidosis

$HCO_3$- < 22 mEq/L and pH > 7.40 indicate renal compensation for a respiratory alkalosis

$HCO_3$- > 26 mEq/L and pH > 7.40 indicate metabolic alkalosis

$HCO_3$- > 26 mEq/L and pH < 7.40 indicate renal compensation for respiratory acidosis

### STEP 5
### Interpret the $PaO_2$ and $SaO_2$

Normal: $PaO_2$ 80 – 100 mm Hg at sea level with $SaO_2$ > 95%

Mild hypoxemia: $PaO_2$ 60 – 79 mm Hg; $SaO_2$ 90% – 95% (if no shift in oxyhemoglobin curve)

Moderate hypoxemia: $PaO_2$ 40 – 59 mm Hg; $SaO_2$ 60% – 90% (if no shift in oxyhemoglobin curve)

Severe hypoxemia: $PaO_2$ < 40 mm Hg; $SaO_2$ < 60% (if no shift in oxyhemoglobin curve)

## Reference Values in Hematology

| | Conventional Units | SI Units |
|---|---|---|
| **Erythrocytes** | | |
| Adult males | $4.3 - 5.6 \times 10^6$/ml | $4.3 - 5.6 \times 10^{12}$/L |
| Adult females | $4.0 - 5.2 \times 10^6$/ml | $4.0 - 5.2 \times 10^{12}$/L |
| **Leukocytes** | | |
| Total | $3.54 - 9.06 \times 10^3$/mm³ | $3.54 - 9.06 \times 10^9$/L |
| **Differential Blood Count** | | |
| Neutrophils | 0.40 – 0.70 | 40 – 70% |
| Lymphocytes | 0.20 – 0.50 | 20 – 50% |
| Monocytes | 0.04 – 0.08 | 4 – 8% |
| Eosinophils | 0.00 – 0.06 | 0 – 6% |
| Basophils | 0.00 – 0.02 | 0 – 2% |
| **Platelet Count** | $165 - 415 \times 10^3$/mm³ | $165 - 415 \times 10^9$/L |
| **Partial Thromboplastin Time (PTT)** | 26.3 – 39.4 sec | 26.3 – 39.4 sec |
| **Hematocrit** | | |
| Adult males | 0.388 – 0.464 | 38.8 – 46.4% |
| Adult females | 0.354 – 0.444 | 35.4 – 44.4% |
| **Hemoglobin** | | |
| Adult males | 13.3 – 16.2 gm/dL | 133 – 162 gm/dL |
| Adult females | 12.0 – 15.8 gm/dL | 120 – 158 gm/dL |

## Reference Values in Clinical Chemistry

| | Conventional Units | | SI Units |
|---|---|---|---|
| **Serum Cholesterol** | | | |
| Total | < 200 mg/dL | Desirable | < 5.17 mmol/L |
| | 200 – 239 mg/dL | Borderline | 5.17 – 6.20 mmol/L |
| | > 240 mg/dL | High | ≥ 6.21 mmol/L |
| LDL cholesterol | < 100 mg/dL | Optimal | < 2.59 mmol/L |
| | 100 – 129 mg/dL | Near optimal | 2.59 – 3.35 mmol/L |
| | 130 – 159 mg/dL | Borderline | 3.36 – 4.12 mmol/L |
| | 160 – 189 mg/dL | High | 4.13 – 4.90 mmol/L |
| | ≥ 190 mg/dL | Very high | ≥ 4.91 mmol/L |
| HDL cholesterol | < 40 mg/dL | Low | < 1.03 mmol/L |
| | ≥ 60 mg/dL | High | ≥ 1.55 mmol/L |
| Triglyceride | < 150 mg/dL | Desirable | < 1.70 mmol/L |
| | 150 – 199 mg/dL | Borderline | 1.70 – 2.25 mmol/L |
| | 200 – 499 mg/dL | High | 2.26 – 5.63 mmol/L |
| | ≥ 500 mg/dL | Very high | > 5.64 mmol/L |

The values are for illustrative purposes. Each clinical laboratory establishes its own reference values.

Data are from: Kratz A, Pesce MA, Fink DJ. Reference Values for Laboratory Tests. In: Fauci A, Braunwald E, Kasper D, Hauser, Longo D, Jameson J, Loscalzo J. Harrison's Manual of Medicine, 17th ed. New York, NY: McGraw-Hill Medical; 2009 http://0-www.accessmedicine.com.lilac.une.edu/Pontent.aspx?aID=2904604. Accessed January 3, 2011.

### Partial Thromboplastin Time (PTT) and Prothrombin Time (PT)[15]

PTT and PT tests measure how quickly the blood clots. The tests are commonly used to monitor oral anticoagulant therapy or to screen for selected bleeding disorders. The tests examine all of the clotting factors of the intrinsic pathway with the exception of platelets. Partial thromboplastin time is more sensitive than prothrombin time in detecting minor deficiencies.

# Common Diagnostic Procedures

### Ambulatory Electrocardiography[5]

Also known as Holter monitoring, ECG electrodes are placed on the chest and attached to a small battery-operated recording monitor carried in a pocket or in a small pouch around the neck (Fig. 6-8). The ECG is recorded for 24 to 48 hours or longer to evaluate cardiac rhythm, the efficacy of medications, and pacemaker function. It is then correlated with a diary of the patient's symptoms and activities.

Fig. 6-8: Woman wearing a Holter monitor.

### Angiography[15]

A radiologic examination that injects a contrast medium into the blood vessels. Coronary angiograms are part of the group of procedures known as cardiac catheterization. An angiogram can show the location of plaques in the coronary arteries and the extent of occlusion.

### Bronchoscopy[15]

A procedure for direct visualization of the bronchial tree performed for diagnostic and therapeutic purposes. A bronchoscope is a fiberoptic instrument that transmits an image to an eyepiece or video camera and can identify tumors, bronchitis, foreign bodies, and bleeding. Tissue specimens may be removed from the lungs by biopsy or bronchoalveolar lavage.

### Cardiac Catheterization[5]

A thin catheter inserted into an artery in the leg or arm is advanced to the coronary arteries where a contrast dye is injected. The test can evaluate narrowing or occlusion of the coronary arteries and measure blood pressure in the heart and oxygen in the blood. Some treatments, such as coronary angioplasty, are performed using cardiac catheterization.

### Carotid Ultrasound[5]

A procedure that uses sound waves to examine and visualize the structure and function of the carotid arteries. The purposes are to screen for blockages that may indicate an increased risk of stroke and to evaluate the placement of a stent or the function of the artery after carotid endarterectomy.

### Chest Radiograph[5]

Chest radiographs are used to visualize the location, size, and shape of the heart, lungs, blood vessels, ribs, and bones of the spine. Chest radiographs can also reveal fluid in the lungs or pleural space, pneumonia, emphysema, cancer, and other conditions.

### Computed Tomography (CT scan)[5]

A CT scan is a diagnostic test that uses an x-ray machine that rotates around a patient lying on a table. A computer processes the information from the scanner and creates a picture of the organ and surrounding structures. The pictures are slices of the body called tomograms and each picture is called a computed tomograph. The newest models of CT scanners allow pictures of the coronary arteries to be taken without the need, in some cases, for catheterization.

## Echocardiography[5]

An echocardiogram uses high frequency sound waves non-invasively to evaluate the functioning of the heart via real time images. An echocardiogram can provide information on the size and function of the ventricles, thickness of the septums, and function of the walls, valves, and chambers of the heart. Transthoracic echocardiography (TTE) is a noninvasive procedure using a handheld ultrasound transducer placed on the chest. In transesophageal echocardiography (TEE), the ultrasound transducer is passed into the esophagus. The transducer provides a more detailed image of the heart because the esophagus lies in extremely close proximity.

## Electrophysiologic Testing[5]

An electrophysiology study evaluates the rhythm or electrical conduction abnormalities of the heart using three to five catheters inserted into a blood vessel and threaded to the heart. The recordings help to locate abnormal tissue that causes cardiac arrhythmias.

## Fluoroscopy[5]

A continuous x-ray procedure that shows the heart and lungs. Because fluoroscopy involves a relatively high dose of radiation, it has been largely replaced by echocardiography and other diagnostic tests. It is still a component of cardiac catheterization and electrophysiological testing.

## Invasive Hemodynamic Monitoring[14]

Continuous monitoring of cardiovascular status is performed by intraarterial catheters and intravenous lines that measure pressure, volume, and temperature. A balloon catheter, also known as a Swan-Ganz catheter, is placed in the pulmonary artery to obtain the pulmonary artery wedge pressure and left atrial pressure. A thermodilution catheter can be used to measure cardiac output. A central venous pressure (CVP) line measures pressure in the vena cava or right atrium.

## Magnetic Resonance Imaging (MRI)[15]

MRI uses a magnetic field and radio waves to create 3-D images of the heart and blood vessels to assess the size and function of the chambers, thickness and movement of the walls, extent of damage caused by myocardial infarction or heart disease, structural problems in the aorta (e.g., aneurysms, dissections), and the presence of plaques and blockages in blood vessels. MRI is also used to image masses located in the mediastinum, but is of limited value for imaging the lungs.

## Myocardial Perfusion Imaging (MPI)[16]

Also known as radionuclide stress test and nuclear stress test, the test shows how well the heart muscle is perfused at rest and under exercise stress. A radionuclide agent is injected into the blood at rest and at a maximum level of exercise. Images of the heart reveal areas that have reduced blood supply due to narrowing of one or more coronary arteries.

## Pharmacologic Stress Test[16]

A diagnostic procedure in which cardiovascular stress is induced by pharmacologic agents when contraindications to a routine exercise stress test exist, or when the patient is unable to exercise due to injury or another debilitating condition. It is used in combination with imaging modalities such as radionuclide imaging and echocardiography. Pharmacologic agents used include adenosine, dipyridamole, and dobutamine.

## Phonocardiography[17]

A diagnostic test that creates a graphic record, or phonocardiogram, of the sounds produced by the heart and great vessels. The phonocardiogram supplements auscultation and improves the detection of S3 and S4 heart sounds in the diagnosis of heart failure.

## Pleuroscopy[3]

A procedure that includes examination of the lung surfaces, pleura, and pleural space using a small video camera inserted between the ribs into the pleural space. A tissue sample may be taken to biopsy.

## Positron Emission Tomography (PET)[15]

A PET scan is an imaging test in which a small amount of radioactive material is injected, inhaled or swallowed, depending on the organ or tissue being studied. Increased radioactive material tends to accumulate in areas with high levels of chemical activity corresponding to areas of disease. This presents as a different color or brighter spots on the scan. A PET scan is useful in evaluating heart disease and cancer.

## Thoracentesis[3]

A procedure that includes removal of fluid from the pleural space with a needle for microbiologic and cytologic studies.

## Venography[3]

A radiopaque dye is injected into a vein while an x-ray procedure creates an image of the vein to detect a clot or blockage.

## Ventilation–Perfusion Scan[15]

Also known as a lung scan or V/Q scan, the study uses small amounts of radioactive material to study airflow and blood flow within the lungs. It is used most commonly in the diagnosis of pulmonary embolism.

# Pharmacological Management of Heart and Vascular Diseases

## Alpha Adrenergic Antagonist Agents[18,19]

**Action:** Alpha adrenergic antagonist agents reduce peripheral vascular tone by blocking alpha-1-adrenergic receptors. This action causes dilation of arterioles and veins and decreases blood pressure.

**Indications:** hypertension, benign prostatic hyperplasia

**Side effects:** dizziness, palpitations, orthostatic hypotension, drowsiness

**Implications for PT:** Use caution when rising from a sitting or lying position due to the risk of dizziness and/or orthostatic hypotension. Closely monitor patient during exercise.

**Examples:** Cardura (doxazosin), Minipress (prazosin), Hytrin (terazosin)

## Angiotensin-Converting Enzyme (ACE) Inhibitor Agents[18,19]

**Action:** ACE inhibitor agents decrease blood pressure and afterload by suppressing the enzyme that converts angiotensin I to angiotensin II.

**Indications:** hypertension, congestive heart failure

**Side effects:** hypotension, dizziness, dry cough, hyperkalemia, hyponatremia

**Implications for PT:** Avoid sudden changes in posture due to the risk of dizziness and fainting from hypotension. Patients with heart failure should avoid rapid increases in physical activity.

**Examples:** Capoten (captorpril), Vasotec (enalapril), Prinivil (lisinopril), Altace (ramipril)

## Angiotensin II Receptor Antagonist Agents[18,19]

**Action:** Angiotensin II receptor antagonists block angiotensin II receptors which limit vasoconstriction and stimulation of vascular tissue.

**Indications:** hypertension, congestive heart failure

**Side effects:** dizziness, back and leg pain, angina pectoris

**Implications for PT:** Minimal implications for physical therapy.

**Examples:** Cozaar (losartan), Atacand (candesartan), Diovan (valsartan)

## Antiarrhythmic Agents[18,19]

**Action:** Antiarrhythmic agents are divided into four classes. **Class I** (sodium channel blockers) - control cardiac excitation and conduction. **Class II** (beta blockers) - inhibit sympathetic activity by blocking ß-adrenergic receptors. **Class III** - prolong repolarization by inhibiting both potassium and sodium channels and are often considered the most effective antiarrhytmic agent. **Class IV** (calcium channel blockers) - depress depolarization and slow conduction through the AV node.

**Indications:** cardiac arrhythmias

**Side effects:** unique to the specific antiarrhythmic agent; exacerbation of cardiac arrhythmias, dizziness, hypotension

**Implications for PT:** Encourage patients to adhere to the prescribed dosing schedule and immediately report any adverse reactions to a healthcare professional.

**Examples:** Sodium channel blockers: quinidine (generic), Xylocaine (lidocaine); Beta blockers: Tenormin (atenolol); Prolonged repolarization: Cordarone (amiodarone); Calcium channel blockers: Cardizem (diltiazem)

## Anticoagulant Agents[18,19]

**Action:** Anticoagulant agents inhibit platelet aggregation and thrombus formation.

**Indications:** post percutaneous transluminal coronary angioplasty and coronary artery bypass graft surgery, prevention of venous thromboembolism and cardioembolic events in patients with atrial fibrillation and prosthetic heart valves

**Side effects:** hemorrhage, increased risk of bleeding, gastrointestinal distress with oral medication

**Implications for PT:** A therapist must be careful to avoid injury secondary to the risk of excessive bleeding or bruising. Patient education regarding common side effects is also indicated to protect the patient.

**Examples:** Heparin, Coumadin (warfarin), Lovenox (enoxaparin)

## Antihyperlipidemia Agents[18,19]

**Action:** There are five categories of lipid-modifying agents. The most commonly used drugs, the statins, inhibit enzyme action in cholesterol synthesis, break down low density lipoproteins, decrease triglyceride levels, and increase HDL levels. The other categories are bile acid sequestrants, nicotinic acid, cholesterol absorption inhibitors, and fibric acid derivatives.

**Indications:** hyperlipidemia, atherosclerosis, prevent coronary events in patients with existing coronary disease, diabetes or peripheral vascular disease

**Side effects:** headache, gastrointestinal distress, myalgia, rash

**Implications for PT:** Aerobic exercise can increase high density lipoproteins and maximize the effects of drug therapy.

**Examples:** Lipitor (atorvastatin), Zocor (simvastatin), Tricor (fenobibrate)

## Antithrombotic (Antiplatelet) Agents[18,19]

**Action:** Antithrombotic agents inhibit platelet aggregation and clot formation.

**Indications:** post-myocardial infarction, atrial fibrillation, prevent arterial thrombus formation

**Side effects:** hemorrhage, thrombocytopenia, potential liver toxicity with the use of aspirin, gastrointestinal distress

**Implications for PT:** A therapist must be careful to avoid injury secondary to the risk of excessive bleeding. Patient education regarding common side effects is also indicated to protect the patient.

**Examples:** Bayer (aspirin), Plavix (clopidogrel), Persantine (dipyridamole)

## Beta Blocker Agents (Beta-Adrenergic Blocking Agents)[18,19]

**Action:** Beta blocker agents decrease the myocardial oxygen demand by decreasing heart rate and contractility by blocking ß-adrenergic receptors.

**Indications:** hypertension, angina, arrhythmias, heart failure, migraines, essential tremor

**Side effects:** bradycardia, cardiac arrhythmias, fatigue, depression, dizziness, weakness, blurred vision

**Implications for PT:** Heart rate and blood pressure response to exercise will be diminished. Rate of perceived exertion may be used to monitor exercise intensity. Closely monitor patients during positional changes due to an increased risk for orthostatic hypotension.

**Examples:** Tenormin (atenolol), Lopressor (metoprolol), Inderal (propanolol)

## Calcium Channel Blocker Agents[18,19]

**Action:** Calcium channel blocker agents decrease the entry of calcium into vascular smooth muscle cells resulting in diminished myocardial contraction, vasodilation, and decreased oxygen demand of the heart.

**Indications:** hypertension, angina pectoris, arrhythmias, congestive heart failure

**Side effects:** dizziness, headache, hypotension, peripheral edema

**Implications for PT:** Heart rate and blood pressure response to exercise will be diminished. Monitor patient closely when moving to an upright position secondary to dizziness and/or orthostatic hypotension. Observe the patient for signs and symptoms of congestive heart failure such as worsening peripheral edema, dyspnea or weight gain.

**Examples:** Norvasc (amlodipine), Procardia (nifedipine), Calan (verapamil), Cardizem (diltiazem)

## Diuretic Agents[18,19]

**Action:** Diuretic agents increase the excretion of sodium and urine. This causes a reduction in plasma volume which decreases blood pressure. Classifications include thiazide, loop, and potassium sparing agents.

**Indications:** hypertension, edema associated with heart failure, pulmonary edema, glaucoma

**Side effects:** dehydration, hypotension, electrolyte imbalance, polyuria, increased low-density lipoproteins, arrhythmias

**Implications for PT:** Positioning changes can increase the risk of dizziness and falls due to decreased blood pressure. Monitor patients closely for signs and symptoms of electrolyte imbalance and muscle weakness or cramping.

**Examples:** Thiazide: Diuril (chlorothiazide); Loop: Lasix (furosemide); Potassium sparing: Dyrenium (triamterene)

## Nitrate Agents[18,19]

**Action:** Nitrate agents decrease ischemia through smooth muscle relaxation and dilation of peripheral vessels.

**Indications:** angina pectoris

**Side effects:** headache, dizziness, orthostatic hypotension, reflex tachycardia, nausea, vomiting

**Implications for PT:** Patients must be educated to come to a standing position slowly to minimize the risk of orthostatic hypotension. Sublingual administration of nitroglycerin is the preferred method to treat an acute angina attack.

**Examples:** Nitrostat (nitroglycerin), Isordil (isosorbide dinitrate), Amyl nitrite solution for inhalation

## Positive Inotropic Agents[18,19]

**Action:** Positive inotropic agents increase the force and velocity of myocardial contraction, slow the heart rate, decrease conduction velocity through the AV node, and decrease the degree of activation of the sympathetic nervous system.

**Indications:** heart failure, atrial fibrillation

**Side effects:** cardiac arrhythmias, gastrointestinal distress, dizziness, blurred vision

**Implications for PT:** Therapists should monitor heart rate during activity, teach the patient and family to take the patient's pulse, and seek health care provider's advice for rates less than 60 beats/minute or more than 100 beats/minute

**Examples:** Lanoxin (digoxin)

## Thrombolytic Agents[18,19]

**Action:** Thrombolytic agents facilitate clot dissolution through conversion of plasminogen to plasmin. Plasmin breaks down clots and allows occluded vessels to reopen to maintain blood flow.

**Indications:** acute myocardial infarction, pulmonary embolism, ischemic stroke, arterial or venous thrombosis

**Side effects:** hemorrhage (specifically intracranial in certain populations), allergic reaction, cardiac arrhythmia

**Implications for PT:** Therapists must be careful to avoid situations that may cause trauma due to altered clotting activity.

**Examples:** Linlytic (urokinase), Activase (alteplase)

# Medical Procedures for Heart and Vascular Diseases

## Atherectomy[8]

A surgical procedure similar to angioplasty except that the catheter has a rotating shaver to cut away plaque from the artery and increase blood flow.

## Automatic Implantable Cardioverter-Defibrillator (AICD)[15]

A surgically implanted device similar to a pacemaker that continuously monitors the heart rhythm and delivers electrical shocks to restore a normal heart rhythm when necessary.

## Balloon Angioplasty[15]

Angioplasty involves temporarily inserting a small balloon-tipped catheter into a stenotic artery and expanding the balloon at the site of blockage to help widen a narrowed artery (Fig. 6-9). Angioplasty is usually combined with implantation of a small metal coil called a stent in the narrowed artery to help prop it open and decrease the chance of restenosis.

Fig. 6-9: Balloon Angioplasty.

## Balloon Valvuloplasty[3]

This surgical procedure uses cardiac catheterization to treat stenotic heart valves. A balloon-tipped catheter is threaded through the veins to the faulty heart valve, then inflated to open the narrowed valve and increase blood flow.

## Cardiac Ablation[15]

A surgical procedure that uses radiofrequencies or chemicals to destroy areas of the myocardium that have been identified by electrophysiologic testing to be causing cardiac arrhythmia. Ablation is an option for patients with tachyarrhythmias that cannot be controlled by medication or who have arrhythmias that respond well to ablation, such as Wolff-Parkinson-White syndrome.

## Cardiac Pacemaker[14]

A pacemaker is a surgically implanted battery-powered device placed under the skin, usually in the left anterior chest wall. Pacemakers are a standard treatment for conditions affecting the electrical conduction system including a slow heart rate and arrhythmias. By preventing a slow heart rate, pacemakers can treat fatigue, lightheadedness, and fainting.

Pacemaker modes and functions are described by a 5-position format known as the NBG code.

## Cardioversion[15]

Cardioversion is performed to restore a normal heart rhythm for tachyarrhythmias that do not respond to medication. Electrical shocks are delivered by a defibrillator through electrodes on the chest.

## Coronary Artery Bypass Graft Surgery (CABG)[15]

CABG surgery is performed to treat coronary arteries that are narrowed or occluded in an attempt to revascularize the myocardium. In this procedure, blood is rerouted around the affected artery joining the patient's own saphenous vein, internal thoracic/mammary artery, or radial artery to connect the affected artery above and below the occlusion.

## Enhanced Extracorporeal Counterpulsation (EECP)[14]

A noninvasive procedure in which inflation of pressure cuffs on the lower extremities compresses the veins and assists with venous return to the heart.

## Heart Transplant[15]

A surgical procedure in which a failing, diseased heart is replaced with a healthier donor heart. A heart transplant is reserved for patients with end-stage heart failure for whom other treatments have not been successful (e.g., patients with cardiomyopathy, coronary artery disease, valvular disease, and congenital heart disease).

## Intraaortic Balloon Counterpulsation (IABP)[14]

Inflation and deflation of a balloon surgically placed in the aorta provides circulatory assistance for patients after infarction or with cardiogenic shock.

## Valve Replacement[14]

A surgical procedure in which a prosthetic valve is implanted in the heart to replace a leaky or narrowed heart valve. Prosthetic valves may be either mechanical (e.g., ball-in-cage, tilting disc, bileaflet) or tissue grafts from the same patient, a cadaver or a pig.

| | | NBG Pacemaker Code | | |
|---|---|---|---|---|
| **I** | **II** | **III** | **IV** | **IV** |
| Chamber paced | Chamber sensed | Response sensed | Rate modulation | Multisite pacing |
| V=Ventricle<br>A= Atrium<br>D=Dual (A+V)<br>O=None | V=Ventricle<br>A= Atrium<br>D=Dual (A+V)<br>O=None | T=Triggered<br>I=Inhibited<br>D=Dual (A+V)<br>O=None | R=Rate modulation<br>O=None | V=Ventricle<br>A= Atrium<br>D=Dual (A+V)<br>O=None |

## Ventricular Assist Devices (VAD)[15]

A VAD is a miniature pump that is implanted in the chest to provide mechanical support to the ventricle. A right ventricular device (RVAD) attaches to the right atrium and pulmonary artery, bypassing the right ventricle. A left ventricular device (LVAD) attaches to the left atrium, bypassing the left ventricle. With a biventricular device (BiVAD), both ventricles are bypassed. VADs are commonly used as a temporary treatment for people waiting for a heart transplant and increasingly as a permanent treatment for heart failure.

# Pharmacological Management of Airway and Lung Diseases

## Antihistamine Agents[18,19]

**Action:** Antihistamine agents block the effects of histamine resulting in a decrease in nasal congestion, mucosal irritation, and symptoms of the common cold, sinusitis, conjunctivitis, and allergies.

**Indications:** respiratory seasonal allergies, rhinitis and sneezing from the common cold, allergic conjunctivitis, motion sickness, and Parkinson's disease

**Side effects:** arrhythmias, postural hypotension, gastrointestinal distress, dizziness, drowsiness, headache, blurred vision, fatigue, nausea, thickening of bronchial secretions

**Implications for PT:** Increase guarding when rising from a sitting or lying position due to the risk of orthostatic hypotension. Closely monitor patient during exercise.

**Examples:** Benadryl (diphenhydramine), Allegra (fexofenadine), Zyrtec (cetirizine HCL), Claritin (loratadine)

## Anti-Inflammatory Agents[18,19]

**Action:** Inhaled corticosteroids, leukotriene modifiers, and mast cell stabilizers help prevent inflammatory-mediated bronchoconstriction by inhibiting production of inflammatory cells, suppressing release of inflammatory mediators (cytokines, prostaglandins, leukotrienes), and reversing capillary permeability, in turn reducing airway edema.

**Indications:** bronchospasm, asthma

**Side effects:** Corticosteroid: systemic side effects are decreased with the inhaled form of corticosteroids, but may include damage of supporting tissues, skin breakdown, osteoporosis, decreased bone density, glaucoma, and delayed growth. Local effects include nasal irritation and dryness, sneezing, and bloody mucus; Leukotriene modifier: liver dysfunction; Mast-cell stabilizer: bronchospasm, throat and nasal irritation, cough, gastrointestinal distress.

**Implications for PT:** Instruct the patient in the correct use of the inhaler and to rinse their mouth with water after use to avoid irritation of local mucosa. Advise the patients that these agents are not bronchodilators and should not be used to treat acute episodes of asthma. Inform patients to contact their health care provider immediately if they experience signs and/or symptoms of liver dysfunction (e.g., fatigue, flu-like symptoms, jaundice, lethargy).

**Examples:** Corticosteroid: Qvar (beclomethasone dipropionate), Pulmicort (budesonide), AeroBid (flunisolide); Leukotriene modifier: Zyflo (zileuton); Mast-cell stabilizer: Nasalcrom (cromolyn sodium)

## Bronchodilator Agents[18,19]

**Action:** Bronchodilator agents relieve bronchospasm by stimulating the receptors that cause bronchial smooth muscle relaxation or by blocking the receptors that trigger bronchoconstriction. Primary classifications of bronchodilators include anticholinergic, sympathomimetics, and xanthine derivatives.

**Indications:** bronchospasm, wheezing, and shortness of breath in asthma and COPD

**Side effects:** (depending on class of drug) paradoxical bronchospasm, dry mouth, gastrointestinal distress, chest pain, palpitations, tremor, nervousness. Long-acting sympathomimetics, including salmeterol, increase the risk of asthma-related death.

**Implications for PT:** Therapists should advise patients to take their bronchodilator medication as prescribed before therapy and to bring their short acting sympathomimetics (rescue medications) with them. Cardiac or vision abnormalities may indicate toxicity, and the physician should be notified immediately.

**Examples:** Anticholinergic: Atrovent (ipratropium); Spiriva (tiotropium); Sympathomimetics: Ventolin (albuterol), Primatene mist (epinephrine), Serevent (salmeterol); Xanthine derivative: Theo-Dur (theophylline), Aminophylline.

## Expectorant Agents[18,19]

**Action:** Expectorant agents increase respiratory secretions which help to loosen mucus. Reducing the viscosity of secretions and increasing sputum volume improves the efficiency of the cough reflex and of ciliary action in removing accumulated secretions.

**Indications:** cough associated with respiratory tract infections and related conditions such as sinusitis, pharyngitis, bronchitis, and asthma, when complicated by tenacious mucus or mucus plugs and congestion

**Side effects:** gastrointestinal distress, drowsiness

**Implications for PT:** Therapists can exploit the effects of expectorant agents by performing airway clearance interventions within

one hour after drug administration. Therapists should encourage the patient to take the medication with a glass of water.

**Examples:** Mucinex (guaifenesin), terpin hydrate

## Mucolytic Agents [18,19]

**Action:** Mucolytic agents decrease the viscosity of mucus secretions by altering their composition and consistency, making them easier to expectorate. They are administered by a nebulizer.

**Indications:** viscous mucus secretions due to pneumonia, emphysema, chronic bronchitis, and cystic fibrosis

**Side effects:** pharyngitis, oral mucosa inflammation, rhinitis, chest pain

**Implications for PT:** Therapists can exploit the effects of mucolytic agents by performing airway clearance interventions within one hour after drug administration. Patients should be instructed in the proper use and maintenance of the nebulizer and compressor system used in its delivery.

**Examples:** Pulmozyme (dornase alpha), Mucosil or Mucomyst (acetylcysteine)

# Medical Procedures for Airway and Lung Diseases

## Airway Adjuncts[14]

A variety of devices are used to maintain or protect the airway, to provide mechanical ventilation or to promote airway clearance.

**Oral pharyngeal airway:** A plastic tube shaped to fit the curvature of the soft palate and tongue that holds the tongue away from the back of the throat and maintains the patency of the airway.

**Nasal pharyngeal airway:** A latex or rubber tube inserted through the nose to allow for nasotracheal suctioning.

**Endotracheal tube:** A plastic tube inserted in the trachea from the mouth or nose to provide an airway and to allow for mechanical ventilation.

**Tracheostomy tube:** An artificial airway inserted into the trachea from an incision in the neck below the vocal cords used in patients needing prolonged mechanical ventilation.

## Airway Suctioning[14]

Suctioning is the mechanical aspiration of secretions from the nasopharynx, oropharynx, and trachea using a suction catheter. Endotracheal suctioning refers to the mechanical aspiration of pulmonary secretions from a patient with an artificial airway in place. Nasotracheal suctioning refers to the insertion of a suction catheter through the nasal passage and pharynx into the trachea without a tracheal tube or tracheostomy to aspirate accumulated secretions or foreign material. Indications for suctioning include increased or thickened secretions and inadequate cough. The frequency of suctioning is dependent on the amount of secretion produced.

## Bullectomy[3]

A surgical procedure in which one or more of the large air spaces called bullae that form when the alveoli are destroyed by emphysema are removed. The procedure can improve breathing.

## Lobectomy[3]

Surgical removal of a lobe of one lung.

## Lung Transplant[3]

A surgical procedure to replace one or both diseased or failing lungs with healthy donor lungs. A lung transplant is reserved for patients with end-stage COPD, interstitial pulmonary fibrosis, cystic fibrosis, and other serious lung diseases, but who do not have serious comorbidities.

## Lung Volume Reduction Surgery[3]

A surgical procedure in which a portion of lung tissue damaged by emphysema is removed. This creates extra space in the chest so that the remaining lung tissue and the diaphragm work more efficiently, enabling the patient to breathe more easily.

## Mechanical Ventilation[14]

Patients with severe pulmonary dysfunction may need assistance to breathe from a positive pressure mechanical ventilator or breathing machine. The positive pressure from the ventilator provides the force that delivers air into the lungs by increasing intrathoracic pressure. Mechanical ventilation involves an automatic cycling ventilator connected to a tracheostomy tube or mask to assist or breathe for the patient.

## Oxygen Therapy[14]

Liquid or gaseous oxygen is indicated for the treatment of acute and chronic hypoxemia in patients with a $PaO_2$ ≤ 55 mm Hg, or an oxygen saturation ≤ 88% while seated at rest, or a $PaO_2$ of 56 to 59 mm Hg, or oxygen saturation of 89% in the presence of cor pulmonale or polycythemia. A number of devices are available to deliver the supplemental oxygen to the patient including nasal cannula, simple face mask, partial rebreathing mask, nonrebreathing mask, aerosol face mask, Venturi mask, and transtracheal catheter.

## Thoracotomy[20]

A surgical incision cutting the chest wall to access the heart, great vessels, lungs, esophagus, and diaphragm for diagnostic and therapeutic purposes. The incision may be made under the arm (axillary thoracotomy), through the sternum (median sternotomy), from the back to the side (posterolateral thoracotomy) or under the breast (anterolateral thoracotomy).

## Tracheostomy[15]

A surgically created hole through the neck into the trachea below the level of the vocal cords. The term for the surgical procedure to create the opening is tracheotomy. There are two primary indications for tracheostomy: airway obstruction at or above the level of the larynx and respiratory failure requiring prolonged mechanical ventilation. The tracheostomy can be surgically closed when it is no longer needed.

# Physical Therapy Tests and Measures

## Angina Pain Scales

A number of pain scales are used to grade the severity of angina pectoris.[21,22] One of the more commonly used angina scales rates angina pain from one to four.

| Rating | Description |
|--------|-------------|
| 1 | Mild, barely noticeable |
| 2 | Moderate, bothersome |
| 3 | Moderately severe, very uncomfortable |
| 4 | Most severe or intense pain ever experienced |

## Ankle-Brachial Index (ABI)[15]

Also known as the ankle-arm index, the ABI compares systolic blood pressures at the ankle and arm to check for peripheral artery disease.

### Procedure

- Systolic blood pressures are measured in both brachial arteries and both tibialis posterior arteries with a sphygmomanometer and a handheld Doppler ultrasound device.
- The ABI is calculated by dividing the higher of the two blood pressure measurements in the ankles by the higher of the two systolic blood pressure measurements at the arms.

### Interpretation

| | |
|--|--|
| ≥ 1.30 | Indicates rigid arteries and the need for an ultrasound test to check for peripheral artery disease |
| 1.0 – 1.30 | Normal; no blockage |
| 0.8 – 0.99 | Mild blockage; beginnings of peripheral artery disease |
| 0.4 – 0.79 | Moderate blockage; may be associated with intermittent claudication during exercise |
| < 0.4 | Severe blockage suggesting severe peripheral artery disease; may have claudication pain at rest |

## Arterial Blood Pressure[6]

Noninvasive measurement of arterial blood pressure (BP) with a pneumatic cuff and sphygmomanometer is considered one of the "vital signs" and an important indicator of health (Fig. 6-10). Deviations from normal pressure provide important information regarding a variety of cardiovascular conditions.

**Fig. 6-10:** Checking blood pressure at the brachial artery with a sphygmomanometer and stethoscope.

## Procedure

- Use the appropriate sphygmomanometer cuff for the size of the body part. The bladder inside the cuff should encircle 80% of the arm in adults and 100% of the arm in children younger than 13 years old. If the bladder is too small, false high readings may result. If in doubt, use a larger cuff.

- The brachial artery is occluded by a sphygmomanometer cuff wrapped snugly around the upper arm and inflated to above the anticipated systolic pressure.

- As the cuff is slowly deflated (no more than 2-3 mm Hg per second), pulsatile blood flow is re-established and accompanied by sounds that can be detected by a stethoscope held over the artery.

- The sounds, known as Korotkoff sounds, originate from a combination of turbulent blood flow and oscillations of the arterial wall. As the pressure is reduced, the sounds change in quality and intensity.

  **Phase I** - first appearance of clear tapping sounds corresponding to the appearance of a palpable pulse; Phase I corresponds to systolic blood pressure (SBP)

  **Phase II** - sounds become softer and longer

  **Phase III** - sounds become crisper and louder

  **Phase IV** - sounds become muffled and softer

  **Phase V** - sounds disappear completely; the diastolic pressure (DBP) is the pressure at the last audible sound

## Interpretation

- **In children ages 3 – 17:** BP is classified by SBP and DBP percentiles for age, sex, and height.

  **Normal BP:** SBP and DBP <90th percentile

  **Prehypertension:** SBP or DBP ≥ 90th percentile to < 95th percentile

  **Stage 1 Hypertension:** SBP and/or DBP ≥ 95th percentile to ≤ 99th percentile plus 5 mm Hg

  **Stage 2 Hypertension:** SBP and/or DBP > 99th percentile plus 5 mm Hg

- **In adults:**

  **Normal BP:** < 120 mm Hg SBP and < 80 mm Hg DBP

  **Prehypertension:** 120 – 139 mm Hg SBP or 80 – 89 mm Hg DBP

  **Stage 1 Hypertension:** 140 – 159 mm Hg SBP or 90 – 99 mm Hg DBP

  **Stage 2 Hypertension:** ≥ 160 mm Hg SBP or ≥ 100 mm Hg DBP

### Auscultation of Heart Sounds[23]

Listening to the intensity and quality of heart sounds over the surface of the chest can provide useful information about the condition and function of the heart. Although considered an advanced skill, with supervised practice, the therapist should be able to differentiate normal heart sounds from blatantly abnormal sounds such as loud murmurs and gallops.

## Procedure

The bell or diaphragm of the stethoscope is held directly on the patient's bare skin with enough pressure to provide a skin seal while the patient breathes quietly through the nose.

- Listen over four designated auscultatory areas (Fig. 6-11):

  **Aortic area** – 2nd intercostal space at the right sternal border

  **Pulmonic area** – 2nd intercostal space at the left sternal border

  **Mitral area** – 5th intercostal space, medial to the left midclavicular line

  **Tricuspid area** – 4th intercostal space at the left sternal border

- Listen to the overall rate and rhythm of the heart sounds.

- Listen separately to each sound and each pause in the cardiac cycle for as many beats as necessary to evaluate the sounds in one area before moving to the next area.

- Listen for extra sounds or murmurs while concentrating on systole and diastole.

2nd ICS
Aortic area

2nd ICS
Pulmonic area

Left sternal border
3rd, 4th and 5th ICS
Tricuspid area

ICS = Intercostal space

Apex
Usually in the 5th ICS, midclavicular line
Mitral area

**Fig. 6-11:** Four areas to auscultate for heart sounds generated from the aortic, pulmonic, tricuspid, and mitral valves.

## Interpretation

**S1 (lub)**

- 1st heart sound - closure of the mitral and tricuspid (atrioventricular) valves at the onset of ventricular systole.

- High frequency sound with lower pitch and longer duration than S2.

**S2 (dub)**

- 2nd heart sound - closure of the aortic and pulmonic (semilunar) valves at the onset of ventricular diastole.

- High frequency sound with higher pitch and shorter duration than S1 (Fig. 6-12).

## S3

- 3rd heart sound - vibrations of the distended ventricle walls due to passive flow of blood from the atria during the rapid filling phase of diastole.
- Normal in healthy young children; termed "physiologic" 3rd heart sound.
- Abnormal in adults, may be associated with heart failure; often called "ventricular gallop."

## S4

- 4th heart sound - pathological sound of vibration of the ventricular wall with ventricular filling and atrial contraction.
- May be associated with hypertension, stenosis, hypertensive heart disease or myocardial infarction; often called an "atrial gallop".

### Murmurs

- Heart murmurs are vibrations of longer duration than the heart sounds and are often due to disruption of blood flow past a stenotic or regurgitant valve; the sounds are variably described as soft, blowing or swishing.
- When the leaflets of the heart valves are thickened, the forward flow of blood is restricted; when the leaflets lose competency and fail to close tightly, blood can flow backwards (regurgitation).

## Auscultation of Lung Sounds[24]

Movement of air in the tracheobronchial tree produces sounds that can be heard with a stethoscope. Auscultation of lung sounds and voice sounds is performed to assist in diagnosis and to evaluate the effects of treatment. Lung or breath sounds are characterized by pitch, intensity, quality, and the duration of the inspiratory and expiratory phases.

Fig. 6-13: Auscultation of lung sounds from the posterior thorax.

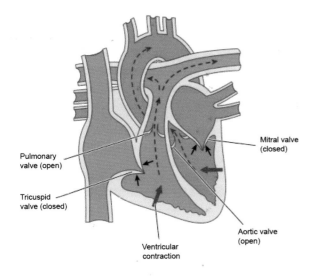

The first heart tone (S1), is caused by the closure of the mitral and tricuspid valves at the beginning of ventricular contraction (systole).

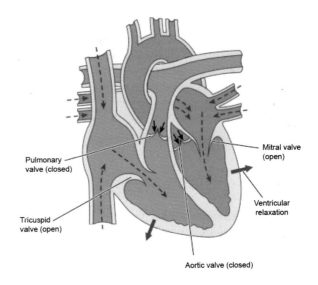

The second heart tone (S2), is caused by the closure of the aortic and pulmonary valves at the end of ventricular systole

Fig. 6-12: Origin of the first and second heart sounds, S1 and S2, respectively.

Fig. 6-14: Areas to auscultate for lung or breath sounds on the anterior thorax. Listen to at least one breath sound in each bronchopulmonary segment comparing the sounds from the left and right sides.

Fig. 6-15: Areas to auscultate for lung sounds on the posterior thorax.

## Procedure

- Place the diaphragm of the stethoscope in firm contact with the patient's unclothed chest wall (Fig. 6-13).
- Start at the apices and work downward, comparing symmetrical points sequentially (Figs. 6-14, 6-15).
- Have the patient breathe in and out through the mouth, a little deeper than normal.
- Listen to at least one cycle of inspiration and expiration in each pulmonary segment.

## If abnormal sounds are suspected:

- Compare the intensity, pitch, and quality of the sounds heard on one side with sounds heard in the same location on the other side.
- Identify the breath sounds as vesicular, bronchovesicular, bronchial or absent by the duration of inspiration and expiration, and by the quality and pitch.
- Note the presence or absence of adventitious (extra) sounds.

## Interpretation

### Normal breath sounds

- Tracheal and bronchial sounds
  - Loud, tubular sounds normally heard over the trachea.
  - Inspiratory phase is shorter than the expiratory phase and there is a slight pause between them.

    Note: Bronchial sounds heard over distal airways are abnormal and represent consolidation or compression of lung tissue that facilitates transmission of sound.
- Vesicular breath sounds
  - High pitched, breezy sounds normally heard over the distal airways in healthy lung tissue.

  - Inspiratory phase is longer than expiratory phase and there is no pause between them.

### Abnormal breath sounds

These are sounds that are heard outside of their normal location or phase of respiration.

### Adventitious breath sounds

Abnormal breath sounds heard with inspiration and/or expiration that can be continuous or discontinuous.

### Crackle (formerly rales)

- An abnormal, discontinuous, high-pitched popping sound heard more often during inspiration. May be associated with restrictive or obstructive respiratory disorders.
- Typically represents the movement of fluid or secretions during inspiration (wet crackles) or occurs from the sudden opening of closed airways (dry crackles). Crackles that occur during the latter half of inspiration typically represent atelectasis, fibrosis, pulmonary edema or pleural effusion. Crackles due to the movement of secretions are usually low-pitched and can be heard during inspiration and/or expiration like the sound of hairs being rubbed together between the thumb and forefinger.
- Pulmonary edema may produce fine crackles as air bubbles through fluid in the distal small airways.
- Often heard in the bases of lungs with interstitial lung disease, atelectasis, pneumonia, bronchiectasis, and pulmonary edema.

### Pleural friction rub

- Dry, crackling sound heard during both inspiration and expiration.
- Occurs when inflamed visceral and parietal pleurae rub together.
- Heard over the spot where the patient feels pleuritic pain.

## Rhonchi

- Continuous low-pitched sounds described as having a "snoring" or "gurgling" quality that may be heard during both inspiration and expiration.
- Caused by air passing through an airway which is obstructed by inflammatory secretions or liquid, bronchial spasm or neoplasms in the smaller (sibilant rhonchi) or larger (sonorous rhonchi) airways.

## Stridor

- Continuous high-pitched wheeze heard with inspiration or expiration.
- Indicates upper airway obstruction.

## Wheeze

- Continuous "musical" or whistling sound composed of a variety of pitches.
- Heard during both inspiration and/or expiration, but variable from minute to minute and area to area.
- Arise from turbulent airflow and the vibrations of the walls of small airways due to narrowing by bronchospasm, edema, collapse, secretions, neoplasm or foreign body.

## Bronchial breath sounds

Abnormal breath sounds when heard in locations where vesicular sounds are normally present. Pneumonia may produce these sounds.

## Decreased or diminished sounds

A less audible sound may indicate severe congestion, emphysema or hypoventilation.

## Absent breath sounds

Absent lung sounds may indicate pneumothorax or lung collapse.

## Voice Sounds

In the normal lung, transmission of spoken sounds is usually muffled; whispered words are faint and the syllables are not distinct, except over the main bronchi. Increases in loudness and distinctness indicate consolidation, atelectasis or fibrosis, all of which improve transmission of vibrations through lung tissue. Whispered and spoken voice sounds are somewhat more valuable than breath sounds in detecting pulmonary consolidation, infarction, and atelectasis.

### Bronchophony:

Increased vocal resonance with greater clarity and loudness of spoken words (e.g., "99").

### Egophony:

A form of bronchophony in which the spoken long "E" sound changes to a long, nasal-sounding "A."

### Whispered pectoriloquy:

Recognition of whispered words "1, 2, 3."

## Body Mass Index (BMI)[25]

BMI describes relative weight for height and is a measurement used to identify increased risk for mortality and morbidity due to excess weight and obesity. It can also monitor changes in body weight from treatment. Although BMI can be used for most men and women, it may overestimate body fat in athletes and others who have a muscular build and underestimate body fat in older persons and others who have lost muscle.

### Procedure

- Measure the subject's standing height and body weight.
- BMI = weight [kg] ÷ height [m²] OR BMI = weight [lb] ÷ height [in²] x 703

### Interpretation

| Adult BMI | Classification |
|---|---|
| < 18.5 | Underweight |
| 18.5 – 24.9 | Normal |
| 25.0 – 29.9 | Overweight |
| 30.0 – 34.9 | Obesity (Class 1) |
| 35.0 – 39.9 | Obesity (Class 2) |
| ≥ 40.0 | Extreme obesity (Class 3) |

Classifications do not apply to children and adolescents as BMI changes with age and sex.

- BMI between the 85th and 95th percentile for age and sex is considered at risk for becoming overweight.
- BMI ≥ the 95th percentile is considered overweight or obese.

## Capillary Refill Time[23]

The time it takes the capillary bed to refill after it is occluded by pressure is an indicator of impaired perfusion to the extremities.

### Procedure

- Apply firm pressure over a nail bed or bony prominence (e.g., chin, forehead, or sternum) until the nail or skin blanches.
- Release the pressure.
- Observe the time for the nail or skin to regain its full color.

### Interpretation

- Normal – Full color returns in < 2 seconds
- Abnormal – Refill time is > 2 seconds; indicates capillary blood flow is compromised (e.g., arterial occlusion, hypovolemic shock, hypothermia)

## Circumferences for Limb Edema[26]

Circumference measurements made at a number of points along the limb at specified distances from an anatomical landmark are an accepted technique to detect limb enlargement and to provide a quantitative assessment of changes in limb size due to edema, lymphedema, and joint effusion.

### Procedure

- Measurements should be made on a measuring board.

- Measurements should be from a standard point of reference on the extremity that is replicable (e.g., every 5 or 10 centimeters along the extremity or a specified distance from a bony prominence).

- Seven circumferences are recommended for the upper and lower extremities to deduce that the fluid has been removed and not just redistributed.

### Interpretation

The opposite limb, when available, is used for comparison. A difference of two or three centimeters between four comparative circumferences on bilateral upper extremities is evidence of lymphedema.

### Classification for lymphedema[27]

**Mild:** < 3 centimeters difference between the affected and unaffected limbs

**Moderate:** 3 to 5 centimeters difference between the affected and unaffected limbs

**Severe:** > 5 centimeters difference between the affected and unaffected limbs

## Claudication Test[28]

Claudication is a cardinal symptom of peripheral artery disease. Claudication occurs when skeletal muscle oxygen demand during exercise exceeds blood oxygen supply. This results from stimulation of local sensory receptors by accumulating lactate or other metabolites. It is characterized by pain, aches, cramping, sense of fatigue or other discomfort in the affected muscle group, which limit the ability to exercise.

### Procedure

Patient walks on a flat track at maximum speed or on a treadmill at 2.0 mph at a constant grade between 0 - 12%.

### Interpretation

**Scoring:**

- Initial claudication distance (ICD) = pain-free walking distance

- Absolute claudication distance (ACD) = maximum distance walked when test is terminated due to pain

- Speed of walking

**Grading scale for claudication pain:**[21]

- Grade 1 - Definite discomfort or pain, but only of initial or modest levels

- Grade 2 - Moderate discomfort or pain from which the patient's attention can be diverted

- Grade 3 - Intense pain from which the patient's attention cannot be diverted

- Grade 4 - Excruciating and unbearable pain

**The location of the symptoms often corresponds to the site of the most proximal stenosis:**

- Pain in the buttock, hip or thigh occurs with obstruction of the aorta and iliac arteries

- Pain in the calf occurs with stenosis of the femoral and popliteal arteries

- Pain in the ankle or foot occurs with disease of the tibial or peroneal arteries

## Dyspnea Scales

Dyspnea is an uncomfortable awareness of breathing that may result from decreased oxygenation, hypoventilation, hyperventilation, or increased work of breathing due to changes in respiratory mechanics or anxiety. A number of scales are available to rate dyspnea.[21, 29-31]

| Borg Dyspnea Scale[29] | |
|---|---|
| 0 | No breathlessness at all |
| 0.5 | Very, very slight |
| 1 | Very slight |
| 2 | Slight breathlessness |
| 3 | Moderate |
| 4 | Somewhat severe |
| 5 | Severe breathlessness |
| 6 | |
| 7 | Very severe breathlessness |
| 8 | |
| 9 | Very, very severe breathlessness |
| 10 | Maximal |

## Electrocardiogram (ECG)[32]

The ECG is a graphic representation of the heart's electrical activity recorded from electrodes on the surface of the body. The ECG provides insight into the electrical behavior of the heart and its modification by physiologic, pharmacologic, and pathologic events. A 12-lead ECG provides 12 views of the heart. It is used to assess cardiac rhythm, to diagnose the location, extent, and acuteness of myocardial ischemia and infarction, and to evaluate changes with activity (Fig. 6-16).

### Procedure

The resistance between skin and electrode is reduced by removing skin oils and cutaneous debris with an alcohol-saturated gauze pad, then abrading the skin sites to remove the superficial layer of skin.

**Fig. 6-16:** Anatomic locations of limb and chest electrodes for a 12-lead ECG recording.

**Apply ECG electrodes to the anatomic locations.**

- Anatomic locations of limb electrodes for limb leads:

    Right arm (RA) - Infraclavicular fossa medial to the right deltoid muscle

    Left arm (LA) - Infraclavicular fossa medial to the left deltoid muscle

    Left leg (LL) - Left side of the abdomen below the rib cage

    Right leg (RL) - Right side of the abdomen (ground electrode)

- Anatomic locations of chest electrodes for precordial leads:

    V1 - 4th intercostal space at right sternal border

    V2 - 4th intercostal space at left sternal border

    V3 - Midway between V2 and V4

    V4 - 5th intercostal space at left midclavicular line

    V5 - Left anterior axillary line at V4 level

    V6 - Left midaxillary line at V4 and V5 levels

Connect the electrodes to their corresponding lead wires to form three bipolar limb leads, three augmented unipolar limb leads, and six unipolar leads.

| Location of Electrodes and Lead Connections for 12-Lead ECG | | |
|---|---|---|
| **Lead** | **Positive Input** | **Negative Input** |
| **Bipolar Limb Leads** | | |
| Lead I | Left arm | Right arm |
| Lead II | Left leg | Right arm |
| Lead III | Left leg | Left arm |
| **Augmented Unipolar Limb Leads** | | |
| aVR | Right arm | Left arm and left leg |
| aVL | Left arm | Right arm and left leg |
| aVF | Left leg | Right arm and left arm |
| **Unipolar Precordial Leads** | | |
| V1 | 4th intercostal space at right sternal border | Central terminal* |
| V2 | 4th intercostal space at left sternal border | Central terminal |
| V3 | Midway between V2 and V4 | Central terminal |
| V4 | 5th intercostal space at left midclavicular line | Central terminal |
| V5 | Left anterior axillary line at V4 level | Central terminal |
| V6 | Left midaxillary line at V4 and V5 levels | Central terminal |

*Negative or reference input is composed of a compound electrode formed by electrically combining the output of the left arm, right arm, and left leg electrodes.

Interpretation

## Waveforms and Intervals (Fig. 6-17)

- **P wave:** Atrial depolarization
- **PR interval:** Time for atrial depolarization and conduction from the SA node to the AV node. Normal duration is 0.12 to 0.20 seconds
- **QRS complex:** Ventricular depolarization and atrial repolarization. Normal duration is 0.06 to 0.10 seconds
- **QT interval:** Time for both ventricular depolarization and repolarization. Normally ranges from 0.20 to 0.40 seconds, depending on heart rate
- **ST segment:** Isoelectric period following QRS when the ventricles are depolarized
- **T wave:** Ventricular repolarization

## Sinus Node Rhythms

- **Normal sinus rhythm:** Atrial depolarization begins in the SA node and spreads normally throughout the electrical conduction system with a heart rate between 60 and 100 beats/minute
- **Sinus bradycardia:** Sinus rhythm with a heart rate less than 60 beats/minute (in adults)
- **Sinus tachycardia:** Sinus rhythm with a heart rate more than 100 beats/minute (in adults)
- **Sinus arrhythmia:** A sinus rhythm, but with quickening and slowing of impulse formation in the SA node resulting in a slight beat-to-beat variation of the rate
- **Sinus arrest:** A sinus rhythm, except with intermittent failure of either SA node impulse formation or AV node conduction that results in the occasional complete absence of P or QRS waves

## Atrial Dysrhythmias

### Premature atrial contractions (PAC)

- Occur when an ectopic focus in the atrium initiates an impulse before the SA node
- The P wave is premature with abnormal configuration

**Clinical Significance:**

- PACs are very common and generally benign, but may progress to atrial flutter, tachycardia or fibrillation
- May occur with a normal heart (from caffeine, stress, smoking, alcohol) and any type of heart disease

### Atrial flutter

- An ectopic, very rapid atrial tachycardia
- Atrial rate of 250–350 beats per minute; ventricular rate dependent upon AV node conduction
- Saw-tooth shaped P waves (also known as flutter waves) are characteristic

**Clinical Significance:**

- Occurs with valvular disease (especially mitral), ischemic heart disease, cardiomyopathy, hypertension, acute myocardial infarction, chronic obstructive lung disease, and pulmonary emboli
- Signs and symptoms include palpitations, lightheadedness, and angina due to a rapid rate
- Stagnation of blood may predispose to thrombi in the atria

### Atrial fibrillation

- A common arrhythmia where the atria are depolarized between 350 and 600 times/min
- ECG shows characteristically irregular undulations of ECG baseline without discrete P waves

**Clinical Significance:**

- Occurs in healthy hearts and in patients with coronary artery disease, hypertension, and valvular disease
- Symptoms may include palpitations, fatigue, dyspnea, lightheadedness, syncope, and chest pain
- Stagnation of blood may predispose to thrombi in the atria

## Atrioventricular Conduction Blocks

### 1st degree atrioventricular block

- PR interval is longer than 0.2 seconds, but relatively constant from beat to beat

**Clinical Significance:**

- No symptoms or significant change in cardiac function
- PR interval may become prolonged for many reasons including medications that suppress AV conduction

### 2nd degree atrioventricular block

- AV conduction disturbance in which impulses between the atria and ventricles fail intermittently
- Two major types: Mobitz type I block (also called Wenckebach block) and Mobitz type II block

**Clinical significance**

- Mobitz I – progressive prolongation of PR interval until one impulse is not conducted (generally benign)
- Mobitz II – consecutive PR intervals are the same and normal followed by nonconduction of one or more impulses (a more serious condition). If heart rate is slow, cardiac output will decrease with the blocked impulse. Also, 2nd degree AV block may progress to 3rd degree AV block

### 3rd degree atrioventricular block (complete heart block)

- All impulses are blocked at the AV node and none are transmitted to the ventricles
- The atria and ventricles are paced independently; atrial rate > ventricular rate

**Clinical Significance:**

- Considered a medical emergency, requiring a pacemaker

- If the ventricular rate is too slow, the cardiac output drops and the patient may faint

- Common causes include degenerative changes of the conduction systems, digitalis, heart surgery, and acute MI

## Ventricular Arrhythmias

### Premature ventricular complex (PVC)

- Premature depolarization arising in the ventricles due to an ectopic focus

- Unifocal PVCs arise from the same ectopic focus and have the same configuration

- Multifocal PVCs arise from different ectopic foci and have different configurations

- On ECG, the P wave is usually absent and the QRS complex has a wide and aberrant shape

- Bigeminy – Normal sinus impulse is followed by a PVC

- Trigeminy – PVC occurs after every two normal sinus impulses

**Clinical Significance:**

- A common arrhythmia that occurs in healthy and diseased hearts

- Patient may be asymptomatic or have palpitations

- Common causes include anxiety, caffeine, stress, smoking, and all forms of heart disease

### Ventricular tachycardia (v-tach)

- 3 or more consecutive PVCs at a ventricular rate of > 150 beats/minute

- P waves are absent and QRS complexes are wide and aberrant in appearance

**Clinical Significance:**

- V-tach longer than 30 seconds is a life-threatening arrhythmia and requires immediate medical intervention

- Patients are not able to maintain an adequate blood pressure and eventually become hypotensive

- V-tach may degenerate into ventricular fibrillation causing cardiac arrest

- Common causes include: MI, cardiomyopathy, and valvular disease

### Ventricular fibrillation (v-fib)

- Ventricles do not beat in a coordinated fashion, but fibrillate or quiver asynchronously and ineffectively

- No cardiac output; patient becomes unconscious

- ECG shows characteristic fibrillatory waves with an irregular pattern that is either coarse or fine

**Clinical Significance:**

- A lethal tachyarrhythmia requires immediate defibrillation

- Additional measures include medications to support the circulation and intravenous antiarrhythmic agents

- Common causes include heart disease of any type, MI, and cocaine use

### Ventricular asystole

- Ventricular standstill with no rhythm

- ECG records a straight-line pattern

**Clinical Significance:**

- Requires immediate defibrillation and/or medications to stimulate cardiac activity

- Common causes include acute MI, ventricular rupture, cocaine use, lightning strikes, and electrical shock

## Signs of Myocardial Ischemia and Infarction

### ST segment depression

- A depressed ST segment is a sign of subendocardial ischemia, but also can be due to digitalis toxicity or hypokalemia

- The segment is evaluated relative to isoelectric baseline at 0.08 seconds after the J point (junction between the end of the QRS complex and the beginning of the ST segment)

- Deviations from the isoelectric baseline are expressed as ST segment depression of 1 mm, 2 mm, etc.

### ST segment elevation

- Earliest sign of acute transmural infarction

- Can also indicate a benign early repolarization pattern in a normal heart

- Deviations from the isoelectric baseline are expressed as ST segment elevation of 1 mm, 2 mm, etc.

### Q wave

- A characteristic marker of infarction; signifies the loss of positive electrical voltages due to necrosis

- A significant or abnormal Q wave is longer than 0.04 msec and larger than 1/3 the amplitude of the R wave

### T wave inversion

- Occurs hours or days after an MI as the result of a delay in repolarization produced by the injury

- May also occur with right and left bundle branch blocks, after a CVA, and as a normal juvenile T wave pattern in children and some adults

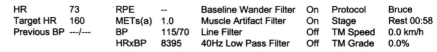

| HR | 73 | RPE | -- | Baseline Wander Filter | On | Protocol | Bruce |
|---|---|---|---|---|---|---|---|
| Target HR | 160 | METs(a) | 1.0 | Muscle Artifact Filter | On | Stage | Rest 00:58 |
| Previous BP | ---/--- | BP | 115/70 | Line Filter | Off | TM Speed | 0.0 km/h |
| | | HRxBP | 8395 | 40Hz Low Pass Filter | Off | TM Grade | 0.0% |

**Fig. 6-17:** Example of a normal 12-lead ECG recorded after 58 seconds of resting just prior to a graded exercise test using a Bruce protocol.

## Exercise Stress Testing[21]

Exercise stress tests are used to assess the patient's ability to tolerate increasing intensity of exercise while ECG, BP, HR, and symptoms are monitored for evidence of myocardial ischemia, abnormal electrical conduction, or other abnormal signs and symptoms of exertion. They may be used to evaluate disease severity and prognosis and to determine functional capacity, especially for exercise prescription and counseling. A number of exercise protocols are available using a treadmill, cycle ergometer or upper extremity ergometer.

### Procedure

- Generally, the patient is required to exercise at progressively greater increments of work, by varying the speed and grade of the treadmill, or the speed and resistance to pedaling an upper extremity or cycle ergometer.

- HR, BP, ECG, RPE, and signs and symptoms are monitored before, during, and after the test

- Absolute indications for terminating an exercise test:

  - Drop in SBP > 10 mm Hg from baseline despite increase in workload with other evidence of ischemia

  - Moderately severe angina (three on a scale of four)

  - Increasing nervous system symptoms (e.g., ataxia, dizziness)

  - Signs of poor perfusion (cyanosis, pallor)

  - Sustained ventricular tachycardia

  - 1.0 mm ST elevation in leads without diagnostic Q waves

- Relative indications for terminating an exercise test:

  - Drop in SBP > 10 mm Hg from baseline despite increase in workload without other evidence of ischemia

  - > 2 mm ST segment depression

  - Arrhythmias other than sustained ventricular tachycardia, including multifocal PVCs, supraventricular tachycardia, heart block or bradyarrhythmias

  - Fatigue, shortness of breath, wheezing, leg cramps, and claudication

  - Development of bundle branch block or intraventricular conduction delay

  - Increasing chest pain

  - Hypertensive response (SBP > 250 mm Hg and/or DBP > 115 mm Hg)

## Consider This

### Systematic Approach for Analyzing ECG Rhythm Strips[14]

| | |
|---|---|
| 1. Scan rhythm strip | • Is rate unusually slow or fast?<br>• Does rhythm appear to be regular?<br>• Are there any abnormal looking beats? |
| 2. Determine the heart rate | • Regular rhythm: divide 300 by number of large squares (including fraction of a square) between two consecutive P waves<br>• Irregular rhythm: count the number of QRS complexes in a 6 second strip; multiply by 10 |
| 3. Evaluate the rhythm by comparing R to R intervals | • Regular rhythm: R to R intervals are within 0.04 seconds<br>• If irregular, is there a pattern, or is it totally irregular? |
| 4. Evaluate P waves | • Present versus absent<br>• Identical in shape? Upright in leads I, II, and III?<br>• Each P wave followed by a QRS complex? |
| 5. If P waves are present, measure PR interval to evaluate for conduction blocks | • Normal: 0.12 to 0.20 seconds |
| 6. Examine QRS complexes to determine if conduction is normal through the ventricles | • Normal: QRS width is 0.04 to 0.10 seconds in all leads<br>• Identical in shape? |
| 7. Assess ST segment 0.08 seconds after the J point | • Is segment at isoelectric baseline, depressed, or elevated? |

### Interpretation

A negative test indicates a low probability of coronary artery disease; a positive test indicates a high probability of coronary artery disease.

Prognosis can be assessed using various multivariate indices (e.g., Duke Treadmill Test score and Veteran's Administration Score).

An aerobic exercise prescription can be determined from performance on the exercise test (see also Physical Therapy Procedural Interventions - Cardiac Rehabilitation).

### Homan's Sign for Deep Vein Thrombosis[33]

Homan's sign is a test to detect deep vein thrombosis (DVT) in the lower leg.

#### Procedure

Passively dorsiflex the foot at the ankle with the knee straight.

### Interpretation

Homan's sign is positive for DVT if the maneuver produces pain in the calf or popliteal space.

Clinical findings alone are insensitive and nonspecific and cannot be relied on to confirm or exclude the diagnosis of DVT.

Despite the lack of specificity, a positive Homan's sign warrants further evaluation.

### Mediate Percussion[23]

Mediate percussion is the act of tapping the surface of the body to identify areas of altered density.

#### Procedure

• Percuss the back with the patient sitting and the anterior chest with the patient sitting or supine

• Facing the patient, place the palmar surface of the middle finger of one hand firmly against the chest wall in the intercostal space parallel to the ribs; other fingers remain off the chest.

- Strike this finger with a quick, sharp blow using the middle finger of the other hand.

- Two or three consecutive blows are struck in one place, before moving the finger to another intercostal space.

- Compare the sounds from each space from left and right sides.

### Interpretation

Percussion sounds are evaluated for loudness (intensity) and pitch. Unilateral abnormalities are easier to identify than bilateral abnormalities because there will be a difference in the sounds from side to side in unilateral disease.

The percussion sounds progress from tissues of high density to tissues of low density in the following sequence:

- **Flat or dull** – sound elicited by percussion of the thigh muscles; in the upper lung, suggests neoplasm, atelectasis or consolidation of the lung.

- **Resonance** – percussion sound from the normal air-filled lung.

- **Hyperresonance** – intermediate sound between resonance and tympany; percussion note emitted by the emphysematous lung; suggests pulmonary emphysema or pneumothorax.

- **Tympany** – hollow sound vaguely resembling a drumbeat; occurs almost exclusively with a large pneumothorax.

## Palpation of Peripheral Arterial Pulses

The peripheral pulse is a periodic fluctuation in the flow of blood through a peripheral artery caused by the ejection of blood with each heartbeat. Normal pulses are strong and regular. The pulse will be irregular with a cardiac arrhythmia and weak and difficult to palpate in peripheral artery disease. A higher intensity pulse will be present when stroke volume is increased (e.g., exercise, fever).

### Procedure

- Heart rate and rhythm, as well as blood flow in the extremity, are assessed by palpating over the artery with the tip of the index or middle finger with enough pressure to feel the pulse, but without obstructing blood flow.

- Common arteries used include brachial, carotid, dorsal pedal, femoral, popliteal, posterior tibial, radial, and temporal.

- Note the time between pulsations.

- For regular rhythms (i.e., time between pulsations is approximately equal), count the pulses in 15 seconds and multiply by four.

- For irregular rhythms (i.e., time between pulsations is not equal), count the pulses in 60 seconds.

- Note the volume and quality of the pulse and any differences between the pulses in the two limbs.

### Pulse Points of Selected Peripheral Arteries

| Artery | Pulse Point |
|---|---|
| **Carotid** | The medial aspect of the sternocleidomastoid muscle in the lower half of the neck (Fig. 6-18) |
| **Brachial** | Medial to the biceps tendon and lateral to the medial epicondyle of the humerus |
| **Radial** | At the wrist, lateral to the flexor carpi radialis tendon (Fig. 6-19) |
| **Ulnar** | At the wrist, between the flexor digitorum superficialis and the flexor carpi ulnaris tendons |
| **Femoral** | In the upper thigh, one-third of the distance from the pubis to the anterior superior iliac spine |
| **Popliteal** | In the popliteal space of the posterior knee |
| **Posterior tibial** | In the space between the medial malleolus and the Achilles tendon, above the calcaneus |
| **Dorsalis pedis** | Near the center of the long axis of the foot, between the first and second metatarsal bones (Fig. 6-20) |

**Fig. 6-18:** Palpating the carotid artery.

**Fig. 6-19:** Palpating the radial artery.

**Fig. 6-20:** Palpating the dorsalis pedis artery.

## Procedure

- While maintaining an upright posture, the subject exhales into the spirometer mouthpiece as hard and as fast as possible for six seconds until no more air can be expelled.
- An adequate FVC test requires three acceptable maneuvers.
- Modern spirometers calculate "predicted normal" values, (i.e., the test value the patient should normally attain based on age, sex, height, weight, and race).

## Interpretation

### Characterize the heart rate

| | |
|---|---|
| **Normal infant** | 100 to 130 beats/minute |
| **Normal child** | 80 to 100 beats/minute |
| **Normal adult** | 60 to 100 beats/minute |
| **Bradycardia** | < 60 beats/minute |
| **Tachycardia** | > 100 beats/minute |

### Characterize the volume or amplitude of the pulse[34]

| | |
|---|---|
| **3+** | = large or bounding pulsation |
| **2+** | = normal or average pulsation |
| **1+** | = small or reduced pulsation |
| **0** | = absence of pulsation |

**Fig. 6-21:** Performing a pulmonary function test with a bedside digital spirometer.

## Interpretation[36]

**Obstructive ventilatory impairment**

- Characterized by decreased expiratory flows.
- Airway narrowing during exhalation causes a disproportionate reduction of maximal air flow compared to the maximal volume displaced from the lungs.
- $FEV_1/FVC$ < 70% is the primary indicator of an obstructive impairment.

## Pulmonary Function Testing (PFT)[35]

Pulmonary function testing measures the volume or flow of air during inhalation and exhalation (Fig. 6-21). The measurements include, but are not limited to, forced vital capacity (FVC), and other forced expiratory flow measurements such as peak expiratory flow (PEF), the forced expiratory volume in the first second ($FEV_1$), and the mid-expiratory flow (FEF 25-75%).

| Obstruction can be classified as: | |
|---|---|
| > 100% | = possible normal variant |
| 70 – 100% | = mild obstruction |
| 60 – 70% | = moderate obstruction |
| 50 – 60% | = moderate to severe obstruction |
| < 50% | = severe obstruction |

- Pathologies include asthma, emphysema, and chronic bronchitis

Restrictive ventilatory impairment

- Characterized by reduced lung volumes (total lung capacity, FVC, FEV₁) and relatively normal expiratory flow rates.
- Inferred from spirometry when FVC is reduced and FEV₁/FVC is normal or > 80%.
- Pathologies include interstitial lung disease, tumors, pleural diseases, chest wall deformities, obesity, pregnancy, neuromuscular disease, and tumor.

## Pulse Oximetry[37]

A pulse oximeter estimates the percent of arterial oxygen saturation of hemoglobin by placing a sensor on the finger or earlobe (Fig. 6-22). The sensor measures the differential absorption of light by oxygenated and nonoxygenated hemoglobin. This estimate is denoted as $SpO_2$, which is an indication of the partial pressure of oxygen in arterial blood.

### Procedure

- Apply the sensor to the earlobe or finger tip.
- Assess the strength of the waveform or pulse amplitude to assure that the oximeter is detecting adequate arterial blood flow.
- Holding the finger dependent and motionless and covering the finger sensor to occlude ambient light improves the quality of readings.

Fig. 6-22: A pulse oximeter.

### Interpretation

$SpO_2$ is only an estimate of the arterial $O_2$ saturation; actual arterial oxygen saturation is ± 4% of $SpO_2$. A number of factors limit the accuracy of oximeter readings:

- Motion artifact
- Abnormal hemoglobin
- Intravascular dyes
- Exposure of probe to ambient light during measurement
- Poor cutaneous perfusion at the measurement site due to hypotension, hypothermia, low cardiac output or vasoconstrictor medications
- Skin pigmentation
- Nail polish or nail coverings (with finger probe)

If $SpO_2$ < 90% in acutely ill patients or < 85% in patients with chronic lung disease, activity should be stopped and a discussion with the physician should take place to consider adding or increasing supplemental oxygen.

## Rate Pressure Product (RPP)[14]

RPP, or double-product, is an index of myocardial oxygen consumption and coronary blood flow. RPP provides an easy to measure physiologic correlate to the onset of angina pectoris or the development of ECG abnormalities in patients with heart disease. These signs and symptoms of myocardial ischemia generally occur at a reproducible RPP value.

### Procedure

- Measure SBP and heart rate (HR) during the same exercise workload
- RPP = HR x SBP
- RPP is usually reported as a two digit number x $10^3$ (e.g., if HR = 150 and SBP = 170, RPP = 25.5 · $10^3$).

### Interpretation

In patients with fixed-threshold angina:

- A relatively constant level of activity will precipitate angina.
- RPP obtained during an exercise test may be used to guide the exercise prescription.
- Keeping the intensity of exercise below the RPP value will reduce the risk of developing angina.

## Rating of Perceived Exertion (RPE)[38]

The RPE is used to quantify the subject's overall sense of effort during activity. The reported RPE provides the therapist with an idea of the amount of strain or level of exertion the patient is experiencing.

### Procedure

- There are two RPE scales that are widely used: the original 6 – 20 scale and the revised 0 – 10 scale. These scales are often referred to as the Borg Scale.
- Recommended instructions for administering the RPE scale:[29]

*"While doing physical activity, we want you to rate your perception of exertion. This feeling should reflect how heavy and strenuous the exercise feels to you, combining all sensations and feelings of physical stress, effort, and fatigue. Do not concern yourself with any one factor such as leg pain or shortness of breath, but try to focus on your total feeling of exertion."*

*"Choose the number that best describes your level of exertion. This will give you a good idea of the intensity level of your activity. Try to appraise your feeling of exertion as honestly as possible, without thinking about what the actual physical load is. Your own feeling of effort and exertion is important, not how it compares to other people's."*

| Original RPE Scale | | Revised RPE Scale | |
|---|---|---|---|
| 6 | | 0 | Nothing at all |
| 7 | Very, very light | 0.5 | Very, very weak |
| 8 | | 1 | Very weak |
| 9 | Very light | 2 | Weak |
| 10 | | 3 | Moderate |
| 11 | Fairly light | 4 | Somewhat strong |
| 12 | | 5 | Strong |
| 13 | Somewhat hard | 6 | |
| 14 | | 7 | Very strong |
| 15 | Hard | 8 | |
| 16 | | 9 | |
| 17 | Very hard | 10 | Very, very strong |
| 18 | | | • Maximal |
| 19 | Very, very hard | | |
| 20 | | | |

## Interpretation

RPE of 13 - 14 represents about 70% of maximum heart rate during exercise on a treadmill or cycle ergometer. RPE of 11 - 13 corresponds to the upper limit of prescribed training heart rates early in cardiac rehabilitation. RPE can substitute for HR in prescribing the intensity of exercise when:[39]

- Ability to monitor HR is compromised (e.g., sensory deficits)
- Patients begin an exercise-based rehabilitation program without a preliminary exercise test

- The HR response to exercise is altered (e.g., cardiac transplant)
- Physical activities other than cardiorespiratory endurance activity are assessed
- Clinical status or medical therapy changes

Ratings can be influenced by psychological state, environmental conditions, mode of exercise, and age.

## Respiratory Rate, Rhythm, and Pattern

A complete assessment of respiration considers four parameters: rate, rhythm, depth, and character. Respiratory rate is the number of breaths per minute. Rhythm refers to the regularity of inspirations and expirations. Depth of respiration refers to the volume of air exchanged with each breath. The character of respirations refers to the effort and sound produced during breathing.

### Procedure

- Observe the patient's breathing at rest for 60 seconds (an alternate method is to place your hand over the patient's upper thorax or abdomen and observe and feel movement with each respiration).
- Document the rate, rhythm, depth, and character of respiration.

### Interpretation

Resting respiratory rates for healthy individuals[40]

- **Newborn:** 33 - 45 breaths/minute
- **1 year:** 25 - 35 breaths/minute
- **10 years:** 15 - 20 breaths/minute
- **Adult:** 12 - 20 breaths/minute

Respiratory rhythm

- **Normal:** Inspiration (I) is half as long as expiration (E); I:E ratio is 1:2
- **COPD:** I:E ratio reflects a longer expiration phase; 1:3 or 1:4

Depth of respiration

- Characterized as deeper or shallower than normal tidal volume

Character of respiration

- Normal breathing is quiet and effortless
- Labored breathing is evident by the use of accessory muscles of respiration
- Wheezes and crackles are abnormal sounds produced by changes in the airways

## Common Breathing Patterns[23]

| | |
|---|---|
| **Apnea** | absence of spontaneous breathing |
| **Biot's** | irregular breathing; breaths vary in depth and rate with periods of apnea; often associated with increased intracranial pressure or damage to the medulla |
| **Bradypnea** | slower than normal respiratory rate; < 12 breaths/minute in adults; may be associated with neurologic or electrolyte disturbance, infection or high level of cardiorespiratory fitness |
| **Cheyne-Stokes (periodic)** | decreasing rate and depth of breathing with periods of apnea; can occur due to central nervous system damage |
| **Eupnea** | normal rate and depth of breathing |
| **Hyperpnea** | increased rate and depth of breathing |
| **Hypopnea** | decreased rate and depth of breathing |
| **Kussmaul's** | deep and fast breathing; often associated with metabolic acidosis |
| **Paradoxical** | chest wall moves in with inhalation and out with exhalation; due to chest trauma or paralysis of the diaphragm |
| **Tachypnea** | faster than normal respiratory rate; > 20 breaths/minute in adults |

## Six-Minute Walk Test (6MWT)[41]

The 6MWT is used to measure functional status and to document treatment outcomes in patients with heart and lung disease as well as healthy and older adults.

### Procedure

- Walk on a measured "track" at least 100 feet (30 meters) in length.

- Subjects may self-administer any medications ordinarily taken before activity, may use supplemental $O_2$ at their prescribed flow rate for exercise, and may use any assistive device for walking.

- Three walks are recommended with at least 15 minutes of rest between each walk.

- BP, HR, RR, RPE, and $O_2$ saturation may be measured before and immediately after the test.

- Standard instructions are given:

    *"The purpose of this test is to find out how far you can walk in six minutes. You will start from this point and follow the hallway to the marker at the end, then turn around and walk back. You will go back and forth as many times as you can in the six-minute period. You may stop and rest, if you need to, just remain where you are until you can go on again. The most important thing is that you cover as much ground as you possibly can during the six minutes. I will tell you the time, and I will let you know when the six minutes are up. When I say 'stop', stand right where you are."*

- Standard words of encouragement are provided at regular intervals (e.g., "you're doing well," "keep up the good work," "you have three minutes to go").

### Interpretation

The therapist should record the distance walked and the number of rest stops.

## Waist Circumference[25]

Waist circumference is a practical anthropometric measurement for assessing abdominal fat before and during weight loss treatment. Monitoring changes in waist circumference may be helpful, in addition to measuring BMI, since it can provide an estimate of decreased abdominal fat even in the absence of a change in BMI. The measurement of waist-to-hip ratio provides no advantage over waist circumference alone.

### Procedure

- With the subject standing, a measuring tape is placed snugly in a horizontal plane around the abdomen at the level of the iliac crest at the end of a normal exhalation.

- It is not necessary to measure waist circumference in individuals with BMI ≥ 35 $kg/m^2$ since it adds little to the predictive power of the disease risk classification of BMI.

### Interpretation

- An increased risk for type 2 diabetes, dyslipidemia, hypertension, and cardiovascular disease is associated with a circumference > 102 centimeters (> 40 inches) for men and > 88 centimeters (> 35 inches) for women.

- Individuals with waist circumferences greater than these values should be considered one risk category above that defined by their BMI.

# Physical Therapy Procedural Interventions

## Aerobic Exercise Prescription[21,39]

Aerobic exercise, or cardiorespiratory endurance exercise, refers to submaximal, rhythmic repetitive exercise of large muscle groups during which adenosine triphosphate is synthesized primarily by the long-term energy system and the utilization of inspired oxygen.

### Indications

Reduced cardiorespiratory endurance

Primary and secondary prevention of cardiovascular disease

### Precautions/Contraindications

Appropriate screening or health appraisal should be performed prior to beginning exercise training to identify known diseases, risk factors for coronary artery disease, and other factors that will optimize adherence, minimize risk, and maximize benefits.

Avoid Valsalva maneuver

### Procedure

Effective aerobic exercise training and improvement in $VO_{2max}$ is directly related to the intensity, frequency, and duration of aerobic activity interacting with the two major principles of exercise training: overload and specificity. The overload principle states that to improve its function, a tissue or organ must be exposed to a stress or load greater than that which it normally encounters. The principle of specificity states that the long-term adaptations to the metabolic and physiologic systems derived from exercise are specific to the exercises performed and the muscles involved.

### Mode

- Rhythmic activities that use large muscle groups and can be performed continuously and safely (e.g., walking, hiking, running, jogging, bicycling, cross-country skiing, aerobic dance/calisthenics, rope skipping, rowing, skating, stair climbing, swimming, and various endurance game activities).

### Intensity

A target heart rate (THR) zone is established from lower and upper heart rate limits calculated using different percentage training intensities depending on the individual's age, fitness level, health status, and goals.

- **Method 1:** Percent of maximum heart rate (HRmax)

    Lower THR = HRmax x 55%

    Upper THR = HRmax x 90%

- **Method 2:** Heart rate reserve (HRR) or Karvonen formula

    Lower THR = [(HRmax – HRrest) x 40%] + HRrest

    Upper THR = [(HRmax – HRrest) x 85%] + HRrest

    – HRmax = maximum heart rate measured during a graded exercise test or estimated by 220 - age

    – HRrest = resting heart rate

### Duration

Duration is dependent on the intensity of the activity.

20 – 60 minutes of continuous or intermittent activity (minimum of 10-minute bouts accumulated throughout the day).

Lower intensity activity should be performed over a longer period of time (≥ 30 minutes).

Higher intensity activity should be performed for 20 minutes or longer.

Moderate intensity activity of longer duration is recommended for adults not training for athletic competition due to the potential hazards and adherence problems associated with high-intensity activity.

### Frequency

3 – 5 days per week

### Expected outcomes

The therapist should be aware of the normal cardiorespiratory responses to aerobic exercise as well as the chronic adaptations that occur from a successful long-term aerobic exercise training program.

### Normal Cardiorespiratory Response to Acute Aerobic Exercise

- Increased oxygen consumption due to increased cardiac output, increased blood flow, and oxygen utilization in the exercising skeletal muscles.
- Linear increase in SBP with increasing workload (8 to 12 mm Hg per MET)
- No change or moderate decrease in DBP
- Increased respiratory rate and tidal volume

### Chronic Adaptations to Aerobic Exercise

- $VO_{2max}$: increased at maximal exercise
- HR: no change or decrease at maximal exercise; decreased at submaximal exercise
- Arteriovenous oxygen difference: increased at maximal exercise; no change at submaximal exercise
- SBP and DBP: no change or slight increase at maximal exercise; no change or slight decrease at submaximal exercise
- Blood lactate: increased at maximal exercise; decreased at submaximal exercise
- Oxidative capacity of muscle: increase in mitochondrial number and size, capillary density, and oxidative enzymes
- Maximal voluntary ventilation: increased at maximal exercise
- Plasma volume: increased
- Skeletal muscle blood flow: increase at maximum exercise; no change at submaximal exercise

- Reduced body mass and body fat and increase in fat free body mass
- Improved body heat transfer due to larger plasma volume and more responsive thermoregulatory mechanisms
- Psychological benefits: reduced anxiety, stress, and depression; improved mood, and self-esteem

## Airway Clearance Techniques

Airway clearance techniques are intended to manage or prevent the consequences of impaired mucociliary transport or the inability to protect the airway (e.g., impaired cough). The techniques may include breathing strategies, manual and mechanical techniques, and postural drainage.

### Indications for airway clearance[42]

- Retained secretions in the central airways
- Prophylaxis against postoperative pulmonary complications
- Obtain sputum for diagnostic analysis
- Difficulty clearing secretions
- Atelectasis caused by or suspected of being caused by mucus plugging

### Active cycle of breathing

The active cycle of breathing (ACB) technique was developed under the name "forced expiratory technique" to assist secretion clearance in patients with asthma. The name of the technique was changed to "active cycle of breathing" to emphasize that ACB always couples breathing exercise with the huff cough. It includes three phases: breathing control, thoracic expansion exercises, and forced expiratory technique.[43]

### Procedure

- Breathing control:
  - Gentle, relaxed breathing (may be diaphragmatic breathing at patient's tidal volume and resting respiratory rate for 5 – 10 seconds, or as long as the patient needs in order to prepare for the next phase).
- Thoracic expansion exercise:
  - Three to four deep, slow, relaxed inhalations to inspiratory reserve with passive exhalation
  - Chest percussion, vibration or shaking may be combined with exhalation
- Forced expiratory technique:
  - One or two huffs at mid to low lung volumes with the glottis open into the expiratory reserve volume
  - A brisk adduction of the upper arms may be added to self-compress the thorax.

### Precautions/Contraindications

- Splinting postoperative incisions to achieve adequate expiratory force
- Bronchospasm or hyperreactive airways

### Autogenic drainage (AD)

AD uses controlled breathing to mobilize secretions by varying expiratory airflow without using postural drainage positions or coughing. The theory is to improve airflow in small airways to facilitate the movement of mucus. AD requires patience to learn, so this may not be suitable for young children and patients who are not motivated or easily distracted. Because AD does not require the assistance of another person or equipment, it can be performed anywhere and during activities of daily living.[43]

### Procedure

- The patient is sitting upright in a chair with back support.
- Controlled breathing at three lung volumes
  - "Unsticking phase": slowly breathe in through the nose at low-lung volumes followed by a two to three second breath-hold to allow collateral ventilation to get air behind the secretions, then exhale down into the expiratory reserve volume
  - "Collecting phase": breathe at tidal volume, interspersed by two to three second breath-holds
  - "Evacuating phase": deeper inspirations from low-to-mid inspiratory reserve volume, with breath holding followed by a huff.
- Exhalation through pursed-lips may be used to control expiratory flow rate.
- An average treatment is 30 to 45 minutes.

### Precautions/Contraindications

- Requires motivation and concentration to learn

### Directed cough and huffing[44]

A directed cough tries to compensate for the patient's physical limitations to elicit a maximum forced exhalation.

Huffing is a forced expiratory maneuver performed with the glottis open. The maneuver is similar to fogging a pair of glasses with your breath. Although a huff does not produce the same airflow velocity as a cough, the potential for airway collapse is less. Huffing may be reinforced by a quick adduction of the arms to self-compress the chest wall.

### Procedure

### Cough

- Inhale maximally, close the glottis and hold breath for two to three seconds.
- Contract the expiratory muscles to produce increased intrathoracic pressure against the closed glottis.
- Cough sharply two to three times through a slightly open mouth.
- Post-surgical patients may need to splint the chest or abdomen by applying pressure over the incision with a pillow or blanket roll.

### Huff

- Inhale deeply through an open mouth.
- Contract the abdominal muscles during a rapid exhalation with the glottis open, saying, "Ha, ha, ha."

## Precautions/Contraindications

- Inability to control possible transmission of infection from patients suspected or known to have pathogens transmittable by droplets
- Elevated intracranial pressure or known intracranial aneurysm
- Reduced coronary artery perfusion (e.g., acute myocardial infarction)
- Acute unstable head, neck or spine injury
- Potential for regurgitation/aspiration
- Acute abdominal pathology, abdominal aortic aneurysm, hiatal hernia or pregnancy
- Untreated pneumothorax
- Osteoporosis
- Flail chest

## High-frequency airway oscillation[43]

The Acapella® and Flutter® are handheld devices that combine positive expiratory pressure and high frequency airway vibrations to mobilize mucus secretions in the airways.

### Procedure

- Place the device in the mouth with the lips firmly sealed around the mouthpiece
- Inhale slowly to 75% of a full breath
- Hold the breath for two to three seconds
- Exhale through the device for three to four seconds
- Repeat 10 to 20 breaths
- Remove the device and perform two or three coughs or huffs to raise secretions

### Precautions/Contraindications

- Patient tolerance of increased work of breathing (acute asthma, COPD)
- Intracranial pressure >20 mm Hg
- Hemodynamic instability
- Recent facial, oral, or skull surgery or trauma
- Acute sinusitis
- Nosebleed
- Esophageal surgery
- Active hemoptysis
- Nausea
- Known or suspected tympanic membrane rupture or other middle ear pathology
- Untreated pneumothorax

## Postural drainage, percussion, and vibration[42]

Postural drainage consists of positioning the patient so that gravity will help drain bronchial secretions from specific lung segments toward the central airways where they can be removed by cough or mechanical aspiration.

Percussion, also known as cupping and clapping, is the rhythmic clapping or striking of the thorax with a cupped hand or mechanical percussor directly over the lung segment being drained. This rhythmic sequence should last for several minutes and should not be painful.

Vibration is the application of a fine, tremulous action on the chest wall over the lung segment being drained in the direction the ribs move during exhalation. It may be performed manually or with a mechanical vibrator. Vibration should be performed during exhalation.

### Procedure for postural drainage

- The patient assumes the appropriate position for the affected lung segment (Figs. 6-23, A-J).
- Standard positions may be modified as the patient's condition and tolerance warrant.
- Maintain each position for two to three minutes.

### Precautions/Contraindications

All positions are contraindicated for:

- Intracranial pressure > 20 mm Hg
- Head and neck injury until stabilized
- Active hemorrhage with hemodynamic instability
- Recent spinal surgery (e.g., laminectomy) or acute spinal injury
- Active hemoptysis
- Empyema
- Bronchopleural fistula
- Pulmonary edema associated with congestive heart failure
- Large pleural effusion
- Pulmonary embolism
- Confused or anxious patients who do not tolerate position changes
- Rib fracture, with or without flail chest
- Surgical wound or healing tissue

Trendelenburg position is contraindicated for:

- Uncontrolled hypertension
- Distended abdomen
- Esophageal surgery
- Recent gross hemoptysis related to lung carcinoma treated surgically or with radiation therapy
- Uncontrolled airway at risk for aspiration (e.g., tube feeding or recent meal)

# Postural Drainage Positioning

**Fig. 6-23A: Apical segments right and left upper lobes:** The patient is in a sitting position, leaning back 30-40 degrees. Percussion and vibration are performed above the clavicles.

**Fig. 6-23B: Posterior segment right upper lobe:** The patient is turned ¼ from prone on the left side with the bed horizontal and the head and shoulders raised on a pillow. Percussion and vibration are performed around the medial border of the right scapula.

**Fig. 6-23C: Posterior segment left upper lobe:** The patient is turned ¼ from prone on the right side with the head of the bed elevated 45 degrees and the head and shoulders raised on a pillow. Percussion and vibration are performed around the medial border of the left scapula.

**Fig. 6-23D: Lingula left upper lobe.** The patient is turned ¼ from supine on the right side with the foot of the bed elevated 12 inches. Percussion and vibration are performed over the left chest between the axilla and the left nipple.

**Fig. 6-23E: Anterior segments right and left upper lobes:** The patient is in supine with the bed horizontal. Percussion and vibration are performed below the clavicles.

**Fig. 6-23F: Right middle lobe:** The patient is turned ¼ from supine on the left side with the foot of the bed elevated 12 inches. Percussion and vibration are performed over the right chest between the axilla and the right nipple.

**Fig. 6-23G: Superior segments left and right lower lobes:** The patient is prone with the bed horizontal. Percussion and vibration are performed below the inferior border of the left and right scapulae.

**Fig. 6-23H: Anterior basal segments left and right lower lobes:** The patient is in supine with the foot of the bed elevated 18 inches. Percussion and vibration are performed over the lower ribs on the left and right side.

**Fig. 6-23I: Posterior basal segments left and right lower lobes:** The patient is in prone with the foot of the bed elevated 18 inches. Percussion and vibration are performed over the lower ribs on the left and right side of the chest.

**Fig. 6-23J: Lateral basal segments lower lobes:** The patient is in sidelying with the foot of the bed elevated 18 inches. Percussion and vibration performed over the lower ribs. The image shows the position for the lateral segment of the left lower lobe with the patient lying on the right side. For the lateral segment of the right lower lobe, the patient lies on the left side.

## Procedure for percussion and vibration

- Place the patient in the appropriate postural drainage position.
- Cover the skin overlying the affected segment with a thin material (towel, t-shirt, hospital gown).
- Therapist rhythmically strikes the chest with a cupped hand for two to three minutes per lung segment (Fig. 6-24).
- Therapist places one hand on top of the other over affected area or one hand on each side of the rib cage.
- Vibrate the chest wall as the patient exhales by tensing the muscles of the hands and arms while applying moderate pressure downward.
- The maneuver is performed in the direction in which the ribs move on expiration.
- Encourage the patient to cough or huff after two or three vibrations.

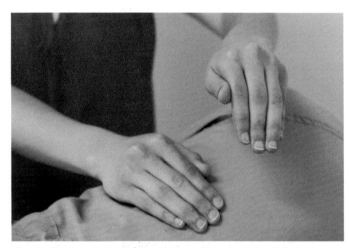

**Fig. 6-24:** Percussion of the thorax during postural drainage.

## Precautions/Contraindications

- All contraindications listed for postural drainage
- Subcutaneous emphysema
- Recent epidural spinal infusion or spinal anesthesia
- Recent skin grafts, or flaps, on the thorax
- Burns, open wounds, and skin infections of the thorax
- Recently placed transvenous or subcutaneous pacemaker
- Suspected pulmonary tuberculosis
- Lung contusion
- Bronchospasm
- Osteomyelitis of the ribs
- Osteoporosis
- Complaint of chest wall pain

## Expected outcomes of airway clearance

- Easier clearance of secretions and increased volume of secretions during and after treatments
- Improved breath sounds in the lungs being treated
- Increase in sputum production
- Change in vital signs - moderate changes in respiratory rate and/or pulse rate are expected
- Resolution or improvement of atelectasis and localized infiltrates observed with chest x-ray
- Improvement in arterial blood gas values or oxygen saturation

## Breathing Exercises

### Diaphragmatic breathing (DB)[45,46]

DB involves breathing predominantly with the diaphragm while minimizing the action of accessory muscles and motion of the upper rib cage during inspiration (Fig. 6-25).

#### Indications

- Post-surgical patient with pain in the chest wall or abdomen, or restricted mobility
- Patient learning active cycle of breathing or autogenic drainage airway clearance techniques
- Dyspnea at rest or with minimal activity
- Inability to perform ADLs due to dyspnea or inefficient breathing pattern

#### Precautions/Contraindications

- Moderate to severe COPD and marked hyperinflation of the lungs without diaphragmatic movement
- Patients with paradoxical breathing patterns, or who demonstrate increased inspiratory muscle effort, and increased dyspnea during DB

#### Procedure

- Semi-Fowler's position is a good starting position.
- Sniffing can be used to facilitate contraction of the diaphragm.
- Have the patient place one hand on the upper chest and the other just below the rib cage.
- Instruct the patient to:

*"Breathe in slowly through your nose so that your stomach moves out against your hand. The hand on your chest should remain as still as possible. Feel your abdomen gently rise into your hand. Exhale through pursed lips, let the hand on your abdomen descend, while the hand on your upper chest remains still."*

**Fig. 6-25:** A physical therapist teaches diaphragmatic breathing.

## Expected outcomes

- Decrease respiratory rate
- Decrease use of accessory muscles of inspiration
- Increase tidal volume
- Decrease respiratory flow rate
- Subjective improvement of dyspnea
- Improve tolerance for activity

### Inspiratory muscle training (IMT)[45,47,48]

IMT attempts to strengthen the diaphragm and intercostal muscles. Two different IMT devices provide different modes of training: flow resistive breathing and threshold breathing. During flow resistive breathing, the patient inspires through a mouthpiece and adapter with an adjustable diameter. Decreasing the diameter increases the resistance to breathing, provided that breathing rate, tidal volume, and inspiratory time are kept constant. Threshold loading requires a buildup of negative pressure before flow occurs through a valve that opens at a critical pressure. Threshold breathing provides consistent and specific pressure for IMT, regardless of how quickly or slowly patients breathe.

### Indications

- Impaired inspiratory muscle strength and/or a ventilatory limitation to exercise performance

### Precautions/Contraindications

- Clinical signs of inspiratory muscle fatigue (in characteristic order of appearance)
  - Tachypnea
  - Reduced tidal volume
  - Increased $PaCO_2$
  - Bradypnea and decreased minute ventilation

## Procedure

- Measure the patient's maximum inspiratory pressure (MIP) with a manometer. Use the measured MIP to calculate the training load.

### Using the Threshold® Inspiratory Muscle Trainer

- Have the patient place the mouthpiece in his or her mouth and inhale with enough force to open the valve.
- Adjust the spring tension by turning the control knob to adjust the pressure indicator to the prescribed setting.
- The device is marked every 2 centimeters $H_2O$. The higher the setting the greater the effort needed.
- Begin training with the setting that elicits 30% to 40% of the patient's MIP.
- The patient breathes against that resistance at resting respiratory rate and tidal volume for 5 to 15 minutes, two to three times daily, as tolerated.
- Resistance can be increased in small increments by adjusting the tension on the spring until the training load reaches 40 to 60% of MIP over a four to six week period.

### Using the PFLEX® Inspiratory Muscle Trainer

- Have the patient place the PFLEX® in his or her mouth and breathe at tidal volume.
- Turn the dial selector to regulate the resistance to breathing - setting 1 provides the least resistance.
- Begin training with the setting that elicits the 30% to 40% level of MIP for 10 to 15 minutes daily, gradually increasing to 20 to 30 minutes, three to five days per week.
- Once the patient can easily tolerate 30 minutes at one resistance, increase the resistance to the next setting.

### Expected outcomes

- Increase inspiratory muscle strength and endurance
- Decrease dyspnea at rest and during exercise
- Increase functional exercise capacity

### Paced breathing and exhale with effort[45]

Paced breathing is a strategy to decrease the work of breathing and prevent dyspnea during activity. It allows anyone who experiences shortness of breath to become less fearful of activity and exercise.

Exhale with effort is a breathing strategy employed during activity to prevent a patient from holding their breath. The technique breaks any activity into one or more breaths with inhalation during the resting or less active phase of the activity and exhalation during the movement or more active phase of the activity.

### Indications

- Patients with dyspnea at rest or with minimal activity
- Inability to perform activity due to pulmonary limitation
- Inefficient breathing pattern during activity

## Precautions/Contraindications

- Avoid Valsalva maneuver during activity

## Procedure

- Perform activity at a tempo that does not exceed the patient's breathing limitations.
- Find a comfortable inspiration to expiration (I:E) time to synchronize with the exertion phase of activity.
- Synchronize breathing with components of the activity:
  - inhale before or during the easier component of the activity
  - exhale during the more vigorous component of the activity
- Do not hold breath or rush through the activity.

## Walking:

- Inhale through the nose while walking two steps and then pause; exhale through pursed lips while walking four steps.

## Climbing stairs:

- Inhale through the nose while standing
- Exhale through pursed lips while stepping up (or down) one or two stairs
- Remain on the step until breathing control is restored

## Lifting:

- Inhale through the nose while standing or sitting; exhale through pursed lips while bending to reach the object
- Pause
- Inhale through the nose while grabbing the object; exhale through pursed lips while standing up

## Expected outcomes

- Complete activity without dyspnea
- Decrease patient's fear of becoming short of breath during activity

## Pursed-lip breathing (PLB)[49]

PLB is a simple technique to reduce respiratory rate, reduce dyspnea, and maintain a small positive pressure in the bronchioles, which may help prevent airway collapse in patients with emphysema. Any patient who is short of breath may use this technique.

## Indications

- Tachypnea
- Dyspnea

## Precautions/Contraindications

- Forcing exhalation

## Procedure

- Semi-Fowler's is a good position to initiate the breathing technique.

- Instruct the patient to:

*"Breathe in slowly through your nose with the mouth closed for two counts. Pucker, or purse your lips as if you were going to whistle, then gently breathe out through pursed lips, as if trying to make a candle flame flicker, for a four count. Do not blow with force."*

## Expected outcomes

- Decrease respiratory rate
- Relieve dyspnea
- Reduce arterial partial pressure of carbon dioxide ($PaCO_2$)
- Improve tidal volume
- Improve oxygen saturation
- Prevent airway collapse in patients with emphysema
- Increase activity tolerance

## Segmental breathing[45,50]

Segmental breathing, also known as localized breathing or thoracic expansion exercise, is intended to improve regional ventilation and prevent and treat pulmonary complications after surgery. It is based on the presumption that asymmetrical chest wall motion may coincide with underlying pathology (e.g., pneumonia, pleuritic chest wall pain, retained secretions) and that inspired air can be directed to a particular area by facilitation or inhibition of chest wall movement through proper hand placements, verbal cues or coordination of breathing.

## Indications

- Decreased intrathoracic lung volume
- Decreased chest wall lung compliance
- Increased flow resistance from decreased lung volume
- Ventilation:perfusion mismatch

## Precautions/Contraindications

- None

## Procedure

- Position the patient:
  - Sitting position for basal atelectasis
  - Sidelying with affected lung uppermost
  - Postural drainage positions with affected lung uppermost to assist with secretion removal
- Therapist applies firm pressure at the end of exhalation to the patient's chest wall overlying the area to be expanded.
- Patient inhales deeply and slowly expanding the rib cage under the therapist's hands.
- Therapist reduces hand pressure during the patient's inhalation.

## Expected outcomes

- Increase chest wall mobility
- Expand collapsed alveoli via airflow through collateral ventilation channels
- Assist with secretion removal

## Sustained maximal inhalation with incentive spirometer[51]

In a sustained maximal inspiration (SMI), a maximal inspiratory effort is held for three or more seconds at the point of maximum inspiration before exhalation. Many airway clearance techniques include SMI to compensate for asynchronous ventilation, to promote air passage past mucus obstructions in airways, and to maximize alveolar expansion. SMI is also called incentive spirometry when using a device that provides visual or other feedback to encourage the patient to take long, slow, deep inhalations (Fig. 6-26).

Fig. 6-26: Incentive spirometer.

### Indications

- Decreased intrathoracic lung volume
- Decreased chest wall lung compliance
- Increased flow resistance from decreased lung volume
- Ventilation:perfusion (V:Q) mismatch
- Atelectasis or risk of atelectasis due to thoracic and upper abdominal surgery
- Restrictive lung defect associated with quadriplegia and/or dysfunctional diaphragm

### Precautions/Contraindications

- Patient is not cooperative or is unable to understand or demonstrate proper use of the incentive spirometer.
- Patient is unable to deep breathe effectively (e.g., with vital capacity less than 10 mL/kg or inspiratory capacity less than one-third of predicted).
- Patients with moderate to severe COPD with increased respiratory rate and hyperinflation.

### Procedure

- Hold the incentive spirometer in a vertical position.
- Have the patient exhale completely, then seal his lips around the mouthpiece.
- Breathe in slowly and deeply through the mouth, raising the ball or piston of the spirometer.
- Encourage the patient to move the diaphragm and expand the lower chest, not the upper chest.
- Hold the breath for at least three seconds and note the highest level the piston reaches.
- Perform SMI independently five to ten breaths per hour when awake.

### Expected outcomes

- Absence of or improvement in signs of atelectasis
- Decreased respiratory rate
- Resolution of fever
- Normal pulse rate
- Normal chest x-ray
- Improved $PaO_2$
- Increased forced vital capacity and peak expiratory flows

## Positions to Relieve Dyspnea

A number of positions may be used to provide relief from dyspnea. The choice of position will depend on the circumstances at the time. The forward leaning position often provides relief of dyspnea to patients with lung disease.

Forward leaning with arm support optimizes the length-tension relationship of the diaphragm and allows the pectoralis minor and pectoralis major muscles to assist in elevating the rib cage during inspiration. The positions may be combined with other breathing techniques.

### Reverse Trendelenburg position

The opposite of the Trendelenburg position, the reverse Trendelenburg position places a person in supine with their head above their trunk and lower extremities, decreasing the weight of the abdominal contents on the diaphragm and reducing the resistance to movement during breathing.

### Semi-Fowler's position

The semi-Fowler's position places a patient in supine with the head of the bed elevated to 45 degrees and pillows under the knees for support and maintenance of a proper lumbar curve. This position is used often for patients with congestive heart failure or other cardiac conditions.

## Cardiac Rehabilitation[21,52,53]

Cardiac rehabilitation services are multidisciplinary, long-term programs involving medical evaluation, prescribed exercise, cardiac risk factor modification, education, and counseling. The goals are to limit the physiological and psychological effects of cardiac illness; reduce the risk for sudden death or reinfarction, control cardiac symptoms, stabilize or reverse the atherosclerotic process, and enhance the psychosocial and vocational status of selected patients. Services are provided along a continuum of care, beginning with early assessment and mobilization in the inpatient setting, through early outpatient rehabilitation, to long-term maintenance and follow-up.

### Clinical indications for inpatient and outpatient cardiac rehabilitation

- Medically stable post-myocardial infarction
- Stable angina pectoris
- Coronary artery bypass surgery
- Percutaneous transluminal coronary angioplasty (PTCA)
- Compensated heart failure
- Cardiomyopathy
- Heart transplant
- Other cardiac surgery (e.g., valve repair, pacemaker)
- Peripheral arterial disease
- High risk for coronary artery disease with diagnosis of diabetes mellitus, dyslipidemia, hypertension or obesity
- End-stage renal disease

### Clinical contraindications for inpatient and outpatient cardiac rehabilitation

- Unstable angina
- Resting systolic pressure > 200 mm Hg or resting diastolic pressure > 110 mm Hg
- Orthostatic blood pressure drop of > 20 mm Hg with symptoms
- Critical aortic stenosis
- Acute systemic illness or fever
- Uncontrolled atrial/ventricular arrhythmias
- Third-degree atrial ventricular block without pacemaker
- Active pericarditis or myocarditis
- Recent embolism
- Thrombophlebitis
- Resting ST segment depression or elevation > 2 mm
- Uncompensated congestive heart failure
- Orthopedic or metabolic conditions that would prohibit exercise

### Physical therapist role in cardiac rehabilitation

- Develop an individualized exercise prescription considering mode, intensity, duration, and frequency.
- Monitor heart rate, blood pressure, ECG, RPE, and signs and symptoms.
- Supervise exercise and promote proper technique and breathing patterns (Fig. 6-27)

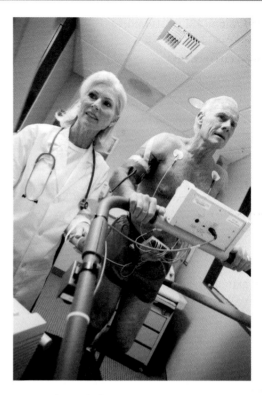

**Fig. 6-27:** A physical therapist monitoring a patient during cardiac rehabilitation.

### Inpatient Cardiac Rehabilitation (Phase I)

Phase I begins with the physician referral to cardiac rehabilitation when the patient is medically stable. Phase I consists of patient and family education, self-care evaluation, continuous monitoring of vital signs, group discussions, and low-level exercise. Exercise activities include active range of motion, ambulation, and self-care. Exercise intensity is often prescribed according to heart rate and by rating on a perceived exertion scale. The trend toward early hospital discharge following a cardiac event has resulted in Phase I programs averaging three to five days.

#### Procedure

#### Medical evaluation

- A patient may begin rehabilitation when considered medically stable by the referring physician:
  - No new or recurrent chest pain in eight hours
  - No new signs of uncompensated heart failure (e.g., dyspnea at rest with bilateral basilar crackles)
  - No new significant, abnormal heart rhythm or ECG changes in eight hours
  - Stable creatine kinase and troponin levels

#### Monitoring and safety

- Ask patient to report any chest discomfort, dyspnea or faintness that occurs during activity
- Discontinue exercise for any of the following adverse responses:

- Heart rate > 130 beats/minute or > 30 beats/minute above resting heart rate
- DBP ≥ 110 mm Hg
- Decrease in SBP > 10 mm Hg
- Significant ventricular or atrial dysrhythmias
- 2nd or 3rd degree heart block
- Signs or symptoms including angina, marked dyspnea, and ECG changes suggestive of ischemia

### Active exercise

- Active upper and lower extremity exercises may begin 24 hours after bypass graft surgery and two days after infarction.
- Active exercises progress from sitting to standing (1 – 4 METs).
- Upper extremity exercise should not stress the incisions of post-surgical patients.

### Aerobic exercise[21,52]

- Mode:
  - Progressive, supervised level walking (2 – 3 METs) to walking up and down steps or treadmill walking (3 – 4 METs).
- Intensity:
  - RPE < 13 (6-20 scale)
  - Post infarction: heart rate < 120 beats/minute OR < 20 beats/minute above resting heart rate
  - Post surgery: < 30 beats/minute above resting heart rate
- Duration:
  - Intermittent bouts of three to five minutes, progressing to 10 to 15 minutes of continuous activity.
- Frequency:
  - First three days: three to four times per day
  - After three days: two times per day with increased duration
- Progression:
  - Progress varies according to patient tolerance and risk stratification
  - Activity may be progressed provided:
    - Adequate increase in heart rate
    - Adequate rise in systolic blood pressure (10 – 40 mm Hg)
    - No new dysrhythmias or ST changes on the ECG
    - No cardiac symptoms are observed (e.g., palpitations, dyspnea, angina, excessive fatigue)

### Expected outcomes of inpatient cardiac rehabilitation

- Prevent the harmful physiological and psychological effects of bed rest during hospitalization
- Walk 5 to 10 minutes continuously, or 1000 feet, four times daily

- Walk down and up one flight of stairs independently
- Know safe heart rate and RPE limits for exercise
- Recognize abnormal signs and symptoms suggesting intolerance to activity
- Promote a more rapid and safe return to activities of daily living within the limits imposed by their disease
- Prepare the patient and home support system to optimize recovery following discharge

### Immediate Outpatient (Phase II)

Outpatient cardiac rehabilitation is a comprehensive program that includes prescribed exercise, cardiac risk factor modification, education, and counseling about diet and disease management. A Phase II program can begin immediately after hospitalization and last up to 12 weeks.

### Procedure

#### Medical evaluation

An exercise test with ECG is recommended for patients entering an outpatient program, and as changes in the patient's condition warrant, to assess:

- Heart rate and rhythm
- Signs and symptoms
- ST segment changes
- Exercise capacity
- Risk stratification
- Target heart rate for exercise
- Initial level of work for exercise

Before beginning formal physical activity, a physical examination of the patient should include:

- Medical history
- Cardiovascular disease risk profile
- Body mass index or waist-hip ratio
- Resting ECG and blood pressure
- Auscultation of lung sounds
- Palpation and inspection of extremities for arterial pulses, edema, and skin integrity
- Examination of chest and leg wounds in patients after CABG or PTCA
- Orthopedic and neuromuscular status (e.g., ROM, strength, posture, balance, activities of daily living)

#### Monitoring and safety

- For low risk patients with known stable coronary artery disease, 6 to 12 sessions of ECG and BP monitoring and medical supervision are recommended to ascertain desirable exercise levels.
- For patients at moderate to high risk and/or unable to self-regulate or to understand recommended activity levels, continuous ECG and BP monitoring and medical supervision are recommended until safety is established, usually ≥ 12 sessions.

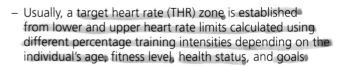

# Spotlight on Safety

## Activity Guidelines for the Patient with Angina Pectoris

A rating of one on the angina scale is the recommended endpoint to cease activity during inpatient and outpatient cardiac rehabilitation.

Individuals who experience angina during activity should discontinue the activity immediately and rest in a sitting or recumbent position until the discomfort is resolved.

Individuals with medication for angina should be encouraged to use the medication as directed.

If angina is not relieved by termination of activity or by three sublingual nitroglycerin tablets (one taken every five minutes), transport the individual to the nearest emergency center.

The exercise target heart rate for aerobic exercise training should be ≥ 10 beats/minute below the known ischemic or anginal threshold.

- Discontinue exercise for any of the following adverse responses:
  - Plateau or decrease in HR with increase in work
  - SBP plateaus or falls with increase in work or > 250 mm Hg
  - DBP > 115 mm Hg
  - ST segment depression > 1 mm
  - 2nd or 3rd degree heart block
  - Ventricular dysrhythmias
  - Angina or other symptoms of cardiovascular insufficiency

## Aerobic exercise

### Mode

- Rhythmic activities that use large muscle groups and can be performed continuously and safely (e.g., walking, hiking, running, jogging, bicycling, cross-country skiing, aerobic dance/calisthenics, rope skipping, rowing, skating, stair climbing, swimming, and various endurance game activities).

### Intensity

- Intensity can be prescribed based on heart rate, METs, and RPE.
- Heart rate (HR)
  - For patients without an entry exercise test, an exercise HR equal to standing resting heart rate + 20 beats/minute may be used with caution. A period of continuous ECG monitoring is recommended with the intensity gradually increased provided there are no symptoms, abnormal hemodynamics, ventricular dysrhythmias or ECG changes indicative of myocardial ischemia.

- Usually, a target heart rate (THR) zone is established from lower and upper heart rate limits calculated using different percentage training intensities depending on the individual's age, fitness level, health status, and goals.
  - Percent of maximum heart rate (HRmax)
    Lower THR = HRmax x 55%
    Upper THR = HRmax x 90%
  - Heart rate reserve (HRR) or Karvonen formula
    Lower THR = [(HRmax − HRrest) x 40%] + HRrest
    Upper THR = [(HRmax − HRrest) x 85%] + HRrest
    HRmax = maximum heart rate measured during a graded exercise test or estimated by 220 - age.
    HRrest = resting heart rate

- Metabolic equivalents (METs)
  - 1 MET is the energy expended while sitting quietly (3.5 mLO$_2$ /kg/min or 1 kcal/kg/h)
  - To establish a MET level training zone, maximum METs must be measured during an exercise test. Lower and upper MET limits are calculated using the same percentage training intensities as the Karvonen formula
    Lower METs = [(MaxMETs − RestMETs) x 40%] + RestMETs
    Upper METs = [(MaxMETs − RestMETs) x 85%] + RestMETs

## Rating of perceived exertion (RPE)

- RPE is a useful guide for rating exercise intensity, especially when heart rate cannot be used to regulate intensity (e.g., after heart transplant, patients taking beta blockers, individuals who do not have an exercise test prior to entering cardiac rehabilitation, individuals who cannot feel their pulse, and for patients whose clinical status or medical therapy changes).
- An RPE rating of 12 to 16 ("somewhat hard" to "hard") on the 6 - 20 scale corresponds to 40% to 85% of maximal capacity.
- RPE of 11 to 13 ("fairly light " to "somewhat hard") is an appropriate upper limit during the initial phases of outpatient cardiac rehabilitation.
- RPE of 14 to 16 may be appropriate for higher intensity training later in cardiac rehabilitation if there are no signs or symptoms of ischemia or serious dysrhythmias.
- RPE is specific to the mode of exercise.

## Duration

- 15 to 20 minutes of continuous or intermittent exercise during the first month (initial training phase).
- 25 to 30 minutes during the next three or four months (improvement stage).
- 40 minutes or longer after six months (maintenance phase).
- Interval training (exercise bouts of three to five minutes duration followed by equal rest periods) may be appropriate for patients who cannot exercise continuously.

# Consider This

## MET Values of Common Physical Activities[14]

Once the appropriate MET levels for exercise are determined for the patient, activities with the desired aerobic requirement can be selected from a published table of MET values.

| Light (< 3 METs) | Moderate (3 - 6 METs) | Vigorous (> 6 METs) |
|---|---|---|
| **Walking, Jogging, Running** | | |
| Walking slowly at home or office = 2.0 | Walking 3 mph = 3.0 – 4.0 | Walking 4.5 mph = 6.3 |
| | Walking 4 mph = 4.5 – 7.0 | Jogging 5 mph = 8.0 |
| | | Running 7 mph = 11.5 |
| **Self-care, Household, and Occupation** | | |
| Toileting = 1.0 – 2.0 | Washing windows or car = 3.0 | Shoveling = 7.0 |
| Driving a car = 1.0 – 2.0 | Sweeping, vacuuming = 3.0 – 3.5 | Carrying heavy loads = 7.5 |
| Working at a computer or desk = 1.5 | Light gardening = 3.0 – 4.0 | Heavy farm work = 8.0 |
| Making bed, washing dishes = 2.0 | Carrying, stacking wood = 5.5 | Digging ditches = 9.5 |
| Bathing = 2.0 – 3.0 | Power lawn mowing = 5.5 | |
| Cooking = 2.0 – 3.0 | | |
| **Leisure Time and Sports** | | |
| Playing cards, arts, and crafts = 1.5 | Slow dancing = 3.0 | Backpacking = 5.0 – 11.0 |
| Playing musical instrument = 2.0 – 2.5 | Table tennis = 4.0 | Basketball game = 8.0 |
| Fishing (sitting) = 2.5 | Fast dancing = 4.5 | Bicycling (flat) 12 – 14 mph = 8.0 |
| | Basketball shooting around = 4.5 | Bicycling (flat) 14 – 16 mph = 10.0 |
| | Sexual intercourse = 4.0 – 5.0 | |
| | Golf (walking) = 4.0 – 7.0 | |
| | Swimming = 4.0 – 8.0 | |
| | Tennis doubles = 5.0 | |
| | Bicycling (flat) = 10 – 12 mph = 6.0 | |

# Spotlight on Safety
Environmental Considerations for Exercise[21]

Physical therapists should be aware of the special problems encountered during exercise in hot and cold environments and at high altitudes.

### Exercise in Hot Environments

Activity in hot environments should be modified to include access to fluids, increased frequency/duration of rest breaks, and shorter exercise time.

Moderate dehydration (loss of ≥ 6% of body weight) contributes to a drop in exercise performance and increases the risk of heat illness. To maintain hydration, measure body weight before and after exercise and drink at least one pint of fluid for each pound of body weight lost.

Wear clothing with a high wicking capacity to assist in evaporative heat loss. Remove clothing and equipment to permit heat loss, especially head gear.

#### Signs and symptoms of heat-related illnesses:

**Heat stroke:** disorientation, dizziness, apathy, headache, nausea, vomiting, hyperventilation, dry skin

**Heat exhaustion:** low blood pressure, elevated heart rate and respiratory rate, wet and pale skin, weakness, dizziness

**Heat syncope:** decreased heart rate and respiratory rate, pale skin, weakness, vertigo, nausea

**Heat cramps:** localized muscle spasms progressing to debilitating muscle cramps

### Exercise in Cold Environments

Exercise in the cold may lower the angina threshold and increase the risk of death or injury in individuals with heart disease. Inhalation of cold air may exacerbate asthma.

#### Signs and symptoms of cold-related illnesses:

**Frostbite:** Loss of feeling and a white or pale appearance in fingers, toes, ear lobes, and the tip of the nose

**Hypothermia:** Body temperature < 97° Fahrenheit, shivering, confusion, disorientation, incoherence, poor coordination, slurred speech

Hypothermia develops when heat loss exceeds heat production. Factors that increase the risk of developing hypothermia include water immersion, rain, wet clothing, low body fat, age ≥ 60 years, and hypoglycemia.

Clothing should be adjusted during activity to minimize sweating and reduce sweat accumulation.

### Exercise in High-Altitude Environments

The decreased atmospheric pressure at ≥ 5000 feet reduces the partial pressure of oxygen in the air, resulting in decreased arterial oxygen levels. The immediate compensatory responses include increases in ventilation and heart rate and a decrease in performance.

Acclimatization to altitude is the best prevention and treatment for altitude-related illness. Staging, or living at a moderate elevation for as long as one week before ascending to the final elevation, minimizing activity, and maintaining hydration and food intake reduce risk and facilitate recovery. If severe signs and symptoms persist, descending to a lower altitude is effective.

#### Signs and symptoms of altitude-related illnesses:

**Acute mountain sickness:** headache, nausea, fatigue, poor appetite and sleep, mild swelling in hands, feet or face

**High altitude pulmonary edema:** crackles/rales in the lungs, cyanosis of lips and nail beds

- As fitness improves and the patient gains confidence, increase the duration of the exercise periods.

## Frequency

- Three to five days per week

## Expected outcomes of outpatient cardiac rehabilitation

- Promote an active lifestyle through increased participation in domestic, occupational, and recreational activities
- Improved functional capacity through enhanced aerobic capacity, muscular endurance and strength, flexibility, and weight management
- Lower cardiovascular risk factors
- Improve symptoms and physiological responses to physical challenges
- Modification of unhealthy behaviors and psychosocial characteristics
- Improve patient understanding of safety issues during exercise

## Pulmonary Rehabilitation[55-57]

Pulmonary rehabilitation is a medically supervised, multi-disciplinary program for patients with chronic respiratory impairment. Comprehensive services include exercise training, education, psychosocial and behavioral interventions, nutritional therapy, and outcome assessment to assist the patient to manage and cope with progressive dyspnea.

### Clinical indications for pulmonary rehabilitation

Pulmonary rehabilitation is indicated in the presence of respiratory impairments including dyspnea at rest or with exertion, hypoxemia, hypercapnia, reduced exercise tolerance or a decline in the ability to perform activities of daily living due to:

- Chronic bronchitis
- Emphysema
- Asthma
- Interstitial lung disease (sarcoidosis, occupational or environmental lung disease)
- Bronchiectasis
- Cystic fibrosis
- Lung cancer
- Chest wall disease
- Neuromuscular disease (Parkinson's, amyotrophic lateral sclerosis, multiple sclerosis)
- Preoperative and postoperative lung resection, transplantation or volume reduction
- Ventilator dependency

### Clinical contraindications/precautions for pulmonary rehabilitation

- Ischemic cardiac disease
- Congestive heart failure
- Acute cor pulmonale
- Severe pulmonary hypertension
- Significant hepatic dysfunction
- Metastatic cancer
- Renal failure
- Severe cognitive deficit that interferes with memory and compliance
- Visual, hearing or orthopedic impairments are not contraindications, but may require the exercise program to be modified

### Physical therapist role in pulmonary rehabilitation

- Administer a Six-minute walk test or other appropriate exercise tests
- Develop an individualized exercise prescription considering mode, intensity, duration, and frequency
- Monitor heart rate, blood pressure, dyspnea, and signs and symptoms
- Supervise exercise and promote proper technique and breathing patterns
- Perform airway clearance and breathing exercises, as needed
- Instruct patient in energy conservation techniques

### Procedure

### Medical evaluation[56]

- Before beginning formal physical activity, a patient examination should include:
  - Medical history
  - Nutritional assessment
  - Spirometry
  - Resting arterial blood gas
  - Arterial oxygen saturation by pulse oximeter
  - Chest x-ray
  - Resting ECG
  - Exercise test (e.g., Six-minute walk test or graded exercise test)
  - Complete blood count
  - Height and weight
  - Resting blood pressure, heart rate, and respiratory rate
  - Temperature
  - Breathing pattern
  - Auscultation of lung sounds
  - Auscultation of breath sounds

– Palpation and inspection of extremities for arterial pulses, edema, and skin integrity

– Orthopedic and neuromuscular status (ROM, strength, posture)

– Functional status

– Anxiety and depression

### Monitoring and safety

- Remind patients not to hold their breath during exercise and to exhale during the exertion phase of the activity.

- Clinical monitoring during exercise includes:

  – Signs and symptoms of exercise intolerance

  – Heart rate and blood pressure

  – ECG, if the patient has heart disease

  – RPE and dyspnea

  – Oxygen saturation via pulse oximeter

### Aerobic exercise

- Mode

  – Rhythmic activities that use large muscle groups and can be performed continuously and safely (e.g., walking, hiking, running, jogging, bicycling, cross-country skiing, aerobic dance/calisthenics, rope skipping, rowing, skating, stair climbing, swimming and various endurance games).

- Intensity

  – Target heart rate ranges used by healthy individuals or in cardiac rehabilitation generally are not applicable to patients with chronic lung disease who stop exercise at low heart rates due to ventilatory limits

  – There is no known threshold exercise intensity for training; intensity is determined primarily by patient tolerance and safety

  – Guidelines for exercise intensity include:

    - ≥ 50% of peak oxygen consumption determined from an exercise test

    - Using a dyspnea rating reported at a submaximal exercise level during an exercise test

    - 60% to 80% of the peak work rate achieved determined from an exercise test

    - A RPE of 4 to 6 on the 0 – 10 scale, or 12 to 16 on the 6 – 20 scale

    - Maintaining oxygen saturation > 90% as measured by pulse oximetry

- Duration

  – A minimum of 30 minutes of accumulated exercise per session is recommended

  – Interval training (exercise bouts of 30 seconds to three minutes followed by equal rest periods) may be appropriate for patients who cannot exercise continuously

  – As fitness improves and the patient gains confidence, increase the duration of the exercise periods

- Frequency

  – Three to five days per week

### Expected outcomes of pulmonary rehabilitation

- Increase exercise tolerance

- Increase peak oxygen uptake

- Increase endurance time during submaximal testing

- Increase functional walking distance

- Increase muscle strength and endurance

- Reduce exertional dyspnea

- Improve ability to perform activities of daily living

- Improve health-related quality of life

- Reduce anxiety and depression

# Spotlight on Safety

Summary of Key Basic Life Support Components for Adults, Children, and Infants

| Component | Adults | Children | Infants |
|---|---|---|---|
| Recognition | Unresponsive (all ages) | | |
| | No breathing or no normal breathing (i.e., only gasping) | No breathing or only gasping | |
| | No pulse palpated within 10 seconds for all ages (HCP only) | | |
| CPR sequence | Compression – Airway – Breathing | | |
| Compression rate | At least 100/min | | |
| Compression depth | At least 2 inches (5 cm) | At least 1/3 AP depth About 2 inches (5 cm) | At least 1/3 AP depth About 1.5 inches (4 cm) |
| Chest wall recoil | Allow complete recoil between compressions HCPs rotate compressors every 2 minutes | | |
| Compression interruptions | Minimize interruptions in chest compressions Attempt to limit interruptions to <10 seconds | | |
| Airway | Head tilt–chin lift (HCP suspected trauma: jaw thrust) | | |
| Compression-to-ventilation ratio (until advanced airway placed) | 30:2 1 or 2 rescuers | 30:2 Single rescuer 15:2 2 HCP rescuers | |
| Ventilations: when rescuer is untrained or trained and not proficient | Compressions only | | |
| Ventilations with advanced airway (HCP) | 1 breath every 6-8 seconds (8-10 breaths/minute) Asynchronous with chest compressions About 1 second per breath Visible chest rise | | |
| Defibrillation | Attach and use an AED as soon as available. Minimize interruptions in chest compressions before and after shock. Resume CPR beginning with compressions immediately after each shock. | | |
| AED = automated external defibrillator; AP = anterior-posterior; CPR = cardiopulmonary resuscitation; HCP = healthcare provider | | | |

From: Highlights of the 2010 American Heart Association Guidelines for CPR and ECC. American Heart Association Web site. http://static.heart.org/eccguidelines/pdf/90-1043_ECC_2010_Guidelines_Highlights_noRecycle.pdf. Accessed: January 12, 2011

# Cardiovascular/Pulmonary and Lymphatic Systems Essentials

1. The components of the cardiac conduction system include the sinoatrial (SA) node, internodal tracts, atrioventricular (AV) node, common AV bundle or bundle of His, right and left bundle branches, and Purkinje fibers.

2. Sympathetic nerves stimulate the heart to beat faster (chronotropic effect) and with greater force of contraction (inotropic effect). Parasympathetic nerves slow the heart rate (chronotropic effect) primarily through their influence on the SA node.

3. The Valsalva maneuver produces increased intrathoracic pressure, increased central venous pressure, and decreased venous return and should be avoided, especially by patients with heart, blood vessel or lung disease.

4. Ventricular systole denotes contraction of the ventricles; ventricular diastole denotes the relaxation phase.

5. Cardiac output is the product of heart rate and stroke volume. It is approximately 5.0 – 5.5 L/min in resting adults, but can increase fivefold during exercise.

6. The components of blood are plasma, red blood cells, white blood cells, and platelets.

7. Oxygen is both dissolved in the blood plasma and chemically combined to hemoglobin in red blood cells. Only about 0.3 mL $O_2$ is dissolved in 100 mL of arterial blood; the rest is attached to hemoglobin.

8. The diaphragm is the primary muscle of inspiration. Secondary muscles of inspiration are the internal and external intercostals, sternocleidomastoids, and scalenes.

9. The bronchopulmonary segments are the topographic units of the lungs. There are ten bronchopulmonary segments in the right lung and eight in the left lung.

10. The most common sign of a heart attack in both men and women is chest pain or discomfort.

11. Hypertension in adults is defined as sustained elevation of systolic blood pressure ≥ 140 mm Hg or diastolic blood pressure ≥ 90 mm Hg.

12. Pulmonary edema can be fatal if not treated. Seek immediate emergency medical assistance if the signs or symptoms of acute pulmonary edema develop including extreme shortness of breath or difficulty breathing, a feeling of suffocating or drowning, wheezing or gasping for breath, anxiety, restlessness or a sense of apprehension or a cough that produces frothy sputum tinged with blood.

13. Arterial blood gases evaluate acid–base status (pH), ventilation ($PaCO_2$), and oxygenation ($PaO_2$). Mean arterial blood gas values in adults at sea level are: pH = 7.4; $PaCO_2$ = 40 mm Hg; $PaO_2$ = 97 mm Hg; $HCO_3-$ = 24 mEq/L.

14. A complete blood count (CBC) measures red blood cell count, total white blood cell count, white blood cell differential, platelets, hemoglobin, and hematocrit.

15. Antihypertensive medications include diuretics, calcium channel blockers, ACE inhibitors, angiotensin II blockers, ß-adrenergic blockers, and alpha adrenergic antagonists.

16. Bronchodilator agents work to relieve bronchospasm by stimulating the receptors that cause bronchial smooth muscle relaxation or by blocking the receptors that trigger bronchoconstriction. Primary classifications of bronchodilators include anticholinergic, sympathomimetics, and xanthine derivatives.

17. BMI describes relative weight for height and is a useful measurement for identifying adults at increased risk for mortality and morbidity due to being overweight and obese. BMI = weight [kg] ÷ height [$m^2$].

18. Normal heart sounds are S1 (closing of the mitral and tricuspid valves) and S2 (closing of the aortic and pulmonic valves).

19. ST segment depression on the ECG may indicate ischemia of the myocardium.

20. Adventitious inspiratory or expiratory breath sounds include crackles, pleural friction rub, rhonchi, stridor, and wheeze.

21. Pulmonary function tests help to differentiate obstructive and restrictive forms of lung dysfunction. Obstructive defects are characterized by decreased expiratory flows ($FEV_1$/FVC < 70%). Restrictive defects are characterized by reduced lung volumes and relatively normal expiratory flow rates (FVC is reduced and $FEV_1$/FVC is normal or increased).

# Cardiovascular/Pulmonary and Lymphatic Systems Essentials

22. If the percent of arterial oxygen saturation of hemoglobin falls below 90% in acutely ill patients or below 85% in patients with chronic lung disease, activity should be stopped and a discussion with the physician should take place to consider adding or increasing supplemental oxygen.

23. The rate pressure product (RPP), the product of heart rate and systolic blood pressure, is a clinical index of myocardial oxygen consumption that provides an easy to measure physiologic correlate to the onset of angina pectoris or the development of ECG abnormalities in patients with previous heart disease.

24. Active cycle of breathing and autogenic drainage are breathing techniques that patients can perform independently to assist with airway clearance.

25. Huffing is a forced expiratory maneuver performed with the glottis open that can be used instead of a cough.

26. Pursed-lip breathing helps to reduce respiratory rate, reduce dyspnea, and prevent airway collapse in patients with emphysema. Any patient who is short of breath may use this technique.

27. An incentive spirometer provides visual or other feedback to encourage the patient to take long, slow, deep inhalations, which is especially important after thoracic and abdominal surgery.

28. Intensity of aerobic exercise can be regulated by heart rate, MET level, and RPE.

29. During inpatient cardiac rehabilitation, exercise intensity is usually limited to:

    – RPE < 13 (6 - 20 scale)
    – Exercise heart rate < 120 beats/minute OR < 20 beats/minute above resting heart rate for patients post infarction.
    – Exercise heart rate < 30 beats/minute above resting heart rate for patients after heart surgery

30. The target heart rate zone for exercise can be calculated using the Karvonen formula:

    – Lower THR = [(HRmax – HRrest) x 40%] + HRrest
    – Upper THR = [(HRmax – HRrest) x 85%] + HRrest

31. The exercise target heart rate should be ≥ 10 beats/minute below the patient's known anginal threshold.

32. One MET is the energy expended while sitting quietly (3.5 mLO$_2$/kg/min or 1kcal/kg/h).

33. The target MET zone for exercise can be calculated using the Karvonen formula:

    – Lower METs = [(MaxMETs – RestMETs) x 40%] + RestMETs
    – Upper METs = [(MaxMETs – RestMETs) x 85%] + RestMETs

34. RPE of 11 - 13 corresponds to the upper limit of prescribed training heart rates for patients in the early phase of outpatient cardiac rehabilitation.

35. There is no optimal exercise intensity for the aerobic exercise training of patients in pulmonary rehabilitation. Intensity is determined primarily by patient tolerance and safety.

# Cardiovascular/Pulmonary & Lymphatic Systems Proficiencies

## 1. Heart Anatomy

Identify the appropriate term for each of the specified locations. Answers must be selected from the Word Bank and can be used only once.

**Word Bank:** inferior vena cava, left ventricle, left atria, left pulmonary veins, left pulmonary arteries, left subclavian artery, left cardiac vein, left common carotid artery, right pulmonary veins, right atria, right coronary artery, superior vena cava

**2. Heart Circulation**

Identify the appropriate term for each of the specified locations. Answers must be selected from the Word Bank and can be used only once.

**Word Bank:** aortic valve, deoxygenated blood from body, deoxygenated blood to left lung, deoxygenated blood to right lung, left atria, left ventricle, mitral valve, oxygenated blood from left lung, oxygenated blood to body, pulmonary valve, right atria, right ventricle, tricuspid valve

**Cardiovascular/Pulmonary & Lymphatic Systems Proficiencies**

## 3. Vessels of the Heart

Identify the appropriate vessel of the heart based on the described function. Answers must be selected from the Word Bank and can each be used only once.

**Word Bank:** aorta, inferior vena cava, pulmonary arteries, pulmonary veins, superior vena cava

| Great Vessel | Description |
|---|---|
| a | returns blood to the right atrium from the head, neck and arms |
| b | takes blood away from the right ventricle to the left and right lungs |
| c | returns blood from the left and right lungs to the left atrium |
| d | takes blood away from the left ventricle |
| e | returns blood to the right atrium from the lower body and viscera |

## 4. Heart Valves

Identify the areas associated with each valve. Answers must be selected from the Word Bank. Answers can be used more than once.

**Word Bank:** aorta, left atrium, left ventricle, pulmonary artery, right atrium, right ventricle

a. The tricuspid valve controls blood flow between the _____ and the _____ .

b. The pulmonary valve controls blood flow between the _____ and the _____ .

c. The aortic valve controls blood flow between the _____ and the _____ .

d. The mitral valve controls blood flow between the _____ and the _____ .

## 5. Lung Capacities

Identify the components of each of the listed lung capacities. The sum of the identified components must equal the stated capacity. A list of possible components is provided in the Word Bank. The components can be used more than once.

**Word Bank:** Expiratory Reserve Volume (ERV), Functional Residual Capacity (FRC), Inspiratory Capacity (IC), Inspiratory Reserve Volume (IRV), Residual Volume (RV), Tidal Volume (TV), Vital Capacity (VC)

| Measure | Components |
|---|---|
| functional residual capacity | a |
| inspiratory capacity | b |
| total lung capacity | c |
| vital capacity | d |

# Cardiovascular/Pulmonary & Lymphatic Systems Proficiencies

## 6. Lung Volumes and Capacities

Identify the volumes and capacities most closely associated with the supplied descriptions. Answers must be selected from the Word Bank and can each be used only once.

**Word Bank:** anatomic dead space volume, expiratory reserve volume, forced vital capacity, functional residual capacity, inspiratory capacity, inspiratory reserve volume, residual volume, tidal volume, total lung capacity, vital capacity

| Volumes and Capacities | Description |
|---|---|
| a | The maximal volume of air that can be inspired after a normal tidal exhalation. |
| b | The volume of air in the lungs after normal exhalation. |
| c | The maximal volume of air that can be exhaled after a normal tidal exhalation. |
| d | The volume change that occurs between maximal inspiration and maximal expiration. |
| e | The volume of air in the lungs after a maximal inspiration; the sum of all lung volumes. |
| f | The volume of gas remaining in the lungs at the end of a maximal expiration. |
| g | The volume of air expired during a forced maximal expiration after a forced maximal inspiration. |
| h | Total volume inspired and expired with each breath during quiet breathing. |
| i | The volume of air that occupies the non-respiratory conducting airways. |
| j | The maximal volume of air inspired after normal tidal volume inspiration. |

## 7. Pathology of the Cardiovascular and Pulmonary Systems

Identify the appropriate medical condition based on the supplied descriptions. Answers must be selected from the Word Bank and can each be used only once.

**Word Bank:** acute respiratory distress syndrome, angina pectoris, asthma, atelectasis, atherosclerosis, bronchitis, cor pulmonale, cystic fibrosis, endocarditis, myocarditis, pulmonary edema, rheumatic fever

| Pathology | Description |
|---|---|
| a | hypertrophy of the right ventricle caused by altered structure or function of the lungs |
| b | an inflammatory disease that can develop as a complication of strep throat |
| c | inflammation of the bronchi characterized by hypertrophy of the mucus secreting glands |
| d | fluid collects in the alveoli in the lungs making it difficult to breathe |
| e | a transient precordial sensation of pressure or discomfort resulting from myocardial ischemia |
| f | one or more areas of the lungs collapse or fail to properly inflate |
| g | inflammation of the endothelium that lines the heart and cardiac valves |
| h | a slow progressive accumulation of fatty plaques on the inner walls of arteries |
| i | chronic inflammation of the airways caused by increased airway sensitivity to various stimuli |
| j | inflammation and weakness of the heart muscle |
| k | an autosomal recessive genetic disease of the exocrine glands |
| l | respiratory failure due to fluid accumulation in the alveoli |

# QUIZ Cardiovascular/Pulmonary & Lymphatic Systems Proficiencies

## 8. Arterial Blood Gas Values

Identify the appropriate arterial blood gas measure for each of the supplied values. Answers must be selected from the Word Bank and can each be used only once.

**Word Bank:** $HCO_3$-, $PaCO_2$, $PaO_2$, pH, $SaO_2$

| Measure | Value |
|---|---|
| a | 7.35 - 7.45 |
| b | 40 mm Hg |
| c | 97 mm Hg |
| d | 24 mEq/L |
| e | 95-98% |

## 9. Arterial Blood Gas Analysis

Identify the anticipated change in pH, $PaCO_2$, and $HCO_3$- based on the listed medical conditions. Place an ↑ or ↓ in each of the provided spaces.

| Partially Compensated | pH | $PaCO_2$ | $HCO_3$- |
|---|---|---|---|
| respiratory acidosis | a | b | c |
| respiratory alkalosis | d | e | f |
| metabolic acidosis | g | h | i |
| metabolic alkalosis | j | k | l |

## 10. Pharmacology of the Cardiovascular and Pulmonary Systems

Identify the appropriate medication based on the supplied descriptions. Answers must be selected from the Word Bank and can each be used only once.

**Word Bank:** alpha adrenergic antagonist agents, angiotensin-converting enzyme inhibitor agents, anticoagulant agents, anti-inflammatory agents, beta blocker agents, calcium channel blockers, diuretics, expectorant agents, nitrates, positive inotropic agents

| Drug | Action |
|---|---|
| a | decrease the entry of calcium into vascular smooth muscle cells |
| b | increase the excretion of sodium and urine |
| c | decrease blood pressure and afterload by suppressing a specific enzyme |
| d | decrease ischemia through smooth muscle relaxation and dilation of peripheral vessels |
| e | reduce peripheral vascular tone causing dilation of arterioles and veins resulting in decreased blood pressure |
| f | decrease myocardial oxygen demand by decreasing heart rate and contractility |
| g | increase respiratory secretions which help to loosen mucus |
| h | inhibit platelet aggregation and thrombus formation |
| i | prevent inflammatory-mediated bronchoconstriction |
| j | increase the force and velocity of myocardial contraction, slow the heart rate, and decrease conduction through the AV node |

# QUIZ Cardiovascular/Pulmonary & Lymphatic Systems Proficiencies

## 11. Hypertension

Next to each value state whether the BP is normal, prehypertensive, stage 1 hypertension, or stage 2 hypertension. Answers must be selected from the Word Bank and can each be used more than once.

**Word Bank:** normal, prehypertensive, stage 1 hypertension, stage 2 hypertension

| Blood Pressure Value | Classification |
|---|---|
| 125/89 mm Hg | a |
| 170/105 mm Hg | b |
| 155/95 mm Hg | c |
| 110/75 mm Hg | d |
| 142/105 mm Hg | e |
| 135/82 mm Hg | f |

## 12. Heart Sounds

Identify the appropriate heart sounds for each of the supplied descriptions. Answers must be selected from the Word Bank and can each be used only once.

**Word Bank:** S1, S2, S3, S4, murmur

| Heart Sound | Definition |
|---|---|
| a | closure of the aortic and pulmonic valves at the onset of diastole |
| b | closure of the mitral and tricuspid valves at the onset of systole |
| c | pathological sound of vibration of the ventricle walls with ventricular filling and atrial contraction |
| d | vibrations of the distended ventricle walls due to passive flow of blood from the atria during diastole |
| e | vibrations of longer duration than the heart sounds due to disrupted blood flow past a stenotic or regurgitant valve |

## 13. Abnormal Breath Sounds

Identify the appropriate abnormal breath sound for each of the supplied descriptions. Answers must be selected from the Word Bank and can each be used only once.

**Word Bank:** crackle, pleural friction rub, rhonchi, stridor, wheeze

| Breath Sound | Definition |
|---|---|
| a | dry, crackling sound heard during inspiration and expiration |
| b | continuous low-pitched sounds resembling snoring or gurgling during inspiration and expiration |
| c | continuous high-pitched wheeze heard with inspiration or expiration |
| d | discontinuous high-pitched popping sound heard during inspiration |
| e | continuous musical or whistling sound composed of a variety of pitches |

# QUIZ Cardiovascular/Pulmonary & Lymphatic Systems Proficiencies

## 14. Waveforms and Intervals for an Electrocardiogram

Identify the appropriate waveform or interval for each of the supplied descriptions. Answers must be selected from the Word Bank and can each be used only once.

**Word Bank:** P Wave, PR Interval, QRS Complex, QT Interval, ST Segment, T Wave

| Segment | Electrical Activity |
|---|---|
| a | time for both ventricular depolarization and repolarization |
| b | ventricular repolarization |
| c | atrial depolarization |
| d | time for atrial depolarization and conduction from the SA node to the AV node |
| e | isoelectric period following the QRS complex |
| f | ventricular depolarization and atrial repolarization |

## 15. Peripheral Pulses

Identify the appropriate artery based on the supplied descriptions. Answers must be selected from the Word Bank and can each be used only once.

**Word Bank:** brachial, carotid, dorsalis pedis, femoral, popliteal, posterior tibial, radial, ulnar

| Artery | Pulse Location |
|---|---|
| a | the medial aspect of the sternocleidomastoid muscle in the lower half of the neck |
| b | at the wrist, lateral to the flexor carpi radialis tendon |
| c | in the upper thigh, one-third of the distance from the pubis to the anterior superior iliac spine |
| d | in the space between the medial malleolus and the achilles tendon, above the calcaneus |
| e | medial to the biceps tendon and lateral to the medial epicondyle of the humerus |
| f | at the wrist, between the flexor digitorum superficialis and the flexor carpi ulnaris tendons |
| g | in the popliteal space of the posterior knee |
| h | near the center of the long axis of the foot, between the first and second metatarsal bones |

## 16. Cardiovascular and Pulmonary Systems Basics

Mark each statement as True or False. If the statement is False correct the statement in the space provided.

| True/False | Statement |
|---|---|
| a | Cardiac output refers to the volume of blood ejected by each contraction of the left ventricle. |

**QUIZ** Cardiovascular/Pulmonary & Lymphatic Systems Proficiencies

| True/False | Statement |
|---|---|
| **Correction:** | |
| b | Preload refers to the tension in the ventricular wall at the end of diastole. |
| **Correction:** | |
| c | The radial artery is assessed at the wrist, medial to the flexor carpi radialis tendon. |
| **Correction:** | |
| d | The dorsalis pedis artery is assessed near the center of the long axis of the foot, between the second and third metatarsals. |
| **Correction:** | |
| e | White blood cells, also known as leukocytes, protect the body from infection by ingesting bacteria and debris. |
| **Correction:** | |
| f | Minute volume ventilation is calculated by multiplying total lung capacity and respiratory rate. |
| **Correction:** | |
| g | The pulmonic area of the heart is auscultated by placing the diaphragm of the stethoscope over the fourth intercostal space at the left sternal border. |
| **Correction:** | |
| h | A body mass index of 27.5 would be classified as normal. |
| **Correction:** | |

# QUIZ  Cardiovascular/Pulmonary & Lymphatic Systems Proficiencies

| True/False | Statement |
|---|---|
| i | When observing an electrocardiogram, the P wave represents atrial depolarization. |
| Correction: | |
| j | A drop in systolic blood pressure greater than 5 mm Hg from baseline would warrant terminating an exercise stress test. |
| Correction: | |
| k | A rating of 14 on a rate of perceived exertion scale represents approximately 50% of the maximum heart rate during exercise on a treadmill. |
| Correction: | |
| l | Eupnea refers to the absence of spontaneous breathing. |
| Correction: | |
| m | When performing pursed lip breathing, the inspiratory phase is twice as long in duration as the expiratory phase. |
| Correction: | |
| n | Activities requiring 3-6 metabolic equivalents would be considered moderate level activity. |
| Correction: | |
| o | A compression rate of greater than or equal to 100 compressions per minute should be used when performing cardiopulmonary resuscitation on an adult. |
| Correction: | |

**Cardiovascular/Pulmonary & Lymphatic Systems Answer Key**

## 1. Heart Anatomy
a. superior vena cava
b. right pulmonary veins
c. right atria
d. right coronary artery
e. inferior vena cava
f. left ventricle
g. left cardiac vein
h. left atria
i. left pulmonary veins
j. left pulmonary arteries
k. left subclavian artery
l. left common carotid artery

## 2. Heart Circulation
a. deoxygenated blood from body
b. deoxygenated blood to right lung
c. right atria
d. pulmonary valve
e. tricuspid valve
f. right ventricle
g. aortic valve
h. left ventricle
i. mitral valve
j. left atria
k. oxygenated blood from left lung
l. deoxygenated blood to left lung
m. oxygenated blood to body

## 3. Vessels of the Heart
a. superior vena cava
b. pulmonary arteries
c. pulmonary veins
d. aorta
e. inferior vena cava

## 4. Heart Valves
a. The tricuspid valve controls blood flow between the right atrium and the right ventricle.
b. The pulmonary valve controls blood flow between the right ventricle and the pulmonary artery.
c. The aortic valve controls blood flow between the left ventricle and the aorta.
d. The mitral valve controls blood flow between the left atrium and the left ventricle.

## 5. Lung Capacities
a. $FRC = ERV + RV$
b. $IC = TV + IRV$
c. $TLC = RV + VC$ or $TLC = FRC + IC$
d. $VC = TV + IRV + ERV$

## 6. Lung Volumes and Capacities
a. inspiratory capacity
b. functional residual capacity
c. expiratory reserve volume
d. vital capacity
e. total lung capacity
f. residual volume
g. forced vital capacity
h. tidal volume
i. anatomic dead space volume
j. inspiratory reserve volume

## 7. Pathology of the Cardiovascular and Pulmonary Systems
a. cor pulmonale
b. rheumatic fever
c. bronchitis
d. pulmonary edema
e. angina pectoris
f. atelectasis
g. endocarditis
h. atherosclerosis
i. asthma
j. myocarditis
k. cystic fibrosis
l. acute respiratory distress syndrome

## 8. Arterial Blood Gas Values
a. pH
b. $PaCO_2$
c. $PaO_2$
d. $HCO_3-$
e. $SaO_2$

# Cardiovascular/Pulmonary & Lymphatic Systems Answer Key

## 9. Arterial Blood Gas Analysis

a. pH ↓
b. $PaCO_2$ ↑
c. $HCO_3$- ↑
d. pH ↑
e. $PaCO_2$ ↓
f. $HCO_3$- ↓
g. pH ↓
h. $PaCO_2$ ↓
i. $HCO_3$- ↓
j. pH ↑
k. $PaCO_2$ ↑
l. $HCO_3$- ↑

## 10. Pharmacology of the Cardiovascular and Pulmonary Systems

a. calcium channel blockers
b. diuretics
c. angiotensin-converting enzyme inhibitor agents
d. nitrates
e. alpha adrenergic antagonist agents
f. beta blocker agents
g. expectorant agents
h. anticoagulant agents
i. anti-inflammatory agents
j. positive inotropic agents

## 11. Hypertension

a. prehypertensive
b. stage 2 hypertension
c. stage 1 hypertension
d. normal
e. stage 2 hypertension
f. prehypertensive

## 12. Heart Sounds

a. S2
b. S1
c. S4
d. S3
e. murmur

## 13. Abnormal Breath Sounds

a. pleural friction rub
b. rhonchi
c. stridor
d. crackle
e. wheeze

## 14. Waveforms and Intervals for an Electrocardiogram

a. QT Interval
b. T Wave
c. P Wave
d. PR Interval
e. ST Segment
f. QRS Complex

## 15. Peripheral Pulses

a. carotid
b. radial
c. femoral
d. posterior tibial
e. brachial
f. ulnar
g. popliteal
h. dorsalis pedis

## 16. Cardiovascular and Pulmonary Systems Basics*

a. FALSE: Correction - Stroke volume refers to the volume of blood ejected by each contraction of the left ventricle.
b. TRUE
c. FALSE: Correction - The radial artery is assessed at the wrist, lateral to the flexor carpi radialis tendon.
d. FALSE: Correction - The dorsalis pedis artery is assessed near the center of the long axis of the foot, between the first and second metatarsal.
e. TRUE
f. FALSE: Correction - Minute volume ventilation is calculated by multiplying tidal volume and respiratory rate.
g. FALSE: Correction - The tricuspid area of the heart is auscultated by placing the diaphragm of the stethoscope over the fourth intercostal space at the left sternal border.
h. FALSE: Correction - A body mass index of 18.5 - 24.9 would be considered normal.
i. TRUE

# Cardiovascular/Pulmonary & Lymphatic Systems Answer Key

j.  FALSE: Correction - A drop in systolic blood pressure greater than 10 mm Hg from baseline would warrant terminating an exercise stress test.

k.  FALSE: Correction - A rating of 14 on a rate of perceived exertion scale represents approximately 70% of the maximum heart rate during exercise on a treadmill.

l.  FALSE: Correction - Apnea refers to the absence of spontaneous breathing. Eupnea refers to the normal rate and depth of breathing.

m.  FALSE: Correction - When performing pursed lip breathing, the expiratory phase is twice as long in duration as the inspiratory phase.

n.  TRUE

o.  TRUE

   *The correction presented for each false statement is an example of several possible corrections.

## Cardiovascular/Pulmonary and Lymphatic Systems References

1. Components of Blood. The Merck Manuals Online Medical Library. http://www.merckmanuals.com/home/sec14/ch169/ch169b.html#sec14-ch169-ch169b-4. Updated August 2006. Accessed January 3, 2011.

2. DePalo VA, McCool F D. Pulmonary Anatomy & Physiology. In: Hanley ME, Welsh CH, eds. **CURRENT Diagnosis & Treatment in Pulmonary Medicine**. New York, NY: McGraw-Hill; 2003. http://0-www.accessmedicine.com.lilac.une.edu/content.aspx?aID=575000. Accessed January 3, 2011.

3. Diseases and Conditions. Mayo Clinic Web site. http://www.mayoclinic.com/health/DiseasesIndex/DiseasesIndex. Accessed January 3, 2011.

4. Lawrence EC, Brigham KL. Chronic Cor Pulmonale. In: Fuster V, O'Rourke RA, Walsh RA, Poole-Wilson P, eds. **Hurst's the Heart**, 12th ed. New York, NY: McGraw-Hill; 2008. http://0-www.accessmedicine.com.lilac.une.edu/content.aspx?aID=3070848. Accessed January 13, 2011.

5. Diagnostic tests and procedures. American Heart Association Web site. http://www.heart.org/HEARTORG/Conditions/HeartAttack/SymptomsDiagnosisofHeartAttack/Diagnostic-Tests-Procedures_UCM_303929_Article.jsp. Updated November 3, 2010. Accessed January 2, 2011.

6. Chobanian AV, Bakris GL, Black HR, et al. Seventh report of the joint national committee on prevention, detection, evaluation, and treatment of high blood pressure: the JNC 7 complete report. **Hypertension**. 2003; 42: 1206–1252.

7. The Seventh Report of the Joint National Committee on Prevention, Detection, Evaluation, and Treatment of High Blood Pressure (JNC 7). National Heart Lung and Blood Institute Web site. http://www.nhlbi.nih.gov/guidelines/hypertension/jnc7full.pdf. Accessed January 3, 2011.

8. Cardiac procedures and surgeries. American Heart Association Web site. http://www.heart.org/HEARTORG/Conditions/HeartAttack/PreventionTreatmentofHeartAttack/Cardiac-Procedures-and-Surgeries_UCM_303939_Article.jsp. Updated November 3, 2010. Accessed January 2, 2011.

9. ACC/AHA 2005 Practice guidelines for the management of patients with peripheral arterial disease (lower extremity, renal, mesenteric, and abdominal aortic) **Circulation** 2006; 113:1474-1547.

10. Valve disease. Texas Heart Institute Web site. http://www.texasheartinstitute.org/HIC/Topics/Cond/valvedis.cfm Updated July 2010. Accessed January 3, 2011.

11. Asthma. American Lung Association website. http://www.lungusa.org/lung-disease/asthma/. Accessed January 3, 2011.

12. Diseases and conditions index. National Heart Lung and Blood Institute Web site. http://www.nhlbi.nih.gov/health/dci/index.html. Updated June 2010. Accessed January 3, 2010.

13. About cystic fibrosis. Cystic Fibrosis Foundation Web site. http://www.cff.org/AboutCF/. Accessed January 3, 2011.

14. 14. Watchie J. **Cardiovascular and Pulmonary Physical Therapy. A Clinical Manual.** 2nd ed. St. Louis, MO: Saunders Elsevier; 2010.

15. Tests and procedures. Mayo Clinic Web site. http://www.mayoclinic.com/health/tests-and-procedures/Test Procedure Index. Accessed January 3, 2011.

16. Fuster V, O'Rourke RA, Walsh RA, Poole-Wilson P. Nuclear Cardiology. In: Fuster V, O'Rourke RA, Walsh RA, Poole-Wilson P, eds. Hurst's The Heart, 12th ed. New York, NY: McGraw-Hill; 2008. http://0-www.accessmedicine.com.lilac.une.edu/content.aspx?aID=3059284. Accessed January 13, 2011.

17. Chang AM, Maisel AS, Hollander JE. Diagnosis of heart failure. **Heart Failure Clinics**. 2009; 5:25-35.DOI: 10.1016/j.hfc.2008.08.013.

18. Drug Facts and Comparison. Facts and Comparisons Web site. http:www.factsandcomparisons.com. Accessed January 3, 2011.

19. Monographs A-Z. Clinical Pharmacology Web site. http://www.clinicalpharmacology.com/?epm=2_1. Accessed January 3, 2011.

20. Nason KS, Maddaus MA, Luketich JD. Chest Wall, Lung, Mediastinum, and Pleura. In: Brunicardi FC, Andersen DK, Billiar TR, Dunn DL, Hunter JG, Matthews JB, Pollock RE, eds. **Schwartz's Principles of Surgery**, 9th ed. New York, NY: McGraw-Hill; 2010. http://0-www.accessmedicine.com.lilac.une.edu/content.aspx?aID=5016069. Accessed January 3, 2010.

21. American College of Sports Medicine. **ACSM's Guidelines of Exercise Testing and Prescription**. 8th ed. Philadelphia PA: Lippincott Williams & Wilkins; 2010.

22. Campeau L. The Canadian Cardiovascular Society grading of angina pectoris revisited 30 years later. **Can J Cardiol**. 2002:18:371-9.

23. Seidel HM, Ball JW, Dains JE, Benedict GW. **Mosby's Guide to Physical Examination**. 4th ed. St. Louis, MO: Mosby; 1999.

24. LeBlond RF, DeGowin RL, Brown DD. Cardiovascular and Respiratory Signs. DeGowin's Diagnostic Examination. 9th ed. New York: McGraw-Hill Medical; 2009. http://0-www.accessmedicine.com.lilac.une.edu/content.aspx?aID=3661627. Accessed January 3, 2011.

25. Assessing your weight and health risk. National Heart Lung and Blood Institute website. http://www.nhlbi.nih.gov/health/public/heart/obesity/lose_wt/risk.htm. Accessed January 3, 2011.

26. Zuther JE. Lymphedema Management. **The Comprehensive Guide for Practitioners**. New York, NY: Thieme; 2005

## Cardiovascular/Pulmonary and Lymphatic Systems References

27. *Guide to Physical Therapist Practice*. 2nd ed. Phys Ther. 2001; 81:583.

28. Wullink M, Stoffers HE, Kuipers H. A primary care walking exercise program for patients with intermittent claudication. *Med Sci Sports Exerc*. 2001; 33:1629-1634.

29. Borg G. Borg's Perceived Exertion and Pain Scales. Champaign IL: Human Kinetics; 1998.

30. Prasad SA, Randall SD, Balfour-Lynn IM. Fifteen-count breathlessness score: an objective measure for children. *Pediatr Pulmonol*. 2000 30(1):56-62.

31. American Thoracic Society. Dyspnea. Mechanisms, assessment, and management: A consensus statement. *Am J Respir Crit Care Med*. 1999; 159:3321-340.

32. Goldberger AL. *Clinical Electrocardiography: A Simplified Approach*. 7th ed. Philadelphia, PA: Mosby Elsevier; 2006.

33. American Thoracic Society. The diagnostic approach to acute venous thromboembolism. Clinical practice guideline. *Am J Respir Crit Care Med*. 1999; 160:1043-1066.

34. O'Rourke RA, Shaver JA, Silverman ME. The History, Physical Examination, and Cardiac Auscultation. In: Fuster V, O'Rourke RA, Walsh RA, Poole-Wilson P, eds. *Hurst's The Heart*, 12th ed. New York, NY: McGraw-Hill; 2008. http://0-www.accessmedicine.com.lilac.une.edu/content.aspx?aID=3057120. Accessed January 3, 2011.

35. Miller MR, Hankinson J, Brusasco V, Burgos R, et al. Standardisation of spirometry. *Eur Respir J.* 2005; 26: 319-338.

36. American Thoracic Society. Lung function testing: Selection of reference values and interpretative strategies. *Am Rev Respir Dis*. 1991; 144:1202-1218.

37. AARC Clinical Practice Guideline: Exercise testing for evaluation of hypoxemia and/or desaturation. *Respir Care*. 1992; 37: 907-912.

38. Borg GAV: Psychophysical bases of perceived exertion. *Med Sci Sports Exerc.* 1982;14:377.

39. Wallace J. Principles of cardiorespiratory endurance programming. In: *ACSM's Resource Manual for Guidelines for Exercise Testing and Prescription*. Philadelphia, PA: Lippincott Williams & Wilkins; 2006; 336-349.

40. Krider SJ. Vital Signs. In: Wilkins RL, Krider SJ, Sheldon RL, eds. *Clinical Assessment in Respiratory Care*, 4th ed. St. Louis, MO: Mosby; 2000.

41. ATS statement: Guidelines for the six-minute walk test. *Am J Respir Crit Care Med*. 2002; 166:111-117.

42. AARC Clinical Practice Guideline. Postural drainage therapy. *Respir Care*. 1991; 36:1418-1426

43. Hardy KA. A review of airway clearance: new techniques, indications and recommendations. *Respir Care*. 1994; 39:440.

44. AARC Clinical Practice Guideline. Directed cough. *Respir Care*. 1993; 38:495-499

45. Levenson CR. Breathing exercises. In: *Pulmonary Management in Physical Therapy*. In: Zadai CC. Ed. New York, NY; 1992: 135-155.

46. Cahalin LP, Braga M, Matsuo Y, Hernandez ED. Efficacy of diaphragmatic breathing in persons with chronic obstructive pulmonary disease: a review of the literature. *J Cardiopulm Rehabil.* 2002; 22:7-21.

47. Shekleton M, Berry JK, Covey MK. Respiratory muscle weakness and training. In: Frownfelter D, Dean E, eds. *Principles and Practice of Cardiopulmonary Physical Therapy*. 3rd ed. St. Louis, Mo: Mosby; 1996: 443-452.

48. Lotters F, van Tol B, Kwakkel G, Gosselink R. Effects of controlled inspiratory muscle training in patients with COPD: a meta-analysis. *Eur Respir*. 2002; 20:570-576.

49. Gosselink R. Controlled breathing and dyspnea in patients with chronic obstructive pulmonary disease (COPD) *J Rehabil Res Dev.* 2003;40(5): Suppl 2:25-33.

50. Humberstone N, Tecklin JS. Respiratory treatment. In: Irwin S, Tecklin JS, eds. *Cardiopulmonary Physical Therapy*. 3rd ed. St. Louis, Mo: Mosby; 1995; 356-374.

51. AARC Clinical Practice Guideline. Incentive spirometry. *Respir Care*. 1991; 36:1402-1405.

52. American Association of Cardiovascular & Pulmonary Rehabilitation. *Guidelines for Cardiac Rehabilitation and Secondary Prevention Programs.* 4th ed. Champaign,IL: Human Kinetics; 2004.

53. Balady GJ, Ades PA, Comoss P, Limacher M, et al. Core components of cardiac rehabilitation/secondary prevention programs: A statement for healthcare professionals from the American Heart Association and the American Association of Cardiovascular and Pulmonary Rehabilitation. *Circulation*. 2000;102:1069-1073.

54. Keteyian SJ, Brawner CA. Cardiopulmonary Adaptations to Exercise. In: Kaminsky LA, ed. ACSM's *Resource Manual for Guidelines for Exercise Testing and Prescription*. 5th ed. Baltimore, MD: Williams & Wilkins; 2006.

55. AARC Clinical Practice Guideline Pulmonary Rehabilitation. *Respir Care* 2002; 47:617-625.

56. American Association of Cardiovascular & Pulmonary Rehabilitation. *Guidelines for Pulmonary Rehabilitation Programs*. 3rd ed. Champaign, IL: Human Kinetics; 2004.

57. Troosters T, Casaburi R, Gosselink R, Decramer M. Pulmonary rehabilitation in chronic obstructive pulmonary disease. Am J Respir Crit Care Med 2005:172:19-38.

# 7

## OTHER SYSTEMS

**Therese Giles**
**Scott Giles**
**Danielle Cowan**
**Ryan Bailey**

Other Systems represents approximately 15.5% (31 questions) of the National Physical Therapy Examination.

The actual number of questions in this category can range from 28 to 40 questions.

313 Integumentary System

333 Metabolic System

337 Endocrine System

346 Gastrointestinal System

354 Genitourinary System

360 Obstetrics

364 System Interactions

364 Oncology

374 Psychological Disorders

378 Bariatrics

381 Nutrition

385 Essentials

388 Proficiencies

SCOREBUILDERS

# Integumentary System

## Foundational Science: Integumentary System

The integumentary system (or skin) is the body's largest organ consisting of stratified dermal and epidermal layers, hair follicles, nails, sebaceous glands, and sweat glands. The avascular epidermis is the most superficial layer of skin. The dermis, known as the true skin, is well vascularized, and is characterized as elastic, flexible, and tough (Fig. 7-1).[1]

### Key Functions of the Integumentary System

- Protection
- Sensation
- Thermoregulation
- Excretion of sweat
- Vitamin D synthesis

### Phases of Normal Wound Healing[1,2]

Normal wound healing occurs as damaged tissues move through distinct yet overlapping phases of repair. In chronic wounds, this progression is either interrupted or delayed causing the wound to become "stuck" in a particular phase of healing.

### Inflammatory Phase (1 to 10 days)[3,4]

Inflammation is the immune system's initial response to a wound. Temporary repair mechanisms rapidly re-establish hemostasis through platelet activation and the clotting cascade. Debris and necrotic tissue are removed and bacteria are killed by mast cells, neutrophils, and leukocytes. Processes occurring in the inflammatory phase establish a clean wound bed which signals tissue restoration and permanent repair processes to begin. Re-epithelialization typically begins within 24 hours at the wound borders, though visible signs are usually not observed earlier than three days after injury.

### Proliferative Phase (3 to 21 days)[3,4]

The formation of new tissue signals the beginning of the proliferative phase. Capillary buds and granulation tissue begin to fill the wound bed creating a support structure for the migration

of epithelial cells. Keratinocytes, endothelial cells, and fibroblasts are active and the collagen matrix is formed. Skin integrity is restored in the proliferative phase with wound closure occurring through epithelialization and wound contraction.

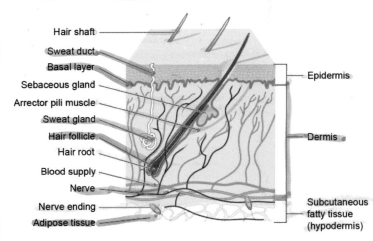

**Fig. 7-1:** Anatomy of the skin.

### Maturation Phase (7 days to 2 years)[3,4]

The maturation, or remodeling phase is initiated when granulation tissue and epithelial differentiation begin to appear in the wound bed. As the maturation phase progresses, mechanisms of fiber reorganization and contraction shrink and thin the scar. An immature scar will appear red, raised, and rigid while a mature scar will appear pale, flat, and pliable. Scar tissue is remodeled and strengthened through the processes of collagen lysis and synthesis. Newly repaired tissues have approximately 15% of pre-injury tensile integrity and should be protected to prevent re-injury. Over time, tensile integrity may increase to as much as 80% of the pre-injury strength. Hypertrophic scarring, especially in relation to burn injuries, can significantly impact maturation phase progression. A burn without hypertrophic scarring will typically mature within four to eight weeks; burns with hypertrophic scarring, however, may require up to two years to reach maturity.

## Consider This

### The Inflammatory Phase and Chronic Wounds[2]

An abnormal inflammatory response (e.g., chronic or delayed) is believed to be the most significant factor in delayed wound healing and chronicity. Re-injury, infection, poor tissue perfusion or the body's failure to initiate appropriate responses may prolong the inflammatory phase. Inflammation that persists chronically for weeks or months interferes with the initiation of proliferative phase processes and increases the risk of infection.

Anti-inflammatory or immunosuppressive medications, arterial insufficiency or conditions that alter immune responses (e.g., diabetes mellitus, alcoholism, AIDS) can limit the body's response to a wound. This can occur to the extent that the healing process is never truly initiated, resulting in a chronic wound. Differing from chronically inflamed wounds, chronic wounds show little if any of the usual inflammatory phase characteristics and fail to progress.

## Healing by Intention[2,4]

### Primary Intention

Healing by primary intention most commonly occurs in acute wounds with minimal tissue loss. Smooth clean edges are reapproximated and closed with sutures, staples or adhesives to facilitate re-epithelialization. Superficial partial thickness wounds, such as abrasions or blisters, also heal by primary intention with epithelial migration over the wound bed frequently completed within 72 hours. Wounds healing by primary intention typically have minimal scarring and heal quickly in an uncomplicated and orderly progression (e.g., surgical incision, laceration, puncture, and superficial and partial-thickness wounds).

### Secondary Intention

Healing by secondary intention permits wounds to close on their own without superficial closure. Wounds with characteristics such as significant tissue loss or necrosis, irregular or nonviable wound margins that cannot be reapproximated, infection or debris contamination typically heal by secondary intention. These wounds are often associated with pathology such as diabetes, ischemic conditions, pressure damage or inflammatory disease. A layer of granulation tissue will gradually fill the wound bed to the level of the surrounding skin, with closure occurring by wound contraction and scar formation. Wounds healing by secondary intention require ongoing wound care and have significantly larger scars than those healing by primary intention (e.g., neuropathic, arterial, venous or pressure ulcers, most full-thickness wounds, and chronically inflamed wounds).

### Tertiary Intention

Healing by tertiary intention may also be referred to as delayed primary intention healing. Wounds at risk for developing complications, such as sepsis or dehiscence, may be temporarily left open. Once risk factors have been alleviated (e.g., wounds with significant edema, contamination from debris, at high risk for infection or with questionable vascular integrity) the wound is closed by the usual primary intention methods.

## Factors Influencing Wound Healing

There are a variety of factors, not inherent to the wound itself, which can significantly impact the rate and degree of wound healing. Physical therapists should encourage patients to make positive changes with modifiable factors and assist them in compensating for unmodifiable factors.

**Age:** The epidermis thins and flattens as part of the aging process, making it more fragile and susceptible to injury from friction and shear. Decreased metabolism in older adults is also correlated with a decrease in the overall rate of wound healing.[2,4]

**Co-morbidities:** Medical co-morbidities such as cardio-pulmonary disease, vascular conditions, and diabetes mellitus can significantly delay wound healing. This is often attributed to poor tissue perfusion which limits the wound's ability to sustain cellular activity. Co-morbidities which suppress or compromise the immune system can result in altered inflammatory responses and increased risk of infection.[1,2]

**Edema:** Some degree of edema is considered a normal part of the body's inflammatory response to a wound. However, increased tissue pressure from excessive edema, such as with venous insufficiency or lymphedema, can negatively impact both tissue perfusion and the removal of cellular waste. This alteration in hemodynamics decreases the availability of oxygen and nutrients thus delaying healing and increasing the risk of infection.[1,2]

**Harsh or Inappropriate Wound Care:** Failure to use appropriate technique or best-practice interventions in wound care can contribute to wound healing delays. Vigorous wound irrigation, aggressive debridement, prolonged whirlpool exposure or the use of harsh cleansing techniques and agents can impair healing by further damaging peripheral and granulating tissues.[4]

**Infection:** Wound infection negatively impacts the restorative processes necessary for wound healing. Immune responses become overwhelmed as infectious bacteria compete with the body's own cells for available nutrients. Infectious bacteria can also release toxins into the wound causing further tissue damage and increasing the rate of cellular necrosis.[1,2]

**Lifestyle:** Regular physical activity and good nutrition facilitate wound healing by enhancing tissue perfusion and the availability of nutrients needed to sustain cellular activity. In contrast, smoking dramatically impedes wound healing by limiting the blood's oxygen carrying capacity. The resulting wound hypoxia slows healing and creates an ideal environment for anaerobic bacteria growth, thereby increasing the risk of wound infection.[1,2]

**Medication:** Medications from a variety of pharmacological classes can negatively impact wound healing. Common classes include anti-inflammatory, immunosuppressive, anti-coagulant, anti-neoplastic, steroid, and oral contraceptive agents. Undesirable physiologic effects may include a poor or prolonged in-

flammatory response, reduced blood supply, delayed collagen synthesis, and decreased tensile strength of repaired tissues.[1,2]

**Obesity:** Obesity is associated with numerous medical co-morbidities in addition to various inherent factors that may negatively impact wound healing. Poor periwound skin quality is susceptible to fissuring, which increases the risk of wound infection. Increased skin tension heightens the risk of skin tears and limits options for reapproximation. Large skin folds create moist, warm environments contributing to skin maceration and bacterial growth which may lead to both the onset and perpetuation of wounds in skin crevasses.[2,5]

## Consider This

### Contaminated, Colonized or Infected?[4]

**Contamination:** The presence of non-replicating bacteria on a wound surface that causes no additional tissue injury and does not stimulate an inflammatory immune response.

**Colonization:** The presence of replicating bacteria on a wound surface that does not invade or further injure tissues and does not stimulate an inflammatory immune response. Colonization can delay wound healing, however, colonized bacteria occasionally benefit wound healing by preventing more virulent organisms from proliferating in the wound bed.

**Infection:** The presence of replicating bacteria that invades viable tissue beyond the wound surface causing a visible inflammatory immune response. Infection will significantly delay wound healing and, if untreated, can progress to sepsis, osteomyelitis, and gangrene.

# Wound Types

### Acute Wounds[2]

**Abrasion:** An abrasion is a wound caused by a combination of friction and shear forces, typically over a rough surface, resulting in the scraping away of the skin's superficial layers.

**Avulsion:** A soft tissue avulsion, sometimes referred to as degloving, is a serious wound resulting from tension that causes skin to become detached from underlying structures.

**Incisional wound:** An incisional wound is most often associated with surgery and is created intentionally by means of a sharp object such as a scalpel or scissors.

**Laceration:** A laceration is a wound or irregular tear of tissues, often associated with trauma. Lacerations can result from shear, tension or high force compression with the resultant wound characteristics dependent on the mechanism of injury.

**Penetrating:** A penetrating wound can result from various mechanisms of injury and is described as a wound that enters the interior of an organ or cavity.

**Puncture:** A puncture wound is made by a sharp pointed object as it penetrates the skin and underlying tissues. Typically, there is relatively little tissue damage beyond the wound tract, however, the risks of contamination and infection can be significant.

**Skin tear:** A skin tear often results from trauma to fragile skin such as bumping into an object, adhesive removal, shear or friction forces. The severity of a skin tear can range from a flap-like tear, that may or may not remain viable, to full-thickness tissue loss.

### Ulcers

### Arterial Insufficiency Ulcers[1,2]

Wounds resulting from arterial insufficiency occur secondary to inadequate circulation of oxygenated blood (e.g., ischemia) often due to complicating factors such as atherosclerosis.

**General Recommendations:**

- Rest
- Limb protection
- Risk reduction education
- Inspect legs and feet daily
- Avoid unnecessary leg elevation
- Avoid using heating pads or soaking feet in hot water
- Wear appropriately sized shoes with clean, seamless socks

## Consider This

### Assessing Protective Sensation[4]

The loss of protective sensation in individuals with peripheral neuropathy can significantly increase the risk of tissue damage. Monofilament testing is a reliable method of assessing and documenting changes in protective sensation. Monofilament testing kits contain a variety of filament thicknesses which are applied perpendicular to the skin and held in place for one second with enough force to bend the filament into a "C" shape (Fig. 7-2).

Failure to perceive the application of a 10 gm monofilament indicates a loss of protective sensation (e.g., inability to feel a small pebble in a shoe or a developing blister) and places a patient at increased risk for developing a neuropathic ulcer. Failure to perceive a 75 gm monofilament indicates that an area is insensate.[4]

**Fig. 7-2:** A monofilament applied perpendicular to the target area.

## Venous Insufficiency Ulcers[1,2]

Wounds resulting from venous insufficiency occur secondary to impaired functioning of the venous system resulting in inadequate circulation and eventual tissue damage and ulceration.

**General Recommendations:**

- Limb protection
- Risk reduction education
- Inspect legs and feet daily
- Compression to control edema
- Elevate legs above the heart when resting or sleeping
- Attempt active exercise including frequent range of motion
- Wear appropriately sized shoes with clean, seamless socks

## Neuropathic Ulcers[1,2]

Neuropathic ulcers are a secondary complication usually associated with a combination of ischemia and neuropathy. Neuropathic ulcers are often associated with diabetes mellitus, however, any form of peripheral neuropathy poses an increased risk of wound development.

**General Recommendations:**

- Limb protection
- Risk reduction education
- Inspect legs and feet daily
- Inspect footwear for debris prior to donning
- Wear appropriately sized off-loading footwear with clean, cushioned, seamless socks

## Pressure Ulcers[1,2]

Pressure ulcers, also referred to as decubitus ulcers, result from sustained or prolonged pressure on tissue at levels greater than that of capillary pressure. Skin covering bony prominences is particularly susceptible to localized ischemia and tissue necrosis due to pressure. Pressure injuries to deeper tissues may initially present as bruising or purple blisters under intact skin before opening to reveal full-thickness damage. Factors contributing to pressure ulcers include shearing forces, moisture, heat, friction, medications, muscle atrophy, malnutrition, and debilitating medical conditions. Valid and reliable pressure injury risk assessment tools are readily available (e.g., Braden Scale, Norton Scale) and typically include intervention recommendations based on the level of risk assessed.

**General Recommendations:**

- Repositioning every two hours in bed
- Management of excess moisture
- Off-loading with pressure relieving devices
- Inspect skin daily for signs of pressure damage
- Limit shear, traction, and friction forces over fragile skin

| | Characteristics of Lower Extremity Ulcers[1,2,4] | | |
|---|---|---|---|
| | **Arterial Insufficiency Ulcers** | **Venous Insufficiency Ulcers** | **Neuropathic Ulcers** |
| **Location** | Lower one-third of leg, toes, web spaces (distal toes, dorsal foot, lateral malleolus) | Proximal to the medial malleolus | Areas of the foot susceptible to pressure or shear forces during weight bearing |
| **Appearance** | Smooth edges, well defined; lack granulation tissue; tend to be deep | Irregular shape; shallow | Well-defined oval or circle; callused rim; cracked periwound tissue; little to no wound bed necrosis with good granulation |
| **Exudate** | Minimal | Moderate/heavy | Low/moderate |
| **Pain** | Severe | Mild to moderate | None, however dysesthesia may be reported |
| **Pedal Pulses** | Diminished or absent | Normal | Diminished or absent; unreliable ankle-brachial index with diabetes |
| **Edema** | Normal | Increased | Normal |
| **Skin Temperature** | Decreased | Normal | Decreased |
| **Tissue Changes** | Thin and shiny; hair loss; yellow nails | Flaking, dry skin; brownish discoloration | Dry, inelastic, shiny skin; decreased or absent sweat and oil production |
| **Miscellaneous** | Leg elevation increases pain | Leg elevation lessens pain | Loss of protective sensation |

**Additional detail regarding pressure ulcer characteristics and the National Pressure Ulcer Advisory Panel (NPUAP) descriptions are found in the Wound Assessment section.

# Wound Assessment

## Wound Classification by Depth of Injury[4]

Wounds that are not categorized as pressure or neuropathic ulcers (e.g., skin tears, surgical wounds, venous stasis ulcers) are classified based on the depth of tissue loss.

### Superficial wound

A superficial wound causes trauma to the skin with the epidermis remaining intact, such as with a non-blistering sunburn. A superficial wound will typically heal as part of the inflammatory process.

### Partial-thickness wound

A partial-thickness wound extends through the epidermis and possibly into, but not through, the dermis. Examples include abrasions, blisters, and skin tears. A partial-thickness wound will typically heal by re-epithelialization or epidermal resurfacing depending on the depth of injury.

### Full-thickness wound

A full-thickness wound extends through the dermis into deeper structures such as subcutaneous fat. Wounds deeper than 4 millimeters are typically considered full-thickness and heal by secondary intention.

### Subcutaneous wound

Subcutaneous wounds extend through integumentary tissues and involve deeper structures such as subcutaneous fat, muscle, tendon or bone. Subcutaneous wounds typically require healing by secondary intention.

## Wagner Ulcer Grade Classification Scale

| Grade | Description |
|:-----:|-------------|
| 0 | No open lesion, but may possess pre-ulcerative lesions; healed ulcers; presence of bony deformity |
| 1 | Superficial ulcer not involving subcutaneous tissue |
| 2 | Deep ulcer with penetration through the subcutaneous tissue; potentially exposing bone, tendon, ligament or joint capsule |
| 3 | Deep ulcer with osteitis, abscess or osteomyelitis |
| 4 | Gangrene of digit |
| 5 | Gangrene of foot requiring disarticulation |

## Wagner Ulcer Grade Classification System[1,2]

The Wagner Ulcer Grade Classification System categorizes dysvascular ulcers based on wound depth and the presence of infection. Most commonly associated with the assessment of diabetic foot ulcers, the scale can be appropriately used to categorize most ulcers arising from neuropathic, ischemic or arterial etiology.

## Pressure Ulcer Staging

A pressure ulcer describes a localized injury to the skin and/or underlying tissue usually over a bony prominence, as a result of pressure or pressure in combination with shear and/or friction forces. A number of contributing or confounding factors are also associated with pressure ulcers including excessive moisture, friction, and shear forces.

**Stage I:** Intact skin with non-blanchable redness of a localized area usually over a bony prominence. Darkly pigmented skin may not have visible blanching, but instead present as local coloration differing from the surrounding area. The area may be painful, firm, soft, warmer or cooler as compared to adjacent tissue. Stage I may be difficult to detect in individuals with dark skin tones.

**Stage II:** Partial-thickness tissue loss of the dermis presenting as a shallow open ulcer with a red or pink wound bed. May present as an intact or ruptured serum-filled blister or presents as a shiny or dry shallow ulcer without slough or bruising. This stage should not be used to describe skin tears, tape burns, perineal dermatitis, maceration or excoriation.

**Stage III:** Full-thickness tissue loss. Subcutaneous fat may be visible but bone, tendon or muscle are not exposed. Slough may be present, but does not obscure the depth of tissue loss. May include undermining and tunneling. Bone and tendon are not visible or directly palpable. The depth of a stage III pressure ulcer varies by anatomical location. For example, a stage III ulcer on the bridge of the nose, ear, occiput, and malleolus, where there is not significant subcutaneous tissue, can be quite shallow. In contrast, areas with significant adipose tissue can develop extremely deep stage III pressure ulcers.

**Stage IV:** Full-thickness tissue loss with exposed bone, tendon or muscle that is visible or directly palpable. Slough or eschar may be present on some parts of the wound bed. Undermining and tunneling may be present. The depth of a stage IV pressure ulcer varies by anatomical location. For example, a stage IV pressure ulcer on the bridge of the nose, ear, occiput, and malleolus will have a shallow presentation. Stage IV ulcers can extend into muscle and supporting structures (e.g., fascia, tendon, joint capsule) making osteomyelitis possible.

**Suspected Deep Tissue Injury:** Purple or maroon localized areas of intact skin or blood-filled blister due to damage of underlying soft tissue from pressure and/or shear forces. The area may be preceded by tissue that is painful, firm, mushy, boggy, warmer or cooler as compared to adjacent tissue. Deep tissue injury may be difficult to detect in individuals with dark skin tones. The evolution may include a thin blister over a dark wound bed. The wound may further evolve and become covered by thin eschar. Evolution may be rapid, exposing additional layers of tissue even with optimal treatment.

**Unstageable:** Full-thickness tissue loss in which the base of the ulcer is covered by slough (yellow, tan, gray, green or brown) and/or eschar (tan, brown or black) in the wound bed. Until enough slough and/or eschar is removed to expose the base of the wound, the true depth, and therefore stage, cannot be determined. Stable (dry, adherent, intact without erythema or fluctuating appearance) eschar on the heels serves as "the body's natural (biological) cover" and should not be removed.

Adapted from NPUAP's Pressure Ulcer Staging System, Revised 2007

# Spotlight on Safety
## Integumentary Injury and Autonomic Dysreflexia[3]

Ingrown toenails, burns, pressure ulcers, blisters, and other integumentary trauma can trigger an episode of autonomic dysreflexia when occurring below the level of a patient's spinal cord injury.

Since this is a potentially life-threatening condition, it is important for therapists to recognize signs, symptoms, and causative factors of the condition as well as how to immediately and appropriately intervene. If symptoms do not begin to resolve after the patient has been assisted into a sitting position with catheter obstruction ruled out, the therapist should activate the emergency response system and begin to assess for other potential sources of noxious stimuli.

## Bony Prominences Associated with Pressure Injuries[1]

| Supine | Prone | Sidelying | Sitting (Chair) |
|---|---|---|---|
| Occiput | Forehead | Ears | Spine of the scapula |
| Spine of scapula | Anterior portion of acromion process | Lateral portion of acromion process | Vertebral spinous processes |
| Inferior angle of scapula | Anterior head of humerus | Lateral head of humerus | Ischial tuberosities |
| Vertebral spinous processes | Sternum | Lateral epicondyle of humerus | |
| Medial epicondyle of humerus | Anterior superior iliac spine | Greater trochanter | |
| Posterior iliac crest | Patella | Head of fibula | |
| Sacrum | Dorsum of foot | Lateral malleolus | |
| Coccyx | | Medial malleolus | |
| Heel | | | |

## Exudate Classification[1]

**Serous:** Presents with a clear, light color and a thin, watery consistency. Serous exudate is considered to be normal in a healthy healing wound and is observed during the inflammatory and proliferative phases of healing.

**Sanguineous:** Presents with a red color and a thin, watery consistency. The red appearance of sanguineous exudate is due to the presence of blood which may become brown if allowed to dehydrate. Sanguineous exudate may be indicative of new blood vessel growth or the disruption of blood vessels.

**Serosanguineous:** Presents with a light red or pink color and a thin, watery consistency. Serosanguineous exudate is considered to be normal in a healthy healing wound and is typically observed during the inflammatory and proliferative phases of healing.

**Seropurulent:** Presents as cloudy or opaque, with a yellow or tan color and a thin, watery consistency. Seropurulent exudate may be an early warning sign of an impending infection and is always considered an abnormal finding.

**Purulent:** Presents with a yellow or green color and a thick, viscous consistency. Purulent exudate is generally an indicator of wound infection and is always considered an abnormal finding.

# Consider This

## Components of Wound Examination and Documentation[4]

There are a number of important areas that therapists must thoroughly assess and document when examining a wound. Each element provides the therapist with potentially useful information that can guide the therapist when developing an individualized plan of care (Fig. 7-3).

- etiology
- location
- wound type and classification
- clinical signs of infection
- area, depth, and shape of wound
- condition of wound margins/edges
- undermining or tunneling
- involvement of underlying structures (e.g., tendon/bone/muscle)
- stage of healing
- color of base
- odor
- exudate type and volume
- chronicity
- response to previous treatment
- surrounding skin/scar assessment
- presence of necrosis

**Fig. 7-3:** Quantifying the area of a wound.

## Necrotic Tissue Types[1,4]

Necrotic tissue is dead tissue resulting from the localized physiological and enzymatic changes associated with cell death. Necrotic tissue is often documented and named by the specific type observed, and may also be referred to as devitalized or nonviable tissue. The color, consistency, and adherence of necrotic tissue varies depending on other wound characteristics such as hydration and bacterial activity.

**Eschar:** Eschar is described as hard or leathery, black/brown, dehydrated tissue that tends to be firmly adhered to the wound bed.

**Gangrene:** Gangrene refers to the death and decay of tissue resulting from an interruption in blood flow to an area of the body. Some types of gangrene are also characterized by the presence of bacterial infection. Gangrene most commonly affects the extremities, but can also occur in muscles and internal organs.

**Hyperkeratosis:** Hyperkeratosis, also referred to as callus, is typically white/gray in color and can vary in texture from firm to soggy depending on the moisture level in surrounding tissue.

**Slough:** Slough is described as moist, stringy or mucinous, white/yellow tissue that tends to be loosely attached in clumps to the wound bed.

# Wound Healing Interventions

## Red-Yellow-Black System[2]

| Red-Yellow-Black System | | |
|---|---|---|
| Color | Wound Description | Goals |
| Red | Pink granulation tissue | Protect wound; maintain moist environment |
| Yellow | Moist, yellow slough | Remove exudate and debris; absorb drainage |
| Black | Black, thick eschar firmly adhered | Debride necrotic tissue |

## Selective Debridement[2]

Selective debridement involves the removal of only nonviable tissues from a wound. Selective debridement is most often performed by sharp debridement, enzymatic debridement or autolytic debridement.

### Sharp Debridement

Sharp debridement requires the use of a scalpel, scissors, and/or forceps to selectively remove devitalized tissue, foreign material or debris from a wound. Sharp debridement is most often used for wounds with large amounts of thick, adherent, necrotic tissue; however, it may also be used in the presence of cellulitis or sepsis. Sharp debridement is the most expedient form of removing necrotic tissue. Physical therapists are permitted to perform sharp, selective debridement as a procedural intervention.

### Enzymatic Debridement

Enzymatic debridement refers to the topical application of an enzymatic preparation to necrotic tissue. Enzymatic debridement can be used on infected and non-infected wounds with necrotic tissue. This type of debridement may be used for wounds that have not responded to autolytic debridement or in conjunction with other debridement techniques. Enzymatic debridement can be slow to establish a clean wound bed and should be discontinued once devitalized tissue is removed to avoid damage to adjacent healthy tissue.

### Autolytic Debridement

Autolytic debridement refers to the use of the body's own mechanisms to remove nonviable tissue. Common methods of autolytic debridement include the use of transparent films, hydrocolloids, hydrogels, and alginates. Autolytic debridement establishes a moist wound environment that rehydrates necrotic tissue and eschar, facilitating enzymatic digestion of the nonviable tissue. This type of debridement is non-invasive and pain-free. Autolytic debridement can be used with any amount of necrotic tissue, however, requires a longer healing period and should not be performed on infected wounds.

## Non-selective Debridement[1,2,4]

Non-selective debridement involves the removal of both viable and nonviable tissues from a wound. Non-selective debridement is often termed "mechanical debridement" and is most commonly performed via wet-to-dry dressings, wound irrigation, and hydrotherapy (whirlpool).

### Wet-to-dry Dressings

Wet-to-dry dressings refer to the application of a moistened gauze dressing over an area of necrotic tissue. The dressing is allowed to dry completely and is later removed, along with any necrotic tissue that has adhered to the gauze. Wet-to-dry dressings are most often used to debride wounds with moderate amounts of exudate and necrotic tissue. This type of debridement should be used sparingly on wounds containing both necrotic and viable tissue since granulation tissue will be traumatized in the process. Removal of dry dressings from granulation tissue may cause bleeding and be extremely painful.

### Wound Irrigation

Wound irrigation removes necrotic tissue from the wound bed using pressurized fluid. Pulsatile lavage is an example of wound irrigation that uses a pressurized stream of irrigation solution. This type of debridement is most desirable for wounds that are infected or have loose debris. Many devices permit variable pressure settings and provide suction for the removal of exudate and debris.

### Hydrotherapy

Hydrotherapy is most commonly employed using a whirlpool tank with agitation directed toward a wound requiring debridement. This process softens and loosens adherent necrotic tissue. Physical therapists must be aware of potential hydrotherapy side effects such as maceration of viable tissue, edema from dependent lower extremity positioning, and systemic effects such as hypotension.

## Modalities and Physical Agents[1,2,5]

### Negative Pressure Wound Therapy (NPWT)

NPWT, also referred to as vacuum-assisted closure (V.A.C.), is a non-invasive wound care modality used to facilitate healing and manage drainage (Fig. 7-4). A sterile foam dressing is placed in the wound and sealed with an airtight secondary dressing which attaches via tubing to a vacuum pump with a reservoir container. Treatment protocols vary depending on wound characteristics.

Fig. 7-4: Negative pressure wound therapy applied to the lower extremity.

### Indications

Chronic or acute wounds which cannot be closed by primary intention such as dehisced surgical incisions, full-thickness wounds, partial-thickness burns, heavily draining granular wounds, flaps, grafts, and most ulcer types.

### Contraindications

Malignancy within the wound, insufficient vascularity to sustain wound healing, large amounts of necrotic tissue with eschar present, untreated osteomyelitis, fistulas to organs or body cavities, exposed arteries or veins, and uncontrolled pain.

### Advantages

- Provides management of wound drainage
- Maintains a moist wound environment
- Decreases interstitial edema
- Decreases bacterial colonization
- Increases capillary blood flow
- Increases granular tissue formation
- Enhances epithelial cell migration

### Disadvantages

- Requires special supplies and training
- Treatment can be painful
- Not reimbursed in acute or long-term care settings

### Hyperbaric Oxygen

Hyperbaric oxygen refers to the inhalation of 100% oxygen delivered at pressures greater than one atmosphere. Hyperbaric oxygen treatment is delivered in a closed chamber typically at pressures two to three times that of the atmosphere, effectively reducing edema and hyperoxygenating tissues.

### Indications

Osteomyelitis, diabetic wounds, crush injuries, compartment syndromes, necrotizing soft tissue infection, thermal burns, radiation necrosis, and compromised flaps and grafts.

### Contraindications

Terminal illness, untreated pneumothorax, active malignancy, pregnancy, seizure disorder, emphysema, and use of certain chemotherapy agents.

### Advantages

- Antibiotic effects
- Stimulation of fibroblast production and collagen synthesis
- Stimulation of growth factor release and epithelialization

### Disadvantages

- Specialized equipment is not widely available
- Cannot be used with active malignancy

### Growth Factors

Growth factors used in wound healing are derived from naturally occurring protein factors. These substances facilitate healing by stimulating the activity of specific cell types (e.g., neutrophils, endothelial cells, fibroblasts). Currently, only a limited number of growth factors have been approved by the Food and Drug Administration for topical wound healing applications.

### Indications

Neuropathic ulcers extending into or through subcutaneous tissue with adequate circulation to sustain wound healing.

### Contraindications

Wounds closed by primary intention, patients with known hypersensitivity to any component of the product or a history of neoplasm at the application site.

### Advantages:

- Adjunct to promote wound healing environment
- Increases growth rate of new tissue
- Promotes cell division

### Disadvantages

- Costly
- Poor reimbursement
- Additional research is needed
- Secondary dressing required
- Requires refrigeration
- Limited number of products have been approved by the Food and Drug Administration

# Consider This

## Therapeutic Modalities with Wound Healing Applications[1]

Therapeutic ultrasound applied at a low intensity with pulsed duty cycle has been shown to enhance all phases of wound healing. During the inflammatory and proliferative phases, fibroblast, endothelial, and white blood cell activity are stimulated by ultrasound. Ultrasound use during these early stages of repair has been shown to enhance the strength and elasticity of scar tissue. Recommended treatment protocols vary depending on the phase of healing and intended outcome (e.g., restarting the inflammatory phase of healing in a chronic ulcer vs. dispersing ecchymosis associated with skin tears or contusions to reduce pain and edema).

High-voltage pulsed current (HVPC) electrical stimulation has been shown to enhance healing in numerous types of wounds including chronic ulcers, burns, and donor and graft sites. The application of monophasic direct current stimulates angiogenesis and epithelial migration, decreases bacterial activity and wound pain, and increases oxygen perfusion and tensile strength. HVPC is typically applied using a sensory or sub-sensory intensity. Treatment protocols vary widely depending on the stage of healing or presence of infection.

## Types of Dressings[1,2,4]

Dressings may be defined as either primary or secondary. A primary dressing is one that comes into direct contact with a wound. A number of primary dressings include a self-adhesive backing and do not require a secondary dressing. Secondary dressings are placed directly over the primary dressing to provide additional protection, absorption, occlusion, and/or to secure the primary dressing in place.

### Hydrocolloids

Hydrocolloid dressings consist of gel-forming polymers (e.g., carboxymethylcellulose, gelatin, pectin) backed by a strong film or foam adhesive. The dressing does not attach to the wound itself but instead anchors to the intact surrounding skin. The dressings absorb exudate by swelling into a gel-like mass and vary in permeability, thickness, and transparency.

#### Indications

Hydrocolloids are useful for partial and full-thickness wounds. The dressings can be used effectively with granular or necrotic wounds.

#### Advantages

- Provides a moist environment for wound healing
- Enables autolytic debridement
- Offers protection from microbial contamination
- Provides moderate absorption
- Does not require a secondary dressing
- Provides a waterproof surface

#### Disadvantages

- May traumatize surrounding intact skin upon removal
- May tend to roll in areas of excessive friction
- Cannot be used on infected wounds

### Hydrogels

Hydrogels consist of varying amounts of water and gel-forming materials such as glycerin. The dressings are typically available in both sheet and amorphous forms.

#### Indications

Hydrogels are moisture retentive and commonly used on superficial and partial-thickness wounds (e.g., abrasions, blisters, pressure ulcers) that have minimal drainage.

#### Advantages

- Provides a moist environment for wound healing
- Enables autolytic debridement
- May reduce pressure and diminish pain
- Can be used as a coupling agent for ultrasound
- Minimally adheres to wound
- Some products have absorptive properties

#### Disadvantages

- Potential for dressings to dehydrate
- Cannot be used on wounds with significant drainage
- Typically requires a secondary dressing

### Foam Dressings

Foam dressings are comprised of a hydrophilic polyurethane base that contacts the wound surface and a hydrophobic outer layer. The dressings allow exudate to be absorbed into the foam through the hydrophilic layer. The dressings are most commonly available in sheets or pads with varying degrees of thickness. Semipermeable foam dressings are produced in adhesive and non-adhesive forms. Non-adhesive forms require a secondary dressing.

### Indications

Foam dressings are used to provide protection and absorption over partial and full-thickness wounds with varying levels of exudate. They can also be used as secondary dressings over amorphous hydrogels.

### Advantages

- Provides a moist environment for wound healing
- Available in adhesive and non-adhesive forms
- Provides prophylactic protection and cushioning
- Encourages autolytic debridement
- Provides moderate absorption

### Disadvantages

- May tend to roll in areas of excessive friction
- Adhesive form may traumatize periwound area upon removal
- Lack of transparency makes inspection of wound difficult

### Transparent Film

Film dressings are thin membranes made from transparent polyurethane with water-resistant adhesives. The dressings are permeable to vapor and oxygen, but are largely impermeable to bacteria and water. They are highly elastic, conform to a variety of body contours, and allow easy visual inspection of the wound since they are transparent.

### Indications

Film dressings are useful for superficial or partial-thickness wounds with minimal drainage (e.g., scalds, abrasions, lacerations).

### Advantages

- Provides a moist environment for wound healing
- Enables autolytic debridement
- Allows visualization of the wound
- Resistant to shearing and frictional forces
- Cost effective over time

### Disadvantages

- Excessive exudate accumulation can result in periwound maceration
- Adhesive may traumatize periwound area upon removal
- Cannot be used on infected wounds

### Gauze

Gauze dressings are manufactured from yarn or thread and are the most readily available dressing used in inpatient environments. Gauze dressings come in many shapes and sizes (e.g., sheets, squares, rolls, packing strips). Impregnated gauze is a variation of woven gauze in which various materials such as petrolatum, zinc or antimicrobials have been added.

### Indications

Gauze dressings are commonly used on infected or non-infected wounds of any size. The dressings can be used for wet-to-wet, wet-to-moist or wet-to-dry debridement.

### Advantages

- Readily available and cost effective short-term dressings
- Can be used alone or in combination with other dressings and topical agents
- Can modify number of layers to accommodate for changing wound status
- Can be used on infected or non-infected wounds

### Disadvantages

- Has a tendency to adhere to the wound bed traumatizing viable tissue on removal
- Highly permeable
- Requires frequent dressing changes
- Prolonged use decreases cost effectiveness
- Increased infection rate compared to occlusive dressings

### Alginates

Alginate dressings are derived from a seaweed extraction, specifically, the calcium salt component of alginic acid. Alginates are highly absorptive, but are also highly permeable and non-occlusive. As a result, they require a secondary dressing. Alginate dressings act as a hemostat and create a hydrophilic gel through the interaction of calcium ions in the dressing and sodium ions in the wound exudate.

### Indications

Alginates are typically used on partial or full-thickness draining wounds, such as pressure or venous insufficiency ulcers. Alginates are often used on infected wounds due to the likelihood of excessive drainage.

### Advantages

- High absorptive capacity
- Enables autolytic debridement
- Offers protection from microbial contamination
- Can be used on infected or non-infected wounds
- Non-adhering to wound

### Disadvantages

- May require frequent dressing changes based on level of exudate
- Requires a secondary dressing
- Cannot be used on wounds with an exposed tendon, joint capsule or bone

## Consider This

### Combination Dressings using Silver and Iodine[1,2]

Silver and iodine are elemental broad-spectrum antimicrobial agents that have become valuable adjuncts to wound healing interventions. First used in topical applications (e.g., powder, ointment, cream), these elements control microorganism activity in wound beds without damaging viable tissue. Many silver and iodine-impregnated dressings also help to maintain a moist wound healing environment. Absorbency and recommended frequency of dressing changes are product dependent with many requiring a secondary dressing.

### Moisture and Occlusion[2,4]

A dry wound bed slows normal metabolic functions, impeding the healing process. Dry peripheral tissues are at risk for developing cracks or fissures that can become open avenues for infection. Conversely, prolonged excessive moisture (e.g., from poorly managed exudate or incontinence) will cause maceration damage and erosion of intact peripheral tissues.

In an appropriately moist wound environment, macrophages appear earlier and in greater numbers helping to reduce the risk of infection. Collagen synthesis and epithelialization rate are enhanced, facilitating more rapid wound closure. In exudating wounds, moisture must be well managed to prevent damage to surrounding tissue. In dry wounds, moisture must be added in order to maintain hydration and sustain cellular activity. Maintaining an appropriately moist wound bed requires a delicate balance often necessitating specialized dressings to appropriately manage exudate and provide some level of occlusion.

Occlusion refers to the ability of a dressing to transmit moisture, vapor or gases between a wound bed and the atmosphere. A fully occlusive substance would be completely impermeable (e.g., latex gloves), while a non-occlusive substance would be completely permeable (e.g., gauze pads). Wound dressings are typically classified according to this occlusion continuum or by their moisture retention properties.

| Dressings from Most Occlusive to Non-Occlusive | Dressings from Most to Least Moisture Retentive |
|---|---|
| Hydrocolloids | Alginates |
| Hydrogels | Semipermeable foams |
| Semipermeable foam | Hydrocolloids |
| Semipermeable film | Hydrogels |
| Impregnated gauze | Semipermeable films |
| Alginates | |
| Traditional gauze | |

## Consider This

### Incontinence and Tissue Injury[5]

Incontinence refers to the inability to control urination or defecation. A patient who is incontinent is at a significantly increased risk of tissue injury or in the presence of existing tissue injury, may experience additional complications including delayed healing.

- Urine and feces are typically acidic in composition and can contribute to tissue irritation and erosion.
- Skin shear and friction are increased in the presence of mild to moderate moisture.
- Macerated skin has decreased epidermal resilience to shear and friction forces.
- Harsh cleansers, hot water, and scrubbing will make delicate tissues more friable.
- Mild cleansers, warm water, and minimal friction should be used when cleansing to minimize irritation.
- Topical agents should be employed both to maintain the skin's natural moisture and act as a barrier to excessive moisture from incontinence.
- Emollient creams and ointments are typically better choices for skin moisturizers than watery lotions as they tend to have higher concentrations of solids and oils requiring less frequent reapplication and providing better barrier protection.

## Skin Care Products[2,3]

**Therapeutic moisturizers:** (e.g., lotion, cream) Lotions are largely water-based and best used to replace skin moisture that has been lost either to the air or as a result of frequent hand washing. Creams are thicker water-based substances with higher concentrations of solids and oils than lotions, making the need for reapplication less frequent. Therapeutic moisturizers are intended to maintain the skin's natural moisture and prevent tissue cracking due to dryness, but do not typically protect the skin from excessive moisture.

**Moisture barriers:** (e.g., ointment) Moisture barriers are designed to adhere to the skin and repel excess moisture from protected areas. They are frequently used to protect surrounding skin from a heavily draining wound or perineal tissues from exposure to incontinence.

**Liquid skin protectants:** (e.g., skin sealant) Liquid skin protectant is applied to skin and when dry it creates a thin plastic film protecting the skin from adhesive-related tissue damage. This thin barrier also offers some degree of moisture protection. Skin protectant application varies slightly depending on packaging (e.g., swab, wipes, tube, bottle). Regardless, once applied to the skin it should be allowed to dry fully before an adhesive product is applied over it.

**Skin cleansers:** Skin cleansers are liquid agents typically intended for use on the skin of patients at risk for breakdown. Ingredients often have a pH balancing component that is especially beneficial for perineal cleansing in patients who are incontinent. Skin cleansers are designed to be less drying to the skin and more effective than usual soap or detergent skin products.

**Wound cleansers:** Wound cleansers vary from simple saline solutions to more complex compositions with cytotoxicity. Many wound cleansers have the potential to cause inflammation, however, this quality is product dependent. Wound cleansers are not typically designed to remove necrotic tissue, but rather associated wound substances such as foreign materials, exudate and dried blood.

# Wound Terminology[1,2,4,5]

**Contusion:** An injury, usually caused by a blow, that does not disrupt skin integrity. The injury is characterized by pain, edema, and discoloration which appears as a result of blood seepage under the surface of the skin.

**Dehiscence:** The separation, rupture or splitting of a wound closed by primary intention. This disruption of previously approximated surfaces may be superficial or involve all layers of tissue.

**Dermis:** The vascular layer of skin located below the epidermis containing hair follicles, sebaceous glands, sweat glands, lymphatic and blood vessels, and nerve endings.

**Desiccated:** The drying out or dehydration of a wound. Desiccation often results from poor dressing selection that does not control the evaporation of wound bed moisture.

**Desquamation:** The peeling or shedding of the outer layers of the epidermis. Desquamation normally occurs in small scales, although certain conditions, injuries, and medications may cause peeling in larger scales or sheets and extend to deeper layers of the skin.

**Ecchymosis:** The discoloration occurring below intact skin resulting from trauma to underlying blood vessels and blood seeping into tissues. The discoloration is typically blue-black, changing in time to a greenish brown or yellow color. An area where ecchymosis is present is commonly referred to as a bruise.

**Epidermis:** The superficial, avascular epithelial layer of the skin that includes flat, scale-like squamous cells, round basal cells, and melanocytes which produce melanin and give skin its color.

**Erythema:** A diffuse redness of the skin often resulting from capillary dilation and congestion or inflammation.

**Friable:** Tissue that readily tears, fragments or bleeds when gently palpated or manipulated.

**Hematoma:** A localized swelling or mass of clotted blood confined to a tissue, organ or space usually caused by a break in a blood vessel.

**Hypergranulation:** Increased thickness of the granular layer of the epidermis that exceeds the surface height of the skin.

**Hyperpigmentation:** An excess of pigment in a tissue that causes it to appear darker than surrounding tissues.

**Hypertrophic scar:** An abnormal scar resulting from excessive collagen formation during healing. A hypertrophic scar is typically raised, red, and firm with disorganized collagen fibers.

**Keloid:** An abnormal scar formation that is out of proportion to the scarring required for normal tissue repair and is comprised of irregularly distributed collagen bands. A keloid scar typically exceeds the boundaries of the original wound appearing red, thick, raised, and firm.

**Maceration:** The skin softening and degeneration that results from prolonged exposure to water or other fluids.

**Normotrophic scar:** A scar characterized by the organized formation of collagen fibers that align in a parallel fashion.

**Turgor:** The relative speed with which the skin resumes its normal appearance after being lightly pinched. Turgor is an indicator of skin elasticity and hydration and normally occurs more slowly in older adults.

**Ulcer:** An open sore or lesion of the skin accompanied by sloughing of inflamed necrotic tissue.

# Burns

## Types of Burns[6]

**Thermal burn:** Caused by conduction or convection. Examples include burns resulting from contact with a hot liquid, fire or steam.

**Electrical burn:** Caused by the passage of electrical current through the body. Typically there is an entrance and an exit wound. Complications can include cardiac arrhythmias, respiratory arrest, renal failure, neurological damage, and fractures. A burn caused by a lightning strike is an example of an electrical burn.

**Chemical burn:** Occurs when certain chemical compounds come in contact with the body. The reaction will continue until the chemical compound is diluted at the site of contact. Compounds that cause chemical burns include sulfuric acid, lye, hydrochloric acid, and gasoline.

**Radiation burn:** Occurs most commonly with exposure to external beam radiation therapy. DNA is altered in exposed tissues and ischemic injury may be irreversible. Complications may include severe blistering and desquamation, non-healing wounds, tissue fibrosis, permanent discoloration, and new malignancies.

## Zones of Injury[3]

**Zone of coagulation:** The area of the burn that received the most severe injury with irreversible cell damage.

**Zone of stasis:** The area of less severe injury that possesses reversible damage and surrounds the zone of coagulation.

**Zone of hyperemia:** The area surrounding the zone of stasis that presents with inflammation, but will fully recover without any intervention or permanent damage.

## Burn Classification[3,6]

The extent and severity of a burn is dependent on gender, age, duration of burn, type of burn, and affected area. Burns are most appropriately classified according to the depth of tissue destruction.

**Superficial Burn:** A superficial burn involves only the outer epidermis. The involved area may be red with slight edema. Healing occurs without peeling or evidence of scarring in two to five days.

**Superficial Partial-Thickness Burn:** A superficial partial-thickness burn involves the epidermis and the upper portion of the dermis. The involved area may be extremely painful and exhibit blisters. Healing occurs with minimal to no scarring in 5-21 days.

**Deep Partial-Thickness Burn:** A deep partial-thickness burn involves complete destruction of the epidermis and the majority of the dermis. The involved area may appear to be discolored with broken blisters and edema. Damage to nerve endings may result in only moderate levels of pain. Hypertrophic or keloid scarring may occur. In the absence of infection, healing will occur in 21-35 days.

## Spotlight on Safety
### Iontophoresis Related Burns[7]

Chemical burns from iontophoresis occur when skin pH increases or decreases beyond the range of normal tolerance. Chemically induced pH levels below 3 or greater than 5 can result in acidic or alkaline reactions, respectively.

Chemical burns are typically more severe under the negative electrode where pooling of the alkaline medium can occur. This can create a pH exceeding 9 which will quickly begin to erode the insulating epidermis. With skin resistance reduced, electrical current delivery increases, further accelerating skin erosion.

Factors contributing to chemical burns from iontophoresis include treatment delivered with excessive current, prolonged duration, and electrode placement over defective skin areas with lower resistance.

Poor iontophoresis electrode placement can contribute to a thermal burn in cases of excessive impedance or poor electrode contact.

**Full-Thickness Burn:** A full-thickness burn involves complete destruction of the epidermis and dermis along with partial damage to the subcutaneous fat layer. The involved area typically presents with eschar formation and minimal pain. Patients with full-thickness burns require grafts and are susceptible to infection. Healing time varies significantly with smaller areas healing in a matter of weeks, with or without grafting, and larger areas requiring grafting and potentially months to heal.

**Subdermal Burn:** A subdermal burn involves the complete destruction of the epidermis, dermis, and subcutaneous tissue. Subdermal burns may involve muscle and bone and as a result, often require multiple surgical interventions and extensive healing time.

## Rule of Nines

Allows for a gross approximation of the percentage of the body affected by a burn. The rule of nines does not account for severity.

### Adult Values

| | |
|---|---|
| Head and neck | 9% |
| Anterior trunk | 18% |
| Posterior trunk | 18% |
| Bilateral anterior arm, forearm, and hand | 9% |
| Bilateral posterior arm, forearm, and hand | 9% |
| Genital region | 1% |
| Bilateral anterior leg and foot | 18% |
| Bilateral posterior leg and foot | 18% |

### Child Values

A child under one year has 9% taken from the lower extremities and added to the head and neck region. Each year of life, 1% is distributed back to the lower extremities until the age of nine when the head is considered to be the same proportion as an adult.

## Anticipated Deformities Based on Burn Location

| Area | Anticipated deformity | Splinting type |
|---|---|---|
| Anterior neck | Flexion with possible lateral flexion | Soft collar, molded collar, Philadelphia collar |
| Anterior chest and axilla | Shoulder adduction, extension, and medial rotation | Axillary or airplane splint, shoulder abduction brace |
| Elbow | Flexion and pronation | Gutter splint, conforming splint, three-point splint, air splint |
| Hand and wrist | Extension or hyperextension of the MCP joints; flexion of the IP joints; adduction and flexion of the thumb; flexion of the wrist | Wrist splint, thumb spica splint, palmar or dorsal extension splint |
| Hip | Flexion and adduction | Anterior hip spica, abduction splint |
| Knee | Flexion | Conforming splint, three-point splint, air splint |
| Ankle | Plantar flexion | Posterior foot drop splint, posterior ankle conforming splint, anterior ankle conforming splint |

# Consider This

## Calculating Burn Severity[6]

Like the rule of nines, the Lund and Browder method also provides an estimated calculation of the extent of body surface area burned based on assigned percentages. This method, however, offers a more detailed calculation for children under the age of seven.

While both the rule of nines and the Lund and Browder method provide a gross surface area burned calculation method, neither offer indications of severity or prognosis. Prognostic burn indexes have been developed as more thorough evaluative tools used to predict medical attention needs, outcomes, and mortality by taking into account both the surface area burned and the severity of burns.

## Scar Management[3,6]

Hypertrophic scarring is the result of an imbalance between collagen synthesis and lysis during healing, and can occur with any integumentary injury. The development of hypertrophic scarring is particularly common in relation to severe burn injuries. Complications of hypertrophic scarring may include contracture, adhesions, hypersensitivity, functional limitation, and poor cosmesis.

**Scar assessment:** Assessment devices, such as a tonometer, and rating scales aid in quantifying scar characteristics. A number of rating scales are available to objectively document observed characteristics. These tend to be more helpful in the assessment and re-assessment of an individual rather than for comparative assessment of a group. General characteristics that should be documented include location, sensation, texture, pigmentation, vascularity, pliability, and height.

**Scar massage:** Friction massage is advocated to loosen adhesions between cutaneous scar tissue and underlying structures. Reported benefits include decreased sensitivity, and improved pliability. Caution should be taken not to begin scar massage too soon or too aggressively due to the risk of causing re-injury or re-initiating the inflammatory phase of healing. Massage techniques should be slow and firm using perpendicular, parallel, circular, and/or rolling strokes to mobilize tissue layers.

**Compression Garments:** Compression therapy to reduce hypertrophic scarring is typically recommended for burns requiring greater than 14 days to heal. The use of sustained compression from 15-35 mm Hg is believed to create an environment that facilitates the balance of collagen synthesis and lysis, improving scar structure. Compression is applied by custom-made garments worn for 22-23 hours per day until the scar has matured. Silicone or foam inserts may be necessary to provide sufficient pressure over small areas or concave surfaces. For optimal effect, it is recommended that the use of compression garments begin between two weeks and two months after wound closure or grafting, continuing for up to two years.

# Consider This

## Desensitization Techniques[8]

As with some patients status post amputation, patients who have sustained severe burns are susceptible to developing hypersensitivity that can become functionally limiting. Incorporating desensitization techniques into the plan of care and a patient's self-care routine can significantly improve a patient's tolerance to variable temperatures, touch, pressure, and vibration, thereby decreasing discomfort and improving functional abilities.

Desensitization interventions typically include variable texture, pressure, and vibratory sensations applied to the affected area by either rubbing, tapping or rolling motions. The use of particle contact (e.g., container of dry beans, popcorn kernels or fluidotherapy) can be beneficial in desensitizing distal extremities. Compression and TENS have also been shown to have clinical applications for desensitization goals.

It is recommended that desensitization interventions be performed for five to ten minutes, three to four times daily. Each session should begin with a sensation that is slightly irritating, but tolerable, and progress to more noxious stimuli. A textural progression may include: feather, cotton ball, chamois cloth, soft terry cloth, corduroy cloth, rough terry cloth, wool.

## Topical Agents Used in Burn Care[9]

| Topical Agent | Advantages | Disadvantages |
|---|---|---|
| Silver Sulfadiazine | Can be used with or without dressings<br>Painless<br>Can be applied to wound directly<br>Broad-spectrum<br>Effective against yeast | Does not penetrate into eschar |
| Silver Nitrate | Broad-spectrum<br>Non-allergenic<br>Dressing application is painless | Poor penetration<br>Discolors, making assessment difficult<br>Can cause severe electrolyte imbalances<br>Removal of dressings is painful |
| Povidone-iodine | Broad-spectrum<br>Antifungal<br>Easily removed with water | Not effective against pseudomonas<br>May impair thyroid function<br>Painful application |
| Mafenide Acetate | Broad-spectrum<br>Penetrates burn eschar<br>May be used with or without occlusive dressings | May cause metabolic acidosis<br>May compromise respiratory function<br>May inhibit epithelialization<br>Painful application |
| Gentamicin | Broad-spectrum<br>May be covered or left open to air | Has caused resistant strains<br>Ototoxic<br>Nephrotoxic |
| Nitrofurazone | Bacteriocidal<br>Broad-spectrum | May lead to overgrowth of fungus and pseudomonas<br>Painful application |

From Trofino, RB: Nursing Care of the Burn-Injured Patient. F.A. Davis Company, Philadelphia 1991, p.46, with permission.

# Skin Graft Terminology[6]

**Allograft (homograft):** A temporary skin graft taken from another human, usually a cadaver, in order to cover a large burned area.

**Autograft:** A permanent skin graft taken from a donor site on the patient's own body.

**Donor site:** A site where healthy skin is taken and used as a graft.

**Escharotomy:** A surgical procedure that opens or removes eschar from a burn site to reduce tension on a surrounding structure, relieve pressure from interstitial edema, and subsequently enhance circulation.

**Full-thickness graft:** A skin graft that contains the dermis and epidermis.

**Heterograft (xenograft):** A temporary skin graft taken from another species.

**Mesh graft:** A skin graft that is altered to create a mesh-like pattern in order to cover a larger surface area.

**Recipient site:** A site that has been burned and requires a graft.

**Sheet graft:** A skin graft that is transferred directly from the unburned donor site to the prepared recipient site.

**Split-thickness graft:** A skin graft that contains only a superficial layer of the dermis in addition to the epidermis.

**Z-plasty:** A surgical procedure to eliminate a scar contracture. An incision in the shape of a "z" allows the contracture to change configuration and lengthen the scar.

# Integumentary Pathology[1,4,10]

## Cellulitis

Cellulitis is a fast spreading inflammation that occurs as a result of a bacterial infection of the skin and connective tissues. It can develop anywhere under the skin, but will typically affect the extremities.

**Etiology** – Cellulitis is caused by particular bacterial infections including streptococci or staphylococci. Predisposing factors to cellulitis include an increased age, immunosuppression, trauma, the presence of wounds or venous insufficiency.

**Signs and Symptoms** – Symptoms may include localized redness that may spread quickly, skin that is warm or hot to touch, local abscess or ulceration, tenderness to palpation, chills, fever, and malaise.

**Treatment** – A patient with suspected cellulitis should be immediately referred to a physician for further assessment. Cellulitis requires pharmacological intervention using systemic antibiotics. Differential diagnosis should attempt to rule out deep vein thrombosis and contact dermatitis. Physical therapy may be warranted for wound care. Cellulitis can lead to sepsis or gangrene if not properly treated.

## Contact Dermatitis

Contact dermatitis is a superficial irritation of the skin resulting from localized irritation (e.g., poison ivy, latex, soap, jewelry sensitivity). This condition can be acute or chronic based on exposure to the precipitating agent. Contact dermatitis is a very common skin disease that can occur at any age.

**Etiology** – Contact dermatitis occurs with exposure to mechanical, chemical, environmental or biological agents. Nickel, rubber, latex, and topical antibiotics are common precipitating agents.

**Signs and Symptoms** – Patients experience intense itching, burning, and red skin in areas corresponding to the location of the topical irritation. Edema may also occur in the area of sensitivity and symptoms can expand beyond the initial point of topical irritation.

**Treatment** – The focus of treatment should be on identifying and removing the source of irritation. Topical steroid application is commonly employed. Acute lesions should resolve with treatment once exposure to the external irritant has been removed.

## Eczema

Eczema, also referred to as dermatitis, is used to describe a group of disorders that cause chronic skin inflammation typically due to an immune system abnormality, allergic reaction or external irritant.

**Etiology** – Eczema's etiology is based on the particular form of the disorder. Infants and children are at higher risk for eczema, however, many outgrow the condition with age. The geriatric population is also at an increased risk for many forms of eczema.

**Signs and Symptoms** – Red or brown-gray, itchy, lichenified skin plaques that may be exacerbated by some topical agents such as soaps and lotions. The younger population will also frequently experience oozing and crusting of the patchy areas of irritation.

**Treatment** – Pharmacological interventions are variable ranging from topical or oral corticosteroids to oral antibiotics and antihistamines. Cold compresses and other modalities may assist with reducing the itching. Stress management techniques and avoidance of extreme temperatures should be employed to avoid potential exacerbations of the condition.

## Gangrene (Dry)

Gangrene is referred to as "dry" when there is a loss of vascular supply resulting in local tissue death. Fingers, toes, and limbs are most often affected. The hardened tissue is not painful, however, there may be significant pain at the line of demarcation. Dry gangrene typically develops slowly and in some cases results in auto-amputation.

**Etiology** – Dry gangrene occurs most commonly in blood vessel disease, such as diabetes mellitus or atherosclerosis. It develops when blood flow to an affected area is impaired, typically as a result of poor circulation. Infection is typically not present in dry gangrene, however, dry gangrene can progress to wet gangrene if infection occurs.

**Signs and Symptoms** – Dry gangrene presents as dark brown or black nonviable tissue that eventually becomes a hardened mass (mummified). The patient may complain of cold or numb skin and they may present with pain.

**Treatment** – Gangrene is a serious medical condition and requires immediate medical intervention. Depending on the severity, gangrene is treated by pharmacological intervention, surgery, and hyperbaric oxygen therapy.

## Gangrene (Wet)

Gangrene is referred to as "wet" if there is an associated bacterial infection in the affected tissue. Gangrene may develop as a complication of an infected untreated wound. Swelling resulting from the bacterial infection causes a sudden stoppage of blood flow.

**Etiology** – Wet gangrene can develop after a severe burn, frostbite or injury and requires immediate treatment since it tends to spread very quickly and can be fatal. There is cessation of blood flow that starts a chain of events including invasion by bacteria at the affected site. As a result of the occluded blood supply, the white blood cells are unable to fight the infection.

**Signs and Symptoms** – swelling and pain at the site of infection, change in skin color from red to brown to black, blisters that produce pus, fever, and general malaise

**Treatment** – Wet gangrene is a serious medical condition and requires immediate medical intervention. Surgical debridement of the gangrene and intravenous antibiotic treatment are typical interventions for wet gangrene. Depending on the severity, gangrene is treated by pharmacological intervention, surgery, and hyperbaric oxygen therapy.

## Onychomycosis

Onychomycosis refers to a fungal infection that primarily affects the toenails and nailbeds. Onychomycosis is divided into subtypes, but are typically medically treated in a similar fashion.

**Etiology** – Acquiring a fungal infection can be a fairly common occurrence. Risk factors include manicures and pedicures with unsterile utensils, possessing nail injuries or deformities, excess skin moisture, wearing closed toe shoes, and an impaired immune response.

**Signs and Symptoms** – yellow or brown nail discoloration, hyperkeratosis and hypertrophy of the nail causing it to partially detach from the nailbed

**Treatment** – Manual debridement of the nail and topical antifungal medications are primary interventions. Fungal infections may return to the nailbeds and in some cases, the nails may have permanent damage.

## Plaque Psoriasis

Plaque psoriasis is a chronic autoimmune disease of the skin and is the most common of the five types of psoriasis. T cells trigger inflammation within the skin and produce an accelerated rate of skin cell growth. The skin cells accumulate in raised red patches on the surface of the skin.

**Etiology** – Some patients have a genetic predisposition to plaque psoriasis. Other factors may trigger psoriasis, such as injury to the skin, insufficient or excess sunlight, stress, excessive alcohol, HIV infection, smoking, and certain medications.

**Signs and Symptoms** – The primary symptom is red raised blotches that typically present in a bilateral fashion for example over both knees or elbows. These plaques can appear anywhere on the body and will tend to itch and flake. Complications can include arthritis, pain, severe itching, secondary skin infections, and side effects secondary to pharmacological interventions.

**Treatment** – The primary goal for treatment of plaque psoriasis is to control the symptoms and prevent secondary infection. Treatment varies widely from topical applications to systemic medications and phototherapy. Plaque psoriasis is a life-long condition that can be effectively managed and controlled through the various stages and exacerbations.

## Tinea Pedis

Tinea pedis, commonly referred to as athlete's foot, is a superficial fungal infection which causes epidermal thickening and a scaly skin appearance. This fungus is opportunistic and will rapidly multiply in a warm and moist environment (e.g., between the toes).

**Etiology** – Risk factors include wearing closed toe shoes that don't allow airflow, prolonged periods of moisture or wetness, excessive sweating, and possessing small nail or skin abrasions. This infection is contagious through direct contact or when making contact with a surface containing the tinea pedis infection.

**Signs and Symptoms** – itching, redness, peeling skin between the toes, pain, odor, and in more severe cases breaks in skin continuity

**Treatment** – Pharmacological intervention includes topical or oral antibiotics depending on the severity of symptoms. Tinea pedis may persist or recur and more long-term management may be required. Prevention includes thorough drying of the feet when bathing or swimming, wearing sandals around public pools or showers, changing socks frequently, proper hygiene, and avoiding shoe wear that creates a moist environment.

# Metabolic and Endocrine Systems

# Metabolic System

## Key Functions of the Metabolic System [11]

The metabolic system governs the chemical and physical changes that take place within the body enabling it to grow and function. Metabolism involves breakdown of the body's complex organic compounds in order to generate energy for all bodily processes. It also generates energy for the synthesis of complex substances that form tissues and organs. During metabolism, organic compounds are broken down by a process called catabolism, while anabolism is the process that combines simple molecules for tissue growth. Many metabolic processes are facilitated by enzymes. The overall speed at which an organism carries out its metabolic processes is termed its metabolic rate (or when the organism is at rest, its basal metabolic rate).

## Metabolic System Pathology

### Inherited Metabolic Disorders [10]

Metabolic disorders are classified by the particular building block that is affected. An enzyme deficiency leads to accumulation of the substrate and a subsequent deficiency in the intended enzyme's product. There are many different disorders that can occur genetically and these are grouped according to the substrate that has been affected (i.e., carbohydrates, amino acids). Inherited metabolic disorders can be diagnosed in utero via amniocentesis or chorionic villus sampling. Many inherited metabolic disorders will produce symptoms in a newborn including lethargy, apnea, poor feeding, tachypnea, vomiting, hypoglycemia, urine changes, and seizures. Symptoms that are immediately apparent indicate a more dangerous disorder.

### Phenylketonuria
### (amino acid/organic acid metabolic disorder) [12]

Phenylketonuria (PKU) is a syndrome that consists of mental retardation as well as behavioral and cognitive issues secondary to an elevation of serum phenylalanine. There is a deficiency in the enzyme phenylalanine hydroxylase. Normally, excessive phenylalanine is converted to tyrosine by phenylalanine hydroxylase. When this process does not occur and there is an excess of phenylalanine, the brain is the primary organ that becomes affected. Children in the United States are tested at birth for PKU and levels greater than 6 mg/dl of phenylalanine require some form of treatment.

**Etiology** – This is an autosomal recessive inherited trait and is most common in Caucasian populations.

**Signs and symptoms** – Symptoms will typically present within a few months of birth as the phenylalanine accumulates. If left untreated, severe mental retardation will occur. These children may also experience gait disturbances, hyperactivity, psychoses, abnormal body odor, and display features that are lighter in coloring when compared to other family members.

**Treatment** – Phenylketonuria is treated through dietary restriction of phenylalanine throughout the person's lifetime. Adequate prevention will avoid all manifestations of the disease.

### Tay-Sachs Disease (lysosomal storage disorder) [10]

Tay-Sachs disease is the absence or deficiency of hexosaminidase A. This produces an accumulation of gangliosides (GM2) within the brain.

**Etiology** – This disease is an autosomal recessive inherited trait and carried primarily in the Eastern European (Ashkenazi) Jewish population.

**Signs and symptoms** – At approximately six months of age, the child will start to miss developmental milestones and will continue to deteriorate in motor and cognitive skills. As symptoms progress, the patient develops significant mental retardation and paralysis, and will usually die by the age of five.

**Treatment** – There is currently no effective treatment for this condition. Genetic testing in high risk populations to identify the carriers prior to pregnancy is important in order to avoid this disorder.

### Mitochondrial Disorders [10]

There are over one hundred different forms of mitochondrial disease and each produces a different spectrum of disability and clinical manifestations.

**Etiology** – Mitochondrial disorders result from genetically inherited or spontaneous mutations in the DNA that lead to impaired function of proteins found within the mitochondria.

**Signs and symptoms** – Symptoms vary depending on the type of mitochondrial disorder, however, can include loss of muscle coordination, muscle weakness, visual and hearing problems, learning disabilities, heart, liver, and kidney disease, respiratory, neurological, and gastrointestinal disorders, and dementia.

**Treatment** – These diagnoses are relatively new and treatment is as varied as the symptomatology and presentation of the disease. Treatment is aimed at alleviating the current symptoms and slowing the progression of the disease process.

### Wilson's Disease (hepatolenticular degeneration) [10]

Wilson's disease is a rare inherited disorder that is most common in eastern Europeans, Sicilians, and southern Italians, but may occur in any group. Wilson's disease typically appears in people under 40 years old and symptoms can develop in children typically between four and six years of age.

**Etiology** – Wilson's disease is an autosomal recessive inherited trait that produces a defect in the body's ability to metabolize copper. The copper accumulates over time within the brain, liver, cornea, kidney, and other tissues.

**Signs and symptoms** – Symptoms typically appear between the ages of four to six and include Kayser-Fleischer rings surrounding the iris of the eye secondary to copper deposits, degenerative changes in the brain (especially within the basal ganglia), hepatitis, cirrhosis of the liver, athetoid movements, and ataxic gait patterns. There may also be emotional and behavioral changes as the copper continues to accumulate. Over time, and with severe disease, there will be deformities of the musculoskeletal system, pathologic fractures, osteomalacia, muscle atrophy, and contractures.

**Treatment** – Treatment consists of continual pharmacological intervention using vitamin B6 and D-penicillamine as both promote the excretion of excess copper from the body. Treatment will also focus on prevention of hepatic disease since a patient will die from hepatic failure if the condition is left untreated.

> ### Rehabilitation Considerations for Patients with Inherited Metabolic Disorders[10]
>
> - Must have an awareness of dietary restrictions
> - Patient and family training to prevent deleterious effects from the metabolic disease
> - Adapt treatment to facilitate developmental milestones within patient tolerance

## Acid-Base Metabolic Disorders[13]

The process of metabolism is regulated by the endocrine and nervous systems. The rate of metabolism can be influenced by body temperature, exercise, hormone activity, and digestion activity. If proper fluid or acid-base balance is compromised, it can alter metabolic function and cause many signs and symptoms of the dysfunction.

## Metabolic Alkalosis[13]

Metabolic alkalosis is a condition that occurs when there is an increase in bicarbonate accumulation or an abnormal loss of acids. As a result, the pH rises above 7.45.

**Etiology** – Metabolic alkalosis commonly occurs when there has been continuous vomiting, ingestion of antacids or other alkaline substances or diuretic therapy. It may also be associated with hypokalemia or nasogastric suctioning.

**Signs and symptoms** – Symptoms include nausea, diarrhea, prolonged vomiting, confusion, muscle fasciculations, muscle cramping, neuromuscular hyperexcitability, convulsions, paresthesias, and hypoventilation. If left untreated the patient can become comatose, experience seizures, and respiratory paralysis.

**Treatment** – The most important interventions include managing the underlying cause, correcting coexisting electrolyte imbalances, and administering potassium chloride to the patient.

## Metabolic Acidosis[13]

Metabolic acidosis is a condition that occurs when there is an accumulation of acids due to an acid gain or bicarbonate loss. As a result, the pH drops below 7.35.

**Etiology** – Metabolic acidosis commonly occurs with conditions such as renal failure, lactic acidosis, starvation, diabetic or alcoholic ketoacidosis, severe diarrhea or poisoning by certain toxins.

**Signs and symptoms** – Symptoms include compensatory hyperventilation, vomiting, diarrhea, headache, weakness and malaise, hyperkalemia, and cardiac arrhythmias. If left untreated the continued increase in acid can induce coma and eventual death.

**Treatment** – Treatment includes managing the underlying cause, correcting any coexisting electrolyte imbalances, and administering sodium bicarbonate.

> ### Rehabilitation Considerations for Patients with Acid-Base Disorders[10,13]
>
> - Recognize higher risk populations for imbalances such as patients with renal, cardiovascular, pulmonary disease; burns, fever, and sepsis; patients on mechanical ventilation; diabetes mellitus; patients currently vomiting with diarrhea or enteric drainage
> - Recognize signs of dehydration in a diabetic patient
> - Injury prevention during involuntary muscular contractions secondary to metabolic alkalosis
> - Recognize that patients using diuretic therapy may be at risk for potassium depletion
> - Recognize that Trousseau's sign during blood pressure measurements may indicate calcium deficiency and the early stages of tetany

## Metabolic Bone Disease[10]

Metabolic bone disease is a classification for particular diagnoses where there has been a disruption in normal metabolism within the skeletal system. The skeletal system houses calcium and phosphorus. It also continuously balances the remodeling of the cortical and trabecular bone in order to optimize the structure of the skeleton. Disruption in the homeostasis of skeletal metabolic processes will result in deformity, bone loss, fracture, softening of the bone, arthritis, and pain.

## Osteomalacia[10]

Osteomalacia is a metabolic condition where bones become soft secondary to a calcium or phosphorus deficiency. There is adequate bone matrix, however, there is insufficient calcification of the matrix due to the deficiency.

**Etiology** – Calcium is typically lost secondary to inadequate intestinal absorption and the phosphorus is lost secondary to an increase in renal excretion. A deficiency in vitamin D will also cause osteomalacia.

## Consider This

### Low Bone Mass[12]

Certain medical conditions may present with low bone mass as an associated clinical feature. A patient may report such conditions while detailing their medical history, but not be aware of the condition's potential influence on bone mass. Physical therapists should be aware of such conditions, regardless of an accompanying osteopenia or osteoporosis diagnosis, in order to best incorporate preventative interventions and education into the plan of care.

Medical conditions which may cause low bone mass include: Cushing's syndrome, osteomalacia, hyperthyroidism, hyperparathyroidism, celiac disease, rheumatoid arthritis, renal failure, hypogonadism, and osteogenesis imperfecta.

---

**Signs and symptoms** – Osteomalacia can include a vague presentation of aching, fatigue, and weight loss. Myopathy and sensory polyneuropathy may also occur along with periarticular tenderness and pain, thoracic kyphosis deformity, and bowing of the lower extremities. The patient may also struggle to perform transfers and assume a standing position.

**Treatment** – Specific intervention will focus on the underlying etiology. Increased nutrition is recommended and pharmacological intervention may include vitamin D or phosphate supplements.

### Osteoporosis[10]

Osteoporosis is a metabolic condition that presents with a decrease in bone mass that subsequently increases the risk of fracture. Osteoporosis primarily affects trabecular and cortical bone where the rate of bone resorption accelerates while the rate of bone formation declines. Declining osteoblast function coupled with the loss of calcium and phosphate salts will cause the bones to become brittle.

**Etiology** – Primary osteoporosis can include idiopathic, post-menopausal or involutional (senile) osteoporosis. Secondary osteoporosis can occur as a result of another primary condition or with use of certain medications.

**Signs and symptoms** – Symptoms include compression and other bone fractures, low thoracic or lumbar pain, loss of lumbar lordosis, deformities such as kyphosis, decrease in height, dowager's hump, and postural changes.

**Treatment** – Management of primary osteoporosis includes vitamin and pharmacological intervention, proper nutrition, assistive and adaptive device prescription, and patient education. Surgical intervention may be required for fracture stabilization.

### Paget's Disease[10]

Paget's disease is a metabolic condition characterized by heightened osteoclast activity. This process of excessive bone formation lacks true structural integrity. The bone appears enlarged, but lacks strength due to the high turnover of bone secondary to abnormal osteoclastic proliferation.

**Etiology** – This disease has a genetic component as well as geographical incidence, and most commonly affects patients over 50 years of age.

**Signs and symptoms** – Symptoms include musculoskeletal pain accompanied by bony deformities (kyphosis, coxa varus, bowing of the long bones, vertebral compression). The skull, clavicle, pelvis, femur, spine and tibia are common sites that will exhibit bony changes. Symptoms of advanced progression of the disease include continued pain, headache, vertigo, hearing loss, mental deterioration, fatigue, increased cardiac output, and heart failure (secondary to an increased cardiac output).

**Treatment** – Management relies heavily on pharmacological intervention using bisphosphonates in order to inhibit bone resorption and improve the quality of the involved bone. Exercise, weight control, and cardiac fitness are all key components in a program to maintain strength and motion.

### Rehabilitation Considerations for Patients with Metabolic Bone Disease[10]

- Must have awareness of signs of compression fracture and of patients at higher risk for all forms of fracture
- Focus on both resistance training and endurance training to build bone density and increase strength
- Avoid treatments that exacerbate the condition or place patients at risk for fracture

### Metabolic System Terminology[10, 14-16]

**Aerobic metabolism:** The ATP producing metabolic processes that are dependent on oxygen transported via the circulatory system. Aerobic metabolic functions typically provide energy for low intensity and/or longer duration activities.

**Anabolism:** The metabolic process in which simple molecules (e.g., nucleic acids, polysaccharides, amino acids) are combined to create the complex molecules (e.g., proteins) needed for tissue and organ growth.

**Anaerobic metabolism:** Metabolic functions that do not require the presence of oxygen and produce energy for high intensity, shorter duration activities.

**Adenosine triphosphate (ATP):** The molecular unit within the body which transports the chemical compounds used for cellular metabolism.

## Consider This

### Osteoporosis Risk Factors and Prevention[12,14,15]

Bone mineral density (BMD) is used to diagnose osteoporosis and other low bone mass disorders. BMD is measured via dual-energy x-ray absorptiometry and expressed in terms of T-score and Z-score. T-score refers to how many standard deviations above or below average healthy young adult norms an individual's BMD is. Z-score refers to how many standard deviations above or below average age and gender adjusted norms an individual's BMD is .5. The World Health Organization reports that in women, a T-score lower than -1 standard deviation (SD) but greater than -2.5 SD is indicative of osteopenia. A score that is -2.5 SD or lower is indicative of osteoporosis, and a score at or below -2.5 SD with one or more related fractures is considered severe osteoporosis.

Physical therapists are often the primary educator with patients who have either sustained or are at risk for osteoporotic fractures. Therapists should therefore have a sound understanding of non-modifiable and modifiable risk factors so that education topics and treatment planning may be adapted to address both.

Non-modifiable risk factors associated with the development of low bone mass include age, early menopause, history of previous fracture, slender build, family history of low bone mass, female gender, and being of either Asian or Caucasian descent. Certain conditions and medications, such as glucocorticoids, may also be considered non-modifiable if discontinuing such medications is medically ill-advised.

Modifiable risk factors associated with the development of low bone mass include insufficient dietary intake of vitamin D and calcium, estrogen deficiency, cigarette smoking, alcohol use in excess of two drinks per day, caffeine intake in excess of two servings per day, and sedentary lifestyle.

Treatment interventions and educational topics are similar for both osteopenia and osteoporosis. Prevention of osteoporosis associated fractures is a primary goal of therapeutic interventions for at-risk individuals of all ages. Specific interventions, however, may be emphasized or excluded depending on the patient's age and associated risk factors.

### Interventions for Children and Adolescents

Osteoporosis prevention is important to begin during childhood by ensuring adequate nutrition, especially with regard to calcium intake, since malnutrition and undernutrition negatively impact bone development. Bone mass density typically peaks during an individual's mid-20's. Younger patients should be encouraged to participate regularly in physical activity to promote bone strength. The adverse effects of smoking and excessive alcohol consumption on bone development should also be addressed with younger patient populations. Adherence to recommendations may be the greatest challenge in addressing osteoporosis in younger populations.

### Interventions for Adults

Once peak BMD has been reached, maintaining this during the processes of ongoing remodeling is paramount in minimizing the eventual imbalance between bone formation and remodeling. Maintaining good nutrition, including recommended calcium and vitamin D intake, is a key factor in managing the risk of osteoporotic fractures. Regular weight bearing exercise is strongly recommended in addition to avoiding smoking and heavy drinking. Postural education and fall prevention activities are also increasingly important during later years when fracture risk is heightened.

**Catabolism:** The metabolic process in which complex materials (e.g., proteins, lipids) are broken down in the body for the purpose of creating and releasing heat and energy.

**DNA (deoxyribonucleic acid):** A double helix molecule that contains the genes that provide the blueprint for all of the structures and functions of a living being.

**Gene:** A fundamental unit of heredity.

**Metabolism:** The physical and chemical processes of cells burning fuel to produce and use energy. Examples include digestion, elimination of waste, breathing, thermoregulation, muscular contraction, brain function, and circulation.

**Mitochondria:** The part of the cell that is responsible for energy production. The mitochondria are also responsible for converting nutrients into energy and other specialized tasks.

**Osteopenia:** A condition presenting with low bone mass that is not severe enough to qualify as osteoporosis. Individuals with osteopenia may not have actual bone loss, but a naturally lower bone density than established norms.

**Osteopetrosis:** A group of conditions characterized by impaired osteoclast function, which causes bone to become thickened but fragile. Osteopetrosis is an inherited condition that can vary widely in symptoms and severity.

**pH:** A measure of the hydrogen ion concentration in body fluid.

# Endocrine System

## Key Functions of the Endocrine System[12]

The endocrine system consists of endocrine glands (specialized ductless glands) that secrete hormones that travel through the bloodstream to signal specific target cells throughout the body. The hormones travel throughout the body to the target organs upon which they act. They will bind selectively to receptor sites on the surface of the receptor cells. The endocrine system and nervous system both function to achieve and maintain stability of the internal environment (homeostasis). The systems are capable of working alone or in concert with each other. The endocrine and nervous systems work together to regulate metabolism, response to stress, sexual reproduction, blood pressure, and water and salt balances.

### Endocrine System

- Secreting cells send hormones through the bloodstream to signal specific target cells
- Hormones diffuse into the blood and travel long distances to virtually every area of the body
- Endocrine effectors consist of virtually all tissues
- Regulatory effects are slow and tend to last for long periods

### Nervous System

- Neurons secrete neurotransmitters to signal nearby cells that have an appropriate receptor site
- Neurotransmitters are sent very short distances across a synapse
- Nervous effectors are limited to muscle and glandular tissue
- Regulatory effects appear rapidly and are often short lived

NEXT EXIT

MOTIVATIONAL MOMENT

See Page 1028

## Glands of the Endocrine System[10,12]

### Hypothalamus

The hypothalamus is part of the diencephalon located below the thalamus and cerebral hemisphere. The hypothalamus connects to the pituitary gland through the infundibular or pituitary stalk. It is responsible for regulation of the autonomic nervous system (body temperature, appetite, sweating, thirst, sexual behavior, rage, fear, blood pressure, sleep) and other endocrine glands through its impact on the pituitary gland.

### Pituitary Gland

The pituitary gland is normally the size of a pea and is located at the base of the brain just beneath the hypothalamus. The pituitary gland consists of two separate glands, the adenohypophysis (anterior) and the neurohypophysis (posterior). The pituitary gland is considered the most important part of the endocrine system since it releases hormones that regulate several other endocrine glands. This "master gland" is influenced by factors such as seasonal changes or emotional stress. The pituitary gland secretes endorphins that act on the nervous system and reduce a person's sensitivity to pain. It also controls ovulation and works as a catalyst for the testes and ovaries to create sex hormones.

### Thyroid Gland

The thyroid gland is located on the anterior and lateral surfaces of the trachea immediately below the larynx and is shaped like a "bow tie" or "butterfly" with two halves (lobes); a right lobe and a left lobe joined by an isthmus. The thyroid produces thyroxine and triiodothyronine that act to control the rate at which cells burn the fuel from food. An increase in thyroid hormones will increase the rate of the chemical reactions within the body.

### Parathyroid Glands

There are four parathyroid glands found on the posterior surface of the thyroid's lateral lobes. These glands produce parathyroid hormone, which functions as an antagonist to calcitonin and is important for the maintenance of normal blood levels of calcium and phosphate. Parathyroid hormone increases the reabsorption of calcium and phosphate from bones to the blood. Secretion of parathyroid hormone is stimulated by hypocalcemia and inhibited by hypercalcemia. Normal clotting, neuromuscular excitability, and cell membrane permeability are dependent on normal calcium levels.

### Adrenal Glands

The two adrenal glands are located on top of each kidney, the outer portion is called the adrenal cortex and the inner portion is called the adrenal medulla. The adrenal cortex and the adrenal medulla secrete different hormones. The adrenal cortex produces corticosteroids that will regulate water and sodium balance, the body's response to stress, the immune system, sexual development and function, and metabolism. The adrenal medulla produces epinephrine that increases heart rate and blood pressure when there is an increase in stress.

## Pancreas

The pancreas is located in the upper left quadrant of the abdominal cavity, extending from the duodenum to the spleen. The pancreas includes both endocrine and exocrine tissues. The islets of Langerhans are the hormone-producing cells of the pancreas. Alpha cells produce glucagon and beta cells produce insulin. These hormones work in combination to ensure a consistent level of glucose within the bloodstream and properly maintain stores of energy within the body.

## Ovaries

The ovaries are located in the pelvic cavity on each side of the uterus. The ovaries provide estrogen and progesterone that contribute to regulation of the menstrual cycle and pregnancy. Estrogen is secreted by the ovarian follicles and is responsible for the development and maintenance of female sex characteristics such as breast development and the cycles of the female reproductive system. Progesterone is produced by the corpus luteum and functions to maintain the lining of the uterus at a level necessary for pregnancy.

## Testes

The testes are located in the scrotum between the upper thighs. The testes secrete androgens (most importantly testosterone) that regulate body changes associated with sexual development and support the production of sperm.

## Classes of Hormones[10, 12, 16]

### Steroid hormones (e.g., prostaglandins)

All cells create prostaglandins from the phospholipids of the cell membrane. They are unique from other hormones since they do not circulate in the blood and instead exert their effects only where they are produced. Prostaglandins are capable of producing a wide variety of effects; some effects as it pertains to rehabilitation are related to inflammation, pain mechanisms, vasodilation, vasoconstriction, nutrient metabolism, and blood clotting.

### Amine hormones (e.g., catecholamines)

Catecholamines (epinephrine, norepinephrine, and dopamine) are synthesized from chromaffin cells within the adrenal medulla. Sympathetic nervous system stimulation releases the catecholamines into the bloodstream. Epinephrine has one of the largest effects on the sympathetic nervous system and creates the "fight or flight" response. The target areas for epinephrine are receptor sites in the cardiovascular and metabolic systems. Other functions of catecholamines include increasing cardiac contraction, constriction of blood vessels, activation of glycogen breakdown, blocking of insulin secretion, increasing metabolic rate, and dilation of the airways within the lungs.

### Peptide hormones (e.g., insulin)

Insulin is a hormone secreted by the beta cells of the islets of Langerhans within the pancreas. Insulin is released when there is an elevation in the level of blood glucose. The insulin produces an increase in cellular uptake of glucose for metabolism. Insulin also stimulates the skeletal muscle and liver to store the glucose and increases amino acid transport across hepatic, muscle, and adipose tissues. Insulin release affects all systems of the body with its primary goal of reducing blood glucose levels.

## Endocrine System: Hormone, Function, and Regulation of Secretion[10,12]

| Hormone | Function | Regulation of Secretion |
|---|---|---|
| **Hypothalamus** | | |
| **Growth hormone-releasing hormone** Target: pituitary gland | Increases the release of growth hormone | Central nervous system feedback; circulating levels of hormones |
| **Growth hormone-inhibiting hormone** Target: pituitary gland | Decreases the release of growth hormone | Central nervous system feedback; circulating levels of hormones |
| **Gonadotropin-releasing hormone** Target: pituitary gland | Increases the release of luteinizing hormone and follicle-stimulating hormone | Central nervous system feedback; circulating levels of hormones |
| **Thyrotropin-releasing hormone** Target: pituitary gland | Increases the release of thyroid-stimulating hormone | Central nervous system feedback; circulating levels of hormones |
| **Corticotropin-releasing hormone** Target: pituitary gland | Increases the release of adrenocorticotropic hormone | Central nervous system feedback; circulating levels of hormones |
| **Prolactin-releasing hormone** Target: pituitary gland | Stimulates the release of prolactin | Central nervous system feedback; circulating levels of hormones |
| **Prolactin-inhibitory factor; dopamine** Target: pituitary gland | Decreases the release of prolactin | Central nervous system feedback; circulating levels of hormones |

| Hormone | Function | Regulation of Secretion |
|---------|----------|-------------------------|
| **Pituitary** | | |
| **Growth hormone**<br>Target: bone and muscle | Promotes growth and development; increases the rate of protein synthesis | Hypothalamus |
| **Follicle-stimulating hormone**<br>Target: ovaries and testes | Promotes follicular development and the creation of estrogen in females; promotes spermatogenesis in males | Hypothalamus |
| **Luteinizing hormone**<br>Target: ovaries and testes | Promotes ovulation along with estrogen/progesterone synthesis from the corpus luteum in females; promotes testosterone synthesis in males | Hypothalamus |
| **Thyroid-stimulating hormone**<br>Target: thyroid gland | Increases the synthesis of thyroid hormones T3 and T4 | Hypothalamus |
| **Adrenocorticotropic hormone**<br>Target: adrenal cortex | Increases cortisol synthesis (adrenal steroids) | Hypothalamus |
| **Prolactin**<br>Target: mammary glands | Allows for the process of lactation | Hypothalamus |
| **Oxytocin**<br>Target: uterus and mammary glands | Increases contraction of uterine muscles; promotes release of milk from mammary glands | Nerve impulses from the hypothalamus; stretching of cervix; nipple stimulation |
| **Antidiuretic hormone**<br>Target: kidneys | Increases water reabsorption; conserves water; increases blood pressure through stimulating contraction of muscles in small arteries | Decreased water content |
| **Adrenal Cortex** | | |
| **Androgen**<br>Target: ovaries and testes | Increases masculinization; promotes growth of pubic hair in males and females | Influenced by the hypothalamic production and release of GnRH and Luteinizing hormone (LH) |
| **Aldosterone (mineralocorticoid)**<br>Target: kidneys | Increases reabsorption of sodium ions by the kidneys to the blood; increases excretion of potassium ions by the kidney into the urine | Low blood sodium level; high blood potassium level |
| **Cortisol (glucocorticoid)**<br>Target: gastrointestinal system | Influences metabolism of food molecules; anti-inflammatory effect in large amounts | Adrenocorticotropic hormone |
| **Adrenal Medulla** | | |
| **Epinephrine**<br>Target: cardiovascular and metabolic systems | Increases heart rate and force of contraction; increases energy production; vasodilation in skeletal muscle | Sympathetic impulses from the hypothalamus in stress situations |
| **Norepinephrine**<br>Target: cardiovascular and metabolic systems | Vasoconstriction in skin, viscera, and skeletal muscles | |
| **Ovaries** | | |
| **Estrogen, progesterone**<br>Target: uterus and mammary glands | Involved in regulation of the female reproductive system and female sexual characteristics | Cyclical rise and fall of hormone levels |

| Hormone | Function | Regulation of Secretion |
|---|---|---|
| **Pancreas** | | |
| **Glucagon** <br> Target: liver | Increases blood glucose by stimulating the conversion of glycogen to glucose | Hypoglycemia |
| **Insulin** <br> Target: all body systems | Decreases blood glucose and increases the storage of fat, protein, and carbohydrates | Hyperglycemia |
| **Parathyroids** | | |
| **Parathormone** <br> Target: bone, kidney, intestinal mucosa | Increases blood calcium | Hypocalcemia |
| **Testes** | | |
| **Testosterone** <br> Target: pituitary gland | Involved in the process of spermatogenesis and male sexual characteristics | Influenced by pituitary release of LH |
| **Thyroid** | | |
| **Thyroxine (T4), Triiodothyronine (T3)** <br> Target: all tissues | Involved with normal development; increases cellular level metabolism | Thyroid-stimulating hormone |
| **Calcitonin** <br> Target: plasma | Increases calcium storage in bone; decreases blood calcium levels | Hypercalcemia |

## Endocrine System Dysfunction General Signs and Symptoms[10,12]

**Neuromuscular**
- Muscle weakness
- Periarthritis
- Myalgia
- Arthralgia
- Stiffness
- Osteoarthritis
- Muscle atrophy
- Adhesive capsulitis

**Systemic**
- Polydipsia
- Growth dysfunction
- Skin pigmentation dysfunction
- Polyuria
- Increased vital signs
- Hair dysfunction
- Nervousness or anxiety

## Endocrine System Pathology[10,12]

The endocrine system is multifaceted and can develop pathology in one or more areas due to hyperfunction or hypofunction of one or more glands. In many instances, it is the hypothalamus or the pituitary gland that affects the function of other endocrine glands when they experience direct or indirect dysfunction.

**Hyperfunction of an endocrine gland:** usually secondary to overstimulation of the pituitary gland. This can also occur due to hyperplasia or neoplasia of the gland itself.

**Hypofunction of an endocrine gland:** usually secondary to understimulation of the pituitary gland. This can also occur from congenital or acquired disorders.

There are other instances where direct damage to the hypothalamus or pituitary gland creates dysfunction:

**Hypothalamus Dysfunction**
- Hypothalamus tumors (i.e., ependymomas)
- Inflammatory processes (i.e., sarcoidosis)
- Surgical transection
- Trauma (i.e., skull fracture)

**Pituitary Dysfunction**
- Pituitary tumors (i.e., adenomas)
- Ischemic necrosis or infarction of the pituitary gland
- Infiltrative disorders (i.e., hemochromatosis)
- Inflammatory processes (i.e., meningitis)
- Iatrogenic (i.e., irradiation)

**Hypopituitarism:** This condition occurs when there is a decreased or absent hormonal secretion from the anterior pituitary gland. This is a rare disorder and symptoms are dependent on the age of the affected person and deficit hormones. Typical disorders may include short stature (dwarfism), delayed growth and puberty, sexual and reproductive disorders, and diabetes insipidus. Treatment is also based on the deficit hormones and usually includes pharmacological replacement therapy.

**Hyperpituitarism:** This condition occurs when there is an excessive secretion of one or more hormones under the pituitary gland's control (frequently growth hormone that produces acromegaly in adults). Disorders and symptoms are dependent on the hormone(s) that are affected. Some disorders include gigantism or acromegaly, hirsutism, galactorrhea (abnormal lactation in males or females), amenorrhea, infertility, and impotence. Treatment is hormone and site dependent and can include tumor resection, surgery, radiation therapy, and hormone suppression or replacement (if gland becomes dysfunctional after treatment).

## Rehabilitation Considerations for Patients with Pituitary Dysfunction[10]

- Ambulation/exercise encouraged within 24 hours of surgery (post tumor/gland removal)
- Must demonstrate increased awareness for signs of hypoglycemia
- Bilateral carpal tunnel syndrome, arthritis, osteophyte formation are common with hyperpituitarism
- Orthostatic hypotension may be present with hypopituitarism
- Bilateral hemianopsia that can occur with hypopituitarism requires special consideration during treatment

## Adrenal Dysfunction

### Addison's Disease[12]

Addison's disease is a form of adrenal dysfunction that presents with hypofunction of the adrenal cortex. Subsequently, there is decreased production of both cortisol (glucocorticoid) and aldosterone (mineralocorticoid).

**Etiology** – When the adrenal cortex produces insufficient cortisol and aldosterone hormones it is termed Addison's disease.

**Signs and symptoms** – Symptoms include a widespread metabolic dysfunction secondary to cortisol deficiency as well as fluid and electrolyte imbalances secondary to aldosterone dysfunction. The person may experience hypotension, weakness, anorexia, weight loss, altered pigmentation, and if left untreated this condition will result in shock and possible death.

**Treatment** – Treatment primarily consists of long-term pharmacological intervention using synthetic corticosteroids and mineralocorticoids.

### Cushing's Syndrome[12]

Cushing's disease is a form of adrenal dysfunction that presents with hyperfunction of the adrenal gland, allowing for excessive amounts of cortisol (glucocorticoid) production.

**Etiology** – When the pituitary gland produces excessive adrenocorticotropic hormone (ACTH) with subsequent hyper cortisolism, it is termed Cushing's disease.

**Signs and symptoms** – Symptoms evolve over years and can include persistent hyperglycemia, growth failure, truncal obesity, purple abdominal striae, "moon shaped face," "buffalo hump" posteriorly at the base of the neck, weakness, acne, hypertension, and male gynecomastia. Mental changes can include depression, poor concentration, and memory loss.

**Treatment** – Treatment may include pharmacological intervention to block the production of the hormones, radiation therapy, chemotherapy or surgery.

## Rehabilitation Considerations for Patients with Adrenal Dysfunction[10]

- Recognize signs of stress or exhaustion and avoid treatments that exacerbate the condition
- Notify the physician with any signs of illness or increased intracranial pressure (e.g., papilledema); medications may need to be altered
- Orthostatic hypotension is common secondary to long-term cortisol therapy
- Report sleep disturbances to the physician
- Increased incidence of osteoporosis, bone fractures, degenerative myopathy, tendon ruptures, ataxic gait
- Delayed wound healing may be common

## Thyroid Dysfunction[11]

**Hypothyroidism:** This condition occurs when there are decreased levels of thyroid hormones in the bloodstream, slowing metabolic processes within the body. Symptoms may include fatigue, weakness, decreased heart rate, weight gain, constipation, delayed puberty, and retarded growth and development. Common causes of hypothyroidism are Hashimoto's thyroiditis or an underdeveloped thyroid gland. Treatment includes oral thyroid hormone replacement therapy.

**Hyperthyroidism:** This condition occurs when there are excessive levels of thyroid hormones in the bloodstream. Symptoms can include an increase in nervousness, excessive sweating, weight loss, increase in blood pressure, exophthalmos, myopathy, chronic periarthritis, and an enlarged thyroid gland. Treatment may include pharmacological intervention, radioactive iodine, and surgery.

## Consider This

### Postpartum Thyroiditis[14]

Postpartum thyroiditis refers to a painless inflammation of the thyroid occurring in some women after childbirth. The presentation of this condition is typically defined by two phases. Initially, a state of hyperthyroidism will present within the first one to four months following childbirth. This is followed by a shift to hypothyroidism four to eight months following delivery.

Signs of the hyperactive phase of postpartum thyroiditis may include tachycardia, unexplained weight loss, anxiety, irritability, fatigue, and heat sensitivity. Unfortunately, the initial signs of this hyperactive thyroid phase may be misinterpreted as typical postpartum symptoms, thereby delaying diagnosis. More frequently, postpartum thyroiditis is detected after the onset of the hypoactive phase. Symptoms in this phase are consistent with other hypothyroidism disorders including dry skin, hoarse voice, depression, cold sensitivity, and poor exercise tolerance. Risk factors for postpartum thyroiditis include a history of autoimmune disorders, thyroid dysfunction, prior postpartum thyroiditis or a family history of thyroid dysfunction. Blood tests are used to confirm a diagnosis in either phase.

Timely diagnosis and treatment of women with postpartum thyroiditis can impact both physical therapy outcomes and the patient's quality of life. Physical therapists should be cautious not to dismiss symptoms of fatigue and irritability as typical postpartum occurrences, especially if other signs of thyroid dysfunction can be identified. Therapists should also be mindful that pharmacological interventions (e.g., beta blockers, thyroid replacement hormones) may further influence a patient's exercise tolerance and anticipated outcomes.

### Graves' Disease[10]

Graves' disease is the most specific cause of hyperthyroidism. Graves' disease is most common in women over age 20, however, it occurs in men as well and can affect any age group.

**Etiology** – Graves' disease is caused by an autoimmune disease in which certain antibodies produced by the immune system stimulate the thyroid gland causing it to become overactive.

**Signs and symptoms** – Symptoms are consistent with hyperthyroid presentation. The classic signs of Graves' disease include mild enlargement of the thyroid gland (goiter), heat intolerance, nervousness, weight loss, tremor, and palpitations.

**Treatment** – Management includes pharmacological intervention and/or removal of the thyroid gland using radiation or surgical intervention.

| Hypothyroidism[17] | Hyperthyroidism[17] |
|---|---|
| Depression and/or anxiety, increased lethargy, fatigue, headache, slowed speech, slowed mental function, impaired short-term memory | Tremors, hyperkinesis, nervousness, increased DTRs, emotional lability, insomnia, weakness, atrophy |
| Proximal muscle weakness, carpal tunnel syndrome, trigger points, myalgia, increased bone density, cold intolerance, paresthesias | Chronic periarthritis, heat intolerance, flushed skin, hyperpigmentation, increased hair loss |
| Dyspnea, bradycardia, CHF, respiratory muscle weakness, decreased peripheral circulation, angina, increase in cholesterol | Tachycardia, palpitations, increased respiratory rate, increase in blood pressure, arrhythmias |
| Anorexia, constipation, weight gain, decreased absorption of food and glucose | Hypermetabolism, increased appetite, increased peristalsis, nausea, vomiting, diarrhea, dysphagia |
| Infertility, irregular menstrual cycle, increased menstrual bleeding | Polyuria, infertility, increased first trimester miscarriage, amenorrhea |

## Rehabilitation Considerations for Patients with Thyroid Dysfunction[10]

- Recognize reduced exercise capacity and fatigue are typical
- Avoid treatments that exacerbate the condition such as exercise in a hot aquatic or gym setting due to heat intolerance (Graves' disease)
- Avoid cardiovascular stress to eliminate secondary complications from hypotension, goiter, Graves' disease
- Provide close monitoring of vital signs
- Recognize the effects of radioiodine therapy
- Recognize the risk of rhabdomyolysis (hypothyroidism)

## Parathyroid Dysfunction[10]

Hypoparathyroidism: This condition occurs due to hyposecretion or low-level production of parathyroid hormone by the parathyroid gland. Symptoms may include hypocalcemia, neurological symptoms such as seizures, cognitive defects, short stature, tetany (life-threatening) muscle spasms, muscle pain, and cramps. Treatment of acute hypoparathyroidism requires rapid elevation in serum calcium levels through intravenous calcium. Long-term treatment includes pharmacological management and dietary modifications.

Hyperparathyroidism: This condition occurs due to excessive levels of hormone production by the parathyroid gland that leads to disruption of calcium, phosphate, and bone metabolism. Symptoms may include renal stones and kidney damage, depression, memory loss, muscle wasting, bone deformity, and myopathy. Acute treatment may include pharmacological intervention that produces an immediate lowering of serum calcium using diuretics or antiresorptive medications. Surgical intervention is usually required to remove the diseased parathyroid gland. Pharmacological intervention may be used prior to surgery or for long-term management.

## Rehabilitation Considerations for Patients with Parathyroid Dysfunction[10]

- Must be familiar with all signs and symptoms of parathyroid dysfunction in order to refer patients to a physician if a change in their status occurs
- Recognize symptoms of excessive or inadequate pharmacological treatment and side effects of the agents
- Avoid treatments that exacerbate the condition
- Recognize effects of hypercalcemia (hyperparathyroidism) and hypocalcemia (hypoparathyroidism)
- Recognize the increased risk for fractures and effects from osteogenic synovitis (Achilles, triceps, and obturator tendons most affected)

| Hypoparathyroidism[17] | Hyperparathyroidism[17] |
| --- | --- |
| Decreased bone resorption | Increased bone resorption |
| Hypocalcemia | Hypercalcemia |
| Elevated serum phosphate levels | Decreased serum phosphate levels |
| Shortened 4th and 5th metacarpals (pseudohypoparathyroidism) | Osteitis fibrosa, subperiosteal resorption, arthritis, bone deformity |
| Compromised breathing due to intercostal muscle and diaphragm spasms | Nephrocalcinosis, renal hypertension, and significant renal damage |
| Cardiac arrhythmias and potential heart failure | Gout |
| Increased neuromuscular activity that can result in tetany | Decreased neuromuscular irritability |

## Pancreas Dysfunction[12]

### Type 1 Diabetes Mellitus (DM)

This form of DM occurs when the pancreas fails to produce enough or any insulin. This form of diabetes is normally diagnosed in childhood, but can occur at any age. It is also known as insulin-dependent diabetes or juvenile diabetes.

**Etiology** – The exact cause is unknown, but genetic predisposition in combination with exposure to a viral or environmental trigger is believed to cause an immune reaction that damages the pancreas with subsequent failure in secretion of endogenous insulin.

**Signs and symptoms** – Symptoms of DM include a rapid onset of symptoms, polyphagia, weight loss, ketoacidosis, polyuria, polydipsia, blurred vision, dehydration, and fatigue.

**Treatment** – Management includes exogenous insulin injections that are required to maintain proper glucose blood levels and avoid complications. Proper nutritional management is also required for blood glucose control. Insulin pumps may be indicated for continuous administration of insulin. Presently, there is no cure for type 1 DM and as a result, the goal is to control the regulation of blood glucose levels (Fig. 7-5).

### Type 2 Diabetes Mellitus (DM)

This form of DM typically occurs in the population over the age of 40, however, there has been an increase in children diagnosed with type 2 DM secondary to a rise in childhood obesity. This form of DM typically retains the ability to produce some endogenous insulin.

**Etiology** – Type 2 DM occurs secondary to an array of dysfunctions resulting from the combination of resistance to insulin action and inadequate insulin secretion. This disorder is characterized by hyperglycemia when the body cannot properly respond to insulin. Obesity is found to contribute to this condition by increasing insulin resistance.

**Signs and symptoms** – Symptoms are relatively the same as with type 1, however, ketoacidosis does not occur since insulin is still typically produced.

**Treatment** – Treatment of type 2 diabetes includes blood glucose control through diet, exercise, oral medications or insulin injections when necessary.

**Fig. 7-5:** Self-monitoring of blood glucose levels.

## Spotlight on Safety
### Blood Glucose Levels – Exercise Response[11,18]

For patients with diabetes mellitus (DM), an awareness of how to manage blood glucose levels is imperative to prevent the potentially life threatening effects of hyper or hypoglycemia. Both patients and physical therapists must be aware of the signs and symptoms of these emergent conditions, how to respond, and how therapy interventions may be either a causative or alleviating factor. According to the American Diabetes Association, recommended blood glucose levels include 70-130 mg/dl prior to a meal and <180 mg/dl after a meal.

### Hyperglycemia

Unaddressed hyperglycemia is a significant factor in the development of DM related complications. In addition to blood glucose measures, early signs of hyperglycemia that can occur when blood glucose is >180-200 mg/dl include increased thirst and frequent urination. Recognition of these early signs is crucial in preventing the dangerous onset of ketoacidosis, often referred to as a "diabetic coma." Most commonly occurring in patients with type 1 DM, ketoacidosis is a life-threatening condition requiring immediate medical attention. Symptoms include dyspnea, a fruity breath odor, dry mouth, nausea, vomiting, confusion, and an eventual loss of consciousness.

### Hypoglycemia

It is equally important to recognize the initial signs of hypoglycemia so that early intervention may prevent more serious symptoms. Early signs of hypoglycemia that may occur when blood glucose is <70 mg/dl include hunger, sweating, shaking, dizziness, clumsiness, and headache. If unaddressed, patients who become hypoglycemic may lose consciousness, at which point immediate medical attention is necessary. Hypoglycemia is often counteracted simply by ingestion of a glucose or carbohydrate-rich substance (e.g., sugar, honey, juice, crackers). Patients with significant hypoglycemic issues may be advised by their physician to carry a glucose source or injectable glucagon with them at all times.

### Exercise Response

A regular exercise program offers numerous benefits to patients with DM. The weight and stress management aspects of exercise are particularly beneficial with regard to controlling blood glucose levels. Physical and mental stressors have been shown to elevate blood glucose levels making long term management more challenging for patients with DM. Exercise provides positive dual influences of aiding stress management and increasing blood glucose uptake by the muscles without significantly impacting insulin levels. Physical therapists, however, must be alert to signs of exercise induced hypoglycemia which may occur with strenuous or prolonged exercise tasks. The risk of symptom onset can often be reduced by ingestion of a carbohydrate snack prior to exercise in order to compensate for increased glucose demands and/or increased insulin absorption.

| Type 1 Diabetes Mellitus[12] (insulin-dependent, juvenile diabetes) | Type 2 Diabetes Mellitus[12] (non-insulin dependent, adult onset diabetes) |
|---|---|
| Onset: usually less than 25 years of age | Onset: usually older than 40 years of age |
| Abrupt onset | Gradual onset |
| 5-10% of all cases | 90-95% of all cases |
| Etiology: destruction of islet of Langerhans cells secondary to possible autoimmune or viral causative factor | Etiology: resistance at insulin receptor sites usually secondary to obesity; ethnic prevalence |
| Insulin production: very little or none | Insulin production: variable |
| Ketoacidosis can occur | Ketoacidosis will rarely occur |
| Treatment includes insulin injection, exercise, and diet | Treatment includes weight loss, oral insulin, exercise, and diet |

### Rehabilitation Considerations for Patients with Diabetes Mellitus[10]

- Recognize the risk for peripheral neuropathies, small vessel angiopathy, tissue ischemia and ulceration, impaired wound healing, tissue necrosis, and amputation
- Recognize acute metabolic changes
- Recognize the signs of sudden hypoglycemia and necessary treatment
- Focus on consistent management of insulin intake, diet, and physical activity
- Provide education for proper skin care, shoe evaluation, and shoe wear

## Testes and Ovaries Dysfunction[10]

In males, the hypothalamus produces gonadotropin-releasing hormone (GnRH) and the pituitary responds by producing luteinizing hormone (LH) and follicle-stimulating hormone (FSH). The Leydig cells of the testes respond to these hormones with the production of testosterone. This cycle normally occurs on a daily basis.

In females, the hypothalamus produces GnRH and the pituitary responds by producing LH and FSH. In the ovaries, LH acts on theca and interstitial cells to produce progestins and androgens, and FSH acts on granulosa cells to stimulate the precursor steroids to estrogen.

**Male hypogonadism:** Primary hypogonadism is defined as a deficiency of testosterone secondary to failure of the testes to respond to FSH and LH (produced by the pituitary and hypothalamus). The most common cause of primary hypogonadism is Klinefelter's syndrome. Secondary hypogonadism occurs when there is a failure of the hypothalamus or pituitary to produce the hormones that will subsequently stimulate the production of testosterone. If a male experiences this prior to puberty, symptoms will include sparse body hair, underdevelopment of skeletal muscles, and long arms and legs secondary to a delay in the closure of the epiphyseal growth plates. Adult-onset testosterone deficiency will present with a decreased libido, erectile dysfunction, infertility, decreased cognitive skills, mood changes, and sleep disturbances. Treatment includes hormone replacement pharmacological intervention.

**Female hypogonadism:** Primary hypogonadism results if the gonad does not produce the amount of sex steroid sufficient to suppress secretion of LH and FSH at normal levels. The most common cause of primary hypogonadism is Turner syndrome. Secondary hypogonadism occurs when there is a failure of the hypothalamus or pituitary to produce the hormones that subsequently stimulate the production of estrogen. If a female experiences this prior to puberty symptoms will include gonadal dysgenesis, a short stature, failure to progress through puberty or primary amenorrhea, and premature gonadal failure. When hypogonadism occurs in postpubescent females, secondary amenorrhea is the primary symptom. Treatment includes hormone replacement pharmacological intervention.

## Pharmacology - Endocrine Management[19]

Endocrine pharmacological intervention will either consist of replacement therapy that will provide the deficient hormones or hyperfunction therapy which inhibits the oversecretion of the target hormones. The following is an overview highlighting only the general process for treatment.

### Hormone Replacement Agents

**Action:** These agents restore normal endocrine function when endogenous production of a particular hormone is deficient or absent.

**Indications:** decrease in endogenous hormone secretion

**Side effects:** Vary by exogenous or synthetic hormone replacement used for treatment

**Implications for PT:** Therapists must be aware of signs and symptoms of hormone deficit and side effects of hormone therapy.

**Examples:** see specific hormone categories, pg. 338-340

### Hyperfunction Agents

**Action:** These agents manage hyperactive endocrine function to allow for inhibition of hormone function. This is accomplished through negative feedback loops or through hormone antagonists.

**Indications:** hyperactive or excessive endocrine function, excessive hormone levels

**Side effects:** Vary depending on the use of exogenous or synthetic hormone therapy

**Implications for PT:** Therapists must be aware of signs of hyperfunction of particular hormones and side effects from agents that attempt to regulate and normalize hormone functioning.

**Examples:** see specific hormone categories, pg. 338-340

### Bone Mineral Regulating Agents

**Action:** Bone mineral regulating agents attempt to enhance and maximize bone mass along with preventing bone loss or rate of bone reabsorption. Typical agents can include estrogens, calcium and vitamin D, bisphosphonates, calcitonin, and anabolic agents.

**Indications:** Paget's disease, osteoporosis, hyperparathyroidism, rickets, hypoparathyroidism, osteomalacia

**Side effects:** (agent dependent) gastrointestinal distress, dyspepsia, dysphagia, anorexia, bone pain, cardiac arrhythmias

**Implications for PT:** Patients with bone mineralization deficit are at risk for fracture and side effects from drug therapy. Therapists must be aware of potential side effects and should attempt to augment drug therapy through ambulation and other weight bearing activities that stimulate bone formation.

**Examples:** Estrogens: Premarin (conjugated estrogen); Calcium and vitamin D: Tums (calcium carbonate), Calderol (calcifediol); Bisphosphonates: Fosamax (alendronate sodium), Boniva (ibandronate); Calcitonin: Cibacalcin (human calcitonin)

## Gastrointestinal System

## Gastrointestinal System

The gastrointestinal system is responsible for the process of digestion. It breaks down food into its components, absorbs nutrients, and discards the waste.

### Gastrointestinal Anatomy and Function[10]

| Upper GI | | Lower GI – Small Intestine | |
|---|---|---|---|
| Mouth | Initiation of mechanical and chemical digestion | Duodenum | Neutralizes acid in food from the stomach and mixes pancreatic and biliary secretions with food |
| Esophagus | Transports food from the mouth to the stomach | Jejunum | Absorbs water, electrolytes, and nutrients |
| Stomach | Grinding of food, secretion of hydrochloric acid and other exocrine functions, secretion of hormones that release digestive enzymes from the liver, pancreas, and gallbladder to assist with digestion | Ileum | Absorbs bile and intrinsic factors to be recycled |

Lower GI – Large Intestine

| | |
|---|---|
| Ascending colon<br>Transverse colon<br>Descending colon<br>Sigmoid<br>Rectum<br>Anus | Continues to absorb water and electrolytes; stores and eliminates undigested food as feces |

Gland Organs

| | |
|---|---|
| Gallbladder | Stores and releases bile into the duodenum to assist with digestion |
| Liver | Bile is produced and is necessary for absorption of lipid soluble substances, assists with red blood cell and vitamin K production, regulates serum level of carbohydrates, proteins, and fats |
| Pancreas | Exocrine - secretes bicarbonate and digestive enzymes into the duodenum; Endocrine - secretes insulin, glucagon, and other hormones into the blood to regulate serum glucose level |

## Gastrointestinal System Pathology

| GI Components | Common Pathologies |
|---|---|
| Esophagus | Hiatal hernia, gastroesophageal reflux disease, esophageal cancer, dysphagia, esophageal varices, Barrett's esophagus |
| Stomach | Gastritis, peptic ulcer disease, gastric cancer, gastrointestinal hemorrhage, motility and emptying disorders |
| Intestines | Malabsorption syndrome, appendicitis, irritable bowel syndrome, Crohn's disease, ulcerative colitis, colon cancer, intestinal hernia, diverticular diseases |
| Rectum and anus | Rectal or anal cancer, hemorrhoids, anorectal fistula, rectal fissure |
| Gallbladder | Gallstones (cholelithiasis), cholecystitis, gallbladder cancer |
| Liver | Cirrhosis, jaundice, hepatitis (A, B, C, D, E, G), ascites, hepatic encephalopathy, liver cancer, hepatomegaly |
| Pancreas | Pancreatitis (acute and chronic), diabetes mellitus, pancreatic cancer |

## Rehabilitation Considerations for Patients with Gastrointestinal Disease[10]

- Recognize electrolyte imbalances from diarrhea, vomiting, and weight loss

- Recognize the potential for orthostatic hypotension secondary to electrolyte imbalances

- Increased risk for muscle cramping secondary to alteration in the sodium-potassium pumps

- Potential for difficulty swallowing secondary to disk protrusion or esophageal pathology

- Recognize that back pain and/or shoulder pain may be secondary to an acute ulcer or GI bleed

- Observation of Kehr's sign indicates free air or blood within the abdominal cavity

## Esophagus

### Gastroesophageal Reflux Disease (GERD)[10,17]

GERD is the result of an incompetent lower esophageal sphincter (LES) that allows reflux of gastric contents. This backwards movement of stomach acids and contents can cause esophageal tissue injury over time as well as other pathology. GERD is estimated to occur in 20-30% of adults and can be found in some newborns or infants.

**Etiology** – The etiologies of GERD include weakness of the LES, intermittent relaxation of the LES, direct damage of the LES through NSAIDs, alcohol, infectious agents, smoking, and certain prescription medications.

**Signs and symptoms** – Clinical symptoms include heartburn, regurgitation of gastric contents, belching, chest pain, hoarseness and coughing, esophagitis, and hematemesis. If GERD is left untreated, the patient may develop esophageal strictures, esophagitis, aspiration pneumonia, asthma, Barrett's esophagitis, and esophageal adenocarcinoma.

**Treatment** – Treatment is primarily through pharmacological intervention.

## Rehabilitation Considerations for Patients with GERD[10,17]

- Avoid certain exercise secondary to an increase in symptoms with activity; recumbency will induce symptoms

- Recognize increased incidence of neck and head discomfort secondary to perception of a lump in the throat and subsequent compensation

- Left sidelying preferred since right sidelying may promote acid flowing into the esophagus

- Recognize conditions such as chronic bronchitis, asthma, and pulmonary fibrosis may all present with GERD

- Recognize that tight clothing, exercise, and constipation may all precipitate GERD

- Consider that certain positioning during postural drainage may encourage acid to move into the esophagus

## Stomach

### Gastritis[10,17]

Gastritis is the inflammation of the gastric mucosa or inner layer of the stomach. Symptoms are similar to GERD, however, they tend to have a higher intensity. Gastritis is classified as erosive or non-erosive based on the level and zone of injury.

### Erosive Gastritis (acute gastritis)[10,17]

**Etiology** – Etiology includes bleeding from the gastric mucosa secondary to stress, NSAIDs, alcohol utilization, viral infection or direct trauma.

**Signs and symptoms** – Symptoms include dyspepsia, nausea, vomiting, and hematemesis. At times, the patient may be asymptomatic.

**Treatment** – Treatment is supportive with removal of the stimulus of the disease process and pharmacological intervention. Surgical procedures may be required if the bleeding continues.

### Non-erosive Gastritis (chronic type B gastritis)[10,17]

**Etiology** – This condition is typically a result of a helicobacter pylori infection (H. pylori).

**Signs and symptoms** – The patient is usually asymptomatic but will show symptoms if the gastritis progresses.

**Treatment** – H. pylori is a carcinogen and must be treated aggressively. Pharmacological intervention is most common and typically includes a proton pump inhibitor and antibiotics.

## Rehabilitation Considerations for Patients with Gastritis[10,17]

- Patients with gastritis secondary to chronic NSAID use may be asymptomatic

- Knowledge of blood in the stool should result in physician referral

- Educate each patient to take medications with food and avoid certain types of food and drink

- The patient should avoid all aspirin-containing compounds

### Peptic Ulcer Disease[10,17]

Peptic ulcer disease is a condition where there is a disruption or erosion in the gastrointestinal mucosa. There is an imbalance between the protective mechanisms of the stomach and the secretion of acids within the stomach.

**Etiology** – Many ulcers are caused by the H. pylori infection and chronic NSAID use. Irritants that increase risk of ulcer include stress, alcohol, particular medications, foods, and smoking.

**Signs and symptoms** – Symptoms are dependent on the location and severity of ulceration (gastric or duodenal) and can include epigastric pain, burning or heartburn, nausea, vomiting, bleeding, bloody stools, and pain that comes in waves that is relieved by eating. Symptoms specific to the etiology of H. pylori can also include halitosis, rosacea, and flushing. Complications can include hemorrhage, perforation, obstruction (secondary to scarring), and malignancy.

**Treatment** – Treatment is primarily through pharmacological intervention, however, in more severe cases, surgical intervention may be required.

## Rehabilitation Considerations for Patients with Peptic Ulcer Disease[10]

- Asymptomatic patients with history of ulcer should be monitored for signs of bleeding
- Fatigue level, pallor, and exercise tolerance must be monitored for signs of bleeding
- Recognize that heart rate increase or blood pressure decrease may be signs of bleeding
- Recognize that back pain is a sign of a perforated ulcer located on the posterior wall of the stomach and duodenum
- Recognize that pain that radiates from the midthoracic area to the right upper quadrant and shoulder may signify blood and acid within the peritoneal cavity secondary to a perforated and bleeding ulcer

## Diarrhea/Constipation[10]

Diarrhea is defined as an abnormal frequency or volume of stool and can appear as a symptom of certain gastrointestinal pathologies. Constipation is defined as the infrequent or difficult passage of stool, secondary to an increase in the hardness of the stool, and can also appear as a symptom of certain gastrointestinal pathologies.

### Pathologies Associated with Diarrhea and Constipation[17]

| Diarrhea | Constipation |
|---|---|
| Irritable bowel syndrome | Multiple sclerosis |
| Hyperthyroidism | Spinal cord tumors |
| Electrolyte imbalance | Irritable bowel syndrome |
| Endocrine disorder | Duchenne muscular dystrophy |
| Incomplete obstruction of the bowel | Endocrine disorder |
| Diverticulitis | CVA |
| Certain medications | Inactivity |
| Caffeine | Bowel obstruction or fecal impaction |
| Diet | Pregnancy |
| Malabsorption | Diet |
| Pelvic inflammatory disease | Certain medications |

## Intestines

### Malabsorption Syndrome[10,17]

Malabsorption syndrome is a condition characterized by a group of pathologies where there is reduced intestinal absorption and inadequate nutrition. Celiac disease, cystic fibrosis, pancreatic carcinoma, pernicious anemia, AIDS, Crohn's disease, and Addison's disease are a few pathologies that may present with malabsorption syndrome.

**Etiology** – Malabsorption syndrome occurs secondary to defects in digestion and/or the inability of the intestinal mucosa to absorb the nutrients from digested food.

**Signs and symptoms** – Although each patient's symptoms are based on the root pathology and co-morbidities that may exist, the primary symptoms are weight loss, chronic diarrhea, and anemia. Other symptoms can include fatigue, abdominal bloating, steatorrhea (oil covered stools), abdominal cramps, indigestion, bone pain, and excessive gas.

**Treatment** – Once diagnosed, treatment includes avoidance of the underlying cause for the malabsorption, probiotics, antibiotics, dietary modification, and nutritional support including vitamins, minerals, and electrolytes.

## Rehabilitation Considerations for Patients with Malabsorption Syndrome[10]

- Recognize increased risk for osteoporosis and pathologic fractures
- Monitor fatigue level, pallor, bone pain, and exercise tolerance
- Recognize weight loss and abdominal bloating
- Recognize increased risk for muscle spasms secondary to electrolyte imbalances
- Recognize increased risk for generalized swelling secondary to protein depletion

### Irritable Bowel Syndrome (IBS)[10,17]

Irritable bowel syndrome consists of recurrent symptoms of the upper and lower gastrointestinal system that interfere with the normal functioning of the colon.

**Etiology** – The etiology is unknown, but one theory believes that the colon or large intestine may be sensitive to certain foods or stress. Other theories hypothesize that the immune system, serotonin, and bacterial infections may all be causative factors. IBS typically occurs in as many as 20% of adults, more commonly in females, and begins prior to the age of 30 in 50% of patients. Females have a slightly higher rate of incidence which may be triggered by food sensitivities, stress, anxiety, caffeine, smoking, alcohol or high fat intake.

**Signs and symptoms** – Symptoms can include abdominal pain, bloating or distention of the abdomen, nausea, vomiting, anorexia, changes in form and frequency of stool, and passing of mucus in the stool.

**Treatment** – IBS is normally a diagnosis of exclusion from other GI diagnoses and treatment is usually multifactorial. Change in lifestyle and nutrition, decrease in stress, pharmacological intervention, adequate sleep, exercise, and psychotherapy may all assist in alleviating symptoms. Patients with IBS should avoid large meals, milk, wheat, rye, barley, alcohol, and caffeine. Although the symptoms can be severe, it does not lead to serious disease. Symptoms can typically be controlled by diet, pharmacological intervention, and stress management.

> **Rehabilitation Considerations for Patients with Irritable Bowel Syndrome[10]**
>
> - Emphasize physical activity to assist with bowel function and relieve stress
> - Emphasize breathing techniques to assist in stress reduction and with breath-holding patterns
> - Recognize that biofeedback training may be beneficial

### Diverticulitis[10,17]

Diverticulitis is the condition of having inflamed or infected diverticula. This occurs in approximately 20-25% of the population that has diverticulosis. Diverticulosis is the condition of having diverticula. These are pouch-like protrusions occurring in the colon. Approximately 10% of the population over 40 years of age develops diverticulosis. Approximately 80% of individuals with diverticulosis are asymptomatic, however, those with symptoms may experience bloating, mild cramping, and constipation. Treatment includes an increased amount of dietary fiber (20-35 grams per day recommended) to avoid diverticulitis.

**Etiology** – The exact etiology of diverticulitis is unknown; however, a dominant theory is that the disease results from a low fiber diet.

**Signs and symptoms** – Abdominal pain is the primary symptom of diverticulitis. Tenderness over the left side of the lower abdomen, cramping, constipation, nausea, fever, chills, and vomiting can also occur.

> **Rehabilitation Considerations for Patients with Diverticular Disease[10]**
>
> - Physical activity assists the bowel function and is extremely important during periods of remission
> - Breathing techniques will assist in stress reduction and with breath-holding patterns
> - Avoid any increase in intra-abdominal pressure with exercise or activity
> - Back pain and/or referred hip pain must be examined for possible medical diseases

**Treatment** – Treatment includes diet modification, controlling the underlying infection, and lowering internal colonic pressure through increased fiber intake. In more severe cases, a nasogas-tric tube may be required to give the intestines a rest. Surgical intervention is indicated for severe obstruction, perforation or necrosis. Complications can include bleeding infections, intestinal blockage, abscess, perforations or tears in the colon, fistulas or peritonitis.

## Liver

### Hepatitis[10,17]

Hepatitis is an inflammatory process within the liver. Viral hepatitis is most common and is classified as hepatitis A, B, C, D, E or G. Hepatitis A, B, and C are the most common and discussed briefly below.

**Etiology** – Many instances of hepatitis are viral in nature. Other etiologies include a chemical reaction, drug reaction or alcohol abuse. Other viruses that can cause hepatitis include Epstein-Barr virus, herpes virus I and II, varicella-zoster virus, and measles.

**Signs and symptoms** – Symptoms of hepatitis include fever, flu symptoms, abrupt onset of fatigue, anorexia, headache, jaundice, darkened urine, lighter stool, enlarged spleen and liver, and intermittent pruritus.

**Treatment** – Acute viral hepatitis usually resolves with medical treatment, but can become chronic in some cases. Chronic hepatitis may result in the need for liver transplant.

#### Hepatitis A (HAV)

Hepatitis A is a virus that affects the liver and its function. Transmission occurs by close personal contact with someone that has the infection or through the fecal-oral route (i.e., contaminated water and food sources). The flu-like symptoms represent an acute infection; this form does not progress to chronic disease or cirrhosis of the liver. Patients usually recover in six to ten weeks. Treatment is supportive and the virus is self-limiting.

#### Hepatitis B (HBV)

Hepatitis B is a virus that affects the liver and its function. Transmission of this virus occurs through the sharing of needles, intercourse with an infected person, exposure to an infected person's blood, semen or maternal-fetal exposure. Approximately 10% of cases progress to chronic hepatitis since the body cannot always rid itself of HBV. Treatment includes hepatitis B immunoglobulin (HBIG) for the unvaccinated patient within 24 hours of exposure. The patient should then receive the vaccination series at one and six months. If the patient is already vaccinated, they may require another dose of the HBV vaccine. Chronic hepatitis is now being treated with interferon alfa-2b, providing remission for some patients.

#### Hepatitis C (HCV)

Hepatitis C is a virus that affects the liver and its function. It is one of the primary etiologies for chronic liver disease and eventual liver failure. Transmission of this virus occurs through the sharing of needles, intercourse with an infected person, exposure to an infected person's blood, semen, body fluids or maternal-fetal exposure. The virus accounts for 90% of post transfusion hepatitis cases. Like hepatitis B, this virus is often asymptomatic and the acute infection can be mild. Patients with hepatitis C have an increased frequency of manifesting conditions such as Hashimoto's thyroiditis, diabetes mellitus, and corneal ulceration. Treatment may include the use of interferon alfa-2b to reduce the inflammation and liver damage but only a small percentage of patients with hepatitis C benefit from the medication. There is no vaccine to prevent this virus and no immunoglobulin fully effective in treating the infection. Chronic hepatitis occurs in 50% of cases and 20% of those cases progress to cirrhosis of the liver.

### Rehabilitation Considerations for Patients with Hepatitis[10]

- Health care workers that are at risk for contact with hepatitis should receive all immunizations for HBV, and if exposed to blood or body fluids of an infected person must receive immunoglobulin therapy immediately

- Standard precautions should be followed at all times for protection

- Enteric precautions are required for patients with hepatitis A and E

- Recognize that arthralgias may be noted, especially in older patients, and will not typically respond to traditional therapeutic intervention

- Energy conservation techniques and pacing skills should be incorporated into therapy

- Balance activities along with periods of rest, avoid prolonged bed rest, and provide patient education regarding signs of relapse or chronic hepatitis

### Cirrhosis of the Liver[10,17]

Cirrhosis of the liver is a condition where the healthy tissue of the liver is replaced with scar tissue that blocks the flow of blood through the organ and prevents the liver from properly functioning.

**Etiology** – The etiology is usually alcoholism or hepatitis C. Alcohol tends to block the normal metabolism of protein, fats, and carbohydrates. This condition will normally occur after a patient has been heavily drinking for more than a decade. Inflammation of the liver secondary to hepatitis C is also a large causative factor for cirrhosis. Persistent inflammation and slow damage to the liver will result in cirrhosis of the liver after several decades of infection. Other causes include hepatitis B and D, certain drugs, infections, and toxins, specific hereditary diseases, nonalcoholic steatohepatitis, and blocked bile ducts.

**Signs and symptoms** – Symptoms include fatigue, decreased appetite, nausea, weakness, abdominal pain, spider angiomas, and weight loss. Common complications from cirrhosis include ascites (water accumulation in the abdomen secondary to decreased production of albumin by the liver), edema in the lower extremities, jaundice, gallstones, increased itching, ecchymosis, bleeding, an increase in sensitivity to medications, accumulation of toxins in the brain, portal vein hypertension, development of varices (enlarged blood vessels in the stomach and esophagus), immune system dysfunction, encephalopathy, and liver cancer.

**Treatment** – Treatment cannot reverse the process or damage, but can slow the process. Treatment is based on the causative factors and is implemented until symptoms cannot be controlled. A liver transplant may be necessary to sustain life.

### Rehabilitation Considerations for Patients with Cirrhosis of the Liver[10]

- Recognize that ascites may develop as well as fluid accumulation in the ankles and feet

- Report any blood loss through nose bleeds, gum bleeds, tarry stools or excessive bruising

- Avoid all activities that produce the Valsalva maneuver (increase in intra-abdominal pressure)

- Adequate rest is required to lower the demands on the liver and improve circulation; avoid unnecessary fatigue with therapeutic or daily activities

### Pancreas

### Diabetes Mellitus

Please refer to the endocrine section on page 337 and the clinical application template on diabetes mellitus on page 600.

### Gallbladder

### Cholecystitis and Cholelithiasis[10,17]

Cholecystitis refers to inflammation of the gallbladder that may be acute or chronic.

**Etiology** – The most common etiology is gallstones (cholelithiasis) that have become impacted within the cystic duct. Gallstones develop from hypomobility of the gallbladder, supersaturation of the bile with cholesterol or crystal formation from bilirubin salts. These stones can also cause infection which exacerbate the condition.

**Signs and symptoms** – Many times gallstones are asymptomatic, however, the most common symptom is right upper quadrant pain. If the gallstone becomes lodged within the cystic duct, then the patient can experience many problems including severe right upper quadrant pain with muscle guarding, tenderness, and rebound pain. These symptoms can radiate to the interscapular region. Other symptoms include jaundice, fever, nausea, vomiting, anorexia, and abdominal rigidity.

**Treatment** – Treatment is not recommended for the patient with asymptomatic gallstones, but a low fat diet can decrease gallbladder stimulation if mild symptoms are present. If patients are symptomatic, a lithotripsy procedure can be used in an attempt to break up and dissolve the stones. Primary treatment is a laparoscopic cholecystectomy to remove the gallbladder and the lodged stones from the ducts. Acute cholecystitis should resolve itself within a week with analgesics, antibiotics, and intravenous alimentary feedings.

## Rehabilitation Considerations for Patients with Cholecystitis and Cholelithiasis[10]

- Must be familiar with all signs and symptoms of cholecystitis in order to refer patients to a physician if a change in their status occurs.
- Post-surgical exercises and ambulation are appropriate post laparoscopic cholecystectomy such as breathing exercises, splinting while coughing, and mobility training.

## Pharmacology - Gastrointestinal Management[19]

Pharmacological intervention is normally related to gastrointestinal disorders that are caused by gastric acid secretion and abnormal food movement through the gastrointestinal tract.

### Antacid Agents

**Action:** Antacid agents are used to chemically neutralize gastric acid and increase the intragastric pH. Primary antacids are classified as aluminum-containing, calcium carbonate-containing, magnesium-containing or sodium bicarbonate-containing.

**Indications:** episodic minor gastric indigestion or heartburn, peptic ulcer, gastroesophageal reflux disease (GERD)

**Side effects:** acid rebound phenomenon, constipation or diarrhea (depending on the antacid), may affect metabolism of other medication, electrolyte imbalances

**Implications for PT:** Since these agents are well tolerated, there are typically no side effects that interfere with physical therapy. Patients are more likely to participate in therapy with effective management of gastrointestinal issues using these agents.

**Examples:** Aluminum-containing: Basaljel (aluminum carbonate gel); Calcium carbonate-containing: Tums (calcium carbonate); Magnesium-containing: Milk of Magnesia (magnesium hydroxide); Sodium bicarbonate-containing: Bromo seltzer (sodium bicarbonate)

### H$_2$ Receptor Blockers

**Action:** H$_2$ receptor blockers bind specifically to histamine receptors to prevent the histamine-activated release of gastric acid normally stimulated during food intake.

**Indications:** dyspepsia, acute and long-term treatment of peptic ulcer, GERD

**Side effects:** headache, dizziness, mild gastrointestinal distress, tolerance, arthralgia, acid rebound with discontinuation of agent

**Implications for PT:** Since these agents are well tolerated there are typically no side effects that interfere with physical therapy. Patients are more likely to participate in therapy with effective management of gastrointestinal issues using these agents.

**Examples:** Tagamet (cimetidine), Pepcid (famotidine), Zantac (ranitidine)

### Proton Pump Inhibitors (PPI)

**Action:** Proton pump inhibitor agents inhibit the H+/K+ -ATPase enzyme that blocks secretions of acid from gastric cells into the stomach. These agents prevent erosive esophagitis and may also possess antibacterial effects against H. pylori.

**Indications:** dyspepsia, GERD

**Side effects:** acid rebound phenomenon when discontinued after prolonged use

**Implications for PT:** Since these agents are well tolerated, there are typically no side effects that interfere with physical therapy. Patients are more likely to participate in therapy with effective management of gastrointestinal issues using these agents.

**Examples:** Prevacid (lansoprazole), Nexium (esomeprazole), Prilosec (omeprazole), Protonix (pantoprazole), AcipHex (rabeprazole)

### Anticholinergics

**Action:** Anticholinergics block the effects of acetylcholine on parietal cells in the stomach and decrease the release of gastric acid.

**Indications:** gastric ulcers

**Side effects:** dry mouth, confusion, constipation, urinary retention

**Implications for PT:** Physical therapists should be aware of potential side effects in order to respond appropriately to changes in cognition or complaints of dry mouth, constipation or urinary retention.

**Examples:** Gastrozepin (pirenzepine), muscarinic cholinergic antagonist

### Antibiotics

**Action:** Antibiotics are prescribed to treat H. pylori infection with the goal of facilitating more rapid healing of associated gastric ulcerations.

**Indications:** H. pylori bacteria

**Side effects:** hypersensitivity, diarrhea, nausea

**Implications for PT:** Physical therapists should be aware of potential side effects in order to respond appropriately especially with regard to severe dermatologic and respiratory reactions which may be associated with hypersensitivity.

**Examples:** metronidazole, tetracycline, clarithromycin, amoxicillin

### Antidiarrheal Agents

**Action:** Antidiarrheal agents are used to slow the serious debilitating effects of dehydration associated with prolonged diarrhea. There are multiple classes of antidiarrheal agents.

**Indications:** prolonged diarrhea

**Side effects:** constipation, abdominal discomfort

**Implications for PT:** Since these agents are well tolerated there are typically no side effects that interfere with physical therapy. Patients are more likely to participate in therapy with effective management of gastrointestinal issues using these agents.

**Examples:** Donnagel (attapulgite), Kapectolin (kaolin), Pepto-Bismol (bismuth subsalicylate), Motofen (difenoxin), Imodium (loperamide)

## Consider This

### Referred Visceral Pain May Mimic Musculoskeletal Conditions[17]

Visceral pain refers to pain caused by pathology in the visceral organs (e.g., organ cancer, small bowel obstruction, kidney stones). Pain originating from organs is often difficult to localize due to the tendency to perceive the pain in locations other than the organ source. Due to the overlap in sensory and visceral nerve pathways, symptoms will often refer to soft tissue within the dermatome that corresponds to the organ's spinal cord innervation. The left arm or jaw pain commonly associated with myocardial infarction is a well known example of referred visceral pain. With lesser known symptoms, however, referred pain patterns may result in a delayed diagnosis. Many referred visceral pain patterns mimic musculoskeletal symptoms. Therefore physical therapists must be diligent in assessing pain of an unknown origin. Since visceral pain is transmitted via the autonomic nervous system, this is especially true when pain is accompanied by autonomic responses such as nausea, vomiting, pallor or sweating.

### Laxative Agents

**Action:** Laxative agents are used to facilitate bowel evacuation and should be used sparingly.

**Indications:** to promote defecation

**Side effects:** nausea, abdominal discomfort, cramping, electrolyte imbalance, dehydration, dependence with prolonged use

**Implications for PT:** If the laxative was recently ingested, physical discomfort may temporarily limit patient participation in therapy interventions. Patients may also express concern about treatment occurring in areas that do not have easy access to restroom facilities.

**Examples:** Citrucel (methylcellulose), Metamucil (psyllium), Colace (docusate), Fleet Glycerin suppository (glycerin), Phillips' Milk of Magnesia (magnesium hydroxide), Correctol (bisacodyl), Senokot (senna)

### Emetic Agents

**Action:** Emetic agents are used to induce vomiting.

**Indications:** to induce vomiting; usually after ingestion of a toxic substance

**Side effects:** dehydration, electrolyte imbalance, and upper GI erosion may occur with inappropriate or prolonged usage

**Implications for PT:** The medical concerns associated with administration of an emetic agent should be addressed prior to initiation or resumption of therapy interventions. Therapy should also be deferred if a patient is actively vomiting.

**Examples:** apomorphine, ipecac

### Antiemetic Agents

**Action:** Antiemetic agents are used to decrease symptoms of nausea and vomiting.

**Indications:** nausea associated with motion sickness, anesthesia, pain or oncology treatments

**Side effects:** side effects are agent dependent, but can include sedation, dysrhythmias, and pain.

**Implications for PT:** Antihistamine antiemetic agents frequently cause sedative effects which can be limiting to physical therapy interventions. Many other antiemetic agents are typically well tolerated and should not significantly interfere with therapy interventions.

**Examples:** Scopolamine (anticholinergic agent), Meclizine (antihistamine agent), Dolasetron (5-HT3 receptor antagonist agent), Phenergan (promethazine hydrochloride)

### Abdominal Pain Quadrant and Potential Etiologies[17,20]

| Left upper quadrant | Right upper quadrant | Left lower quadrant | Right lower quadrant |
|---|---|---|---|
| Gastric ulcer | Hepatomegaly | Perforated colon | Kidney stone |
| Perforated colon | Duodenal ulcer | Ileitis | Ureteral stone |
| Pneumonia | Cholecystitis | Sigmoid diverticulitis | Meckel diverticulum |
| Spleen injury | Pneumonia | Kidney stone | Appendicitis |
| Spleen rupture | Hepatitis | Ureteral stone | Cholecystitis |
| Aortic aneurysm | Biliary stones | Intestinal obstruction | Intestinal obstruction |

# Genitourinary System

## Genitourinary System

The genitourinary system consists of all the reproductive organs and the urinary organs. These are often considered together due to their common embryological origin.

### Genitourinary Anatomy and Function

The genitourinary system is supported by the pelvic floor consisting of muscle, fascia, and ligament.

| Muscles of the Pelvic Floor[20,21] | |
| --- | --- |
| Pelvic diaphragm | Levator ani: pubococcygeus, puborectalis, iliococcygeus, and coccygeus (ischiococcygeus) |
| Urogenital diaphragm | Deep transverse perineal, urethrae sphincter |
| Urogenital triangle | Female: bulbocavernosus, ischiocavernosus, superficial transverse perineal<br>Male: bulbospongiosus, ischiocavernosus, superficial transverse perineal |
| Anal triangle | Internal anal sphincter, external anal sphincter |

### Genital System

The genital system consists of the male and female gonads and associated ducts, external genitalia, and associated hormones that all function for reproduction.

| Female Genital System[20-22] | |
| --- | --- |
| **External genitalia**<br>Mons pubis, labia majora, labia minora, clitoris, vestibule of vagina, bulbs of vestibule, greater vestibular (Bartholin's) glands, Skene's gland | • Provides protection and hydration of vaginal tissue and urethra |
| **Vagina**<br>Musculomembranous tube connected to the cervix | • Receptacle for male sperm<br>• Birth canal<br>• Excretory duct for menstrual fluid |
| **Uterus**<br>Hollow muscular organ | • Houses the fetus during development |
| **Uterine tubes**<br>Extend laterally from the ovaries to the uterus | • Provides transport for the ovum from the ovary for fertilization and implantation within the uterus |
| **Ovaries**<br>Almond-shaped glands suspended in the broad ligaments | • Produce hormones such as estrogen and progesterone<br>• Storage of oocytes prior to ovulation |

| Male Genital System[20] | |
|---|---|
| **Penis** | • External genitalia that expels urine during voiding and semen during the act of copulation |
| **Scrotum** | • Cutaneous fibromuscular external sac for the testes, ductus deferens, epididymis, nerves, and blood vessels |
| **Testes** | • Produce sperm and hormones such as testosterone |
| **Ductus/vas deferens** | • Carries sperm from the testes to the seminal vesicle to form the ejaculatory duct |
| **Epididymis** | • Encased within the scrotum<br>• Stores sperm |
| **Seminal vesicles** | • Internal tubes that secrete a thick fluid to combine with sperm within the ejaculatory duct |
| **Prostate** | • Internal organ lying inferior to the bladder<br>• Produces and secretes fluid to combine with sperm, seminal vesicle fluid, and bulbourethral gland fluid to create semen |

## Renal System

The renal system consists of two kidneys, two ureters, the urinary bladder, and the urethra that function to form and eliminate urine.

| Renal System[20,21] | |
|---|---|
| **Kidneys** | • Remove water, salt, and metabolic waste from the blood through excretion of urine<br>• Contribute to homeostasis including: acid-base balance, regulation of electrolyte concentrations, control of blood volume, and regulation of blood pressure through the control of hormones secreted into the bloodstream |
| **Ureters** | • Muscular tubes connecting the kidneys to the urinary bladder to transport urine |
| **Urinary bladder** | • Temporary muscular reservoir for urine |
| **Urethra** | • Muscular tube for excretion of urine<br>• Semen transport during ejaculation in males |

## Consider This

### Genitourinary System Support Structure[20,21]

The pelvic floor muscles' primary functions include bladder/bowel control and sexual function. In addition, the pelvic floor muscles support the pelvic organs by holding the organs in position in conjunction with ligaments and surrounding fascia. The muscles are made up of two different fiber types, type I (slow twitch) and type II (fast twitch). When the pelvic floor muscles are weak or have poor endurance due to pregnancy, trauma, surgery, repetitive straining or genetics they are not able to support the pelvic organs leading to organ prolapse. Affected structures may include the bladder, uterus, cervix, intestines, and rectum. This may result in urgency, frequency, urinary or fecal incontinence due to the muscle imbalance during increased intra-abdominal pressure.

## Genitourinary System Pathology

| Genital Components | Common Pathologies[20,21] |
|---|---|
| Uterus | Cervical cancer*, endometriosis, uterine prolapse |
| Vagina | Dyspareunia, vulvodynia, vulvovaginal candidiasis (yeast infection) |
| Prostate | Prostatitis, prostate cancer* |
| Penis | Erectile dysfunction |
| Renal Components | Common Pathologies[20,21] |
| Kidneys | Glomerulonephritis, nephrolithiasis, renal failure |
| Bladder | Cystocele, dysuria, hematuria, interstitial cystitis, neurogenic bladder, nocturia, polyuria, urgency, frequency, urinary incontinence, urinary tract infections |

*For more information on cervical and prostate cancer see pages 367-368.

## Uterus

### Endometriosis[21,23]

Endometriosis is the development of endometrial tissue, which normally lines the uterus, in extrauterine locations within the abdomen and pelvis. The most common location of extrauterine endometrial growth occurs at the uterosacral ligaments. The level of pain does not always correlate with the severity of extrauterine tissue growth.

**Etiology** – The exact etiology of endometriosis is unknown. During each menstrual cycle the endometrial tissue bleeds causing subsequent scarring and adhesions.

**Signs and symptoms** – Symptoms can vary, but typically include moderate to severe lower abdominal, pelvic or low back pain before or during menstruation, irregular menstrual cycles, premenstrual spotting, dyspareunia, pain during defecation, and infertility.

**Treatment** – Physical therapy treatment may include manual techniques such as myofascial release, visceral mobilization and soft and deep tissue massage to break up scar tissue and adhesions. Mobility exercises are performed to sustain elongation of tissues. Relaxation exercises such as breathing routines and restorative poses are performed to regulate the pain cycle. TENS is also indicated. Pharmacological intervention may be indicated to alter hormonal balance using oral contraceptives and antigonadotropins. Surgery to remove extrauterine endometrial tissue, scarring, and adhesions; and a total hysterectomy may be recommended when pregnancy is no longer desired.

### Uterine Prolapse[24,25]

Uterine prolapse is the descent of the uterus and cervix into the vagina. The Baden-Walker System is the most widespread classification of prolapse using a five-point grading system ranging from no prolapse to maximum descent of vaginal tissue outside of the body.

**Etiology** – The etiology typically consists of genetics, denervation or direct muscle trauma (i.e., labor and delivery).

**Signs and symptoms** – Primary symptoms vary, but can include pelvic pressure that increases with exertion, urgency, frequency, urinary incontinence, incomplete bladder emptying, discomfort, vaginal dryness or irritation, dyspareunia, and lower back pain that is relieved by lying down.

**Treatment** – Physical therapy treatment may include pelvic floor muscle training using biofeedback, Kegel exercises, core strengthening exercises, body mechanics, and symptom dependent lifestyle modifications. In more severe cases, an intravaginal mechanical support device called a pessary may be indicated. The patient may require reconstructive or obliterative surgery, if conservative treatment fails.

## Prostate

### Prostatitis[24]

Prostatitis is an inflammation of the prostate gland.

**Etiology** – The most common etiologies include bacterial infection or the backup of prostate secretions within the gland. Classification of prostatitis includes acute bacterial prostatitis (I), chronic bacterial prostatitis (II), chronic pelvic pain syndrome (III), and asymptomatic inflammatory prostatitis (IV).

**Signs and symptoms** – Common symptoms include watery urethral discharge, urgency, frequency, discomfort with urination, and pain with ejaculation. Chronic pelvic pain syndrome manifests as pain in the perineum, rectum, prostate, penis, testicles, and abdomen. Asymptomatic inflammatory prostatitis is characterized by prostate inflammation in the absence of genitourinary tract symptoms.

**Treatment** – Management includes lifestyle modifications, biofeedback training, stretching exercises, myofascial techniques, and bladder retraining. Pharmacological intervention such as antibiotics, alpha blockers or nonsteroidal anti-inflammatory medication for pain may be indicated.

## Penis

### Erectile Dysfunction (ED)[10,20,24]

Erectile dysfunction, also known as impotence, is estimated to range from 25-85% in men with diabetes, which makes this population three times more likely than the general population. Onset of ED in individuals with diabetes usually occurs 10-15 years earlier than in men without diabetes.

**Etiology** – There are various causative factors for ED. Diabetes is a primary etiology, while other risk factors include coronary heart disease, hypertension, hypothyroidism, hypopituitarism, multiple sclerosis, psychiatric disorders, excessive alcohol consumption, smoking, vessel disease, kidney disease, pharmacological side effects, and hormonal imbalances.

**Signs and symptoms** – The primary symptom is the consistent inability to maintain an erection adequate for sexual intercourse.

**Treatment** – Treatment varies and includes pharmacological intervention, surgical intervention, injections directly to the penis, and Kegel exercises.

## Kidneys

### Renal Failure[10,24]

Renal failure is a condition where the kidneys experience a decrease in glomerular filtration rate and fail to adequately filter toxins and waste from the blood. There are two forms: acute renal failure and chronic renal failure.

**Etiology** – Renal pathology typically occurs secondary to diabetes mellitus or hypertension, but can also occur from poison, trauma, and genetics. The nephrons are usually damaged and they lose their ability to filter the blood. Renal failure can be classified as:

- Acute (damage occurs quickly)
- Chronic (damage occurs slowly)
- End-stage (nearly total or total renal failure, dialysis required)

## Acute Renal Failure (ARF)

- Sudden decline in renal function
- Increase in BUN and creatinine
- Oliguria, hyperkalemia, sodium retention
- Prerenal etiology is secondary to a decrease in blood flow typically due to shock, hemorrhage, burn or pulmonary embolism
- Postrenal etiology is secondary to obstruction distal to the kidney due to neoplasm, kidney stone or prostate hypertrophy
- Intrarenal etiology is secondary to primary damage of renal tissue due to toxins, intrarenal ischemia or vascular disorders

## Chronic Renal Failure (CRF)

- Progressive deterioration in renal function
- Diabetes mellitus
- Severe hypertension
- Glomerulopathies
- Obstructive uropathy
- Interstitial nephritis
- Polycystic kidney disease

### Stages of Kidney Disease According to the National Kidney Foundation

**Stage 1** kidney damage with normal GFR (90 or greater)

**Stage 2** mild decrease in GFR (60-89)

**Stage 3** moderate decrease in GFR (30-59)

**Stage 4** severe reduction in GFR (15-29)

**Stage 5** kidney failure (GFR less than 15)

**Signs and symptoms** – Symptoms of renal failure vary based on severity of the condition and can include nausea, vomiting, lethargy, weakness, hiccups, anorexia, ulceration within the GI tract, sleep disorders, headache, peripheral neuropathy, anemia, pruritus, osteomalacia, ecchymosis, pulmonary edema, seizures, and coma.

**Treatment** – Treatment of ARF includes management of primary etiology, pharmacological intervention, diuretics, nutritional support, hydration, hemodialysis and/or transfusions if applicable. Treatment of CRF includes conservative management and renal replacement therapy. Conservative management assists with slowing the process and assisting the body in its compensation. Nutritional support, hydration, avoidance of protein, and pharmacological intervention are usually the primary basis of intervention. Renal replacement therapy includes some form of hemodialysis and/or organ transplant. Peritoneal dialysis is a form of renal replacement therapy that uses the peritoneal cavity as a semi-permeable membrane between the dialysate fluid and blood vessels of the abdominal cavity.

## Hemodialysis

Hemodialysis is a treatment process for patients with advanced and permanent kidney failure. Kidney failure creates excess toxic waste, increased blood pressure, retention of excess body fluids, and a decrease in red blood cell production. Hemodialysis removes the blood from the body along with waste, excess sodium, and fluids. The process cleanses the blood and returns it to the body. A patient requires this process on average three times per week and each visit requires three to five hours to complete the treatment. Side effects that may be associated with dialysis include anemia, renal osteodystrophy, pruritus (itching), sleep disorders ("restless legs"), and dialysis-related amyloidosis.

### Rehabilitation Considerations for Patients with Renal Failure/Dialysis[10,24]

- Modify treatment plan based on fluid and electrolyte status
- Standard precautions should be followed at all times for protection
- Recognize patient's abilities post dialysis and potential for dehydration and hypotension
- Monitor vital signs closely, however, avoid placement of the blood pressure cuff over the fistula
- Avoid mobilization activities as they are contraindicated during dialysis
- Energy conservation techniques and pacing skills should be incorporated into therapy

## Bladder

### Neurogenic Bladder[10,24]

Neurogenic bladder is a dysfunction where there is damage to the cerebral control that allows for urinary dysfunction. If the urine cannot be properly released, there may be an increase in urinary tract infections and kidney damage.

**Etiology** – The etiology of neurogenic bladder can include diabetes, diminished bladder capacity, hyperactive detrusor muscle, CVA, other disease processes, infection, and nerve damage.

**Signs and symptoms** – Symptoms include frequent urinary tract infections, leakage of urine, inability to empty the bladder or loss of the urge to urinate when the bladder is full. Diagnosis should include an evaluation by a physician, X-rays, and urodynamics to assist with diagnosis.

**Treatment** – Management is dependent on the actual etiology with a goal of preventing bladder overdistention, UTIs, and renal damage. Patient education, bladder techniques, lower abdominal massage, temporary catheterization, pharmacological intervention, and a timed urination program may be indicated.

### Urinary Incontinence[10,24]

Urinary incontinence is an involuntary loss of urine that is great enough to be problematic for the person and typically occurs when bladder pressure exceeds sphincter resistance. Below are four classifications of urinary incontinence. General treatment includes pelvic floor muscle training using biofeedback, lifestyle modifications, bladder retraining, prompted voiding programs, urge suppression strategies, myofascial release, visceral mobilization, body mechanics, abdominal strengthening, and stretching exercises of surrounding muscles. Pharmacological intervention to address urgency, injection therapy of a "bulking" agent, and surgical intervention for urethral and bladder positioning may also be indicated. These interventions may not apply to all types of urinary incontinence and should be determined on a per patient basis.

### Stress Urinary Incontinence (SUI)

SUI is the loss of urine due to activities that increase intra-abdominal pressure, such as sneezing, coughing, laughing, running, and jumping. *Please refer to clinical application template on page 686 for more information.*

## Consider This

### Lifestyle Modifications to Address Bladder Symptoms[24]

- Daily fluid intake should be 2,500 mL, or 10 cups, to regulate excessively high or low fluid intake.
- Reduce bladder irritants including carbonated, caffeinated, and alcoholic beverages, spicy foods, citric juices, and artificial sweeteners. Caffeine reduction should be tapered slowly to avoid severe headaches.
- Schedule voiding for every 3-4 hours to reduce bladder distention. An average person voids 6-8 times in a 24-hour period. A bladder diary assists with baseline measurements and goal setting.
- Regulate bowel function to prevent constipation and straining during bowel movements by monitoring dietary fiber, fluid intake, and exercise.
- Avoid fluid intake 2-3 hours prior to bedtime to reduce nocturia.
- A smoking cessation program may decrease the occurrence of coughing and subsequent bladder leakage.
- A weight loss program, if moderately obese, may decrease pressure on the pelvic tissues and organs.

## Urge Urinary Incontinence (UUI)

UUI is the loss of urine after a sudden, intense urge to void due to the detrusor muscle of the bladder involuntarily contracting during bladder filling. UUI is the most common incontinence in the geriatric population and among residents in long-term care facilities.

**Etiology** – The most common etiologies are detrusor muscle overactivity, overactive bladder also known as "urgency-frequency" syndrome, changes in the smooth muscle of the bladder, increased afferent activity, increased sensitivity of the detrusor to acetylcholine, and idiopathic. There is also association with the following neurological disorders: multiple sclerosis, spinal cord injury, cardiovascular accident, and Parkinson's disease.

**Signs and symptoms** – For many people, UUI is triggered by certain events due to a conditioned reflex. Two of the most common triggers are "key-in-the-lock" when arriving home and running water.

**Treatment** – Behavior modification is the primary goal of treatment for this condition. Biofeedback, pelvic floor strengthening, and bladder retraining (scheduled voiding) are key components in resolving UUI. Pharmacological intervention may also be warranted.

## Overflow Urinary Incontinence (OUI)

OUI is the loss of urine when the intra-bladder pressure exceeds the urethra's capacity to remain closed due to urinary retention.

**Etiology** – This condition is caused by outflow obstruction secondary to a narrowed or obstructed urethra that results from a prolapsed pelvic organ, a stricture, an enlarged prostate, chronic constipation or neurological disease.

**Signs and Symptoms** – Individuals who present with OUI may also experience difficulty initiating the urine stream. Once the stream is initiated, it is weak and presents with post void dribble.

**Treatment** – Treatment will likely include surgical intervention if there is an obstruction. If there is weakness of the detrusor muscles, double voiding is recommended for these patients as well as other strengthening measures. Failed intervention may result in intermittent catheterization.

## Functional Urinary Incontinence (FUI)

FUI is the loss of urine due to the inability or unwillingness of a person to use the bathroom facilities prior to involuntary bladder release.

**Etiology** – A decreased level of mental awareness or a decrease in mobility are the two primary causative factors for FUI. FUI is rarely seen without another bladder issue or neurological involvement.

**Signs and symptoms** – These patients will typically present with impaired cognition and/or mobility and will experience incontinence secondary to the inability to successfully use a bathroom to void.

**Treatment** – Since there is typically no urologic pathology associated with functional incontinence, treatment should be directed to alleviate the underlying issue. Improving mobility, modifying clothing style, increasing independence with ambulation and with function will assist with decreasing functional incontinence. Patients may also require a behavioral toileting schedule or program to decrease incontinence.

## Spotlight on Safety

### Functional Incontinence and At-risk Populations[24]

When working with patients within the acute care, long-term care or home care settings there are many factors contributing to functional incontinence that pose an added safety risk.

- Restricted mobility or dexterity: Patients may have difficulty or the inability to get to the bathroom in a timely fashion due to underlying physical disabilities or limitations such as a spinal cord injury, rheumatoid arthritis or acute illness.

- Environmental barriers: Patients may not be able to reach the restroom or toilet due to stairs, lack of handrails or narrow doorways that do not accommodate wheelchairs or walkers.

- Mental and psychosocial disability: Patients may not realize they have to urinate or may be confused over the location of the restroom.

- Pharmacological intervention: Patients may take medications that affect awareness, mobility, and dexterity.

## Urinary Tract Infections (UTI)[10,24]

Urinary tract infections are very common and occur within the general population, however, there is a higher incidence in women and the geriatric population. UTIs can be classified as uncomplicated, complicated, recurrent or chronic.

**Etiology** – Urinary tract infections (UTI) occur when bacteria infiltrate the urethra (termed urethritis) or further into the bladder itself (cystitis). Untreated, this type of infection can spread and cause a kidney infection (pyelonephritis). Diagnosis is confirmed with urinalysis. Frequent UTIs may require ultrasound, intravenous pyelogram, and cystoscopy to further assess the function of the bladder.

**Signs and symptoms** – Symptoms of a UTI include increased frequency of urination, pain and/or burning with urination, cloudy urine, pressure above the pubic bone in women, shakiness, fever, back pain, and fatigue.

**Treatment** – Early treatment has the best results; delay in treatment may allow for serious infection to occur. Pharmacological treatment includes bacteria-specific antibiotics based on the bacteria found in the bladder. Patients are also encouraged to drink an excess of fluids to assist with treatment of the infection.

## Consider This

### Advanced Physical Therapy Interventions[21,23,24]

Other treatment techniques that are not entry-level for pelvic floor dysfunction may include:

- Perineal massage both by the practitioner and patient
- Scar tissue massage both by the practitioner and patient
- Intravaginal soft tissue massage (also known as Thiele massage)
- Intravaginal trigger point release and myofascial release
- Intravaginal self-stretching techniques including the use of a dilator
- Prostate massage

These techniques may be used for, but are not limited to patients who have dyspareunia, vulvodynia, prostatitis, interstitial cystitis, urgency, urge incontinence, levator ani syndrome, coccydynia, and perineal pain from pregnancy.

## Obstetrics

### Obstetric Musculoskeletal Pathology

#### Coccydynia[21]

After childbirth the joint between the coccyx and sacrum can become hypermobile causing the soft tissue surrounding the coccyx to become painful.

**Etiology** – Subluxation during delivery, adherence to tear or episiotomy scar.

**Signs and symptoms** – Difficulty sitting on hard surfaces, referred pain to the low back, sacroiliac joint, hip, buttock, groin or rectum areas, pain with bowel movements, dyspareunia, and formation of hemorrhoids.

**Treatment** – Treatment may include heat, external joint mobilization, myofascial release, muscle energy techniques, biofeedback for pelvic floor muscle relaxation, postural training, abdominal strengthening exercises, stretching exercises for surrounding muscles, and the use of a cushion for sitting.

#### Diastasis Recti[21,22,25]

Diastasis recti is a separation of the rectus abdominis muscle along the linea alba that can occur during pregnancy. Testing for diastasis recti should be performed on all pregnant women prior to prescribing exercises that require the use of the abdominals.

**Etiology** – The exact cause is unknown, however, theories indicate biomechanical and hormonal changes in women may cause the separation. The therapist must note how many fingers fit into the separation and modify treatment accordingly.

**Signs and symptoms** – A patient is considered to have diastasis recti if the therapist detects a separation greater than the width of two fingers when the woman lifts her head and shoulders off the plinth (Figs. 7-6, 7-7).

**Treatment** – Treatment will include stabilization and support with abdominal strengthening exercises, postural awareness exercises, and body mechanics training. A newborn can also have

diastasis recti secondary to incomplete development, however, in infants this condition usually resolves itself without intervention.

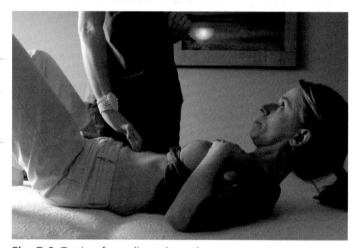

Fig. 7-6: Testing for a diastasis recti.

Fig. 7-7: A three finger separation at the linea alba.

## Piriformis Syndrome[21]

Piriformis syndrome refers to a persistent, severe radiating low back and buttock pain spanning from the sacrum to the hip and posterior thigh. However, controversy exists over piriformis syndrome's efficacy as an accurate diagnosis.

**Etiology** – During pregnancy the piriformis may shorten or spasm due to postural changes and hip lateral rotation while walking.

**Signs and symptoms** – The primary symptom is sciatic paresthesia due to nerve entrapment as the sciatic nerve passes under or through the piriformis muscle.

**Treatment** – Manual techniques for correcting pelvic or sacral alignment such as muscle energy techniques, joint mobilization, self-correction techniques for alignment, heat application, deep tissue massage, myofascial release, strain-counterstrain, abdominal strengthening, stretching exercises for both the piriformis and surrounding muscles, body mechanics, and postural education.

## Symphysis Pubis Pain[21]

To prepare for delivery, the symphysis pubis joint becomes mobile in order to allow the joint to slightly separate during delivery.

**Etiology** – Postural adaptations, ligamentous laxity, and complications during delivery or birthing of a large infant can result in more severe injury to the soft tissues surrounding the joint.

**Signs and symptoms** – Severe pain in the symphysis pubis and sacroiliac joints as well as blood in the urine due to injury to the urethra or bladder neck.

**Treatment** – Medical treatment includes pharmacological intervention for pain and surgical intervention based on the degree of separation in the joint. Treatment may also include heat or ice if acute, manual techniques for correcting pelvic or sacral alignment such as muscle energy techniques, self-correction techniques for alignment, education on positioning, postural training, gait training, pelvic and lumbar stabilization exercises, and the use of a lumbo-pelvic brace or binder.

## Physiological and Postural Changes during Pregnancy[21,22,25]

- Weight gain between 25 and 35 pounds; anemia may occur

- Uterus ascends into the abdominal cavity becoming an abdominal organ

- Ribs expand to accommodate the uterine ascent; respiratory diaphragm elevates four centimeters

- Increased depth of respiration, tidal volume, and minute ventilation

- Increased oxygen consumption (15-20%), blood volume (40-50%), and cardiac output (30-60%)

- Hypotension in supine position during pregnancy from pressure on the inferior vena cava

- Abdominals become overstretched; ligaments become lax secondary to hormonal changes

- Joints may become hypermobile

## Exercise & Pregnancy[21,22,25-27]

Pregnant women are encouraged to continue with exercise activity at a moderate rate during a low risk pregnancy. Guidelines permit women to remain at 50-60% of their maximal heart rate for approximately thirty minutes per session. Women must monitor their heart rate intermittently to ensure that they are maintaining their target heart rate. Non-weight bearing activities are preferred due to the continuous change in the center of gravity and balance. Loose clothing is advised to allow for adequate heat loss, and adequate fluids are required during exercise. Women should avoid becoming overtired and should not exercise in the supine position after the first trimester.

## Pelvic Floor Muscle Exercises[21,25]

Once the pelvic floor muscles have been assessed for strength, an exercise routine can be created based on the findings. Some factors to consider are: position, endurance, and repetitions. Introduce new positions transitioning from gravity-assisted to standing as the strength and awareness of the pelvic floor muscles increase. The goal is for the patient to be able to perform the contractions with functional tasks.

## Consider This

### Back Pain During Pregnancy[21,22]

Back pain has been reported in 70% of pregnant women, ranging from minor strain to significant structural deformities. Back pain is often caused by physical changes associated with pregnancy including weight gain, altered muscle tone, increased lordosis, changes in center of gravity and laxity within pelvic ligaments. Typically excessive bending, lifting and walking can produce back pain especially if there is a history of prior back pain or obesity.

Minor back pain can be relieved through education related to body mechanics, postural awareness, and stretching and strengthening exercises to provide balance within musculature. More severe pain should not be dismissed as simply a side effect of pregnancy. Etiology of severe back pain may include pregnancy-induced osteoporosis, disk disease or herniated disk, vertebral osteoarthritis, and septic arthritis. Patients with both minor and severe back pain should be examined to determine if the source of the pain is mechanical, muscular, joint or discogenic.

Recommendations vary from 80-100 contractions per day combining quick, long hold, and functional contractions. Quick contractions are important to withstand increased intra-abdominal pressure. The patient typically begins with three sets of ten quick contractions daily, holding for two seconds and resting for four seconds. Long hold contractions are for endurance training and are important for maintaining proper posture and pelvic support. The patient typically begins with three sets of five long hold contractions daily, holding for five seconds and resting for ten seconds, gradually increasing the contraction time to ten seconds. Make sure the patient fully relaxes after each contraction. Variations of contractions will depend on each patient's diagnosis, awareness, and ability.

## Spotlight on Safety

### Contraindications to Exercise During Pregnancy[27]

Participating in a wide range of recreational activities and exercise appears to be safe during and after pregnancy. Exercise programs are designed to minimize impairments and help maintain function during pregnancy. Certain circumstances exist where exercise is not safe during pregnancy. Below is a list of relative and absolute contraindications to exercise.

**Relative**

- Severe anemia
- Unevaluated maternal cardiac dysrhythmia
- Chronic bronchitis
- Poorly controlled type 1 diabetes
- Extreme morbid obesity
- Extreme underweight (BMI <12)
- History of extremely sedentary lifestyle
- Intrauterine growth restriction in current pregnancy
- Poorly controlled hypertension
- Orthopedic limitations
- Poorly controlled seizure disorder
- Poorly controlled hyperthyroidism
- Heavy smoker

**Absolute**

- Hemodynamically significant heart disease
- Restrictive lung disease
- Incompetent cervix/cerclage
- Multiple gestation at risk for premature labor
- Persistent second or third trimester bleeding
- Placenta previa after 26 weeks of gestation
- Premature labor during the current pregnancy
- Ruptured membranes
- Preeclampsia/pregnancy-induced hypertension

## American College of Obstetricians and Gynecologists (ACOG) Recommendations for Exercise in Pregnancy and Postpartum[27]

1. During pregnancy, women can continue to exercise and derive health benefits even from mild to moderate exercise routines. Regular exercise (at least three times per week) is preferable to intermittent activity.

2. Women should avoid exercise in the supine position after the first trimester. Such a position is associated with decreased cardiac output in most pregnant women. Since the remaining cardiac output will be preferentially distributed away from splanchnic beds (including the uterus) during vigorous exercise, such regimens are best avoided during pregnancy. Prolonged periods of motionless standing should be avoided.

3. Women should be aware of the decreased oxygen available for aerobic exercise during pregnancy. They should be encouraged to modify the intensity of their exercise according to maternal symptoms. Pregnant women should stop exercising when fatigued and not exercise to exhaustion. Weight bearing exercises may, under some circumstances, be continued at intensities similar to those prior to pregnancy throughout pregnancy. Non-weight bearing exercises, such as cycling or swimming, will minimize the risk of injury and facilitate the continuation of exercise during pregnancy.

4. Morphologic changes in pregnancy should serve as a relative contraindication to types of exercise in which loss of balance could be detrimental to maternal or fetal well-being, especially in the third trimester. Further, any type of exercise involving the potential for even mild abdominal trauma should be avoided.

5. Pregnancy requires an additional 300 kcal/day in order to maintain metabolic homeostasis. Thus, women who exercise during pregnancy should be particularly careful to ensure an adequate diet.

6. Pregnant women who exercise in the first trimester should augment heat dissipation by ensuring adequate hydration, appropriate clothing, and optimal environmental surroundings during exercise.

7. Many of the physiological and morphological changes of pregnancy persist 4 to 6 weeks postpartum. Thus, pre-pregnancy exercise routines should be resumed gradually based upon a woman's physical capability.

From American College of Obstetricians and Gynecologists. Exercise During Pregnancy and the Postpartum Period. (Technical Bulletin No. 189). Washington, DC, copyrights ACOG, February 1994, with permission.

# Spotlight on Safety

**Management Guidelines and Precautions for High-Risk Pregnancies[25]**

A pregnancy is designated as high-risk based on complications from disease or pathology that place the mother and fetus at risk for illness or death. Medical intervention is focused on prevention of preterm delivery through the prescription of bed rest, activity restriction, and medications.

Physical therapy can enhance the well-being and quality of life of the pregnant woman with a high-risk pregnancy. The physical therapist should closely monitor the patient during all activities, reassess after each treatment, and develop an individualized exercise program addressing the patient's needs. The patient should also be instructed in self-monitoring techniques during activities to avoid adverse reactions.

The following guidelines can assist in working with high-risk patients:

- Left sidelying is the position of choice to reduce the pressure on the inferior vena cava, maximize cardiac output to enhance maternal and fetal circulation, and reduce the risk of incompetent cervix.
- Abdominal exercises may stimulate uterine contractions. The therapist should modify or discontinue the exercises.
- Keep exercises simple, slow, smooth, and with minimal exertion.
- Avoid the Valsalva maneuver by discontinuing activities that increase intra-abdominal pressure.
- Provide instruction on proper body mechanics and postural instruction to limit straining during abdominal contractions.
- Encourage maximum muscle efficiency during each movement.
- Educate the women about Cesarean delivery rehabilitation.
- Monitor and report any uterine contraction, bleeding or amniotic fluid loss.

## Pharmacology - Genitourinary Management[19]

Pharmacological intervention is used for treating bladder symptoms related to urgency, frequency, infection, and pain.

### Overactive Bladder Agents

**Action:** Overactive bladder agents relieve the symptoms of an overactive bladder. This condition is noted by involuntary contractions of the bladder (detrusor muscle).

**Indications:** urinary urgency, urinary frequency, urge incontinence, nocturia

**Side effects:** widely vary based on drug classification; typically gastrointestinal distress, nausea, dizziness, photosensitivity, headache, constipation, pulmonary reactions

**Implications for PT:** Therapists should be aware of the adverse effects of these agents, however, these agents do not typically interfere with rehabilitation. A therapist should communicate any signs of pulmonary impairment or distress to the physician.

**Examples:** Ditropan (oxybutynin chloride), Detrol (tolterodine tartrate)

### Urinary Anti-infective Agents

**Action:** Urinary anti-infective agents treat urinary tract infections, but are not traditional antibiotics or sulfonamide agents. These agents can be used independently or in combination to treat urinary infections.

**Indications:** cystitis, urinary urgency, burning with urination, urinary tract infection, nocturia

**Side effects:** widely vary based on drug classification; gastrointestinal distress, nausea, dizziness, photosensitivity, headache, constipation, rash

**Implications for PT:** Therapists should be aware of the adverse effects of these agents, however, these agents do not typically interfere with rehabilitation.

**Examples:** Cinobac (cinoxacin), Furadantin (nitrofurantoin)

### Diuretic Agents

See Cardiac pharmacology

### Hormones

See Metabolic and Endocrine pharmacology

## Genitourinary System Terminology[10,20,24]

**Anuria:** Inadequate urine output in a 24-hour period; less than 100 ml (severe dehydration, shock, end-stage renal disease).

**Benign prostatic hypertrophy:** A non-cancerous enlargement of the prostate gland that is progressive. Common in males over 60 and can interfere with normal voiding.

**Cystocele:** Bulging of the bladder into the vagina.

**Ectopic:** Implantation of a fertilized ovum outside of the uterus (fallopian tube is the most common site of an ectopic pregnancy).

**Endometrium:** The inner lining of the uterus that is shed monthly in response to hormonal influence.

**Glomerular filtration rate:** An estimate of the filtering capacity of the kidneys; volume of filtrate produced per minute by the kidneys.

**Glomerulus:** The specialized tuft of capillaries that are needed for the filtration of fluid as blood passes through the arterioles of the kidneys.

## Consider This

### Hormone Replacement Therapy for Menopausal Symptoms[23]

Hormone replacement therapy (HRT), including estrogen and progestin replacement, has been approved by the Food and Drug Administration (FDA) for treatment of menopausal symptoms and osteoporosis.

The Women's Heath Initiative (WHI) trial of HRT found the benefits for hormone replacement to be reduction in hot flash frequency and severity, improvement in atrophic vaginitis and UTIs, and prevention of osteoporosis and fractures. Studies suggest women going through menopausal transition who are experiencing depression and memory loss may also benefit from HRT, however, this remains a controversial claim.

The risks of participating in HRT include pulmonary embolus, stroke, deep vein thrombosis, gallbladder disease, and a small increase in breast cancer.

Over the past 30 years, there has been an increase in HRT for post-menopausal women who also have cardiovascular disease (CVD). The primary and secondary prevention of CVD using HRT has not been demonstrated in randomized treatment trials leading to much controversy. However, studies also indicate that early initiation of HRT may inhibit the progression of CVD.

The decision to use HRT should be individualized based on the woman's goals for therapy. Each woman should consult her physician to discuss the benefits and risks, and should reevaluate periodically to ensure the benefits continue to favor hormone use.

**Hematuria:** Presence of blood in the urine (cancer, faulty catheterization, serious disease).

**Impotence:** Impairment with ejaculation, orgasm, erection, and/or libido.

**Myometrium:** The muscular outer layer of the uterus.

**Nephrolithiasis:** The condition of developing kidney stones. There are various types of crystal formations that create stones.

**Nocturia:** Urinary frequency at night (diabetes mellitus, congestive heart failure).

**Oliguria:** Inadequate urine output in a 24-hour period; less than 400 ml (acute renal failure, diabetes mellitus).

**Polyuria:** Large volume of urine excreted at one time (diabetes mellitus, chronic renal failure).

**Perimetrium:** The serous peritoneal coat of the uterus.

**Radical mastectomy:** A surgical procedure in which the entire breast, pectoral muscles, axillary lymph nodes, and some skin are removed usually secondary to breast cancer.

**Rectocele:** The bulging of the anterior wall of the rectum into the vagina secondary to weakening of the pelvic supporting structures.

**Seminiferous tubules:** Coiled tubes found within each lobe of the testes where spermatogenesis takes place.

**Urea:** Major nitrogen-containing end product of protein metabolism normally cleared from the blood by the kidney into the urine.

**Urinary frequency:** Voiding more than eight times in a 24-hour period. Etiology may include overactive bladder, reduced bladder capacity, painful bladder syndrome or increased urine output caused by uncontrolled diabetes mellitus.

**Urinary urgency:** The sudden desire to urinate that is stronger than usual and difficult to defer. Etiology may include detrusor overactivity, bladder infection, inflammation or the presence of a foreign body such as stones or tumors. Urgency may lead to urinary urge incontinence.

# System Interactions

## System Interactions

### Oncology[28,29]

Cancer, malignancy, neoplasm, and tumor are all terms referring to abnormal uncontrolled cell growth within the body. There are more than one hundred different cancers of various types and tissue origins currently recognized, including lymphoma and hematologic cancers. Malignant cancer cells are characterized by their ability to grow uncontrollably, invade other tissues, remain undifferentiated, initiate growth at distant sites, and avoid detection and destruction by the body's immune system. The origins of malignant cells vary widely from environmental factors and lifestyle choices to genetic predisposition.

Carcinoma is a malignancy originating from the epithelial cells of organs. Carcinomas in specific organs may be named more specifically depending on the characteristics present. For example, large cell carcinoma, adenocarcinoma, and squamous cell carcinoma are all subsets of lung carcinoma. The American Cancer Society reports that at least 80% of all cancers in the United States are carcinomas.

## Tissue and Tumor Classification[30]

| Tissue Classification | Examples | Tumor Classification |
|---|---|---|
| **Epithelium**<br>Protect, absorb, and excrete | – Skin<br>– Lines internal cavities<br>– Mucous membrane<br>– Lining of bladder | Carcinoma<br><br>Adenocarcinoma (glandular tissue) |
| **Pigmented Cells** | – Moles | Malignant melanoma |
| **Connective Tissues**<br>Elastic, collagen, fibrous | – Striated muscle<br>– Blood vessels<br>– Bone<br>– Cartilage<br>– Fat<br>– Smooth muscle | Sarcoma<br>Fibrosarcoma<br>Liposarcoma<br>Chondrosarcoma<br>Osteosarcoma<br>Hemangiosarcoma<br>Leiomyosarcoma<br>Rhabdomyosarcoma |
| **Nerve Tissues**<br>Neurons, nerve fibers, dendrites, glial cells | – Brain<br>– Nerves<br>– Spinal cord<br>– Retina | Astrocytoma<br>Glioma<br>Neurilemic sarcoma<br>Neuroblastoma<br>Retinoblastoma |
| **Lymphoid Tissues** | – Wherever lymph tissue is present throughout the body<br>– Lymph nodes<br>– Spleen<br>– Can appear in stomach, intestines, skin, CNS, bone, and tonsils | Lymphoma |
| **Hematopoietic Tissues** | – Bone marrow<br>– Plasma cells | Leukemia<br>Myelodysplasia<br>Myeloproliferative syndromes<br>Multiple myeloma |

## Risk Factors[28]

| | |
|---|---|
| • Increasing age | • Poor diet |
| • Tobacco use | • Stress |
| • Alcohol use | • Occupational hazards |
| • Gender | • Ethnic background |
| • Virus exposure | • Genetic influence |
| • Environmental influence | • Sexual/reproductive behavior |

## General Signs and Symptoms of Cancer

C – Change in bowel/bladder routine

A – A sore that will not heal

U – Unusual bleeding/discharge

T – Thickening/lump develops

I – Indigestion or difficulty swallowing

O – Obvious change in wart/mole

N – Nagging cough/hoarseness

Unexplained weight loss, fatigue, anorexia, anemia, pain, and/or weakness are other general symptoms that may indicate cancer.[28]

## Cancer Prevention[28]

| | |
|---|---|
| **Primary Prevention** | • Screening for high risk population<br>• Elimination of modifiable risk factors<br>• Use of natural agents (i.e., teas, vitamins) to prevent cancer<br>• Cancer vaccine |
| **Secondary Prevention** | • Early detection<br>• Selective preventative pharmacological agents (e.g., Tamoxifen)<br>• Multifactorial risk reduction |
| **Tertiary Prevention** | • Prevent disability that can occur secondary to cancer and its treatment<br>• Manage symptoms<br>• Limit complications |

## Spotlight on Safety
### Musculoskeletal Pain and Oncology[30]

Musculoskeletal pain complaints should not be taken lightly in oncology populations. Bony or soft tissue pain complaints can be heralding signs of disease progression or adverse treatment effects.

Bony pain complaints may relate to a primary site of malignancy, such as with osteosarcoma, or new metastasis to a bony area. New back pain complaints of unclear origin, for example, should be evaluated immediately as this pain may be indicative of spinal metastasis which may result in neurological deficits.

Soft tissue complaints may relate to medication side effects or physiological changes in the tissue itself as a result of oncological interventions. Women who have received radiation treatment for breast cancer and develop axillary web syndrome or radiation fibrosis, for example, may experience considerable discomfort along with palpable tissue changes and functional limitations in the affected upper quadrant.

### Diagnostic Tools[28]

| | |
|---|---|
| • Family history | • Pap smear |
| • Physical examination | • Blood tests |
| • Radiography | • Biopsy |
| • CT scan | • Mammography |
| • Bone scan | • Endoscopy |
| • Stool guaiac | • Isotope scan |

### Staging[31,32]

The stage of a malignancy is determined by evaluating the extent of the disease, lymph node involvement, and existence of metastasis. Staging data is utilized in the selection of treatment interventions, to assist in goal setting, and in the prediction of outcomes and prognosis for both oncological and physical therapy interventions. Staging data and responses to treatment are also typically reported to a tumor registry. The aggregate data maintained by a tumor registry supplies medical providers with information regarding treatment outcomes that can be compared nationally. Numerous staging systems exist with some used for many cancer types and others being type specific such as for cancers of the blood or lymphatic system.

The TNM system is one of the most commonly used methods of determining tumor stage. The system describes a malignancy based on the size and extent of the primary tumor (T), lymph node involvement (N), and presence of metastasis (M). For most cancers, the TNM combination will correspond to a stage designation that further defines the severity of the disease. Lower numbered stages are considered to have a better overall prognosis.

### National Cancer Institute Staging[31]

| Stage | Definition |
|---|---|
| Stage 0 | Early malignancy that is present only in the layer of cells in which it began. For most cancers, this is referred to as carcinoma in situ. Not all cancers have a stage 0. |
| Stage I | Malignancy limited to the tissue of origin with no lymph node involvement or metastasis. |
| Stage II | Malignancy spreading into adjacent tissues; lymph nodes may show signs of micrometastases. |
| Stage III | Malignancy that has spread to adjacent tissue showing signs of fixation to deeper structures. The likelihood of metastatic lymph node involvement is high. |
| Stage IV | Malignancy that has metastasized beyond the primary site, for example, to bone or another organ. |

Adapted from National Cancer Institute, www.cancer.gov

**Clinical staging** refers to the estimated extent of malignancy present based on the findings of a patient's physical examination, laboratory values, imaging tests, and biopsy. Clinical staging is a key component in determining a patient's optimal course of treatment and also establishes a baseline for comparison used in assessing the response to treatment.

**Pathologic staging** refers to staging based on the pathology findings of tissue samples obtained during surgery. Often surgery is performed to remove a malignant mass and/or nearby lymph nodes, or for an exploratory assessment and tissue sample removal. In some cases, the pathologic stage may differ from the clinical stage (e.g., if surgery reveals that the cancer has spread more than expected in relation to the clinical staging). The pathological stage gives the health care team more precise information which can be used to more definitively predict treatment responses and prognosis.

# Consider This

## Lymphedema: Interventions and Risk Factors[33]

Lymphedema is a chronic, incurable condition caused by the accumulation of lymph fluid in the body. The result is edema that typically presents in the extremities, but can occur anywhere in the body including the face, neck, abdomen, genitalia, and trunk. Lymphedema is categorized as either primary or secondary lymphedema based on etiology. Primary lymphedema is attributed to a poorly developed lymphatic system that cannot effectively manage the body's normal lymphatic load. Secondary lymphedema occurs when a condition (e.g., infection, tumor growth, inflammation, scarring) or procedure (e.g., lymph node excision) blocks or damages lymph nodes and/or vessels to such a degree that the remaining local system cannot compensate for the damage and maintain normal lymphatic flow.

Secondary lymphedema, as related to oncology diagnoses, is perhaps most often discussed in relation to breast cancer and axillary node dissection. While the incidence of lymphedema is significant in the breast cancer population, any patient undergoing lymph node dissection, chemotherapy or radiation has some risk of developing lymphedema. At risk patients should be counseled regarding the use of prophylactic compression, especially during high-risk activities such as air travel, skin protection, and signs and symptoms of lymphedema so that early interventions can be initiated at the first sign of symptoms. The severity of symptoms in patients who have been diagnosed with lymphedema can vary widely. Once a diagnosis is made, regardless of severity, formal intervention is recommended in order to assist patients in managing their symptoms at the lowest possible level. Early, appropriate intervention and ongoing self-care significantly decrease the risk of infection and other negative sequelae associated with poor symptom management.

Treatment for lymphedema is referred to as complete decongestive therapy (CDT). CDT consists of a combination of manual lymphatic drainage, compression bandaging/garments, education, skin care, and exercise. CDT Phase 1 is considered the intensive acute treatment phase typically provided in an outpatient setting by a trained clinician 4-5 days per week for 4-6 weeks. CDT Phase 2 refers to the long-term management of symptoms utilizing various components of CDT modified for a self-care model. It is not expected that a patient with lymphedema only undergo one course of CDT phase 1 in their lifetime, but rather return for intensive treatment periodically whenever a significant change in symptoms is noted.

The Lymphology Association of North America and the National Lymphedema Network advocate that to ensure patient safety and avoid undue complications, lymphedema treatment should only be provided by a certified lymphedema therapist.

## Oncology Pathology

### Brain Cancer[10,32]

Brain cancer may occur as a primary tumor arising from astrocytes, meninges, nerve cells, or tissues within the brain. Metastatic brain cancer occurs when a brain tumor develops as a consequence of cancer in another primary area of the body.

**Etiology** – Most primary cancers outside of the brain metastasize to the brain during progression of the cancer.

**Signs and symptoms** – Symptoms are dependent on the location of the tumor and typically progress rapidly. Symptoms include headache, seizures, increased intracranial pressure, cognitive and emotional impairment, and decreased motor and sensory function.

**Treatment** – Surgical resection along with radiation or other combined therapies are typically indicated.

### Breast Cancer[10,32]

Breast cancer is the most common female malignancy, but can also occur in men. The majority of cases are classified as adenocarcinoma and it is the second leading cause of female death from cancer. Common metastases are found in the lymph nodes, lungs, bones, skin, and brain. If the cancer recurs, it is usually within two years of the initial diagnosis.

**Etiology** – Risk factors include genetics, gender, age, menstrual history, and geography.

**Signs and symptoms** – Breast cancer presents as a lump and is usually found by the woman. The mass is typically firm, irregular, and non-painful. The patient may also present with signs including nipple discharge, erythema or a change in breast shape.

**Treatment** – Treatment may include surgery, radiation, chemotherapy or hormonal manipulation. It is curable if diagnosed prior to metastases; survival rate decreases as the stage of the cancer increases. The current 5-year survival rate for localized tumors is 92%; this drops substantially if there is nodal involvement.

### Cervical Cancer[10,32]

Cervical cancer starts in the cells on the surface of the cervix, typically squamous cells. This precancerous condition is called dysplasia and is easily treatable. Annual cervical screening is recommended; diagnosis is made through a Pap test (smear). Prognosis is good with timely intervention. If dysplasia goes undetected, changes can develop into cervical cancer and metastasize to the bladder, intestines, lungs, and liver.

**Etiology** – The human papilloma virus (HPV) is the primary cause of cervical cancer; it is slow growing. Risk factors include smoking, maternal use of diethylstilbestrol (DES), African American ethnicity, oral contraceptive use, and certain sexually transmitted diseases.

**Signs and symptoms** – Asymptomatic during the early stages; however, symptoms can include abnormal bleeding, pelvic and low back pain, impairment with bladder and bowel function.

**Treatment** – Treatment is dependent on staging of the cancer and may include laser therapy, excision, cryotherapy or hysterectomy with adjunct chemotherapy or radiation.

## Colorectal Cancer[10,32]

Colorectal cancer accounts for approximately 15% of cancer deaths annually. Adenocarcinoma and primary lymphoma account for the majority of intestinal cancers.

**Etiology** – Risk factors include increasing age, history of polyps, ulcerative colitis, Crohn's disease, family history, and a diet high in fat and low in fiber.

**Signs and symptoms** – Colon cancer does not provide early signs of disease and the most prominent symptom is a continuous change in bowel habits. Bright red blood from the rectum is another prominent sign of colon cancer. The patient may experience symptoms of fatigue, weight loss, anemia, and overt rectal bleeding.

**Treatment** – Treatment is based on the type and staging of the cancer and may include surgical resection of the tumor and potentially a portion of the bowel, with subsequent radiation therapy and/or chemotherapy; colostomy may be required. Prognosis is good for early diagnosis if the cancer is contained; prognosis is poor if it has metastasized.

## Lung Cancer[10,32]

Lung cancer is cancer of the epithelium within the respiratory tract. It is the most frequent cause of death from all cancers. Rapid metastasis can occur through the pulmonary vascular system, adrenal gland, brain, bone, and liver.

**Etiology** – Risk factors include smoking, environment, geography, occupational hazards, age, and family history.

**Signs and symptoms** – Early symptoms include cough, sputum, and dyspnea. Progression may include symptoms of adventitious breath sounds, chest pain, and hemoptysis.

**Treatment** – There is a poor prognosis secondary to expedited metastasis (less than 14% for a five-year survival rate). Surgical intervention along with combination therapies may be required.

## Lymphoma (Hodgkin's disease, non-Hodgkin's disease)[10,32]

Lymphoma is classified as cancer found in the lymphatic system and lymph tissues; lymphomas are categorized as Hodgkin's disease or non-Hodgkin's lymphoma.

**Etiology** – Risk factors for Hodgkin's disease include association with Epstein-Barre virus, drug abuse, immunosuppressant use, obesity, chronic or autoimmune diseases. Risk factors for non-Hodgkin's lymphoma include exposure to benzene (i.e., cigarette smoke), auto emissions, and pollution.

**Signs and symptoms** – A painless lump is typically the first sign. Hodgkin's disease is distinguished by the presence of Reed-Sternberg cells and Hodgkin's disease can metastasize to extralymphatic sites including the liver, spleen, and lungs.

**Treatment** – Hodgkin's disease is one of the most curable cancers depending on age, disease stage, overall health, and responsiveness to treatment. Treatment options are based on the patient's age and staging classification and include chemotherapy, radiation, stem cell transplant, and highly active antiretroviral therapy. Non-Hodgkin's progression varies based on classification, co-morbidities, and treatment response.

## Pancreatic Cancer[10,32]

Pancreatic cancer is a prominent type of cancer with an extremely high mortality rate. Cancer of the exocrine cells within the ducts is the most common form of pancreatic cancer. It will metastasize to the liver, lungs, pleura, colon, stomach, and spleen.

**Etiology** – Risk factors include tobacco use, gender, increasing age, and cholecystectomy.

**Signs and symptoms** – Symptoms are very vague during the initial stages of the disease which often results in delayed diagnosis. Common symptoms include weight loss, jaundice, and epigastric pain that can radiate to the thoracic region. Advanced cancer may present with severe pain that may indicate the cancer has metastasized.

**Treatment** – Treatment is usually directed to assist in the relief of symptoms. Pancreatic cancer has a very poor survival rate with a mortality rate of almost 100%. Surgical resection along with chemotherapy and radiation assist to relieve symptoms.

## Prostate Cancer[10,32]

Adenocarcinoma is the most common type of prostate cancer. Prostate cancer typically affects men over 50 years old; it is the second highest cause of death from cancer in men. Diagnosis is found through prostate biopsy and prognosis is good with appropriate treatment. There is an approximate 10% fatality from this diagnosis.

**Etiology** – Risk factors include increased age, high fat diet, genetic predisposition, African American descent, and exposure to cadmium.

**Signs and symptoms** – Most times this is asymptomatic until the cancer reaches the advanced stages. Symptoms include urinary obstruction, pain, urgency, and decreased stream/flow of urine.

**Treatment** – Treatment varies and may include surgical incision of the prostate gland, radiation, or hormonal therapy; can metastasize to the bladder, musculoskeletal system, lungs, and lymph nodes.

## Skin Cancer[10,32]

### Basal Cell Carcinoma

Basal cell carcinoma is a slow growing form of skin cancer that rarely metastasizes. It originates from the epidermis and is the most common form of skin cancer.

**Etiology** – Sun exposure is a common cause, with risk factors including frequent sun exposure, light eyes, and fair skin.

**Signs and symptoms** – Open sores that can bleed or crust and remain for three or more weeks, reddish patches of skin, a shiny bump on the skin that is often pink, or a scar-like area that has poorly defined borders.

**Treatment** – Prognosis is good; basal cell carcinoma can routinely be cured. Surgical excision may be required to remove the cancer cells.

### Malignant Melanoma

Malignant melanoma originates from melanocytes and can be classified as: superficial spreading, nodular, lentigo maligna or acral lentiginous melanomas. Peak incidence is between 40-60 years of age. Early diagnosis is vital to prognosis, as it can spread and metastasize quickly. Areas of metastases include the brain, lungs, liver, bone, and skin.

## Consider This

### Exercise Guidelines for Patients Undergoing Cancer Treatment[30]

The combination of surgical, medical, and radiation oncology interventions can produce a variety of unpleasant symptoms which may significantly impact a patient's quality of life during treatment. Common side effects include pain, fatigue, depression, anxiety, altered body image, sleep disturbances, lymphedema, and gastrointestinal distress. With therapeutic exercise, physical therapists have the ability to positively impact both symptoms and quality of life. In planning exercise interventions, therapists should consider the following:

- Always check physician orders prior to treating a patient with bone metastases to verify weight bearing status and clearance to perform mobility

- Monitor a patient's blood values daily, especially platelet and hematocrit counts, to ensure that it is safe for the patient to participate in therapy activities

- Exercise should be conducted at a range of 40-65% of the peak heart rate, heart rate reserve, and $VO_2$ max or below the anaerobic threshold

- During exercise, perceived exertion should not exceed a 12 using the Borg's Rating of Perceived Exertion Scale

- Treatment visits should be scheduled during the time of day when the patient's energy is at peak levels

- Treatment should be modified as needed to accommodate any side effects of medical treatment

---

**Etiology** – Risk factors for malignant melanoma include a history of blistering sunburns prior to 20 years of age, family history, immunosuppression, light eyes, fair skin, and a previous history of cancer.

**Signs and symptoms** – Lesions can be elevated on the surface of the skin and appear keratotic or scaly. Other symptoms when observing the skin or a mole may include asymmetry, irregular borders, varied color, and a diameter of greater than six millimeters.

**Treatment** – This form of cancer is 100% curable with early diagnosis. Excision may solely be required with early treatment. If melanoma has metastasized, surgical intervention along with combination therapies may be required.

## Pediatric Oncology Pathology[34,35]

### Astrocytoma

Astrocytoma is a classification that accounts for approximately fifty percent of pediatric brain tumors. The etiology of pediatric cancers is usually unknown.

**Etiology** – Etiology includes genetic predisposition, environmental influence, radiation and toxin exposure, and association with certain childhood disorders.

**Signs and symptoms** – There are two types of astrocytoma with characteristics as follows:

**Cerebellar** - clumsiness, ataxic gait, headache, change in personality, and vomiting

**Supratentorial** - headache, seizures, change in personality, visual impairments, and vomiting

**Treatment** – Surgical resection of cerebellar tumors offers an 80-90% cure rate. Supratentorial tumors also require surgery to resect the tumor with radiation and/or chemotherapy.

### Leukemia

Leukemia is a cancer of the blood that occurs when leukocytes change into malignant cells. These immature cells proliferate, accumulate in bone marrow, and ultimately cease the production of normal cells. This process will spread to lymph nodes, liver, spleen, and other areas of the body.

**Etiology** – The exact etiology is unknown, however, causative factors include environmental, chemical or toxin exposure, genetic predisposition, and viral association. There are many types of leukemia with acute lymphoblastic leukemia (ALL) and acute myelogenous leukemia (AML) occurring most frequently in children.

**Signs and symptoms** – Characteristics include an abrupt onset with high fever, bleeding, enlarged lymph nodes and spleen, progressive weakness, fatigue, and painful joints. Blood work will indicate anemia, a leukocyte count greater than 500,000 $mm^3$ and thrombocytopenia.

**Treatment** – Treatment will vary based on the type and degree of leukemia. Options include immunotherapy, cytotoxic agents, chemotherapy or radiation, and bone marrow transplant. Over 90% of patients with ALL achieve complete remission with treatment, while 70-80% of patients with AML achieve complete remission with treatment.

### Neuroblastoma

A neuroblastoma is a tumor that initiates from primitive ectodermal cells of the neural plate and is found within the sympathetic nervous system, primarily seen in the adrenal glands or paraspinal ganglias. This is the most common malignant tumor seen in children.

**Etiology** – The etiology remains unknown, but causative factors include genetic predisposition, familial incidence, environmental influence, radiation and toxin exposure or viral association.

**Signs and symptoms** – Characteristics vary with the site and include an abdominal mass, change in personality, anemia, sweating, pain, and diarrhea.

**Treatment** – Treatment includes surgical resection, chemotherapy, and radiation. Prognosis is best for children diagnosed in the first year of life. A neuroblastoma will spontaneously regress in rare cases.

### Osteogenic Sarcoma

An osteogenic sarcoma is a cancer that occurs at the epiphyses of long bones. Osteogenic sarcoma is the most common form of bone cancer in children with a peak incidence between the ages of 10 and 20.

**Etiology** – Exact etiology is unknown, however, there is a correlation between immunoincompetence and rate of tumor progression. Osteogenic sarcoma can metastasize quickly.

**Signs and symptoms** – Characteristics include presence of a mass, rapid metastases, and associated pain. Diagnosis can be made with a biopsy.

**Treatment** – Treatment includes amputation with proximal resection to ensure proper removal of affected tissue or surgical procedures that attempt to resect the tumor and salvage the limb. Chemotherapy is beneficial, however, radiation is not effective with this type of tumor.

### Wilms' Tumor

Wilms' tumor is an embryonal adenomyosarcoma found in the kidney. Most cases are diagnosed between one and four years of age.

**Etiology** – Etiology includes genetic inheritance as an autosomal dominant disease or a non-inherited form with an unknown etiology.

**Signs and symptoms** – Characteristics include an abdominal mass, pain, hematuria, fever, nausea, and vomiting.

**Treatment** – Treatment includes resection of the kidney and the associated lymphatic tissue followed by chemotherapy and/or radiation. Dactinomycin is also administered due to the drug's antitumor properties. The five-year cure rate is approximately 75%.

## Oncology Treatment Options[28,36,37]

### Surgery

Surgery is often used to resect and excise a defined area of malignancy, but may be indicated for prophylactic, diagnostic, curative or palliative goals. Surgical interventions usually require a combination of other treatment modalities secondary to the potential for metastases. These adjunct therapies function to destroy any residual malignant cells. Common side effects include fatigue, pain, deformity, scar tissue formation, and infection.

### Radiation

Radiation is administered as either ionizing radiation or particle radiation and can be delivered by teletherapy (external beam), brachytherapy (a sealed and/or implanted source) or system therapy (unsealed source). Radiation destroys the hydrogen bonds between the DNA strands of malignant cells. Radiation may be curative, adjuvant or palliative in its use. It may be used prior to surgical intervention, palliatively to shrink a malignant mass or post-surgically to ensure destruction of residual malignant cells. Radiation is most useful with localized malignancy. Common side effects include headache, bone marrow suppression, skin reactions, neuropathy, visual disturbances, nausea, vomiting, urinary frequency, diarrhea, delayed wound healing, and infection.

## Consider This

### Chemotherapy Related Altered Blood Counts[38]

Many chemotherapeutic agents include side effects that alter a patient's normal blood count which may result in conditions such as anemia, thrombocytopenia, and neutropenia. These conditions are diagnosed based on the laboratory results from a complete blood count.

Anemia refers to hemoglobin and hematocrit levels below normal gender specific laboratory reference values. In severe cases, a blood transfusion may be necessary. Symptoms may include dyspnea, heart palpitations, and dizziness. Patients who are anemic are advised to change positions slowly, rest frequently during activity, and allow themselves full nights of sleep.

Thrombocytopenia refers to platelet levels below normal reference laboratory values. Patients with thrombocytopenia will bruise very easily. Other symptoms may include petechiae, epistaxis, bleeding gums, and black or bloody stool. Patients with thrombocytopenia are advised to consult a physician before using over the counter medications that may further affect platelets such as aspirin and ibuprofen. Other precautions include avoiding contact sports, working with or around sharp objects, and tight fitting clothing or accessories.

Neutropenia refers to a neutrophil count below normal laboratory reference values placing a patient at risk for developing a serious infection. The severity of neutropenia may be categorized as mild, moderate or severe. An individual's risk of infection is typically a factor of the severity and duration of neutropenia. Patients who are neutropenic do not typically present with observable signs or symptoms. In hospitals, patients with neutropenia are typically assigned a private room with precautions instituted to decrease a patient's risk of exposure to infection from visitors, staff or unhygienic conditions. Patients with neutropenia who are not in medical facilities are advised to maintain excellent hand and body hygiene, closely self monitor for signs and symptoms of infection, wear shoes even in the home, and avoid exposure to potentially infectious environmental factors (e.g., crowds or people with illnesses, litter boxes, bird cages, fish tanks, flowers and plants, stagnant water, manicures/pedicures, jacuzzis/hot tubs).

## Spotlight on Safety

**Rehabilitation Considerations for Patients Undergoing Chemotherapy and Radiation[30]**

- Strenuous activity should be initially avoided following implantation of radioactive seeds utilized for brachytherapy. Communication with the radiation oncologist and/or referring physician is imperative as further activity contraindications or precautions may be advised depending on the individual case.

- Skin tattoos are used to guide beam alignment with external beam radiation. Physical therapists must be cautious and defer interventions which may alter the position of alignment tattoos (e.g., taping interventions, certain soft tissue or myofascial mobilizations).

- Irradiated skin requires special care to protect tissues prone to erythema, rash, and dry desquamation, as well as more painful wet desquamation and superficial burns.

- Massage and heat are contraindicated over irradiated areas for a minimum of 12 months.

- Certain chemotherapy agents may cause the patient to have a level of toxicity that requires staff and visitors to take additional precautions before making physical contact.

- Patient vomiting during therapy should be reported to the nurse/physician, especially if the patient is taking antiemetic medication to control nausea and vomiting.

### Chemotherapy

Chemotherapy consists of a group of drugs that are administered to destroy malignant cells. Chemotherapeutic agents include alkylating agents, antimetabolite agents, steroid hormones, plant alkaloid agents, interferons, and antitumor antibiotics. Each class of chemotherapeutic agents has a different mechanism of action to destroy malignant cells. Chemotherapy is most useful with widespread and metastatic malignancies, but is also used to induce remission, cure and/or eradicate residual malignant cells. The drugs may be administered orally, subcutaneously, intramuscularly, intravenously or intracavitary. Common side effects include nausea, vomiting, electrolyte imbalance, sexual dysfunction, hair loss, pain, and a decrease in platelet, red, and white blood cell counts.

### Biotherapy (Immunotherapy)

Biotherapy utilizes various agents and/or techniques to change the relationship between the malignancy and its host. Biologic response modifiers are commonly utilized for biotherapy and act to strengthen a patient's biological response to the malignant cells. Common agents or procedures used with this treatment include interferons, interleukin-2, bone marrow transplant, stem cell transplant, monoclonal antibodies, hormonal therapy, and colony-stimulating factors. Common side effects include fever, chills, nausea, vomiting, anorexia, central nervous system impairment, inflammatory reactions, leukopenia, and fatigue.

### Antiangiogenic Therapy

Antiangiogenic therapy focuses on the use of thalidomide and its suppression of blood supply formation. It has had initial success in the treatment of multiple myeloma. There is research that supports blocking the process of growth, as opposed to destruction of an already formed mass, as a means of inhibiting growth of primary malignant masses.

### Other Pharmacologic Therapies

Hormone therapy is a systemic intervention that is utilized with some types of cancer which rely on a particular hormone to grow (e.g., estrogen). Prescribed agents typically alter the body's production or action of specific hormones, preventing malignant cells from using the hormone they need to grow. Examples of hormone types used in oncology interventions include anti-estrogens, aromatase inhibitors, progestins, estrogens, anti-androgens, and corticosteroids. Targeted therapies refer to drugs designed to specifically target cancer cells. More specific in their action than systemic chemotherapeutic agents, targeted therapies attack mutated versions of a gene or the cells carrying the mutation. Targeted therapies may be a part of the primary oncological interventions or used to help maintain remission.

## Spotlight on Safety

**Modalities and Palliative Care[39]**

Numerous electrotherapeutic, thermal, and mechanical modalities are considered to be contraindicated for use with the oncology population. Physical therapists should be aware of the specifics of these contraindications in order to avoid limiting appropriate treatment options. For example, most heat and electrotherapeutic modalities are contraindicated for use over an active malignancy, but are not necessarily contraindicated for use elsewhere on the body. The therapist's ability to interpret information with respect to an individual's disease status, and when appropriate to seek physician guidance, is imperative when treating patients undergoing oncological interventions.

The use of heat and electrical modalities are typically contraindicated for direct use over malignancies due to the potential for facilitating growth of a malignant mass or hematogenous spread. With physician guidance, these contraindications often may be overlooked in lieu of palliative goals for terminally ill patients. This is especially true in hospice environments where curative efforts have been discontinued and end of life is imminent. However, therapists are advised to be mindful of and adhere to contraindications which may cause a terminally ill patient additional discomfort (e.g., the potential for neuromuscular electrical stimulation causing a pathological fracture in a patient with bone metastasis).

## Palliative Treatment[39,40]

Palliative treatment emphasizes symptom management as opposed to curative efforts. Palliative oncology interventions may include radiation, chemotherapy, physical therapy, chiropractic, acupuncture, alternative and homeopathic medicines, relaxation, biofeedback, pharmacological intervention, and hospice. Palliative treatment may be provided at any time in the disease process with goals of maintaining comfort and dignity through appropriate symptom management. Palliative services can be differentiated into patient support and caregiver support. Patient focused goals may include pain management, emotional and spiritual support, and management of symptoms such as confusion, fatigue, dyspnea, nausea, weakness, and bowel/bladder concerns. Caregiver support may include respite care, education, assistance with transportation, home management, and accessing social services.

## Pharmacology - Oncology Management[19,41]

### Alkylating Agents

**Action:** Alkylating agents bind the DNA strands together to prevent replication. If the DNA cannot untwist, then it cannot divide and replicate its genetic code. These agents initiate cell death by disrupting DNA function and releasing enzymes that destroy the cell.

**Indications:** various malignancies

**Side effects:** vary by class of drugs and by specific agent; multisystem involvement with mild to severe side effects, however, potential risks are typically warranted secondary to the diagnosis of malignancy

**Implications for PT:** Therapists must be aware of the chemotherapy regimen and modify treatment based on the patient's symptoms and side effects from cancer treatment. Extreme fatigue, gastrointestinal distress, cancer pain, and blood disorders are common. Therapists must provide support and encouragement without pushing the patient beyond their abilities.

**Examples:** Mustargen (mechlorethamine), Busulfex (busulfan), Leukeran (chlorambucil)

### Antimetabolite Agents

**Action:** Antimetabolite agents impair biosynthesis of genetic material and interrupt the cellular pathways that synthesize DNA and RNA. These agents create an impostor to the endogenous metabolites within the body to form a nonfunctional genetic product that is incapable of reproduction.

**Indications:** various malignancies, particularly rapidly dividing neoplastic cells

**Side effects:** vary by class of drugs and by specific agent; multisystem involvement with mild to severe side effects, however, potential risks are typically warranted secondary to the diagnosis of malignancy

**Implications for PT:** Therapists must be aware of the chemotherapy regimen and modify treatment based on the patient's symptoms and side effects from cancer treatment. Extreme fatigue, gastrointestinal distress, cancer pain, and blood disorders are common. Therapists must provide support and encouragement without pushing the patient beyond their abilities.

**Examples:** Leustatin (cladribine), Adrucil (fluorouracil), Fludara (fludarabine), Trexall (methotrexate)

### Antibiotic Agents

**Action:** Certain antibiotic agents are used with treatment of cancer due to their high toxicity and ability to interfere with DNA and RNA synthesis and subsequent cell division.

**Indications:** various malignancies

**Side effects:** vary by class of drugs and by specific agent; multisystem involvement with mild to severe side effects, however, potential risks are typically warranted secondary to the diagnosis of malignancy; shortness of breath, dysrhythmias, blood disorders, myelosuppression, pedal edema

**Implications for PT:** Therapists must be aware of the chemotherapy regimen and modify treatment based on the patient's symptoms and side effects from cancer treatment. Extreme fatigue, gastrointestinal distress, cancer pain, and blood disorders are common. Therapists must provide support and encouragement without pushing the patient beyond their abilities.

**Examples:** Adriamycin (doxorubicin), Mithracin (plicamycin), Cosmegen (dactinomycin)

### Plant Alkaloid Agents (Mitotic Inhibitors)

**Action:** Agents in this classification are nitrogen-based and largely derived from plants. They directly target the replication process prior to and during mitosis to inhibit cell division. This limits cell division and cancer growth in various types of malignancy.

**Indications:** various malignancies

**Side effects:** vary by class of drugs and by specific agent; multisystem involvement with mild to severe side effects, however, potential risks are typically warranted secondary to the diagnosis of malignancy

**Implications for PT:** Therapists must be aware of the chemotherapy regimen and modify treatment based on the patient's symptoms and side effects from cancer treatment. Extreme fatigue, gastrointestinal distress, cancer pain, and blood disorders are common. Therapists must provide support and encouragement without pushing the patient beyond their abilities.

**Examples:** Oncovin (vincristine sulfate), Taxotere (docetaxel), Taxol (paclitaxel)

### Hormones

**Action:** Certain hormones can exacerbate or facilitate proliferation of particular forms of cancer while other hormones can attenuate particular cancers. Hormones are typically used as adjunct therapy along with other forms of treatment specific to the malignancy.

**Indications:** various malignancies, particularly hormone sensitive neoplasms

## Consider This

### "Chemo Brain": Cognitive Changes Associated with Cancer Treatment[42]

Many patients and medical professionals recognize that treatment related cognitive changes in the oncology population are common occurrences. Referred to as "chemo brain" or "chemo fog," these colloquial names are misleading as research has not definitively connected impaired cognition with chemotherapy interventions. A number of factors make defining "chemo brain" difficult. For example, many patients still perform well on formal cognitive assessments, and most do not undergo baseline cognitive testing prior to beginning cancer treatment. Likewise, it is difficult for researchers to truly delineate if cognitive changes are due to the disease process itself, the treatment interventions or side effects of treatment (e.g., depression, fatigue, hormonal changes, altered blood counts, stress).

Regardless, the collection of symptoms commonly associated with "chemo brain" are openly acknowledged in the medical community and anecdotally supported by millions of patients. Physical therapists must be aware of and sensitive to these potential cognitive changes so that they may alter treatment interventions and teaching methods appropriately.

Common "chemo brain" complaints may include feelings of "foggy cognition," confusion, fatigue, limited attention span or short-term memory, and an unusual degree of difficulty with concentration, word finding, multi-tasking, and organization.[28]

---

**Side effects:** vary by class of drugs and by specific agent; multi-system involvement with mild to severe side effects, however, potential risks are typically warranted secondary to the diagnosis of malignancy; masculinization in women, hot flashes, general catabolic effects

**Implications for PT:** Therapists must be aware of the chemotherapy regimen and modify treatment based on the patient's symptoms and side effects from cancer treatment. Extreme fatigue, gastrointestinal distress, cancer pain, and blood disorders are common. Therapists must provide support and encouragement without pushing the patient beyond their abilities.

**Examples:** Nolvadex (tamoxifen citrate), Lupron (leuprolide acetate), Casodex (bicalutamide)

### Biologic Response Modifier Agents

**Action:** Biologic response modifier agents include interferons, interleukin-2, and monoclonal antibodies that are responsible for enhancing the body's own ability to respond to neoplastic growth. These agents are not cytotoxic, but facilitate the patient's immune response to destroy malignant tissues.

**Indications:** various malignancies, particularly leukemias, lymphomas, Kaposi sarcoma, organ and tissue malignancies

**Side effects:** vary by class of drugs and by specific agent; multi-system involvement with mild to severe side effects, however, potential risks are typically warranted secondary to the diagnosis of malignancy

**Implications for PT:** Therapists must be aware of the chemotherapy regimen and modify treatment based on the patient's symptoms and side effects from cancer treatment. Extreme fatigue, gastrointestinal distress, cancer pain, and blood disorders are common. Therapists must provide support and encouragement without pushing the patient beyond their abilities.

**Examples:** Proleukin (aldesleukin), Avastin (bevacizumab), Intron-A (interferon alfa-2b)

### Heavy Metal Compounds

**Action:** Heavy metal compounds used as antineoplastic agents are also known as platinum coordination complexes. They act as alkylating agents that inhibit DNA translation and replication.

**Indications:** various malignancies; particularly epithelial malignancies, ovarian cancer, testicular cancer, bladder cancer

**Side effects:** vary by class of drugs and by specific agent; multi-system involvement with mild to severe side effects, however, potential risks are typically warranted secondary to the diagnosis of malignancy

**Implications for PT:** Therapists must be aware of the chemotherapy regimen and modify treatment based on the patient's symptoms and side effects from cancer treatment. Extreme fatigue, gastrointestinal distress, cancer pain, and blood disorders are common. Therapists must provide support and encouragement without pushing the patient beyond their abilities.

**Examples:** Platinol (cisplatin), Paraplatin (carboplatin), Eloxatin (oxaliplatin)

### Oncology Terminology[16,31,32]

**Adjuvant:** Treatment provided, in addition to other cure-focused interventions, with the intention of preventing cancer recurrence.

**Benign neoplasm:** An abnormal cell growth that is usually slow growing and harmless, closely resembling the composition of adjacent tissues.

**Cancer:** A group of diseases characterized by uncontrolled cell proliferation with mutation and spreading of the abnormal cells. The etiology is based on the type and location of the cancer. The most common causes include cigarette smoking, diet and nutrition, chemical agents, physical agents, environmental causes, viral causes, and genetics.

**Differentiated cells:** Cells that have matured from a less specific to a more specific cell type.

**Dysplasia:** An abnormal development of cells or tissue that is often an early sign of neoplasia.

**Hyperplasia:** An increase in cell number that may be normal or abnormal depending on additional characteristics.

**Malignant neoplasm:** An abnormal uncontrolled cell growth that invades and destroys adjacent tissues and may metastasize to other sites and systems of the body.

**Metaplasia:** A change in a cell from one type to another that may be normal or abnormal.

**Neoadjuvant:** Chemotherapy or radiation given prior to surgical oncology intervention.

**Tumor (neoplasm):** An abnormal new growth of tissue that increases the overall tissue mass. Tumors are benign (non-cancerous) or malignant (cancerous) as well as primary or secondary. Primary tumors form from cells that belong to the area of the tumor. Secondary tumors grow from cells that have metastasized (spread) from another affected area within the body. Tumor classification is defined by cell type, tissue of origin, amount of differentiation, benign versus malignant, and anatomic site.

**Undifferentiated cells:** Cells which have not differentiated into a specific type (e.g., primitive, embryonic) or have no special structure or function.

# Psychological Disorders[10,32,43]

## Affective Disorders

Affective disorders are classified by disturbances in mood or emotion. States of extreme happiness or sadness occur and mood can alternate without cause. These extreme emotions can become intense and unrealistic.

### Depression

- Slower mental and physical activity; poor self-esteem
- Immobilized from everyday activities; sadness, hopelessness, and helplessness
- Desire to withdraw; delusions in severe cases

### Mania

- Constantly active
- Impulses immediately expressed
- Unrealistic activity
- Elation and self-confidence
- Disagreement with a patient may produce patient aggression
- Disorganized thoughts and speech
- Very few patients are diagnosed with only a manic disorder

### Bipolar

- Alternating periods of depression and mania
- Females are at greater risk; typically begins in a patient's twenties

## Neuroses Disorders

Neuroses refer to a group of disorders that are characterized by individuals exhibiting fear and maladaptive strategies in dealing with stressful or everyday stimuli. Patients with neuroses are not dealing with psychosis, do not have delusions, and usually realize that they have a problem.

### Obsessive-compulsive Disorder

- Obsessions – persistent thoughts that will not leave
- Compulsions – repetitive ritual behaviors the patient cannot stop performing
- Thoughts or ritual behaviors that interfere with daily living
- Unable to control irrational behavior
- Most commonly begins in young adulthood

### Anxiety Disorder

- Constant high tension; overreacts in certain instances
- Presents with apprehension and chronic worry
- Acute anxiety attacks
  - Lasts a few minutes in duration
  - Excitation of the sympathetic autonomic nervous system
  - Fear of impending doom or death
  - Shortness of breath, heart palpitations, dizziness, nausea
  - Initiated by unconscious and internal mechanisms

### Phobia Disorder

- Excessive fear of objects, occurrences or situations that is considerably out of proportion/irrational
- Fear creates difficulty in everyday life
- Subclassifications include agoraphobia, social phobia, and simple phobia; simple phobia is easiest to treat
- May develop from traumatic experiences, observation, classical conditioning

## Dissociative Disorders

Dissociative disorders develop when a person unconsciously dissociates (separates) one part of the mind from the rest.

### Psychogenic Amnesia

- Produced by the mind with no physical cause
- Forgets all aspects of the past

## Multiple Personality

- A rare dissociative disorder, includes two or more independent personalities
- Each personality may or may not know about the other
- Causative factors are not understood, believed to allow a person to engage in behaviors that are against the patient's morality and normally produce guilt

## Somatoform Disorders

Somatoform disorders are classified based on the physical symptoms present in each disorder.

### Somatization Disorder

- Primarily in women, has familial association, and often chronic and long lasting
- Complaints of symptoms with no physiological basis
- Symptoms usually lead to medications and medical visits and alter the patient's life
- Resembles hypochondriasis disorder

### Conversion Disorder

- Physical complaints of neurological basis with no underlying cause
- Paralysis is the most common finding; other findings include deafness, blindness, paresthesia
- Freud believed this is mental anxiety transformed into physical symptoms
- Diagnosis can be made once testing is negative for physical ailments

### Hypochondriasis Disorder

- Excessive fear of illness
- Believes that minor illnesses or medical problems indicate a serious or life threatening disease

## Schizophrenia Disorders

Schizophrenia disorders are psychotic in nature and present with disorganization of thought, hallucinations, emotional dysfunction, anxiety, and perceptual impairments. Causative factors include traumatic events, genetic inheritance, biochemical imbalances, and environmental influence.

### Catatonic Schizophrenia

- Motor disturbances with rigid posturing
- Episodes consist of uncontrolled movements, however, patients remain aware during episodes
- Medications are required to regulate episodes

### Paranoid Schizophrenia

- Delusions of grandeur; delusions of persecution
- May believe they possess special powers

### Disorganized Schizophrenia

- Usually progressive and irreversible with inappropriate emotional responses; mumbled talking

## Personality Disorders

A personality disorder is classified by observing a patient's pattern of behavior, dysfunctional view of society, and level of sadness. Personality disorders are usually ongoing patterns of dysfunctional behavior.

### Psychopathic Personality

- Low morality, poor sense of responsibility, no respect for others
- Impulsive behavior for immediate gratification; high frustration
- Little guilt or remorse for all actions; inability to alter behavior, even with punishment
- Expert liar

### Antisocial Behavior

- Results from particular causes (e.g., need for attention or involvement in a gang)
- Typically has some concern for others
- Blames other institutions (e.g., family, school) for their actions
- Symptoms are typically seen before 16 years of age
- Violates the rights of others; lacks responsibility and emotional stability

### Narcissistic Behavior

- Incapable of loving others
- Self-absorbed; obsessed with success and power
- Unrealistic perception of self-importance

### Borderline Behavior

- Instability in all aspects of life
- Can identify self from others
- Uses projection, denial, defensiveness; unpredictable mood or behavior
- Intense and uncontrolled anger; chronic feelings of emptiness

## Pharmacology - Psychiatric Management[19,43]

### Antianxiety Agents

**Action:** Antianxiety agents collectively target the CNS through facilitating the effects of GABA or targeting dopamine and serotonin within the brain. Benzodiazepines, azapirones, and certain selective serotonin reuptake inhibitor (SSRI) antidepressants treat various anxiety disorders.

**Indications:** general anxiety disorder, social anxiety, panic disorder, obsessive-compulsive disorder, post-traumatic stress syndrome

**Side effects:** drowsiness, sedation, withdrawal symptoms including rebound anxiety

**Implications for PT:** Similar concerns as with sedative-hypnotic agents; therapists can also implement alternate methods to decrease stress and anxiety including exercise and physical activity, massage, relaxation techniques, and stress management education.

**Examples:** Benzodiazepines: Xanax (alprazolam), Valium (diazepam), Ativan (lorazepam); Azapirones: BuSpar (buspirone); SSRIs: Effexor (venlafaxine), Paxil (paroxetine)

### Antidepressant Agents (Tricyclic, SSRI, MAOI, Other)

**Action:** Antidepressant agents are classified as tricyclic, monoamine oxidase inhibitors (MAOI), and selective serotonin reuptake inhibitors (SSRI), as well as miscellaneous agents that attempt to increase aminergic transmission and normalize neurotransmission activity.

**Indications:** depression, certain agents also treat anxiety disorders

**Side effects:** vary by class of drugs and by specific agent; sedation, blurred vision, tachycardia, dry mouth, insomnia, weight gain, sexual dysfunction

**Implications for PT:** Therapists should typically see improvement in a patient's affect with pharmacological treatment for depression. Therapists must be aware of side effects such as sedation, fatigue, hypertension or orthostatic hypotension. Therapists must also look for any signs of further depression or suicidal tendencies.

**Examples:** Tricyclics: Elavil (amitriptyline), Pamelor (nortriptyline); MAOIs: Nardil (phenelzine); SSRIs: Wellbutrin (bupropion), Prozac (fluoxetine), Paxil (paroxetine)

### Antipsychotic Agents (Neuroleptic Agents)

**Action:** Most antipsychotic agents block dopamine receptors and reduce the overactivity of dopamine typically transmitted in areas such as the limbic system. The agents will bind to the dopamine receptors, but will not allow for activation. There are traditional and newer "atypical" antipsychotic agents used for schizophrenia and other various psychosis disorders.

**Indications:** schizophrenia, various psychotic disorders, Alzheimer's disease (certain cases)

**Side effects:** traditional agents produce increased extrapyramidal (motor) side effects, tardive dyskinesia, pseudoparkinsonism, akathisia, sedation, constipation, dry mouth; atypical agents can produce substantial weight gain, diabetes mellitus, hyperlipidemia

**Implications for PT:** These agents assist patients to participate in physical therapy by decreasing their symptoms of psychoses and allowing for an increased attention span, diminished agitation and restlessness, improved sense of reality, and an overall normalization of their behavior and affect. The largest barrier is the influence of extrapyramidal effects on therapy. Early detection of these effects can allow for prompt medical and pharmacological management.

**Examples:** Traditional: Haldol (haloperidol), Thorazine (chlorpromazine); Atypical: Risperdal (risperidone), Abilify (aripiprazole)

# Spotlight on Safety
### Respectful Management of Escalating Patient Behaviors[32]

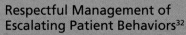

Patients with or without a psychiatric diagnosis may exhibit escalating behaviors from time to time. The financial, social, physical, and mental stress that accompanies injury or illness can be frustrating enough to cause even mild mannered patients to become agitated or combative. When dealing with patients in these challenging situations, physical therapists should be respectful in their de-escalation attempts, but also mindful of maintaining a safe environment for everyone involved.

Many health care facilities offer training in non-verbal de-escalation techniques which are helpful in defusing a potentially threatening situation. Guiding principles for safe use of these techniques include an understanding that attempting to reason with an escalating patient may make matters worse, and that calm reasoning in a threatening situation is counterintuitive to our own "fight or flight" response. Successful non-verbal de-escalation requires the provider to maintain self-control and a protective yet non-threatening physical presence while facilitating the de-escalation conversation.

Tips for interacting with an escalating patient:

- Be empathetic when setting boundaries
- Use a low, calm tone of voice when speaking
- Do not respond defensively to patient comments
- Offer choices, options or small concessions if appropriate
- Do not force constant eye contact, allow the patient to look away
- Be respectful and acknowledge the patient's complaints or frustration
- When speaking, wait for the patient to pause rather than raising your voice to be heard
- Be aware of your supportive resources, including the option to leave the area if necessary
- Avoid physical contact
- Do not turn your back to an agitated or escalating patient
- Do not allow an agitated or escalating patient to block your exit route
- Maintain more space than usual between yourself and the patient for safety
- Stand at an angle facing the patient so that it is easier to sidestep if necessary
- Always stay at the same eye level as the patient (e.g., both standing, both sitting)
- Keep hands out of your pockets both for self-protection and to avoid the appearance of concealment

## Pharmacology-Systems Side Effects

### Review of Systems: Side Effects/Subjective Complaints
#### (In Order of Most Common Occurrence)

**Gastrointestinal Distress:** dyspepsia, heartburn, nausea, vomiting, abdominal pain, constipation, diarrhea, bleeding

- Salicylates
- Skeletal muscle relaxants
- Antiarrhythmic agents
- Theophylline
- Calcium-channel blockers
- Cholesterol-lowering agents
- Antidepressants (TCAs and MAOIs, lithium)

- Opioids
- ACE inhibitors
- Neuroleptics
- NSAIDs
- Diuretics
- Estrogens and progestins

- ß-Blockers
- Nitrates
- OCAs
- Corticosteroids
- Digoxin
- Antiepileptic agents

**Pulmonary:** bronchospasm, shortness of breath, respiratory depression

- Salicylates
- NSAIDs

- Opioids
- ß-Blockers

- ACE inhibitors

**Central Nervous System:** dizziness, drowsiness, insomnia, headaches, hallucinations, confusion, anxiety, depression, muscle weakness

- NSAIDs
- Nitrates
- Antiepileptic agents
- Corticosteroids
- Antianxiety agents

- Opioids
- Digoxin
- Estrogens and progestins
- Calcium-channel blockers
- Neuroleptics

- ß-Blockers
- Antidepressants (TCAs and MAOIs)
- Skeletal muscle relaxants
- ACE inhibitors
- OCAs

**Dermatologic:** skin rash, itching, flushing of face

- NSAIDs
- Nitrates
- Antiepileptics
- ACE inhibitors
- Estrogens and progestins

- ß-Blockers
- Antiarrhythmic agents
- Corticosteroids
- Cholesterol-lowering agents

- Calcium-channel blockers
- OCAs
- Opioids
- MAOIs and lithium

**Musculoskeletal:** weakness, fatigue, cramps, arthritis, decreased exercise tolerance, osteoporosis

- Corticosteroids
- Antianxiety agents
- ACE inhibitors
- Neuroleptic agents

- Calcium-channel blockers
- Antidepressants
- Digoxin

- Diuretics
- ß-Blockers
- Antiepileptic agents

**Cardiac:** bradycardia, ventricular irritability, AV block, CHF, PVCs, ventricular tachycardia

- Opioids
- TCAs
- Calcium-channel blockers

- ß-Blockers
- Oral antiasthmatic agents
- Antiarrhythmic agents

- Digoxin
- Diuretics
- Neuroleptics

**Vascular:** claudication, hypotension, peripheral edema, cold extremities

- NSAIDs
- Nitrates
- Corticosteroids
- Antidepressants (TCAs and MAOIs)

- Diuretics
- Neuroleptics
- ß-Blockers
- OCAs

- Calcium-channel blockers
- Estrogens and progestins
- ACE inhibitors

**Genitourinary:** sexual dysfunction, urinary retention, urinary incontinence

- Opioids
- OCAs
- Neuroleptics

- ß-Blockers
- Diuretics
- Antidepressants (TCAs and MAOIs)

- Estrogens and progestins
- Antiarrhythmic agents

**HEENT:** tinnitus, loss of taste, headache, lightheadedness, dizziness

- Salicylates
- Calcium-channel blockers
- Antiepileptic agents
- Nitrates
- Antidepressants (TCAs and MAOIs)

- Opioids
- Digoxin
- NSAIDs
- ACE inhibitors

- ß-Blockers
- Antianxiety agents
- Skeletal muscle relaxants
- Antiarrhythmic agents

**Abbreviations:** ACE, angiotensin-converting enzyme; MAOIs, monoamine oxidase inhibitors; NSAIDs, nonsteroidal anti-inflammatory drugs; OCAs, oral contraceptive agents; TCAs, tricyclic antidepressants.— From Boissonnault, WG: Examination in Physical Therapy Practice: Screening for Medical Disease. W.B. Saunders Company, Philadelphia 1995, p.350-351, with permission.

## Bipolar Disorder Agents

**Action:** Bipolar disorder agents focus on the prevention of manic episodes in order to avoid the extreme mood swings that follow. The primary agent used in this treatment is lithium. Certain antiseizure and antipsychotic medications may assist as mood stabilizers with bipolar disorder.

**Indications:** bipolar or manic-depressive disorders

**Side effects:** in general, gastrointestinal distress, tardive dyskinesia, fatigue, confusion, ataxia, nystagmus, lethargy, tremor, parkinsonism, seizures, diabetes insipidus, toxicity, coma, risk of death

**Implications for PT:** Therapists should become familiar with the side effects of medications that treat bipolar disorder, especially symptoms of toxicity as it relates to lithium. Long-term use of lithium may result in osteoporosis which will impact the physical therapy plan of care.

**Examples:** Lithobid (lithium); Antipsychotics: Clozaril (clozapine), Risperdal (risperidone); Antiseizures: Tegretol (carbamazepine), Neurontin (gabapentin)

## Sedative-hypnotic Agents (Benzodiazepine and Non-benzodiazepine)

**Action:** Sedative agents produce a calming and relaxation while hypnotic agents induce sleep. Benzodiazepines have properties to promote sleep through increasing inhibitory effects at the CNS synapses where GABA (gamma-aminobutyric acid) is found. Non-benzodiazepines include barbiturates and other drugs that also provide CNS depression through the inhibitory effects of GABA.

**Indications:** anxiety, preoperative sedation, insomnia

**Side effects:** residual effects can produce drowsiness and decreased motor performance, anterograde amnesia, tolerance, dependency, rebound insomnia with withdrawal; barbiturates are highly addictive and can be fatal

**Implications for PT:** Therapists may find it beneficial to treat a patient when peak blood levels of the agent exist so that the patient is calm, relaxed, and can focus on the treatment regimen, however, this may become problematic if the patient experiences side effects of drowsiness and impairments in motor control. The risk of falling increases with use of these agents.

**Examples:** Benzodiazepine: Halcion (triazolam), Dalmane (flurazepam); Non-benzodiazepine: Luminal (phenobarbital), Sonata (zaleplon), Ambien (zolpidem)

# Bariatrics[44-46]

Obesity refers to the state of excessive adipose tissue accumulation in the body contributing to a variety of chronic conditions that negatively impact multiple body systems and overall health. Obesity is most commonly the result of a prolonged imbalance between an individual's energy intake through diet and energy expenditure through activity and metabolic functions. The prevalence of obesity has reached pandemic proportions and has in recent years become viewed as a chronic progressive disease. Obesity is a modifiable morbidity and mortality risk factor second only to smoking.

## Risk Factors for Developing Obesity[44-46]

| | |
|---|---|
| • Sedentary lifestyle | • Medications that increase appetite or food cravings |
| • High glycemic diet | • Genetic or familial predisposition |
| • Environmental and lifestyle factors: smoking cessation, stress, history of abuse | • Underlying illness (e.g. hypothyroidism, polycystic ovary syndrome, Cushing syndrome, Prader-Willi syndrome) |

## Anatomic and Physiologic Changes Commonly Associated with Obesity[45]

| | |
|---|---|
| Cardiac | Cardiomyopathy (e.g., heart failure), abnormal ventricular remodeling (e.g., hypertrophy), atrial fibrillation, dysrhythmias |
| Pulmonary | Asthma, obstructive sleep apnea, hypoventilation syndrome |
| Kidneys | Decreased renal perfusion |
| Genitourinary | Urinary incontinence, infertility |
| Integumentary | Infection, hyperkeratosis, acanthosis nigricans |
| Vascular | Increased total blood volume, altered stroke volume and cardiac output, hypertension, venous insufficiency, varicosities |
| Musculoskeletal | Osteoarthritis, altered mobility patterns |
| Adipose tissue | Increased production of adipokines (e.g., leptin, interleukin-6, angiotensinogen) |
| Liver | Non-alcoholic fatty liver disease, non-alcoholic steatohepatitis |
| Pancreas | Insulin resistance, type 2 diabetes mellitus |

# Consider This

## Childhood Obesity

The behaviors and systemic changes associated with childhood obesity can set children and adolescents on an unfortunate path toward lifelong health problems. The rise of childhood obesity has had a significant impact on the development of co-morbidities and risk factors previously associated only with adults (e.g., hypertension, type 2 diabetes mellitus, sleep disorders, metabolic syndrome). Adding to the physical health concerns of the condition, children and adolescents that are obese have also been shown to be at increased risk for a number of social and emotional issues including bullying, low self-esteem, depression, and behavioral problems.[47,48]

Because of the rapid developmental changes and variations in body type associated with this younger population, health care providers and caregivers must be cautious not to assume that all children who appear to be carrying extra weight are truly overweight or obese. At various points in normal development children and adolescents are expected to carry differing proportions of body fat. For parents, a conversation with their child's pediatrician is usually the best way to determine if the appearance of extra weight is truly a long term health concern. In general, a child is considered overweight if their age-appropriate BMI is between the 85th and 94th percentiles. Childhood obesity is characterized by an age-appropriate BMI greater than or equal to the 95th percentile.[49,50]

Behavioral risk factors for developing childhood obesity are similar to those in adult populations. Increased dietary intake, decreased activity levels, and psychological factors such as stress and boredom are most frequently attributed to childhood obesity. Some children may be more susceptible to weight gain due to genetic factors, however, genetic predisposition is often erroneously blamed for childhood obesity. Prader-Willi syndrome is an example of a condition where children are more likely to become obese. However, given the prevalence of childhood obesity, the greater influence of diet, activity, behavioral habits, and environmental factors must be both clearly acknowledged and addressed.[49,50]

## Diagnostic Tools[2,35]

Body Mass Index (BMI) estimates an individual's body fat percentage and weight related health risks based on a calculation using height and weight measures. An adult would be considered underweight with a BMI less than 18.5, of desirable weight between 18.5 and 24.9, and obese with a BMI greater than 30. There are some limitations in correlating BMI with potential health risks, for example, an individual who is very muscular may have a BMI over 30 despite being extremely fit and healthy. Because of this, therapists cannot rely solely on BMI when characterizing a patient's weight related health risks. Other important factors in determining these risks are the patient's morphological distribution of body fat, waist circumference, and hip-to-waist ratio. These additional factors are primarily utilized as indicators of visceral fat distribution.

A peripheral fat distribution, also referred to as pear shape or gluteofemoral obesity, is more common in women and typically associated with a lower relative incidence of obesity related risk factors. A central fat distribution, also referred to as apple shape or abdominal obesity, is much more highly correlated with significant risk factors such as cardiovascular disease and type 2 diabetes mellitus. This is in part attributed to the presence of a much higher percentage of metabolically active visceral fat.

Research suggests that waist circumference measures may be better predictors of diabetes and cardiovascular risks than BMI alone, even though waist circumference measures are correlated with BMI. Waist measurements greater than 40 inches for adult males and greater than 36 inches for adult females are considered to be indicative of central obesity. Waist to hip ratio has also been found to show positive correlation to obesity related risks of death and disease; a ratio of greater than 1.0 in males and greater than 0.85 in females is suggestive of central obesity.

## Bariatric Interventions[45,46]

**Medical Management:** Due to the multi-system health risks associated with obesity, physician involvement is imperative for support on many levels. With physician monitoring, patients are more likely to have appropriate medical management of co-morbidities as well as access to education or program referrals which may assist in weight loss goals. For patients who do not elect to attempt weight loss, the physician role typically becomes more focused on the medical management of co-morbidities. Most bariatric surgical teams include a physician specialist, often an internist, responsible for the medical assessment and monitoring of patients throughout the weight loss process.

**Behavioral Therapy:** Typically there is some degree of psychological influence associated with the behaviors that lead to obesity. Identifying and addressing these influences can significantly improve long-term outcomes that could otherwise be limited by underlying issues of motivation and compliance. Behavioral therapy may be provided in individualized or support group formats with topics including stimulus control, goal setting and problem solving strategies, social support, and/or strategies to improve self-monitoring of dietary intake and physical activity. Patients hoping to undergo bariatric surgery are typically required to participate in some form of behavioral counseling prior to surgery.

**Increased Activity:** Increased activity levels are essential for long term weight loss and weight management. For obese individuals, increased activity in the first six months of weight loss efforts has not been shown to significantly impact weight reduction. Patient education and support should be offered so as to prevent frustration and diminished motivation in attempts to make long-term modifications in activity level. Patients should be advised to begin increasing activity levels with gentle modes

## Consider This

### Obesity, Lipedema or Both?[33,46]

Lipedema is a disease with undefined etiology that affects the physical size and distribution of adipose cells in the body. The condition is most simply described as a bilateral, symmetrical, soft swelling most frequently appearing in the lower extremities of women. Many times a hereditary trend can be identified. Initial symptoms tend to present at times of significant hormonal change (e.g., menarche, menopause or during pregnancy). Women affected earlier in life often comment that their "big legs" have always seemed disproportionate to their body.

Patients with lipedema are often frustrated by the failure of weight loss efforts to alter the general shape and proportion of their affected lower extremities. This frustration can be compounded by the failure of health care professionals to recognize lipedema and instead continue to advise weight loss to patients who, in the absence of lipedema, would likely be of normal weight. In obese populations, weight loss is a reasonable expectation that does positively impact lipedema symptoms. However, patients should be educated regarding realistic outcome expectations so as not to assume that weight loss will "fix" their overall morphological proportions.

Signs and symptoms of lipedema include exquisite tenderness to palpation in the affected extremities, column-like or "riding breeches" fat distribution in the lower extremities, and increased edema as the day progresses which subsides overnight. Ongoing healthy weight management and complete decongestive therapy interventions are most often recommended to patients with lipedema as symptom management options.

of exercise, such as walking or swimming, performed at a tolerable pace. A general target of thirty minutes of increased activity daily is recommended and may be spread out into smaller intervals over the course of a day. Caution should be taken to prevent injury as intensity level and exercise duration increase. Research suggests that increased activity levels can positively influence the body's insulin sensitivity and fasting blood glucose to a measurable degree even in the absence of weight loss.

**Dietary Modifications:** In obese populations, a 500-1000 kcal/day reduction in dietary intake is usually sufficient to produce a 1-2 pounds per week weight loss. This rate can typically be maintained for six months before slowing or plateauing. Patients often have the misconception that reducing fat intake alone will produce the desired weight loss result. While this is a component of dietary modification, reduction of carbohydrate intake and overall calories are equally important. It is recommended that patients who are obese and wish to lose weight consult both a physician and dietician to ensure a medically safe and nutritionally sound approach to weight loss.

**Pharmacology:** The Food and Drug Administration (FDA) has approved a number of pharmacological weight loss agents for short-term adjunct use with diet, activity, and behavioral modifications. Classes of approved medications include appetite suppressants and lipase inhibitors. Appetite suppressants function to either reduce feelings of hunger or increase feelings of fullness. Lipase inhibitors decrease the body's ability to absorb dietary fats, thereby decreasing overall caloric intake. Though not specifically approved for weight loss by the FDA, some antidepressant, seizure, and diabetes medications are prescribed for short-term use to assist weight loss goals.

**Community Resources:** A variety of community-based weight loss programs are in existence, each with their own structured approach. Program commonalities include advocating increased activity and decreased caloric intake. Patients often cite geographical, philosophical or financial concerns as barriers

to participating in a formal program. Well known community-based programs include Weight Watchers, Jenny Craig, Take Off Pounds Sensibly (TOPS), and Food Addicts Anonymous.

**Bariatric Surgery:** Bariatric surgery is a consideration for some patients who are morbidly obese and is often considered the intervention of last resort. Pre-operatively, patients must meet a number of requirements in order to be considered a surgical candidate. This typically includes a BMI greater than 40, or greater than 35 with additional co-morbidities, and evidence that other weight loss interventions have been largely unsuccessful. Most bariatric programs require a pre-operative commitment to support group attendance or individual counseling as well as some degree of substantive weight loss by more traditional methods. Pre- and post-operatively a multidisciplinary team is responsible for providing support and assessing a number of pre-operative factors (e.g., co-morbidities, behavioral history, extent of adiposity). This bariatric specialty team commonly includes an internist, surgeon, psychologist, dietician, and program coordinator.

Bariatric surgical procedures may be classified as restrictive, malabsorptive or a combination of the two. The most common bariatric procedure is the invasive Roux-en-Y gastric bypass which facilitates weight loss through a combination of restriction and malabsorption. Due to the nature of the procedure, the risk of both post-operative and long-term complications is high. In contrast, the most common restrictive procedure is also the least invasive. Laparoscopic gastric banding, often referred to as a "lap-band" procedure, has a low risk of complications and can be adjusted or removed as needed.

## Consider This

### Eating Disorders - The Other End of the Weight Spectrum[44]

Weight related health risks are not exclusive to overweight and obese populations. The Centers for Disease Control and Prevention consider individuals with a BMI of less than 18.5 to be underweight. While some patients may be naturally more slender, physical therapists should be cognizant of the signs, symptoms, and health concerns associated with eating disorders. Due to the significant roles of both physical and psychological factors in low-weight eating disorders, treatment in a partial-hospitalization or inpatient program is often recommended.

Bulimia nervosa refers to a binge-purge cycle that can cause chemical and enzyme imbalances that can lead to multiple organ dysfunction. Major health concerns include heart failure due to electrolyte imbalance, gastric rupture during purging, esophageal inflammation and tooth decay due to frequent vomiting, dehydration, peptic ulcers, pancreatitis, and bowel irregularity.

Anorexia nervosa refers to a self-imposed starvation that forces the body to either slow or shut down normal systemic processes. Major health concerns include heart failure due to slowed heart rate and decreased blood pressure, kidney failure due to dehydration, osteoporosis, and muscle atrophy.

## Nutrition[10,19,32]

### Vitamins

Vitamins are essential non-caloric nutrients that are required in small amounts for certain metabolic functions and cannot be manufactured by the body. Vitamins are most often classified as fat-soluble or water-soluble.

### Fat-Soluble Vitamins

Fat-soluble vitamins include vitamins A, D, E, and K. After being absorbed by the intestinal tract, the vitamins are stored in the liver and fatty tissues. Fat-soluble vitamins require protein carriers to move through body fluids and excesses are stored in the body. Since they are not water-soluble, it is possible that the vitamins may reach toxic levels.

### Vitamin A

Vitamin A is essential to the eyes, epithelial tissue, normal growth and development, and reproduction.

- Common food sources containing vitamin A include green, orange, and yellow vegetables, liver, butter, egg yolks, and fortified margarine.
- Symptoms of deficiency include night blindness, rough and dry skin, and growth failure.
- Symptoms of toxicity include appetite loss, hair loss, and enlarged liver and spleen.

### Vitamin D

Vitamin D increases the blood flow levels of minerals, notably calcium and phosphorus.

- Common food sources containing vitamin D include fortified milk, fish oils, and fortified margarine.
- Symptoms of deficiency include faulty bone growth, rickets, and osteomalacia.
- Symptoms of toxicity include calcification of soft tissues and hypercalcemia.

### Vitamin E

Vitamin E functions as an antioxidant in cell membranes and is especially important for the integrity of cells that are constantly exposed to high levels of oxygen such as the lungs and red blood cells.

- Common food sources containing vitamin E include vegetable oils, wheat germ, nuts, and fish.
- Symptoms of deficiency include breakdown of red blood cells, however, this is relatively rare in adults.
- Symptoms of toxicity include decreased thyroid hormone levels and increased triglycerides.

### Vitamin K

Vitamin K is necessary for the synthesis of at least two of the proteins involved in blood clotting.

- Common food sources containing vitamin K include dark green leafy vegetables, cheese, egg yolks, and liver.
- Symptoms of deficiency include hemorrhage and defective blood clotting.
- Toxicity has not been reported.

### Water-Soluble Vitamins

Water-soluble vitamins are not stored in the body in any significant amount and therefore need to be included in the diet on a daily basis. Toxicity is less common than with fat-soluble vitamins.

### Vitamin B2 (Riboflavin)

Vitamin B2 facilitates selected enzymes involved in carbohydrate, protein, and fat metabolism.

- Common food sources containing vitamin B2 include milk, green leafy vegetables, eggs, and peanuts.

- Symptoms of deficiency include inflammation of the tongue, sensitive eyes, and scaling of the skin.
- Toxicity has not been reported.

### Vitamin B3 (Niacin)

Vitamin B3 facilitates several enzymes that regulate energy metabolism.

- Common food sources containing vitamin B3 include meats, whole grains, and white flour.
- Symptoms of deficiency include pellagra and gastrointestinal disturbances.
- Symptoms of toxicity include abnormal glucose metabolism, nausea, vomiting, and gastric ulceration.

### Vitamin B6 (Pyridoxine)

Vitamin B6 is essential in the metabolism of proteins, amino acids, carbohydrates, and fat.

- Common food sources containing vitamin B6 include liver, red meats, whole grains, and potatoes.
- Symptoms of deficiency include peripheral neuropathy, convulsions, and depression.
- Symptoms of toxicity include sensory damage, numbness of the extremities, and ataxia.

### Vitamin B12 (Cobalamin)

Vitamin B12 is essential for the functioning of all cells and aids in hemoglobin synthesis.

- Common food sources containing vitamin B12 include meats, whole eggs, and egg yolks.
- Symptoms of deficiency include pernicious anemia and various psychological disorders.
- Toxicity has not been reported.

### Vitamin C

Vitamin C assists the body to combat infections and facilitates wound healing. The vitamin is necessary for the development and maintenance of bones, cartilage, connective tissue, and blood vessels.

- Common food sources containing vitamin C include citrus fruits, tomatoes, and cantaloupe.
- Symptoms of deficiency include anemia, swollen gums, loose teeth, and scurvy.
- Symptoms of toxicity include urinary stones, diarrhea, and hypoglycemia.

### Biotin

Biotin is necessary for the action of many enzyme systems.

- Common food sources containing biotin include liver, meats, and milk.
- Symptoms of deficiency include anemia, depression, and muscle pain.
- Toxicity has not been reported.

## Spotlight on Safety

### Adverse Effects of Complimentary and Alternative Medications (CAM)[19]

Patients have ready access to countless vitamin, mineral, herbal, and other natural supplements. Often these supplements are sought out for preventative means, to support or to replace more traditional pharmacological interventions. While the use of many of these substances cause mild to no side effects, some supplements can reach toxic levels or impact the actions of other medications causing significant adverse effects. More specifically, some natural supplements interfere with the metabolism, absorption, and excretion of prescription medications. This is typically due to interference with liver function, which can prevent drugs from reaching therapeutic levels or cause them to metabolize either too quickly or too slowly. Given the prevalence and underreporting of CAM use it is important for physical therapists to address this topic when taking a patient's history and be aware of potential interactions.

**Garlic:** reported to exacerbate bleeding issues for patients who are taking prescription anticoagulants

**Ginkgo biloba:** reported to increase the risk of hemorrhage in patients using other anticoagulants

**Ginseng:** reported to reduce the effects of anticoagulants and exaggerate the effects of medications such as insulin and oral antidiabetic medications

**Kava:** reported to cause liver toxicity

**St. John's wort:** reported to accelerate metabolism of some medications (e.g., warfarin, cyclosporine) and prevent numerous others from reaching therapeutic levels

### Choline

Choline is a component of compounds necessary for nerve function and lipid metabolism.

- Choline is synthesized from methionine which is an amino acid.
- Symptoms of deficiency only occur when intake of methylamine is low.
- Toxicity has not been reported.

### Folacin (Folic acid)

Folacin is involved in the formation of red blood cells and in the functioning of the gastrointestinal tract.

- Common food sources containing folacin include yeast, dark green leafy vegetables, and whole grains.
- Symptoms of deficiency include impaired cell division and alteration of protein synthesis.
- Toxicity has not been reported.

## Pantothenic Acid

Pantothenic acid is an integral component of complex enzymes involved in the metabolism of fatty acids.

- Common food sources containing pantothenic acid include liver, eggs, and whole grains.
- Symptoms of deficiency include headache, fatigue, and poor muscle coordination.
- Symptoms of toxicity include diarrhea.

## Minerals[10,19,32]

Minerals are organic elements that fulfill essential roles in the metabolic process.

### Major Minerals

### Calcium (Ca)

Calcium facilitates muscle contraction and relaxation, builds strong bones and teeth, and aids in coagulation.

- Common food sources containing calcium include milk, green leafy vegetables, and soy products.
- Calcium deficiency may lead to poor bone growth, rickets, osteomalacia, and osteoporosis.
- Symptoms of toxicity include kidney stones.

### Chloride (Cl)

Chloride facilitates the maintenance of fluid and acid-base balance.

- Common food sources containing chloride include table salt, fish, and vegetables.
- Chloride deficiency may lead to a disturbance of acid-base balance.
- Toxicity has not been reported.

### Magnesium (Mg)

Magnesium builds strong bones and teeth, activates enzymes, and helps regulate heartbeat.

- Common food sources containing magnesium include raw dark vegetables, nuts, soybeans, milk, and cheese.
- Symptoms of deficiency include confusion, apathy, muscle weakness, and tremors.
- Symptoms of toxicity include increased calcium excretion.

### Phosphorus (P)

Phosphorus strengthens bones, assists in the oxidation of fats and carbohydrates, and aids in maintaining acid-base balance.

- Common food sources containing phosphorus include milk, milk products, meats, whole grains, and soft drinks.
- Symptoms of deficiency include weakness, stiff joints, and fragile bones.
- Symptoms of toxicity include muscle spasms.

### Potassium (K)

Potassium maintains fluid and acid-base balance.

- Common food sources containing potassium include apricots, bananas, oranges, grapefruit, and milk.
- Symptoms of deficiency include impaired growth, hypertension, and diminished heart rate.
- Symptoms of toxicity include hyperkalemia and cardiac disturbances.

### Sodium (Na)

Sodium facilitates the maintenance of acid-base balance, transmits nerve impulses, and helps control muscle contractions.

- Common food sources containing sodium include salt and milk.
- Deficiency and toxicity have not been reported.

### Sulfur (S)

Sulfur facilitates enzyme activity and energy metabolism.

- Common food sources containing sulfur include meat, eggs, milk, and cheese.
- Deficiency is extremely rare.
- Toxicity has not been reported.

### Trace Minerals

### Chromium (Cr)

Chromium controls glucose metabolism.

- Common food sources containing chromium include whole grains, meats, and cheese.
- Symptoms of deficiency include weight loss and central nervous system abnormalities.
- Symptoms of toxicity include liver damage.

### Cobalt (Co)

Cobalt is an essential component of vitamin B12 and functions to activate enzymes.

- Common food sources containing cobalt include figs, cabbage, and spinach.
- Symptoms of deficiency include pernicious anemia.
- Symptoms of toxicity include polycythemia and increased blood volume.

### Copper (Cu)

Copper facilitates hemoglobin synthesis and lipid metabolism.

- Common food sources containing copper include shellfish, liver, meat, and whole grains.
- Symptoms of deficiency include anemia, central nervous system abnormalities, and abnormal electrocardiograms.
- Symptoms of toxicity include Wilson's disease.

### Fluorine (F)

Fluorine aids in the formation of bones and teeth and prevents osteoporosis.

- Common food sources containing fluorine include fish and water.
- Symptoms of deficiency include increased susceptibility of dental cavities.
- Symptoms of toxicity include fluorosis.

### Iodine (I)

Iodine assists with the regulation of cell metabolism and basal metabolic rate.

- Common food sources containing iodine include iodized salt and seafood.
- Symptoms of deficiency may include goiters.
- Toxicity has not been reported.

### Iron (Fe)

Iron assists in oxygen transport and cell oxidation.

- Common food sources containing iron include red meats and liver.
- Symptoms of deficiency include anemia.
- Symptoms of toxicity include hemochromatosis.

### Manganese (Mn)

Manganese facilitates proper bone structure and functions as an enzyme component in general metabolism.

- Common food sources containing manganese include cereals and whole grains.
- There are no known symptoms of deficiency.
- Toxicity has not been reported.

### Selenium (Se)

Selenium is a synergistic antioxidant with vitamin E.

- Common food sources containing selenium include meat, eggs, milk, seafood, and garlic.
- Symptoms of deficiency include Keshan's disease.
- Symptoms of toxicity include physical defects of fingernails and toenails, nausea, and abdominal pain.

### Molybdenum (Mo)

Molybdenum is a component of three enzymes in particular, that are necessary for normal cell functioning.

- Common food sources containing molybdenum include meats, whole grains, and dark green vegetables
- Symptoms of deficiency include vomiting and tachypnea.
- Toxicity has not been reported.

### Zinc (Zn)

Zinc aids in immune function and cell division.

- Common food sources containing zinc include seafood, liver, milk, cheese, and whole grains.
- Symptoms of deficiency include depressed immune functions and impaired skeletal growth.
- Symptoms of toxicity include anemia, nausea, and vomiting.

# Other Systems Essentials

## Integumentary System

1. The integumentary system or "skin" is the largest organ of the body and consists of dermal and epidermal layers, hair follicles, nails, sebaceous glands, and sweat glands.

2. The normal phases of healing are overlapping and progressive beginning with an inflammatory response and ending with scar maturity.

3. Healing can occur through primary, secondary or tertiary intention. Most wounds requiring formal wound care interventions will heal by secondary intention.

4. Maintaining the balance of moisture in and around healing wounds is paramount. A wound that is too dry will have delayed healing; a wound with excessive moisture is at risk for additional tissue deterioration.

5. Infection is the most common cause of wound chronicity.

6. Certain types of wound exudate typically occur during the various stages of wound healing while others may be signs of impending infection or other complications.

7. Ulcers have primary classification as arterial, venous, neuropathic or pressure. Causative factors are ulcer specific and treatment is dependent on classification and severity of the ulcer.

8. Wounds that are not classified as pressure or neuropathic can be classified by depth of tissue loss.

9. Wound color, depth, exudate, and infection status must be considered in order to select the most appropriate wound dressing for a patient.

10. Wagner Ulcer Grade Classification System categorizes dysvascular ulcers based on wound depth and the presence of infection.

11. Pressure ulcer staging typically includes stage I, II, III, IV, Suspected Deep Tissue Injury, and Unstageable.

12. Exudate is typically classified as serous, sanguineous, serosanguineous, seropurulent, and purulent.

13. Physical therapists provide selective debridement through sharp, enzymatic or autolytic debridement interventions. Non-selective debridement typically includes wet-to-dry dressings, hydrotherapy, and wound irrigation interventions.

14. Modalities and physical agents such as negative pressure wound therapy, hyperbaric oxygen, and growth factors promote and facilitate healing, improve oxygenation and blood flow, increase collagen synthesis, minimize edema, and decrease drainage from the wound.

15. Therapeutic modalities such as ultrasound and high-voltage pulsed current have clinical applications and parameters which can assist through all stages of healing.

16. A fully occlusive substance would be completely impermeable while a non-occlusive dressing permits bacteria and fluid contamination of the wound bed increasing the risk for infection and delaying the healing process.

17. Classification of dressings includes hydrocolloids, hydrogels, foam dressings, transparent film, gauze, and alginates. Each dressing classification has advantages and disadvantages and is used based on the wound characteristics and goals for the dressing.

18. The major classifications of burn injury include thermal, electrical, chemical, and radiation burns. The extent of burn-related tissue damage in each zone of injury will significantly impact the overall healing prognosis.

19. The level of pain secondary to a burn varies based on the depth of the burn with superficial partial-thickness burns typically exhibiting the highest level of pain.

20. The Rule of Nines is well recognized for its use in estimating the amount of total surface area damaged by a burn injury. However, this calculation does not reflect wound severity and therefore cannot predict prognosis or outcomes.

21. Numerous scar assessment scales are available to assess characteristics such as scar height, thickness, pliability, banding/adherence, color, vascularity, texture, and size.

22. Burns sustained in proximity to joints are at particular risk for developing limiting contractures as patients will tend to assume a position of comfort. Splints should be used to support limbs in a neutral or slight stretch position to prevent deformity.

23. Principles of burn scar management, such as scar massage and desensitization techniques, are valuable tools for managing non-burn related scars that may be painful or otherwise restrictive.

## Metabolic and Endocrine

24. The metabolic system is responsible for generating the energy required to fuel all bodily functions.

25. Catabolism refers to metabolic processes which provide heat and energy to the body while anabolism refers to processes involved with tissue growth and repair.

26. Inherited metabolic disorders, though present at birth, may not immediately show symptoms.

**SCORE**BUILDERS

## Other Systems Essentials

27. Metabolic acidosis occurs when the body's pH drops below 7.35 as a result of an acid and bicarbonate imbalance which allows acid to accumulate.

28. Metabolic alkalosis occurs when the body's pH rises above 7.45 as a result of a bicarbonate and acid imbalance which allows bicarbonate to accumulate.

29. Osteoporosis or osteopenia may be an underlying clinical feature of various other metabolic or systemic disorders.

30. A diagnosis of osteopenia may not be due to bone loss, but rather a naturally occurring bone density that is lower than established norms.

31. General classes of hormones controlled by the endocrine system include prostaglandins, catecholamines, and insulin.

32. Endocrine pathology most commonly relates to either hyper or hypofunction of endocrine glands and the effect of their targeted hormone secretions.

33. Patients with hyperthyroidism may present with exercise limitations associated with heat intolerance caused by hypermetabolism.

34. Patients with hypothyroidism often present with limited exercise tolerance due to a hypofunctioning metabolism and subsequent energy deficits.

35. Untreated, both hyperglycemia and hypoglycemia are life threatening conditions.

36. Type 1 diabetes mellitus occurs when the pancreas fails to produce insulin to regulate blood glucose levels in the body.

37. Type 2 diabetes mellitus occurs when the body becomes insulin resistant and is unable to effectively utilize the insulin that is present to control blood glucose levels.

38. Patients with diabetes mellitus must be cautious to avoid becoming hypoglycemic with exercise as a result of increased glucose uptake with increased muscle activity.

39. Patients with type 1 diabetes mellitus are at the greatest risk for becoming hyperglycemic and developing life threatening ketoacidosis.

### Gastrointestinal

40. The gastrointestinal system is responsible for the process of digestion. It breaks down food into its components, absorbs nutrients, and discards the waste.

41. Diverticula, or pouch-like protrusions that occur in the colon, can become infected causing diverticulitis. A high fiber diet will help to avoid this condition.

42. The hepatitis B vaccine is administered in three doses and may be used prophylactically or as treatment for an unvaccinated patient who has been exposed.

43. Health care workers that are at risk for contact with hepatitis should receive all immunizations for HBV, and if exposed to blood or body fluids of an infected person must receive immunoglobulin therapy immediately.

44. Physical therapists must be diligent in assessing pain of an unknown origin. This is especially true when pain is accompanied by autonomic responses such as nausea, vomiting, pallor or sweating.

45. For numerous gastrointestinal disorders, lifestyle changes are the primary intervention recommended for symptom management.

### Genitourinary

46. The pelvic floor complex attaches to the pelvis and serves the genitourinary system through three primary functions: support, sphincteric function, and sexual function.

47. The genitourinary system consists of female and male genital organs and the urinary organs.

48. Physical therapy intervention for all bladder pathologies includes behavioral modification to address healthy bladder habits.

49. A woman's body transitions through multiple physiological and postural changes during pregnancy that may lead to impairments and functional limitations.

50. Relative and absolute contraindications need to be considered when developing an exercise program for a pregnant woman.

51. The goal of pelvic floor muscle strengthening exercises is to be able to perform a contraction during functional tasks.

### Oncology

52. Cancers are typically named based on the cell type involved and the tissue of origin.

53. A significant percentage of cancer related risk factors are modifiable.

54. The American Cancer Society names cancer as the leading cause of death in the United States.

55. Musculoskeletal pain in patients with cancer may be indicative of metastasis and should be promptly evaluated.

56. Physical therapists should be aware of the general signs and symptoms of cancer and refer patients back to the

# Other Systems Essentials

referring physician when signs and symptoms are observed in patients without a cancer diagnosis.

57. Staging of a malignancy is most commonly based on factors relating to the size of the primary tumor, lymph node involvement, and the presence of metastasis.

58. Staging assists multidisciplinary care providers to establish an optimal plan of care with appropriate goals and interventions.

59. Patients being treated for a cancer diagnosis with chemotherapy, radiation, and/or surgical interventions are at an increased risk for developing lymphedema.

60. Palliative treatment emphasizes symptom relief and may be provided in any care setting at any time during the course of a disease process.

61. Hospice care includes palliative interventions and goals, but is specifically reserved for patients at the end of life when curative efforts are no longer being pursued.

62. The usual modality contraindications relating to a cancer diagnosis may be occasionally disregarded in lieu of palliative goals for some patients at the end of life.

63. Cognitive changes related to oncological interventions are widely recognized and acknowledged despite limited definitive research on the subject.

64. The prevention of infection in patients who are neutropenic is imperative to prevent potentially life threatening complications.

## Psychological Disorders

65. Affective disorders relate to changes in mood or emotion and include depression, mania, and bipolar disorder.

66. Neuroses disorders are characterized by irrational fears or maladaptive responses to everyday stimuli and include phobias, psychogenic amnesia, multiple personality, obsessive-compulsive, anxiety, and dissociative disorders.

67. Somatoform disorders are classified by the presenting physical characteristics and include somatization, conversion, and hypochondriasis disorders.

68. Schizophrenic disorders are psychotic in nature and vary widely in presentation. Classifications of schizophrenia include catatonic, paranoid, disorganized, and undifferentiated.

69. Personality disorders are classified based on behavior patterns and include psychopathic, antisocial, narcissistic, and borderline personalities.

70. The side effects of numerous medications can have a significant impact on a patient's willingness and ability to effectively participate in physical therapy treatment.

## Bariatric

71. The morphological distribution of a patient's adipose tissue often correlates to their overall health risk factors.

72. Therapists may be the first health care providers to initiate a conversation about weight loss with a patient and should therefore be well informed of both appropriate community and medical resources so that a referral may be made as needed.

73. Waist-to-hip ratio measures are highly correlative to body mass index and indicators of central obesity.

74. Failure to address psychological influences associated with obesity, or eating disorders of any kind, will limit the potential for positive long-term success.

75. Significant weight loss cannot be achieved or maintained in a healthful way through a single mode of intervention.

76. With regard to weight loss, an individual's readiness and commitment to altering behavior is a significant factor in predicting long-term outcomes and success.

77. Options for bariatric surgical interventions vary from minimally invasive, reversible procedures to highly invasive procedures which significantly impact the body's anatomy and gastrointestinal function.

78. When initiating an exercise program for a morbidly obese patient special care should be taken to prevent injury and ensure safe, appropriate systemic responses.

## Nutrition

79. Vitamins are commonly classified as either fat-soluble or water-soluble.

80. Fat-soluble vitamins are more likely to reach toxic levels in the body.

81. Water-soluble vitamins are not stored in significant amounts within the body.

82. Some complimentary and alternative medicine supplements can interfere with the action of pharmaceutical agents and reach toxic levels within the body.

83. Minerals and vitamins are necessary to support the body's metabolic functions.

## Other Systems Proficiencies

### 1. Integumentary Anatomy

Select the appropriate term for each of the specified locations. Answers must be selected from the Word Bank and can be used only once.

**Word Bank:** adipose tissue, arrector pili muscle, blood supply, dermis, epidermis, hair follicle, nerve, nerve ending, sebaceous gland, subcutaneous fatty tissue, sweat duct, sweat gland

Hair shaft

a

Basal layer

b

c

d

e

Hair root

f

g

h

i

l

k

j

### 2. Ulcer Characteristics

Identify the type of ulcer that is most associated with the supplied description. Answers must be selected from the Word Bank and can be used more than once.

**Word Bank:** arterial, neuropathic, venous

| Type of Ulcer | Clinical Finding |
|---|---|
| a | ulcer located proximal to the medial malleolus |
| b | normal pedal pulse |
| c | leg elevation diminishes pain |
| d | absence of pain |
| e | evidence of increased edema |
| f | evidence of hair loss in tissue |

QUIZ

# Other Systems Proficiencies

## 3. Ulcer Staging

Identify the stage of ulcer that is most associated with the supplied description. Answers must be selected from the Word Bank and can be used more than once.

**Word Bank:** I, II, III, IV

| Stage | Clinical Finding |
|---|---|
| a | slough is present, but does not obscure depth of tissue loss |
| b | subcutaneous fat is visible, but bone, tendon or muscles are not exposed |
| c | extends into the joint capsule |
| d | intact skin with non-blanchable redness |
| e | tunneling with muscle visible |
| f | intact serum filled blister |
| g | shallow ulcer with a red wound bed |

## 4. Pressure Injuries

Identify the position or positions, most likely to cause a pressure injury over the identified bony prominence. The number of desired responses for each bony prominence is identified in parentheses.  Answers must be selected from the Word Bank and can be used more than once.

**Word Bank:** sidelying, sitting, supine, prone

| Bony Structure | Position(s) | |
|---|---|---|
| patella | a | (1) |
| dorsum of foot | b | (1) |
| ear | c | (1) |
| ischial tuberosity | d | (1) |
| vertebral spinous process | e | (2) |
| sternum | f | (1) |
| head of fibula | g | (1) |
| anterior superior iliac spine | h | (1) |

# QUIZ  Other Systems Proficiencies

## 5. Debridement

Classify each of the debridement techniques as selective or non-selective debridement.

| Type of Debridement | Classification |
|---|---|
| autolytic | a |
| enzymatic | b |
| hydrotherapy | c |
| sharp debridement | d |
| wet-to-dry | e |
| wound irrigation | f |

## 6. Wound Terminology

Identify the wound terminology most closely associated with the supplied description. Answers must be selected from the Word Bank and can be used only once.

**Word Bank:** contusion, dehiscence, desiccated, ecchymosis, erythema, friable, hematoma, keloid, maceration, turgor

| Terminology | Description |
|---|---|
| a | The separation, rupture or splitting of a wound closed by primary intention. |
| b | Tissue that readily tears, fragments or bleeds when gently palpated or manipulated. |
| c | A diffuse redness of the skin often resulting from either capillary dilation and congestion or inflammation. |
| d | Skin softening and degeneration that results from prolonged exposure to water or other fluids. |
| e | The drying out or dehydration of a wound. |
| f | A localized swelling or mass of clotted blood confined to a tissue, organ or space usually caused by a break in a blood vessel. |
| g | The discoloration occurring below intact skin resulting from trauma to underlying blood vessels and blood seeping into tissue. |
| h | An abnormal scar formation that is out of proportion to the scarring required for normal tissue repair. |
| i | The relative speed with which the skin resumes its normal appearance after being lightly pinched. |
| j | An injury, usually caused by a blow, that does not disrupt the skin integrity. |

# QUIZ   Other Systems Proficiencies

Identify the percentage of the total body surface affected based on the description of the area involved. Answers must be selected from the Word Bank and can be used more than once. Not all answers will be used.

**Word Bank:** 10%, 18%,19%, 22.5%, 23.5%, 28%, 36%, 54%, 55%, 63%, 64%

| % of Body | Areas Affected |
|---|---|
| a | anterior right arm, forearm, and hand; anterior trunk |
| b | bilateral legs and feet |
| c | anterior trunk, genital region, bilateral legs and feet |
| d | posterior head and neck; posterior trunk |
| e | bilateral arms, forearms, and hands; entire trunk |
| f | genital region, anterior left leg and foot |

## 8. Integumentary System Basics

Mark each statement as True or False. If the statement is False, correct the statement in the space provided.

| True/False | Statement |
|---|---|
| a | A patient with a deep partial-thickness burn would typically experience more pain than a patient with a superficial partial-thickness burn. |
| Correction: | |
| b | Patients with venous insufficiency ulcers should avoid unnecessary leg elevation. |
| Correction: | |
| c | Enzymatic debridement refers to the use of the body's own mechanisms to remove nonviable tissue. |
| Correction: | |

## Other Systems Proficiencies

| True/False | Statement |
|---|---|
| d | The epidermis thickens as part of the aging process, making it more resilient and therefore less susceptible to injury from friction and shear. |
| Correction: | |
| e | Healing by primary intention permits wounds to close on their own without superficial closure. |
| Correction: | |
| f | Patients with arterial insufficiency ulcers should avoid heating pads or soaking their feet in hot water. |
| Correction: | |
| g | A full-thickness burn involves complete destruction of the epidermis and dermis, along with partial damage to the subcutaneous fat layer. |
| Correction: | |
| h | The goal of treatment with a wound classified as "Red" using the Red-Yellow-Black System is to remove exudate and debris. |
| Correction: | |
| i | A superficial partial-thickness burn involves the epidermis and the upper portion of the dermis. |
| Correction: | |
| j | A grade of 3 on the Wagner Ulcer Grade Classification scale is indicative of a superficial ulcer not involving subcutaneous tissue. |
| Correction: | |

# QUIZ   Other Systems Proficiencies

## 9. Pathology of the Metabolic and Endocrine Systems

Identify the appropriate medical condition based on the supplied descriptions. Answers must be selected from the Word Bank and can only be used once.

**Word Bank:** Cushing's syndrome, Graves' disease, Klinefelter's syndrome, osteoporosis, Paget's disease, phenylketonuria, diabetes mellitus-type 1, Wilson's disease

| Pathology | Description |
|---|---|
| a | Adrenal dysfunction that produces excessive cortisol as well as a "moon-shaped face" and "buffalo hump." |
| b | Metabolic bone disease that affects trabecular and cortical bone resulting in decreased bone mass and increased risk for fracture. |
| c | Hypofunction of the pancreas where there is failure to produce adequate endogenous insulin. |
| d | Primary hypogonadism that presents with a deficiency of testosterone secondary to a failure of the testes to respond to follicle stimulating and luteinizing hormones. |
| e | Autosomal recessive inherited trait in which an enzyme deficiency permits excessive phenylalanine accumulation within the brain. |
| f | Autosomal recessive inherited trait that produces a defect in the body's ability to metabolize copper allowing it to accumulate in the brain and other tissues. |
| g | Autoimmune disease that produces thyroid hypersecretion resulting in heat intolerance, tremor, weight loss, and nervousness. |
| h | Metabolic bone disease characterized by heightened osteoclast activity resulting in excessive bone formation that lacks true structural integrity. |

## 10. Metabolic Acidosis versus Metabolic Alkalosis

Identify characteristics of each condition. Answers must be selected from the Word Bank and can be used only once.

**Word Bank:** <7.35, >7.45, compensatory hyperventilation, continuous vomiting, potassium chloride, renal failure, slowed breathing, sodium bicarbonate

| Metabolic Acidosis | | Metabolic Alkalosis |
|---|---|---|
| a | **Possible etiologies** | e |
| b | **pH** | f |
| c | **Symptoms** | g |
| d | **Treatment** | h |

# Other Systems Proficiencies

## 11. Glands of the Endocrine System and Hormones Secreted

Identify the endocrine gland or associated hormones. Answers must be selected from the Word Bank and can be used only once.

**Word Bank:** adrenal gland, estrogen and progesterone, glucagon and insulin, parathyroid gland, testes, thyroxine and triiodothyronine

| Endocrine Gland | Associated Hormones |
|---|---|
| a | testosterone and other androgens |
| ovaries | b |
| thyroid | c |
| pancreas | d |
| e | parathyroid hormone |
| f | corticosteroids and epinephrine |

## 12. Diabetes: Type 1 or Type 2

Identify the characteristic as Type 1 or Type 2 Diabetes mellitus. Answers must be selected from the Word Bank and can be used more than once.

**Word Bank:** Type 1, Type 2

| Type | Characteristic |
|---|---|
| a | treatment includes insulin injections or insulin pump |
| b | etiology unclear, but a genetic predisposition with a viral or environmental trigger is believed to facilitate onset |
| c | typically controlled through diet, exercise, and oral medications |
| d | obesity contributes to the condition by increasing insulin resistance |
| e | increased incidence in children due to rise in childhood obesity |
| f | typically there is some ongoing production of endogenous insulin |
| g | exogenous insulin injections are typically required |
| h | ketoacidosis rarely occurs |
| i | 5-10% of all cases of diabetes mellitus |
| j | gradual onset |
| k | destruction of the islet of Langerhans cells |

# Other Systems Proficiencies

## 13. Other Systems Basics

Mark each statement as True or False.  If the statement is False, correct the statement in the space provided.

| True/False | Statement |
| --- | --- |
| a | Catabolism is the process that combines simple molecules for tissue growth. |
| **Correction** | |
| b | Hormones secreted by endocrine glands travel through the bloodstream and signal specific target organs in order to maintain homeostasis of the internal environment. |
| **Correction** | |
| c | Norepinephrine is the catecholamine that creates the "fight or flight" response. |
| **Correction** | |
| d | Gastroesophageal reflux disease occurs as the result of an incompetent lower esophageal sphincter and allows for backwards movement of stomach acids into the esophagus. |
| **Correction** | |
| e | Diverticulitis is a condition with inflamed diverticula (pouch-like protrusions within the colon). |
| **Correction** | |
| f | Cirrhosis of the liver is a condition where the blood vessels dilate and allow for excess blood flow within the liver. |
| **Correction** | |
| g | The ovaries provide storage of oocytes prior to ovulation and secrete both estrogen and progesterone. |
| **Correction** | |

# Other Systems Proficiencies

| True/False | Statement |
|---|---|
| h | Hemodialysis is a treatment for patients with end-stage renal disease in order to cleanse the blood and is typically performed one time per week. |
| **Correction** | |
| i | Functional urinary incontinence is the loss of urine secondary to increased intra-abdominal pressure from activities such as sneezing or coughing. |
| **Correction** | |
| j | Diastasis recti is the separation of the rectus abdominis along the linea alba. |
| **Correction** | |
| k | Hypertension in supine during late pregnancy is secondary to compression of the inferior vena cava. |
| **Correction** | |
| l | Incompetent cervix, placenta previa, restrictive lung disease, and preeclampsia are absolute contraindications for exercise during pregnancy. |
| **Correction** | |
| m | A melanoma is a malignancy originating from connective tissues such as fat, cartilage, bone or muscle. |
| **Correction** | |
| n | Affective disorders include diagnoses such as obsessive-compulsive, anxiety, and phobia disorders. |
| **Correction** | |
| o | A body mass index of greater than 30 is indicative of obesity. |
| **Correction** | |

# Other Systems Proficiencies

## 14. Other Systems Terminology

Identify the term most closely associated with the supplied description. Answers must be selected from the Word Bank and can be used only once.

**Word Bank:** anorexia nervosa, anuria, cystocele, erectile dysfunction, gastritis, gene, glomerular filtration rate, hypoglycemia, insulin, lymphoma, mitochondria, neoplasm, osteopenia, pH, seminiferous tubules, urgency

| Terminology | Description |
|---|---|
| a | bulging of the bladder into the vagina |
| b | self-imposed starvation that results in impairment or "shut down" of systemic processes |
| c | the measure of the hydrogen ion concentration in body fluid |
| d | a fundamental unit of heredity |
| e | a group of oncology diagnoses referring to cancers that involve uncontrolled lymphocyte proliferation in the lymph nodes |
| f | a part of the cell that is responsible for energy production |
| g | synonymous with impotence |
| h | an abnormal new growth of tissue that can be classified as benign or malignant |
| i | a condition that presents with decreased bone mass, but not severe enough to be classified as osteoporosis |
| j | an estimate of the volume of filtrate produced per minute by the kidneys |
| k | a condition where blood sugar levels decrease below 70 mg/dL |
| l | the sudden strong desire to urinate that is difficult to defer |
| m | inflammation of the gastric mucosa of the inner layer of the stomach |
| n | hormone secreted by the islets of Langerhans within the pancreas |
| o | inadequate urine output in a 24-hour period of less than 100 ml |
| p | coiled tubes found within each lobe of the testes where spermatogenesis occurs |

## QUIZ    Other Systems Proficiencies

### 15. Staging of Cancer

Identify the appropriate sequence of staging based on the supplied description. Answers must be selected from the Word Bank and can be used only once.

**Word Bank:** 0, I, II, III, IV

| Stage | Description |
|---|---|
| a | Malignancy that has spread to adjacent tissue showing signs of fixation to deeper structures. The likelihood of metastatic lymph node involvement is high. |
| b | Malignancy that has metastasized beyond the primary site, for example, to bone or another organ. |
| c | Malignancy spreading into adjacent tissues; lymph nodes may show signs of micrometastases. |
| d | Early malignancy that is present only in the layer of cells in which it began. For most cancers, this is referred to as carcinoma in situ. |
| e | Malignancy limited to the tissue of origin with no lymph node involvement or metastasis. |

### 16. Pharmacology for Other Systems

Identify the appropriate medication based on the supplied descriptions. Answers must be selected from the Word Bank and can be used only once.

**Word Bank:** antacid agents, antimetabolite agents, bipolar disorder agents, bone mineral regulating agents, chemotherapy, emetic agents, endocrine hyperfunction agents, insulin, laxative agents, proton pump inhibitors

| Drug | Action |
|---|---|
| a | prevents histamine-activated release of gastric acid |
| b | administered to destroy malignant cells |
| c | administered as mood stabilizers preventing manic episodes and extreme swings in mood |
| d | facilitate bowel evacuation |
| e | administered via injection to maintain blood glucose levels |
| f | used to induce vomiting |
| g | promote inhibition of hormone function |
| h | chemically neutralize gastric acid and increase the intragastric pH |
| i | impair biosynthesis of genetic material by interrupting cellular pathways that synthesize DNA and RNA |
| j | enhance and maximize bone mass while preventing bone loss or rate of bone reabsorption |

# Other Systems Proficiencies

## 17. Vitamins and Potential Food Sources

Identify the appropriate vitamin based on the supplied potential food sources. Answers must be selected from the Word Bank. Each answer can be used only once.

**Word Bank:** A, B12, C, D, E, K

| Vitamin | Potential Food Sources |
|---------|------------------------|
| a | fortified milk, fish oils, salmon |
| b | green, orange, yellow vegetables, liver |
| c | citrus fruits, tomatoes, cantaloupe |
| d | vegetable oils, nuts, fish |
| e | meats, whole eggs |
| f | dark green leafy vegetables, cheese, egg yolks |

## 18. Minerals and their Function

Identify the appropriate mineral based on the supplied function. Answers must be selected from the Word Bank. Each answer can be used only once.

**Word Bank:** calcium, chromium, copper, iodine, iron, sodium, sulfur, zinc

| Mineral | Function |
|---------|----------|
| a | assists with glucose metabolism |
| b | facilitates the maintenance of acid-base balance, transmits nerve impulses, and assists to control muscle contractions |
| c | facilitates muscle contraction and relaxation, builds strong bones, aids in coagulation |
| d | facilitates enzyme activity and energy metabolism |
| e | assists with regulation of cell metabolism and basal metabolic rate |
| f | facilitates hemoglobin synthesis and lipid metabolism |
| g | assists in oxygen transport and cell oxidation |
| h | aids in immune function and cell division |

# Other Systems Answer Key

## 1. Integumentary Anatomy

a. sweat duct
b. sebaceous gland
c. arrector pili muscle
d. sweat gland
e. hair follicle
f. blood supply
g. nerve
h. nerve ending
i. adipose tissue
j. subcutaneous fatty layer
k. dermis
l. epidermis

## 2. Ulcer Characteristics

a. venous
b. venous
c. venous
d. neuropathic
e. venous
f. arterial

## 3. Ulcer Staging

a. III
b. III
c. IV
d. I
e. IV
f. II
g. II

## 4. Pressure Injuries

a. prone
b. prone
c. sidelying
d. sitting
e. supine, sitting
f. prone
g. sidelying
h. prone

## 5. Debridement

a. selective
b. selective
c. non-selective
d. selective
e. non-selective
f. non-selective

## 6. Wound Terminology

a. dehiscence
b. friable
c. erythema
d. maceration
e. desiccated
f. hematoma
g. ecchymosis
h. keloid
i. turgor
j. contusion

## 7. Rule of Nines

a. 22.5%
b. 36%
c. 55%
d. 22.5%
e. 54%
f. 10%

## 8. Integumentary System Basics*

a. FALSE: Correction - A patient with a deep partial-thickness burn would typically experience less pain than a patient with a superficial partial-thickness burn.

b. FALSE: Correction - Patients with venous insufficiency ulcers should elevate the legs when possible.

c. FALSE: Correction - Autolytic debridement refers to the use of the body's own mechanisms to remove nonviable tissue.

d. FALSE: Correction - The epidermis thins as part of the aging process, making it less resilient and therefore more susceptible to injury from friction and shear.

e. FALSE: Correction - Healing by secondary intention permits wounds to close on their own without superficial closure.

f. TRUE

g. TRUE

h. FALSE: Correction - The goal of treatment with a wound classified as "Red" using the Red-Yellow-Black System is to protect the wound and maintain a moist wound environment.

i. TRUE

j. FALSE: Correction - A grade of 3 on the Wagner Ulcer Grade Classification scale is indicative of a deep ulcer with osteitis, abscess or osteomyelitis.

*The correction presented for each false statement is an example of several possible corrections.

# Other Systems Answer Key

**9. Pathology of the Metabolic and Endocrine Systems**

a. Cushing's syndrome
b. osteoporosis
c. diabetes mellitus - type 1
d. Klinefelter's syndrome
e. phenylketonuria
f. Wilson's disease
g. Graves' disease
h. Paget's disease

**10. Metabolic Acidosis versus Metabolic Alkalosis**

a. renal failure
b. <7.35
c. compensatory hyperventilation
d. sodium bicarbonate
e. continuous vomiting
f. >7.45
g. slowed breathing
h. potassium chloride

**11. Glands of the Endocrine System and Hormones Secreted**

a. testes
b. estrogen and progesterone
c. thyroxine and triiodothyronine
d. glucagon and insulin
e. parathyroid gland
f. adrenal gland

**12. Diabetes: Type 1 or Type 2**

a. Type 1
b. Type 1
c. Type 2
d. Type 2
e. Type 2
f. Type 2
g. Type 1
h. Type 2
i. Type 1
j. Type 2
k. Type 1

**13. Other Systems Basics**

a. FALSE: Correction - Catabolism is the process of breaking down organic compounds during metabolism.
b. TRUE

c. FALSE: Correction - Epinephrine is the catecholamine that creates the "fight or flight" response.
d. TRUE
e. TRUE
f. FALSE: Correction - Cirrhosis of the liver is a condition where tissue of the liver is replaced with scar tissue that blocks blood flow within the liver resulting in decreased functioning.
g. TRUE
h. FALSE: Correction - Hemodialysis is a treatment for patients with end-stage renal disease in order to cleanse the blood and is typically performed three times per week.
i. FALSE: Correction - Stress urinary incontinence is the loss of urine secondary to increased intra-abdominal pressure from activities such as sneezing or coughing.
j. TRUE
k. FALSE: Correction - Hypotension in supine during late pregnancy is secondary to compression of the inferior vena cava.
l. TRUE
m. FALSE: Correction - A sarcoma is a malignancy originating from connective tissues such as fat, cartilage, bone or muscle.
n. FALSE: Correction - Neuroses disorders would include diagnoses such as obsessive-compulsive, anxiety, and phobia disorders. Affective disorders include depression, mania, and bipolar disorders.
o. TRUE

*The correction presented for each false statement is an example of several possible corrections.

**14. Other Systems Terminology**

a. cystocele
b. anorexia nervosa
c. pH
d. gene
e. lymphoma
f. mitochondria
g. erectile dysfunction
h. neoplasm
i. osteopenia
j. glomerular filtration rate
k. hypoglycemia
l. urgency
m. gastritis
n. insulin
o. anuria
p. seminiferous tubules

# Other Systems Answer Key

### 15. Staging of Cancer

a.  III

b.  IV

c.  II

d.  0

e.  I

### 16. Pharmacology for Other Systems

a.  proton pump inhibitors

b.  chemotherapy

c.  bipolar disorder agents

d.  laxative agents

e.  insulin

f.  emetic agents

g.  endocrine hyperfunction agents

h.  antacid agents

i.  antimetabolite agents

j.  bone mineral regulating agents

### 17. Vitamins and Potential Food Sources

a.  D

b.  A

c.  C

d.  E

e.  B12

f.  K

### 18. Minerals and their Function

a.  chromium

b.  sodium

c.  calcium

d.  sulfur

e.  iodine

f.  copper

g.  iron

h.  zinc

## Other Systems References

1.  Sussman C, Bates-Jensen B. **Wound Care: A Collaborative Practice Manual for Health Professionals**. Third Edition. Wolters Kluwer Health/Lippincott Williams & Wilkins, 2007.

2.  Irion G. **Comprehensive Wound Management**. Second Edition. SLACK Inc., 2010.

3.  O'Sullivan SB, Schmitz TJ. **Physical Rehabilitation**. Fifth Edition. F.A. Davis Company, 2007.

4.  Baranoski S, Ayello EA. **Wound Care Essentials: Practice Principles.** Second Edition. Lippincott Williams & Wilkins, 2008.

5.  Milne CT, Corbett LQ, Dubuc DL. **Wound, Ostomy, and Continence Nursing Secrets**. Hanley & Belfus, 2003.

6.  Herdon DN. **Total Burn Care**. Third Edition. Saunders Elsevier, 2007.

7.  Prentice WE. **Therapeutic Modalities in Rehabilitation**. Third Edition. McGraw-Hill Companies Inc., 2005.

8.  Stanley BG, Tribuzi SM. **Concepts in Hand Rehabilitation**. F.A. Davis Company, 1992.

9.  Trofino RB. **Nursing Care of the Burn-Injured Patient**. FA Davis Company, 1991.

10. Goodman CC, Fuller KS. **Pathology Implications for the Physical Therapist**. Third Edition. Saunders Elsevier, 2009.

11. Gould BE, Dyer RM. **Pathophysiology for the Health Professions**. Fourth Edition. Saunders Elsevier, 2011.

12. McDermott MT. **Endocrine Secrets**. Fifth Edition. Mosby Elsevier, 2009.

13. **Fluids & Electrolytes: An Incredibly Easy Pocket Guide**. Lippincott WIlliams & Wilkins, 2006.

14. About Osteoporosis. National Osteoporosis Foundation Website. http://www.nof.org/aboutosteoporosis. Updated 2010. Accessed September 15, 2010.

15. About Osteoporosis. International Osteoporosis Foundation Website. http://www.iofbonehealth.org/health-professionals/about-osteoporosis.html. Updated 2010. Accessed September 15, 2010.

16. **Stedman's Medical Dictionary**. 27th Edition. Lippincott Williams & Wilkins, 2000.

17. Goodman CC, Snyder TEK. **Differential Diagnosis for Physical Therapists: Screening for Referral**. Fourth Edition. Saunders Elsevier, 2007.

18. Blood Glucose Control. American Diabetes Association Website. http://www.diabetes.org/living-with-diabetes/treatment-and-care/blood-glucose-control/?utm_source=WWW&utm_medium=DropDownLWD&utm_content=BGC&utm_campaign=CON. Accessed October 4, 2010.

# Other Systems References

19. Ciccone CD. *Pharmacology in Rehabilitation*. Fourth Edition. F.A. Davis Company, 2007.

20. Moore K, Dalley A. *Clinically Oriented Anatomy*. Fourth Edition. Lippincott Williams & Wilkins, 1999.

21. Stephenson R, O'Connor L. *Obstetric and Gynecologic Care in Physical Therapy*. Second Edition. Slack Inc., 2000.

22. Cunningham FG, Leveno KJ, Bloom SL, Hauth JC, Rouse DJ, Spong CY. *Williams Obstetrics*. 23rd Edition. McGraw Hill Medical, 2010.

23. Gibbs RS, Karlan BY, Kaney AF, Nygaard I. *Danforth's Obstetrics and Gynecology*. Tenth Edition. Lippincott Williams & Wilkins, 2008.

24. Newman DK, Wein AJ. *Managing and Treating Urinary Incontinence*. Second Edition. Health Professions Press, 2009.

25. Kisner C, Colby LA. *Therapeutic Exercise Foundations and Techniques*. Fourth Edition. F.A. Davis Company, 2002.

26. American College of Sports Medicine: *ACSM's Guidelines for Exercise Testing and Prescription*. Seventh Edition. Lippincott Williams & Wilkins, 2006.

27. American College of Obstetricians and Gynecologists: Exercise During Pregnancy and the Postpartum Period, ACOG Committee Opinion No. 267. Obstet Gynecol 2002; 99: 171-173.

28. Gates RA, Fink RM. *Oncology Nursing Secrets*. Third Edition. Mosby Elsevier; 2008.

29. Disease Information. Leukemia and Lymphoma Society Website. http://www.leukemia-lymphoma.org/all_toplevel. adp?item_id=4187. Accessed September 24, 2010.

30. Schneider CM, Dennehy CA, Carter SD. *Exercise and Cancer Recovery*. Human Kinetics Publishing, 2003.

31. Staging: Questions and Answers. National Cancer Institute Website. http://www.cancer.gov/cancertopics/factsheet/ Detection/staging. Reviewed September 22, 2010. Accessed September 29, 2010.

32. *The Merck Manual*. 18th Edition. Merck Research Laboratories, 2006.

33. Foldi M, Foldi E. *Foldi's Textbook of Lymphology for Physicians and Lymphedema Therapists*. Second Edition. Mosby Elsevier, 2006.

34. Tecklin J. *Pediatric Physical Therapy*. Fourth Edition. Lippincott Williams & Wilkins, 2007.

35. Campbell S. *Physical Therapy for Children*. Third Edition. WB Saunders Company, 2006.

36. Paz J, West MP. *Acute Care Handbook for Physical Therapists*. Third Edition. Saunders, 2008.

37. Cancer Facts and Figures 2010. American Cancer Society Website. http://www.cancer.org/acs/groups/content/@ epidemiologysurveilance/documents/document/acspc-026238.

pdf. Reviewed 2010. Accessed September 24, 2010.

38. Understanding Your Complete Blood Count. Clinical Center National Institute of Health Website. http://www.cc.nih.gov/ ccc/patient_education/pepubs/cbc97.pdf. Updated November 2008. Accessed September 26, 2010.

39. Cooper J. *Occupational Therapy in Oncology and Palliative Care*. Second Edition. John Wiley & Sons, 2007.

40. JAMA Patient Page: Palliative Care. Journal of the American Medical Association Website. http://jama.ama-assn.org/cgi/ reprint/296/11/1428.pdf. Updated September 20, 2006. Accessed September 26, 2010.

41. Chemotherapy Principles: An Indepth Discussion. American Cancer Society Website. http://www.cancer.org/Treatment/ TreatmentsandSideEffects/TreatmentTypes/Chemotherapy/ ChemotherapyPrinciplesAnIn-depthDiscussionoftheTechnique sanditsRoleinTreatment/index. Updated September 28, 2010. Accessed October 1, 2010.

42. Chemo Brain. Mayo Clinic Website. http://www.mayoclinic. com/health/chemo-brain/DS01109. Updated October 10, 2010. Accessed October 15, 2010.

43. Bickley L, Szilagyi P. *Bates' Guide to Physical Examination and History Taking*. Tenth Edition. Lippincott Williams & Wilkins, 2009.

44. American College of Sports Medicine. *Resource Manual for Guidelines for Exercise Testing and Prescription*. Sixth Edition. Wolters Kluwer/Lippincott Williams & Wilkins, 2010.

45. Alvarez A, Brodsky JB, Lemmens HJM, Morton JM. *Morbid Obesity: Peri-operative Management*. Second Edition. Cambridge University Press, 2010.

46. Clinical Guidelines on the Identification, Evaluation, and Treatment of Overweight and Obesity in Adults: The Evidence Report. National Heart, Lung, and Blood Institute Website. http://www.nhlbi.nih.gov/guidelines/obesity/ob_gdlns.pdf. 1998.

47. Childhood Obesity: Risk Factors. Mayo Clinic Website. http:// www.mayoclinic.com/health/childhood-obesity/DS00698/ DSECTION=risk%2Dfactors. Reviewed October 9, 2010. Accessed October 14, 2010.

48. Childhood Overweight and Obesity. Centers for Disease Control Website. http://www.cdc.gov/obesity/childhood/index. html. Reviewed March 31, 2010. Accessed October 9, 2010.

49. Childhood Obesity. Mayo Clinic Website. http://www. mayoclinic.com/health/childhood-obesity/DS00698. Updated October 9, 2010. Accessed October 11, 2010.

50. Childhood Overweight and Obesity. Centers for Disease Control and Prevention Website. http://www.cdc.gov/obesity/ childhood/index.html. Updated March 31, 2010. Accessed September 24, 2010.

# 8

# EQUIPMENT AND DEVICES; THERAPEUTIC MODALITIES

## Scott Giles

Equipment and Devices represents approximately 2.5% (5 questions) of the National Physical Therapy Examination.

The actual number of questions in this category can range from 5 to 6 questions.

## Scott Giles

Therapeutic Modalities represents approximately 3.5% (7 questions) of the National Physical Therapy Examination.

The actual number of questions in this category can range from 6 to 8 questions.

405 Mobility

408 Wheelchairs

416 Ambulation

416 Assistive Devices

420 Medical Equipment

422 Diagnostic Tests

426 Cryotherapy

430 Superficial Thermotherapy

434 Deep Thermotherapy

440 Hydrotherapy

444 Traction

446 Compression

448 Electrotherapy

462 Essentials

465 Proficiencies

SCOREBUILDERS

# Mobility

### Preparation for Treatment

In order to create an effective and successful treatment environment, the patient must be informed regarding all expectations of the upcoming treatment as well as have all questions answered prior to initiating the actual hands-on intervention. The therapist must obtain informed consent from the patient and document consent in the patient's chart. The therapist must also determine if there are any potential limitations to treatment due to a patient's religious or cultural beliefs. The patient must be notified as to appropriate clothing for therapy, and subject areas such as draping must also be discussed prior to the initiation of therapy in order to ensure a patient's comfort during treatment.

### Draping

Draping is a technique utilized by health care providers to ensure the patient's privacy and modesty when treating particular areas of the body. Draping assists to keep the patient warm during treatment, adequately expose the area of treatment, and protect open areas, wounds, scars, and the patient's personal belongings from being soiled or injured during treatment. Draping materials may include gowns, towels, and sheets that must be secured in a manner that will properly expose the area of the body that requires treatment, while maintaining a patient's modesty and overall level of comfort during treatment.

## Bed Mobility Guidelines[1,2]

- A patient that is dependent must be repositioned in bed at least every two hours
- Skin should be inspected for redness or breakdown with each position change
- A dependent patient must be lifted when changing positions in order to avoid shearing of the skin across the bed
- Use pillows, towels or blankets when positioning a patient in order to support and maintain a particular position
- A patient should always be encouraged to participate in all mobility and positioning
- Practice moving segmentally from one side of the bed to the other
- Utilize the "bridging" position of hip flexion and knee flexion with feet flat on the surface to assist with movement and rolling
- Move from a supine to sitting position by rolling into sidelying and placing the feet over the edge; with assist as needed
- All components of bed mobility are complete only when the patient ends in a comfortable and safe position

## Transfers

### Communication During Transfers

The patient should be informed about the transfer itself and their responsibility during the transfer. The explanation should be understood by the patient and should occur prior to performing the transfer.

Commands and counts are used to synchronize the actions of the participants involved in the transfer. The therapist at the head of the patient should give the commands during transfers when more than one person is involved (Fig. 9-1).

### Levels of Physical Assistance[1,3]

**Independent:** The patient does not require any assistance to complete the task.

**Supervision:** The patient requires a therapist to observe throughout completion of the task.

**Contact Guard:** The patient requires the therapist to maintain contact with the patient to complete the task. Contact guard is usually needed to assist if there is a loss of balance.

**Minimal Assist:** The patient requires 25% assist from the therapist to complete the task.

**Moderate Assist:** The patient requires 50% assist from the therapist to complete the task.

**Maximal Assist:** The patient requires 75% assist from the therapist to complete the task.

**Dependent:** The patient is unable to participate and the therapist must provide all of the effort to perform the task.

## Transfer Guidelines

- Evaluate the patient's level of cognition and mobility
- When in doubt, utilize a second person to maintain patient/therapist safety
- Obtain all appropriate equipment prior to initiating the transfer
- Utilize a safety belt
- Educate the patient regarding the expectations and transfer sequence through verbal explanation and demonstration
- Instruct the patient in smaller segments of the transfer, if necessary, prior to performing the entire transfer all at once
- Position yourself correctly around the patient and maintain a large base of support; use proper body mechanics throughout the transfer

Fig. 9-1: The therapist at the head verbally initiates the transfer.

Fig. 9-2: The therapists lift the patient from the wheelchair in a coordinated fashion.

- Vary the amount of assistance as needed
- Utilize manual contacts with the patient to direct their participation during the transfer
- Complete the transfer with the patient positioned comfortably and safely

## Types of Transfers[1,3]

### Dependent Transfers

#### Three-person carry/lift

The three-person carry or lift is used to transfer a patient from a stretcher to a bed or treatment plinth. Three therapists carry the patient in a supine position; one therapist supports the head and upper trunk, the second therapist supports the trunk, and the third supports the lower extremities. The therapist at the head is the one to initiate commands. The therapists flex their elbows that are positioned under the patient and roll the patient on their side towards them. The therapists then lift on command and move in a line to the destination surface, lower, and position the patient properly.

#### Two-person lift

The two-person lift is used to transfer a patient between two surfaces of different heights or when transferring a patient to the floor. Standing behind the patient, the first therapist should place their arms underneath the patient's axilla. The therapist should grasp the patient's left forearm with their right hand and grasp the patient's right forearm with their left hand. The second therapist places one arm under the mid to distal thighs and the other arm is used to support the lower legs. The therapist at the head usually initiates the command to lift and transfer the patient out of the chair to the destination surface (Figs. 9-1, 9-2, 9-3, 9-4).

#### Dependent squat pivot transfer

The dependent squat pivot transfer is used to transfer a patient who cannot stand independently, but can bear some weight through the trunk and lower extremities. The therapist should position the patient at a 45-degree angle to the destination surface. The patient places their upper extremities on the therapist's shoulders, but should not be allowed to pull on the therapist's neck. The therapist should position the patient at the edge of the surface, hold the patient around the hips and under the

Fig. 9-5: A therapist prepares to initiate a dependent squat pivot transfer.

Fig. 9-6: The therapist moves the patient from the chair to a supported squatting position. The patient can bear some weight through the lower extremities.

**Fig. 9-3:** The patient is slowly lowered to the mat table.

**Fig. 9-4:** The patient must be in a comfortable and safe position before the therapist concludes the transfer.

buttocks, and block the patient's knees in order to avoid buckling while standing. The therapist should utilize momentum, straighten their legs, and raise the patient or allow the patient to remain in a squatting position. The therapist should then pivot and slowly lower the patient to the destination surface (Figs. 9-5, 9-6, 9-7, 9-8).

### Hydraulic lift

The hydraulic lift is a device used for dependent transfers when a patient is obese, there is only one therapist available to assist with the transfer or the patient is totally dependent. The hydraulic lift needs to be locked in position before the transfer. The therapist positions a webbed sling under the patient and attaches the S-ring to the bars on the lift. Once all attachments are checked, the therapist should pump the handle on the device in order to elevate the patient. When the patient is elevated, the therapist can navigate the lift with the patient to the destination surface. The chains should be removed once the patient has been transferred, however, the webbed sling should remain in place in preparation for the return transfer.

### Assisted Transfers

#### Sliding board transfer

The sliding board transfer is used for a patient who has some sitting balance, some upper extremity strength, and can adequately follow directions. The patient should be positioned at the edge of the wheelchair or bed and should lean to one side while placing one end of the sliding board sufficiently under the proximal thigh. The other end of the sliding board should be positioned on the destination surface. The patient should not hold onto the end of the sliding board in order to avoid pinching the fingers. The patient should place the lead hand four to six inches away from the sliding board and use both arms to initiate a push-up and scoot across the board. The therapist should guard in front of the patient and assist as needed as the patient performs a series of push-ups across the board. The therapist should be careful to avoid direct contact between the patient's skin and the sliding board to avoid shearing force and potential skin breakdown.

**Fig. 9-7:** The therapist blocks the patient's knees in order to provide additional stability during the transfer.

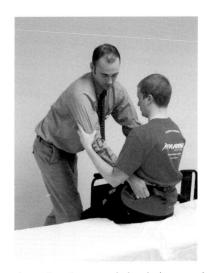

**Fig. 9-8:** The therapist pivots and slowly lowers the patient to the plinth.

### Stand pivot transfer

The stand pivot transfer is used when a patient is able to stand and bear weight through one or both of the lower extremities. The patient must possess functional balance and the ability to pivot. Patients with unilateral weight bearing restrictions or hemiplegia may utilize this transfer and lead with the uninvolved side. The transfer may also be used therapeutically, leading with the involved side for a patient post CVA. A patient should be positioned at the edge of the wheelchair or bed to initiate the transfer. The therapist can assist the patient to keep their feet flat on the floor while bringing the head and trunk forward. The therapist should assist the patient as needed with their feet. The therapist must guard or assist the patient through the transfer and instruct the patient to reach back for the surface before they begin to sit down. Once the stand pivot is performed, the therapist should assist as needed to ensure control with lowering the patient to the destination surface.

### Stand step transfer

The stand step transfer is used with a patient who has the necessary strength and balance to weight shift and step during the transfer. The patient requires guarding or supervision from the therapist and performs the transfer as a stand pivot transfer, except the patient actually takes a step to maneuver and reposition their feet instead of a pivot.

## Wheelchairs

Wheelchairs can be manually propelled or externally powered. Manual wheelchairs require patients to possess sufficient strength to propel the wheelchair independently (Fig. 9-9). Powered wheelchairs are propelled by an external energy source, usually a battery, that provides stored energy to one or more belts that propel the wheelchair (Fig. 9-10). Considerations when selecting an appropriate wheelchair include the patient's physical needs, physical abilities, cognition, coordination, and endurance.

Fig. 9-9: A manual wheelchair.

Fig. 9-10: A powered wheelchair.

### Wheelchair Measurements[4]

**A** = total height
**B** = seat depth
**C** = armrest height
**D** = seat height from floor
**E** = seat and back width
**F** = back height

Fig. 9-11: Common wheelchair measurements.[4]

## Standard Wheelchair Measurements for Proper Fit[1]

| Measurement | Instructions | Average Adult Size |
|---|---|---|
| **Seat Height Leg Length** | Measure from the user's heel to the popliteal fold and add 2 inches to allow clearance of the footrest. | 19.5 to 20.5 inches |
| **Seat Depth** | Measure from the user's posterior buttock, along the lateral thigh to the popliteal fold; then subtract approximately 2 inches to avoid pressure from the front edge of the seat against the popliteal space. Fig. 9-12: A therapist assesses the depth of a wheelchair. | 16 inches |
| **Seat Width** | Measure the widest aspect of the user's buttocks, hips or thighs and add approximately 2 inches. This will provide space for bulky clothing, orthoses or clearance of the trochanters from the armrest side panel. Fig. 9-13: A therapist assesses the width of a wheelchair. | 18 inches |
| **Back Height** | Measure from the seat of the chair to the floor of the axilla with the user's shoulder flexed to 90 degrees and then subtract approximately 4 inches. This will allow the final back height to be below the inferior angles of the scapulae. (Note: This measurement will be affected if a seat cushion is to be used. The person should be measured while seated on the cushion or the thickness of the cushion must be considered by adding that value to the actual measurement.) | 16 to 16.5 inches |
| **Armrest Height** | Measure from the seat of the chair to the olecranon process with the user's elbow flexed to 90 degrees and then add approximately 1 inch. (Note: This measurement will be affected if a seat cushion is to be used. The person should be measured while seated on the cushion or the thickness of the cushion must be considered by adding that value to the actual measurement.) | 9 inches above the chair seat |

From Pierson, FM: Principles and Techniques of Patient Care. W.B. Saunders Company, Philadelphia 2002, p.168, with permission.

| Common Components of Wheelchair Prescription[5-8] | |
|---|---|
| **Wheelchair Component** | **Clinical Indication** |
| **Wheelchair Frame** | |
| Ultralight frame | Patient is highly active with no need for postural supports; used for sports |
| Standard or lightweight frame | Patient is able to self propel using both upper extremities; adequate lower extremity ROM and sitting ability for comfortable seating |
| Hemi frame | Patient is able to self propel using lower extremities |
| One-hand drive frame | Patient is able to self propel using one upper extremity |
| Amputee frame | Patient is able to self propel, but center of gravity is shifted posteriorly due to amputation |
| Power wheelchair | Patient is not able to self propel, but is able to safely operate a power mobility device; patient may have transfer, sitting and/or upper extremity functional limitations |
| Geri chair | Patient is not able to self propel or safely operate a power mobility device; requires assistance for seated mobility |
| Reclining frame | Patient is unable to perform weight shifting tasks and/or is unable to sit upright for extended periods; moderate to severe trunk involvement |
| Backward tilt-in-space frame | Patient is unable to sit upright or perform weight shifts, but also has issues with sliding or extensor tone |
| **Headrest** | |
| Planar (flat) posterior | Patient uses a reclining or tilt-in-space frame or patient tends to maintain a hyperextended head/neck position in upright sitting |
| Curved headrest | Patient tends to maintain backward listing and/or lateral head and neck position in sitting; side panels may be indicated for more aggressive support |
| **Back Inserts** | |
| Sling back | Patient requires no postural support and has no neuromuscular deficits; not typically intended for long term use |
| Planar back insert | Patient requires mild to moderate trunk support due to tone, strength or deformity related postural concerns |
| Curved back insert | Patient requires moderate trunk support due to tone, strength or deformity related postural concerns |

| Common Components of Wheelchair Prescription[5-8] | |
|---|---|
| Wheelchair Component | Clinical Indication |
| Custom molded insert | Patient requires significant trunk support due to severe postural concerns |
| Removable back insert | Wheelchair must be able to fold |
| Back height below inferior angle of scapula | Patient is able to self propel and has good trunk control |
| Back height above inferior angle of scapula | Patient is either able to self propel, but requires some spinal support or uses a power mobility device with or without poor trunk control. |
| **Seat Inserts** | |
| Sling seat | Patient requires no postural support and has no neuromuscular deficits; not typically intended for long term use. |
| Planar seat | Patient has no seated deformity |
| Curved seat | Patient requires mild to aggressive supportive curvature to provide increased contact between the lower body and seat |
| Custom molded seat | Patient requires customized seat support to correct for pelvic obliquity or a fixed asymmetrical deformity |
| Removable seat insert | Wheelchair must be able to fold |
| Bevel (undercut) front edge of seat | Patient self propels using lower extremities |
| **Trunk Supports** | |
| Planar lateral supports | Patient requires mild to moderate lateral support due to listing or scoliosis |
| Contoured or curved lateral supports | Patient requires total contact lateral support for significant lateral listing or scoliosis |
| Chest strap | Patient requires trunk support to correct for anterior listing |
| Chest harness | Patient requires both trunk and shoulder support to correct for anterior listing |

## Common Components of Wheelchair Prescription[5-8]

| Wheelchair Component | Clinical Indication |
|---|---|
| **Armrests** | |
| Removable | Patient transfers via slide board or two person maximal assist; patient requires access to wheels for propulsion |
| No armrests | Patient does not require any upper extremity or trunk support |
| Full length arms | Patient performs sit to stand transfers; patient requires additional postural support; patient utilizes a lap board |
| Tubular or single posted arms | Patient requires minimal support for the upper extremities; patient requires easy access to wheels for propulsion; patient requires easy removal of arms |
| Fixed/non-removeable | Patient requires durable upper extremity support |
| **Wheel locks/brakes** | |
| Toggle/lever brakes (push or pull) | Patient has coordinated motor ability to operate brakes |
| Brake extension | Patient requires additional leverage to operate a toggle/lever break; patient has limited ability to reach brake mechanism |
| Attendant operated brakes | Patient does not possess the ability to safely or independently operate breaks |
| **Handrims** | |
| Small diameter | Patient has adequate strength to efficiently propel chair without adaptation; typically suggested for patients requiring speed for tasks |
| Large diameter | Patient has some degree of weakness in the upper extremities; typically suggested for patients requiring the ability to propel with more power |
| Rim projections | Patient has grip deficits or hand deformity which limits the ability to functionally grip rims |
| Covered rims | Patient requires assist for adequate grasp or friction when hands are in contact with wheel rims |
| **Footrests** | |
| Standard | Patient has full ROM available through feet and ankles |

## Common Components of Wheelchair Prescription[5-8]

| Wheelchair Component | Clinical Indication |
|---|---|
| Adjustable angle | Patient has some degree of deformity in feet and/or ankles |
| One-piece footboard | Patient requires a supportive surface to maximize strength and/or stability; patient requires additional lateral foot support |
| Custom foot box | Patient's lower extremities are not aligned with body midline as with a windswept deformity; individualized height, angle or support needs are identified |
| **Power Mobility Controls** | |
| Joystick control | Joysticks options vary widely and can be adapted for operation by numerous body parts (e.g., hand, chin, foot) |
| Proportional control | Allows user to modulate speed of device based on the displacement of the joystick; 360 degree directionality |
| Non-proportional control | Device moves at a pre-set speed regardless of joystick displacement; user must release joystick in order to change directions |
| Sip-and-puff control | A switch based system often used for patients with high level spinal cord injuries; patient controls direction based on the force of inhalation/exhalation into a small tube positioned near the patient's mouth |
| Head control | Head controls may be proportional or non-proportional and operate via an electronic switch system; configurations vary |
| **Other Considerations** | |
| Bariatric wheelchair | Bariatric wheelchairs are available in a variety of weight ratings and dimensions to accommodate patient needs. Weight limits for bariatric wheelchairs typically range between 300 and 1,000 pounds. |
| Solid cushions (viscoelastic, polyurethane or honeycomb foam) | Solid cushions vary greatly in density and stiffness depending on the product selected. Solid cushions are typically lightweight, however, can produce high shear forces. Examples include Sunmate, Stimulite, and T-foam cushions. |
| Liquid cushions (gel or water filled) | Liquid cushions vary greatly in the density and stiffness depending on the product selected. Liquid cushions are typically heavier than other alternatives, but serve to limit shear forces. Examples include Jay, Flo-fit, Avanti, and Action cushions. |
| Air filled cushions | Air filled cushions vary in average shear forces depending on the product selected. Common characteristics include being lightweight with pressure influenced by altitude. Air filled cushions require diligent monitoring of inflation levels. Examples include the Roho and Bye Bye Decubiti cushions. |

**Fig. 9-14:** A therapist tips a wheelchair backwards.

**Fig. 9-15:** The wheelchair is moved forward until the rear wheels come in contact with the curb.

## Wheelchair Mobility[1,3]

### Ascending a curb with a forward approach

1. Elevate the front casters of the wheelchair by tipping the wheelchair backwards (Fig. 9-14).
2. Move the wheelchair forward until the rear wheels are in contact with the curb and the casters are above the curb (Fig. 9-15).
3. Lower the casters on the elevated surface and ascend the curb with the real wheels until the rear wheels and the casters are in contact with the elevated surface (Figs. 9-16, 9-17).

### Ascending a curb with a backward approach

1. Position the patient facing away from the curb.
2. Standing on the upper surface, lift and roll the rear wheels backward up the curb.
3. Continue to roll the wheelchair backwards until the casters are in contact with the upper surface.

### Descending a curb with a forward approach

1. Position the casters close to the elevated edge of the curb.
2. Tip the wheelchair backwards and slowly roll the wheelchair forward until the rear wheels are in contact with the lower surface.
3. Gently lower the casters to the lower surface.

### Descending a curb with a backward approach

1. Position the patient facing away from the curb.
2. Move the wheelchair backwards and slowly lower the rear wheels to the lower surface maintaining contact with the curb.
3. Continue to roll the wheelchair backwards and gently lower the casters to the lower surface.

**Fig. 9-16:** The casters are lowered and the rear wheels ascend the curb.

**Fig. 9-17:** The rear wheels and casters are positioned on the elevated surface.

# Consider This

## Equipment for Activities of Daily Living[9]

Physical therapists should be aware of equipment available to assist patients to perform activities of daily living as effectively and efficiently as possible. The most appropriate equipment for each patient will depend on the patient's medical status and their current living condition.

A listing of some of the more commonly used equipment for activities of daily living is presented.

**Bed safety rails** - Externally applied rails assist patients with bed mobility.

**Button hook** - A device that allows individuals with limited dexterity to button clothing using a hand held device. Individuals unable to utilize the device effectively can use Velcro instead of buttons.

**Commode chair** - A chair with a cut out seat for personal hygiene and a removable pan for commode use. The device is elevated above the level of a standard commode and the armrests increase safety during transfers.

**Door knob extenders** - A device that increases leverage when opening and closing doors making it easier for individuals with diminished strength and dexterity to function independently.

**Grab bars** - Stable, mounted bars designed to provide individuals with a handgrip for added stability during functional tasks.

Fig. 9-18: Grab bars positioned around a commode.

**Handwriting aids** - Writing devices can be enlarged using a triangular grip or cylindrical foam. This adaptation makes it easier for patients with limited dexterity and pinch strength to write.

**Long straw** - A long plastic straw enables individuals to drink from a glass without lifting the glass from the surface.

**Reacher** - The device consists of a long, lightweight aluminum surface with a trigger which activates a grip closure enabling an individual to reach upward or downward without excessive bending.

Fig. 9-19: A patient using a reacher to retrieve a shoe.

**Rocker knife** - This type of knife has a curved blade with an enlarged handle which allows an individual to cut food using a rocking motion.

**Sock aids/shoe aids** - Devices designed to assist individuals to independently apply socks and shoes using some type of a plastic or wire frame. The devices work by maintaining the sock in an open position or providing a funnel for the patient to use when placing the foot into a shoe.

**Tub bench** - A bench that allows an individual to sit on a firm, stable surface when bathing.

Fig. 9-20: A tub bench positioned in a bath tub.

**Zipper pull** - A device that allows individuals with inadequate strength in the arms and fingers to pull a zipper using a loop.

SCOREBUILDERS

# Ambulation

## Assistive Devices

Primary indications for using an assistive device during ambulation include:

- Decreased weight bearing on the lower extremities
- Muscle weakness of the trunk or lower extremities
- Decreased balance or impaired kinesthetic awareness
- Pain

## Assistive Device Selection[1,3,10]

### Parallel Bars

Parallel bars provide maximum stability and security for a patient during the beginning stages of ambulation or standing. Proper fit includes bar height that allows for 20–25 degrees of elbow flexion while grasping on the bars approximately four to six inches in front of the body. A patient must progress out of the parallel bars as quickly as possible to increase overall mobility and decrease dependence using the parallel bars.

### Walker

A walker can be used with all levels of weight bearing. The walker has a significant base of support and offers good stability (Fig. 9-21). The walker should allow for 20–25 degrees of elbow flexion to ensure proper fit. The standard walker has many variations including rolling, hemi, reciprocal, folding, or adjustable walker with brakes, upper extremity attachments and/or a seat platform. The walker is used with a three-point gait pattern.

**Fig. 9-21:** A standard walker.

**Fig. 9-22:** Axillary crutches.

### Axillary Crutches

Axillary crutches can be used with all levels of weight bearing, however, require higher coordination for proper use (Fig. 9-22). Proper fit includes positioning with the crutches six inches in front and two inches lateral to the patient. The crutch height should be adjusted no greater than three finger widths from

**Fig. 9-23:** A therapist assesses crutch height by determining the distance from the top of the crutch to the base of the axilla.

the axilla (Fig. 9-23). The handgrip height should be adjusted to the ulnar styloid process and allow for 20–25 degrees of elbow flexion while grasping the handgrip (Fig. 9-24). A platform attachment can be utilized with this device. Axillary crutches can be used with two-point, three-point, four-point, swing-to, and swing-through gait patterns.

**Fig. 9-24:** The handgrip of an axillary crutch should be at the approximate level of the ulnar styloid process.

## Lofstrand (forearm) Crutches

Lofstrand crutches can be used with all levels of weight bearing, however, require the highest level of coordination for proper use (Fig. 9-25). Proper fit includes 20–25 degrees of elbow flexion while holding the handgrip with the crutches positioned six inches in front and two inches lateral to the patient's foot. The arm cuff should be positioned one to one and one half inches below the olecranon process so it does not interfere with elbow flexion. A platform attachment can be utilized with this device if necessary. The Lofstrand crutches can be used with two-point, three-point, four-point, swing-to, and swing-through gait patterns.

**Fig. 9-25:** Lofstrand crutches.

## Cane

A cane provides minimal stability and support for patients during ambulation activities. The straight cane provides the least support and is used primarily for assisting with balance. A straight cane should not be utilized for patients that are partial weight bearing. The small base and large base quad canes provide a larger base of support and can better assist with limiting weight bearing on an involved lower extremity and improving balance on unlevel surfaces, curbs, and stairs. The cane is typically used on the opposite side of an involved lower extremity. Proper fit includes standing the cane at the patient's side and adjusting the handle to the level of the wrist crease at the ulnar styloid (Fig. 9-26). The patient should have 20–25 degrees of elbow flexion while grasping the handgrip. The straight cane can be used with the two-point, four-point, modified two-point, and modified four-point gait patterns.

**Fig. 9-26:** The handle of a cane should be at the approximate level of the ulnar styloid process.

**Non-weight bearing (NWB):** A patient is unable to place any weight through the involved extremity and is not permitted to touch the ground or any surface. An assistive device is required.

**Toe touch weight bearing (TTWB):** A patient is unable to place any weight through the involved extremity, however, may place the toes on the ground to assist with balance. An assistive device is required.

**Partial weight bearing (PWB):** A patient is allowed to put a particular amount of weight through the involved extremity. The amount of weight bearing is expressed as allowable pounds of pressure or as a percentage of total weight. A therapist must monitor the amount of actual weight transferred through the involved foot during partial weight bearing (Fig. 9-27). An assistive device is required.

**Fig. 9-27:** A patient using a scale to determine the approximate amount of weight bearing.

**Weight bearing as tolerated (WBAT):** A patient determines the proper amount of weight bearing based on comfort. The amount of weight bearing can range from minimal to full. An assistive device may or may not be required.

**Full weight bearing (FWB):** A patient is able to place full weight on the involved extremity. An assistive device is not required at this level, but may be used to assist with balance.

## Guarding

### Guarding During Ambulation

A therapist must consider the patient's size, weight, and level of impairment prior to initiating ambulation activities. The following are general guarding recommendations:

- Stand to the side (usually the affected side) and slightly behind the patient.
- Grasp the safety belt with one hand; place the other hand on the patient's shoulder.

- Avoid grasping the arm since it can interfere with the patient's ability to use the extremity.

- Move the lead foot forward when the patient moves; the back leg should advance as the patient ambulates.

- Attempt to anticipate potential hazards during ambulation and take appropriate precautions when possible.

- Utilize a second therapist when needed.

## Gait Patterns[1,3]

An appropriate gait pattern is determined by the amount of weight bearing permitted and the severity of the patient's overall condition. Commonly used gait patterns include two-point, three-point, four-point, swing-to, and swing-through.

### Two-point gait

This is a pattern in which a patient uses two crutches or canes. The patient ambulates moving the left crutch forward while simultaneously advancing the right lower extremity and vice versa. Each step is one point and a complete cycle is two points.

### Three-point gait

This pattern can be seen with a walker or crutches. It involves one injured lower extremity that may have decreased weight bearing. The assistive device is advanced followed by the injured lower extremity and then the uninjured lower extremity. The assistive device and each lower extremity are considered separate points.

### Four-point gait

This pattern is very similar to the two-point pattern. The primary difference is that the patient does not move the lower extremities simultaneously with the device, but rather waits and advances the opposite leg once the crutch/cane has been advanced. This gait pattern may be prescribed when a patient exhibits impaired coordination, balance or significant strength deficits. Each advancement of the crutch or cane as well as the bilateral lower extremities indicates a single point, thus allowing for a four-point gait pattern.

### Swing-to gait

A gait pattern where a patient with trunk and/or bilateral lower extremity weakness, paresis or paralysis, uses crutches or a walker and advances the lower extremities simultaneously only to the point of the assistive device.

### Swing-through gait

A gait pattern where the patient performs the same sequence as a swing-to gait pattern, however, advances the lower extremities beyond the point of the assistive device.

## Guarding During Curbs and Stairs[1,11]

### Ascending

- When using a handrail, stand to the opposite side and behind the patient.

- When a handrail is not available, stand behind the patient slightly toward the affected side (Fig. 9-29).

- Grasp the safety belt with one hand and have the opposite hand available to support the trunk as needed.

- The therapist should position one foot on the step the patient is starting from and the other on the step below. The therapist should maintain a wide base of support.

- Remain static when the patient is moving, then advance keeping the feet in stride position.

### Descending

- When using a handrail, stand to the opposite side and in front of the patient.

- When a handrail is not available, stand in front of the patient slightly toward the affected side.

- Grasp the safety belt with one hand and have the opposite hand available to support the trunk as needed.

- The therapist should position one foot on the step the patient will step to and the other on the step below. The therapist should maintain a wide base of support.

- Remain static when the patient is moving, then advance keeping the feet in stride position.

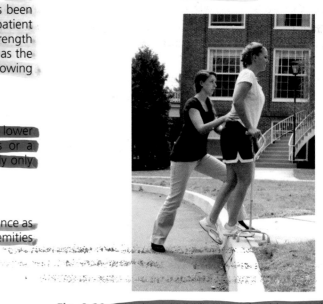

Fig. 9-29: A patient ascending a curb with a quad cane.

# Consider This

## Ascending and Descending Stairs with an Assistive Device[1,11]

Patients can ascend and descend stairs with a number of different assistive devices. Regardless of the specific assistive device utilized, when ascending stairs the patient should place the uninvolved lower extremity on the higher stair since it will generate the force needed to propel the body. The involved lower extremity and the assistive device then move to the same stair. When descending stairs, the uninvolved lower extremity generates the force needed to lower the involved extremity with the assistive device to the next step.

Additional factors for therapists to consider when using various assistive devices on stairs are listed.

### Walker

**Ascending** - The patient should place the walker on the opposite side of the handrail and turn the walker sideways. The patient should then grasp the handrail with one hand and the top of the walker's handpiece with the other hand. Using the handrail and walker for stability, the patient takes a step up with the uninvolved extremity. The involved extremity is then advanced to the same step and the walker follows.

**Descending** - The walker is positioned in a similar manner as described previously. The patient uses the handrail and top of the walker for stability while lowering the involved lower extremity. The uninvolved lower extremity is then lowered and the walker follows.

### Axillary Crutches

**Ascending** - The patient should use the handrail and turn the crutch sideways. This will result in the patient grasping the handrail and the crutch with the same hand. The patient should use the handrail and advance the uninvolved lower extremity to the next step. The patient will then advance the involved lower extremity followed by the crutches.

**Descending** - The patient uses the handrail and turns the crutch sideways as described previously. The patient lowers the involved lower extremity and the crutch to the next step followed by the uninvolved extremity.

The patient may alternately elect to ascend and descend stairs holding the handrail with one hand and the two crutches in the other hand.

Fig. 9-28: A patient ascending stairs with axillary crutches using the alternate method.

### Cane

**Ascending** - The patient should use the handrail and turn the cane sideways. This will result in the patient grasping the handrail and the cane with the same hand. The patient should use the handrail and advance the uninvolved lower extremity to the next step. The patient will then advance the involved lower extremity.

**Descending** - The patient uses the handrail and turns the cane sideways as described previously. The patient lowers the involved lower extremity to the next step followed by the uninvolved extremity.

# Spotlight on Safety
## Loss of Balance During Stair Training[1]

Physical therapists take many precautions to avoid unnecessary safety risks when instructing patients in a variety of functional activities. Despite these precautions, on occasion adverse events still occur. In these instances, therapists must be prepared to take immediate action to avoid or minimize the potential impact of an adverse event.

The most appropriate therapist action when a patient experiences a loss of balance during stair training is described. The descriptions are based on the therapist being positioned behind the patient when ascending the stairs and in front of the patient when descending the stairs.

### Forward loss of balance

**Ascending:** Pull backwards on the safety belt and attempt to move the trunk backwards with the opposing hand. If the patient cannot regain balance, transition the patient toward the handrail or lower the patient slowly toward the stairs.

**Descending:** Use one hand to apply a posterior directed force to the patient's trunk. The therapist may elect to use both hands to stabilize the patient or may use one hand to grasp the handrail while stabilizing the trunk with the opposing hand. If the patient cannot regain balance, the therapist should attempt to move them to a sitting position.

### Backward loss of balance

**Ascending:** Attempt to stabilize the patient's trunk by applying an anterior directed force while maintaining a wide base of support. If the patient cannot regain balance, transition the patient toward the handrail or lower the patient slowly toward the stairs.

**Descending:** Pull forwards on the safety belt using one hand to grasp the handrail. If the patient cannot regain balance, transition the patient toward the handrail or attempt to move them to a sitting position.

### Sideways loss of balance toward the therapist

**Ascending:** Use one hand or your trunk to stabilize the patient and use the other hand to grasp the handrail. If the patient cannot regain balance, transition the patient toward the handrail or lower the patient slowly toward the stairs.

**Descending:** Use one hand or your trunk to stabilize the patient and use the other hand to grasp the safety belt or handrail. If the patient cannot regain balance, transition the patient toward the handrail or attempt to move them to a sitting position.

### Sideways loss of balance away from the therapist

**Ascending:** Use one hand to pull the safety belt toward you and use the other to stabilize the trunk or grasp the handrail. If the patient cannot regain balance, transition the patient toward the handrail or lower the patient slowly toward the stairs.

**Descending:** Use one hand to pull the safety belt toward you and use the other to stabilize the trunk or grasp the handrail. If the patient cannot regain balance, transition the patient toward the handrail or attempt to move them to a sitting position.

# Medical Equipment

## Feeding Devices[1,12]

### Nasogastric tube (NG tube)

A nasogastric tube is a plastic tube inserted through a nostril that extends into the stomach. The device is commonly used for short-term liquid feeding, medication administration or to remove gas from the stomach. The position of the tube in the nostril and back of the throat can inhibit a cough and be irritating for the patient.

### Gastric tube (G tube)

A gastric tube is a tube inserted through a small incision in the abdomen into the stomach. The tube can be used for long-term feeding in the presence of difficulty with swallowing due to an anatomic or neurologic disorder or to avoid the risk of aspiration.

### Jejunostomy tube (J tube)

A jejunostomy tube is a tube inserted through endoscopy into the jejunum via the abdominal wall. The tube can be used for long-term feeding for patients that are unable to receive food by mouth.

### Intravenous system (IV)

An intravenous system consists of a sterile fluid source, a pump, a clamp, and a catheter to insert into a vein (Fig. 9-30). An intravenous system can be used to infuse fluids, electrolytes, nutrients, and medication. Intravenous lines are most commonly inserted into superficial veins such as the basilic, cephalic or antecubital. Intravenous infusion lines permit nutirents to be introduced when the gastrointestinal tract is not able to digest and absorb food.

**Fig. 9-30:** An intravenous system.

## Monitoring Devices[1,12,13]

### Arterial line

An arterial line is a monitoring device consisting of a catheter that is inserted into an artery and attached to an electronic monitoring system. An arterial line is used to measure blood pressure or to obtain blood samples. The device is considered to be more accurate than traditional measures of blood pressure and does not require repeated needle punctures. If an arterial line is displaced, a therapist should apply direct pressure to limit blood loss and call for assistance.

### Central venous pressure catheter

A central venous pressure catheter is used for measuring pressures in the right atrium or the superior vena cava by means of an indwelling venous catheter and a pressure manometer. It is used to evaluate the right ventricular function, right atrial filling pressure, and circulating blood volume. The use of the catheter significantly reduces the need for repeated venipuncture.

### Indwelling right atrial catheter (Hickman)

An indwelling right atrial catheter is inserted through the cephalic or internal jugular vein and threaded into the superior vena cava and right atrium. The catheter is used for long-term administration of substances into the venous system such as chemotherapeutic agents, total parenteral nutrition, and antibiotics.

### Intracranial pressure monitor

An intracranial pressure monitor measures the pressure exerted against the skull using pressure sensing devices placed inside the skull. Excessive pressure can be produced by a closed head injury, cerebral hemorrhage, overproduction of cerebrospinal fluid or brain tumor. Types of intracranial pressure monitors include epidural sensor, subarachnoid bolt, and intraventricular catheter.

### Oximeter

An oximeter is a photoelectric device used to determine the oxygen saturation of blood. The device is most commonly applied to the finger or the ear. Oximetry is often used by therapists to assess activity tolerance. Therapists should monitor changes in oxygen saturation during exercise and position changes.

### Pulmonary artery catheter (Swan-Ganz catheter)

A pulmonary artery catheter is a soft, flexible catheter that is inserted through a vein into the pulmonary artery. The device is used to provide continuous measurements of pulmonary artery pressure. The patient should avoid excessive movement of the head, neck, and extremities to avoid disrupting the line at the insertion site.

## Oxygen Therapy[1,12]

### Nasal cannula

A nasal cannula consists of tubing extending approximately one centimeter into each of the patient's nostrils. The tubing is connected to a common tube that is attached to an oxygen source. This method of oxygen therapy is capable of delivering up to six liters of oxygen per minute.

### Oronasal mask

An oronasal mask consists of a facepiece designed to cover the nose and mouth with small vent holes to expel exhaled air along with a breathing tube and connector. The device is used most often for oxygen therapy, however, can be used to administer medications, mucolytic detergents, or humidity, by the use of an accessory nebulizer.

### Tent

An oxygen tent refers to a canopy placed over the head and shoulders or the entire body for the purpose of delivering oxygen at a higher level than normal.

### Tracheostomy mask

A tracheostomy mask is placed over a stoma or tracheostomy for the purpose of administering supplemental oxygen. The mask is held in place by an elastic strap placed around the patient's neck.

## Skeletal Traction[12]

### Balanced suspension

Balanced suspension traction requires pins, screws, and wires to be surgically inserted into bone for the purpose of applying a traction force using an externally applied weight. This type of traction is most often utilized with comminuted femur fractures. Balanced suspension traction requires prolonged immobilization and therefore increases the incidence of secondary complications such as contractures or skin breakdown.

### External fixation

External fixation refers to a surgical procedure where holes are drilled into uninjured areas of bone surrounding the fracture. The fracture is then set in the desired anatomical configuration using specialized wires, pins, bolts, and screws. An external frame is used to maintain the bony fragments in the desired alignment (Fig. 9-31). External fixation enhances stability and allows for earlier mobility while maintaining the desired alignment.

**Fig. 9-31:** An external fixation device applied to a tibial fracture sustained in a motor vehicle accident.

### Internal fixation

Internal fixation refers to a surgical procedure that attempts to promote the healing process of bone without appliances being applied external to the skin. Common types of internal fixation include metal plates, rods, wires, screws, and nails. Internal fixation is often employed with comminuted or displaced fractures. The procedure provides needed stability to healing joints which allows earlier mobility and less postoperative complications.

## Urinary Catheters[1,12]

### External catheter

An external catheter is applied over the shaft of the penis and is held in place by a padded strap or adhesive tape.

### Foley catheter

A Foley catheter is an indwelling urinary tract catheter that has a balloon attachment at the indwelling end. The balloon which is filled with air or sterile water must be deflated before the catheter can be removed.

### Suprapubic catheter

A suprapubic catheter is an indwelling urinary catheter that is surgically inserted directly into the patient's bladder. Insertion of a suprapubic catheter is performed under general anesthesia.

## Miscellaneous[1,12]

### Chest tube

A chest tube is a flexible plastic tube that is inserted through an incision into the side of the chest. The tube uses a suction system to remove air, fluid or pus from the intrathoracic space. A chest tube can cause significant discomfort and result in inhibition of a cough, deep breathing, and mobility.

### Mechanical ventilator

A mechanical ventilator produces a controlled flow of gas into a patient's airways. The flow of gas provides positive pressure that produces lung inflation. Patients with acute illness, trauma, and severe chronic illness may require mechanical ventilation. The most common type of ventilators include volume cycled and pressure cycled. Volume cycled ventilators deliver a predetermined amount of gas based on the patient's needs during the inspiratory phase. This type of ventilation is most commonly used for patients that require long-term support. Pressure cycled ventilators deliver a predetermined maximum pressure of gas during respiration. When the established pressure is reached, the inspiratory phase ends. The expiratory phase is passive with both volume cycled and pressure cycled ventilators.

### Ostomy device

An ostomy device provides a method for collection of waste from a surgically produced opening in the abdomen. The removal of the waste occurs through a stoma extending into the small intestine. The waste is collected in a plastic bag or pouch covering the stoma. Ostomy systems are typically air and water-tight and allow the user to lead an active normal lifestyle.

## Diagnostic Tests[14,15]

### Arteriography

Arteriography refers to a radiograph that visualizes injected radiopaque dye in an artery. The test can be used to identify arteriosclerosis, tumors or blockages.

### Arthrography

Arthrography is an invasive test utilizing a contrast medium to provide visualization of joint structures through radiographs. Soft tissue disruption can be identified by leakage from the joint cavity and capsule. The test is commonly used at peripheral joints such as the hip, knee, ankle, elbow, and wrist.

### Bone Scan

A bone scan is an invasive test that utilizes isotopes to identify stress fractures, infection, and tumors. Bone scans can identify bone disease or stress fractures with as little as 4-7% bone loss.

### Computed Tomography

Computed tomography produces cross-sectional images based on x-ray attenuation. A computerized analysis of the changes in absorption produces a detailed reconstructed image (Fig. 9-32). The test is commonly used to diagnose spinal lesions and in diagnostic studies of the brain.

### Doppler Ultrasonography

Doppler ultrasonography is a non-invasive test that evaluates blood flow in the major veins, arteries, and cerebrovascular system. The test relies on the transmission and reflection of high frequency sound waves to produce cross-sectional images in a variety of planes. Doppler ultrasonography is safer, less expensive, and requires a shorter time period than more invasive tests such as arteriography and venography.

**Fig. 9-32:** Images of the pelvis and abdomen obtained through computed tomography.

**Fig. 9-33:** A magnetic resonance imaging machine.

### Electrocardiography

Electrocardiography is the recording of the electrical activity of the heart. The test identifies three distinct waveforms: P wave (atrial depolarization), QRS complex (ventricular depolarization), and the T wave (ventricular repolarization). Electrocardiography is used to help identify conduction abnormalities, cardiac arrhythmias, and myocardial ischemia.

### Electroencephalography

Electroencephalography is the recording of the electrical activity of the brain. The electrical activity is collected by examining the difference between the electrical potential of two electrodes placed at different locations on the scalp. Electroencephalography is used to assess seizure activity, metabolic disorders, and cerebellar lesions.

### Electromyography

Electromyography is the recording of the electrical activity of a selected muscle or muscle groups at rest and during voluntary contraction. Electromyography is performed by inserting a needle electrode percutaneously into a muscle or through the use of surface electrodes. The test is commonly used to assess peripheral nerve injuries and to differentiate between various neuromuscular disorders.

### Fluoroscopy

Fluoroscopy is designed to show motion in joints through x-ray imaging. The technique permits objects placed between a fluorescent screen and a roentgen tube to become visible. Fluoroscopy is not used commonly due to excessive radiation exposure.

### Magnetic Resonance Imaging

Magnetic resonance imaging is a non-invasive technique that utilizes magnetic fields to produce an image of bone and soft tissue (Fig. 9-33). The test is valuable in providing images of soft tissue structures such as muscles, menisci, ligaments, tumors, and internal organs (Fig. 9-34). Magnetic resonance imaging requires the patient to remain still for prolonged periods of time and is extremely expensive.

**Fig. 9-34:** Images of the knee obtained through magnetic resonance imaging.

### Myelography

Myelography is an invasive test that combines fluoroscopy and radiography to evaluate the spinal subarachnoid space. The test utilizes a contrast medium that is injected into the epidural space by spinal puncture. Myelography is used to identify bone displacement, disk herniation, spinal cord compression or tumors.

### Venography

Venography refers to a radiograph that visualizes injected radiopaque dye in a vein. The test can be used to identify tumors or blockages in the venous network.

**X-ray**

X-ray is a radiographic photograph commonly used to assist with the diagnosis of musculoskeletal problems such as fractures, dislocations, and bone loss. X-ray produces planar images and as a result often requires images to be taken in multiple planes in order to visualize a lesion's location and size (Fig. 9-35).

**Fig. 9-35:** X-ray images of the knee using an anteroposterior and lateral view.

NEXT EXIT

MOTIVATIONAL MOMENT

See Page 1030

# Therapeutic Modalities

Therapeutic modalities is a broad term describing a variety of agents used in the rehabilitation of patients. Therapeutic modalities include thermal agents (e.g., hot pack, ultrasound), mechanical agents (e.g., traction, compression), and electromagnetic agents (e.g., electrical stimulation, diathermy). In a rehabilitation program, therapeutic modalities are primarily used as adjuncts to other interventions, such as therapeutic exercise.

## Indications for Therapeutic Modalities[16,17,18]

**Inflammation and repair:** Modalities can alter circulation, chemical reactions, flow of body fluids, and cell function throughout all phases of healing. Modalities can enhance and accelerate the healing process and reduce the risk of adverse effects associated with inflammation.

**Pain:** Modalities can assist with controlling pain by altering the origin of the pain or altering the process of pain perception.

**Restriction in motion:** Modalities are used to enhance extensibility of collagen to allow for greater range of motion and tolerance to stretch.

**Abnormal tone:** Modalities can influence tonal abnormalities that are due to pain, musculoskeletal pathology or neurological pathology. Alterations in nerve conduction, pain, and biomechanical properties of muscle can normalize tone and enhance functional outcomes.

## Principles of Heat Transfer[16,18]

Therapeutic modalities result in the transfer of heat to or from a patient's body. Heating agents transfer heat to the body, while cooling agents transfer heat away from the body. Methods of heat transfer include conduction, convection, conversion, evaporation, and radiation.

### Conduction

Conduction refers to the gain or loss of heat resulting from direct contact between two materials at different temperatures. Heat is conducted from a material of higher temperature to a material of lower temperature. Heat transfer continues until the temperature and speed of molecular movement of both materials become equal. The rate of heat transfer will accelerate when there is a large temperature difference between a heating or cooling agent and the body part being treated. Materials with high thermal conductivity transfer heat faster than those with low thermal conductivity. For example, water transfers heat faster than air since it possesses higher thermal conductivity. Metal has extremely high thermal conductivity, which is the rationale for removing all metal jewelry prior to initiating treatment with a conductive thermal agent.

Examples of modalities that utilize conduction include hot pack, cold pack, paraffin, ice massage, and Cryo Cuff.

### Convection

Convection refers to the gain or loss of heat resulting from air or water moving in a constant motion across the body. Since the thermal agent is in motion and new parts of the agent are constantly coming into contact with the target area, heating by convection is capable of transferring large amounts of heat. For example, blood circulating in the body maintains body temperature by convection. As a result, when circulation is compromised, the relative risk of thermal injury significantly increases.

Examples of modalities that utilize convection include fluidotherapy, hot whirlpool, and cold whirlpool.

### Conversion

Conversion refers to heating that occurs when nonthermal energy (e.g., mechanical, electrical) is absorbed into tissue and transformed into heat. The rate of heat transfer with conversion is determined by the power of the energy source. For example, the power of ultrasound would be determined by the selected intensity. Heating by conversion is not affected by the temperature of the thermal agent as it is with conduction and convection. Heat transfer does not require direct contact between the thermal agent and the target area, however, it does require a medium that allows transmission of the particular type of energy. In the case of ultrasound, the medium may be gel, lotion or water.

Examples of modalities that utilize conversion include diathermy and ultrasound.

### Evaporation

Evaporation refers to the transfer of heat that occurs as a liquid absorbs energy and changes form into a vapor. In the case of a vapocoolant spray, the liquid spray is applied to a patient's body. The vapocoolant spray is then heated by the warmer skin of the body, causing the liquid to change into a vapor. The evaporation of sweat is another example of this cooling phenomenon.

An example of a modality that utilizes evaporation is vapocoolant spray.

### Radiation

Radiation refers to the direct transfer of heat from a radiation energy source of higher temperature to one of cooler temperature. In order for heating by radiation to occur, there must be a difference in temperature between the energy source and the target area. This difference must exist without the energy source being in direct contact with the target area. The rate of heat transfer will be influenced by a number of factors including the intensity and size of the energy source, the target area, the angle of the radiation in relation to the target area, and the distance between the energy source and the target area.

Examples of modalities that utilize radiation include infrared lamp, laser, and ultraviolet light.

## Examples of Heat Transfer by Category

| Conduction | Convection | Conversion | Evaporation | Radiation |
|---|---|---|---|---|
| Cold pack | Cold whirlpool | Diathermy | Vapocoolant spray | Infrared lamp |
| Cryo Cuff | Fluidotherapy | Ultrasound | | Laser |
| Ice massage | Hot whirlpool | | | Ultraviolet light |
| Hot pack | | | | |
| Paraffin | | | | |

## Cryotherapy

Cryotherapy refers to the local or general use of low temperatures in rehabilitation. Cryotherapy generates therapeutic effects by influencing hemodynamic (e.g., blood flow), metabolic (e.g., metabolic rate), and neuromuscular processes (e.g., nerve conduction velocity). Common examples of modalities used for cryotherapy include ice massage, cold pack, cold bath, controlled cold compression unit, Cryo Cuff, and vapocoolant spray. The type of cryotherapeutic agent selected is influenced by numerous variables including the size of the target area, anatomical location, desired magnitude of cooling, and the patient's medical history.

### Therapeutic Effects[16,18]

- Decreased blood flow to the treatment area
- Decreased edema
- Decreased local temperature
- Decreased metabolic rate
- Decreased nerve conduction velocity
- Decreased tone
- Increased pain threshold

### Indications[16,18]

- Abnormal tone
- Acute or chronic pain
- Acute or subacute inflammation
- Bursitis
- Muscle spasm
- Musculoskeletal trauma
- Myofascial trigger points
- Tendonitis
- Tenosynovitis

### Contraindications[16,18]

- Cold intolerance
- Cold urticaria
- Cryoglobulinemia
- Infection
- Over an area of compromised circulation
- Over regenerating peripheral nerves
- Paroxysmal cold hemoglobinuria
- Peripheral vascular disease
- Raynaud's phenomenon
- Skin anesthesia

## Ice Massage

Ice massage is typically performed by freezing water in a paper cup and then applying the ice directly to the treatment area. A wooden tongue depressor can be frozen in water to form an ice popsicle. Ice massage is ideal for small or contoured areas and is easily integrated into a home exercise program. In addition to the anti-inflammatory effects, ice massage can be used as a stimulus to facilitate a desired motor response in patients with impaired motor control. In this scenario, ice is applied with direct pressure over a muscle belly for 3-5 seconds or quickly stroked over the targeted muscle belly to enhance contraction.[16]

**Fig. 9-36:** Using a towel to absorb excess water during ice massage.

Ice massage should be applied with the patient in a relaxed and comfortable position. Clothing and jewelry should be removed from the treatment area. The top third of the paper cup should be removed leaving the base of the cup covered for the therapist or patient to grip. A towel should be used to absorb dripping water as melting occurs. Ideally, the body part to be treated should also be elevated (Fig. 9-36).

The ice should be applied using small, overlapping circles or strokes. An area 10 cm by 15 cm can be covered in 5-10 minutes (Fig. 9-37).[17] Patients will typically progress through a series of unique sensations during ice massage including intense cold, burning, aching, and analgesia.[17] These sensations are thought to be caused by increased stimulation of thermal receptors and pain receptors, followed by blocking of sensory nerve conduction as the tissue temperature decreases.

Fig. 9-37: Ice massage being self administered.

Ice massage should continue until the patient reports analgesia. The exact amount of time for analgesia to occur will depend largely on the size of the treatment area, however, 5-10 minutes is typically adequate.[17] Maintaining skin temperature above 59 degrees Fahrenheit will minimize the risk of damaging tissue or producing frostbite.[16]

Ice massage typically cools tissues more rapidly than other types of cryotherapy, including an ice pack or ice bag. The therapist should inspect the skin during treatment and after the completion of treatment. Normally, the skin should appear to be red or dark pink. An abnormal response is most often noted by the presence of wheals or a rash.[16]

## Cold Pack

A cold pack typically contains silica gel and is available in a variety of shapes and sizes. The gel remains in a semisolid form even at relatively low temperatures, which allows the cold pack to conform to the contour of the body. Cold packs are typically

Fig. 9-38: A specialized cooling unit containing cold packs and cups for ice massage. Courtesy Chattanooga, a DJO Global Company.

stored in a specialized cooling unit at approximately 25 degrees Fahrenheit (Fig. 9-38).[17] Cold packs should be cooled for at least 30 minutes between uses and for two or more hours prior to the initial use.[17]

The therapist should thoroughly inspect the targeted area prior to initiating treatment. Clothing and jewelry should be removed from the treatment area. If edema is present, the involved extremity can be elevated. The cold pack should be applied over a moist, cold towel to increase the initial magnitude of cooling. (Fig. 9-39). The moist towel increases the conduction by minimizing the influence of air, which is a poor conductor.[17] Warm water can be used to moisten the towel when using a cold pack on a patient who is sensitive to cold, since it allows for a more gradual onset of cold. The cold pack can be applied using an elastic wrap to increase the surface contact between the cold pack and the target area. The patient should be given a bell or another type of call device in the event they need assistance during treatment.

A cold pack should be applied for approximately 20 minutes.[18] Applying a cold pack for this duration reduces the temperature of the skin and subcutaneous tissues up to two centimeters in depth. Additional treatment time may be necessary when applying the cold pack over bandages or other types of wraps to

Fig. 9-39: Application of a cold pack to a patient's shoulder.

allow the cold to adequately penetrate through the additional layers. The therapist should inspect the skin during and after the completion of treatment. Normally, the skin should appear red or dark pink. An abnormal response is most often noted by the presence of wheals or a rash.[16]

Cold packs can be applied every one to two hours for the reduction of inflammation and pain control. Patients can use a variety of substitute cryotherapeutic agents at home, such as a bag of frozen vegetables or a plastic bag filled with crushed ice.

Application may extend to 30 minutes if the treatment goal is spasticity reduction.[17] In this scenario, the skin would require inspection every ten minutes. Treatment beyond 20 minutes may require replacing the original cold pack.

## Cold Bath

A cold bath is commonly used for the immersion of the distal extremities. Unlike many other forms of cryotherapy, a cold bath allows for circumferential contact with the cooling agent. In the presence of edema, therapists should be mindful of the influence of a gravity-dependent position on the involved extremity during treatment.

A cold bath requires water temperature ranging from 55-64 degrees Fahrenheit.[19] A whirlpool or container of water with crushed ice can be used (Fig. 9-40). The body part should be immersed for 15-20 minutes to attain the desired therapeutic effects.[19] The lower the temperature selected, the shorter the duration of treatment. The intervention is often used as a component of a home exercise program.

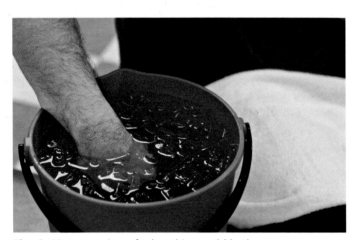

Fig. 9-40: Immersion of a hand in a cold bath.

## Controlled Cold Compression Unit

A controlled cold compression unit circulates cooled water through a sleeve that is applied to an extremity. The water can be maintained at temperatures ranging from 50-77 degrees Fahrenheit.[19] Compression is applied intermittently by inflating the sleeve with air with the goal of controlling inflammation and reducing edema in the extremity. In post-operative situations, the sleeve may be placed on the patient's involved extremity immediately after surgery. The combined use of cold and compression is more effective than cold or compression alone in controlling inflammation.[18]

## Cryo Cuff

A Cryo Cuff is a cold water circulating unit that combines the benefits of cold with compression. The Cryo Cuff consists of a nylon sleeve that is connected to a specialized gallon container via a plastic tube. Water from the container flows via gravity into the sleeve when the gallon container is elevated approximately 15-18 inches above the level of the sleeve (Fig. 9-41). This action provides cooling from the cold water and compression from the increased pressure in the sleeve. The water is drained from the sleeve via gravity by placing the container below the level of the sleeve (Fig. 9-42). The water in the container must be recooled periodically in order to maintain the desired therapeutic temperature.

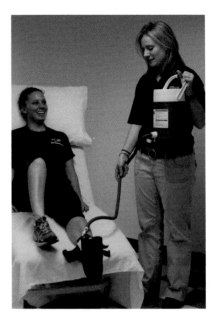

Fig. 9-41: Filling an ankle Cryo Cuff.

The device can provide hours of mild cooling at levels far below the intensity of other cryotherapeutic agents, such as ice massage or cold packs.[20] The Cryo Cuff is most commonly used on the knee, however, it is available for a number of other areas of the body including the shoulder and the ankle. The device is commonly employed post-operatively with the goal of decreasing pain and the need for analgesic medications.

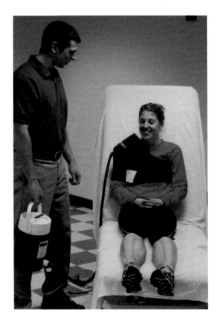

Fig. 9-42: Draining water from a shoulder Cryo Cuff.

# Consider This

## Cryotherapy Agents - Advantages and Disadvantages[16,17,18]

There are a variety of cryotherapy agents that provide similar therapeutic effects. Therapists should consider the nuances associated with the patient's current condition, as well as the advantages and disadvantages of each cryotherapy agent, when selecting an appropriate mode of intervention.

The following table illustrates several advantages and disadvantages of commonly used cryotherapy agents.

| Cryotherapy Agent | Advantages | Disadvantages |
|---|---|---|
| Ice massage | Effective for small or irregular areas<br>Target area can be observed during treatment<br>Short duration of treatment<br>Available for home use | Intensity of cooling may not be tolerated by the patient<br>Time consuming for large areas<br>Requires active participation from the therapist or patient |
| Cold pack | Covers moderate to large areas<br>Can be applied in conjunction with elevation<br>Available for home use | May not maintain good contact on small or severely contoured areas<br>Patient may not tolerate the weight of the pack<br>Difficult to observe target area directly during treatment |
| Cold bath | Effective for cooling the distal extremities<br>Allows for circumferential contact with water<br>Available for home use | Requires the extremity to remain in a gravity-dependent position |
| Controlled cold compression unit | Allows simultaneous application of cold and compression<br>Temperature and compression force can be accurately controlled<br>Can be combined with other interventions, such as electrotherapy | Difficult to observe target area directly during treatment<br>Limited to extremity use |
| Cryo Cuff | Allows simultaneous application of cold and compression<br>Provides hours of mild cooling<br>Available for home use | Difficult to precisely control temperature and compression force |
| Vapocoolant spray | Localized area of application<br>Brief duration of cooling<br>Effectively treats trigger points<br>Increases range of motion | Difficult to apply spray uniformly<br>Risk of frostbite if skin is not rewarmed between repeated treatments<br>Limited in scope of use |

## Vapocoolant Spray[16,18,20]

A vapocoolant spray produces rapid cooling through evaporation, with temperature changes occurring superficially in the epidermis. This therapeutic modality is most commonly used in the treatment of trigger points, which are described as deep and hypersensitive, localized spots in a muscle that cause a referred pain pattern. Vapocoolant sprays produce a counter-irritant stimulus to the cutaneous thermal afferent nerves that overlay the muscles. This causes a reduction in motor neuron activity and a decrease in the resistance to stretch. This may break the pain cycle and allow the muscle to be stretched to its normal length.

The use of vapocoolant spray to treat trigger points is often termed "spray and stretch" based on the work of Janet Travell. When using spray and stretch, therapists should identify the trigger point and make three to four sweeps with the spray in the direction of the muscle fibers. The spray must be applied in one direction only and not in a back and forth motion. Special care must be taken to cover the patient's eyes, nose, and mouth if spraying near the face. The spray should be applied at a 30 degree angle at a distance of 12-18 inches from the skin.

Stretching should begin while applying the spray and continue after the spray has been applied (Fig. 9-43).[18] Repeated applications during the same treatment are safe if the skin is rewarmed between applications.

When using vapocoolant sprays to increase range of motion without the presence of trigger points, the spray is applied along the muscle from the proximal to the distal attachment. Clinical conditions that may respond to treatment with vapocoolant sprays include torticollis, neck or low back pain caused by muscle spasm, acute bursitis, and hamstrings tightness.

**Fig. 9-43:** Vapocoolant spray applied to the right upper quadrant.

## Superficial Thermotherapy

Superficial thermotherapy refers to the local or general use of high temperatures in rehabilitation with the goal of increasing skin temperature and superficial subcutaneous tissue to depths of up to two centimeters. Superficial thermotherapy generates therapeutic effects by influencing hemodynamic (e.g., blood flow), metabolic (e.g., metabolic rate), and neuromuscular pro-

cesses (e.g., nerve conduction velocity). Common examples of modalities used for superficial thermotherapy include hot packs, warm water baths, fluidotherapy, infrared lamp, and paraffin. Relative changes in skin temperature and superficial subcutaneous tissue will be influenced by the intensity of the heating agent, duration of the exposure, and thermal conductivity of the tissues.

### Therapeutic Effects[16,18]

- Decreased muscle spasm
- Decreased tone
- Increased blood flow to the treatment area
- Increased capillary permeability
- Increased collagen extensibility

- Increased local temperature
- Increased metabolic rate
- Increased muscle elasticity
- Increased nerve conduction velocity
- Increased pain threshold

### Indications[16,18]

- Abnormal tone
- Decreased range of motion
- Muscle guarding
- Muscle spasm

- Myofascial trigger points
- Subacute or chronic pain
- Subacute or chronic inflammatory conditions

### Contraindications[16,18]

- Acute musculoskeletal trauma
- Arterial disease
- Bleeding or hemorrhage
- Over an area of compromised circulation

- Over an area of malignancy
- Peripheral vascular disease
- Thrombophlebitis

## Hot Packs

A hot pack consists of a canvas or nylon-covered pack filled with bentonite, a hydrophilic silicate gel that provides a moist heat. The size and shape of the hot pack varies depending on the size and contour of the treatment area. A standard size hot pack measures 12 inches by 12 inches and is used for the majority of body segments. A double size hot pack measures 24 inches by 24 inches and is generally used for the low back or buttocks. A cervical hot pack measures 6 inches by 18 inches.

Hot packs transmit heat to the body through conduction, since hot packs have a much higher temperature than the surface of the skin. The primary therapeutic effects include decreased pain, increased tissue extensibility, and reduced muscle spasm. A hot pack is easy to use, inexpensive, and can cover large areas. Limitations of hot packs include the need for close monitoring of the skin, the inability to maintain total contact in contoured areas, and the patient's inability to move during treatment.

Hot packs are stored in water between 158 and 167 degrees Fahrenheit.[16] The water is housed in a thermostatically controlled container that maintains the water at a relatively constant

Fig. 9-44: Hot pack removal from a hydrocollator unit using tongs.

temperature. The hot pack should be removed from the container with tongs due to the high water temperature (Fig. 9-44). The therapist should thoroughly inspect the target area prior to initiating treatment. Clothing and jewelry should be removed from the target area. Application requires six to eight layers of towels between the hot pack and skin.[16] If commercial hot pack covers are used, they typically are equivalent to two to three layers of towels.

The hot pack should be applied on top of the treatment area. The therapist should not permit the patient to lie on top of the hot pack since this action tends to remove some of the water from the hot pack, which can result in an accelerated rate of heating and an increased risk for burns. In addition, lying directly on the hot pack can reduce local circulation through compression of vessels resulting in reduced circulatory convective cooling.[17] If a patient cannot tolerate the weight of the hot pack directly on the target area (e.g., the low back while positioned in prone), the hot pack can be applied in sidelying with a strap or tied sheet.

The patient should feel a mild to moderate heating sensation from the hot pack.[17] Skin checks for excessive redness, blistering or other signs of a burn are required after five minutes (Fig. 9-45). The treatment area of fair-skinned individuals may turn bright pink or red, while darker-skinned individuals may exhibit areas of lighter or darker color. The maximum surface temperature is reached within 6-8 minutes, making it critical to perform frequent skin checks during the first 10 minutes of treatment.[17] The patient should be given a bell or another type of call device in the event that they need assistance during treatment.

Hot packs require approximately 15-20 minutes to achieve the desired effects.[18] If a patient reports that the heat is too intense, the therapist may elect to add towel layers. If the patient reports insufficient warming, the therapist may elect to remove towels prior to administering a hot pack at the next treatment session.

Towels should not be removed during the current session since the increased skin temperature may diminish the patient's thermal sensitivity and the ability to accurately assess the intensity of the heat. A hot pack can take up to two hours to initially heat in the hydrocollator unit and 30 minutes to reheat after use.

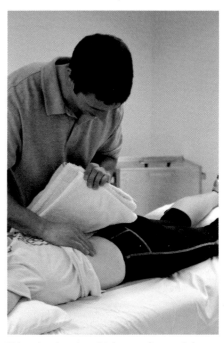

Fig. 9-45: Skin checks should be performed frequently when using hot packs.

## Fluidotherapy

Fluidotherapy consists of a container that circulates warm air and small cellulose particles (Fig. 9-46). The superficial heating modality generates dry heat through forced convection. The dry cellulose medium does not irritate the skin and allows for higher treatment temperatures than hydrotherapy. Fluidotherapy units come in a variety of sizes and shapes and are most often used to treat the distal extremities.

The therapist must thoroughly inspect the area to be treated and have the patient remove all clothing and jewelry. The extremity is placed into the container and a protective shield is applied to prevent the escape of the cellulose particles. Direct contact between the skin and the cellulose particles is desired since this will maximize heat transfer. Open wounds should be covered with a plastic barrier to prevent the cellulose particles from becoming embedded in the wound bed.

The fluidotherapy unit contains a separate portal that provides the therapist with access to the extremity during treatment. The temperature should be set between 100-118 degrees Fahrenheit.[16] The maximum temperature rise during treatment occurs after approximately 15 minutes. Treatment time is usually 15-20 minutes.[18] The level of agitation (i.e., air speed) can be controlled for patient comfort or for use as part of a desensitization program. Some units provide other treatment options including the ability to preheat or select a pulse mode. The therapeutic effects of fluidotherapy include the promotion of tissue healing, skin desensitization, and edema management.

**Fig. 9-46:** A fluidotherapy unit. Courtesy Chattanooga, a DJO Global Company.

Heated air is circulated in the unit causing cellulose particles to become suspended and move rapidly within the unit. The result is a fluidized bed of cellulose particles that take on the properties of a liquid. Patients often report that the body part feels like it is suspended in a moving liquid. Patients can perform active exercise of the distal extremity during treatment, however, therapists should avoid placing the extremity in a gravity-dependent position whenever possible.[19]

### Infrared Lamp

An infrared lamp produces superficial heating of tissue through radiant heat. Infrared radiation has a wavelength that lies between visible light and microwaves on the electromagnetic spectrum. Infrared lamps used in the clinical setting have a wavelength ranging from 780 to 1500 nanometers.[16] The majority of infrared radiation is absorbed within the first few millimeters of human tissue. Human skin allows maximum penetration of infrared radiation with a wavelength of 1200 nm.[16]

Infrared allows for constant observation of the skin since it does not require contact with the treatment area. The main therapeutic effect is the enhancement of soft tissue healing. The amount of tissue temperature increase is directly proportional to the amount of radiation that penetrates the tissue. The amount of radiation is influenced by the power and wavelength of the radiation, the distance of the radiation source from the target area, the angle of incidence, and the absorption coefficient of the target area.[16]

The therapist must thoroughly inspect the area to be treated and have the patient remove all clothing and jewelry. Opaque goggles should be worn by the therapist and the patient to avoid potential irradiation of the eyes. The patient should be positioned approximately 20 inches from the source to produce a comfortable level of warmth.[18] Protective toweling should be applied to tissues outside of the target area. Optimal absorption occurs when the infrared radiation strikes perpendicular to the target area. Darker tissue absorbs more radiation than lighter tissue.

The therapist should record the distance from the infrared lamp to the target area. The patient should be periodically monitored during the session and instructed to avoid moving closer or further away from the lamp since this will alter the amount of radiation reaching the target area. Treatment duration is generally 15-30 minutes and is influenced by the distance from the infrared lamp to the target area.[16] Infrared radiation tends to dry the skin more than other superficial heating agents and results in uneven heating when the target area is nonuniform.

### Paraffin

Paraffin wax is a commonly used heating source for the distal extremities. There are several internal characteristics of paraffin that make it an effective superficial heating agent. Paraffin has a low melting point that can be lowered further by adding mineral oil. As a result, paraffin can provide a more even distribution of heat to areas, such as the fingers and toes. Secondly, paraffin has a low specific heat, that enhances a patient's ability to tolerate heat from paraffin compared to heat from water at the same temperature.

Therapists must have patients remove jewelry and thoroughly wash the body part being treated to minimize the chance of paraffin bath contamination. Paraffin cannot be applied to areas with open wounds or infected skin lesions. The temperature of the paraffin mixture should be maintained between 113 and 122 degrees Fahrenheit.[16]

There are three methods of paraffin application: dip-wrap, dip-reimmersion, and paint application.

**Fig. 9-47:** Application of a plastic wrap to the hand following paraffin application.

**Dip-wrap:** The patient is required to maintain a static position as the distal extremity dips into the paraffin bath and is removed. After waiting briefly for the paraffin to harden, the extremity should be redipped 6-10 times and then immediately placed into a plastic bag (Fig. 9-47).[16] A towel should be wrapped around the bag to slow the paraffin cooling. The paraffin should be left in place for 10-15 minutes.[16]

**Dip-reimmersion:** After the initial 6-10 dips, the distal extremity should remain in the paraffin bath for the duration of treatment. The paraffin unit should be turned off during the treatment session to prevent the sides and the bottom of the unit from becoming too hot. It may also be necessary to use a temperature closer to the lower limit (i.e., 113 degrees Fahrenheit) since the affected extremity will remain in the bath for up to 20 minutes.[16]

**Paint application:** The paint method is used for body parts that cannot be immersed into the paraffin bath. A layer of paraffin is painted on the body with a brush. After a few seconds, 6-10 additional layers are applied. The area is then covered by a plastic bag or plastic wrap with a towel wrapped around it as described in the dip-wrap method. The paraffin should be left in place for approximately 20 minutes.[16]

Removal of the paraffin is the same for all forms of application. Paraffin should be peeled off after treatment and either placed back into the container to melt or discarded.[18] A paraffin bath can be reused unless it becomes contaminated. Some paraffin units have the ability to elevate the temperature to 212 degrees Fahrenheit, which will destroy bacteria that can grow in the paraffin.[18] In the absence of contamination, the contents of the paraffin bath must be changed at least every six months.

# Consider This

## Documentation of Therapeutic Modalities

The primary purpose of physical therapy patient care documentation is to communicate relevant information to other health care providers who are concurrently treating the same patient. The failure to document relevant patient care information in a clear, objective, and timely manner can result in professional negligence.

Documentation of therapeutic modalities must provide other health care providers with a clear understanding of the intervention performed and the associated parameters used. Appropriate documentation will allow another therapist treating the same patient to perform the identical intervention.

**Relevant information when documenting therapeutic modalities includes:**

- Body part to be treated (e.g., knee, anterior thigh, low back)
- Modality used (e.g., ultrasound, TENS)
- Patient position (e.g., supine with legs elevated, prone with two pillows under the waist)
- Treatment duration (e.g., 10 minutes, 20 minutes)
- Parameters (e.g., intensity, duty cycle, pulse rate)
- Patient response to treatment (e.g., skin color, pain level, sensitivity)
- Outcome measure (e.g., goniometry, circumferential measurements, visual analog pain scale)

**The following is an example of a documented ultrasound treatment in S.O.A.P. note format. Abbreviations were not used in the S.O.A.P. note below to increase clarity.**

**S:** Patient reports the absence of knee pain during a recent exercise session.

**O:** Ultrasound to the anterior midline of the knee over the peri-patellar tendon region at 0.5 W/cm$^2$, pulsed 20% duty cycle, 7 minutes.

**A:** Patient tolerated treatment without adverse effects.

**P:** Continue ultrasound treatment as described for three additional sessions. Continue to increase the intensity of exercise activities.

## Deep Thermotherapy

Deep thermotherapy refers to the local or general use of energy (i.e., sound, electromagnetic) in rehabilitation with the goal of increasing tissue temperature.[16,18] Deep heating agents are capable of heating to depths of three to five centimeters.[21] Deep thermotherapy generates therapeutic effects by influencing mechanical (e.g., microstreaming), muscular (e.g., muscle heating), connective tissue (e.g., tendon, ligament), hemodynamic (e.g., blood flow), metabolic (e.g., metabolic rate), and neuromuscular processes (e.g., nerve conduction velocity).[16,18] Common examples of modalities used for deep thermotherapy include ultrasound and diathermy.

Relative changes in tissue temperature will be influenced by the intensity of the heating agent, the duration of the exposure, and the thermal conductivity of the tissues.

## Ultrasound

Ultrasound is a common deep heating agent that transfers heat through conversion, and elevates tissue temperature to depths up to five centimeters (Fig. 9-48). The modality uses high frequency acoustic mechanical vibrations to produce thermal and nonthermal effects. Ultrasound has a frequency above 20,000 hertz (Hz).[16] Therapeutic ultrasound typically has a frequency between 0.75 and 3 megahertz (MHz).[18]

Fig. 9-48: An ultrasound machine. Courtesy Chattanooga, a DJO Global Company.

An ultrasound machine uses an alternating electrical current, generated at the same frequency as the crystal resonance, to create a mechanical vibration of the piezoelectric crystal located in the transducer. This action converts electrical energy to acoustic energy and generates ultrasound at the desired frequency.

### Thermal effects[16,18]

Thermal effects of ultrasound include acceleration of metabolic rate, modulation of pain, reduction of muscle spasm, decreased joint stiffness, alteration of nerve conduction velocity, increased circulation, and increased soft tissue extensibility. The extent of the thermal effects are dependent on the intensity, duration, and frequency selected.

### Nonthermal effects[16,18]

Nonthermal effects of ultrasound include increased cell and skin membrane permeability, increased intracellular calcium levels, facilitation of tissue repair, and promotion of normal cell function. The nonthermal effects occur as a result of cavitation and acoustic microstreaming.

## Indications[16,18]

- Acute and post-acute conditions (ultrasound with nonthermal effects)
- Calcium deposits
- Chronic inflammation
- Delayed soft tissue healing
- Dermal ulcers
- Joint contracture
- Muscle spasm
- Myofascial trigger points
- Pain
- Plantar warts
- Scar tissue
- Tissue regeneration

## Contraindications[16,18]

- Acute and post-acute conditions (ultrasound with thermal effects)
- Areas of active bleeding
- Areas of decreased temperature sensation
- Areas of decreased circulation
- Deep vein thrombosis
- Infection
- Malignancy
- Over breast implants
- Over carotid sinus or cervical ganglia
- Over epiphyseal areas in young children
- Over eyes, heart, and genitalia
- Over methylmethacrylate cement or plastic
- Over pelvic, lumbar or abdominal areas in pregnant women
- Over a pacemaker
- Thrombophlebitis
- Vascular insufficiency

Fig. 9-49: Coupling agents used with ultrasound.

Cavitation refers to the formation of gas-filled bubbles that expand and compress secondary to pressure changes caused by ultrasound.[18] Cavitation can be classified as stable or unstable. During stable cavitation, the bubbles oscillate in size in response to pressure changes, but do not burst. During unstable cavitation, the bubbles change in size over several cycles and then suddenly burst. Unstable cavitation is possible with high intensity, low frequency ultrasound, however, it does not typically occur with therapeutic ultrasound. Acoustic microstreaming refers to the unidirectional movement of fluids along the boundaries of cell membranes caused by ultrasound.[18]

## Ultrasound Parameters

### Technique

A transducer housing a piezoelectric crystal is used to administer ultrasound. Transducers vary in size, but most often range from 5-10 cm[2]. Ultrasound waves do not travel through air and, as a result, a coupling agent is required. Coupling agents are designed to decrease acoustical impedance by eliminating as much air as possible between the transducer and the target area. Coupling agents can be direct or indirect and include gels, gel pads, mineral oil, water, and lotions (Fig. 9-49).

Direct coupling agents (e.g., gel, lotion) should be applied to the treatment area and the transducer before the power is turned on. The face of the transducer must be parallel with the surface of the skin so that ultrasound waves will be introduced at a 90 degree angle.[18] Failure to maintain the integrity of the transducer-skin interface will result in a large percentage of the ultrasound energy being reflected and may damage the ultrasound's piezoelectric crystal.

**Fig. 9-50:** Ultrasound applied to the dorsal surface of the forearm.

Indirect coupling agents are often employed when the treatment area is excessively small, irregularly shaped or unable to tolerate direct pressure from the transducer. Water immersion is an indirect coupling method requiring the treatment area to be immersed in a basin of water (Fig. 9-52). The basin should be made of rubber or plastic to minimize the amount of reflection present with metals. The transducer should be moved parallel to the treatment surface at a distance of 0.5 - 3.0 centimeters away from the skin.[21] Air bubbles occurring on the transducer and the patient's skin should be wiped away by the therapist since they

will interfere with ultrasound transmission.[17] Increased intensity, as much as 50%, may be necessary when using the underwater technique due to dispersion and ultrasound energy absorption by the water. Other methods of indirect coupling include gel or water-filled bladders and gel pads. This type of indirect coupling is often referred to as "cushion contact."

Administration of ultrasound can occur with a stationary or moving (i.e., dynamic) technique (Fig. 9-50). The stationary technique is used sparingly in clinical practice due to the potential for uneven heating and other undesirable effects, such as subjective reports of pain or tissue damage. Justification for use of the stationary technique may include a very small treatment area or when pulsed ultrasound is used with low intensity. When using a moving technique the transducer should be moved slowly in a small, rhythmical pattern. Longitudinal stroking or overlapping circular motions are the most common application method (Fig. 9-51). The transducer should be moved at an approximate rate of 4 centimeters per second.[16]

### Intensity

Intensity measures the quantity of energy delivered per unit area. The power generated from ultrasound is not uniform and therefore, some portions of the ultrasound beam are more intense than others as it leaves the transducer. Effective radiating area (ERA) refers to the area of the transducer that transmits ultrasound energy.[16] The ERA is always smaller than the total size of the transducer head. Spatial-averaged intensity refers to the intensity of the ultrasound beam averaged over the area of the transducer.[18] It is computed by dividing the power output in watts by the total effective radiating area of the soundhead in cm[2]. Spatial-averaged intensity is labeled as intensity on an ultrasound unit and is expressed in watts per square centimeter (W/cm[2]). Spatial-peak intensity refers to the intensity of the ultrasound beam at its highest point.[18]

**Fig. 9-51:** Ultrasound applied to the posterior knee region combined with gravity assisted passive stretching.

Beam nonuniformity ratio (BNR) is the ratio between the spatial-peak intensity and spatial-averaged intensity. The BNR is derived from the intrinsic factors and quality of the piezoelectric crystal. The higher the quality of the crystal, the lower the BNR. A lower BNR is more favorable since patients will be less likely to experience hot spots and discomfort during treatment.[20] The BNR of an ultrasound unit is required to be listed on the device for consumer education and awareness. BNR values should range between 2:1 and 8:1, however, most devices often fall in the 5:1 or 6:1 range.[1] The higher the beam nonuniformity ratio, the more critical it is to move the transducer more rapidly to avoid undesirable effects, such as pain, caused by periosteal irritation.[16]

### Frequency

Frequency is the primary determinant in the depth of ultrasound penetration. Attenuation is a term that describes the inevitable decrease in energy intensity as the ultrasound travels through various tissues. Tissues that are high in water content, such as blood plasma, have a low rate of absorption while more dense tissues high in protein, such as bone, have a high rate of absorption.[18]

Ultrasound delivered at a higher frequency is absorbed more rapidly than ultrasound delivered at a lower frequency. As a result, ultrasound at higher frequencies affects more superficial tissues, and ultrasound at lower frequencies affects deeper tissues. A frequency setting of 1 MHz is used for deeper tissues (up to five centimeters) while a setting of 3 MHz is used for more superficial tissues (one to two centimeters).[18]

### Duty Cycle

Ultrasound can be administered using a continuous or pulsed mode. In continuous mode, ultrasound intensity remains constant throughout the treatment. In pulsed mode, the ultrasound intensity is periodically interrupted. The portion of treatment time that ultrasound is generated during the entire treatment is referred to as the duty cycle.

$$\text{Duty cycle} = \frac{\text{on time}}{\text{on time} + \text{off time}} \quad (*100)$$

Duty cycle is calculated by dividing the time sound is delivered (on time) by the total time (on time + off time).[17] For example, if the on time was 1 msec and the off time was 4 msec, the duty cycle would be 20%.

Continuous ultrasound (i.e., 100% duty cycle) generates constant ultrasound waves producing thermal effects at higher intensities and nonthermal effects at lower intensities. Continuous ultrasound is more effective in elevating tissue temperature, while pulsed ultrasound minimizes the thermal effects.

Pulsed ultrasound with a duty cycle of 20% generates ultrasound 20% of the total treatment time (on time + off time). Pulsed ultrasound results in a reduced average heating of the tissues and is therefore used primarily for nonthermal effects. When using pulsed ultrasound for nonthermal effects, most resources recommend a 20% or lower duty cycle.

The duty cycle impacts the total quantity of energy generated. Ultrasound using a pulsed mode requires an intensity measure that takes the duty cycle into consideration. Spatial-temporal averaged intensity refers to the ultrasound beam averaged over the on time and off time of the pulse.[16] This measure allows therapists to compare energy outputs between continuous and pulsed ultrasound, however, it is not frequently used in clinical practice. Instead, therapists often describe the intensity based on the spatial-averaged intensity and then specify a duty cycle.

**Fig. 9-52:** Ultrasound applied to the dorsal surface of the foot using water immersion.

### Duration

Duration of ultrasound is determined based on a number of variables including the size of the treatment area, the depth of penetration, and the desired therapeutic effects. An area two to three times the size of the transducer typically requires a duration of five minutes.[17,18] Longer duration may be necessary when using lower intensities or lower frequencies or when the therapeutic objective is higher tissue temperatures. Ultrasound should not be used to treat areas larger than four times the effective radiating area (ERA) of the transducer. Areas larger than this would require excessively long treatment times making the application of ultrasound impractical.

### Number of Treatments

The number of ultrasound treatments is primarily dependent on the established therapeutic objectives, the level of acuity, and the patient response. Ultrasound using thermal effects is usually applied later in the healing process and is most commonly administered two to three times a week. Ultrasound using nonthermal effects is usually applied earlier in the healing process, as frequently as once a day. A positive response to ultrasound should be evident within three sessions. Failure to observe a desired response within this time frame provides justification to change the ultrasound parameters or select an alternate intervention. Research has indicated that more than 14 ultrasound treatments within a single episode of care can reduce red and white blood cell counts.[18]

### Patient Safety and Effectiveness

Safe and effective ultrasound treatment is dependent on the therapist's ability to identify relevant contraindications to ultrasound and select appropriate treatment parameters. The therapist must comfortably position the patient and seek feedback from the patient throughout the course of treatment. The therapist should periodically inspect the patient's skin during treatment and attempt to determine the relative effect of the intervention. The effectiveness of ultrasound can be assessed through a variety of subjective and objective measures. Examples of positive findings include decreased pain, diminished tenderness to palpation, increased range of motion, and enhanced functional levels.

Ultrasound units must be inspected by qualified personnel at the manufacturer's recommended interval or minimally on an annual basis. Many of the parameters, including intensity output, must conform to established performance standards.

### Phonophoresis

Phonophoresis describes the use of ultrasound for the transdermal delivery of medication. Ultrasound enhances the distribution of medication through the skin, provides a high concentration of the drug directly to the treatment site, and avoids risks that may be associated with the injection of medication.[18] Medications regularly used in phonophoresis include anti-inflammatory agents and analgesics. Phonophoresis can be used with both continuous and pulsed techniques. Phonophoresis is not likely to produce burns or damage skin since the technique transports whole molecules instead of ions into the body's tissue (i.e., iontophoresis). Therapists using phonophoresis must carefully select coupling agents that are effective conductors of acoustic energy and are compatible with the medication selected. There is a limited amount of evidence in the literature that supports the efficacy of phonophoresis.

## Diathermy

Diathermy is a deep heating agent that converts high frequency electromagnetic energy into therapeutic heat (Fig. 9-53). Electrical energy produces a molecular vibration within tissue that generates heat and elevates tissue temperature.

**Fig. 9-53:** A diathermy unit. Courtesy Chattanooga, a DJO Global Company.

## Therapeutic Effects[16,18]

- Altered cell membrane function
- Increased collagen extensibility
- Increased edema
- Increased metabolic rate
- Increased muscle elasticity
- Increased nerve conduction velocity
- Increased pain threshold
- Increased temperature
- Vasodilation

## Indications[16,18]

- Bursitis
- Chronic inflammation
- Chronic inflammatory pelvic disease
- Decreased collagen extensibility
- Degenerative joint disease
- Increased metabolism
- Joint stiffness
- Muscle guarding
- Myofascial trigger points
- Pain
- Peripheral nerve regeneration
- Tissue healing

## Contraindications[16,18]

- Acute infection
- Acute inflammation
- Cardiac pacemaker
- Hemophilia
- Internal and external metal objects
- Intrauterine device
- Ischemic tissue
- Low back, abdomen or pelvis of a pregnant woman
- Malignant area
- Moist wound dressing
- Over a hemorrhagic region
- Over the eyes
- Over the testes
- Pain and temperature sensory deficits

Shortwave diathermy can be delivered in a continuous or pulsed mode. A pulsed mode is typically utilized to attain nonthermal effects while a continuous mode is used for thermal effects. Pulsed diathermy is produced by discontinuing the output of continuous shortwave diathermy at regular intervals. The output during the on time is adequate to produce tissue heating, however, the length of the off time allows the heat to dissipate.

The most common frequency used for shortwave diathermy is 27.12 MHz.[17] Shortwave diathermy can utilize a capacitance technique or inductance technique. Capacitive plate applicators produce a high frequency electrical current that alternates between the plates. The patient becomes part of the electrical circuit and the oscillation of ions increases tissue temperature.

Inductive coil applicators utilize a coil that generates alternating electric current, creates a magnetic field perpendicular to the coil, and produces eddy currents within the tissues. Eddy currents cause the oscillation of ions that increase tissue temperature. Inductive coil applicators are bundled as cables that wrap around an extremity or as a drum applicator.

# Consider This

## Heating Agents - Advantages and Disadvantages[16,17,18]

Therapists should consider the nuances associated with the patient's current condition and the advantages and disadvantages of each heating agent when selecting an appropriate intervention.

The following table illustrates several advantages and disadvantages of commonly used heating agents.

| Heating Agent | Advantages | Disadvantages |
|---|---|---|
| Fluidotherapy | Temperature and agitation of the dry particles can be controlled<br>Patient can perform active exercise during treatment<br>Minimal pressure applied to the treatment area<br>Can be used for desensitization of distal extremities | Constant heat source can result in overheating<br>Some patients are intolerant of the dry particles and the enclosed container<br>Some units require the extremity to be in a dependent position |
| Hot pack | Moist, comfortable heat<br>Variety of shapes and sizes<br>Available for home use | May not maintain good contact on small or contoured areas<br>Patient may not tolerate the weight of the pack<br>Difficult to observe target area directly during treatment |
| Infared lamp | Target area can be observed during treatment<br>Does not require direct contact with the treatment area | Difficult to ensure uniform heating in all treatment areas<br>Difficult to localize to a specific treatment area<br>Tends to dry the skin more than other superficial heating agents |
| Paraffin | Low specific heat allows for application at higher temperatures than water<br>Low thermal conductivity allows for slower heating of tissues which reduces the risk of overheating<br>Maintains good contact with contoured areas<br>Oils used in the wax add moisture to the skin | Effective only in distal extremities<br>Risk of cross-contamination if the paraffin is reused<br>Cannot be used over an open skin lesion |
| Diathermy | Capable of reaching deeper tissues<br>Can produce thermal and nonthermal effects<br>Covers large areas<br>Heat is applied in a more uniform fashion since the application is performed statically<br>Rate of tissue cooling is slower than other deep heating agents | Difficult to target small treatment areas effectively<br>Requires patient to subjectively classify their heat sensation response<br>Relatively large number of contraindications |
| Ultrasound | Capable of reaching deeper tissues<br>Can produce thermal and nonthermal effects<br>Amount of energy delivered per unit area can be quantified<br>Covers small areas effectively<br>Short duration of treatment | May not maintain good contact on small or contoured areas causing uneven heating<br>Patient may not tolerate direct contact with the ultrasound transducer<br>Rate of tissue cooling is faster than other deep heating agents |

## Capacitive Plate Method[16]

- Metal encased in a plastic housing produces an electric field from one plate to the other
- Field radiation consists of a strong electrical field and a weak magnetic field
- Heating pattern is superficial with the majority of energy absorbed within the skin
- Application is generally over areas of low fat content

## Inductive Coil Method[16]

- Rigid metal encased coil produces a magnetic field perpendicular to the coil
- Field radiation consists of a strong magnetic field and a weak electrical field
- Heating pattern is deeper with the majority of energy absorbed within the deeper structures (i.e., tissues with the highest electrical conductivity, such as muscle and synovial fluid)
- Application is generally over areas of high water content

A therapist should first select the most appropriate diathermy technique and device based on patient examination. The patient must remove all metal and jewelry in the area surrounding the treatment site. The therapist should position the patient and clean and dry the patient's skin thoroughly. Nonmetal clothing does not need to be removed before treatment since the magnetic fields will penetrate through clothing, however, when using continuous mode, clothes should be removed so that sweat can be absorbed with towels.

When using an inductive applicator, the therapist must wrap the coils around the extremity that has been covered by a towel. When using a drum, the therapist should place the drum directly over the treatment area. When using a capacitive applicator, place the two plates over both sides of the treatment area ensuring equal distance from the plates to the skin (2-10 centimeters).[16] The patient must remain in the same position throughout treatment for complete and consistent heating.

The amount of energy delivered and corresponding temperature increase can be variable with continuous diathermy. As a result, therapists need to rely on the patient's subjective heat sensation response. The following dosage guidelines are commonly used in clinical practice.

**Dose I** – No sensation of heat

**Dose II** – Mild heating sensation

**Dose III** – Moderate heating sensation

**Dose IV** – Vigorous heating that is tolerable below the pain threshold

The patient should have a call bell and should be checked within the first few minutes of treatment. Treatment time with diathermy is approximately 20 minutes for thermal effects and may last as long as 30-60 minutes for nonthermal effects.[16]

Diathermy is not used as commonly as other therapeutic modalities, however, there are several scenarios where the use of diathermy may be particularly beneficial. These include when an increase in temperature is required at tissue depths greater than those achieved with superficial heating agents and when the target area will not tolerate direct contact from a thermal agent.

Diathermy also offers several potential advantages compared to ultrasound. Diathermy can effectively heat surfaces of up to 25 times the size of a typical ultrasound transducer.[18] Heat is applied to the target area in a more uniform fashion with diathermy since the application is performed statically. In addition, the rate of tissue cooling following heating with diathermy is significantly slower than the rate of tissue cooling with ultrasound. As a result, the therapist has additional time to perform interventions that are enhanced by the increased tissue temperature (e.g., stretching).

## Additional Physical Agents

## Ultraviolet Light

Ultraviolet light is a form of energy that is used therapeutically and is divided into UV-A, UV-B, and UV-C according to wavelength and location on the electromagnetic spectrum.[17] Ultraviolet light is absorbed one to two millimeters into the skin and is most commonly used to treat skin disorders.

## Therapeutic Effects[16,18]

- Bacteriocidal effects
- Exfoliation
- Facilitate healing
- Increased pigmentation
- Thickening of the epidermis
- Vitamin D production

## Indications[16,18]

- Acne
- Chronic ulcer/wound
- Osteomalacia
- Psoriasis
- Sinusitis
- Vitamin D deficiency

## Contraindications[16,18]

- Areas receiving radiation
- Diabetes mellitus
- Herpes simplex
- Pellagra
- Photosensitive medications
- Skin cancer
- Systemic lupus erythematosus
- Tuberculosis

## Ultraviolet Dosage

The ultraviolet dosage is classified according to the patient's response. Dosage categories include:[16]

| Dose | Description |
|---|---|
| Suberythemal dose | The absence of erythema 24 hours after ultraviolet exposure. |
| Minimal erythemal dose | The smallest dose that produces erythema that appears in 1-8 hours and fades without trace within 24 hours. |
| First-degree erythemal dose | A dose that results in erythema that lasts 1-3 days with clear redness and mild desquamation. The dose is approximately 2.5 times the minimal erythemal dose and should be used only if the target area is less than 20% of the total body surface. |
| Second-degree erythemal dose | A dose that results in intense erythema, edema, peeling, pigmentation, and itching. The dose is approximately five times the minimal erythemal dose. |
| Third-degree erythemal dose | A dose that results in erythema with severe blistering, peeling, and exudation. The dose is approximately 10 times the minimal erythemal dose and should be used on areas less than 10 square inches. |

Treatment parameters are based on diagnosis, desired effects, and minimal erythemal dose. Sensitivity to radiation varies greatly from person to person and is primarily influenced by age, pigmentation, prior exposure to ultraviolet radiation, and the use of photosensitive medications.

The therapist must thoroughly inspect the area to be treated and have the patient remove all jewelry. Polarized goggles should be worn by the therapist and the patient. A therapist should initially determine the patient's minimal erythemal dose (MED). The MED is tested by placing a piece of paper with five one-inch cut outs over a patient's anterior forearm. The patient should have all other non-treatment areas covered. Once the lamp is warmed up it should be positioned at a 90-degree angle to the area of treatment (for maximum absorption) and at a distance between 24 and 40 inches from the forearm.[18] The squares should be exposed sequentially in 15 second increments for 15, 30, 45, 60, and 75 seconds.[18] Visual inspection after an 8-hour period will determine the MED. The MED for patients being treated with psoralen-based topical and systemic drugs should be determined after the patient has taken psoralen orally or bathed in psoralen.

Parameters including distance from the lamp, position of the lamp at a 90-degree angle to the treatment site, and the MED must remain consistent over the course of treatment. The treatment time should increase each consecutive treatment day. Patients will build up tolerance to ultraviolet radiation with repeated exposure due to darkening of the skin with tanning and thickening of the skin caused by epidermal hyperplasia. Instead of increasing the treatment time, the therapist may elect to move the lamp closer to the target area. The intensity of the radiation reaching the target area increases as the lamp moves closer according to the inverse square law. For example, the intensity of the radiation increases by a multiple of four if the distance from the lamp to the target area is halved.

The therapist should utilize a stopwatch and continue with ongoing visual inspection during all treatment sessions. The response to ultraviolet radiation must be reassessed if an alternate lamp is used in a subsequent session since even a slight difference in the frequency of the radiation can significantly change the patient response.

## Hydrotherapy

Hydrotherapy transfers heat through conduction or convection and is administered in tanks of varying size, ranging from extremity whirlpools to Olympic size pools. The main therapeutic effects of hydrotherapy include wound care, unloading of weight, and reduction of edema. The specific equipment and parameters used depend on the treatment objectives and site of the pathology.

### Therapeutic Effects[16,18]

- Decreased abnormal tone
- Increased blood flow
- Increased core temperature
- Pain relief
- Relaxation
- Vasodilation
- Wound debridement

### Indications[16,18]

- Arthritis
- Burn care
- Edema
- Decreased range of motion
- Desensitization of residual limb
- Joint stiffness
- Muscle spasm/spasticity
- Muscle strain
- Pain
- Sprain
- Wound care

### Contraindications[16,18]

- Advanced cardiovascular or pulmonary disease
- Active bleeding
- Diminished sensation
- Gangrene
- Impaired circulation
- Incontinence
- Maceration
- Peripheral vascular disease
- Renal infection
- Severe infection
- Severe mental disorders

# Consider This

## Outcome Assessment

Physical therapists must continually assess the effectiveness of selected interventions, including therapeutic modalities. There are a variety of subjective and objective measures that can assist the therapist to determine the relative value of each intervention.

Consider the following scenarios:

### Scenario 1

A physical therapist administers continuous ultrasound at 1.4 W/cm$^2$ for seven minutes to the right shoulder of a patient diagnosed with adhesive capsulitis.

Possible measures to evaluate the effectiveness of the intervention:

1. Administer a visual analog pain scale prior to and at the conclusion of treatment.
2. Perform periodic shoulder goniometric measurements to quantify the relative change in range of motion.

### Scenario 2

A physical therapist administers an ice pack to the knee of a patient positioned in supine with the lower extremity elevated. The patient is two weeks status post anterior cruciate ligament reconstruction.

1. Perform circumferential measurements at predetermined knee landmarks at regular intervals.
2. Administer a visual analog pain scale prior to and at the conclusion of treatment.

It is often difficult to discern the effectiveness of a given intervention in isolation since, in most cases, patients are treated with several interventions addressing the same therapeutic objective. Despite this fact, it remains important for therapists to attempt to assess the relative effectiveness of selected interventions.

## Properties of Water[22]

### Buoyancy

Archimedes' principle of buoyancy states that there is an upward force on the body when immersed in water equal to the amount of water that has been displaced by the body.

### Resistance

Water molecules tend to attract to each other and provide resistance to movement of the body in water. The resistance of water increases in proportion to the speed of motion.

### Specific Gravity

The specific gravity of water is equal to 1.0. The human body varies based on size and somatotype, but typically it has a specific gravity of less than 1.0 (average .974). Therefore, a person will generally float when fully submerged in water.

### Specific Heat

The specific heat is the measure of the ability of a fluid to store heat. This is calculated as the amount of thermal energy required to increase the fluid's temperature by one unit. Water has a specific heat of 1.0 calorie/gram while air has a specific heat of .001 calorie/gram. Water, therefore, retains heat 1,000 times more than an equivalent volume of air.

### Total Drag Force

The total drag force is comprised of profile drag, wave drag, and surface drag forces. This is a hydromechanic force exerted on a person submerged in water that normally opposes the direction of the body's motion.

### Viscosity

Viscosity refers to the magnitude of the cohesive forces between the molecules specific to the fluid. The greater the viscosity of the fluid, the greater the force required to create movement in the fluid.

## Water Motion

The primary determinants of water motion include speed, viscosity, and turbulence. The movement of water includes laminar flow and turbulent flow. Laminar flow occurs when each particle of a fluid follows a smooth path without crossing paths. Typically, laminar flow rates are slow since when water moves quickly even minor oscillations create uneven flow. Turbulent flow occurs when fluids flow in erratic, small whirlpool-like circles called eddy currents or eddies. Movement in water at rest will encounter minimal turbulence. Movement against turbulent water will encounter greater resistance.

## Types of Hydrotherapy Equipment

### Extremity tank[17]

An extremity tank is used for a distal upper or lower extremity. Approximate dimensions for an extremity tank are a depth of 18-24 inches, a length of 28-32 inches, and a width of 15 inches (10-45 gallons).

### Lowboy tank[17]

A lowboy tank is used for larger parts of the extremities and permits long sitting with water up to the midthoracic level (Fig. 9-54). Approximate dimensions for a lowboy tank are a depth of 18 inches, a length of 52-65 inches, and a width of 24 inches (90-105 gallons).

### Highboy tank[17]

A highboy tank is used for larger parts of the extremities and the trunk. This tank permits sitting in chest-high water with the hips and knees flexed. Approximate dimensions for the highboy tank are a depth of 28 inches, a length of 36-48 inches, and a width of 20-24 inches (60-105 gallons).

### Hubbard tank[16]

The Hubbard tank is used for full-body immersion. Approximate dimensions for the Hubbard tank are a depth of four feet, a length of eight feet, and a width of six feet. Contraindications specific to full-body immersion include unstable blood pressure and incontinence. The temperature should not exceed 100 degrees Fahrenheit (425 gallons).

### Therapeutic pool[16]

A therapeutic pool is used for exercising in a water medium. The temperature should range from 79-97 degrees Fahrenheit depending on patient age, health status, and goals.

| Treatment Temperature Guidelines | |
|---|---|
| **Degrees F** | **Purpose** |
| 32 - 79 °F | Acute inflammation of distal extremities |
| 79 - 92 °F | Exercise |
| 92 - 96 °F | Wound care, spasticity |
| 96 - 98 °F | Cardiopulmonary compromise, treatment of burns |
| 99 - 104 °F | Pain management |
| 104 - 110 °F | Chronic rheumatoid or osteoarthritis, increased range of motion |

Adapted from Cameron M: *Physical Agents in Rehabilitation: From Research to Practice*, Third Edition, WB Saunders Company, 2008.

## Whirlpool

A whirlpool consists of a tank that holds water with an attached motor, called a turbine, that provides agitation and aeration to create the "whirlpool effect." The turbine assembly typically allows the height and the lateral position of the turbine to be adjusted. This feature allows the therapist to direct the flow of water directly toward or away from the body part being treated. Whirlpools come in a variety of sizes and can accommodate an isolated body part or the entire body.

Prior to treatment the therapist should explain the sensations the patient will experience during treatment. Water temperature should be selected based on the patient diagnosis and goals. The therapist should assist the patient into a comfortable position and turn on the turbine. The patient's vital signs and reported level of comfort should be periodically assessed. Treatment time ranges between 10 and 30 minutes.[17] Exercise can be performed during whirlpool treatment as indicated. After treatment, dry and inspect the treated area. The tank must be thoroughly cleaned after each use with a disinfectant and antibacterial agent.

Fig. 9-54: A patient immersed in a whirlpool tank.

## Pool Therapy

Advantages of pool therapy include decreased weight bearing due to buoyancy, improved therapist handling, enhanced control over the amount of resistance during exercise, and diminished risk of falling with activity. The therapist should assist the patient as needed into the pool and throughout treatment. The therapist must remain with the patient and monitor vital signs and tolerance to activity. Recommended populations for pool therapy include patients with arthritis, musculoskeletal injuries, neurological deficits, spinal cord injury, CVA, multiple sclerosis, and selected cardiopulmonary diagnoses.

# Spotlight on Safety
## Safety Considerations with Hydrotherapy

All physical therapy interventions, including hydrotherapy, have inherent safety risks. It is essential for therapists to be aware of potential risks in order to ensure patient safety and limit any potential liability. This section identifies specific risks associated with hydrotherapy and offers proactive strategies to assist therapists to minimize their level of risk.

### Drowning

Personnel in charge of therapeutic pools should be trained in personal water safety techniques, as well as current cardiopulmonary resuscitation and first aid. The pool area should be equipped with emergency equipment including a spine board, blanket, life ring, and resuscitation devices. The entire staff should be aware of the facility's emergency action plan and be aware of the supervisory needs of each patient.

### Electrical safety

All electrical equipment should be inspected by qualified personnel according to the manufacturer's recommendations. Ground fault circuit interrupters (GFCI) are required for all hydrotherapy units. GFCIs are designed to cut off electrical supply to equipment when any form of leakage or ground-fault is identified. Whirlpool tanks should be properly grounded and should use a hospital grade plug for the turbine.

### Burns

Therapists must carefully screen patients to identify any potential contraindications to hydrotherapy. Therapists treating patients with a warm or hot whirlpool must correctly determine an appropriate temperature range to achieve the established therapeutic objectives. Prior to immersing the body part in water, the therapist must measure the temperature of the water. Therapists must be aware of medical and environmental conditions that may compromise a patient's ability to adequately dissipate heat.

### Fainting

Patients are at an increased risk for fainting due to hypotension when large body areas are immersed in warm or hot water. This risk can be exaggerated in an aquatic environment due to the relative increase in ambient temperature. Patients taking antihypertensive medications such as beta blockers are also at an increased risk for becoming hypotensive. To minimize this risk, therapists should closely monitor patients during hydrotherapy and only immerse body parts in water that require treatment.

### Falls

The presence of water on floors can result in a slippery surface that places patients at an increased risk of falling. Therapists should be diligent to dry any wet surfaces once they are identified.

## Contrast Bath

A contrast bath utilizes alternating heat and cold in order to decrease edema in a distal extremity (Fig. 9-55). The alternating vasodilation and vasoconstriction is theorized to allow the benefits of heat, such as decreased pain and increased flexibility, while avoiding the risk of increased edema. The technique provides good contact over irregularly shaped areas, allows for movement during treatment, and assists with pain management. Limitations of contrast baths include potential intolerance to cold, dependent positioning, and a lack of credible research supporting the efficacy of contrast baths.

The therapist should position the patient so that both baths are easily accessible for the patient. The treatment should begin with the patient's distal extremity immersed in the hot bath with a temperature between 104-106 degrees Fahrenheit for 3-4 minutes.[17] The patient should then place the distal extremity into the cold bath with a temperature between 50 and 60 degrees Fahrenheit for one minute.[17] The patient should repeat this hot/cold sequence for 25-30 minutes.[16] The degree of temperature increase desired often determines whether the treatment ends in the hot or cold water.

Contrast baths are utilized primarily with arthritis of the smaller joints, musculoskeletal sprains and strains, reflex sympathetic dystrophy, and residual limb desensitization.

**Fig. 9-55:** A patient immersing their hand in hot water as part of a contrast bath.

## Mechanical Agents

### Traction

Traction is a modality that applies forces to the body to separate joint surfaces and decrease pressure. The force can be applied manually by the therapist, passively by the patient or mechanically by a machine. Types of traction include manual traction, mechanical traction, positional traction, gravity-assisted traction, and inversion traction. Traction is indicated for many diagnoses and allows for variation and adjustment of the established protocol based on individual patient needs. Traction affects many of the body's systems and requires ongoing monitoring and reassessment of treatment parameters.

### Therapeutic Effects[16,18]

- Decreased disk protrusion
- Decreased pain
- Increased joint mobility
- Increased muscle relaxation
- Increased soft tissue elasticity
- Promote arterial, venous, and lymphatic flow

### Indications[16,18]

- Disk herniation
- Joint hypomobility
- Muscle guarding
- Muscle spasm
- Narrowing of the intervertebral foramen
- Nerve root impingement
- Osteophyte formation
- Spinal ligament and other connective tissue contractures
- Subacute joint inflammation
- Subacute pain

### Contraindications[16,18]

- Acute inflammation
- Acute sprains or strains
- Aortic aneurysm
- Bone diseases
- Cardiac or pulmonary problems
- Conditions where movement significantly increases symptoms
- Conditions where movement is contraindicated
- Dislocation
- Fracture
- Hiatal hernia
- Increased pain or radicular symptoms with traction
- Infections in bones or joints
- Meningitis
- Osteoporosis
- Peripheralization of symptoms
- Positive alar ligament test*
- Positive vertebral artery test*
- Pregnancy**
- Rheumatoid arthritis– advanced*
- Subluxation
- Temporomandibular joint pain or dysfunction (use of halter)*
- Trauma–if diagnostic tests have not ruled out other medical conditions
- Tumors
- Vascular conditions
- Vertebral joint instability

* Cervical traction only   **Lumbar traction only

## Mechanical Lumbar and Cervical Traction Procedures

### Lumbar Traction

**Procedure for mechanical lumbar traction**

### 1. Determine the patient position

Mechanical lumbar traction is performed with the patient in a supine or prone position. The position chosen is often based on the medical diagnosis and patient tolerance. A flexed position of the spine (i.e., traction in supine) results in greater separation of the posterior structures including the facet joints and intervertebral foramen.[18] An extended position of the spine (i.e., traction in prone) results in greater separation of the anterior structures including the disk spaces.[18]

Traction is most often performed in the supine position, however, the prone position offers the therapist the opportunity to apply other modalities simultaneously and assess the amount of spinous process separation.

Certain medical diagnoses are characteristically treated in a specific position. For example, spinal stenosis is most often treated with a flexed spine since this position increases the intervertebral foramen opening.[17] Disk protrusions are most often treated with the patient positioned in prone since the spine can extend and the forces on the disk are directed anteriorly.[17] This is beneficial since the majority of disk herniations occur in a posterolateral direction.

**Fig. 9-56:** Application of a traction harness.

### 2. Apply the traction harness

Mechanical lumbar traction requires the use of a traction harness. The harness is necessary to stabilize the trunk while the lumbar spine is placed under traction. The non-slip belt surface should be applied directly on the patient's skin in a standing position (Fig. 9-56).[18] This will allow the harness to better adhere to the skin and allow the therapist to adequately secure the harness with minimal active patient participation. The traction harness can also be applied by placing it on the traction table and having the patient lie on top of it. Once secured, the traction harness should be connected to the traction unit (Fig. 9-57).

**Fig. 9-57:** A therapist setting the parameters for mechanical lumbar traction.

### 3. Select the traction parameters

#### Static versus intermittent traction

Traction can be applied in a static or intermittent form. Static refers to consistent force being applied throughout the treatment. Static traction may be desirable if the patient's symptoms are slightly exaggerated by movement.[17] Intermittent refers to varying force applied throughout the treatment. Intermittent traction may be desirable for joint mobilization or for patients who cannot tolerate static traction.[17] Intermittent traction requires the therapist to select the amount of force used during the hold and relax periods. The maximum force is applied during the hold period and the minimum force is applied during the relax period. The force during the relax period usually approximates 50% of the force used during the hold period.[16] There is little evidence to guide the timing of the hold and relax periods. The relax period should be relatively short, but must provide a sufficient interval to allow the patient to feel relaxed prior to the next traction cycle.

#### Force

The force of lumbar traction is dependent on the goals of treatment and is influenced by a number of variables including friction. Friction refers to the force that arises to oppose motion. The amount of friction when performing lumbar traction can be approximated by using the coefficient of friction, which refers to the constant frictional forces when applying traction between surfaces. The coefficient of friction of the human body on a mattress is 0.5.[17] The amount of friction can be estimated by multiplying the percentage of the body weight below L3 (i.e., 50%) and the coefficient of friction (0.5). The result is 25%, meaning that a force of approximately 25% of the patient's body weight is necessary to overcome the force of friction.[17]

The use of a split traction table can eliminate the majority of friction between the patient's body and the treatment table. When the two sections of the split traction table are unlocked and traction is applied, the lower portion of the table slides away from the upper portion. If intermittent traction is used, the table should be split during the second or third hold period

when the traction approaches its maximum force.[16]

The literature varies in the exact amount of force necessary when performing mechanical lumbar traction. The majority of sources indicate that a maximum of 30 pounds should be used for the initial traction session.[18] A force of 25% of total body weight may be adequate to stretch soft tissue and treat muscle spasm or disk protrusion.[16] A force of approximately 50% of the body weight is required for actual separation of the vertebrae.[18]

Many traction units provide therapists with the option to progressively increase or decrease the traction force in a series of predetermined steps. The gradual increase or decrease in pressure may be more comfortable for a patient since it allows the patient to gradually accommodate to the traction force and therefore, stay more relaxed throughout the duration of treatment.

#### Duration

The research does not offer specific guidance on the duration of lumbar traction. In general, treatment times vary from 5-30 minutes.[16] When treating disk-related symptoms, treatment time is generally 10 minutes or less and may extend up to 30 minutes with other spinal conditions.[18] Patient tolerance and changes in symptoms are the primary determining factors when selecting the duration of traction.

## Cervical Traction

### Procedure for mechanical cervical traction

#### 1. Determine the patient position

Mechanical cervical traction is performed with the patient in a supine or sitting position. The position chosen is often based on the medical diagnosis and patient tolerance. A supine position is used more often since the traction force does not have to overcome the force exerted by gravity and the position allows the patient to attain a more relaxed state, minimizing the opposition to force. A flexed position of the spine results in greater separation of the posterior structures including the facet joints and intervertebral foramen.[16] An extended position of the spine results in greater separation of the anterior structures including the disk spaces.[16]

In a supine position, the therapist can adjust cervical flexion, rotation, and sidebending to focus on a specific target area and to promote comfort. In sitting, the amount of cervical flexion and extension can be controlled to a limited extent by the direction the patient is positioned in relation to the traction force. A patient positioned toward the traction force will exhibit more flexion than a patient positioned away from the traction force.

The relative amount of flexion in the cervical spine allows therapists to target specific spinal levels: upper cervical spine = 0-5 degrees of flexion; midcervical spine = 10-20 degrees of flexion; lower cervical spine = 25-35 degrees of flexion.[17]

#### 2. Apply the head halter

Mechanical cervical traction requires the use of a head halter or padded board attached to a frictionless trolley that moves up and down a bar attached to the traction unit. The head halter is necessary to stabilize the head while the cervical spine is placed under traction (Fig. 9-58). The head halter should be applied so that the majority of traction pull is placed on the occiput and not the chin.[16] Therapists must be extremely careful when using the head halter since the device can place considerable force on the temporomandibular joints.

**Fig. 9-58:** A mechanical cervical traction unit.

### 3. Select the traction parameters

#### Static versus intermittent traction

The therapist should select static or intermittent traction. Intermittent traction may be more effective for reducing pain and increasing cervical range of motion.

#### Force

The force of cervical traction is dependent on the goals of treatment and is influenced by a number of variables including patient position. The literature varies as to the exact amount of force necessary when performing mechanical cervical traction. The majority of sources indicate that a force of up to 10 pounds should be used for the initial traction session.[16] A force of 7-10% of a patient's body weight (11-15 pounds) may be adequate to stretch soft tissue or treat muscle spasm and disk protrusion.[16] A force of 13-20% of a patient's body weight (20-30 pounds) may be necessary for joint distraction.[16] A traction force applied to the cervical spine should typically not exceed 30 pounds.

#### Duration

The research does not offer specific guidance on the duration of mechanical cervical traction. In general, treatment time varies from 5-30 minutes.[16] When treating disk-related symptoms, treatment time is generally 10 minutes or less, but may extend up to 30 minutes with other spinal conditions.[18] Patient tolerance and changes in symptoms are the primary determining factors when deciding the duration of traction.

#### Patient safety for mechanical lumbar and cervical traction

The therapist should assess the patient's initial response to traction within the initial five minutes of treatment. If the patient's symptoms worsen or peripheralize, the traction should be temporarily discontinued. The therapist may attempt to modify the traction parameters, however, if undesirable symptoms persist, traction is not likely a viable treatment option.

The patient should be supplied with a call bell or safety switch to turn off the traction in the event that traction increases symptoms or becomes uncomfortable.

## Compression

Compression refers to the application of a mechanical force to increase pressure on the treated body part. Compression works to keep venous and lymphatic flow from pooling in the venous system and interstitial space.

### Therapeutic Effects[16,18]

- Control of peripheral edema
- Management of scar formation
- Prevention of deep vein thrombosis
- Promote lymphatic and venous return
- Shaping of the residual limb

### Indications[16,18]

- Edema
- Hypertrophic scarring
- Lymphedema
- New residual limb
- Risk for deep vein thrombosis
- Stasis ulcers

### Contraindications[16,18]

- Circulatory obstruction
- Deep vein thrombosis
- Heart failure
- Infection of treated area
- Malignancy of treated area
- Unstable or acute fracture
- Pulmonary edema

### Static Compression

Static compression can be used to shape residual limbs, control edema, prevent abnormal scar formation, and reduce the risk of deep vein thrombosis. Examples of static compression devices include compression bandages and compression garments.

#### Compression bandages

Compression bandages increase external pressure on a body part by exerting resting pressure and working pressure. Resting pressure is produced when an elastic bandage is placed on stretch.[16] Pressure can be exerted when the patient is active or at rest. Working pressure is produced by an active muscle contracting against an inelastic bandage.[16] Pressure is only exerted when the patient is active.

Compression bandages are designed to offer greater pressure distally than proximally and must be applied using a figure-eight pattern. The bandages should not be applied in a circular pattern since this can result in uneven pressure and may actually inhibit edema management. In some instances, a liner may be applied under the bandages to minimize the probability of the bandages slipping on the skin.

There are a variety of different types of compression bandages including:

**Long-stretch bandages** provide the greatest resting pressure and are capable of applying 60-70 mm Hg of pressure.[16] The elasticity of the bandage allows them to extend up to 200% of their pre-stretch length.[16] This type of bandage provides very little working pressure since the bandages stretch when the muscles expand. Long-stretch bandages are most often used to apply compression in patients who are immobile.

**Short-stretch bandages** produce low pressure at rest and high working pressure when the muscles expand. These bandages can be moderately effective while a patient is active or at rest since they produce both resting and working pressure. Short-stretch bandages are most often used during exercise.[16] Patients must have a functional calf muscle and a functional gait pattern to maximally benefit from short-stretch bandages in the lower extremities.[16] The bandages are not effective in a flaccid or inactive limb.

**Multi-layered bandages** produce moderate to high resting pressure through the use of several bandages containing elastic and inelastic layers. The multiple layers of bandages provide protection, absorption, and compression. Multi-layered bandages are most commonly used to treat venous stasis ulcers.[16]

**Semirigid bandages** most often consist of treated gauze applied to a distal extremity. The treated gauze is initially wet and later dries into a hardened form. The bandages are often used in the treatment of venous stasis ulcers. An Unna's boot is an example of a semirigid bandage made of zinc oxide impregnated gauze. The boot is capable of providing a sustained compression force of 35-40 mm Hg.[16]

### Compression garments

Compression garments provide varying degrees of resting pressure and working pressure through elasticity. Compression garments are most often used to control edema, limit scar formation after burns, and improve venous circulation in active patients.[16,23] The garments consist of off-the-shelf and custom fit offerings for all parts of the body. Off-the-shelf garments (e.g., antiembolism stockings) provide a compression force of 16-18 mm Hg and are used to prevent deep vein thrombosis in patients on bedrest.[16] The stockings should be worn at all times unless bathing. Compression garments offering 20-30 mm Hg pressure are used for scar tissue control while 30-40 mm Hg pressure is typically required for edema control.[23]

Compression garments should be fit when the level of edema is minimal. An appropriately fit compression garment will fit tightly to the affected body part and can be challenging for some patients to don and doff without assistance. The average life expectancy of a compression garment is six months, although changes may be required sooner if there is a significant change in the size of the limb.[16]

## Intermittent Compression

Intermittent compression refers to the use of compression at specified cyclical intervals to control edema. Intermittent compression is most often delivered using an intermittent pneumatic compression pump.

**Fig. 9-59:** An intermittent compression unit. Courtesy Chattanooga, a DJO Global Company.

### Intermittent Pneumatic Compression Pump

Intermittent compression with a pneumatic device is primarily used to reduce chronic or post-traumatic edema. The therapist has the ability to adjust treatment parameters including inflation pressure, on/off ratio, and total treatment time (Fig. 9-59).

The therapist must ask the patient to remove all jewelry and ensure appropriate fit of the compression sleeve prior to treatment. The patient should be placed in a comfortable position with the extremity elevated. Blood pressure and girth measurements should be recorded. The therapist should then apply a stockinette over the extremity and adjust the compression sleeve. The literature provides little definitive guidance on parameters such as on/off time, inflation time, and deflation time. As a result, patient comfort and the desired therapeutic effects are often the most important variables to consider.

Inflation pressure generally ranges from 30-80 mm Hg and typically should not exceed the patient's diastolic blood pressure.[16] Arterial capillary pressure is approximately 30 mm Hg, and therefore, inflation pressure below this value will not typically have any significant therapeutic value. Inflation pressure greater than the patient's systolic blood pressure may restrict arterial blood flow and create a medical emergency.

Treatment of the upper extremities generally requires 30-60 mm Hg of inflation pressure while treatment of the lower extremities generally requires 40-80 mm Hg of inflation pressure.[16] Treatment time varies from 30 minutes to four hours based on diagnosis. Intermittent compression is utilized from three times per week up to four times per day.[16] The extended treatment times are often utilized when treating primary lymphedema.[18] The patient should have a call bell and be monitored throughout treatment. When treatment is complete, the therapist should reassess the extremity and measure blood pressure. Girth measurements should be recorded and compared to the values obtained before treatment.

Compression may be coupled with therapeutic cold and electrical stimulation.[18] When using electrical stimulation in combination with compression, the current intensity should be adjusted only after the sleeve is fully inflated since this can significantly impact electrode contact with the skin.

## Continuous Passive Motion Machine

The continuous passive motion machine (CPM) is a mechanical device designed to provide continuous motion for a particular joint using a predetermined range and speed (Fig. 9-60). Robert Salter first developed this device based on research that continuous passive motion had beneficial healing effects for injured joints and surrounding soft tissues. Subsequent studies examining the efficacy of using a CPM versus not using a CPM vary in conclusion.[23] Some studies show no significant difference in short-term outcomes for CPM use versus alternate forms of early motion. Others show benefits from using CPM including earlier motion of joints resulting in shorter hospitalizations. The primary indication for CPM is to improve range of motion that may have been impaired secondary to a surgical procedure. Any joint may be indicated for CPM, however, the knee is the most commonly treated.

**Fig. 9-60:** A continuous passive motion machine. Courtesy Chattanooga, a DJO Global Company.

### Therapeutic Effects

- Decrease post-operative pain
- Improve the rate of recovery
- Increase range of motion
- Lessen the debilitating effects from immobilization
- Reduce edema by assisting venous and lymphatic return
- Stimulate tissue healing

### Indications

- Pain
- Limited range of motion
- Edema
- Susceptibility to contractures or adhesions
- Muscle or joint stiffness

### Contraindications

- Increase in pain after use
- Particular anticoagulants may increase the risk for intracompartment hematoma
- Unwanted translation of opposing bones

A continuous passive motion machine is often utilized immediately after surgery. The patient's joint must be aligned with the fulcrum of the CPM in order to receive effective and safe treatment. Proximal and distal stabilization straps stabilize the patient's upper and lower leg in the device and assist to maintain the desired alignment. The patient must be instructed in the use of the CPM and all associated safety information.

Specific protocols apply for each individual joint regarding time of use and degrees of motion. Initially, a small arc of motion is utilized and patients gradually increase the range of motion as tolerated or as allowed based on their current medical status. A rate of two cycles per minute typically allows patients to tolerate the CPM without difficulty. CPMs may be utilized at home after discharge from the hospital. A patient or caregiver must be independent with the CPM protocol for home use.

## Electrotherapy

Electrotherapy is a commonly used therapeutic modality capable of producing a wide variety of therapeutic effects including muscle strengthening, pain management, muscle re-education, and stimulation of denervated muscle. Therapists must possess a thorough understanding of the mechanism by which electrical stimulation affects tissue as well as the advantages and disadvantages of the various electrotherapeutic agents available.

### Therapeutic Effects[16,17,18,21]

- Decreased edema
- Decreased pain
- Eliminate disuse atrophy
- Facilitate bone repair
- Facilitate wound healing
- Improved range of motion
- Increased local circulation
- Muscle re-education
- Muscle strengthening
- Relaxation of muscle spasm

### Indications[16,17,18,21]

- Bell's palsy
- Decreased range of motion
- Facial neuropathy
- Fracture
- Idiopathic scoliosis
- Joint effusion
- Labor and delivery
- Muscle atrophy
- Muscle spasm
- Muscle weakness
- Open wound/ulcer
- Pain
- Stress incontinence
- Shoulder subluxation

### Contraindications[16,17,18,21]

- Cardiac arrhythmia
- Cardiac pacemaker
- Malignancy
- Osteomyelitis
- Over a pregnant uterus
- Over carotid sinus
- Patient with a bladder stimulator
- Phlebitis
- Seizure disorders

## Muscle and Nerve Cell Excitation

Physical therapists must possess a thorough understanding of muscle and nerve cell membranes and their response to electrical stimulation. Muscles and nerve cells are excitable because of the ability to produce action potentials. Action potentials refer to the recorded change in the electrical potential between the inside and outside of a nerve cell.[18] The muscle and nerve cell membranes regulate the exchange of substances between the inside of the cell and the environment outside of the cell. The potential difference in the concentration and permeability of sodium and potassium ions is termed the resting potential. Creating an impulse in a muscle or nerve cell requires the resting potential to be reduced below a threshold level causing changes in the membrane's permeability. The described change creates an action potential that results in depolarization. For an action potential to be evoked using electrical stimulation, the amplitude of the stimulus and pulse duration must be sufficient to overcome the established threshold.

## Principles of Electricity

**Current** (i.e., electrical) refers to the directed flow of charge from one place to another. In order to produce electrical current, there must be a source of electrons, a material that allows passage of the electrons (i.e., conductor), and a driving force of electrons (i.e., electromotive force).[17,18] Current is measured in amperes. One ampere is equal to $6.25 \times 10^{18}$ electrons per second. A milliampere is one thousandth of an ampere, while a microampere is one millionth of an ampere.[18]

**Voltage** is a measure of electromotive force or the electrical potential difference.[17,18] Electrons will only flow between two points when there is a difference in the quantity of electrons between the two points. The magnitude of the difference between the positive and negative poles is the voltage. Voltage is measured in volts.

**Resistance** describes the ability of a material to oppose the flow of ions through it. Resistance is measured in ohms.[17,18] The resistance of a material can be calculated using Ohm's law.

$$\text{Resistance} = \frac{\text{Voltage}}{\text{Current}}$$

Ohm's law states that the current in a conductor varies in proportion to the voltage and inversely with the resistance.[17] An electromotive force of one volt is required to drive one ampere of current across a resistance of one ohm.

## Therapeutic Currents

### Direct Current[17,18]

Direct current is characterized by a constant flow of electrons from the anode (i.e., positive electrode) to the cathode (i.e., negative electrode) for a period of greater than one second without interruption (Fig. 9-61). Polarity remains constant and is determined by the therapist based on treatment goals. Direct current can be modulated for therapeutic use by interrupting the current flow after one second, reversing the polarity or gradually

increasing or decreasing the amplitude. Clinically, direct current is most often used with iontophoresis.

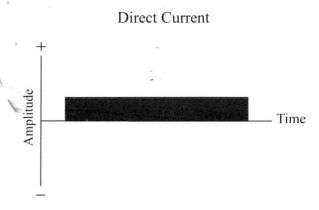

**Fig. 9-61:** Direct current is characterized by a constant flow of electrons from the anode to the cathode.

### Alternating Current[17,18]

Alternating current is characterized by polarity that continuously changes from positive to negative with the change in direction of current flow (Fig. 9-62). Alternating current is biphasic, symmetrical or asymmetrical, and is characterized by a waveform that is sinusoidal in shape. The frequency of cycles of alternating current is measured in cycles per second or Hertz. Alternating current is used most frequently in a modulated form as burst or time-modulated.

**Fig. 9-62:** Alternating current is characterized by a continuous bidirectional flow of current.

### Pulsatile Current[17,18]

Pulsatile current is characterized by the non-continuous flow of direct or alternating current. A pulse is defined as a discrete electrical event separated from other pulses by a period of time in which no electrical activity exists. Most pulse waveforms are either monophasic or biphasic. Monophasic pulsed current has one phase for each pulse and therefore, the waveform is either positive or negative (Fig. 9-63). Monophasic pulsed current produces a polarity effect since the current flows through the tissues in only one polarity (i.e., positive or negative) for a given period of time. Biphasic pulsed current has two phases, one which is positive and one which is negative (Fig. 9-64). Biphasic waveforms can be described as symmetric or asymmetric and balanced or unbalanced (Fig. 9-65).

### Monophasic Pulsatile Current

**Fig. 9-63:** Monophasic pulsatile current has one phase for each pulse.

### Biphasic Pulsatile Current

**Fig. 9-64:** Biphasic pulsatile current has two phases for each pulse.

### Balanced and Unbalanced Current

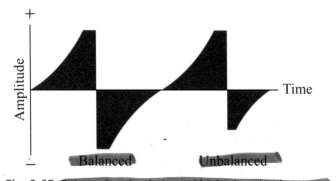

**Fig. 9-65:** Balanced and unbalanced biphasic pulsatile current.

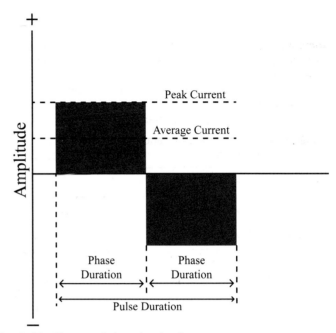

**Fig. 9-66:** Characteristics of pulsatile current.

## Waveforms of Therapeutic Currents[18]

An oscilloscope can be used to create a graphical representation of the shape, direction, amplitude, duration, and pulse frequency of the electrical current being produced by an electrotherapeutic device. On an oscilloscope, an individual waveform is referred to as a pulse. Waveforms of monophasic, biphasic, and pulsatile currents include sine, square, rectangular or spiked (Fig. 9-67).

### Waveforms

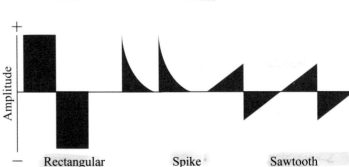

**Fig. 9-67:** Common types of electrical waveforms.

## Electrodes

Administering electrical current to a body requires the use of at least two electrodes of opposing charges. When direct current or a monophasic pulsed waveform is used, one electrode will remain the cathode (negative) and the other the anode (positive) throughout the treatment. In an alternating current, the cathode and anode are constantly changing.

Proper cleaning of the skin and electrode application will facilitate conductance and limit impedance. Prior to applying the electrodes, the patient's skin must be thoroughly cleansed with soap and water or a suitable cleansing wipe. Ideally, hair should be removed from the identified treatment area, however, this is not required.

Electrodes are typically flexible with a self-adhesive gel coating and are intended for one time use. Reusable electrodes are typically made of carbon-silicon rubber. This type of electrode requires application of a gel or coupling spray to ensure appropriate contact. Since they are not self-adhesive, reusable electrodes must be secured on the patient with tape or elastic straps. Therapists should closely monitor the patient's skin since it is fairly common to develop irritation under the electrodes. Some patients may also exhibit an allergic reaction to the material or selected polymers from an electrode.[16] In these instances, the therapist may elect to utilize a different type of electrode, modify the location of the electrode placement or discontinue treatment.

Small electrodes are used for electrotherapy treatments for small areas of the body or small muscles that require relatively low levels of stimulation. Large electrodes are used for larger areas of the body or larger muscles of the body that require high levels of stimulation.[17] Current density is influenced by the size of the electrodes and the distance they are apart. When the same size electrodes are used, the current density under each electrode is the same. When unequal size electrodes are used, the current will be more concentrated in the smaller electrode. Current density can also refer to the concentration of current within the tissues.[20] If the electrodes are in close proximity, the current is more dense in the superficial tissues. If the electrodes are relatively farther apart, the current is more dense in the deeper tissues.[20]

### Characteristics of Electrical Current Based on Electrode Size

| Small Electrodes | Large Electrodes |
| --- | --- |
| Increased current density | Decreased current density |
| Increased impedance | Decreased impedance |
| Decreased current flow | Increased current flow |

## Electrode Placement

The two primary methods of electrode placement are monopolar and bipolar.

**Monopolar technique:** The stimulating or active electrode is placed over the target area. A second dispersive electrode is placed at another site away from the target area. Typically, the active electrode is smaller than the dispersive electrode. This technique is used with wounds, iontophoresis, and in the treatment of edema.[24]

**Bipolar technique:** Two active electrodes are placed over the target area. Typically, the electrodes are equal in size. This technique is used for muscle weakness, neuromuscular facilitation, spasms, and range of motion.[24]

## Parameters of Electrical Stimulation

The law of Dubois Reymond specifies that the effectiveness of a current to target specific excitable tissue is dependent on three major factors:[20]

1. Adequate intensity to reach the threshold (i.e., amplitude)
2. Current onset fast enough to reduce accommodation (i.e., rise time)
3. Duration long enough to exceed the capacitance of the tissue (i.e., phase duration)

The specific parameters selected for electrotherapy determine the anticipated therapeutic effects. Common parameters available on most electrotherapy devices include:

### Amplitude[16,18]

Amplitude refers to the magnitude of current. Average amplitude refers to the average amount of current supplied over a period of time, while peak amplitude refers to the maximum positive or negative point from zero where the pulse is maintained.[20] The peak amplitude must be large enough to exceed the threshold for the nerve or muscle cell. Amplitude controls are often labeled intensity or voltage and can be expressed in volts, microvolts or millivolts. The higher the amplitude, the greater the peak amplitude.

### Rise time[16,18]

Rise time is the time it takes for the current to move from zero to the peak intensity within each phase (Fig. 9-69). Fast rise times are necessary with low capacitance tissues, such as large motor nerves. Rise times are typically very short, ranging from nanoseconds to milliseconds. By observing the graphical representation of a given pulse generated from an oscilloscope, therapists can gain a general sense of the rise time. For example, a sine wave would exhibit a more gradual increase in amplitude compared to a rectangular wave which has an almost instantaneous increase in amplitude. Decay time is the time it takes for the current to move from the peak intensity to zero.

### Phase duration[16,18]

Phase duration is the amount of time it takes for one phase of a pulse. The phase begins when the current departs from the zero line and ends as the current returns to the zero line. Pulse duration is the amount of time it takes for two phases of a pulse with biphasic current (Fig. 9-66). In monophasic current, the phase duration and the pulse duration are the same. If the current is biphasic, there are two phase durations for each pulse. The length of the phase duration must be sufficient to exceed the capacitance of the targeted nerve in order to cause an action potential. Phase duration is typically measured in microseconds. The interpulse interval is the time between two successive phases of a pulse.

### Frequency[16,18]

Frequency determines the number of pulses delivered through each channel per second. Frequency controls are often labeled as rate and are expressed in pulses per second or Hertz. The frequency affects the number of action potentials elicited during the stimulation. Although the same number of fibers are recruited, a higher frequency causes them to fire at a more rapid rate.

### Current modulation[18,24]

Current modulation refers to any alteration in the amplitude, duration or frequency of the current during a series of pulses or cycle.

## Ramping

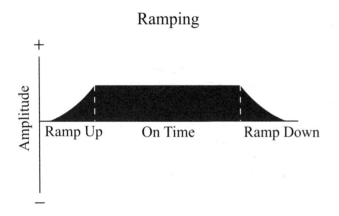

**Fig. 9-68:** Current modulation using a ramp.

Common categories of modulation include bursts, interrupted pulses, and ramps (Fig. 9-68). Bursts occur when pulsed current flows for several milliseconds and then ceases to flow for several milliseconds in a repeated cycle. The minimal length of the interruptions is too short to allow for a true interruption of muscle contraction. Interrupted pulses allow for a true

## Time Dependent Characteristics

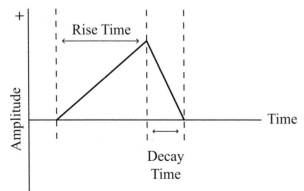

**Fig. 9-69:** Determining rise time and decay time.

interruption by using an on time and off time. This type of modulation is commonly used with muscle strengthening due to the necessity for a rest period. Ramps allow current amplitude to gradually increase to a preset maximum and then gradually decrease. Ramping is commonly used to make the onset of stimulation more comfortable and is frequently utilized with muscle strengthening.[24]

## Neuromuscular Electrical Stimulation

Neuromuscular electrical stimulation (NMES) is a technique used to facilitate skeletal muscle activity (Fig. 9-70). Stimulation of an innervated muscle occurs when an electrical stimulus of appropriate intensity and duration is administered to the corresponding peripheral nerve. Electrical stimulation of a denervated muscle has been used in an attempt to maintain the muscle, however, there is little documented evidence that supports this treatment option. Functional electrical stimulation (FES) uses electrical stimulation to create or enhance the performance of a functional activity.[17] An example of FES is the stimulation of the anterior tibialis to produce dorsiflexion during the swing phase of gait.

**Fig. 9-70:** A neuromuscular electrical stimulation unit. Courtesy Chattanooga, a DJO Global Company.

NMES is a commonly used therapeutic technique to facilitate the return of controlled functional muscular activity or to maintain postural alignment until recovery occurs. When performing NMES the patient should be positioned comfortably (Fig. 9-71). The therapist should place the electrodes over the muscle to be stimulated so that the electrodes are aligned in parallel. This alignment will allow the current to travel parallel to the direction of the muscle fibers. Ideally, one of the electrodes should be placed over the muscle's motor point since this will produce the strongest contraction with the least amount of current. The electrodes should be separated by a minimum of two inches.[17]

### Parameters for Applying NMES for Muscle Strengthening

**Current amplitude:** The amount of current amplitude is dependent on the desired strength of the contraction (Fig. 9-72). For example, a therapist would want a much more forceful muscle contraction for a patient participating in general muscle strengthening than for a patient recovering from a recent surgery.

**Fig. 9-71:** A therapist discussing the use of a neuromuscular electrical stimulation unit with a patient.

**Pulse duration:** The pulse duration should be high enough to overcome the relatively low capacitance of motor nerve fibers. Despite the low capacitance, the relative depth of the muscle fibers requires a high pulse duration.[20] Patients often find shorter pulse durations more comfortable when targeting smaller muscles and longer pulse durations more comfortable when treating larger muscles.[17] Therapists should recognize that as the pulse duration is shortened, a greater current amplitude will be required to produce the same strength of contraction.

**Frequency:** The frequency should be sufficient to produce a tetanus contraction. A smooth tetanic contraction is usually produced at a frequency of 35-50 pulses per second.[20] Higher frequencies will not produce a stronger contraction, but instead will promote more rapid fatigue.

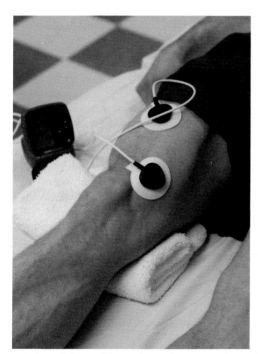

**Fig. 9-72:** A forceful quadriceps femoris contraction using a neuromuscular electrical stimulation unit.

**Duty cycle:** A duty cycle must be used when applying NMES to provide the muscle with relaxation time and limit the influence of fatigue. On time should range from 6-10 seconds while off time should be approximately five times longer.[20] The therapist may elect to decrease the length of the off time in subsequent sessions based on patient progress.

**Ramp time:** A ramp allows current amplitude to gradually increase to a preset maximum and then gradually decrease. Ramping is commonly used to make the onset of stimulation more comfortable when performing muscle strengthening. Based on an on time of 6-10 seconds, a ramp up time of 1-4 seconds would be recommended.

**Treatment time:** Patients should complete a minimum of 10 contractions and a maximum of 20 contractions. Based on typical on and off times, performing 10 contractions would take approximately 10 minutes while 20 contractions would take 20 minutes. Treatment should ideally take place a minimum of three times per week.[18]

## Transcutaneous Electrical Nerve Stimulation (TENS)

Transcutaneous electrical nerve stimulation is widely used for acute and chronic pain management. Areas of use include obstetrics, temporomandibular joint pain, and post-operative pain. The main therapeutic effects of TENS include pain relief through the gate control theory of pain or the endogenous opiate pain control theory. TENS units are portable and indicated for home use (Fig. 9-73). The most commonly used modes of TENS include conventional, acupuncture-like, brief intense, and noxious.[16,25]

### Conventional TENS[17,21,24]

Conventional TENS is characterized by delivery of electrical pulses having short duration and high frequency with low current amplitude. The current amplitude should be sufficient to generate a sensory response, but should be below the motor threshold. Electrodes should be placed over the painful area. The majority of patients report a mild tingling sensation under and between the electrodes. Pain relief is usually brief and only occurs when the current is being generated. Conventional TENS is most often used to relieve pain during activities of daily living. Treatment time is highly variable depending on the duration of the activity.

### Acupuncture-like TENS[17,21,22]

Acupuncture-like TENS is characterized by the delivery of electrical pulses that have long duration and low frequency with moderate current amplitude. The current amplitude should be sufficient to generate muscle twitching. Electrodes should be placed over the area of pain or a related area, such as an acupuncture point. The majority of patients report the stimulus as uncomfortable or burning. Pain relief can last for several hours after stimulation. Acupuncture-like TENS is most often used for patients requiring longer lasting pain relief. It is not often used during activities of daily living since the muscle twitching can interfere with functional tasks. Treatment time is usually 20-45 minutes.

| **Common TENS Techniques and Recommended Parameters**[17] | | | | |
|---|---|---|---|---|
| Technique | Amplitude | Pulse Frequency | Pulse Duration | Treatment Time |
| Conventional | Sufficient for a sensory response | High (30-150 pps) | Short (50-100 µsec) | Variable based on the duration of the activity |
| Acupuncture-like | Sufficient to produce muscle twitching | Low (2-4 pps) | Long (100-300 µsec) | 20-45 minutes |
| Brief Intense | Sufficient for strong paresthesia or a motor response | High (60-200 pps) | Long (150-500 µsec) | 15 minutes |
| Noxious | Highest tolerated stimulus | High or Low | Long (250 µsec up to 1 second) | 30-60 seconds for each point |

Adapted from Michlovitz S: *Thermal Agents in Rehabilitation*, Fourth Edition, FA Davis Company, 2005

**This table demonstrates a typical range for each type of TENS, however, there are discrepancies that exist from author to author regarding the appropriate settings for TENS. Given this fact, it is more important to have a basic understanding of TENS parameters (e.g., short, long, low, high) than it is to memorize an exact pulse frequency or pulse duration.

### Brief Intense TENS[17,21,24]

Brief intense TENS is characterized by delivery of electrical pulses having long duration and high frequency with moderate current amplitude. This mode of TENS is referred to as brief intense TENS since the application is shorter and the current amplitude is higher than some of the other presented modes. The current amplitude should be sufficient for strong paresthesia or a motor response. Brief intense TENS is often used to minimize pain during therapeutic activities that may be painful. Treatment time is usually 15 minutes.

**Fig. 9-73:** A transcutaneous electrical nerve stimulation unit. Courtesy Chattanooga, a DJO Global Company.

### Noxious TENS[17,24]

Noxious TENS is characterized by high density current that is described by patients as uncomfortable or painful. This mode of TENS is administered with a small probe type applicator or electrode. Stimulation is delivered in 30-60 second intervals to motor, acupuncture or trigger points. Noxious level stimulation

should be applied to patients only after the therapist has thoroughly explained the expected sensation.[17]

The waveforms used are monophasic pulsatile current or biphasic pulsatile current with a spiked, square, rectangular or sine waveform. Electrode placement may be based on sites of nerve roots, trigger points, acupuncture sites or key points of pain and sensitivity.[24] Net polarity is normally equal to zero. If the waveform is unbalanced there will be an accumulation of charges that will lead to skin irritation under the electrodes.

## Interferential Current

Interferential current combines two medium frequency alternating waveforms that are biphasic. The two waveforms are delivered through two sets of electrodes from separate channels of the same stimulator. When the currents intersect, they produce a higher amplitude when both currents are in the same phase and a lower current when they are in opposite phases. This continuous sequence produces envelopes of pulses known as beats.[16] Interferential current is often comfortable for patients since a low amplitude current is delivered through the skin and a higher amplitude current is delivered to deeper tissues. Interferential current is most often used for pain relief, increased circulation, and muscle stimulation.[20]

### Methods of Interferential Current Delivery

#### Bipolar delivery[20]

Bipolar delivery utilizes two electrodes connected to a single channel with two medium sinusoidal currents. The interference between the two currents creates an amplitude modulated interferential current with a beat frequency (beats per second). The beat frequency is the net difference between the two currents. The bipolar method allows for the interferential current to be modulated prior to delivery of the current to the electrodes. Bipolar delivery creates an oval-shaped field of interferential current.

## Quadripolar delivery[20]

Quadripolar delivery utilizes four electrodes with each pair connected to a single channel. The interference between the currents using this method occurs at the level of the treatment area within the targeted tissues. When the currents intersect at a 90 degree angle, the maximum resultant amplitude occurs halfway between the two lines of current. The current treatment area creates a four-leaf clover shaped treatment field within the area between all four electrodes (Fig. 9-74).

## Quadripolar with automatic vector scan[21]

The quadripolar method with automatic vector scan is used when there is a need to increase the size of the field of current that is created by the quadripolar method. One of the circuits is allowed to vary in amplitude and this allows the field pattern to automatically rotate between the two lines of current. The field is circular in shape, as opposed to the cloverleaf, and allows for an overall larger field of current.

Some interferential units include suction electrodes that attach to the skin surface through mild suctioning. This feature can be desirable since the electrodes stay in place throughout treatment without having to be strapped to the body surface. Interferential current can be used in combination with other modalities, such as ice or heat. Treatment time is variable and is primarily influenced by the established goals (e.g., pain relief, increased circulation, muscle stimulation).

### Interferential Current

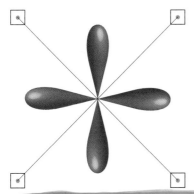

**Fig. 9-74:** Interaction of two medium frequency alternating waveforms using interferential current with a quadripolar technique.

## Iontophoresis

Iontophoresis is the process by which ions are introduced into the body through the skin by means of continuous direct current electrical stimulation (Fig. 9-75). Iontophoresis is based on the theory that like charges repel and, as a result, ions in a solution of similar charge will move away from the electrical source and into the body. Positively charged ions are carried into the body's tissue from the positive pole (anode) and negatively charged ions are carried into the body's tissue from the negative pole (cathode). The rate of ion delivery is determined by the concentration of the ion, the pH of the solution, the current density, and the duration of the treatment.[18] The specific therapeutic effects of iontophoresis are determined based on the the ion selected.

## Spotlight on Safety

### Safety Considerations with Electrotherapy[18,21,24]

Electrical equipment used in health care can pose a significant potential risk to both the patient and therapist. Therapists should be aware of these potential risks in order to ensure safety and limit any potential liability. This section identifies several safe practices that minimize risk when using electrotherapy.

- All electrotherapy equipment should be inspected by qualified personnel at or before the manufacturer's suggested service dates.
- Any electrotherapy equipment that may have been damaged (e.g., dropped on the floor) or is functioning improperly should be inspected by qualified personnel before subsequent use.
- Ensure all line-powered equipment has a testing seal (maximum leakage of a current < 1 milliampere).
- A sticker should be placed on equipment noting the last inspection/maintenance date.
- Maintain an updated log for all equipment used in the physical therapy department.
- Maintain electrotherapy equipment operation manuals in an accessible location for staff members to use as a resource.
- Electrotherapy equipment should only be used by qualified personnel who have read the operating manual and are familiar with how to properly operate the equipment.
- All electrotherapy devices should have a hospital grade three-pronged plug that has a safety ground attached to an earth ground.
- Electrical outlets should be equipped with ground fault circuit interrupters (GFCIs). GFCIs are designed to cut off electrical supply to equipment when any form of leakage or ground-fault is identified.
- Extension cords or multiple adapters should not be used.
- Plugs should be removed from the wall by gripping and pulling the plug and not by pulling the cable.
- Unplug all powered-line devices at the end of each day.
- Always turn the intensity dial to zero before unplugging electrotherapy equipment.
- Instruct patients to avoid all contact with the controls of an electrotherapy devices unless otherwise instructed.
- Thoroughly instruct patients on the type of sensations typically experienced with a specific electrotherapy device.
- Avoid placing containers of liquid (e.g., coffee, soda) on top of the casing of electrical equipment.
- Keep electrotherapy equipment 3-5 meters from each other when in use to minimize the possibility of electrical interference.

## Indications[16,17,18]

- Pain
- Calcium deposits
- Fungal infection
- Hyperhidrosis
- Inflammation
- Ischemia
- Keloids
- Muscle spasm
- Myositis ossificans
- Plantar warts
- Scar tissue
- Wounds

## Contraindications[16,17,18]

- Drug allergies
- Skin sensitivity reactions to specific ions

The amount of electricity used when performing iontophoresis is measured in milliamp minutes (mA-min). This value is often termed "dosage" and is determined by multiplying current amplitude and time. Dosage ranges from 40-80 mA-min with iontophoresis.[16,17]

A dosage of 40 mA-min could be delivered in 10 minutes with a current amplitude of 4.0 mA. The same dosage could be delivered using a lower current amplitude with a longer duration. A lower current amplitude and a longer duration will be less likely to cause skin irritation or burns.[17]

The current amplitude should be adjusted to be comfortable for the patient. Current amplitudes typically range from 1.0-4.0 mA.[16,17] Once the current amplitude is determined, the therapist can select an appropriate amount of time to ensure the appropriate mA-min dosage level. Many iontophoresis units will automatically calculate the duration of the treatment session based on the preset dosage and the current amplitude.

### Iontophoresis Procedures

The therapist must identify any known patient allergies or the potential for adverse reactions based on the ion used. The skin should be thoroughly cleaned with soap or isopropyl alcohol. The patient should be positioned comfortably, but should not lie on top of the electrodes. The unit should be set to continuous direct current. Polarity should be set to the same polarity as the ion solution.[16] The ion solution is placed into a small chamber located on a self-adhesive electrode placed at the treatment site.

The electrode containing the ion solution is referred to as the active electrode.[18] A second electrode, referred to as the dispersive electrode, is placed away from the active electrode. The recommended spacing between the active and dispersive electrodes should be minimally equivalent to the diameter of the active electrode.[18] As the spacing between the electrodes increases, the current density in the superficial tissues decreases, resulting in a diminished risk for burns. Smaller electrodes have higher current density and are often used to treat a specific lesion, while larger electrodes are used when the treatment area is less well defined.[18]

The therapist should make sure the electrodes are appropriately secured and slowly increase the intensity towards a maximum of four milliamperes. Treatment should last 10-20 minutes.[18]

Additional time may be required for treatment at an intensity of less than four milliamperes. The therapist must monitor the patient every 3-5 minutes during treatment to ensure that the patient is not exhibiting signs of skin irritation or burns under the electrode.[18]

**Acidic reaction:** A patient may have an acidic reaction from the iontophoresis treatment as a result of hydrochloric acid forming under the positive electrode (anode).[18]

**Alkaline reaction:** A patient may have an alkaline reaction from the iontophoresis treatment as a result of sodium hydroxide forming under the negative electrode (cathode).

Acidic and alkaline reactions often cause significant discomfort, skin irritation or chemical burns.[18]

The likelihood of a burn can be decreased by increasing the size of the cathode relative to the anode, decreasing the current density, and increasing the space between the electrodes.[18]

Upon completion of treatment, the therapist must slowly decrease the intensity and remove the electrodes. It is common for patients to have redness of the skin under the active electrode. In some cases, the active electrode can be left in place for 12-24 hours after treatment to facilitate further diffusion of ions through the skin.

Fig. 9-75: An electrode with an integrated battery for iontophoresis drug delivery.

The frequency of treatment depends on the ion selected, the underlying condition, patient tolerance, and the relative effectiveness of the treatment.[17] Iontophoresis should be applied no more frequently than every other day due to the potential side effects from using direct current.[17] A therapist should be able to make a relative determination of the effectiveness of iontophoresis within three to five treatment sessions.

## Ions Used with Iontophoresis[16,17,18]

| Medication | Indications | Polarity |
|---|---|---|
| Acetic acid | Calcific deposits, myositis ossificans | Negative |
| Calcium chloride | Scar tissue, keloids, muscle spasms | Negative |
| Copper sulfate | Fungal infection | Positive |
| Dexamethasone | Inflammation | Negative |
| Iodine | Scars, adhesive capsulitis | Negative |
| Lidocaine | Analgesia, inflammation | Positive |
| Magnesium sulfate | Muscle spasms, ischemia | Positive |
| Salicylates | Muscle and joint pain, plantar warts | Negative |
| Zinc oxide | Healing, dermal ulcers, wounds | Positive |

## Electromyography

Electromyography (EMG) is the science of evaluating motor units (the anterior horn cell and its axon, neuromuscular junctions, and muscle fibers innervated by the unit) through the use of intramuscular needle electrodes or surface electrodes. EMG involves the recording of action potentials from muscle fibers during voluntary movement and potentially spontaneous action potentials from muscle fibers at rest.[24] Indwelling electrodes (i.e., intramuscular EMG) are used for small or deep muscles or when there is a need to record a single motor unit potential. Surface electrodes (i.e., biofeedback) are used to monitor larger muscle groups.

### Intramuscular EMG

Intramuscular EMG involves insertion of a needle electrode into the muscle by a trained professional, most often a neurologist, physiatrist or physical therapist. In some licensing jurisdictions, physical therapists may not be able to perform intramuscular EMG due to the established practice act.

The area of skin over the muscle to be tested should be thoroughly cleaned. The needle is inserted into the muscle at rest while the oscilloscope is observed. The insertional irritability should last only a few milliseconds. A normal relaxed muscle should exhibit electrical silence (i.e., no electrical potentials).[26] Spontaneous potentials during rest are abnormal findings and may indicate nerve or muscle damage.[26] When the muscle is voluntarily contracted, action potentials begin to appear. The size, shape, and frequency of the motor unit potentials should be assessed. As the strength of the contraction increases, a greater number of muscle fibers produce action potentials. During full muscle contraction, a disorderly group of action potentials of varying rates and amplitudes is observed. A nerve conduction velocity test is often performed in conjunction with an EMG.

### Abnormal Potentials

#### Spontaneous[24]

**Fibrillation potentials:** indicative of lower motor neuron disease

**Positive sharp wave:** denervated muscle disorders at rest, primary muscle disease such as muscular dystrophy

**Fasciculations:** irritation/degeneration of anterior horn cell, nerve root compression or muscle spasms

**Repetitive discharges:** myopathies, lesion of anterior horn cells and peripheral nerves

#### Voluntary[24]

**Polyphasic potentials:** myopathies, muscle or peripheral nerve involvement

Abnormal results from intramuscular EMG can be associated with a variety of medical conditions including amyotrophic lateral sclerosis, carpal tunnel syndrome, Duchenne muscular dystrophy, Guillain-Barre syndrome, myasthenia gravis, peripheral neuropathy, and poliomyelitis.

## Common Muscles used for Insertion of Needle Electrodes

| Upper Extremity | | Lower Extremity | |
|---|---|---|---|
| C5-6 | Lateral deltoid | L2, 3, 4 | Vastus medialis |
| C5-6 | Biceps brachii | L4-5 | Tibialis anterior |
| C6-7 | Triceps brachii | L4-5, S1 | Tensor fasciae latae |
| C6-7 | Flexor carpi radialis | L5-S1 | Peroneus longus |
| C7-8 | Extensor indicis proprius | L5, S1-2 | Gluteus maximus |
| C8-T1 | Abductor pollicis brevis | L5, S1-2 | Hamstrings |
| C8-T1 | First dorsal interossei | S1-2 | Gastrocnemius |

### Biofeedback

Biofeedback refers to the use of instrumentation to bring specific events to conscious awareness (Fig. 9-76). Biofeedback can be utilized to receive information related to motor performance, kinesthetic performance or physiological response.[16] Electromyographic biofeedback is the most commonly used biofeedback modality in the clinical setting. Biofeedback allows patients to make small changes in performance and receive immediate feedback. By successfully rewarding small changes incrementally, larger changes can potentially be achieved.

Biofeedback does not measure muscle contraction, but rather the electrical activity associated with muscle contraction. There is not a standard measurement scale when reporting electrical activity using a biofeedback unit. The electrical activity is most commonly presented as visual and/or auditory feedback. Visual feedback is often presented as a series of colored lights that go on and off in a linear fashion based on the strength of the incoming signal. Auditory feedback is often presented as a buzzing, clicking or beeping sound that changes in intensity as the strength of the incoming signal increases or decreases.

Prior to treatment the therapist should ensure that the patient's skin is clean and dry. Biofeedback requires the use of surface electrodes which provide less specific information than indwelling electrodes, however, surface electrodes are more effective in quantifying muscle activity in several muscles or a group of muscles. The electrodes can be disposable or non-disposable. Disposable electrodes typically are designed with the appropriate amount of gel and an adhesive that allows the electrode to firmly adhere to the skin. Non-disposable electrodes require gel and need to be adequately secured to the skin by the therapist.

## Therapeutic Effects[18,20]

- Decreased accessory muscle use
- Decreased muscle spasm
- Decreased pain
- Improved muscle strength
- Muscle relaxation
- Neuromuscular control

## Indications[18,20]

- Bowel incontinence
- Cerebral palsy
- Hemiplegia
- Impaired motor control
- Muscle spasm
- Muscle weakness
- Pain
- Spinal cord injury
- Urinary incontinence

## Contraindications[18,20]

- Conditions where muscle contraction is detrimental
- Skin irritation at the electrode site

The two active electrodes should be placed parallel to the muscle fibers and close to each other.[18] The reference or ground electrode can be placed anywhere on the body, but is often secured between the two active electrodes. The signals are transmitted to a differential amplifier and information is conveyed through visual and auditory feedback. The described setup can minimize "noise," which refers to the extraneous electrical activity not produced by the contraction of the muscle.

The therapist can control the relative signal sensitivity during treatment. A high sensitivity will detect extremely small amounts of electrical activity while a low sensitivity setting will detect only large amounts of electrical activity. As a result, high sensitivity settings are used when the treatment objective is relaxation and low sensitivity settings are used when the treatment objective is muscle re-education.[18]

### Muscle Relaxation

The treatment for muscle relaxation requires a high sensitivity setting with active electrodes initially positioned close to each other. As the patient improves with relaxation, the electrodes should be placed further apart and the sensitivity setting should be increased. A decrease in audio or visual feedback would be considered a positive sign. The patient may also benefit from adjunct relaxation techniques, such as imagery. Treatment duration of 10-15 minutes is usually adequate to attain relaxation.

### Muscle Re-education

The treatment for muscle re-education should begin with the patient performing a maximal muscle contraction. The sensitivity of the biofeedback unit should be set at a low sensitivity setting and adjusted so that the patient can perform the repetitions at a ratio of two-thirds of the maximal muscle contraction. Isometric contractions should continue for 6-10 seconds with relaxation in between each contraction. An increase in audio or visual feedback would be considered a positive sign. Treatment duration for a single muscle group is 5-10 minutes.[18] As the patient is able to demonstrate greater recruitment of the target muscle, more complex activities are added to the program.

## Massage

Massage is a manual therapeutic modality that produces physiologic effects through different types of stroking, rubbing, and pressure (Fig. 9-77). Massage is capable of producing mechanical and reflexive effects.

**Fig. 9-76:** A biofeedback unit. Courtesy Chattanooga, a DJO Global Company.

## Therapeutic Effects[27,28,29]

- Altered pain transmission
- Decreased anxiety and tension
- Decreased muscle atrophy
- Decreased muscle spasm
- Facilitate healing
- Improved circulation
- Increased lymphatic circulation
- Loosen adhesions
- Reduction of edema
- Relaxation
- Removal of metabolic waste
- Stimulate reflexive effects

## Indications[27,28,29]

- Adhesion
- Bursitis
- Decreased range of motion
- Edema
- Intermittent claudication
- Lactic acid excess
- Migraine or headache
- Muscle spasm and cramping
- Pain
- Raynaud's syndrome
- Scar tissue
- Tendonitis
- Trigger point

## Contraindications[27,28,29]

- Acute injury
- Arteriosclerosis
- Cancer
- Cellulitis
- Embolus
- Infection
- Thrombus

## Massage Parameters[28]

There are a variety of different massage techniques described in the literature. Each technique varies in relation to a number of important variables.

**Direction** – The general movement pattern of the massage stroke. Direction can be described as centrifugal or centripedal. Centrifugal is moving from the center of the body out. Centripedal is moving in from the extremities toward the center of the body.

**Duration** – The length of time a massage technique is performed. Duration is highly variable depending on the characteristics of the massage technique, established therapeutic objectives, and patient tolerance.

**Frequency** – The rate at which the massage technique repeats itself in a given time frame. The variety of massage techniques are repeated several times prior to transitioning to a different technique.

**Pressure** – The relative amount of compressive stress applied to the body. Pressure is usually described by terms such as light, moderate, deep or variable (Fig. 9-78).

**Rhythm** – The relative regularity of the massage technique. A massage technique applied at regular consistent intervals would be considered rhythmic. If the technique was applied at inconsistent intervals, it would be considered non-rhythmic.

**Speed** – The general rate the therapist's hands move. Speed is usually described as slow, moderate, fast or variable.

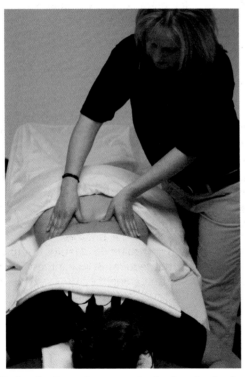

**Fig. 9-77:** Application of massage to the low back of a properly draped patient.

**Fig. 9-78:** Massage applied to the upper back of a patient in supported sitting.

## Massage Techniques[27,28,29]

### Effleurage

Effleurage is a massage technique that is characterized by a light stroke that produces a reflexive response. The technique is performed at the beginning and end of a massage to allow the patient to relax. Strokes should be directed towards the heart. Effleurage can also be applied as a deep stroke to produce both a mechanical and a reflexive response.

### Friction

Friction is a massage technique that incorporates small circular motions over a trigger point or muscle spasm. This is a deep massage technique that penetrates into the depth of a muscle and attempts to reduce edema, loosen adhesions, and relieve muscle spasm. Friction massage is used frequently with chronic inflammation or with overuse injuries (Fig. 9-79).

**Fig. 9-79:** Transverse friction massage applied to the patellar tendon.

### Petrissage

Petrissage is a massage technique described as kneading, where the muscle is squeezed and rolled under the therapist's hands. The goal of petrissage is to loosen adhesions, improve lymphatic return, and facilitate removal of metabolic waste from the treatment area. Petrissage should be performed in a distal to proximal sequence. Petrissage can be performed with two hands over larger muscle groups or with as few as two fingers over smaller muscles.

### Tapotement

Tapotement is a massage technique that provides stimulation through rapid alternating movements such as tapping, hacking, cupping, and slapping. The primary purpose of tapotement is to enhance circulation and stimulate peripheral nerve endings.

### Vibration

Vibration is a massage technique that places the therapist's hands or fingers firmly over an area and utilizes a rapid, shaking motion that causes vibration to the treatment area. The therapist initiates this motion from the forearm while maintaining firm contact on the treatment area. Vibration is used primarily for relaxation.

## Massage Parameters

Prior to initiating massage, a therapist must obtain patient consent. Components of consent when performing massage would minimally include:

1. A description of the proposed massage.

2. The relative risks and benefits.

3. The expectations of the patient during the massage.

4. The opportunity to consent to or refuse the proposed intervention.

Massage should occur in a room with air temperature of 72-75 degrees Fahrenheit.[28] This temperature range will allow the patient to relax and minimize undesired muscular tension. The patient should be comfortably positioned and properly draped prior to the initiation of treatment. Standard bed linens are most often used for draping. The therapist should attempt to leave only the area of the body being massaged exposed, while the remainder of the body should be draped. Pillows, towels, bolsters, foam, and blankets can be used to ensure patient comfort.

The therapist's hands must be clean, dry, and warm. A therapist will typically use a lubricant to reduce friction on the skin during massage. The primary exception to using lubricant would be when performing friction massage. The lubricant should be applied to the therapist's hands and gently warmed by rubbing the hands together prior to patient application.

The therapist must be positioned in an efficient posture during treatment to maintain the required pressure and rhythm based on the goals of treatment. The massage should start with the effleurage technique. The amount of time required for each treatment is dependent on the body part and therapeutic goal. Generally, the back requires 15 minutes as opposed to a smaller area or joint that requires 8-10 minutes. The intensity should progressively increase and then decrease, using effleurage again to end the treatment session.

# Equipment and Devices; Therapeutic Modalities Essentials

## Equipment and Devices

1. Communication between the therapist and patient is essential in performing safe and effective mobility tasks.

2. A patient who is dependent should be repositioned at least every two hours to prevent skin breakdown.

3. Shear and friction forces should be minimized during mobility and transfer tasks to prevent integumentary injury.

4. The level of physical assistance required during a mobility or transfer task is a function of the amount of assistance the therapist must provide in order for the patient to safely complete the task.

5. Levels of physical assistance for transfers include independent, supervision, contact guard, minimal assist, moderate assist, maximal assist, and dependent.

6. Dependent transfers may be performed either with physical assistance from staff or a mechanical lift device.

7. Dependent transfers include three-person carry/lift, two-person lift, dependent squat pivot transfer, and hydraulic lift.

8. Assisted transfers include sliding board transfer, stand pivot transfer, and stand step transfer.

9. The adult standard wheelchair seat specifications are 18 inches wide, 16 inches deep, and 20 inches high.

10. A patient's physical and mental abilities and limitations must be considered when making recommendations for wheelchair prescription.

11. Parallel bars provide the most stable environment for patients who are beginning to initiate standing and ambulation activities.

12. Levels of weight bearing include non-weight bearing, toe touch weight bearing, partial weight bearing, weight bearing as tolerated, and full weight bearing.

13. An appropriately fit walker, crutches or cane requires 20-25 degrees of elbow flexion.

14. A straight cane is not appropriate for patients who are partial weight bearing.

15. When using an assistive device, the gait pattern utilized should be dependent on the patient's weight bearing status and overall condition.

16. Gait patterns include two-point, three-point, four-point, swing-to, and swing-through.

17. Guidelines for guarding a patient during ambulation activities may require modification or the assist of a second therapist depending on the patient's size, impairments, and abilities.

18. During stair training, the physical therapist should be positioned behind the patient while ascending and in front of the patient when descending.

19. An arterial line is a monitoring device consisting of a catheter that is inserted into an artery. The device is used to measure blood pressure or to obtain blood samples.

20. A nasal cannula is a commonly used device for oxygen therapy, capable of delivering up to six liters of oxygen per minute.

21. A suprapubic catheter is an indwelling urinary catheter that is surgically inserted directly into the patient's bladder.

22. Doppler ultrasonography is a non-invasive test that evaluates blood flow in the major veins, arteries, and cerebrovascular system.

23. Magnetic resonance imaging is a non-invasive technique that utilizes magnetic fields to produce an image of bone and soft tissue.

## Therapeutic Modalities

24. Methods of heat transfer include conduction, convection, conversion, evaporation, and radiation.

25. Ice massage should be applied using small, overlapping circles or strokes. An area 10 centimeters by 15 centimeters can be covered in 5 to 10 minutes.

26. Patients typically progress through a series of different sensations during ice massage including intense cold, burning, aching, and analgesia.

27. Ice massage typically cools tissues more rapidly than other types of cryotherapy such as an ice pack or ice bag. The cold pack should be applied over a moist cold towel to increase the initial magnitude of cooling.

28. Cold baths allow for circumferential contact with the cooling agent, however, they require the lower extremity to be in a gravity-dependent position.

29. Controlled cold compression units combine cryotherapy and compression. The units allow therapists to precisely control the temperature of the cold and the amount of compression.

30. A Cryo Cuff is a commercially available device used to provide mild cooling and compression. The device consists of a nylon sleeve connected to a container using a plastic tube.

# Equipment and Devices; Therapeutic Modalities Essentials

31. Vapocoolant sprays produce very rapid cooling through evaporation with temperature changes occurring only in the epidermis. The primary use of vapocoolant sprays is to treat trigger points.

32. Relative changes in surface tissue temperature will be influenced by the intensity of the heating agent, time of the exposure, and thermal conductivity of the tissues.

33. Superficial heating agents produce the largest temperature elevation within 0.5 centimeters from the skin surface.

34. Application of a hot pack requires six to eight towel layers. If commercial hot pack covers are used, they typically are equivalent to two or three layers of towels.

35. A patient should not lie on top of a hot pack since this tends to remove water from the hot pack. This can result in an accelerated rate of heating and an increased risk of burns.

36. Fluidotherapy is a superficial heating agent that generates dry heat through forced convection by circulating warm air and small cellulose particles.

37. An infrared lamp produces superficial heating of tissue through radiant heat. Optimal absorption occurs when the infrared radiation strikes the target area perpendicularly.

38. Paraffin has a low specific heat which enhances a patient's ability to tolerate heat compared to heat from water at the same temperature.

39. Paraffin can be applied using the dip-wrap method, dip-reimmersion method or paint application method.

40. Thermal effects of ultrasound include acceleration of metabolic rate, modulation of pain, reduction of muscle spasm, decreased joint stiffness, alteration of nerve conduction velocity, increased circulation, and increased soft tissue extensibility.

41. Nonthermal effects of ultrasound include increased cell and skin membrane permeability, increased intracellular calcium levels, facilitation of tissue repair, and promotion of normal cell function.

42. A frequency setting of 1 MHz when using ultrasound is used for deeper tissues (up to five centimeters) while a setting of 3 MHz is used for more superficial tissues (one to two centimeters).

43. An area two to three times the size of the ultrasound transducer typically requires a duration of five minutes.

44. The duty cycle of ultrasound is calculated by dividing the time during which sound is delivered (on time) by the total time (on time + off time) and multiplying the result by 100.

45. Phonophoresis is not likely to produce burns or damage skin since the technique transports whole molecules instead of ions into the body's tissue.

46. Shortwave diathermy can be delivered in a continuous or pulsed mode. A pulsed mode is typically utilized to attain nonthermal effects while a continuous mode is used for thermal effects.

47. The patient's subjective heat sensation response is used to estimate the amount of energy delivered and corresponding temperature increase with continuous diathermy.

48. The minimal erythemal dose refers to the smallest dose of ultraviolet light needed to produce an area of mild redness within eight hours of ultraviolet exposure that disappears within 24 hours after exposure.

49. The properties of water essential for physical therapists to understand include buoyancy, resistance, specific gravity, specific heat, total drag force, and viscosity.

50. Hydrotherapy can be administered using a variety of equipment including an extremity tank, lowboy tank, highboy tank, Hubbard tank, and therapeutic pool.

51. A flexed position of the spine results in greater separation of the posterior structures including the facet joints and intervertebral foramen when using mechanical lumbar traction. An extended position of the spine results in greater separation of the anterior structures including the disk spaces.

52. Static traction may be desirable for more acute conditions or if the patient's symptoms are slightly exaggerated by movement.

53. Intermittent traction may be desirable for joint mobilization or for patients who cannot tolerate static traction.

54. A force of 25% of a patient's body weight may be adequate to treat muscle spasm, disk protrusion, and stretch soft tissue when using mechanical lumbar traction. A force of up to 50% of the body weight is required for actual separation of the vertebrae.

55. A supine position is used more often for cervical traction since the traction force does not have to overcome the force exerted by gravity.

56. A force of 7-10% of a patient's body weight (11-15 pounds) may be adequate to treat muscle spasm, stretch soft tissue, and reduce disk protrusion using cervical traction.

# Equipment and Devices; Therapeutic Modalities Essentials

57. A force of 13-20% of a patient's body weight (20-30 pounds) may be necessary for joint distraction using cervical traction.

58. Compression garments are most often used to control edema, limit scar formation after burns, and improve venous circulation in active patients.

59. An intermittent pneumatic compression pump is primarily used to reduce chronic or post-traumatic edema and requires adjusting the parameters of inflation pressure, on/off ratio, and total treatment time.

60. A patient's joint must be aligned correctly with the axis of the CPM to receive safe and effective treatment. A rate of two cycles per minute allows most patients to tolerate the CPM without difficulty.

61. For an action potential to be evoked using electrical stimulation, the amplitude of the stimulus and pulse duration must be sufficient to overcome the established threshold.

62. Direct current is characterized by a constant flow of electrons from the anode to the cathode (for a period of greater than one second) without interruption.

63. Alternating current is characterized by polarity that continuously changes from positive to negative with a change in direction of current flow.

64. Pulsatile current is characterized by the non-continuous flow of direct or alternating current.

65. Small electrodes exhibit increased current density, increased impedance, and decreased current flow. Large electrodes exhibit decreased current density, decreased impedance, and increased current flow.

66. The effectiveness of a current to target specific excitable tissue is dependent on adequate intensity to reach the threshold, current onset fast enough to reduce accommodation (i.e., rise time), and duration long enough to exceed the capacitance of the tissue (i.e., phase duration).

67. Neuromuscular electrical stimulation (NMES) is a technique used to facilitate skeletal muscle activity. Functional electrical stimulation (FES) uses electrical stimulation to create or enhance the performance of a functional activity.

68. The most commonly used modes for TENS include conventional, acupuncture-like, brief intense, and noxious.

69. Interferential current combines two medium frequency alternating waveforms that are biphasic. Interferential current is most often used for pain relief, increased circulation, and muscle stimulation.

70. Iontophoresis is based on the theory that like charges repel and as a result, ions in a solution of similar charge will move away from the electrical source and into the body. The rate of ion delivery is determined by the concentration of the ion, the pH of the solution, the current density, and the duration of the treatment.

71. The likelihood of a burn using iontophoresis can be decreased by increasing the size of the cathode relative to the anode, decreasing the current density, and increasing the space between the electrodes.

72. Indwelling electrodes (i.e., intramuscular EMG) are used for small or deep muscles or when there is a need to record a single motor unit potential. Surface electrodes (i.e., biofeedback) are used to monitor larger muscle groups.

73. Biofeedback can be utilized to receive information related to motor performance, kinesthetic performance or physiological response. A high sensitivity setting will detect extremely small amounts of electrical activity while a low sensitivity setting will detect only large amounts of electrical activity.

74. Descriptive characteristics of massage techniques include direction, duration, frequency, pressure, rhythm, and speed.

75. Commonly used massage techniques include effleurage, friction, petrissage, tapotement, and vibration.

# Equipment and Devices; Therapeutic Modalities Proficiencies

## Equipment and Devices Proficiencies

### 1. Levels of Physical Assistance

Identify the level of physical assistance associated with each of the descriptions. Answers must be selected from the Word Bank and can be used only once.

**Word Bank:** dependent, independent, maximal assist, minimal assist, moderate assist, supervision

| Level | Description |
|---|---|
| a | The patient requires a therapist to observe throughout the completion of the task. |
| b | The therapist exerts all of the effort to perform the task. |
| c | The patient requires 50% assist from the therapist to complete the task. |
| d | The patient does not require any assistance to complete the task. |
| e | The patient requires 25% assist from the therapist to complete the task. |
| f | The patient requires 75% assist from the therapist to complete the task. |

### 2. Wheelchair Measurements

Identify the most appropriate wheelchair component associated with each of the obtained measurements. Answers must be selected from the Word Bank and can be used only once. Secondly, identify the final value in inches for each component based on the obtained measurement.

**Word Bank:** armrest height, back height, seat depth, seat height, seat width

| Component | Obtained Measurement | Final Value |
|---|---|---|
| a | 7 inches from the seat of the chair to the olecranon process with the elbow flexed to 90 degrees. | b |
| c | 18 inches from the user's heel to the popliteal fold. | d |
| e | 18 inches from the posterior buttock, along the lateral thigh to the popliteal fold. | f |
| g | 20 inches from the seat of the chair to the floor of the axilla with the user's shoulder flexed to 90 degrees. | h |
| i | 17 inches represents the widest aspect of the user's buttocks, hips or thighs. | j |

# Equipment and Devices; Therapeutic Modalities Proficiencie

## Equipment and Devices Proficiencies

### 3. Levels of Weight Bearing

Identify the level of weight bearing associated with each of the descriptions. Answers must be selected from the Word Bank and can be used only once.

**Word Bank:** full weight bearing, non-weight bearing, partial weight bearing, toe touch weight bearing, weight bearing as tolerated

| Level | Description |
|-------|-------------|
| a | A patient using axillary crutches is able to transmit approximately 25% of their weight through the involved lower extremity. |
| b | A patient uses a single cane during ambulation. |
| c | A patient is permitted to vary the amount of weight bearing based on their relative comfort level and the amount of pain present. |
| d | A patient is unable to transmit weight through the involved lower extremity, but may place a portion of the involved foot on the ground to assist with balance. |
| e | A patient is unable to transmit weight through the involved extremity or have the foot come in contact with the floor. |

### 4. Assistive Device Selection

Identify the most appropriate assistive device for each patient based on the supplied description. Answers must be selected from the Word Bank and can be used only once.

**Word Bank:** axillary crutches, cane, Lofstrand crutches, parallel bars, walker

| Level | Description |
|-------|-------------|
| a | A 34-year-old male in an acute care hospital prepares to ambulate for the first time following a compound tibia fracture treated with internal fixation. |
| b | An 83-year-old female that often experiences transient periods of dizziness while walking in the home. |
| c | A 21-year-old female that is toe touch weight bearing following a grade II knee sprain. |
| d | A 74-year-old female that experiences subtle balance changes when walking on uneven ground. |
| e | A 28-year-old male that is partial weight bearing on the right ankle following an ankle sprain. The patient is unable to tolerate pressure in the axillary region due to recent removal of a benign cyst. |

# Equipment and Devices; Therapeutic Modalities Proficiencies

## Equipment and Devices Proficiencies

### 5. Wheelchair Frame

Identify the most appropriate wheelchair frame for each patient based on the supplied description. Answers must be selected from the Word Bank and can be used only once.

**Word Bank:** amputee frame, hemi frame, one-hand drive frame, power wheelchair frame, reclining frame, ultralight frame

| Frame | Description |
|---|---|
| a | Patient is able to independently propel the wheelchair, however, the center of gravity is shifted posteriorly. |
| b | Patient is able to independently propel the wheelchair using one or both of the lower extremities. |
| c | Patient is involved in sports activities without the need for postural supports. |
| d | Patient is able to independently propel the wheelchair using one upper extremity. |
| e | Patient is unable to independently propel the wheelchair. |
| f | Patient is unable to sit upright for extended periods of time. |

# Equipment and Devices; Therapeutic Modalities Proficiencie

## Equipment and Devices Proficiencies

### 6. Equipment and Devices Basics

Mark each statement as True or False. If the statement is False, correct the statement in the space provided.

| | True/False | Statement |
|---|---|---|
| a | | A dependent squat pivot transfer is used to transfer a patient who cannot stand independently and is unable to bear any weight through the lower extremities. |
| | Correction: | |
| b | | The standard adult wheelchair has 16 inches of seat width, 18 inches of seat depth, and 20 inches of seat height. |
| | Correction: | |
| c | | Wheelchair seat depth is determined by measuring from the posterior buttock, along the lateral thigh to the popliteal fold and adding two inches. |
| | Correction: | |
| d | | An appropriately fit axillary crutch should result in the patient having 20-25 degrees of elbow flexion when grasping the hand grip. |
| | Correction: | |
| e | | A custom molded wheelchair seat is warranted for patients with pelvic obliquity or fixed asymmetrical deformity. |
| | Correction: | |

# Equipment and Devices; Therapeutic Modalities Proficiencies

## Equipment and Devices Proficiencies

| True/False | Statement |
|---|---|
| f | A cane can be used to improve balance in patient's that are partial weight bearing. |
| Correction: | |
| g | Lofstrand crutches can be used with a variety of gait patterns including four-point, swing-to, and swing-through. |
| Correction: | |
| h | A gastric tube is a plastic tube inserted through a nostril that extends into the stomach. |
| Correction: | |
| i | A suprapubic catheter is applied over the shaft of the penis and is held in place by a padded strap or adhesive tape. |
| Correction: | |
| j | Myelography utilizes a contrast medium that is injected into the epidual space by spinal puncture. |
| Correction: | |

## Equipment and Devices; Therapeutic Modalities Proficiencie

# Therapeutic Modalities Proficiencies

### 7. Heat Transfer

Identify the type of heat transfer utilized by each therapeutic modality. Answers should be selected from the Word Bank. Answers can be used more than once.

**Word Bank:** conduction, convection, conversion, evaporation, radiation

| Modality | Heat Transfer |
|----------|---------------|
| fluidotherapy | a |
| paraffin | b |
| vapocoolant spray | c |
| hot pack | d |
| whirlpool | e |
| ultrasound | f |
| diathermy | g |
| ice massage | h |
| ultraviolet light | i |

### 8. Therapeutic Effects of Cryotherapy

Potential therapeutic effects of cryotherapy are listed. Mark each statement as True or False.

| True/False | Effects |
|------------|---------|
| a | increased metabolic rate |
| b | decreased nerve conduction velocity |
| c | decreased tone |
| d | decreased pain threshold |
| e | decreased blood flow to the treatment area |

QUIZ

# Equipment and Devices; Therapeutic Modalities Proficiencies

## Therapeutic Modalities Proficiencies

### 9. Indications/Contraindications of Cryotherapy

Mark each condition as an indication or contraindication of cryotherapy.

| Indication/Contraindication | | Condition |
|---|---|---|
| a | | bursitis |
| b | | infection |
| c | | cold urticaria |
| d | | tendonitis |
| e | | tenosynovitis |
| f | | skin anesthesia |
| g | | Raynaud's phenomenon |
| h | | muscle spasm |

### 10. Cooling Agents Matching

Assign each of the descriptions to the most appropriate cooling agent. More than one of the descriptions may apply to each cooling agent. The number of desired responses for each cooling agent is identified in parentheses.

1. Effective for small and irregular contoured areas
2. Allows simultaneous application of cold and compression
3. Short duration time (i.e., 10 minutes or less)
4. Unable to observe target area during treatment
5. Difficult to apply spray uniformly
6. Requires the extremity to be in a gravity dependent position

| Cooling Agent | Description | |
|---|---|---|
| cold bath | a | (1) |
| controlled cold compression unit | b | (2) |
| Cryo cuff | c | (2) |
| ice massage | d | (2) |
| vapocoolant spray | e | (1) |

## QUIZ Equipment and Devices; Therapeutic Modalities Proficiencie

# Therapeutic Modalities Proficiencies

### 11. Therapeutic Effects of Superficial Thermotherapy

Potential therapeutic effects of superficial thermotherapy are listed. Mark each statement as True or False.

| | True/False | Effects |
|---|---|---|
| a | | increased tone |
| b | | decreased collagen extensibility |
| c | | increased pain threshold |
| d | | decreased nerve conduction velocity |
| e | | increased metabolic rate |

### 12. Indications/Contraindications of Superficial Thermotherapy

Mark each condition as an indication or contraindication of superficial thermotherapy.

| | Indication/Contraindication | Condition |
|---|---|---|
| a | | decreased range of motion |
| b | | over an area of malignancy |
| c | | subacute or chronic pain |
| d | | muscle spasm |
| e | | arterial disease |
| f | | subacute or chronic inflammatory conditions |
| g | | peripheral vascular disease |
| h | | thrombophlebitis |

# QUIZ Equipment and Devices; Therapeutic Modalities Proficiencies

## Therapeutic Modalities Proficiencies

### 13. Heating Agents Matching

Assign each of the descriptions to the most appropriate heating agent. More than one of the descriptions may apply to each heating agent. The number of desired responses for each heating agent is identified in parentheses.

1. Can produce thermal and nonthermal effects
2. Provides a moist, comfortable heat
3. Tends to dry skin
4. Useful for desensitization of the distal extremities
5. Does not require direct contact with the treatment area
6. May serve to moisturize the skin
7. Capable of reaching deeper tissues

| Heating Agent | Description | |
|---|---|---|
| diathermy | a | (2) |
| fluidotherapy | b | (1) |
| hot pack | c | (1) |
| infrared lamp | d | (2) |
| paraffin | e | (1) |
| ultrasound | f | (2) |

# QUIZ Equipment and Devices; Therapeutic Modalities Proficiencie

## Therapeutic Modalities Proficiencies

### 14. Parameters and Procedures

Mark each statement as True or False. If the statement is False, correct the statement in the space provided.

| True/False | Statement |
|---|---|
| a | The Cryo Cuff should be held approximately 6-8 inches above the level of the sleeve during filling. |
| **Correction:** | |
| b | A vapocoolant spray should be applied perpendicular to the direction of the muscle fibers. |
| **Correction:** | |
| c | 6-8 layers of towels are necessary for hot pack application. |
| **Correction:** | |
| d | Ultrasound frequency of 3 MHz heats deep tissue (up to 5 cm), while 1 MHz heats superficial tissue (1-2 cm). |
| **Correction:** | |
| e | The temperature of a paraffin bath should be maintained between 107 and 112 degrees Fahrenheit. |
| **Correction:** | |
| f | A 20% duty cycle with an on time of 1 second would have an off time of 5 seconds. |
| **Correction:** | |
| g | An area two to three times the size of the ultrasound transducer typically requires a treatment duration of five minutes. |
| **Correction:** | |

## QUIZ Equipment and Devices; Therapeutic Modalities Proficiencies

### Therapeutic Modalities Proficiencies

| True/False | Statement |
|---|---|
| h | A patient's subjective heat sensation response is an important factor when determining the amount of energy delivered with diathermy. |
| Correction: | |
| i | The minimal erythemal dose is characterized by a dose that results in erythema that lasts 1-3 days with clear redness and mild desquamation. |
| Correction: | |
| j | Buoyancy refers to the magnitude of the cohesive forces between the molecules specific to the fluid. |
| Correction: | |
| k | Hot packs are required to be in place for 5-10 minutes to achieve the desired therapeutic effects. |
| Correction: | |
| l | An infrared lamp's primary therapeutic effect is the enhancement of deep tissue healing. |
| Correction: | |
| m | During application of fluidotherapy, patients can perform active exercises of the distal extremity. |
| Correction: | |
| n | The rate of tissue cooling following heating with diathermy is significantly slower than the rate of tissue cooling with ultrasound. |
| Correction: | |
| o | Ultraviolet light is absorbed 1-2 centimeters into the skin. |
| Correction: | |

# QUIZ Equipment and Devices; Therapeutic Modalities Proficiencie

## Therapeutic Modalities Proficiencies

### 15. Electrotherapy Terminology

Identify the electrotherapy term most closely associated with the supplied description. Answers must be selected from the Word Bank and can be used only once.

**Word Bank:** alternating current, current, direct current, frequency, phase duration, pulsatile current, pulse duration, resistance, rise time, voltage

| Terminology | Description |
|---|---|
| a | The time it takes for the current to move from zero to the peak intensity within each phase. |
| b | Characterized by a constant flow of electrons from the anode (i.e., positive electrode) to the cathode (i.e., negative electrode) for a period of greater than one second without interruption. |
| c | The number of pulses delivered through each channel per second. |
| d | The ability of a material to oppose the flow of ions through it. |
| e | Characterized by polarity that continuously changes from positive to negative with the change in the direction of current flow. |
| f | The amount of time it takes for two phases of a pulse with biphasic current. |
| g | A measure of the electromotive force or the electrical potential difference. |
| h | Characterized by the non-continuous flow of direct or alternating current. |
| i | The directed flow of charge from one place to another. |
| j | The amount of time it takes for one phase of a pulse. |

## Therapeutic Modalities Proficiencies

### 16. Electrical Current and Electrode Size

Identify the relevant influence of small electrodes versus large electrodes on selected elements of electrical current. Place the word "increased" or "decreased" in each of the blank cells.

|  | Small Electrodes | Large Electrodes |
|---|---|---|
| current density | a | b |
| impedance | c | d |
| current flow | e | f |

### 17. TENS Parameters

Identify the specific TENS technique most closely associated with the supplied description. The specific technique should be selected from the Word Bank. A specific technique can be used more than once or not at all.

**Word Bank:** acupuncture-like, brief intense, conventional, noxious

| Technique | Description |
|---|---|
| a | characterized by high pulse frequency and short pulse duration |
| b | often administered with a small probe applicator |
| c | the duration is 30-60 seconds for each point |
| d | the amplitude is sufficient for strong paresthesia |
| e | characterized by high density current that is described as uncomfortable or painful |
| f | the amplitude is sufficient for a sensory response |
| g | characterized by high pulse frequency and long pulse duration with moderate current amplitude |

# Equipment and Devices; Therapeutic Modalities Proficiencie

# Therapeutic Modalities Proficiencies

## 18. Iontophoresis

Complete the blank cells with the correct information related to each medication. Answers should be selected from the Word Bank and can be used more than once. The number of desired responses is indicated in parentheses.

**Word Bank: Indications:** analgesia, calcific deposits, dermal ulcers, fungal infection, inflammation, muscle and joint pain
**Polarity:** positive, negative

| Medication | Indications | | Polarity | |
|---|---|---|---|---|
| acetic acid | a | (1) | b | (1) |
| copper sulfate | c | (1) | d | (1) |
| dexamethasone | e | (1) | f | (1) |
| lidocaine | g | (2) | h | (1) |
| salicylates | i | (1) | j | (1) |
| zinc oxide | k | (1) | l | (1) |

## 19. Massage Techniques

Identify the specific massage technique most closely associated with the supplied description. Answers must be selected from the Word Bank and can be used only once.

**Word Bank:** effleurage, friction, petrissage, tapotement, vibration

| Technique | Description |
|---|---|
| a | A technique described as kneading, where the muscle is squeezed and rolled under the therapist's hands. |
| b | A technique that provides stimulation through rapid alternating movements such as tapping, hacking, cupping, and slapping. |
| c | A technique characterized by a light stroke that produces a reflexive response. |
| d | A technique that incorporates small circular motions over a trigger point or muscle spasm. |
| e | A technique that places the therapist's hands or fingers firmly over an area and utilizes a rapid, shaking motion. |

# Equipment and Devices; Therapeutic Modalities Answer Key

## Equipment and Devices

### 1. Levels of Physical Assistance
a.  supervision
b.  dependent
c.  moderate assist
d.  independent
e.  minimal assist
f.  maximal assist

### 2. Wheelchair Measurements
a.  armrest height
b.  8 inches
c.  seat height
d.  20 inches
e.  seat depth
f.  16 inches
g.  back height
h.  16 inches
i.  seat width
j.  19 inches

### 3. Levels of Weight Bearing
a.  partial weight bearing
b.  full weight bearing
c.  weight bearing as tolerated
d.  toe touch weight bearing
e.  non-weight bearing

### 4. Assistive Device Selection
a.  parallel bars
b.  walker
c.  axillary crutches
d.  cane
e.  Lofstrand crutches

### 5. Wheelchair Frame
a.  amputee frame
b.  hemi frame
c.  ultralight frame
d.  one-hand drive frame
e.  power wheelchair frame
f.  reclining frame

### 6. Equipment and Devices Basics*
a.  FALSE: Correction: A dependent squat pivot transfer is used to transfer a patient who cannot stand independently, but is able to bear some weight through the trunk and lower extremities.
b.  FALSE: Correction: The standard adult wheelchair has 18 inches of width, 16 inches of depth, and 20 inches of height.
c.  FALSE: Correction: Wheelchair seat depth is determined by measuring from the posterior buttock, along the lateral thigh to the popliteal fold and subtracting two inches.
d.  TRUE
e.  TRUE
f.  FALSE: Correction: A cane can be used to improve balance, however, does not permit partial weight bearing.
g.  TRUE
h.  FALSE: Correction: A gastric tube is a tube inserted through a small incision in the abdomen into the stomach.
i.  FALSE: Correction: A suprapubic catheter is an indwelling urinary catheter that is surgically inserted directly into a patient's bladder.
j.  TRUE

*The correction presented for each false statement is an example of several possible corrections.

## Therapeutic Modalities

### 7. Heat Transfer
a.  convection
b.  conduction
c.  evaporation
d.  conduction
e.  convection
f.  conversion
g.  conversion
h.  conduction
i.  radiation

### 8. Therapeutic Effects of Cryotherapy
a.  FALSE
b.  TRUE
c.  TRUE
d.  FALSE
e.  TRUE

## Equipment and Devices; Therapeutic Modalities Answer Key

### 9. Indications/Contraindications of Cryotherapy

a. indication
b. contraindication
c. contraindication
d. indication
e. indication
f. contraindication
g. contraindication
h. indication

### 10. Cooling Agents Matching

a. 6
b. 2,4
c. 2,4
d. 1,3
e. 5

### 11. Therapeutic Effects of Superficial Thermotherapy

a. FALSE
b. FALSE
c. TRUE
d. FALSE
e. TRUE

### 12. Indications/Contraindications of Superficial Thermotherapy

a. indication
b. contraindication
c. indication
d. indication
e. contraindication
f. indication
g. contraindication
h. contraindication

### 13. Heating Agents Matching

a. 1,7
b. 4
c. 2
d. 3,5
e. 6
f. 1,7

### 14. Parameters and Procedures*

a. FALSE - Correction: The Cryo Cuff should be held 15-18 inches above the level of the sleeve during filling.
b. FALSE - Correction: A vapocoolant spray should be applied parallel to the direction of the muscle fibers.
c. TRUE
d. FALSE - Correction: Ultrasound frequency of 3 MHz heats superficial tissue (1-2 cm), while 1 MHz heats deep tissue (up to 5 cm).
e. FALSE - Correction: The temperature of a paraffin bath should be maintained between 113 and 122 degrees Fahrenheit.
f. FALSE - Correction: A 20% duty cycle with an on time of 1 second would have an off time of 4 seconds (duty cycle = on time / on + off time x 100).
g. TRUE
h. TRUE
i. FALSE - Correction: First-degree erythemal dose is characterized by a dose that results in erythema that lasts 1-3 days with clear redness and mild desquamation.
j. FALSE - Correction: The supplied definition describes viscosity. The principle of buoyancy states that there is an upward force on the body when immersed in water equal to the amount of water that has been displaced by the body.
k. FALSE - Correction: Hot packs are required to be in place for 15-20 minutes to achieve desired therapeutic effects.
l. FALSE - Correction: An infrared lamp's main therapeutic effect is the enhancement of superficial tissue healing.
m. TRUE
n. TRUE
o. FALSE - Correction: Ultraviolet light is absorbed 1-2 millimeters into the skin.

*The correction presented for each false statement is an example of several possible corrections.

# Equipment and Devices; Therapeutic Modalities Answer Key

### 15. Electrotherapy Terminology
a. rise time
b. direct current
c. frequency
d. resistance
e. alternating current
f. pulse duration
g. voltage
h. pulsatile current
i. current
j. phase duration

### 16. Electrical Current and Electrode Size
a. increased
b. decreased
c. increased
d. decreased
e. decreased
f. increased

### 17. TENS Parameters
a. conventional
b. noxious
c. noxious
d. brief intense
e. noxious
f. conventional
g. brief intense

### 18. Iontophoresis
a. calcific deposits
b. negative
c. fungal infection
d. positive
e. inflammation
f. negative
g. analgesia, inflammation
h. positive
i. muscle and joint pain
j. negative
k. dermal ulcers
l. positive

### 19. Massage Techniques
a. petrissage
b. tapotement
c. effleurage
d. friction
e. vibration

## Equipment and Devices; Therapeutic Modalities References

### Equipment and Devices References

1. Pierson F. *Principles and Techniques of Patient Care*. Fourth Edition. WB Saunders Company, 2008.

2. *Nurse's 3-Minute Clinical Reference*. Second Edition. Lippincott Williams & Wilkins, 2007.

3. Minor M, Minor S. *Patient Care Skills*. Fifth Edition. Appleton & Lange, 2006.

4. Rothstein J, Roy S, Wolf S. *The Rehabilitation Specialist's Handbook*. Third Edition. F.A. Davis Company, 2005.

5. Batavia M. *The Wheelchair Evaluation: A Clinician's Guide*. Second Edition. Jones and Bartlett Publishers, 2010.

6. Cook AM, Hussey SM, Polgar JM. *Cook & Hussey's Assistive Technologies: Principles and Practice.* Mosby Elsevier, 2008.

7. Olson DA, DeRuyter F. *A Clinician's Guide to Assistive Technology*. Mosby Elsevier, 2002.

8. Tan JC. *Practical Manual of Physical Medicine and Rehabilitation*. Second Edition. Mosby Inc., 2005.

9. Pendleton H, Schultz-Krohn W. *Occupational Therapy Practice Skills for Physical Dysfunction*. Sixth Edition. Mosby, 2006.

10. Cameron M, Monroe L. *Physical Rehabilitation: Evidence-Based Examination, Evaluation, and Intervention*. Saunders, 2007.

11. Prentice W, Voight M. *Techniques in Musculoskeletal Rehabilitation*. McGraw-Hill Inc., 2008.

12. Paz J, West MP. *Acute Care Handbook for Physical Therapists*. Third Edition. Saunders, 2008.

13. Hillegass E, Sadowsky S. *Essentials of Cardiopulmonary Physical Therapy*. Second Edition. W.B. Saunders Company, 2001.

14. Magee D. *Orthopedic Physical Assessment*. Fifth Edition. W.B. Saunders Company, 2007.

15. Dutton M. *Orthopaedic Examination, Evaluation, and Intervention*. Second Edition. McGraw-Hill Inc., 2008.

# Equipment and Devices; Therapeutic Modalities References

## Therapeutic Modalities References

16. Cameron M. *Physical Agents in Rehabilitation: From Research to Practice*. Third Edition. WB Saunders Company, 2008.

17. Michlovitz S. *Thermal Agents in Rehabilitation*. Fourth Edition. FA Davis Company, 2005.

18. Prentice W. *Therapeutic Modalities for Physical Therapists*. Third Edition. McGraw-Hill Inc., 2005.

19. Bracciano A. *Physical Agent Modalities. Theories and Application for the Occupational Therapist*. Second Edition. Slack Inc., 2008.

20. Denegar C. *Therapeutic Modalities for Musculoskeletal Injuries*. Second Edition. Human Kinetics, 2005.

21. Belanger AY. *Evidence-Based Guide to Therapeutic Physical Agents*. Lippincott Williams & Wilkins, 2003.

22. Ruoti RG, Morris DM. *Aquatic Rehabilitation*. Lippincott Williams & Wilkins, 1997.

23. Cameron M, Monroe L. *Physical Rehabilitation: Evidence-Based Examination, Evaluation, and Intervention*. Saunders, 2007.

24. Nelson R, Hayes K, Currier D. *Clinical Electrotherapy*. Third Edition. Appleton & Lange, 1999.

25. Kitchen S. *Electrotherapy. Evidence-Based Practice*. Churchill Livingstone. 2002.

26. Robinson A, Snyder-Mackler L. *Clinical Electrophysiology*. Third Edition. Williams & Wilkins, 2007.

27. De Domenico G, Wood E. *Beard's Massage*. Fifth Edition. WB Saunders Company, 2007.

28. Fritz S. *Mosby's Fundamentals of Therapeutic Massage*. Second Edition. Mosby, Inc., 2000.

29. Houglum P. *Therapeutic Exercise for Athletic Injuries*. Human Kinetics, 2001.

# 9

# SAFETY & PROTECTION; PROFESSIONAL RESPONSIBILITIES; RESEARCH

## Scott Giles
## Therese Giles

Safety and Protection represents approximately 2.5% (5 questions) of the National Physical Therapy Examination.

The actual number of questions in this category can range from 4 to 5 questions.

## Scott Giles

Professional Responsibilities represents approximately 2.0% (4 questions) of the National Physical Therapy Examination.

The actual number of questions in this category can range from 3 to 4 questions.

## Michael Fillyaw

Research represents approximately 2.0% (4 questions) of the National Physical Therapy Examination.

The actual number of questions in this category can range from 4 to 5 questions.

487 Infection Control

490 Accessibility

492 Documentation

500 Ethics

504 Health Care Professionals

512 Health Insurance

514 Teaching and Learning

514 Health Behavior Models

519 Research

523 Data and Measurement

524 Sampling

529 Descriptive Statistics

530 Inferential Statistics

533 Essentials

536 Proficiencies

SCOREBUILDERS

# Safety and Protection

## Ergonomic Guidelines[1]

### Workstation Recommendations

- ✓ 18-20 inch monitor
- ✓ Easily adjustable monitor to angle or tilt
- ✓ Split keyboard preferred
- ✓ Adjustable feet for the keyboard
- ✓ Monitor display should be directed ten degrees below the horizontal
- ✓ Monitor should be placed at least twenty inches away from the eyes
- ✓ Chair should swivel 360 degrees for easy access
- ✓ Wrist rests should match the front edge of the keyboard in order to maximize comfort
- ✓ Hands-free telephone set preferred
- ✓ Use a mouse that contours to the hand
- ✓ 30 second exercise break every hour while at a desk
- ✓ Space under the desk should be at least 30 inches wide, 19 inches deep, and 27 inches in height; there should be 2-3 inches between the top of the thighs and the desk

### Workstation Posture

**Head:** level, facing forward, in line with trunk

**Shoulders:** relaxed, arms at side

**Elbows:** remain close to trunk, bent 90-120 degrees

**Forearms, wrists, hands:** parallel to the floor, straight

**Trunk:** maintain normal curves of the spine with appropriate lumbar support, shoulders and pelvis are level

**Hips, thighs:** well supported with contoured seat, parallel to the floor

**Knees:** maintain a level position with a 90 degree angle of flexion, knees generally at the same height as the hips

**Feet:** place feet flat on the floor or supported in a slight incline

## Body Mechanics[2,3]

A therapist must consistently use proper body mechanics when treating patients and avoid unnecessary stress and strain by maintaining proper alignment within the musculoskeletal system.

### Principles of Proper Body Mechanics

- Use the shortest lever arm possible
- Stay close to the patient when possible
- Use larger muscles to perform heavy work
- Maintain a wide base of support
- Avoid any rotary movement when lifting
- Attempt to maintain your center of gravity and the patient's center of gravity within the base of support

## Lifting Guidelines[2,3]

- ✓ Always attempt to increase your base of support
- ✓ Maintain a proper lumbar curve as you lift
- ✓ Pivot your feet when lifting; do not twist your back to turn
- ✓ Maintain a slow and consistent speed while lifting
- ✓ Only lift an object as a last resort

### Deep Squat Lift (Figs. 9-1, 9-2, 9-3)

1. Begin with the hips below the level of the knees
2. Assume a wide base of support
3. Straddle the object
4. Grasp the object from each side or from beneath
5. The trunk should remain vertical
6. Maintain a lumbar lordosis and anterior pelvic tilt

### Half-Kneeling Lift (Figs. 9-4, 9-5, 9-6, 9-7)

1. Begin in a half-kneel position
2. The bottom leg should be positioned behind and to the side of the object
3. Maintain a normal lumbar lordosis
4. Lift the object onto the knee and draw it closer to the trunk
5. Continue the lift by holding the object close as you assume a standing position

**Fig. 9-1:** A patient begins a deep squat lift with the hips below the knees.

**Fig. 9-2:** The patient lifts the container while maintaining the trunk in a vertical position.

**Fig. 9-3:** The patient completes the lift by achieving a fully erect position.

## One Leg Stance Lift

1. Used for lifting light objects that can be lifted with one extremity
2. Face the object in a lunge position
3. Shift weight onto the forward extremity
4. Flex the forward extremity and lower to reach the object
5. The hind leg rises off the ground to counterbalance the shift in weight
6. Maintain a neutral spine throughout the lift

## Power Lift

1. Begin with the hips above the level of the knees
2. Assume a wide base of support behind the object with the feet parallel to each other
3. Grasp the object from each side or from underneath
4. The trunk should remain in a vertical position
5. Maintain a lumbar lordosis and anterior tilt

## Traditional Lift

1. Begin with the lower extremities in a full squat facing the object
2. The feet should be positioned in an anterior-posterior manner on each side of the object
3. Grasp the object and flex the upper extremities to initiate the lift
4. Use bilateral lower extremities to provide the work of the lift
5. Keep the object close to the trunk during the lift
6. Maintain normal lumbar lordosis
7. Do not lift with the back

## Pushing or Pulling an Object

✓ Use a semi-squat position to push or pull
✓ Apply the force parallel to the surface that the object should be moved upon
✓ Exert an initial force that is adequate to overcome the counterforce of inertia and friction
✓ Attempt to push, pull, slide or roll the object prior to lifting or carrying an object

**Fig. 9-4:** The patient begins a half-kneeling lift while grasping the box in a half-kneeling position.

**Fig. 9-5:** The patient lifts the box onto the knee while maintaining normal lordosis.

**Fig. 9-6:** The patient gradually assumes a standing position.

**Fig. 9-7:** The patient completes the lift by achieving a fully erect position.

# Infection Control

## Infectious Disease

Infectious disease is defined as a condition where an organism invades a host and develops a parasitic relationship with the host. The invasion and multiplication of the microorganisms produces an immune response with subsequent signs and symptoms.

### Potential Symptoms of Infectious Disease

- Fever, chill, malaise
- Rash, skin lesion
- Bleeding from gums
- Joint effusion
- Diarrhea
- Frequency, urgency
- Cough, sore throat
- Nausea, vomiting
- Headache
- Stiff neck
- Myalgia
- Convulsions
- Confusion
- Tachycardia
- Hypotension

### Chain of Transmission for Infection

1. Causative agent, bacteria, pathogen, virus
2. Reservoir of humans, animals, inanimate objects
3. Portal of exit through blood, intestinal tract, respiratory tract, skin/mucous membrane, open lesion, excretions, tears or semen
4. Transmission through airborne, contact, vector, vehicle or droplet modes
5. Portal of entry through non-intact skin, blood, mucous membrane, inhalation, ingestion or percutaneous injection
6. Susceptible host regarding age, health status, nutrition, and environmental status

## Standard Precautions[3,4]

Standard Precautions are revised guidelines that update Universal Precautions and are designed for the care of all patients in hospitals regardless of infection or diagnosis.

These precautions combine Universal and body substance isolation precautions and apply to all blood/body fluids, secretions, and excretions.

## Hand Washing

✓ Use plain soap for routine hand washing; use an antimicrobial agent for specific incidences based on the established infection control policy (Fig. 9-8).

**Fig. 9-8:** A therapist washing his hands prior to initiating treatment.

## Gloves

✓ Wear gloves when touching all body fluids, blood secretions, excretions, and contaminated items.

✓ Change gloves between tasks with a patient after coming in contact with infectious material. Remove gloves immediately, avoid touching non-contaminated items, and wash hands at that time.

## Mask

✓ Wear a mask/eye protection/face shield for protection during activities that are at risk for splashing of any body fluids.

## Gown

✓ Wear a gown for protection during activities that are at risk for splashing of any body fluids. Remove gown immediately and wash hands.

## Patient Care Equipment

✓ Handle all patient equipment in a manner that prevents transfer of microorganisms.

✓ Ensure that all reusable equipment is properly sanitized prior to reuse.

## Occupational Health and Bloodborne Pathogens

✓ Vigilance is required when handling/disposing of sharp instruments. Never recap needles or remove syringes by hand. All sharps disposals should use puncture-resistant containers.

✓ Mouthpieces, resuscitation bags, and ventilation devices should be used as an alternative to mouth-to-mouth resuscitation.

### Transmission-based Precautions[3,4]

Transmission-based precautions are updated guidelines for the particular care of specified patients infected with epidemiologically important pathogens transmitted by airborne, droplet or contact modes. These are additional precautions that should be implemented in addition to Standard Precautions.

### Airborne Precautions

Airborne precautions reduce the risk of airborne transmission of infectious agents through evaporated droplets in air or dust particles containing infectious agents.

- Private room with monitored air pressure
- Six to twelve air changes within the room per hour
- Room door should remain closed with patient remaining within the room
- Respiratory protection worn when entering the room
- Limit patient's transport outside of the room for only essential purposes; patient should wear a mask during transport

#### Examples

Measles, varicella, tuberculosis

### Droplet Precautions

Droplet precautions reduce the risk of droplet transmission of infectious agents through contact of the mucous membranes of the mouth and nose, contact with the conjunctivae, and through coughing, sneezing, talking or suctioning. This transmission requires close contact, as the infectious agents do not suspend in the air and travel only three feet or less.

- Private room
- May share a room with a patient that has an active infection of the same microorganism
- Maintain at least three feet between the patient and any contact (patient, staff, visitor)
- Room door may remain open
- Wear a mask when working within three feet of the patient
- Limit the patient's transport outside of the room for only essential purposes; patient should wear a mask during transport

#### Examples

**Bacterial include:** Hemophilus influenza (including meningitis, pneumonia, sepsis), Neisseria meningitidis (including meningitis, pneumonia, sepsis), diphtheria, mycoplasma pneumonia, pertussis, streptococcal (group A)

**Viral include:** Adenovirus, influenza, mumps, parovirus B19, rubella

### Contact Precautions

Contact precautions reduce the risk of transmission of infectious agents through direct or indirect contact. Direct contact involves skin-to-skin transmission; indirect contact involves a contaminated intermediate object, usually within the patient's environment.

- Private room
- May share a room with a patient that has an active infection of the same microorganism
- Use of gloves when entering the room
- Change of gloves after direct contact with infectious material
- Take gloves off prior to leaving the room and perform proper hand washing technique
- Wear a gown if you will have substantial close contact with the patient and remove the gown prior to leaving the room
- Limit patient's transport outside of the room for essential purposes only
- Dedicate non-critical patient care equipment to one patient, do not share between patients or disinfect properly prior to using the equipment again

#### Examples

Gastrointestinal, respiratory, skin or wound infections, multi-drug resistant bacteria, Clostridium difficile, enterohemorrhagic Escherichia coli, Shigella, hepatitis A (for incontinence/diapered), parainfluenza virus or enteroviral infection (infants/young children), diphtheria, herpes simplex virus, impetigo, pediculosis, scabies, zoster, viral hemorrhagic infections (Ebola)

### Nosocomial Infections[4]

A term used to describe an infection that is acquired during a hospitalization. The primary factor in the prevention of nosocomial infections is proper hand washing. Staff must also follow standard precautions and all infection control procedures at all times.

*The CDC Guidelines for Isolation Precautions in Hospitals* is a document that outlines the guidelines from collaboration between the Centers for Disease Control and Prevention (CDC) and the Hospital Infection Control Practices Advisory Committee (HICPAC). This document describes infection control within the hospital setting and provides strategies for surveillance, prevention, and control of nosocomial infections within the hospital setting.

## Application of Sterile Protective Garments[3]

### Gowns

✓ Hold gown firmly away from the sterile field
✓ Shake gown open so it unfolds and keep hands above waist level
✓ Touch only the inside of the gown as you place both arms into the sleeves
✓ Stop when hands reach the sleeve cuff
✓ The gown is tied in back

### Sterile Gloves

✓ Use the gown's sleeve cuffs as mittens and open the glove pack
✓ The sterile glove has a fold at the wrist where the inside (exposed) of the glove is not sterile
✓ Grasp the right glove with the left hand (still using the sleeve cuff as a mitten) and pull it on over the open end of the gown sleeve
✓ The first three fingers of the right hand should reach under the fold (touching the sterile portion of the left glove) and hold the glove while the left hand positions inside the glove
✓ Once both gloves are donned, the left glove can unfold the right glove's cuff

### Cap and Mask

✓ Wash hands
✓ Avoid contact with the hair while applying the cap
✓ All hair must be contained within the cap
✓ Apply a mask, if necessary, by first positioning the mask over the bridge of the nose
✓ The mask should fit securely over the nose and mouth
✓ Secure the upper ties behind the head and the lower ties behind the neck

## Sterile Field Guidelines[3]

✓ All items on a sterile field must be (and remain) sterile
✓ The edges of all packaging of sterile items become non-sterile once the package is opened
✓ Sterile gowns are only considered sterile in the front from the waist level upwards, including the sleeves

✓ Only the top surface of the table or sterile drape is considered sterile, with the outer one-inch of the field considered non-sterile
✓ Avoid all unnecessary activity around the sterile field
✓ Do not talk, sneeze or cough, as it will contaminate the sterile field
✓ Do not turn your back to a sterile field as the back of the gown is not sterile; constant observation of the sterile field is required
✓ If an object on the sterile field becomes contaminated, the field is considered non-sterile and should be discarded
✓ Sterile fields should never be left unattended and should be prepared as close to the treatment time as possible in order to further avoid contamination
✓ Any item that positions or falls below waist level is considered contaminated

## Infection Control Terminology

**Asepsis:** The elimination of the microorganisms that cause infection and the creation of a sterile field.

**Contamination:** A term used to describe an area, surface or item coming in contact with something that is not sterile. Contamination assumes an environment that contains microorganisms.

**Hand washing:** Hand washing is an important technique for asepsis. Guidelines for acceptable hand washing are as follows:

✓ Use warm water
✓ Remove all jewelry
✓ Wash hands with soap for at least 30 seconds (the time it takes to sing "Happy Birthday" twice)
✓ Avoid touching any contaminated surface
✓ Rinse thoroughly
✓ Use a paper towel barrier when turning off the water

**Medical asepsis:** A technique that attempts to contain pathogens to a specific area, object or person. A primary goal is to reduce the spread of pathogens. Example: A patient with tuberculosis is hospitalized and kept in isolation.

**Personal protective equipment (PPE):** Items that are worn and used as barriers to protect someone who is assisting a patient with a potentially infectious disease. Personal protective equipment includes gowns, lab coats, masks, gloves, goggles, spill kits, and mouthpieces.

**Sterile field:** A sterile field is used to maintain surgical asepsis. A sterile field is a designated area that is considered void of all contaminants and microorganisms. There are standard and required protocols that must be followed in order to develop and maintain a sterile field.

**Surgical asepsis:** A state in which an area or object is without any microorganisms. Example: A sterile field.

# Professional Responsibilities

## Accessibility

### Americans with Disabilities Act[1,2]

The Americans with Disabilities Act is designed to provide a clear and comprehensive national mandate for the elimination of discrimination. The Americans with Disabilities Act is federal legislation that was signed into law on July 26, 1990.

The Americans with Disabilities Act is divided into five titles:

| Title I | Employment |
| --- | --- |
| Title II | Public Services |
| Title III | Public Accommodations |
| Title IV | Telecommunications |
| Title V | Miscellaneous |

The Americans with Disabilities Act applies primarily, but not exclusively, to "disabled" individuals. An individual is "disabled" if they meet at least one of the following criteria:

- They have a physical or mental impairment that substantially limits one or more of their major life activities.
- They have a record of such an impairment.
- They are regarded as having such an impairment.

The Employment provisions (Title I) apply to employers of fifteen employees or more. The Public Accommodations provisions (Title III) apply to all businesses, regardless of the number of employees.

Employers are required to make reasonable accommodations for qualified individuals with a disability, who are defined by the Americans with Disabilities Act as individuals who satisfy the job-related requirements of a position held or desired, and who can perform the "essential functions" of such position with or without reasonable accommodation. The Americans with Disabilities Act does not require employers to make accommodations that pose an "undue hardship." "Undue hardship" is defined as significantly difficult or expensive accommodations.

## Consider This

### Ramps[1,2]

Individuals unable to utilize stairs often rely on ramps. A ramp should possess twelve inches of horizontal run for each inch of vertical rise which is equivalent to an 8.3% grade (Fig. 9-9).

### Ramp Specifications

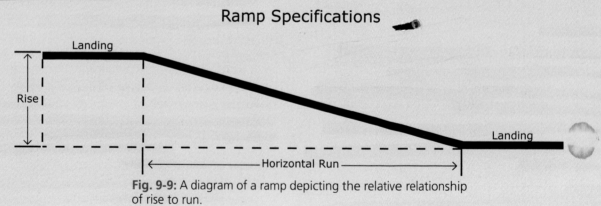

Fig. 9-9: A diagram of a ramp depicting the relative relationship of rise to run.

Percent grade reflects the angle of inclination. A percent grade of 100% would be completely vertical and a percent grade of 0% would be completely horizontal. The percent grade is determined by taking the rise, dividing the value by the run, and then multiplying the number by 100 to convert the value to a percentage.

A ramp should be a minimum of 36 inches wide and should be equipped with handrails if the ramp has a rise of greater than 6 inches or a horizontal run of greater than 72 inches. The ramp should have a level landing at the top and bottom. If a ramp changes direction, the landing area must be a minimum of five feet by five feet (i.e., 60 inches x 60 inches).

## Accessibility Requirements[1,2,5]

| | |
|---|---|
| **Doorway** (Fig. 9-10) | Minimum 32 inch width<br>Maximum 24 inch depth |
| **Threshold** | Less than ¾ inch for sliding doors<br>Less than ½ inch for other doors |
| **Carpet** | Requires ½ inch pile or less |
| **Hallway clearance** (Fig. 9-10) | 36 inch width |
| **Wheelchair turning radius (U-turn)** (Fig. 9-11) | 60 inch width<br>78 inch length |
| **Forward reach in wheelchair** (Fig. 9-12) | Low reach 15 inches<br>High reach 48 inches |
| **Side reach in wheelchair** | Reach over obstruction to 24 inches |
| **Bathroom sink** | Not less than 29 inch height<br>Not greater than 40 inches from floor to bottom of mirror or paper dispenser<br>17 inch minimum depth under sink to back wall |
| **Bathroom toilet** | 17-19 inches from floor to top of toilet<br>Not less than 36 inch grab bar length<br>Grab bars should be 1¼ - 1½ inches in diameter<br>1½ inch spacing between grab bars and wall<br>Grab bar placement 33-36 inches up from floor level |
| **Hotel** | Approximately 2% total rooms must be accessible |
| **Parking space** | 96 inch width<br>240 inch length<br>Approximately 2% of the total spaces must be accessible |

**Fig. 9-10:** An overhead image of the minimum required doorway width and hallway width.

**Fig. 9-11:** An overhead image of the minimum required width for turning a wheelchair.

**Fig. 9-12:** A patient in a wheelchair activating an automatic door opener.

# Documentation[6,7]

## Purpose of Documentation

- Communicate with other treating professionals
- Assistance with discharge planning
- Reimbursement
- Assistance with utilization review
- A legal document regarding the course of therapy

## Types of Documentation

### Record

- An increase in specialization of care and multidisciplinary treatment increases the need for medical records to serve as a means of communication among clinicians.
- Progress notes and referrals related directly to patient care are examples of clinical records.
- Departmental statistics and records are examples of administrative records.

### Referral

- Acceptable forms of referral range from a signed prescription form to a highly structured checklist. The referral must include the name of the patient and be signed and dated by the referring physician.
- Referrals commonly include some indication as to the number and frequency of treatments desired and any special precautions or instructions.

### Progress Note

- Improvement of patient care is the most important function of progress notes.
- Progress notes allow members of all health services to know what the patient is accomplishing in each given area.
- Progress notes should contain patient identification, the date, and the signature of the therapist.
- Progress notes should be written when the patient's condition changes during the course of treatment.
- Specific frequency of progress notes is usually dictated by department policy.
- Appropriate forms of documentation include diagrams, videotapes, and flow sheets as well as many other less frequently used media.

### S.O.A.P. Note

A commonly used record to write daily notes is the S.O.A.P. note. S.O.A.P. stands for:

- **S:** Subjective
- **O:** Objective
- **A:** Assessment
- **P:** Plan

**Subjective:** Refers to information the patient communicates to the therapist. This could include social or medical history not previously recorded. It could also include the patient's statements or complaints.

**Objective:** Refers to information the therapist observes. Common examples include range of motion measurements, muscle strength, and functional abilities. It also includes manual techniques and equipment used during treatment.

**Assessment:** Allows the therapist to express their professional opinion. Changes in the treatment program are often expressed in this section.

**Plan:** Includes ideas for future physical therapy sessions. Frequency and expected duration of physical therapy services can also be incorporated into this section.

### Discharge Summary

A discharge summary should provide a capsule view of the patient's progress during therapy. The discharge summary is usually conducted on the day of the patient's last therapy session.

## Guidelines: Physical Therapy Documentation Of Patient/Client Management[8]

### Preamble

The American Physical Therapy Association (APTA) is committed to meeting the physical therapy needs of society, to meeting the needs and interests of its members, and to developing and improving the art and science of physical therapy, including practice, education, and research. To help meet these responsibilities, APTA's Board of Directors has approved the following guidelines for physical therapy documentation. It is recognized that these guidelines do not reflect all of the unique documentation requirements associated with the many specialty areas within the physical therapy profession. Applicable for both handwritten and electronic documentation systems, these guidelines are intended to be used as a foundation for the development of more specific documentation guidelines in clinical areas, while at the same time providing guidance for the physical therapy profession across all practice settings. Documentation may also need to address additional regulatory or payer requirements.

Finally, be aware that these guidelines are intended to address documentation of patient/client management, not to describe the provision of physical therapy services. Other APTA documents, including APTA Standards of Practice for Physical Therapy, Code of Ethics and Guide for Professional Conduct, and the Guide to Physical Therapist Practice, address provision of physical therapy services and patient/client management.

## APTA Position On Documentation

### Documentation Authority For Physical Therapy Services

Physical therapy examination, evaluation, diagnosis, prognosis, and plan of care (including interventions) shall be documented, dated, and authenticated by the physical therapist who performs the service. Interventions provided by the physical therapist or selected interventions provided by the physical therapist assistant under the direction and supervision of the physical therapist are documented, dated, and authenticated by the physical therapist or, when permissible by law, the physical therapist assistant.

Other notations or flow charts are considered a component of the documented record but do not meet the requirements of documentation in or of themselves.

Students in physical therapist or physical therapist assistant programs may document when the record is additionally authenticated by the physical therapist or, when permissible by law, documentation by physical therapist assistant students may be authenticated by a physical therapist assistant.

## Operational Definitions

### Guidelines

APTA defines a "guideline" as a statement of advice.

### Authentication

The process used to verify that an entry is complete, accurate and final. Indications of authentication can include original written signatures and computer "signatures" on secured electronic record systems only.

The following describes the main documentation elements of patient/client management: 1) initial examination/evaluation, 2) visit/encounter, 3) reexamination, and 4) discharge or discontinuation summary.

### Initial Examination/Evaluation

Documentation of the initial encounter is typically called the "initial examination," "initial evaluation," or "initial examination/evaluation." Completion of the initial examination/evaluation is typically completed in one visit, but may occur over more than one visit. Documentation elements for the initial examination/evaluation include the following:

**Examination:** Includes data obtained from the history, systems review, and tests and measures.

**Evaluation:** Evaluation is a thought process that may not include formal documentation. It may include documentation of the assessment of the data collected in the examination and identification of problems pertinent to patient/client management.

**Diagnosis:** Indicates level of impairment, activity limitation and participation restriction determined by the physical therapist. May be indicated by selecting one or more preferred practice patterns from the Guide to Physical Therapist Practice.

**Prognosis:** Provides documentation of the predicted level of improvement that might be attained through intervention and the amount of time required to reach that level. Prognosis is typically not a separate documentation element, but the components are included as part of the plan of care.

**Plan of care:** Typically stated in general terms, includes goals, interventions planned, proposed frequency and duration, and discharge plans.

### Visit/Encounter

Documentation of a visit or encounter, often called a progress note or daily note, documents sequential implementation of the plan of care established by the physical therapist, including changes in patient/client status and variations and progressions of specific interventions used. Also may include specific plans for the next visit or visits.

### Reexamination

Documentation of reexamination includes data from repeated or new examination elements and is provided to evaluate progress and to modify or redirect intervention.

### Discharge or Discontinuation Summary

Documentation is required following conclusion of the current episode in the physical therapy intervention sequence to summarize progression toward goals and discharge plans.

## General Guidelines

Documentation is required for every visit/encounter.

- All documentation must comply with the applicable jurisdictional/regulatory requirements.

- All handwritten entries shall be made in ink and will include original signatures. Electronic entries are made with appropriate security and confidentiality provisions.

- Charting errors should be corrected by drawing a single line through the error and initialing and dating the chart or through the appropriate mechanism for electronic documentation that clearly indicates that a change was made without deletion of the original record.

- All documentation must include adequate identification of the patient/client and the physical therapist or physical therapist assistant:

  - The patient's/client's full name and identification number, if applicable, must be included on all official documents.

  - All entries must be dated and authenticated with the provider's full name and appropriate designation:

    - Documentation of examination, evaluation, diagnosis, prognosis, plan of care, and discharge summary must be authenticated by the physical therapist who provided the service.

    - Documentation of intervention in visit/encounter notes must be authenticated by the physical therapist or physical therapist assistant who provided the service.

    - Documentation by physical therapist or physical therapist assistant graduates or other physical therapists and physical therapist assistants pending receipt of an unrestricted license shall be authenticated by a licensed physical therapist, or, when permissible by law, documentation by physical therapist assistant graduates may be authenticated by a physical therapist assistant.

– Documentation by students (SPT/SPTA) in physical therapist or physical therapist assistant programs must be additionally authenticated by the physical therapist or, when permissible by law, documentation by physical therapist assistant students may be authenticated by a physical therapist assistant.

- Documentation should include the referral mechanism by which physical therapy services are initiated. Examples include:
  - Self-referral/direct access
  - Request for consultation from another practitioner
- Documentation should include indication of no shows and cancellations.

## Initial Examination/Evaluation

### Examination (History, Systems Review, and Tests and Measures)

**History:**

Documentation of history may include the following:

- General demographics
- Social history
- Employment/work (job/school/play)
- Growth and development
- Living environment
- General health status (self-report, family report, caregiver report)
- Social/health habits (past and current)
- Family history
- Medical/surgical history
- Current condition(s)/chief complaint(s)
- Functional status and activity level
- Medications
- Other clinical tests

**Systems Review:**

Documentation of systems review may include gathering data for the following systems:

**Cardiovascular/Pulmonary**

- Blood pressure
- Edema
- Heart rate
- Respiratory rate

**Integumentary**

- Pliability (texture)
- Presence of scar formation
- Skin color
- Skin integrity

**Musculoskeletal**

- Gross range of motion
- Gross strength
- Gross symmetry
- Height
- Weight

**Neuromuscular**

- Gross coordinated movement (e.g., balance, locomotion, transfers, and transitions)
- Motor function (motor control, motor learning)

Documentation of systems review may also address communication ability, affect, cognition, language, and learning style:

- Ability to make needs known
- Consciousness
- Expected emotional/behavioral responses
- Learning preferences (e.g., education needs, learning barriers)
- Orientation (person, place, time)

**Tests and Measures:**

Documentation of tests and measures may include findings for the following categories:

**Aerobic Capacity/Endurance**

Examples of examination findings include:

- Aerobic capacity during functional activities
- Aerobic capacity during standardized exercise test protocols
- Cardiovascular signs and symptoms in response to increased oxygen demand with exercise or activity
- Pulmonary signs and symptoms in response to increased oxygen demand with exercise or activity

**Anthropometric Characteristics**

Examples of examination findings include:

- Body composition
- Body dimensions
- Edema

**Arousal, Attention, and Cognition**

Examples of examination findings include:

- Arousal and attention
- Cognition
- Communication
- Consciousness
- Motivation
- Orientation time, person, place, and situation
- Recall

## Assistive and Adaptive Devices

Examples of examination findings include:

- Assistive or adaptive devices and equipment use during functional activities
- Components, alignment, fit, and ability to care for the assistive or adaptive devices and equipment
- Remediation of impairments, activity limitations and participation restrictions with use of assistive or adaptive devices and equipment
- Safety during use of assistive or adaptive devices and equipment

## Circulation (Arterial, Venous, Lymphatic)

Examples of examination findings include:

- Cardiovascular signs
- Cardiovascular symptoms
- Physiological responses to position change

## Cranial and Peripheral Nerve Integrity

Examples of examination findings include:

- Electrophysiological integrity
- Motor distribution of the cranial nerves
- Motor distribution of the peripheral nerves
- Response to neural provocation
- Response to stimuli, including auditory, gustatory, olfactory, pharyngeal, vestibular, and visual
- Sensory distribution of the cranial nerves
- Sensory distribution of the peripheral nerves

## Environmental, Home, and Work (job/school/play) Barriers

Examples of examination findings include:

- Current and potential barriers
- Physical space and environment

## Ergonomics and Body Mechanics

Examples of examination findings for ergonomics include:

- Dexterity and coordination during work
- Functional capacity and performance during work actions, tasks, or activities
- Safety in work environments
- Specific work conditions or activities
- Tools, devices, equipment, and workstations related to work actions, tasks, or activities

Examples of examination findings for body mechanics include:

- Body mechanics during self-care, home management, work, community, or leisure actions, tasks, or activities

## Gait, Locomotion, and Balance

Examples of examination findings include:

- Balance during functional activities with or without the use of assistive, adaptive, orthotic, protective, supportive, or prosthetic devices or equipment
- Balance (dynamic and static) with or without the use of assistive, adaptive, orthotic, protective, supportive, or prosthetic devices or equipment
- Gait and locomotion during functional activities with or without the use of assistive, adaptive, orthotic, protective, supportive, or prosthetic devices or equipment
- Gait and locomotion with or without the use of assistive, adaptive, orthotic, protective, supportive, or prosthetic devices or equipment
- Safety during gait, locomotion, and balance

## Integumentary Integrity

Examples of examination findings include:

- Activities, positioning, and postures that produce or relieve trauma to the skin
- Assistive, adaptive, orthotic, protective, supportive, or prosthetic devices and equipment that may produce or relieve trauma to the skin
- Skin characteristics

## Wound

Examples of examination findings include:

- Activities, positioning, and postures that aggravate the wound or scar or that produce or relieve trauma
- Burn
- Signs of infection
- Wound characteristics
- Wound scar tissue characteristics

## Joint Integrity and Mobility

Examples of examination findings include:

- Joint integrity and mobility
- Joint play movements
- Specific body parts

## Motor Function

Examples of examination findings include:

- Dexterity, coordination, and agility
- Electrophysiological integrity
- Hand function
- Initiation, modification, and control of movement patterns and voluntary postures

## Muscle Performance

Examples of examination findings include:

- Electrophysiological integrity
- Muscle strength, power, and endurance
- Muscle strength, power, and endurance during functional activities
- Muscle tension

## Neuromotor Development and Sensory Integration

Examples of examination findings include:

- Acquisition and evolution of motor skills
- Oral motor function, phonation, and speech production
- Sensorimotor integration

## Orthotic, Protective, and Supportive Devices

Examples of examination findings include:

- Components, alignment, fit, and ability to care for the orthotic, protective, and supportive devices and equipment
- Orthotic, protective, and supportive devices and equipment use during functional activities
- Remediation of impairments, activity limitations, and participation restrictions with use of orthotic, protective, and supportive devices and equipment
- Safety during use of orthotic, protective, and supportive devices and equipment

## Pain

Examples of examination findings include:

- Pain, soreness, and nociception
- Pain in specific body parts

## Posture

Examples of examination findings include:

- Postural alignment and position (dynamic)
- Postural alignment and position (static)
- Specific body parts

## Prosthetic Requirements

Examples of examination findings include:

- Components, alignment, fit, and ability to care for prosthetic device
- Prosthetic device use during functional activities
- Remediation of impairments, activity limitations, and participation restrictions with use of the prosthetic device
- Residual limb or adjacent segment
- Safety during use of the prosthetic device

## Range of Motion (including muscle length)

Examples of examination findings include:

- Functional ROM
- Joint active and passive movement
- Muscle length, soft tissue extensibility, and flexibility

## Reflex Integrity

Examples of examination findings include:

- Deep reflexes
- Electrophysiological integrity
- Postural reflexes and reactions, including righting, equilibrium, and protective reactions
- Primitive reflexes and reactions
- Resistance to passive stretch
- Superficial reflexes and reactions

## Self-care and Home Management (including activities of daily living and instrumental activities of daily living)

Examples of examination findings include:

- Ability to gain access to home environments
- Ability to perform self-care and home management activities with or without assistive, adaptive, orthotic, protective, supportive, or prosthetic devices and equipment
- Safety in self-care and home management activities and environments

## Sensory Integrity

Examples of examination findings include:

- Combined/cortical sensations
- Deep sensations
- Electrophysiological integrity

## Ventilation and Respiration

Examples of examination findings include:

- Pulmonary signs of respiration/gas exchange
- Pulmonary signs of ventilatory function
- Pulmonary symptoms

## Work (job/school/play), Community, and Leisure Integration or Reintegration (including instrumental activities of daily living)

Examples of examination findings include:

- Ability to assume or resume work (job/school/play), community, and leisure activities with or without assistive, adaptive, orthotic, protective, supportive, or prosthetic devices and equipment
- Ability to gain access to work (job/school/play), community, and leisure environments
- Safety in work (job/school/play), community, and leisure activities and environments

## Evaluation

Evaluation is a thought process that may not include formal documentation. However, the evaluation process may lead to documentation of impairments, activity limitations, and participation restrictions using formats such as:

- A problem list
- A statement of assessment of key factors (e.g., cognitive factors, comorbidities, social support) influencing the patient/client status

## Diagnosis

Documentation of a diagnosis determined by the physical therapist may include impairment, activity limitation, and participation restrictions.

Examples include:

- Impaired Joint Mobility, Motor Function, Muscle Performance, and Range of Motion Associated With Localized Inflammation (4E)
- Impaired Motor Function and Sensory Integrity Associated With Progressive Disorders of the Central Nervous System (5E)
- Impaired Aerobic Capacity/Endurance Associated With Cardiovascular Pump Dysfunction or Failure (6D)
- Impaired Integumentary Integrity Associated With Partial-Thickness Skin Involvement and Scar Formation (7C)

## Prognosis

Documentation of the prognosis is typically included in the plan of care.

## Plan of Care

Documentation of the plan of care includes the following:

- Overall goals stated in measurable terms that indicate the predicted level of improvement in functioning
- A general statement of interventions to be used
- Proposed duration and frequency of service required to reach the goals
- Anticipated discharge plans

## Visit/Encounter

Documentation of each visit/encounter shall include the following elements:

- Patient/client self-report (as appropriate)
- Identification of specific interventions provided, including frequency, intensity, and duration as appropriate

Examples include:

- Knee extension, three sets, ten repetitions, 10 pound weight
- Transfer training bed to chair with sliding board
- Equipment provided

- Changes in patient/client impairment, activity limitation, and participation restriction status as they relate to the plan of care
- Response to interventions, including adverse reactions, if any
- Factors that modify frequency or intensity of intervention and progression of goals, including patient/client adherence to patient/client related instructions
- Communication/consultation with providers/patient/client/family/significant other
- Documentation to plan for ongoing provision of services for the next visit(s), which is suggested to include, but not be limited to:
  - The interventions with objectives
  - Progression parameters
  - Precautions, if indicated

## Reexamination

Documentation of reexamination shall include the following elements:

- Documentation of selected components of examination to update patient's/client's functioning, and/or disability status
- Interpretation of findings and, when indicated, revision of goals
- When indicated, revision of plan of care, as directly correlated with goals as documented

## Discharge/Discontinuation Summary

Documentation of discharge or discontinuation shall include the following elements:

- Current physical/functional status
- Degree of goals achieved and reasons for goals not being achieved
- Discharge/discontinuation plan related to the patient's/client's continuing care

Examples include:

- Home program
- Referrals for additional services
- Recommendations for follow-up physical therapy care
- Family and caregiver training
- Equipment provided

BOD G03-05-16-41 Updated: 12/14/2009 American Physical Therapy Association, web site 2011

## Consider This

### Documentation Recommendations[9]

Physical therapists are responsible for completing daily documentation on patients throughout the episode of care. Documentation should be completed in a timely manner and accurately describe the patient's status, physical therapy management, and outcome of care.

The American Physical Therapy Association provides therapists with insight on how to improve physical therapy documentation and promote reimbursement from third party payers.

**Top 10 Tips for Defensible Documentation**

1. Limit use of abbreviations
2. Date and sign all entries
3. Document legibly
4. Report progress towards goals regularly
5. Document at the time of the visit when possible
6. Clearly identify note types (e.g., progress reports, daily notes)
7. Include all related communications
8. Include missed or cancelled visits
9. Demonstrate skilled care
10. Demonstrate discharge planning through the episode of care

**Top 10 Payer Complaints Regarding Documentation**

1. Poor legibility
2. Incomplete documentation
3. No documentation for date of service
4. Abbreviations, too many, cannot understand
5. Does not demonstrate skilled care
6. Documentation does not support the billing code
7. Does not support medical necessity
8. Does not demonstrate progress
9. Repetitious daily notes showing no change in patient status
10. Interventions with no clarification of time, frequency, duration

### Symbols Commonly Used in Clinical Practice

| | | | |
|---|---|---|---|
| = | Equal | ± | Very slight trace or reaction, indefinite |
| ≠ | Unequal | + | Slight trace or reaction, positive, plus excess, acidic reaction |
| > | Greater than | ++ | Trace or notable reaction |
| < | Less than | +++ | Moderate amount of reaction |
| ↑ | Increase | ++++ | Large amount or pronounced reaction |
| ↗ | Increasing | # | Number, pound, has been given or done |
| ↓ | Decrease | → | Yields, leads to |
| ↘ | Decreasing | ← | Resulting from or secondary to |
| − | Negative, minus, deficiency, alkaline reaction | 1°, 2° | Primary, secondary |

From Miller-Keane: Encyclopedia and Dictionary of Medicine, Nursing, and Allied Health. W.B. Saunders Company, Philadelphia 1997, p.1802, with permission.

## Military Time

The 24-hour clock (military time) is used to standardize time in the medical record.

| Standard Time | Military Time |
|---|---|
| Noon | 1200 hours |
| 1:00 PM | 1300 hours |
| 2:00 PM | 1400 hours |
| 3:00 PM | 1500 hours |
| 4:00 PM | 1600 hours |
| 5:00 PM | 1700 hours |
| 6:00 PM | 1800 hours |
| 7:00 PM | 1900 hours |
| 8:00 PM | 2000 hours |
| 9:00 PM | 2100 hours |
| 10:00 PM | 2200 hours |
| 11:00 PM | 2300 hours |
| Midnight | 2400 hours |

## Measurement

### Length

| 1 cm | = 0.3937 inch |
|---|---|
| 1 m | = 39.37 inches<br>= 3.28 ft = 1.09 yds |
| 1 km | = 0.62 mile |
| 1 inch | = 2.54 centimeters (cm)<br>= 25.4 millimeters (mm)<br>= 0.0254 meters (m) |
| 1 foot | = 30.48 cm<br>= 304.8 mm = 0.304 m |
| 1 mile | = 5280 ft<br>= 1760 yds = 1609.35 m<br>= 1.61 kilometers (km) |

### Temperature

| 0°C | = 32°F = 273°K |
|---|---|
| 100°C | = 212°F |
| °C | = (°F - 32) x 5/9 |
| °F | = (°C x 9/5) + 32 |

### Weight

| 1 ounce (oz) | = 0.0625 pounds (lb)<br>= 28.35 grams (g)<br>= 0.028 kilograms (kg) |
|---|---|
| 1 pound (lb) | = 16 oz<br>= 454 g = 0.454 kg |
| 1 g | = 0.035 oz<br>= 0.0022 lb<br>= 0.001 kg |
| 1 kg | = 35.27 oz<br>= 2.2 lb<br>= 1000 g |

### Energy and Work

| 1 kcal | = 3086 foot-pounds (ft-lbs)<br>= 426.4 kilogram-meter (kg-m)<br>= 1 kilojoules (kJ) |
|---|---|
| 1 kJ | = 1000 joules (J)<br>= 0.23892 kcal |
| 1 liter O₂ consumed | = 5.05 kcal = 15.575 ft-lbs<br>= 2153 kg-m = 21.237 kJ |
| 1 MET | = 3.5 mL O₂/kg-min = 0.0175 kcal/kg<br>= 0.0732 kJ/kg |
| 1 ft-lb | = 0.1383 kg-m |
| 1 kg-m | = 7.23 ft-lbs |

### Metric versus United States Units of Measure

| 1 inch | = 2.54 centimeters | 1 kilogram | = 2.2 pounds |
|---|---|---|---|
| 1 foot | = 30.5 centimeters | 1 pound | = 4.45 Newtons |
| 1 mile | = 1.61 kilometers | 1 liter | = .2642 gallons |
| 1 meter | = 3.28 feet | 1 milliliter | = .0338 once |
| 1 gram | = .0353 ounce | 1 gallon | = 3.785 liters |
| 1 ounce | = 28.35 grams | 1 calorie | = 4.18 Joule |
| 1 pound | = 454 grams | | |
| °C | = (°F - 32) X 5/9 | Boiling | = 212 °F/100°C |
| °F | = (°C x 9/5) + 32 | Freezing | = 32 °F/0 °C |

# Ethics

"Morality cannot be legislated, but behavior can be regulated. Judicial decrees may not change the heart, but they can restrain the heartless." —*Martin Luther King Jr.*

Ethics is a branch of philosophy that emphasizes morality, justice, honesty, right versus wrong, and free will. Ethics is defined as a principle of good conduct or a body of right principles and specific moral choices. We respond to each instance that we face as health care providers based on specific moral choices. These are specific to each person and are based on cultural, religious, environmental, and personal values.

## Ethical Principles and Terminology[10,11]

**Autonomy:** Requires that the wishes of competent individuals must be honored. Autonomy is often referred to as self-determination.

**Beneficence:** A moral obligation of health care providers to act for the benefit of others.

**Confidentiality:** The holding of professional secrets or discussions. Keeping client information within appropriate limits.

**Duty:** The obligations that individuals have to others in society.

**Fidelity:** Related to confidentiality and is defined as the moral duty to keep commitments that have been promised.

**Justice:** The quality of being just and fair; righteousness.

**Nonmaleficence:** The obligation of health care providers to above all else, do no harm.

**Paternalism:** A term used when someone fails to recognize another individual's rights and autonomy.

**Rights:** The ability to take advantage of a moral entitlement to do something or not to do something.

**Veracity:** Obligation of health care providers to tell the truth.

## Ethical Theories and Issues

### Teleological theory (consequentialism)[10]

This ethical theory believes that the outcome or consequences of a particular action should come from answering the question "What should I do?" The person judges the good and bad outcome based on answering "Which decision would bring the best consequences?" When the decision cannot be made from these questions, a person will choose the course of action that brings the most good and least harm. This theory supports paternalistic behavior if no harm is done. The worth of an action is judged by the consequences and the goal will be that the end result justifies the means.

### Deontologism theory[10]

This ethical theory does not focus on the consequences of an action, but on the action itself and if the action follows moral principles. The theory believes that a person's obligations should determine the ethical course of action. There is a strict following of the principles of ethics (autonomy, nonmaleficence, beneficence, and justice).

## Professional Behaviors

- ✓ Organization
- ✓ Professional presentation
- ✓ Dependability
- ✓ Initiative
- ✓ Empathy
- ✓ Cooperation
- ✓ Clinical reasoning
- ✓ Written communication
- ✓ Verbal communication

**L**- Listen
**E**- Explain
**A**- Acknowledge
**R**- Recommend
**N**- Negotiate

## Malpractice[11]

Claims of malpractice usually stem from the theory of negligence. Negligence describes a substandard level of care for the particular profession. Negligence deals with a particular conduct, not state of mind.

In order to prove malpractice through negligence, there are four elements:

1. A duty to act in a particular manner
2. Conduct that breaches that particular duty
3. Damage that occurs from that conduct
4. Conduct that is substandard, causing injury

## Sexual harassment[12]

This term describes unwanted sexual or gender-based behaviors from one person that has formal or informal power over the other.

In order to qualify as sexual harassment, there are three areas that must be satisfied:

1. The behavior is unwelcome or unwanted
2. The behavior is sexual in nature or related to the gender of the person
3. The behavior must occur in a relationship where the person is being harassed by a superior or a peer; someone who has power over the individual in some respect

Four elements that create a sexual harassment case:

1. Submission or rejection of the conduct is used as a factor in obtaining employment
2. Submission or rejection of the conduct is used to determine the status of a person's employment
3. The conduct must substantially interfere with a person's employment
4. The conduct creates a hostile work environment

# Management

## Quality Management Process[12,13]

- Review selected patient medical records
- Prioritize adverse event outcomes
- Conduct a thorough review of care
- Identify problematic areas of care
- Develop a plan to change identified aspects of care
- Implement the plan
- Monitor the plan
- Determine if the implemented change results in a measurable difference

## Quality Improvement[12,13]

A form of objective self-examination designed to improve the quality of services.

### Agencies Responsible for Quality Improvement

- Joint Commission on Accreditation of Healthcare Organizations (JCAHO)
- Professional Standards Review Organization (PSRO)
- Commission of Accreditation of Rehabilitation Facilities (CARF)
- National Committee for Quality Assurance (NCQA)

Quality measures should assess the structure, process, and outcome of physical therapy care. According to the American Physical Therapy Association structure, process, and outcome are defined as follows:

### Structure

A review of structure is an assessment of organization, staffing and staff qualifications, rules and policies governing physical work, records, equipment, and physical facilities. The assessment may include a judgment of the adequacy as well as the presence of the element of structure being examined.

### Process

Process assessment is based on the degree or extent to which the therapist conforms to accepted professional practices in providing services. The various approaches to care and their application, efficacy, adequacy, and timeliness are considered. A process review requires that considerable attention be given to developing and specifying the standards to be used in the assessment.

### Outcome

Outcome assessment is based on the condition of the patient at the conclusion of care in relation to the goals of treatment. Assessment of outcome provides a means of reviewing the practitioner, the services, and events that led to the results of care. The results of outcome assessment ultimately may lead to the evaluation of the basic treatment procedures and modalities of physical therapy and validation of the approaches to patient care. Outcomes are the ultimate manifestations of effectiveness and quality of care.

# Models of Disability

## The Nagi Model[14]

This model was originally designed in 1965 by a social worker named Saad Nagi as an alternative to the medical model of disease. It describes health status as a product of the relationship between health and function and is defined by four primary concepts:

**Pathology:** An interruption or interference in the body's normal processes and the simultaneous efforts of the systems to regain homeostasis. Pathology occurs at the cellular level.

**Impairment:** The loss or abnormality at the tissue, organ or body system level. This can be of an anatomic, physiologic, mental or emotional nature. Each pathology will present with an impairment, however, impairments can exist without pathology (e.g., congenital defects). Impairments occur at the organ level.

**Functional Limitation:** The inability to perform an action or skill in a normal manner due to an impairment. Functional limitations are at the level of the whole person.

**Disability:** Any restriction or inability to perform a socially defined role within a social or physical environment due to an impairment. Environmental barriers impose disability.

**Example:** A patient with progressive weakness presents with paralysis of the trunk and lower extremities. The patient is diagnosed with a T12 spinal cord tumor. The patient utilizes a wheelchair for mobility and requires assistance with self-care. Prior to hospitalization, the patient worked as a delivery man.

**Pathology:** Spinal cord tumor at T12

**Impairment:** Loss of motor function below T12

**Functional Limitation:** Unable to ambulate

**Disability:** Cannot continue to work as a delivery person

## International Classification of Functioning, Disability and Health (ICF) Model[15]

The International Classification of Functioning, Disability and Health (ICF) is a classification of health and health-related domains. These domains are classified from body, individual, and societal perspectives by means of two lists: one list of body functions and structure and one list of domains of activity and participation. Since an individual's functioning and disability occurs in a context, the ICF also includes a list of environmental factors.

The ICF is the World Health Organization's (WHO) latest framework, endorsed in 2001, for measuring health and disability at both individual and population levels. The WHO's previous model, known as the ICIDH, was defined by the primary concepts of disease, impairment, disability, and handicap. The WHO is also responsible for the creation and implementation of the International Classification of Diseases (ICD-10).

The ICF's constructs acknowledge that every human being can experience some degree of disability. It shifts focus from cause to impact and takes into account the social aspects of disability and acknowledges environmental factors that can impact a person's functioning.

### ICF Primary Concepts:

**Body Functions:** physiological functions of body systems including psychological functions

**Body Structures:** anatomical parts of the body such as organs, limbs and their components

**Impairments:** problems in body function or structure such as a significant deviation or loss

**Activity:** the execution of a task or action by an individual

**Participation:** involvement in a life situation

**Activity Limitations:** difficulties an individual may have in executing activities

**Participation Restrictions:** problems an individual may experience in involvement in life situations

**Environmental Factors:** physical, social, and attitudinal environment in which people live

### Categories that fall under each domain include:

#### Body Function

- Mental functions
- Sensory functions and pain
- Voice and speech functions
- Functions of the cardiovascular, hematological, immunological, and respiratory systems
- Functions of the digestive, metabolic, and endocrine systems
- Genitourinary and reproductive functions
- Neuromuscular and movement-related functions
- Functions of the skin and related structures

#### Body Structure

- Structures of the nervous system
- The eye, ear, and related structures
- Structures involved in voice and speech
- Structures of the cardiovascular, immunological, and respiratory systems
- Structures related to the digestive, metabolic, and endocrine systems
- Structures related to the genitourinary and reproductive systems
- Structures related to movement
- Skin and related structures

### Activities and Participation

- Learning and applying knowledge
- General tasks and demands
- Communication
- Mobility
- Self-care
- Domestic life
- Interpersonal interactions and relationships
- Major life areas
- Community, social, and civic life

### Environmental Factors

- Products and technology
- Natural environment and human-made changes to environment
- Support and relationships
- Attitudes
- Services, systems, and policies

**Example:** A patient status post motor vehicle accident diagnosed with C6 complete tetraplegia is wheelchair dependent for mobility and resides in a town without public transportation. He was very active in his church choir and taught Sunday school prior to his motor vehicle accident.

**Health Condition:** Complete spinal cord injury - tetraplegia

**Impairment:** Paralysis

**Activity Limitation:** Incapable of using public transportation

**Participation Restriction:** Lack of accommodations in public transportation leads to no participation in religious activities

# Legal

## Elements of a Risk Management Program

- Management involvement
- Risk management organization
- Incident reporting and investigation
- Inspections
- Communications

## Recommendations to Avoid Litigation[11]

- Conduct a thorough examination
- Seek consultation when in doubt
- Check the condition of your equipment
- Instruct patients thoroughly
- Keep the referring physician informed
- Obtain proper consent for treatment
- Do not delegate to unqualified individuals
- Keep accurate and timely written records

## Legal Terminology[11]

**Abandonment:** Unacceptable one-sided termination of services by a health care professional without patient consent or agreement.

**Administrative law:** Administrative agencies at the federal and state level develop rules and regulations to supplement statutes and executive orders.

**Common law:** Refers to court decisions in the absence of statutory law. Common law often creates legal precedent in areas where statutes have not been enacted.

**Constitutional law:** Involves law that is derived from the federal Constitution. The United States Supreme Court is responsible for ultimately interpreting and enforcing the Constitution.

**Informed consent:** The patient is required to sign a document and give permission to the health care professional to render treatment. This should be obtained from the patient in accordance with the standards of practice prior to initiation of treatment. The patient has the right to full disclosure of treatment procedures, risks, expected outcomes, and goals.

**Malpractice:** The failure to exercise the skills that would normally be exercised by other members of the profession with similar skills and training. This can include areas of professional negligence, breach of contract issues, and intentional conduct by a health care professional.

**Negligence:** The failure to do what a reasonable and prudent person would ordinarily have done under the same or similar circumstances for a given situation. In order to prove negligence, the plaintiff must prove all of the following:

- There was a duty owed to the plaintiff by the defendant.
- There was a breach of that duty under conditions that constituted negligence and the negligence was the proximate cause of the breach.
- There was damage to the plaintiff's person or property.

**Risk management:** The identification, analysis, and evaluation of risks and the selection of the most advantageous method for treating them.

**Statutory law:** Congress and state legislatures are responsible for enacting statutes. Examples of federal statutes affecting health care include the Americans with Disabilities Act and the Family and Medical Leave Act.

**Tort:** A private or civil wrong or injury, involving omission and/or commission.

# Delegation and Supervision[16]

## Direction and Supervision of the Physical Therapist Assistant

Physical therapists have a responsibility to deliver services in ways that protect the public safety and maximize the availability of their services. They do this through direct delivery of services in conjunction with responsible utilization of physical therapist assistants who assist with selected components of intervention. The physical therapist assistant is the only individual permitted to assist a physical therapist in selected interventions under the direction and supervision of a physical therapist.

Direction and supervision are essential in the provision of quality physical therapy services. The degree of direction and supervision necessary for assuring quality physical therapy services is dependent upon many factors, including the education, experi-

ences, and responsibilities of the parties involved, as well as the organizational structure in which the physical therapy services are provided.

Regardless of the setting in which the physical therapy service is provided, the following responsibilities must be borne solely by the physical therapist:

1. Interpretation of referrals when available.
2. Initial examination, evaluation, diagnosis, and prognosis.
3. Development or modification of a plan of care which is based on the initial examination or reexamination and which includes the physical therapy goals and outcomes.
4. Determination of when the expertise and decision-making capability of the physical therapist requires the physical therapist to personally render physical therapy interventions

and when it may be appropriate to utilize the physical therapist assistant. A physical therapist shall determine the most appropriate utilization of the physical therapist assistant that provides for the delivery of service that is safe, effective, and efficient.

5. Reexamination of the patient/client in light of their goals, and revision of the plan of care when indicated.

6. Establishment of the discharge plan and documentation of discharge summary/status.

7. Oversight of all documentation for services rendered to each patient/client.

The physical therapist remains responsible for the physical therapy services provided when the physical therapist's plan of care involves the physical therapist assistant to assist with selected interventions. Regardless of the setting in which the service is provided, the determination to utilize physical therapist assistants for selected interventions requires the education, expertise, and professional judgment of a physical therapist as described by the *Standards of Practice, Guide to Professional Conduct,* and *Code of Ethics.*

In determining the appropriate extent of assistance from the physical therapist assistant (PTA), the physical therapist considers:

- The PTA's education, training, experience, and skill level.
- Patient/client criticality, acuity, stability, and complexity.
- The predictability of the consequences.
- The setting in which the care is being delivered.
- Federal and state statutes.
- Liability and risk management concerns.
- The mission of physical therapy services for the setting.
- The needed frequency of reexamination.

### Physical Therapist Assistant

**Definition:** The physical therapist assistant is a technically educated health care provider who assists the physical therapist in the provision of physical therapy. The physical therapist assistant is a graduate of a physical therapist assistant associate degree program accredited by the Commission on Accreditation in Physical Therapy Education (CAPTE).

**Utilization:** The physical therapist is directly responsible for the actions of the physical therapist assistant related to patient/client management. The physical therapist assistant may perform selected physical therapy interventions under the direction and at least general supervision of the physical therapist. In general supervision, the physical therapist is not required to be on-site for direction and supervision, but must be available at least by telecommunications. The ability of the physical therapist assistant to perform the selected interventions as directed shall be assessed on an ongoing basis by the supervising physical therapist. The physical therapist assistant makes modifications to selected interventions either to progress the patient/client as directed by the physical therapist or to ensure patient/client safety and comfort.

The physical therapist assistant must work under the direction and at least general supervision of the physical therapist. In all practice settings, the performance of selected interventions by the physical therapist assistant must be consistent with safe and legal physical therapist practice, and shall be predicated on the following factors: complexity and acuity of the patient's/client's needs; proximity and accessibility to the physical therapist; supervision available in the event of emergencies or critical events; and type of setting in which the service is provided.

When supervising the physical therapist assistant in any off-site setting, the following requirements must be observed:

1. A physical therapist must be accessible by telecommunications to the physical therapist assistant at all times while the physical therapist assistant is treating patients/clients.

2. There must be regularly scheduled and documented conferences with the physical therapist assistant regarding patients/clients, the frequency of which is determined by the needs of the patient/client and the needs of the physical therapist assistant.

3. In those situations in which a physical therapist assistant is involved in the care of a patient/client, a supervisory visit by the physical therapist will be made:

    a. Upon the physical therapist assistant's request for a reexamination, when a change in the plan of care is needed, prior to any planned discharge, and in response to a change in the patient's/client's medical status.

    b. At least once a month, or at a higher frequency when established by the physical therapist, in accordance with the needs of the patient/client.

    c. A supervisory visit should include:

        i. An on-site reexamination of the patient/client.

        ii. On-site review of the plan of care with appropriate revision or termination.

        iii. Evaluation of need and recommendation for utilization of outside resources.

HOD P06-05-18-26 Updated: 12/14/2009 American Physical Therapy Association, web site 2011.

## Health Care Professionals[17]

### Audiologists

Audiologists assess patients with suspected hearing disorders. The audiologist can educate patients on how to make the best use of their available hearing and assist them in selecting and fitting appropriate aids. Audiologists are required to possess a master's degree or equivalent. The vast majority of states require audiologists to obtain a license to practice.

### Chiropractors

Chiropractors diagnose and treat patients whose health problems are associated with the body's muscular, nervous, and skeletal systems. Patient care activities include manually adjusting the spine, ordering and interpreting X-rays, performing postural analysis, and administering various physical agents. Chiropractors are required to complete a four-year chiropractic curriculum leading to the Doctor of Chiropractic degree. All states require chiropractors to obtain a license to practice.

## Home Health Aides

Home health aides provide health-related services to the elderly, disabled, and ill in their homes. Patient care activities include performing housekeeping duties, assisting with ambulation or transfers, and promoting personal hygiene. A registered nurse, physical therapist, or social worker is often the health care professional that assigns specific duties and supervises the home health aide. The federal government has established guidelines for home health aides whose employers receive reimbursement from Medicare. The National Association for Home Care offers voluntary national certification for home health aides.

## Licensed Practical Nurses

Licensed practical nurses care for the sick, injured, convalescent, and disabled under the direction of physicians and registered nurses. Patient care activities include taking vital signs, performing transfers, applying dressings, administering injections, and instructing patients and families. In some states, licensed practical nurses can administer prescribed medications or start intravenous fluids. Experienced licensed practical nurses may supervise nursing assistants and aides. Educational programs for licensed practical nurses are approximately one year in length and include classroom study and supervised clinical practice. All states require a license to practice.

## Medical Assistants

Medical assistants perform routine administrative and clinical tasks in a medical office. Administrative duties include answering telephones, updating patient files, completing insurance forms, and scheduling appointments. Clinical duties include taking medical histories, measuring vital signs, and assisting the physician during treatment. Educational programs for medical assistants are typically one to two years in length.

## Occupational Therapists

Occupational therapists help people improve their ability to perform activities of daily living, work, and leisure skills. The educational preparation of occupational therapists emphasizes the social, emotional, and physiological effects of illness and injury. Occupational therapists most commonly work with individuals who have conditions that are mentally, physically, developmentally or emotionally disabling. Occupational therapists can enter the field with bachelors, masters, or doctoral degrees. All states require occupational therapists to obtain a license to practice.

## Occupational Therapy Aides

Occupational therapy aides work under the direction of occupational therapists to provide rehabilitation services to persons with mental, physical, developmental or emotional impairments. Occupational therapy aides often prepare materials and assemble equipment used during treatment and may be responsible for a variety of clerical tasks. The majority of training for occupational therapy aides occurs on the job.

## Occupational Therapy Assistants

Occupational therapy assistants work under the direction of occupational therapists to provide rehabilitation services to persons with mental, physical, developmental or emotional impairments. Occupational therapy assistants perform a variety of rehabilitative activities and exercises as outlined in an established treatment plan. To practice as an occupational therapy assistant, individuals must complete an associate's degree or certificate program from an accredited academic institution. Occupational therapy assistants are regulated in the majority of states.

## Physical Therapists

Physical therapists provide services to help restore function, improve mobility, relieve pain, and prevent or limit permanent physical disabilities of patients suffering from injuries or disease. Physical therapists engage in examination, evaluation, diagnosis, prognosis, and intervention in an effort to maximize patient outcomes. Physical therapists can enter the field with a master's or doctorate degree. As of 2002, all physical therapy programs seeking accreditation were required to offer a minimum of a master's degree. All states require physical therapists to obtain a license to practice.

## Physical Therapy Aides

Physical therapy aides are considered support personnel who may be involved in support services directed by physical therapists. Physical therapy aides receive on the job training under the direction and supervision of a physical therapist and are permitted to function only with continuous on-site supervision by a physical therapist or in some cases, a physical therapist assistant. Support services are limited to methods and techniques that do not require clinical decision making by the physical therapist or clinical problem solving by the physical therapist assistant.

## Physical Therapist Assistants

Physical therapist assistants perform components of physical therapy procedures and related tasks selected and delegated by a supervising physical therapist. Physical therapist assistants may modify an intervention only in accordance with changes in patient status and within the established plan of care developed by the physical therapist. Physical therapist assistants are the only paraprofessionals that perform physical therapy interventions. Typically, physical therapist assistants have an associate's degree from an accredited physical therapist assistant program. The vast majority of states require physical therapist assistants to obtain a license to practice.

## Physicians

Physicians diagnose illnesses and prescribe and administer treatment for people suffering from injury or disease. The term physician encompasses both the Doctor of Medicine (MD) and the Doctor of Osteopathic Medicine (DO). The role of the MD and DO are very similar, however, the DO tends to place special emphasis on the body's musculoskeletal system, preventive medicine, and holistic patient care. All states require physicians to obtain a license to practice.

## Physician Assistants

Physician assistants provide health care services with supervision by physicians. The supervising physician and established state law determine the specific duties of the physician assistant. In the vast majority of states physician assistants may prescribe medication. Physician assistants work with the supervision of a physician. All states require physician assistants to obtain a license to practice.

## Psychologists

Psychologists use various techniques including interviewing and testing to advise people how to deal with problems of everyday life. In the health care setting, psychologists may be involved in counseling programs designed to help people achieve goals such as weight loss or smoking cessation. A doctoral degree is usually required for employment as a licensed clinical or counseling psychologist. All states require psychologists to obtain a license to practice.

## Recreational Therapists

Recreational therapists provide treatment services and recreation activities to individuals with disabilities or illness. In acute care hospitals and rehabilitation hospitals, recreational therapists work closely with other health care professionals to treat and rehabilitate individuals with specific medical conditions. In long-term care settings, recreational therapists function primarily by offering structured group sessions emphasizing leisure activities. Recreational therapists are required to have a bachelor's degree in order to be eligible for certification as certified therapeutic recreation specialists.

## Registered Nurses

Registered nurses work to promote health, prevent disease, and help patients cope with illness. Patient care activities are extremely diverse including tasks such as assisting physicians during treatments and examinations, administering medications, recording symptoms and reactions, and instructing patients and families. Registered nurse programs include associates, bachelors, and diploma programs. All states require registered nurses to obtain a license to practice.

## Respiratory Therapists

Respiratory therapists evaluate, treat, and care for patients with breathing disorders. The vast majority of respiratory therapists are employed in hospitals. Patient care activities include performing bronchial drainage techniques, measuring lung capacities, administering oxygen and aerosols, and analyzing oxygen and carbon dioxide concentrations. Educational programs for respiratory therapists are offered by hospitals, colleges, universities, vocational-technical institutes, and the military. The vast majority of states require respiratory therapists to obtain a license to practice.

## Social Workers

Social workers help patients and their families to cope with chronic, acute or terminal illnesses and attempt to resolve problems that stand in the way of recovery or rehabilitation. A bachelor's degree is often the minimum requirement to qualify for employment as a social worker, however, in the health field, the master's degree is often required. All states have licensing, certification or registration requirements for social workers.

## Speech-Language Pathologists

Speech-language pathologists evaluate speech, language, cognitive-communication, and swallowing skills of children and adults. The majority of practitioners provide direct clinical services to individuals with communication disorders. Speech-language pathologists are required to possess a master's degree or equivalent. The vast majority of states require speech-language pathologists to obtain a license to practice.

# Physical Therapy Practice

## The Elements of Patient/Client Management Leading to Optimal Outcomes[14]

**Examination:** The process of obtaining a history, performing a systems review, and selecting and administering tests and measures to gather data about the patient/client. The initial examination is a comprehensive screening and specific testing process that leads to a diagnostic classification. The examination process also may identify possible problems that require consultation with, or referral to, another provider.

**Evaluation:** A dynamic process in which the physical therapist makes clinical judgments based on data gathered during the examination. This process also may identify possible problems that require consultation with, or referral to, another provider.

**Diagnosis:** Both the process and the end result of evaluating examination data, which the physical therapist organizes into defined clusters, syndromes or categories to help determine the prognosis (including the plan of care) and the most appropriate intervention strategies.

**Prognosis (including plan of care):** Determination of the level of optimal improvement that may be attained through intervention and the amount of time required to reach that level. The plan of care specifies the interventions to be used and their timing and frequency.

**Intervention:** Purposeful and skilled interaction of the physical therapist with the patient/client and, if appropriate, with other individuals involved in the care of the patient/client, using various physical therapy methods and techniques to produce changes in the condition that are consistent with the diagnosis and prognosis. The physical therapist conducts a re-examination to determine changes in patient/client status and to modify or redirect intervention. The decision to re-examine may be based on new clinical findings or on lack of patient/client progress. The process of re-examination also may identify the need for consultation with, or referral to, another provider.

**Outcomes:** Results of patient/client management, which include the impact of physical therapy interventions in the following domains: pathology/pathophysiology (disease, disorder or condition); impairments, functional limitations and disabilities; risk reduction/prevention, health, wellness, and fitness; societal resources; and patient/client satisfaction.

From Guide to Physical Therapist Practice. American Physical Therapy Association, (Phys. Ther. 2001, Vol. 81, Number 1, 43).

## Criteria for Standards of Practice for Physical Therapy[18]

### Preamble

The physical therapy profession's commitment to society is to promote optimal health and function in individuals by pursuing excellence in practice. The American Physical Therapy Association attests to this commitment by adopting and promoting the following *Standards of Practice for Physical Therapy*. These Standards are the profession's statement of conditions and performances that are essential for provision of high quality professional service to society, and provide a foundation for assessment of physical therapist practice.

### I. Ethical/Legal Considerations

#### A. Ethical Considerations

The physical therapist practices according to the *Code of Ethics* of the American Physical Therapy Association.

The physical therapist assistant complies with the *Standards of Ethical Conduct for the Physical Therapist Assistant* of the American Physical Therapy Association.

#### B. Legal Considerations

The physical therapist complies with all the legal requirements of jurisdictions regulating the practice of physical therapy.

The physical therapist assistant complies with all the legal requirements of jurisdictions regulating the work of the assistant.

### II. Administration of the Physical Therapy Service

#### A. Statement of Mission, Purposes, and Goals

The physical therapy service has a statement of mission, purposes, and goals that reflects the needs and interests of the patients and clients served, the physical therapy personnel affiliated with the service, and the community.

The statement of mission, purposes, and goals:

- Defines the scope and limitations of the physical therapy service.
- Identifies the goals and objectives of the service.
- Is reviewed annually.

#### B. Organizational Plan

The physical therapy service has a written organizational plan.

The organizational plan:

- Describes relationships among components within the physical therapy service and, where the service is part of a larger organization, between the service and other components of that organization.
- Ensures that the service is directed by a physical therapist.
- Defines supervisory structures within the service.
- Reflects current personnel functions.

#### C. Policies and Procedures

The physical therapy service has written policies and procedures that reflect the operation, mission, purposes, and goals of the service, and are consistent with the Association's *Code of Ethics*.

The written policies and procedures:

- Are reviewed regularly and revised as necessary.
- Meet the requirements for federal and state law and external agencies.

Apply to, but are not limited to:

- Care of patients/clients, including guidelines
- Clinical education
- Clinical research
- Collaboration
- Collection of patient data
- Competency assessment
- Criteria for access to care
- Criteria for initiation and continuation of care
- Criteria for referral to other appropriate health care providers
- Criteria for termination of care
- Documentation
- Environmental safety
- Equipment maintenance
- Fiscal management
- Improvement of quality of care and performance of services
- Infection control
- Job/position descriptions
- Medical emergencies
- Rights of patients/clients
- Personnel-related policies
- Staff orientation

#### D. Administration

The physical therapist is responsible for the direction of the physical therapy service:

- Ensures compliance with local, state, and federal requirements.
- Ensures compliance with current APTA documents, including *Standards of Practice for Physical Therapy and the Criteria, Guide to Physical Therapist Practice, Code of Ethics, Guide for Professional Conduct, Standards of Ethical Conduct for the Physical Therapist Assistant,* and *Guide for Conduct of the Physical Therapist Assistant*.
- Ensures that services are consistent with the mission, purposes, and goals of the physical therapy service.
- Ensures that services are provided in accordance with established policies and procedures.

- Ensures that the process for assignment of physical therapist staff supports the individual therapist responsibility to their patients and meets their needs.
- Reviews and updates policies and procedures.
- Provides training of physical therapy support personnel that ensures continued competence for their job description.
- Provides for continuous inservice training on safety issues and for periodic safety inspection of equipment by qualified individuals.

### E. Fiscal Management

The director of the physical therapy service, in consultation with physical therapy staff and appropriate administrative personnel, participates in planning for, and allocation of, resources. Fiscal planning and management of the service are based on sound accounting principles.

**The fiscal management plan:**

- Includes a budget that provides for optimal use of resources.
- Ensures accurate recording and reporting of financial information.
- Ensures compliance with legal requirements.
- Allows for cost-effective utilization of resources.
- Uses a fee schedule that is consistent with the cost of physical therapy services and that is within customary norms of fairness and reasonableness.
- Considers option of providing pro bono services.

### F. Improvement of Quality of Care and Performance

The physical therapy service has a written plan for continuous improvement of quality of care and performance of services.

**The improvement plan:**

- Provides evidence of ongoing review and evaluation of the physical therapy service.
- Provides a mechanism for documenting improvement in quality of care and performance.
- Is consistent with requirements of external agencies, as applicable.

### G. Staffing

The physical therapy personnel affiliated with the physical therapy service have demonstrated competence and are sufficient to achieve the mission, purposes, and goals of the service.

**The physical therapy service:**

- Meets all legal requirements regarding licensure and certification of appropriate personnel.
- Ensures that the level of expertise within the service is appropriate to the needs of the patients/clients served.
- Provides appropriate professional and support personnel to meet the needs of the patient/client population.

### H. Staff Development

The physical therapy service has a written plan that provides for appropriate and ongoing staff development.

**The staff development plan:**

- Includes self-assessment, individual goal setting, and organizational needs in directing continuing education and learning activities.
- Includes strategies for lifelong learning and professional career development.
- Includes mechanisms to foster mentorship activities.
- Includes knowledge of clinical research methods and analysis.

### I. Physical Setting

The physical setting is designed to provide a safe and accessible environment that facilitates fulfillment of the mission, purposes, and goals of the physical therapy service. The equipment is safe and sufficient to achieve the purposes and goals of physical therapy.

**The physical setting:**

- Meets all applicable legal requirements for health and safety.
- Meets space needs appropriate for the number and type of patients/clients served.

**The equipment:**

- Meets all applicable legal requirements for health and safety.
- Is inspected routinely.

### J. Collaboration

The physical therapy service collaborates with all disciplines as appropriate.

**The collaboration when appropriate:**

- Uses a team approach for the care of patients/clients.
- Provides instruction to patients/clients and families.
- Ensures professional development and continuing education.

## III. Patient/Client Management

### A. Patient/Client Collaboration

Within the patient/client management process, the physical therapist and the patient/client establish and maintain an ongoing collaborative process of decision making that exists throughout the provision of services.

### B. Initial Examination/Evaluation/Diagnosis/Prognosis

The physical therapist performs an initial examination and evaluation to establish a diagnosis and prognosis prior to intervention.

**The physical therapist examination:**

- Is documented, dated, and appropriately authenticated by the physical therapist who performed it.

- Identifies the physical therapy needs of the patient/client.
- Incorporates appropriate tests and measures to facilitate outcome measurement.
- Produces data that are sufficient to allow evaluation, diagnosis, prognosis, and the establishment of a plan of care.
- May result in recommendations for additional services to meet the needs of the patient/client.

## C. Plan of Care

The physical therapist establishes a plan of care and manages the needs of the patient/client based on the examination, evaluation, diagnosis, prognosis, goals, and outcomes of the planned interventions for the identified impairments, functional limitations, and disabilities.

The physical therapist involves the patient/client and appropriate others in the planning, implementation, and assessment of the plan of care.

The physical therapist, in consultation with appropriate disciplines, plans for discharge of the patient/client taking into consideration achievement of anticipated goals and expected outcomes, and provides for appropriate follow-up or referral.

**The plan of care:**

- Is based on the examination, evaluation, diagnosis, and prognosis.
- Identifies goals and outcomes.
- Describes the proposed intervention, including frequency and duration.
- Includes documentation that is dated and appropriately authenticated by the physical therapist who established the plan of care.

## D. Intervention

The physical therapist provides, or directs and supervises, the physical therapy intervention consistent with the examination, evaluation, diagnosis, prognosis, and plan of care.

**The intervention:**

- Is based on the examination, evaluation, diagnosis, prognosis, and plan of care.
- Is provided under the ongoing direction and supervision of the physical therapist.
- Is provided in such a way that directed and supervised responsibilities are commensurate with the qualifications and the legal limitations of the physical therapist assistant.
- Is altered in accordance with changes in response or status.
- Is provided at a level that is consistent with current physical therapy practice.
- Is interdisciplinary when necessary to meet the needs of the patient or client.
- Documentation of the intervention is consistent with the Guidelines for Physical Therapy Documentation of Patient/Client Management.

- Is dated and appropriately authenticated by the physical therapist or when permissible by law, by the physical therapist assistant.

## E. Re-examination

The physical therapist re-examines the patient/client as necessary during an episode of care to evaluate progress or change in patient/client status and modifies the plan of care accordingly or discontinues physical therapy services.

**The physical therapist re-examination:**

- Is documented, dated, and appropriately authenticated by the physical therapist who performs it.
- Includes modifications to the plan of care.

## F. Discharge/Discontinuation of Intervention

The physical therapist discharges the patient/client from physical therapy when the anticipated goals or expected outcomes for the patient/client have been achieved.

The physical therapist discontinues intervention when the patient/client is unable to continue to progress toward goals or when the physical therapist determines that the patient/client will no longer benefit from physical therapy.

**Discharge documentation:**

- Includes the status of the patient/client at discharge and the goals and functional outcomes attained.
- Is dated and appropriately authenticated by the physical therapist who performed the discharge.
- Includes, when a patient/client is discharged prior to attainment of goals and functional outcomes, the status of the patient/client and the rationale for discontinuation.

## G. Communication/Coordination/Documentation

The physical therapist communicates, coordinates and documents all aspects of patient/client management including the results of the initial examination and evaluation, diagnosis, prognosis, plan of care, interventions, response to interventions, changes in patient/client status relative to the interventions, re-examination, and discharge/discontinuation of intervention and other patient/client management activities.

**Physical therapist documentation:**

- Is dated and appropriately authenticated by the physical therapist who performed the examination and established the plan of care.
- Is dated and appropriately authenticated by the physical therapist who performed the intervention or, when allowable by law or regulations, by the physical therapist assistant who performed specific components of the intervention as selected by the supervising physical therapist.
- Is dated and appropriately authenticated by the physical therapist who performed the re-examination, and includes modifications to the plan of care.
- Is dated and appropriately authenticated by the physical therapist who performed the discharge, and includes the status of the patient/client and the goals and outcomes achieved.

- Includes, when a patient/client is discharged prior to achievement of goals and outcomes, the status of the patient/client and the rationale for discontinuation.
- As appropriate, records patient data using a method that allows collective analysis.

## IV. Education

The physical therapist is responsible for individual professional development. The physical therapist assistant is responsible for individual career development.

The physical therapist and the physical therapist assistant under the direction and supervision of the physical therapist participate in the education of students.

The physical therapist educates and provides consultation to consumers and the general public regarding the purposes and benefits of physical therapy.

The physical therapist educates and provides consultation to consumers and the general public regarding the roles of the physical therapist and the physical therapist assistant.

**The physical therapist:**

- Educates and provides consultation to consumers and the general public regarding the roles of the physical therapist, the physical therapist assistant, and other support personnel.

## V. Research

The physical therapist applies research findings to practice and encourages, participates in, and promotes activities that establish the outcomes of patient/client management provided by the physical therapist.

**The physical therapist:**

- Ensures that his or her knowledge of research literature related to practice is current.
- Ensures that the rights of research subjects are protected and the integrity of research is maintained.
- Participates in the research process as appropriate to promote individual education, experience, and expertise.
- Educates physical therapists, physical therapist assistants, students, other health professionals, and the general public about the outcomes of physical therapist practice.

## VI. Community Responsibility

The physical therapist demonstrates community responsibility by participating in community and community agency activities, educating the public, formulating public policy or providing pro bono physical therapy services.

**The physical therapist:**

- Participates in community and community agency activities.
- Educates the public, including prevention, education, and health promotion.
- Helps formulate public policy.
- Provides pro bono physical therapy services.

BOD S03-06-16-38 Updated: 12/14/2009 American Physical Therapy Association web site 2011.

## Code of Ethics for the Physical Therapist[19]

### Preamble

The Code of Ethics for the Physical Therapist (Code of Ethics) delineates the ethical obligations of all physical therapists as determined by the House of Delegates of the American Physical Therapy Association (APTA). The purposes of this Code of Ethics are to:

1. Define the ethical principles that form the foundation of physical therapist practice in patient/client management, consultation, education, research, and administration.
2. Provide standards of behavior and performance that form the basis of professional accountability to the public.
3. Provide guidance for physical therapists facing ethical challenges, regardless of their professional roles and responsibilities.
4. Educate physical therapists, students, other health care professionals, regulators, and the public regarding the core values, ethical principles, and standards that guide the professional conduct of the physical therapist.
5. Establish the standards by which the American Physical Therapy Association can determine if a physical therapist has engaged in unethical conduct.

No code of ethics is exhaustive nor can it address every situation. Physical therapists are encouraged to seek additional advice or consultation in instances where the guidance of the Code of Ethics may not be definitive.

This Code of Ethics is built upon the five roles of the physical therapist (management of patients/clients, consultation, education, research, and administration), the core values of the profession, and the multiple realms of ethical action (individual, organizational, and societal). Physical therapist practice is guided by a set of seven core values: accountability, altruism, compassion/caring, excellence, integrity, professional duty, and social responsibility. Throughout the document the primary core values that support specific principles are indicated in parentheses. Unless a specific role is indicated in the principle, the duties and obligations being delineated pertain to the five roles of the physical therapist. Fundamental to the Code of Ethics is the special obligation of physical therapists to empower, educate, and enable those with impairments, activity limitations, participation restrictions, and disabilities to facilitate greater independence, health, wellness, and enhanced quality of life.

### Principles

**Principle #1** *Physical therapists shall respect the inherent dignity and rights of all individuals. (Core Values: Compassion, Integrity)*

1A. Physical therapists shall act in a respectful manner toward each person regardless of age, gender, race, nationality, religion, ethnicity, social or economic status, sexual orientation, health condition or disability.

2A. Physical therapists shall recognize their personal biases and shall not discriminate against others in physical therapist practice, consultation, education, research, and administration.

**Principle #2** *Physical therapists shall be trustworthy and compassionate in addressing the rights and needs of patients/clients. (Core Values: Altruism, Compassion, Professional Duty)*

2A. Physical therapists shall adhere to the core values of the profession and shall act in the best interests of patients/clients over the interests of the physical therapist.

2B. Physical therapists shall provide physical therapy services with compassionate and caring behaviors that incorporate the individual and cultural differences of patients/clients.

2C. Physical therapists shall provide the information necessary to allow patients or their surrogates to make informed decisions about physical therapy care or participation in clinical research.

2D. Physical therapists shall collaborate with patients/clients to empower them in decisions about their health care.

2E. Physical therapists shall protect confidential patient/client information and may disclose confidential information to appropriate authorities only when allowed or as required by law.

**Principle #3** *Physical therapists shall be accountable for making sound professional judgments. (Core Values: Excellence, Integrity)*

3A. Physical therapists shall demonstrate independent and objective professional judgment in the patient's/client's best interest in all practice settings.

3B. Physical therapists shall demonstrate professional judgment informed by professional standards, evidence (including current literature and established best practice), practitioner experience, and patient/client values.

3C. Physical therapists shall make judgments within their scope of practice and level of expertise and shall communicate with, collaborate with or refer to peers or other health care professionals when necessary.

3E. Physical therapists shall not engage in conflicts of interest that interfere with professional judgment.

3F. Physical therapists shall provide appropriate direction of and communication with physical therapist assistants and support personnel.

**Principle #4** *Physical therapists shall demonstrate integrity in their relationships with patients/clients, families, colleagues, students, research participants, other health care providers, employers, payers, and the public. (Core Value: Integrity)*

4A. Physical therapists shall provide truthful, accurate, and relevant information and shall not make misleading representations.

4B. Physical therapists shall not exploit persons over whom they have supervisory, evaluative or other authority (e.g., patients/clients, students, supervisees, research participants, or employees).

4C. Physical therapists shall discourage misconduct by health care professionals and report illegal or unethical acts to the relevant authority, when appropriate.

4D. Physical therapists shall report suspected cases of abuse involving children or vulnerable adults to the appropriate authority, subject to law.

4E. Physical therapists shall not engage in any sexual relationship with any of their patients/clients, supervisees, or students.

4F. Physical therapists shall not harass anyone verbally, physically, emotionally, or sexually.

**Principle #5** *Physical therapists shall fulfill their legal and professional obligations. (Core Values: Professional Duty, Accountability)*

5A. Physical therapists shall comply with applicable local, state, and federal laws and regulations.

5B. Physical therapists shall have primary responsibility for supervision of physical therapist assistants and support personnel.

5C. Physical therapists involved in research shall abide by accepted standards governing protection of research participants.

5D. Physical therapists shall encourage colleagues with physical, psychological or substance-related impairments that may adversely impact their professional responsibilities to seek assistance or counsel.

5E. Physical therapists who have knowledge that a colleague is unable to perform their professional responsibilities with reasonable skill and safety shall report this information to the appropriate authority.

5F. Physical therapists shall provide notice and information about alternatives for obtaining care in the event the physical therapist terminates the provider relationship while the patient/client continues to need physical therapy services.

**Principle #6** *Physical therapists shall enhance their expertise through the lifelong acquisition and refinement of knowledge, skills, abilities, and professional behaviors. (Core Value: Excellence)*

6A. Physical therapists shall achieve and maintain professional competence.

6B. Physical therapists shall take responsibility for their professional development based on critical self-assessment and reflection on changes in physical therapist practice, education, health care delivery, and technology.

6C. Physical therapists shall evaluate the strength of evidence and applicability of content presented during professional development activities before integrating the content or techniques into practice.

6D. Physical therapists shall cultivate practice environments that support professional development, lifelong learning, and excellence.

**Principle #7** *Physical therapists shall promote organizational behaviors and business practices that benefit patients/clients and society. (Core Values: Integrity, Accountability)*

7A. Physical therapists shall promote practice environments that support autonomous and accountable professional judgments.

7B. Physical therapists shall seek remuneration as is deserved and reasonable for physical therapist services.

7C. Physical therapists shall not accept gifts or other considerations that influence or give an appearance of influencing their professional judgment.

7D. Physical therapists shall fully disclose any financial interest they have in products or services that they recommend to patients/clients.

7E. Physical therapists shall be aware of charges and shall ensure that documentation and coding for physical therapy services accurately reflect the nature and extent of the services provided.

7F. Physical therapists shall refrain from employment arrangements, or other arrangements, that prevent physical therapists from fulfilling professional obligations to patients/clients.

**Principle #8** *Physical therapists shall participate in efforts to meet the health needs of people locally, nationally or globally. (Core Value: Social Responsibility)*

8A. Physical therapists shall provide pro bono physical therapy services or support organizations that meet the health needs of people who are economically disadvantaged, uninsured, and underinsured.

8B. Physical therapists shall advocate to reduce health disparities and health care inequities, improve access to health care services, and address the health, wellness, and preventive health care needs of people.

8C. Physical therapists shall be responsible stewards of health care resources and shall avoid overutilization or underutilization of physical therapy services.

8D. Physical therapists shall educate members of the public about the benefits of physical therapy and the unique role of the physical therapist.

HOD S06-09-07-12 Updated: October 1, 2009 American Physical Therapy Association, web site 2011.

# Health Insurance

There are three major classifications of health insurance companies. They include private health insurance companies, independent health plans, and government health insurance.

## Private Health Insurance Companies

Private health insurance companies include stock companies, mutual companies, and non-profit insurance plans. Reimbursement for physical therapy services is usually on a fee for service basis.

**Stock companies:** Operated nationally and are owned by independent stockholders.

**Mutual companies:** Operated nationally and are owned by the individual policyholders.

**Non-profit insurance plans:** Operate in a specific geographic region and are subject to specific state regulations. They are classified as tax exempt due to their non-profit status.

## Independent Health Plans[20,21]

Independent health plans are organized into various groups. Health maintenance organizations and self-insurance plans are examples of independent health plans. Reimbursement is typically based on fee for service or a predetermined fixed fee.

**Managed care:** A concept of health care delivery where subscribers utilize health care providers that are contracted by the insurance company at a lower cost. Health maintenance organizations (HMO) and preferred provider organizations (PPO)

are two examples of a managed care system. This concept attempts to attain the highest quality of care at the lowest cost.

**Health maintenance organization:** Subscribers to these insurance plans agree to receive all of their health care services through the predetermined providers of the HMO. The primary physician of the subscriber controls health care access through a referral system. Cost containment is a high priority and subscribers cannot receive care from providers outside of the plan except in an emergency.

**Preferred provider organization:** Subscribers can choose their health care services from a list of providers that contract with the insurance plan. These contracts provide extreme discounts for health care. Subscribers can use a health care provider that is not associated with the PPO, however, they will absorb a greater portion of the cost.

**Consolidated Omnibus Budget Reconciliation Act (COBRA):** A law passed that requires an employer to allow an employee to remain under an employer's group plan for a period of time after the loss of a job, death of a spouse, or a decrease in hours or a divorce. The employee may be required to pay the employer's portion of the premiums for their insurance coverage as well as their own portion.

## Fee for Service versus Managed Care[20,21]

| Fee for Service: | Managed Care: |
|---|---|
| Payers assume primary financial risk | Providers share in financial risk |
| Provides enrollees with freedom of choice | Services provided by a specific pool of providers |
| Unlimited access to specialty providers. | Primary care provider serves as a gatekeeper |
| Co-payments often in the form of 80% / 20% | Provides services for a fixed, prepaid monthly fee. |
| Limited internal/external cost controls | Formal quality assurance and utilization review |
| Minimal emphasis on health promotion and education | Health education and preventive medicine emphasized |

## Government Health Insurance[12,20,21]

Government health insurance programs such as Medicare and Medicaid are administered by the federal government. The government uses private contractors to manage the payment process of each health plan.

### Medicare

Medicare provides health insurance for individuals over 65 years of age and the disabled. Medicare is a nationwide program operated by the Centers for Medicare and Medicaid Services.

Established in 1966, Medicare was the second mandated health insurance program in the United States (Workers' Compensation was the first). In 1972 Medicare coverage was expanded to include certain categories of the disabled, renal dialysis, and transplant patients.

#### Medicare Part A:

Provides benefits for care provided in hospitals, outpatient diagnostic services, extended care facilities, hospice, and short-term care at home required by an illness for which the patient is hospitalized.

Enrollment in Medicare Part A is automatic and funding is through payroll taxes.

#### Medicare Part B:

Provides benefits for outpatient care, physician services, and services ordered by physicians such as diagnostic tests, medical equipment, and supplies.

Enrollment in Medicare Part B is voluntary and funding is through premiums paid by beneficiaries and general federal tax revenues.

The Medicare program requires beneficiaries to share in the costs of health care through deductibles and coinsurance.

- Deductibles require beneficiaries to reach a predetermined amount of personal expenditure each 12 month period before Medicare payment is activated.
- Coinsurance requires that 20% of the costs for hospitalization is covered by the patient.

Medicare sets limits on the total days of hospital care that will be paid based on a lifetime pool of days limit. Medicare payments for post hospital stays in extended care facilities are limited to 100 days.

Providers are reimbursed for Medicare services through intermediaries such as Blue Cross.

### Medicaid

Medicaid provides basic medical services to the economically indigent population who qualify by reason of low income or who qualify for welfare or public assistance benefits in the state of their residence. Medicaid is a jointly funded program through the federal and state governments.

Established in 1965, Medicaid is funded through personal income, corporate, and excise taxes. Federal and state support is shared based on the state's per capita income.

Rate setting formulas, procedures, and policies vary widely among states. All state Medicaid operations must be approved by the Centers for Medicare and Medicaid Services. The Medicaid program reimburses providers directly.

The Medicaid program covers inpatient and outpatient hospital services, physician services, diagnostic services, nursing care for older adults, home health care, preventative health screening services, and family planning services.

### Workers' Compensation

First designed in 1911 to provide protection for employees that were injured on the job. This legislation provides continued income as well as paid medical expenses for employees injured while working. Workers' compensation is a joint federal and state program that is regulated at the state level. Recently, case managers have assisted this process by monitoring the rehabilitation process and controlling potential abuse.

Employers with 10 or more employees or high-risk employers must pay a percentage of each employee salary to the workers' compensation board of the state. The exact payment is based on the risk rating of the job or institution.

## Reimbursement Coding[12]

### Current Procedural Terminology Codes

Current Procedural Terminology (CPT) codes are procedure codes used by physical therapists and other health care professionals to describe the interventions that were provided to a given patient. The majority of codes used by physical therapists are in the CPT 97000 series. Examples of commonly used CPT codes by physical therapists include: 97530 – Therapeutic Activities; 97035 – Ultrasound; 97012 – Traction, mechanical. CPT is a registered trademark of the American Medical Association.

### International Classification of Diseases Codes

The International Classification of Diseases (ICD) codes are designed to describe a patient's infirmity through specific categories based on etiology and affected anatomical systems. The codes consist of five distinct digits (e.g., 755.12). The first three digits indicate the basic diagnosis. The fourth digit and in some cases the fifth digit serve to differentiate the basic diagnosis or anatomical area affected. Physicians are required to make the medical diagnosis, however, in some cases, a physical therapist may need to utilize the ICD manual to determine an appropriate ICD code. This action is within a physical therapist's scope of practice and would not be considered equivalent to making a medical diagnosis.

# Teaching & Learning

## Maslow's Hierarchy of Needs[22]

Maslow's hierarchy of needs hypothesizes that there is a hierarchy of biogenic and psychogenic needs that individuals must progress through. In order to move to a higher level of needs, an individual must attain the objectives associated with the previous level. In essence, an individual must achieve basic or fundamental needs before moving to upper level needs.

**Self-actualization needs:** The need to realize one's full potential as a human being.

**Esteem needs:** The need to feel good about oneself and one's capabilities, to be respected by others, and to receive recognition and appreciation.

**Affiliative needs:** The need for security, stability, and a safe environment.

**Physiological needs:** The need for basic things necessary in order to survive such as food, water, and shelter.

## Classical Conditioning (Pavlov)[22]

Classical conditioning is a process where learning occurs when an unconditioned stimulus (food) is repeatedly preceded by a neutral stimulus (bell); the neutral stimulus serves as a conditioned stimulus and the learned reaction that results is termed the conditioned response. In order to maintain a conditioned response, the conditioned and unconditioned stimuli must occasionally be paired.

## Operant Conditioning (B.F. Skinner)[22]

Operant conditioning is a process where learning occurs when an individual engages in specific behaviors in order to receive certain consequences.

**Positive reinforcement:** Administering desirable consequences to individuals who perform a specific behavior.

**Negative reinforcement:** Removing undesirable consequences from individuals who perform a specific behavior.

**Extinction:** Removing selected variables that reinforce a specific behavior.

**Punishment:** Administering negative consequences to individuals who perform undesirable behaviors.

## Reinforcement Frequency and Schedules

**Continuous reinforcement:** A behavior is reinforced every time it occurs.

**Partial reinforcement:** A behavior is reinforced intermittently.

**Fixed-interval schedule:** The period of time between the occurrences of each instance of reinforcement is fixed or set.

**Variable-interval schedule:** The amount of time between reinforcements varies around a constant average.

# Health Behavior Models[23]

Change in behavior is a complex process that is difficult to attain and sustain. There has been significant research that has resulted in many different models for understanding behavior change and specific interventions. The following are a few commonly used models.

## Health Belief Model

The Health Belief Model is one of the initial theories for behavior change. It is based on the belief that change in behavior depends upon the following factors:

1. **Perceived susceptibility:** one is at risk for the problem
2. **Perceived severity:** the health problem is serious
3. **Perceived benefit:** changing the behavior will reduce the threat
4. **Perceived barriers:** recognize obstacles required to change a behavior
5. **Cues to action:** strategies to activate readiness for change
6. **Self-efficacy:** the ability to change a behavior

The model provides insight as to why patients make health decisions and outlines a process to encourage change. Limitations of this model may include socioeconomic status, previous experiences, and cultural factors.

## Social Cognitive Theory (Social Learning Theory)

This theory assesses the cognitive and emotional aspects of behavior for understanding behavioral change. The Social Cognitive Theory also attempts to explain how patients acquire and continue with particular behavioral patterns as well as providing a basis for intervention strategies. According to this theory, the environment, personal factors, and behavior are constantly influencing each other. The concepts of the Social Cognitive Theory include:

- **Behavior capability:** The process of learning how to make a change in behavior. Possessing the knowledge and skill to perform a given behavior; promote mastery learning through skills training.

- **Emotional coping responses:** Strategies or tactics that are used by a person to deal with emotional stimuli. To provide training in problem solving and stress management.

- **Environment:** Factors physically external to the person. The environment provides opportunities and social support.

- **Expectancies:** The value that is placed on the expected results. The values that the person places on a given outcome or incentives. Expectancies also represent present outcomes of change that have functional meaning.

- **Expectations:** Anticipatory outcomes of a behavior. To model positive outcomes of healthful behavior.

- **Observational learning:** Behavioral acquisition that occurs by watching the actions and outcomes of others' behavior. This will include credible role models of the targeted behavior.

- **Reinforcement:** Responses that are either positive or negative consequences of behavior. These are responses to a person's behavior that increase or decrease the likelihood of reoccurrence. Reinforcement promotes self-initiated rewards and incentives.

- **Reciprocal determinism:** The relationship between an individual and their environment. The dynamic interaction of the person, the behavior, and the environment in which the behavior is performed; consider multiple avenues to behavioral change, including environmental, skill, and personal change.

- **Self-control:** Personal regulation of goal-directed behavior or performance. Self-control will provide opportunities for self-monitoring, goal setting, problem solving, and self-reward.

- **Self-efficacy:** The belief in one's ability to successfully change a behavior. The person's confidence in performing a particular behavior. Approach behavioral change in small steps to ensure success.

- **Situation:** Perception of the environment; correct misperceptions and promote healthful forms.

It is believed that a patient's reality is formed through the interaction of the environment and a person's cognitions (which change with experience and time). Social comparison of a patient's performance to others is also a strong source of self-efficacy. This theory is used when studying a variety of health pathologies, medical management compliance, alcohol abuse, and other health-related issues. A limitation to this theory is that its complexity can make it difficult to use.

## Trans-theoretical Model (Stages of Change)

The Trans-theoretical Model is a model of intentional change. It focuses on the decision making process of the individual. The theory differs from many others in its belief that change implies a process over time, not an isolated event. The process of change includes progressing through five stages:

1. **Precontemplation:** not intending to change

2. **Contemplation:** intending to change behavior in the near future

3. **Preparation:** making a plan to change behavior

4. **Action:** implementing the plan to change behavior

5. **Maintenance:** continuation of behavior change

This process for behavior change is not linear as individuals can enter and exit at any point or may repeat stages several times. The model can be useful to health programs and the process of moving a patient through various stages.

# Patient Education

## Adult Learning

- Therapists must strive to make patient education sessions practical and useful for the patient.

- Failure to identify the relevance of the presented information will promote disinterest and decrease compliance.

### Guidelines to Promote Adult Learning

- Design learning activities that will incorporate the patient's past experiences.

- Encourage the learner to play an active role in their educational program.

- Attempt to demonstrate the relevance of selected learning activities.

- Provide ample opportunities for practice and feedback.

- Recognize skill acquisition or objective improvement in patient performance.

## Domains of Learning

Domains of learning are educational terms that describe various aspects of human behavior. The three most commonly recognized domains of learning are the cognitive, psychomotor, and affective domains. Recognizing the various levels of each of the domains can assist therapists to plan appropriate patient learning activities.

**Affective domain:** The affective domain is primarily concerned with attitudes, values, and emotions.

The domain consists of five specific levels: receiving, responding, valuing, organization, and characterization.

**Cognitive domain:** The cognitive domain is primarily concerned with knowledge and understanding.

The domain consists of six specific levels: knowledge, comprehension, application, analysis, synthesis, and evaluation.

**Psychomotor domain:** The psychomotor domain is primarily concerned with physical action or motor skill.

The domain consists of seven specific levels: perception, set, guided response, mechanism, complex overt response, adaptation, and origination.

## Learning Style

Therapists can often obtain information related to a patient's preferred learning style by asking a few basic questions.

- Do you prefer to learn new information by observing, reading, listening or experiencing?
- Are you more comfortable learning in an active or passive manner?
- What increases your motivation to learn?

## Teaching Methods

### Individual

- Therapists most commonly instruct patients on an individual basis.
- The individual approach allows the therapist to focus on the needs of the learner and is the model of choice when the objectives of the session are unique to an individual patient.
- The individual approach allows the therapist to strengthen the patient/therapist bond and provides additional opportunities for specific feedback.

### Group

- Therapists often instruct patients in a group.
- Group teaching may occur with patients, family members, staff, and support persons.
- Group teaching can be difficult if patients are not supportive of each other or if the learning needs of the group are diverse.
- Some patients may be intimidated by selected group members and tend to withdraw, while others may attempt to take control of the group.
- Since individuals typically receive less individual attention in a group, it is critical for the therapist to regularly assess individual patient progress.
- Group teaching allows participants to support each other in the educational process and permits therapists to effectively use scarce resources such as time or money.
- Patients participating in group activities often feel a sense of camaraderie interacting with others who have similar personal experiences.

## Patient Communication[24,25]

- Verbal commands should focus the patient's attention on specifically desired actions.
- Instruction should remain as simplistic as possible and should not incorporate confusing medical terminology.

- The therapist should describe to the patient the general sequence of events that will occur prior to initiating treatment.
- The therapist should ask the patient questions during treatment in order to establish a rapport with the patient and to provide feedback as to the status of the current treatment.
- The therapist should speak clearly and vary their tone of voice as required by the situation.

## Guidelines for Effective Patient Education[10,25]

- Attempt to establish a positive rapport with the patient.
- Assess the patient's readiness and motivation to learn.
- Attempt to identify the patient's preferred learning style and available resources.
- Identify potential barriers to patient progress.
- Design an individualized education program for the patient based on his/her medical condition and personal goals.
- Coordinate education with the other members of the health care team.
- Focus the majority of available time on the most important concepts.
- Provide clear and succinct communication to the patient.
- Use repetition to improve patient learning.
- Provide frequent feedback to the patient.
- Utilize appropriate teaching resources to facilitate patient learning.
- Assess the effectiveness of patient education.
- Modify the patient education program based on the assessment results.

## Principles of Motivation[25,26]

- Readiness to learn significantly influences motivation.
- Individuals respond differently to selected motivational strategies.
- Success is more motivating than failure.
- Internal motivation has a greater potential to contribute to meaningful and lasting change than external motivation.
- A positive patient/therapist relationship enhances motivation.
- Limited anxiety may serve to motivate, while excessive anxiety may debilitate.
- Affiliation and approval can be motivating.

## Cultural Influences[26]

- Understanding cultural differences in patients can assist therapists to function as more effective educators.
- Patient culture is influenced and shaped by society, community, family, personal values, and attitudes.

- Language barriers, nonverbal communication, and limited personal experience can serve as obstacles when educating patients with significant cultural differences.
- Therapists should embrace cultural diversity and avoid efforts to make patients conform to any particular norm or standard.
- Therapists must be cautious when interpreting specific language or behavior and avoid labeling patients as unmotivated or disinterested.
- Therapists should use available resources such as experienced staff members, interpreters or consultants as necessary to achieve desired outcomes.

## Designing Effective Patient Education Materials

- Design the materials to convey only the necessary information.
- Emphasize essential information.
- Utilize active instructions such as "you" and avoid passive terms such as "patient."
- Larger print may be more desirable than smaller print.
- Avoid long sentences or complex medical terminology.
- Pictures or graphics should be used where appropriate to complement written information.
- Incorporate answers to frequently asked questions.
- Written materials should flow in a logical sequence.
- Written materials should utilize a reading level appropriate for the target audience.

## Teaching Guidelines for Specific Patient Categories[25,26,27]

Therapists often vary their approach when educating patients of various ages and abilities. It is difficult to develop recommendations that apply to all patients in a given category, however, the following represent general guidelines for therapists to consider when treating selected patient categories.

### Infants/Children

- Therapists should try to make therapy sessions with infants/children interactive.
- Sessions should include structured play and should be of relatively short duration.
- Frequent breaks and positive reinforcement will serve to increase the patient's level of participation.

### Adolescents

- Therapists should try to assume the role of an advocate when working with adolescents.

- It is important for therapists to establish patients' trust and incorporate patient goals into the plan of care.
- Adolescents prefer to be treated like adults and may resent the presence of parents during therapy sessions.
- Therapists should provide patients with clear and concise instructions and offer frequent positive reinforcement.

### Adults

- Therapists should involve adults in determining education outcomes.
- The education program should be compatible with the patient's daily routine and goals.
- Emphasizing the relevance of educational activities will serve to increase patient compliance.
- Therapists should be aware of the available patient support system and identify any barriers to progress.

### Elderly

- Therapists may find it necessary to introduce new information gradually when working with the elderly.
- Special attention should be paid to identify signs of hearing loss or visual impairments.
- The elderly population often benefits from the social benefits of group activities.
- Education sessions for the elderly should not be longer in duration, however, the achievement of selected outcomes may require additional sessions.

### Terminally Ill

- Therapists should incorporate patient goals as an integral component of any educational session for patients with terminal illness.
- Family members and other support personnel should be encouraged to participate in the educational session, however, it is important to provide the patient with the opportunity to make independent decisions whenever possible.
- Goals for the terminally ill patient often include maximizing function, safety, and comfort.
- Therapists may alter their teaching methods based on the current mental and physical well-being of the patient.

### Cognitively Impaired

- The therapist should focus on the education of the caregiver and incorporate the patient whenever possible.
- When incorporating the patient in the session, instructions should be clear and concise and should be summarized through demonstration and pictures.
- Therapists should encourage the patient to compensate for any memory deficit.

## Illiteracy

- Therapists should attempt to determine the literacy level of their patients.

- If a patient is determined to be illiterate, the therapist may elect to modify language to use basic wording and short sentences.

- Demonstration, repetition, and pictures should be incorporated into educational sessions.

- Therapists may include more detailed written information in educational sessions if the patient has adequate support at home.

## Stages of Dying[10,24]

Elizabeth Kubler-Ross identified five stages in coming to terms with death after interviewing 500 terminally ill patients. The stages Kubler-Ross identified were denial, anger, bargaining, depression, and acceptance.

### Denial

The denial stage is characterized by a failure of the individual to believe that their condition is terminal. Therapists should attempt to establish trust with a patient in this stage and avoid trying to make the patient accept their condition.

### Anger

The anger stage is characterized by frustration and negative emotional feelings often directed at anyone the individual comes in contact with. Individuals often ask "Why me?" Therapists should avoid taking the anger personally and recognize that expressing anger is often a useful step for the individual to move beyond this stage.

### Bargaining

The bargaining stage is characterized by the individual trying to negotiate with fate. The individual may try to make a deal with a higher being based on good behavior, compliance with an exercise program or dedication of their life to a specific cause. Therapists should facilitate discussion with the patient and serve as a good listener.

### Depression

The depression stage is characterized by the individual expressing the depths of their anguish. The individual is often deeply depressed and may show little interest in any form of medical intervention. Therapists should listen to the individual and exhibit a great deal of patience during this stage.

### Acceptance

The acceptance stage is characterized by the individual coming to terms with their fate. The individual may attempt to resolve any unfinished business and may experience a sense of inner peace. Therapists should encourage the individual and family to ask questions and attempt to spend meaningful time with the individual.

# Education Concepts

## Team Models[28]

**Unidisciplinary:** A single discipline provides patient care services.

**Multidisciplinary:** Several different disciplines are involved in providing patient care, however, the disciplines tend to function independently and communication occurs primarily through the medical record.

**Interdisciplinary:** Several different disciplines are involved in providing patient care. The disciplines function independently, however, they routinely report to each other and may coordinate patient care.

**Transdisciplinary:** Numerous disciplines function as a collective unit to provide patient care services. Team goals are established rather than individual discipline goals and as a result, discipline specific boundaries tend to erode.

NEXT EXIT

MOTIVATIONAL MOMENT

*See Page 1032*

# Research

## Evidence-Based Practice (EBP)

Evidence-based medicine has been defined as the integration of the best clinically relevant research with clinical expertise and patient values.[29] In recognition of the movement's adoption by other health care practitioners, the concept has evolved into evidence-based practice (EBP). The term "practice" recognizes the expansion of the framework to physical therapy, nursing, and other aspects of health care beyond medicine.

Best research evidence refers to clinically relevant, patient-centered clinical research about the accuracy of diagnostic tests, prognostic factors, and the efficacy of interventions. Clinical expertise refers to the clinician's use of past experiences to make clinical judgments. Patient values refer to the preferences and expectations of the patient that are considered in clinical decisions about health care.[29] In physical therapy, the goal of evidence-based practice is to help therapists make sense of knowledge derived from research and use the information as a basis for making decisions about their patients.

## Steps to Practicing Evidence-Based Physical Therapy[29]

1. Identify a problem or area of uncertainty about prevention, diagnosis, prognosis or therapy.

2. Formulate a focused clinical question for a specific patient problem.

3. Search the literature for relevant clinical articles to answer that question.

4. Critically appraise each article to determine its validity (closeness to the truth), impact (size of the effect), and applicability (usefulness in clinical practice).

5. Integrate the relevant findings in clinical practice along with clinical expertise and patient values.

6. Assess the outcomes of the selected action.

## Using P-I-C-O to Ask a Focused Clinical Question

The focused clinical question needs to be directly relevant to the patient's problems and phrased in a way that directs the search of the literature to relevant answers. The focused question makes it relatively easy to combine the appropriate terms to search the databases. A well-built clinical question usually contains four elements that form the acronym PICO.[30]

**Patient or Problem** – What is the target patient population or the problem of interest?

**Intervention** – What intervention or form of therapy needs to be evaluated? Alternatively, if intervention is not the area of interest, the "I" could refer to diagnosis or prognosis.

**Comparison** – What comparison or control treatments (e.g., placebo or other treatments) are being compared to the primary intervention?

**Outcome** – What changes or results would suggest an intervention is effective, a prognostic factor is important, or a diagnostic test is accurate?

## How to Evaluate Individual Studies about Therapy

Individual studies about therapy must be evaluated to determine if the results of the study are valid, important, and applicable to the patient.[31]

1. Determine if the results of the study can be considered valid:

   - Were patients assigned to treatment randomly and was the randomization list concealed?
   - Was the follow-up of patients long enough and complete?
   - Was an intention-to-treat analysis performed?
   - Were patients and clinicians kept blind to patient assignment to group?
   - Except for the experimental therapy, were patients treated equally?
   - Were the groups similar at the start of the study?

2. Determine if the results of the study can be considered important:

   - What is the magnitude of the treatment effect?
   - How precise is the estimate of the treatment effect?

3. Determine if the valid and important results are applicable to the patient?

   - Is the patient so different from those in the study that the results cannot apply?
   - Is the treatment feasible in the clinical setting?
   - What are the potential benefits and harms from the therapy?
   - What are the patient's values and expectations for the treatment?

## Practice Guidelines

Practice guidelines are statements developed by panels of experts to help health care professionals and patients make decisions about screening, prevention or treatment of a specific health condition.[32] These rigorously developed evidence-based guidelines assist health care providers to make the best decision about treatment for a particular patient and to limit potential harm. It is important to remember that guidelines cannot account for individual variation among patients and, therefore, cannot replace clinician judgment with respect to particular patients or special clinical situations.

A number of practice guidelines related to physical therapy may be accessed through "Collections" at the website of *Physical Therapy* – Journal of the American Physical Therapy Association.[33] Also, the Agency for Healthcare Research and Quality of the US Department of Health and Human Services offers a searchable database of clinical practice guidelines online.[34]

## Levels of Evidence for Articles about Therapy/Intervention

The hierarchy of "levels of evidence" refers to how different categories of studies are ranked and should be considered when decisions need to be made about interventions. To evaluate the strength of the different types of clinical evidence, studies or clinical trials are ranked according to the strength of the design (Fig. 9-13).[35] In many cases, it is not possible to find the best level of evidence to answer a particular research question. In these instances, a clinician will need to consider moving down the pyramid to other types of studies, however, clinicians must be aware of the limitations incurred as the strength of the evidence diminishes.

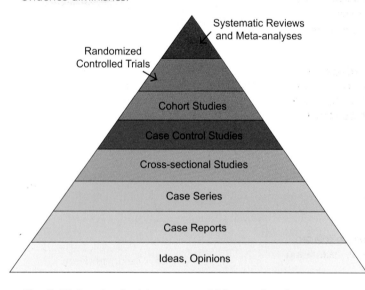

**Fig. 9-13:** Levels of evidence pyramid for studies about interventions.

### Systematic Review

A comprehensive review of the medical literature that uses explicit methods to systematically search, identify, appraise, and summarize all literature on a specific issue. For example, a Cochrane Systematic Review is a type of review aimed at providing evidence specifically in health care and health policy.[29]

### Meta-analysis

A systematic review that uses a statistical technique to derive an estimate of effect size by combining the results of several randomized controlled trials to determine the overall effectiveness of a treatment. This strategy can minimize the problem of small sample size from individual studies since the pooling of trials increases the overall sample size.[36]

### Randomized Controlled Trial (RCT)

A form of experimental research used to assess the relative effect of a specific intervention compared to a control condition. Patients are randomized into a control group and at least one experimental group. The control group receives either no treatment or a standard default treatment. Ideally, the groups will be identical except for the intervention they have been randomized to receive. Random assignment reduces the risk of bias and increases the probability that differences between the groups can be attributed to the intervention.[33]

### Cohort Study

A type of longitudinal, observational study in which individuals with a risk factor or exposure are followed over time to compare the occurrence of a disease in the exposed group to that of the group of unexposed individuals. The measure of association between exposure and disease in cohort studies is the relative risk (i.e., the ratio of the incidence rate of exposed individuals to that of the controls). Cohort studies can be performed prospectively or retrospectively from historical records. Limitations of cohort studies include the excessive length of time a study can take and the influence of other lifestyle variables that invariably result in the two groups being uniquely different.[36]

### Case Control Study

A type of retrospective, observational study in which individuals who already have a particular disease are matched with a comparison group of individuals without the disease. The history of exposure or other characteristics prior to the onset of the disease is recorded through interview and other sources and compared between the two groups. The control group provides an estimate of the frequency and amount of exposure in subjects in the population without the disease being studied. The measure of association between exposure and occurrence of disease in case control studies is the odds ratio (i.e., the ratio of odds of exposure in diseased subjects to the odds of exposure in non-diseased subjects).[36]

### Cross-Sectional Study

A type of observational study where the data or observations are made at only one point in time and all subjects are tested at relatively the same time.[5] A cross-sectional study aims to describe relationships between a disease or condition and factors of interest that exist in a specified population at a given time. These studies can describe the prevalence of disease or conditions and demonstrate associations, but they cannot distinguish between newly occurring and long-established conditions, nor can they identify causal relationships about what may have precipitated the disease or condition.

### Case Report or Case Series

A case report is an in-depth description of an individual's condition or response to treatment. A case series consists of a collection of observations of similar cases. Case reports may be used to generate theories and hypotheses for future research. They cannot test hypotheses or establish cause-and-effect relationships.[36]

## Types of Research

A number of methods are used to classify research. One way is to view research along a continuum reflecting the type of question the research is intended to answer. On this continuum, research is classified as descriptive, experimental or exploratory.[36]

**Descriptive research:** Recording, analyzing, and interpreting conditions that exist for the purpose of classification and understanding a clinical phenomenon. Examples include developmental research, normative research, qualitative research, case report, and case series.

**Experimental research:** Comparing two or more conditions for the purpose of determining cause and effect relationships between independent and dependent variables. Examples include randomized controlled trials, quasi-experimental studies, and single-subject designs.

**Exploratory research:** Examines the dimensions of a phenomenon of interest and its relationships to other factors. Examples include cohort studies, case control studies, historical research, and methodological studies.

Another method of categorizing research is to distinguish it by qualitative and quantitative methods.

## Characteristics of Qualitative and Quantitative Research

| | Qualitative Research | Quantitative Research |
|---|---|---|
| **Definition** | Data are from observation, interviews or verbal interactions and focus on the meanings and interpretations of the participants. | Data are measurements of outcomes that can be subjected to analysis by traditional inferential statistics. |
| **Purpose** | To gain an understanding of underlying reasons and motivations of prevalent trends in thought and opinion. May generate hypotheses for subsequent quantitative research. | To quantify data and generalize results from a sample to a population. |
| **Rationale** | Human behavior must be bound to the context in which the behavior occurs and therefore must be studied in the manner it occurs, rather than being manipulated. | Social reality can be reduced to variables that when tightly controlled, allow researchers to examine how other variables are influenced. |
| **Type of Research Question** | Probing, global | Non-probing, specific |
| **Sample** | A small number of subjects. | A large number of subjects representing the population of interest. |
| **Researcher Role** | Active participant who becomes immersed in the activity for the purpose of maximizing learning. | Objective observer that does not participate in or influence what is being studied. |
| **Data Analysis** | Non-statistical | Statistical |
| **Training of the Researcher** | Background is most often in the social sciences with specialized training and skills in interviewing. | Background is most often in statistics and mathematics. |
| **Outcome** | Exploratory or investigative. Develop an initial understanding for further decision making. Findings are not conclusive and cannot be used to make generalizations about the population. | Used to recommend a final course of action. |

## Ethics of Human Subjects Research

**Assent:** A child's affirmative agreement to participate in research. A child's failure to object should not be construed as agreement.[37]

**Belmont Report:** In 1974, the National Research Act established the National Commission for the Protection of Human Subjects of Biomedical and Behavioral Research. This Commission, in turn, published The Belmont Report which articulated the three ethical principles that guide human subjects' research:[37]

- **Respect for persons:** Refers to the individual's right of self-determination and the right to make decisions about their medical care as an autonomous person. Respect for persons requires that people with diminished autonomy be provided special protection.

- **Beneficence:** Refers to the obligation of the researcher to provide for the well-being of their subjects and to maximize the possible benefits and minimize the possible harm in research.

- **Justice:** Refers to the fair treatment of subjects including the equitable distribution of burdens and benefits in research.

**Confidentiality:** An ethical principle that requires the researcher to not disclose any information revealed by the subject or discovered by the researcher to ensure that data is accessible only to authorized individuals.

**Generalizable knowledge:** Although used in the definition of research, the Code of Federal Regulations does not define the term. Most Institutional Review Boards operationally define it to be information or conclusions of research that have the potential to be applied to individuals and settings beyond those that were the focus of the original research.

**Human subject:** A living individual about whom an investigator conducting research obtains data through intervention or interaction with the individual or identifiable private information.[37]

**Informed consent:** The process by which a person is given important facts about the possible risks, benefits, and limits of the procedure, treatment, trial or testing before deciding whether or not to participate.[37]

**Institutional Review Board (IRB):** A group of scientists and non-scientists charged with protecting the rights and welfare of persons participating in research and authorized to review and approve research involving human subjects.[37]

**Minimal risk:** The probability and magnitude of harm or discomfort anticipated in the research are not greater than those ordinarily encountered in daily living or during the performance of routine physical or psychological examinations or tests.[37]

**Research:** A systematic investigation including research development, testing, and evaluation, designed to develop or contribute to generalizable knowledge.[37]

**Vulnerable populations:** Populations in which a voluntary informed consent process could be compromised are considered "vulnerable." Several populations are typically considered vulnerable including minors (under 18 years of age), subjects with a diminished capacity to consent, pregnant women, human fetuses, neonates and products of labor and delivery, non-English speaking subjects, prisoners or other involuntarily institutionalized persons, and students.[37]

## Consider This
### Informed Consent

In keeping with the principle of Respect for Persons, researchers must obtain the informed consent of the subject or the subject's legally authorized representative under circumstances that provide the opportunity to consider whether or not to participate without undue influence or coercion. Informed consent should contain all of the following:[37]

1. A statement that the study involves research.
2. An explanation of the purpose(s) of the research.
3. A description of the procedures to be followed, including the duration of participation, and identification of any experimental procedures.
4. A description of any reasonably foreseeable risks or discomforts to the subject.
5. A description of any benefits to the subject or to others that may reasonably be expected.
6. A disclosure of any appropriate alternative procedures or treatments that might be advantageous.
7. A description of who will have access to records that identify the subjects, and how confidentiality of those records will be maintained.
8. For research involving greater than minimal risk, an explanation of any compensation and an explanation of any medical treatments that are available if injury occurs, and what they consist of, or where further information may be obtained.
9. Identification of whom to contact for answers to questions about the research and subjects' rights, and whom to contact in the event of a research-related injury to the subject, along with contact information.
10. A statement that participation is voluntary and that the subject may refuse to participate or discontinue participation at any time without penalty.

## Types of Data and Measurement

### Data

Data are the numeric and non-numeric information that represent the quantitative or qualitative attributes of an object, event or person.[38] Types of data include:

**Continuous data:** Data that can assume any value along a continuous scale that covers a range of values without gaps or interruptions. Values are limited by the degree of accuracy of the measuring instrument. Examples of continuous variables are range of motion (degrees), distance (m), weight (kg), and time (s).[36]

**Discrete data:** Data that is measured in whole units.[36] Examples include heart rate, patients diagnosed with cancer, and number of visits to a physical therapy clinic.

**Dichotomous data:** A type of discrete data limited to only two values.[36] Examples include gender (male or female) and smoking status (smoker or non-smoker).

**Qualitative data:** Also known as categorical data, these data represent different categories distinguished by a non-numeric characteristic.[38] Examples include eye color, blood type, and hand dominance.

**Quantitative data:** Data consisting of numbers that represent counts or measurements.[38] A measurement is the numeral assigned to an object, event or person, or the category to which an object, event or person is assigned according to rules.[11]

### Scales of Measurement

**Nominal:** Also known as the classification scale because the values of the variable are mutually exclusive and exhaustive categories, so that each object or person can be assigned to only one category. Nominal scales are qualitative rather than quantitative. Examples of nominal scale measurements in physical therapy include blood type, type of breath sound, and type of arthritis.[39]

**Ordinal:** This scale of measurement is also known as a ranking scale. The data are ranked on the basis of a property of the variable, but the intervals between the ranks may not be equal or known. Examples of ordinal scale measurements in physical therapy include manual muscle test grades, levels of assistance, pain, and joint laxity grades.[39]

**Interval:** A measurement scale where the intervals between adjacent values are equal, but there is no true zero point. Examples of interval scale measurements in physical therapy include temperature (e.g., body, skin, whirlpool) on the Fahrenheit or Celsius scale and some developmental and functional status tests.[39]

**Ratio:** A measurement scale where the intervals between adjacent values are equal and there is a true zero point. Examples of ratio scale measurements in physical therapy include range of motion (degrees), distance walked (m), time to complete an activity (s), and nerve conduction velocity (m/sec).[39]

## Measurement Reliability

Reliability is the reproducibility or repeatability of measurements.[39] Examples of different forms of reliability include:

**Alternate forms reliability:** Also known as parallel forms reliability, it assesses the consistency or agreement of measurements obtained with different forms of a test. Alternate forms reliability is essential if the different forms of the test are to be used interchangeably.[39] For example, different forms of standardized tests like the SAT, GRE, and NPTE can be administered each year as long as the different versions of the tests are considered equivalent measures.

**Internal consistency:** The extent to which items or elements that contribute to a measurement reflect one basic phenomenon or dimension.[39] For example, in physical therapy, a functional assessment scale should only include items that relate to patients' physical function.[36]

**Intrarater reliability:** The consistency or equivalence of repeated measurements made by the same person over time.[39]

**Interrater reliability:** The consistency or equivalence of measurements made by more than one person. Interrater reliability indicates the agreement of measurements taken by different examiners.[39]

**Test-retest reliability:** The consistency or equivalence of repeated measurements made on the same individual on separate occasions.[39] Test-retest reliability can be affected by the interval between tests, effects of fatigue or learning, and changes in the characteristic being measured.[36]

## Measurement Validity

Validity is the degree to which a useful or meaningful interpretation can be inferred from a measurement.[39] Examples of different types of measurement validity include:

**Face validity:** The degree to which a measurement appears to test what it is supposed to.[36] Although face validity is insufficient documentation of validity, it is an important form of validity because patients may not be compliant with repeated testing if they don't see how the measurements derived from the tests relate to their specific problem.

**Content validity:** The degree to which a measurement reflects the meaningful elements of a construct and the items in a test adequately reflect the content domain of interest and not extraneous elements.[39] For example, the McGill Pain Questionnaire may have greater content validity than a visual analog pain scale because, in addition to pain intensity, it assesses the location, quality, and duration of pain.[36]

**Construct validity:** The degree to which a theoretical construct is measured by a test or measurement. Evidence of construct validity is through logical argument based on theoretical and research evidence.[39] For example, manual muscle test (MMT) scores would have construct validity as indicators of innervation status of muscle if there was a relationship between MMT scores and the results of electromyographic testing.

**Criterion-related validity:** The validity of the measurement is established by comparing it to either a different measurement often considered to be a "gold standard" or data obtained by different forms of testing.[39] Examples of criterion-related validity include:

- **Concurrent validity:** A form of criterion-related validity in which an interpretation is justified by comparing a measurement to a "gold standard" measurement at approximately the same time.[39] For example, heart rate measurements made by palpation of peripheral pulses will have concurrent validity if the heart rate measurements by palpation are associated with the heart rates measured simultaneously from an ECG.

- **Predictive validity:** A form of criterion-related validity in which the measurement is considered to be valid because it is predictive of a future behavior or event.[39] For example, the use of a student's GPA or GRE as admission criteria for graduate school is based on their presumed ability to predict future academic success.

- **Prescriptive validity:** A form of criterion-related validity in which the measurement suggests the form of treatment the person should receive. The prescriptive validity of the measurement is judged based on the successful outcome of the treatment.[39] For example, the measurement of asystole on the ECG could be said to have prescriptive validity if patients with this arrhythmia are successfully revived by cardiopulmonary resuscitation techniques.

## Research Subjects and Sampling

**Population:** The complete collection of elements to be studied. The group to which the results of research are intended to be generalized.[38]

**Sample:** A subset of elements drawn from a population to draw conclusions or make estimates about the larger population.[36]

**Sampling error:** The chance difference between the statistic calculated from a sample and the true value of the parameter in the population. Sampling error is inherent in the use of sampling methods.[36]

**Sampling with replacement:** A sampling method in which each unit that is selected for the sample is put back into the population before the next unit is drawn from the sample. This results in each unit truly having an equal chance of being selected throughout the sampling process. This method of sampling is rarely used in research on human subjects.[36]

**Sampling without replacement:** A sampling method in which a unit selected from the population is not returned to the population and therefore, cannot be selected again for the same sample. Thus, the size of the population decreases as the size of the sample increases.[36]

**Probability sampling:** A method of sampling that uses some form of random selection. Every member of the population must have the same probability of being selected for the sample, since the sample should be free of bias and representative of the population.[8] Examples of probability sampling methods include:

- **Simple random sampling:** Subjects have an equal chance of being selected for the sample. The sampling method often relies on a table of random numbers or a random number generator on a computer to determine the sample. However, simple random sampling is not the most statistically efficient method of sampling and may not result in a representative sample, since it is the luck of the draw.[36]

- **Systematic sampling:** Subjects are selected by taking every $n^{th}$ subject from the population. The size of the interval is based on the size of the population and the desired sample size. The greatest advantage associated with this sampling technique is its simplicity.[36]

- **Stratified random sampling:** Also called proportional or quota random sampling, the population is divided into homogenous subgroups (strata) and then a simple random sample is drawn from each. Stratified random sampling assures that the sample will be representative of key subgroups of the population in addition to the overall population.[36]

- **Cluster sampling:** The population is divided into clusters or areas (usually along geographic boundaries) and a random sample of the clusters is selected. Then, all of the units in the selected samples are measured. The sampling technique is less costly and more efficient than simple random sampling, especially when the population is spread across a wide geographic region.[36]

**Non-probability sampling:** Any method of sampling that does not involve random selection of subjects.[36] Examples of non-probability sampling methods include:

- **Convenience sampling:** As the name suggests, the sample is selected from subjects who are convenient or readily available to the researcher.[36]

- **Purposive sampling:** Subjects are deliberately selected based on predefined criteria chosen by the investigators.[36]

- **Quota sampling:** Similar to stratified random sampling, except that subjects from each subgroup are not selected randomly. After identifying the subgroups or strata of interest from the population, the researcher uses convenience sampling to select the required number of subjects from each stratum.[36]

- **Snowball sampling:** Subjects are identified by asking existing subjects to identify the names of other potential participants. Snowball sampling is used when the characteristic to be studied is rare and it would be extremely difficult and costly to identify individuals with this characteristic.[36]

## Experimental Designs

The essence of an experiment is to demonstrate a cause and effect relationship between an intervention or condition (independent variable) and an outcome or response (dependent variable).

**Clinical trial:** A type of research design that tests how well methods of screening, prevention, diagnosis or treatment of a disease work in people.[36]

**Completely randomized design:** A type of research design in which subjects are randomly assigned to different groups and each group receives a unique intervention. The outcomes of the different groups are compared at the end of the trial. This method is also known as a parallel groups design.[36]

**Crossover design:** A type of research design where the subject receives both treatments (e.g., treatment and control) in random order separated by a period of no treatment. In this design, each subject serves as their own control.[36]

**Factorial design:** A type of research design in which two or more independent variables are investigated with different subjects assigned to the various combinations of levels of the independent variables.[36]

**Pretest-posttest control group design:** A type of research design that compares the outcomes of two or more groups formed by random assignment by testing all groups before and after the treatment. This represents the basic format of a randomized controlled trial.[36]

**Posttest only control group design:** A type of research design that compares the outcomes of two or more groups formed by random assignment by testing all groups only after the treatment.[36]

**Randomized controlled trial (RCT):** A clinical trial in which a group of individuals is randomly assigned to an experimental group and a control group.[29]

**Repeated measures design:** A type of research design in which subjects are tested under all conditions, therefore, each person acts as their own control. This is also known as a within-subjects design.[36]

**Sequential clinical trial:** A type of research design in which the data are analyzed as they become available so the trial can be stopped as soon as the evidence is sufficient to show a significant difference between treatments.[36]

**Single-subject design:** A type of research design that permits drawing conclusions about the effects of treatment based on the responses of a single patient. Single-subject designs are characterized by the use of repeated measurement of a response over time and at least two test periods or phases: a baseline phase (A) prior to treatment and an intervention phase (B) after treatment. The baseline and intervention phases may be replicated to create a number of designs (e.g., A-B; A-B-A; A-B-A-B).[36]

**Quasi-experimental design:** A type of research design without a control group, random assignment of subjects to groups, or both.

- **One-group pretest-posttest design:** A type of quasi-experimental research design in which measurements are made on one group of subjects before and after treatment. Time is the independent variable, with two levels (pretest and posttest).[36]

- **One-way repeated measures design over time:** An extension of the one-group pretest-posttest design in which measurements are made on one group of subjects at multiple, prescribed time intervals. The intervention may be administered once or it may be repeated. If more than two measurements are made, trends over time may be evaluated by polynomial contrasts.[36]

- **Time series design:** A type of quasi-experimental research design in which multiple measurements are made before and after treatment to observe patterns or trends during the pretreatment and posttreatment periods.[36]

## Experimental Controls

An experiment is said to have internal validity when there is confidence that the intervention caused the outcome. To achieve this result, the researcher will design the experiment to control extraneous variables and sources of bias that could reduce the validity of the results.[36] There are a number of methods for researchers to help increase the internal validity of an experiment.

**Blinding:** A term used to describe conditions that are imposed to keep groups of individuals from knowing which subjects have or have not received an intervention. Sometimes called masking, blinding is used to reduce bias and the placebo effect. There are several different types of blinding:[36]

- **Single blind:** The subjects are unaware of the research hypothesis and the group to which they were assigned until the end of the study.

- **Double blind:** The subjects and certain members of the research team are unaware of the research hypothesis and the group to which each subject was assigned until the end of the study.

- **Triple blind:** The subject, certain members of the research team, and data analyzers are unaware of the research hypothesis and the group to which each subject was assigned until the end of the study.

**Control group:** In a clinical trial, a group against which the treatment group is compared. The control group should be statistically identical to the treatment group, except for the variable of interest that is being evaluated in the experiment. Control groups are used to help isolate the effect of the independent variable and eliminate the unintended influence of extraneous factors that can confound the results. The two most common forms of control are placebo and active.[36]

- **Active control:** A known effective form of treatment in a clinical trial against which the experimental treatment is compared. When an effective treatment is available, it is unethical to use a placebo control for comparison to the experimental treatment.[36]

- **Placebo control:** An inactive substance or treatment that looks the same as, and is administered in the same way as an active drug or treatment.[36]

**Matching/pairing:** In research, a strategy for attempting to control for differences between subjects. Investigators identify pairs of subjects who have identical characteristics (e.g., weight, age, race) before randomizing them to ensure that the resultant groups are balanced on important variables that may affect the outcome. Using identical twins is a classic example of matching.[36]

**Intention-to-treat analysis:** A method of analysis in which all subjects randomly assigned to one of the treatments are analyzed together, regardless of whether they received or completed that treatment. The method preserves the original balance of subject groups achieved through randomization.[29]

**External validity:** The degree to which results of the research study are generalizable to populations or circumstances beyond those included in the study. Threats to external validity include the interaction of treatment with the specific type of subjects tested and the place (setting) and time (history) in which the experiment is performed.[36]

**Internal validity:** The degree to which an intervention being evaluated (independent variable) is the cause of the outcome measured in the study (dependent variable) and not the result of extraneous factors. Threats to internal validity include history, maturation, attrition, testing, instrumentation, and regression toward the mean.[36]

**Randomization:** A means of assigning subjects to groups in an experiment so that each subject has an equal chance of being assigned to each group. The most robust method of random assignment is accomplished by computer-generated random numbers or random number tables.[36]

**Hawthorne effect:** An untreated subject experiences a change simply from participating in a research study. The tendency for individuals to change their behavior in response to the fact that they are being observed or studied.[36]

**Placebo effect:** A phenomenon in which an inactive treatment or procedure that is intended to mimic a real treatment causes an improvement in the patient's condition simply because the patient has the expectation that it will be helpful.

## Hypothesis Testing

In hypothesis testing, the researcher examines the probability that some estimate calculated from sample data might have occurred by chance.

**Hypothesis:** A tentative statement to explain certain observations or facts that requires further experimentation to be verified.[36]

- **Alternate hypothesis (Ha or H1):** Also known as the experimental hypothesis, the alternate hypothesis is a statement that the population parameter has a value that differs from the null hypothesis. In hypothesis testing, the alternate hypothesis is accepted when the null hypothesis is rejected.[38]

- **Null hypothesis (Ho):** Also known as the statistical hypothesis, the null hypothesis is a statement that the value of a population parameter (e.g., mean, proportion or correlation coefficient) is equal to some claimed value.[38] The null hypothesis is tested statistically by inferential statistics.

**Independent variable:** The variable that is presumed to have caused or influenced the dependent variable. In research, the independent variable is what is controlled or manipulated by the researcher.[36]

**Dependent variable:** The response or outcome assumed to be caused by the effect of the independent variable.[36]

**p-value:** The probability that a particular statistical result could have happened by chance. When the p-value is smaller than the stated value of alpha, or level of significance, the null hypothesis is rejected. When the p-value is larger than the stated value of alpha, or level of significance, the null hypothesis is not rejected.[38]

**Alpha level (a level):** Also known as the significance level, the probability of rejecting the null hypothesis when it is true, or the chance of committing a Type 1 error. Traditional values for alpha are 0.05 and 0.01.[38]

### Steps in Testing a Statistical Hypothesis[38]

1. State the null hypothesis and alternate hypothesis

2. Select the appropriate test statistic

3. Select the level of significance for the statistical test (e.g., $p < 0.05$)

4. Calculate the test statistic from the sample data

5. Interpret the results: Compare the p-value associated with the test statistic to the significance level.

- If the p-value is ≤ the level of significance, reject the null hypothesis in favor of the alternate hypothesis

- If the p-value is > the level of significance, do not reject the null hypothesis

**Type I error (alpha error):** The error the researcher makes when wrongly deciding to reject the null hypothesis, concluding that there is a difference or relationship when there is not. If the level of significance is set at 0.01, there is a 1% chance of a Type I error occurring. A Type I error is a false positive finding.[38]

**Type II error (beta error):** The error the researcher makes when wrongly deciding not to reject the null hypothesis, concluding that there is no difference or relationship when there is. A Type II error is a false negative finding.[38]

**Statistically significant:** A statistical conclusion made when the probability is small that the difference between groups or the relationship between variables happened by chance.[38]

**Statistical power:** Refers to the chance that a statistical test will lead to rejection of a false null hypothesis (i.e., find a "statistically significant" result).[38]

**Effect size (ES):** A measure of the magnitude of the difference between two treatments or the magnitude of the relationship between two variables. The larger the ES, the more likely it will be statistically significant. ES is one of the statistical elements used to estimate sample size and perform a power analysis.[36]

**Effect size index:** A statistic that represents effect size using a standardized value. Generally, the effect size index is calculated by taking the difference between the two groups (e.g., the mean of the treatment group minus the mean of the control group) and dividing it by the standard deviation of one of the groups.

To interpret the resulting index, this general guide is used:[36]

> < 0.1 = trivial effect
>
> 0.1 - 0.3 = small effect
>
> 0.3 - 0.5 = moderate effect
>
> > 0.5 = large effect

**Minimal clinically important difference (MCID):** The smallest difference in a patient's condition that the patient or clinician considers worthwhile and that would, in the absence of side effects and excessive cost, warrant a change in the patient's management. The MCID is an important concept for judging if changes reported in a research study indicate a meaningful or trivial effect on the patient's status. The MCID is also known as the minimal clinically significant difference (MCSD).[36]

**Minimal detectable difference (MDD):** The minimum detectable change in a patient's condition beyond the threshold of measurement error. MDD represents the smallest difference or change that would be statistically significant. The standard error of measurement is a common statistic used to determine the MDD. MDD is also known as minimal detectable change (MDC).[36]

**Parameter:** A numerical measurement describing some characteristic of a population.[38] Parameters are rarely known and usually estimated by statistics computed from a sample. In research publications, Greek letters are used to designate parameters. For example, $\mu$ (mu) is the symbol for the mean of the population and $\sigma$ (sigma) is the symbol for the standard deviation of the population.

**Statistic:** A numerical measurement describing some characteristic of a sample.[38] Statistics are used to estimate population parameters. In research publications, English letters are used to designate statistics. For example, $\bar{x}$ or M is the symbol for the sample mean and s is the symbol for the sample standard deviation.

## Describing Data with Graphs

**Bar graph:** A type of graph used to show the magnitude or frequency of categories of the data. Data in each category are represented by vertical bars, with the length of the bars proportional to the magnitude or frequency on a vertical y-axis (Fig. 9-14).[40]

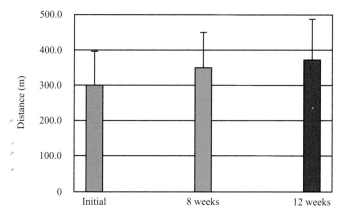

**Fig. 9-14:** Example of a bar graph showing the average distance walked by 31 subjects at three time periods. Values are means +1 standard deviation.

**Box and whisker plot:** A type of graph that illustrates the distribution of values within a group through five numbers: minimum score, lower quartile (Q1), median (Q2), upper quartile (Q3), and maximum score. Outliers are shown as circles (Fig. 9-15).[38]

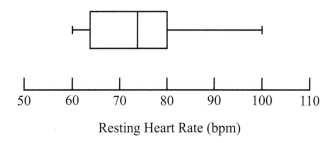

**Fig. 9-15:** Example of a box and whisker plot for 22 subjects. Minimum = 60; lower quartile (Q1) = 64; median (Q2) = 74; upper quartile (Q3) = 80; maximum = 100. No outliers are shown.

**Forest plot:** A type of graph used in a meta-analysis that shows the results of the individual studies as well as a cumulative summary of all studies. The graph plots the point estimate of the measure of effect (e.g., odds ratio, relative risk) for each study as a square along a horizontal line, the width of which represents the confidence interval of the effect. The area of each square is proportional to the study's weight in the meta-analysis. The measure of effect for all studies combined is plotted as a diamond. The center of the diamond represents the point estimate for the cumulative effect and the width of the horizontal line represents the upper and lower confidence limits. A vertical line represents no effect or the null value. A forest plot is also known as a blobbogram (Fig. 9-16).

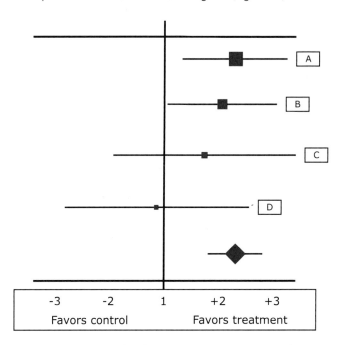

**Fig. 9-16:** Example of a forest plot depicting the odds ratios from four studies (A, B, C, D) and a cumulative summary of all the studies combined (diamond) from a meta-analysis.

**Histogram:** A graphical display of a frequency distribution. Histograms display the distribution of data by plotting the frequency (count or percentages) of observations (y-axis) for each interval represented on the x-axis. Histograms use continuous bars of equal widths determined by the x-axis intervals, where bar height represents frequency (Fig. 9-17).[38]

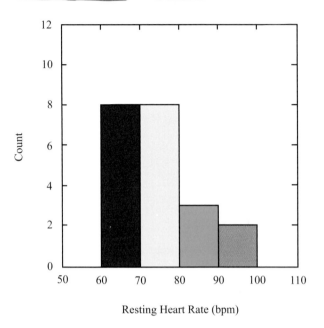

**Fig. 9-17:** Example of a histogram for resting heart rate of 21 subjects.

**Line graphs:** A graph that demonstrates the relationship between two or more quantitative variables. Line graphs usually are designed with the dependent variable on the y-axis and the independent variable on the x-axis and are ideal for showing trends in data over time. The data points are connected by curves (Fig. 9-18).[40]

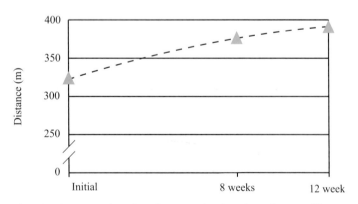

**Fig. 9-18:** Example of a line graph showing the curvilinear increase in average distance walked in a 6-minute walk test performed by 31 patients measured at three time periods.

**Scatter plot:** A graphical display that illustrates the relationship between two quantitative variables. Each paired (x,y) value is plotted on the graph as a single point. A line of best fit generated mathematically may be fitted to the data to show the relationship among the variables (Fig. 9-19).[38]

**Fig. 9-19:** Example of a scatter plot showing the relationship between resting heart rate and post-exercise heart rate in 22 subjects with the linear regression line.

**Stem and leaf plots:** A graphical display which enables the reader to observe the entire distribution of data without losing any information. Most commonly this is done by organizing data into categories (e.g., 20-29, 30-39), and then dividing a number into two digits. The first digit is placed to the left side of a vertical line (stem) and the second digit is placed on the right side of the vertical line (leaves) (Fig. 9-20).[38]

| 5 | 359 |
|---|---|
| 6 | 47888 |
| 7 | 27899 |
| 8 | 1124 |
| 9 | 247 |
| 10 | 23 |

**Fig. 9-20:** Example of a stem and leaf plot showing heart rate data for each of 22 subjects.

## Descriptive Statistics

Descriptive statistics summarize or describe important characteristics of a population. Typically, data from the population are examined for measures of center, distribution, and variation.

## Measures of Center

Values that describe the center of the data.

**Mean:** The arithmetic average; the sum of all the values divided by number of values.[38]

**Median:** The point on a distribution at which 50% of the values fell above and below. It is the 50th percentile. The median is identified by first rank ordering the values. If the number of values is odd, the median is the middle value. If the number of values is even, the median is the mean of the two middle values.[38]

**Mode:** The value that occurs most frequently. A distribution with two modes is termed bimodal. A distribution with more than two modes is termed multimodal.[38]

## Measures of Distribution

Values that describe the shape of the data.

**Kurtosis:** Refers to the "peakedness" of a distribution. It is a measure of whether the data are peaked or flat relative to a normal distribution. A high kurtosis distribution has a sharper peak and longer, fatter tails, while a low kurtosis distribution has a more rounded peak and shorter, thinner tails.[38]

**Normal:** A bell-shaped curve with the majority of data clustered around the mean. The mean, median, and mode are the same (Fig. 9-21).[38]

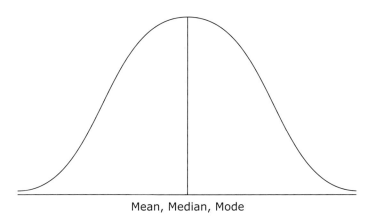

**Fig. 9-21:** Location of the mean, median, and mode in a normal distribution.

- Approximately 68% of all values fall within one standard deviation above and below the mean.

- Approximately 95% of all values fall within two standard deviations above and below the mean.

- Approximately 99% of all values fall within three standard deviations above and below the mean.

(Figs. 9-22, 9-23).

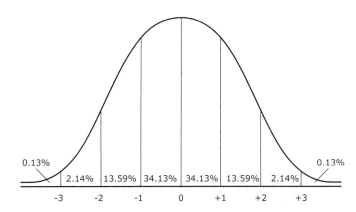

**Fig. 9-22:** Areas under the curve of a normal distribution represented by each standard deviation between -3 and +3.

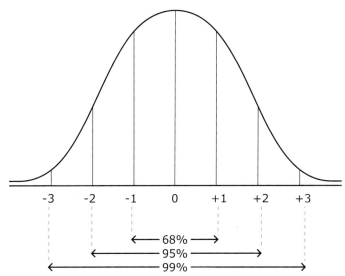

**Fig. 9-23:** The approximate areas of a normal distribution bounded by ±1, ±2, and ±3 standard deviations from the mean.

**Skewness:** Refers to the asymmetry in the shape of a distribution. In a negatively skewed distribution, the mean and median are to the left of the mode, and the left tail is elongated. In a positively skewed distribution, the mean and median are to the right of the mode and the right tail is elongated (Figs. 9-24, 9-25).[38]

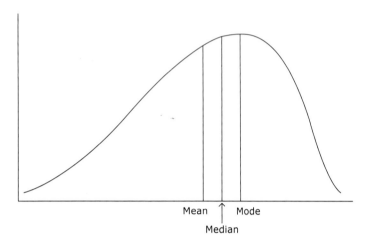

**Fig. 9-24:** Negatively skewed distribution.

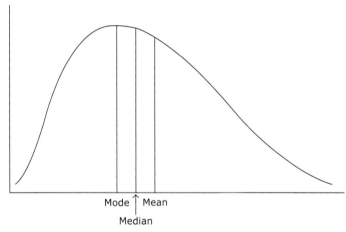

**Fig. 9-25:** Positively skewed distribution.

## Measures of Variation

Values that describe how the data vary.

**Coefficient of variation (CV):** The CV is the ratio of the standard deviation of a distribution to the mean, expressed as a percentage. CV = (s / mean) x 100.[38]

**Percentiles:** The value below which a certain percent of observations within a distribution will fall. For example, the 20th percentile is the value or score below which 20% of scores are found.[38]

**Quartiles:** Quartiles divide the data into four equal parts, so

that each part represents one fourth of the sampled population. The 25th percentile is also known as the first quartile (Q1), the 50th percentile as the median or second quartile (Q2), and the 75th percentile as the third quartile (Q3).[38]

**Range:** The difference between the maximum and minimum values.[38]

**Standard deviation:** A descriptive measure of the spread or dispersion of data; the positive square root of the variance. Describing data by means of standard deviation implies that the data are normally distributed.

**Variance:** The sum of the squared deviations of each data point from the mean, divided by the number of observations in the sample.[38] The variance equals the standard deviation squared, and therefore is expressed as squared units of the data. Because squared units are difficult to make sense of, the variance is often not reported. The formula for the variance ($S^2$) of a sample is:

$$S^2 = \frac{\sum (X-M)^2}{N}$$

where X is a single score, M is the sample mean, and N is the number of scores.

## Inferential Statistics

Inferential statistics are a branch of statistics that use sample data to make inferences about a population. Inferential statistics are used to test hypotheses. Two types of inferential statistics are parametric and nonparametric.

## Parametric Statistics

Parametric statistics assume that samples come from populations that are normally distributed and there is homogeneity of variance. Parametric statistical tests are applied to both interval and ratio level data.[38]

### Analysis of variance (ANOVA)

Analysis of variance is an inferential statistical procedure used to test the equality of means between two or more populations by analyzing sample variances.

**One-way analysis of variance:** A statistical procedure similar to the independent t-test, however, the test is designed to accommodate two or more population means. One-way refers to the fact that the sample data are separated into different groups on the basis of one characteristic or factor; only one independent variable is examined in the analysis.[38]

**Two-way analysis of variance:** A statistical procedure used to compare two or more population means with two or more independent variables. Two-way refers to the fact that the sample data are separated into different groups on the basis of two characteristics or factors. Both independent variables are examined in the analysis, which also examines the interaction of the two independent variables.[38]

**Repeated measures analysis of variance:** An analysis of variance procedure where all individuals are measured under a number of different experimental conditions. It is an appropriate analysis to perform for variables where practice or carryover effects are minimal. Repeated measures ANOVA can also be used when individuals have been matched according to an important characteristic.[36]

**Regression analysis:** A set of statistical procedures to examine the relationship between a dependent variable (Y) and one or more independent predictor variables (X). Regression analysis predicts how a change in one or more of the independent variables affects the dependent variable.[36]

## Confidence intervals

**Confidence interval (CI):** A range of values used to estimate a population parameter. CI is also known as the interval estimate.[38]

**Confidence level:** The probability, usually expressed as a percentage, that the confidence interval actually contains the unknown population parameter. With repeated sampling, the interval would contain the true parameter value with the probability at the stated confidence level. For example, a 95% confidence level means that if the same population is sampled 100 times and CIs are calculated on each sample, 95 of the resulting CIs would be expected to contain the true population parameter.[38]

**Point estimate:** A single value calculated from a sample that best approximates a population parameter of interest. For example, the sample mean is the point estimate for the mean of the population.

## Correlation

A statistical measure of the strength of association among two or more variables. Two variables may be correlated for a number of reasons, so correlation does not imply causation.[36]

**Intraclass correlation (ICC):** A form of correlation coefficient that assesses both the degree of correspondence and agreement among scores. The ICC ranges from 0.0 to 1.0 and is calculated from variance estimates derived from an analysis of variance.[36]

**Pearson product moment correlation (r):** A correlation coefficient that measures the magnitude and direction of the linear relationship of two variables on the interval scale. The test yields a value between -1.0 and +1.0. The sign indicates the direction of the relationship and the number indicates the magnitude of the relationship. A positive sign indicates that the two variables increase or decrease together; a negative sign indicates that an increase in one variable is associated with a decrease in the other. A value of +1.0 or -1.0 indicates that the sample values fall in a straight line, while a value of 0 indicates no relationship.[38]

## t-test

An inferential statistical procedure for estimating a population mean or comparing two means when the population is normally distributed and the population variance is not known.[38]

**Dependent or paired t-test:** A parametric statistical procedure used to compare the means of two groups that are correlated. A paired sample t-test is used when the samples are matched pairs.[38]

**Independent t-test:** A parametric statistical procedure used to compare the means of two independent groups. The groups are considered independent if members of each group are different. For example, the independent sample t-test is appropriate when testing differences between males and females because a person cannot be in both groups.[38]

**One sample t-test:** A statistical procedure used to compare the mean of a sample to an expected or reference mean of the population to make a statistical decision as to whether or not the sample mean is different from the population.[38]

**One-tailed test:** A test of statistical significance in which deviations from the null hypothesis in only one direction are considered. When using a significance level of 0.05, a one-tailed test apportions 0.05 to either the right or left tail of the distribution of the test statistic. This only applies when the test statistic is symmetrically distributed (e.g., z, t). The use of a one-tailed test implies that the intervention could have only one effect (i.e., beneficial or harmful).[38]

**Two-tailed test:** A test of statistical significance in which deviations from the null hypothesis in either direction are considered. When using a significance level of 0.05, a two-tailed test apportions 0.025 to each tail of the distribution of the test statistic. This only applies when the test statistic is symmetrically distributed (e.g., z, t).[38]

## z-test

A statistical procedure for estimating the mean of a population or comparing two means when the population is normally distributed and the population variance is known.[38]

## Nonparametric Statistics

Nonparametric statistics do not assume that samples come from populations that are normally distributed and do not assume homogeneity of variance. Nonparametric statistical tests are commonly applied to nominal or ordinal level data, or interval or ratio data that are not normal.[38]

**Chi-Square test:** A nonparametric statistical procedure for nominal data. The test evaluates the difference between observed and expected frequencies to examine the association or independence between categorical variables.[38]

**Kruskal-Wallis test:** A statistical procedure used to determine if three or more independent samples come from the same population. It is the nonparametric version of the one-way analysis of variance.[38]

**Mann-Whitney test:** A statistical procedure used to compare two independent samples with ordinal level data. It is the nonparametric alternative of the independent t-test and is equivalent to the Wilcoxon signed rank test.[38]

**Spearman rank correlation coefficient:** A type of correlation to test for the association between two variables. The data are ranks (ordinal level) or can be converted to ranks. It is the nonparametric equivalent to the Pearson product moment correlation. The test yields a value between -1.0 and +1.0.[38]

**Wilcoxon Signed Rank test:** A nonparametric statistical procedure used to compare two dependent samples with ordinal level data. It is the nonparametric alternative of the dependent or paired t-test.[38]

## Statistical Measures of Validity for Diagnostic and Screening Tests

**Sensitivity:** When referring to a medical test, sensitivity refers to the percentage of people who test positive for a specific disease among a group of people who have the disease.[36]

**Specificity:** When referring to a medical test, specificity refers to the percentage of people who test negative for a specific disease among a group of people who do not have the disease.[36]

**False negative test:** A test that indicates a person does not have a specific disease or condition when the person actually does have the disease or condition.[36]

**False positive test:** A test that indicates a person has a specific disease or condition when the person actually does not have the disease or condition.[36]

**Negative predictive value:** The ability of a diagnostic test to correctly determine the proportion of patients without the disease from all the patients with negative test results.[29]

**Positive predictive value:** The ability of a diagnostic test to correctly determine the proportion of patients with the disease from all the patients with positive test results.[29]

**SpPin:** A mnemonic used to remember the relationship between a diagnostic or screening test with a high specificity value and the confidence we have in ruling in the diagnosis. In a test with high specificity, a positive diagnostic test rules in the diagnosis.

**SnNout:** A mnemonic used to remember the relationship between a diagnostic or screening test with a high sensitivity value and the confidence we have in ruling out the diagnosis. In a test with high sensitivity, a negative diagnostic test rules out the diagnosis.

## Epidemiology

Epidemiology is the study of the causes, distribution, transmission, and control of disease in groups of people.[36]

**Risk factor:** Something that increases the chance of developing a condition or disease.[36]

### Measures of disease frequency

**Incidence:** The number of new cases of a particular disease or condition in the population at risk during a specified time interval. Often expressed as the number of new cases per 100,000 people at risk.[36]

**Prevalence:** The number of existing cases of a disease or condition at a point in time, including new and pre-existing cases.[36] Often expressed as the number of existing cases per 100,000 people at risk.

### Measures of association and risk

**Relative risk (RR):** A measure of the risk of a certain event happening in one group compared to the risk of the same event happening in another group. Typically, this is the ratio of incidence of disease among individuals exposed to some disease risk factor to the incidence of disease among individuals who were not exposed. Like the odds ratio, a RR of 1.0 means that the event is equally probable in both groups. A RR greater than 1.0 implies that exposure increases the risk and a RR less than 1.0 implies that the exposure decreases the risk. The RR is also known as the risk ratio.[34]

**Odds ratio (OR):** A measure of the odds of an event happening in one group compared to the odds of the same event happening in another group. In research, odds ratios are most often used in case control (backward looking) studies to find out if being exposed to a certain substance or other risk factor increases the risk of developing a certain disease. An OR of 1.0 means that the exposure probably does not increase the risk of developing the disease. An OR > 1.0 means that the exposure may increase the risk of getting the disease, and an OR < 1.0 means that the exposure may reduce the risk. The OR is also known as the relative odds.[34]

**Number needed to treat (NNT):** The number of patients that need to be treated to prevent one bad outcome or result in one additional good outcome.[29] The ideal NNT is one, where everyone improves with treatment. The higher the NNT, the less effective is the treatment.

## Spotlight on Safety
### Laws and Ethics of Research[41]

Institutional policies and procedures on research with human subjects are designed to comply with the Code of Federal Regulations[9] as well as state and local laws to protect individuals involved in research participation.

The Code of Ethics for the Physical Therapist sets forth principles for the ethical practice of physical therapy as determined by the House of Delegates of the American Physical Therapy Association.[13] Principle 5C of the Code of Ethics states: Physical therapists involved in research shall abide by accepted standards governing protection of research participants.

# Safety & Protection; Responsibilities; Research Essentials

## Safety and Protection

1. Standard precautions combine universal precautions and body substance isolation precautions. Standard precautions apply to all blood/body fluids, secretions, and excretions.

2. Transmission-based precautions offer guidelines for the care of specified patients infected with selected pathogens transmitted by airborne, droplet or contact modes.

3. Airborne precautions reduce the risk of airborne transmission of infectious agents through evaporated droplets in air or dust particles.

4. Droplet precautions reduce the risk of droplet transmission of infectious agents through contact of the mucous membranes of the mouth and nose, contact with the conjunctivae, and through coughing, sneezing, talking or suctioning.

5. Contact precautions reduce the risk of transmission of infectious agents through direct or indirect contact. Direct contact involves skin-to-skin transmission; indirect contact involves a contaminated intermediate object, usually within the patient's environment.

6. Personal protective equipment (e.g., gowns, lab coats, masks, gloves, goggles, spill kits, mouthpieces) are used as barriers to protect someone who is assisting a patient with a potentially infectious disease.

7. A sterile field is a designated area that is considered void of all contaminants and microorganisms. Specific protocols are required to develop and maintain the sterile field.

## Professional Responsibilities

8. The Americans with Disabilities Act is federal legislation designed to provide a clear and comprehensive national mandate for the elimination of discrimination.

9. A ramp must possess twelve inches of length for each inch of vertical rise (i.e., 8.3% grade).

10. A S.O.A.P. note is a commonly used format for daily notes. The S.O.A.P. acronym stands for: S = Subjective, O = Objective, A = Assessment, P = Plan.

11. Quality improvement refers to a form of objective self-examination designed to improve the quality of services.

12. The Nagi Model describes health status as a product of the relationship between health and function and is defined by four primary concepts: pathology, impairment, functional limitation, and disability.

13. Negligence refers to the failure to do what a reasonable and prudent person would ordinarily have done under the same or similar circumstances for a given situation.

14. Risk management refers to the identification, analysis, and evaluation of risks and the selection of the most advantageous method for treating them.

15. Responsibilities delegated to support personnel by physical therapists must be commensurate with their qualifications. This includes experience, education, and training of the individuals to whom the responsibilities are being assigned.

16. A physical therapist assistant is a technically educated health care provider who assists the physical therapist in the provision of physical therapy. The physical therapist assistant, under the direction and supervision of the physical therapist, is the only paraprofessional who provides physical therapy interventions.

17. A physical therapy aide is a non-licensed worker who is specifically trained under the direction and supervision of a physical therapist. The physical therapy aide may be involved in the provision of physical therapist directed support services.

18. The Elements of Patient/Client Management Leading to Optimal Outcomes include examination, evaluation, diagnosis, prognosis (including plan of care), intervention, and outcomes.

19. Criteria for Standards of Practice for Physical Therapy serve as the profession's statement of conditions and performances that are essential for provision of high quality professional service to society, and provide a foundation for assessment of physical therapist practice.

20. The Code of Ethics for the Physical Therapist published by the American Physical Therapy Association sets forth principles for the ethical practice of physical therapy. All physical therapists are responsible for maintaining and promoting ethical practice.

21. Medicare provides health insurance for individuals over 65 years of age and the disabled. Medicaid provides basic medical services for individuals with low income or who qualify for welfare or public assistance benefits in the state of their residence.

22. Workers' Compensation provides protection for employees that are injured on the job. This legislation provides continued income as well as paid medical expenses for employees injured while working.

23. Current Procedural Terminology (CPT) codes are procedure codes used by physical therapists and other health care professionals to describe the interventions that were provided to a given patient.

# Safety & Protection; Responsibilities; Research Essentials

24. The International Classification of Diseases (ICD) codes are designed to describe a patient's infirmity through categories based on etiology and affected anatomical systems.

25. Maslow's Hierarchy of Needs includes self-actualization needs, esteem needs, affiliative needs, and physiological needs.

26. Classical conditioning refers to a process where learning occurs when an unconditioned stimulus is repeatedly preceded by a neutral stimulus. The neutral stimulus serves as a conditioned stimulus and the learned reaction that results is termed the conditioned response.

27. Operant conditioning refers to a process where learning occurs when an individual engages in specific behaviors in order to receive certain consequences.

28. Common Health Behavior Models include the Health Belief Model, Social Cognitive Theory (Social Learning Theory), and Trans-theoretical Model (Stages of Change).

29. Domains of learning are educational terms that describe various aspects of human behavior. The three most commonly recognized domains of learning are the cognitive, psychomotor, and affective domains.

30. The Stages of Dying describe five stages in coming to terms with death. The stages include denial, anger, bargaining, depression, and acceptance.

## Research

31. Evidence-based practice refers to the physical therapist's reliance on patient-centered clinical research, clinical expertise and past experiences, and the patient's values when making clinical decisions about the patient's physical therapy plan of care.

32. When searching the literature for patient-centered clinical research, the physical therapist should ask a focused clinical question that is directly relevant to the patient's problems and phrased in a way that directs the search of the literature. A focused clinical question usually contains four elements that form the acronym P-I-C-O.

    **Patient or Problem** – The target patient population or the problem of interest

    **Intervention** – The intervention or form of therapy to evaluate

    **Comparison** – The comparison/control treatments to be compared to the primary intervention

    **Outcome** – The measurements that would suggest the intervention or therapy is effective

33. Before accepting the results of a study about an intervention, therapists should determine if the results of the study are valid, important, and applicable to their patients.

34. There is a hierarchy for the levels of evidence for studies about therapy/intervention, diagnosis, and prognosis. For studies about therapy/interventions, systematic reviews and meta-analyses are considered to be the highest forms of evidence followed by randomized controlled trials.

35. Physical therapists involved in clinical research must adhere to the principles and practices that govern the planning and implementation of research when working with human subjects. These are summarized in the Belmont Report.

36. The three basic ethical principles relevant to research involving human subjects are the principles of respect of persons, beneficence, and justice.

37. Reliability and validity are important properties of measurements. Physical therapists should select tests and measurements which have been investigated for appropriate forms of reliability and validity.

38. Selecting a representative sample of subjects from the population is an important step in the research process to ensure that the results of the research can be generalized to the population of interest.

39. Probability samples involve some form of random selection; non-probability samples do not.

40. A number of different experimental designs are available to test hypotheses in clinical research. The randomized controlled trial (RCT) is considered the gold standard of true experimental designs.

41. Blinding, controls, randomization, and intention-to-treat analysis are important means researchers use to control extraneous variables and sources of bias that could reduce the validity of their results.

42. Researchers use the hypothesis testing procedure to test hypotheses of differences or relationships between variables.

43. When the results of a study report a p-value that is smaller than the stated value of alpha, or level of significance, the null hypothesis is rejected and the result is said to be statistically significant. When the p-value is larger than the stated value of alpha, the null hypothesis is not rejected and the result is not statistically significant.

## Safety & Protection; Responsibilities; Research Essentials

44. When evaluating the effectiveness of interventions, physical therapists must consider the clinical importance in addition to the statistical significance. The minimal clinically important difference (MCID) for the test or measurement, if known, provides a guide to assess the meaningfulness of the change in patient status.

45. Descriptive statistics (e.g., measures of center, distribution, and variability) summarize or describe important characteristics of a population.

46. Inferential statistics are used to test hypotheses and to make inferences from the sample to the population.

47. The t-test and analysis of variance are examples of parametric inferential statistics used to test the significance of the differences in two or more means.

48. The intraclass correlation coefficient and Pearson product moment correlation coefficient are examples of parametric inferential statistics used to test the significance of the relationships between variables.

49. The validity of screening and diagnostic tests are assessed by measures of sensitivity, specificity, negative predictive value, and positive predictive value.

50. The odds ratio and risk ratio are statistical measures used to assess the association between exposure to a risk factor and developing a disease.

## Safety & Protection; Responsibilities; Research Proficiencie

## Safety and Protection; Professional Responsibilities Proficiencies

### 1. Accessibility Requirements

Determine if each provided measurement is consistent with established accessibility standards. If a given measurement satisfies existing standards, it is considered acceptable. If the measurement fails to satisfy existing standards, it is considered unacceptable.

Determine if each measurement is acceptable or unacceptable, and identify the established accessibility standard for each measurement.

**Word Bank:** Acceptable, Unacceptable

| Acceptable/Unacceptable | Measurement |
|---|---|
| a | A ramp with a grade of 9.8%. |
| Standard: | |
| b | A ramp that is 20 feet in length with a 24 inch vertical rise. |
| Standard: | |
| c | A ramp with a width of 36 inches. |
| Standard: | |
| d | A doorway with a width of 34 inches. |
| Standard: | |
| e | A hallway with a width of 32 inches. |
| Standard: | |
| f | A bathroom sink with 30 inches of height from the floor. |
| Standard: | |
| g | A bathroom toilet with 18 inches of height from the floor to the top of the toilet. |
| Standard: | |

# Safety & Protection; Responsibilities; Research Proficiencies

## Safety and Protection; Professional Responsibilities Proficiencies

### 2. S.O.A.P. Notes

Identify the appropriate portion of the S.O.A.P. note for each entry. Answers must be selected from the Word Bank.

**Word Bank:** subjective, objective, assessment, plan

| Section | Entry |
|---|---|
| a | The patient reports hurting the knee after falling down a flight of stairs. |
| b | Right knee active range of motion is 0-126 degrees. |
| c | The patient received instructions for shoulder strengthening using elastic tubing. |
| d | The patient denies pain when coughing. |
| e | The patient may not have exhibited maximal effort during resistive testing. |
| f | The patient exhibits 5/5 strength in the left iliopsoas. |
| g | The patient indicates a desire to return home with her husband after discharge. |
| h | The patient demonstrated appropriate use of pacing techniques during ambulation. |
| i | The patient's cardiac status may diminish the patient's rate of recovery. |
| j | The patient will be referred to a speech-language pathologist. |

### 3. The Nagi Model

Identify the appropriate concept from the Nagi Model based on each description. Answers must be selected from the Word Bank and can be used more than once.

**Word Bank:** disability, impairment, functional limitation, pathology

| Concept | Description |
|---|---|
| a | lateral collateral ligament sprain |
| b | diminished knee range of motion |
| c | difficulty ascending a flight of stairs |
| d | unable to work as a housekeeper |
| e | diminished upper extremity sensation |
| f | unable to propel a wheelchair on level ground |

# Safety & Protection; Responsibilities; Research Proficiencie

## Safety and Protection; Professional Responsibilities Proficiencies

### 4. Scope of Practice

Determine if each described activity is consistent with the scope of practice for the identified health care provider. Appropriate activities should be labeled acceptable and inappropriate activities should be labeled unacceptable.

**Word Bank:** acceptable, unacceptable

| Acceptable/Unacceptable | Entry |
|---|---|
| a | A physical therapist assistant completes a discharge summary. |
| b | A physical therapist instructs a physical therapist assistant to teach an existing patient to utilize axillary crutches. |
| c | A physical therapist assistant describes a patient's exercise tolerance in the medical record. |
| d | A physical therapy aide guards a patient ascending stairs. |
| e | A physical therapist assistant discontinues an existing exercise session due to safety concerns. |
| f | A physical therapist assistant completes a re-examination on a patient. |
| g | A physical therapy aide monitors a patient's vital signs during exercise. |
| h | A physical therapist assistant increases the weight a patient uses on an existing upper extremity progressive resistive exercise. |
| i | A physical therapy aide returns a previously used hot pack to the hydrocollator unit. |

# Safety & Protection; Responsibilities; Research Proficiencies

## Safety and Protection; Professional Responsibilities Proficiencies

### 5. Health Care Disciplines

Identify the health care discipline most closely associated with the supplied description. Answers must be selected from the Word Bank and can be used only once.

**Word Bank:** home health aides, occupational therapists, physical therapist assistants, physical therapists, physical therapy aides, respiratory therapists, social workers, speech-language pathologists

| Discipline | Description |
|---|---|
| a | These individuals provide health related services to the elderly, disabled, and ill in their homes. Patient care activities include performing housekeeping duties, assisting with ambulation or transfers, and promoting personal hygiene. |
| b | These individuals are considered support personnel who may be involved in support services directed by physical therapists. They are permitted to function only with continuous on-site supervision by a physical therapist, or in some cases a physical therapist assistant. |
| c | These individuals evaluate, treat, and care for patients with breathing disorders. Patient care activities include performing bronchial drainage techniques, measuring lung capacities, administering oxygen and aerosols, and analyzing oxygen and carbon dioxide concentrations. |
| d | These individuals help people improve their ability to perform activities of daily living, work, and leisure skills. Educational preparation emphasizes the social, emotional, and physiological effects of illness and injury. |
| e | These individuals provide services to help restore function, improve mobility, relieve pain, and prevent or limit permanent physical disabilities of patients suffering from injuries or disease. |
| f | These individuals evaluate speech, language, cognitive-communication, and swallowing skills of children and adults. |
| g | These individuals perform components of physical therapy procedures and related tasks selected and delegated by a supervising physical therapist. |
| h | These individuals help patients and their families to cope with chronic, acute or terminal illnesses and attempt to resolve problems that stand in the way of recovery or rehabilitation. |

## Safety and Protection; Professional Responsibilities Proficiencies

### 6.  Safety and Professional Roles Basics

Mark each statement as True or False.  If the statement is False, correct the statement in the space provided.

| True/False | Statement |
|---|---|
| a | A computer monitor in a work station should be a minimum of 12 inches away from the eyes. |
| **Correction:** | |
| b | When performing a transfer with a patient that requires assistance, a physical therapist should attempt to be as close to the patient as possible and use a long lever arm. |
| **Correction:** | |
| c | Sterile gowns are only considered sterile in the front from the waist level upwards. |
| **Correction:** | |
| d | If an object on a sterile field becomes contaminated, the entire field is considered non-sterile. |
| **Correction:** | |
| e | A patient with droplet precautions would require a physical therapist to wear a mask if they were within ten feet of the patient. |
| **Correction:** | |
| f | A ramp that is 20 inches in elevation should be a minimum of 20 feet in length. |
| **Correction:** | |

## QUIZ Safety & Protection; Responsibilities; Research Proficiencies

## Safety and Protection; Professional Responsibilities Proficiencies

| True/False | Statement |
|---|---|
| g | A discharge summary should provide a capsule view of the patient's progress during therapy. |
| Correction: | |
| h | One inch is equivalent to 3.28 centimeters. |
| Correction: | |
| i | Autonomy refers to the moral obligation of health care providers to act for the benefit of others. |
| Correction: | |
| j | Prognosis refers to the anticipated level of optimal improvement that may be attained through intervention and the amount of time required to reach that level. |
| Correction: | |
| k | The Consolidated Omnibus Budget Reconciliation Act provides protection for employees that are injured on the job. |
| Correction: | |
| l | Medicare Part A provides benefits for outpatient care, physician services, and services ordered by physicians such as diagnostic tests, medical equipment, and supplies. |
| Correction: | |
| m | International Classification of Diseases Codes are procedure codes used by physical therapists and other health care professionals to describe specific interventions provided to a given patient. |
| Correction: | |

## Safety and Protection; Professional Responsibilities Proficiencies

### 7. Domains of Learning

Identify the appropriate domain of learning for each described activity. Answers must be selected from the Word Bank and can be used more than once.

**Word Bank:** affective, cognitive, psychomotor

| Domain | Description |
|---|---|
| a | A patient lists three postoperative contraindications following total hip arthroplasty. |
| b | A patient reports being fearful that they will reinjure their knee after returning to athletic activities. |
| c | A patient performs a D2 flexion pattern using the right upper extremity. |
| d | A patient verbally summarizes the activities included in a home exercise program with their physical therapist. |
| e | A patient demonstrates a sliding board transfer using the appropriate technique. |
| f | A patient is extremely cautious when weight bearing on the involved lower extremity. |

### 8. Stages of Dying

Identify the appropriate stage of dying for each desciption. Answers must be selected from the Word Bank and can be used only once.

**Word Bank:** acceptance, anger, bargaining, denial, depression

| Stage | Description |
|---|---|
| a | This stage is characterized by an individual trying to negotiate with fate. |
| b | This stage is characterized by frustration and negative emotional feelings often directed at anyone the individual comes in contact with. |
| c | This stage is characterized by the individual expressing the depths of their anguish and showing little interest in any form of medical intervention. |
| d | This stage is characterized by the individual coming to terms with their fate. |
| e | This stage is characterized by a failure of the individual to believe that their condition is terminal. |

**QUIZ**     Safety & Protection; Responsibilities; Research Proficiencies

# Safety and Protection; Professional Responsibilities Proficiencies

## 9. Teaching and Learning Basics

Mark each statement as True or False.  If the statement is False, correct the statement in the space provided.

| True/False | Statement |
|---|---|
| a | According to Maslow's Hierarchy of Needs, esteem needs refer to the need to realize one's full potential as a human being. |
| Correction: | |
| b | Therapists should attempt to identify the patient's preferred learning style and available resources. |
| Correction: | |
| c | Therapists should attempt to design learning activities that will incorporate the patient's past experiences. |
| Correction: | |

# Research Proficiencies

## 10. Levels of Evidence

Assign a number to each category based on the strength of the design. An assignment of "1" would indicate the most desirable or highest level of evidence from the available options while an assignment of "5" would indicate the least desirable or lowest level of evidence.

| Study | Rank |
|---|---|
| randomized controlled trial | a |
| case control study | b |
| systematic review | c |
| cohort study | d |
| case report | e |

## 11. Scales of Measurement

Identify the appropriate scale of measurement for each of the following types of data. Answers must be selected from the Word Bank and can be used more than once.

**Word Bank:** interval, nominal, ordinal, ratio

| Data | Scale |
|---|---|
| range of motion | a |
| body temperature on the Celsius scale | b |
| distance walked | c |
| blood type | d |
| manual muscle test grades | e |
| type of breath sounds | f |
| transfer levels of assistance | g |
| nerve conduction velocity | h |

# Safety & Protection; Responsibilities; Research Proficiencies

## Research Proficiencies

### 12. Validity

Identify the type of validity most closely associated with the supplied definition. Answers must be selected from the Word Bank and can be used only once.

**Word Bank:** face validity, construct validity, content validity, criterion related validity

| Type of Validity | Definition |
|---|---|
| a | The degree to which a measurement reflects the meaningful elements of a construct and the items in a test adequately reflect the content domain of interest and not extraneous elements. |
| b | The degree to which a theoretical construct is measured by a test or measurement. |
| c | The validity of the measurement is established by comparing it to either a different measurement, often considered to be a "gold standard" or data obtained by different forms of testing. |
| d | The degree to which a measurement appears to test what it is supposed to. |

### 13. Sampling

Identify the type of sampling most closely associated with the supplied definition. Answers must be selected from the Word Bank and can be used only once.

**Word Bank:** convenience, purposive, simple random, snowball, stratified random, systematic

| Type of Sampling | Definition |
|---|---|
| a | Subjects are identified by asking existing subjects to identify the names of other potential participants. |
| b | Subjects are selected from those readily available to the researcher. |
| c | Subjects are selected from a population that has been divided into homogenous subgroups or strata and then a simple random sample is drawn from each. |
| d | Subjects have an equal chance of being selected for the sample. |
| e | Subjects are deliberately selected based on predefined criteria chosen by the investigators. |
| f | Subjects are selected by taking every $n^{th}$ subject from the population. |

## Safety & Protection; Responsibilities; Research Proficiencie

## Research Proficiencies

### 14. Testing a Statistical Hypothesis

Identify the appropriate sequence when testing a statistical hypothesis. Assign a "1" for the first step in the process and a "5" for the last step in the sequence.

| Step | Sequence |
|---|---|
| calculate the test statistic from the sample data | a |
| interpret the results | b |
| state the null hypothesis and alternative hypothesis | c |
| select the level of significance for the statistical test | d |
| select the appropriate test statistic | e |

### 15. Statistics

Identify the type of statistic most closely associated with the supplied definition. Answers must be selected from the Word Bank and can be used only once.

**Word Bank:** mean, median, mode, range, standard deviation, variance

| Type of Statistic | Definition |
|---|---|
| a | The sum of the squared deviations of each data point from the mean, divided by the number of observations in the sample. |
| b | The arithmetic average; the sum of all the values divided by the number of values. |
| c | A descriptive measure of the spread or dispersion of data; the positive square root of the variance. |
| d | The point on a distribution at which 50% of the values fall above and below. |
| e | The value that occurs most frequently. |
| f | The difference between the maximum and minimum values. |

**Safety & Protection; Responsibilities; Research Proficiencies**

## Research Proficiencies

### 16. Normal Distribution

Assuming a normal distribution, determine what percentage of values would fall within the specified values. Answers must be selected from the Word Bank and can be used only once.

**Word Bank:** 34%, 50%, 68%, 95%, 99%

| Percentage | Interval |
|---|---|
| a | between plus one and minus one standard deviations |
| b | between the mean and plus one standard deviation |
| c | between plus three and minus three standard deviations |
| d | between the mean and a point beyond three standard deviations above the mean |
| e | between plus two and minus two standard deviations |

### 17. Research Basics

Mark each statement as True or False.  If the statement is False, correct the statement in the space provided.

| True/False | Statement |
|---|---|
| a | A false negative test indicates a person does not have a specific disease or condition when the person actually does have the disease or condition. |
| **Correction:** | |
| b | Specificity refers to the percentage of people who test positive for a specific disease among a group of people who have the disease. |
| **Correction:** | |
| c | Incidence refers to the number of existing cases of a disease or condition at a point in time, including new and pre-existing cases. |
| **Correction:** | |

# Safety & Protection; Responsibilities; Research Proficiencie

## Research Proficiencies

| True/False | Statement |
|---|---|
| d | A two-tailed test is a test of statistical significance in which deviations from the null hypothesis in either direction are considered. |
| Correction: | |
| e | Alpha level refers to the probability of rejecting the null hypothesis when it is true or the chance of committing a type 2 error. |
| Correction: | |
| f | In research, the dependent variable is controlled or manipulated by the researcher. |
| Correction: | |
| g | A single blind study indicates that the subjects are unaware of the research hypothesis and the group to which they were assigned. |
| Correction: | |
| h | Interrater reliability refers to the consistency or equivalence of measurements made by more than one person. |
| Correction: | |
| i | Beneficence refers to the fair treatment of subjects including the equitable distribution of burdens and benefits in research. |
| Correction: | |
| j | Qualitative research typically uses a relatively large number of subjects and data is analyzed using statistical measures. |
| Correction: | |

# Safety & Protection; Responsibilities; Research Answer Key

## Safety and Protection; Professional Responsibilities

### 1. Accessibility Requirements

a. Unacceptable: Guideline - A ramp should have a maximum grade of 8.3%.

b. Unacceptable: Guideline - A ramp should possess twelve inches of horizontal run for each inch of vertical rise.

c. Acceptable: Guideline - A ramp should have a minimum width of 36 inches.

d. Acceptable: Guideline - A doorway should have a minimum width of 32 inches.

e. Unacceptable: Guideline - A hallway should have a minimum width of 36 inches.

f. Acceptable: Guideline - A bathroom sink should have a minimum of 29 inches of height from the floor.

g. Acceptable: Guideline - A bathroom toilet should have 17-19 inches of height from the floor to the top of the toilet.

### 2. S.O.A.P. Notes

a. subjective

b. objective

c. objective

d. subjective

e. assessment

f. objective

g. subjective

h. objective

i. assessment

j. plan

### 3. The Nagi Model

a. pathology

b. impairment

c. functional limitation

d. disability

e. impairment

f. functional limitation

### 4. Scope of Practice

a. unacceptable

b. acceptable

c. acceptable

d. unacceptable

e. acceptable

f. unacceptable

g. unacceptable

h. acceptable

i. acceptable

### 5. Health Care Disciplines

a. home health aides

b. physical therapy aides

c. respiratory therapists

d. occupational therapists

e. physical therapists

f. speech-language pathologists

g. physical therapist assistants

h. social workers

### 6. Safety and Professional Roles Basics*

a FALSE: Correction: A computer monitor of a work station should be a minimum of 20 inches away from the eyes.

b. FALSE: Correction: When performing a transfer with a patient that requires assistance, a physical therapist should attempt to be as close to the patient as possible and use a short lever arm.

c. TRUE

d. TRUE

e. FALSE: Correction: A patient with droplet precautions would require a physical therapist to wear a mask if they were within three feet of the patient.

f. TRUE

g. TRUE

h. FALSE: Correction: One inch is equivalent to 2.54 centimeters.

i. FALSE: Correction: Beneficence refers to the moral obligation to health care providers to act for the benefit of others.

j. TRUE

k. FALSE: Correction: The Consolidated Omnibus Budget Reconciliation Act allows an employee to remain under an employer's group plan for a period of time after the loss of a job, death of a spouse, a decrease in hours or a divorce.

l. FALSE: Correction: Medicare Part B provides benefits for outpatient care, physician services, and services ordered by physicians such as diagnostic tests, medical equipment, and supplies.

m. FALSE: Correction: Current procedural terminology codes are procedure codes used by physical therapists and other health care professionals to describe specific interventions provided to a given patient.

*The correction presented for each false statement is an example of several possible corrections.

# Safety & Protection; Responsibilities; Research Answer Key

## 7. Domains of Learning

a.  cognitive

b.  affective

c.  psychomotor

d.  cognitive

e.  psychomotor

f.  affective

## 8. Stages of Dying

a.  bargaining

b.  anger

c.  depression

d.  acceptance

e.  denial

## 9. Teaching and Learning Basics*

a.  FALSE: Correction: According to Maslow's Hierarchy of Needs, self-actualization refers to the need to realize one's full potential as a human being.

b.  TRUE

c.  TRUE

   *The correction presented for each False Statement is an example of several possible corrections.

## Research

## 10. Levels of Evidence

a.  2

b.  4

c.  1

d.  3

e.  5

## 11. Scales of Measurement

a.  ratio

b.  interval

c.  ratio

d.  nominal

e.  ordinal

f.  nominal

g.  ordinal

h.  ratio

## 12. Validity

a.  content validity

b.  construct validity

c.  criterion-related validity

d.  face validity

## 13. Sampling

a.  snowball

b.  convenience

c.  stratified random

d.  simple random

e.  purposive

f.  systematic

## 14. Testing a Statistical Hypothesis

a.  4

b.  5

c.  1

d.  3

e.  2

## 15. Statistics

a.  variance

b.  mean

c.  standard deviation

d.  median

e.  mode

f.  range

## 16. Normal Distribution

a.  68%

b.  34%

c.  99%

d.  50%

e.  95%

## 17. Research Basics*

a.  TRUE

b.  FALSE: Correction: Sensitivity refers to the percentage of people who test positive for a specific disease among a group of people who have the disease.

c.  FALSE: Correction: Prevalence refers to the number of existing cases of a disease or condition at a point in time, including new and pre-existing cases.

d.  TRUE

# Safety & Protection; Responsibilities; Research Answer Key

e.  FALSE: Correction: Alpha level refers to the probability of rejecting the null hypothesis when it is true or the chance of committing a type 1 error.

f.  FALSE: Correction: In research, the independent variable is controlled or manipulated by the researcher.

g.  TRUE

h.  TRUE

i.  FALSE: Correction: Justice refers to the fair treatment of subjects including the equitable distribution of burdens and benefits in research.

j.  FALSE: Correction: Quantitative research typically uses a relatively large number of subjects and data is analyzed using statistical measures.

  *The correction presented for each false statement is an example of several possible corrections.

## Safety & Protection; Responsibilities; Research References

1. Cameron M, Monroe L. *Physical Rehabilitation: Evidence-Based Examination, Evaluation, and Intervention*. Saunders. 2007.

2. Minor M, Minor S. *Patient Care Skills*. Fifth Edition. Appleton & Lange. 2006.

3. Pierson F. *Principles and Techniques of Patient Care*, Fourth Edition. WB Saunders Company. 2008.

4. Guide to Infection Prevention for Outpatient Settings: Minimum Expectations for Safe Care. Centers for Disease Control and Prevention Web site. http://www.cdc.gov/HAI/settings/outpatient/outpatient-care-gl-standard-precautions.html. Updated July 12, 2011. Accessed August 10, 2011.

5. Rothstein J, Roy S, Wolf S. *The Rehabilitation Specialist's Handbook*. Third Edition, FA Davis Company, 2005.

6. Kettenbach G. *Writing SOAP Notes*. Second Edition. F.A. Davis Company. 1995

7. Shamus E, Stern D. *Effective Documentation for the Physical Therapy Professional*. McGraw-Hill Inc. 2004.

8. Guidelines: Physical Therapy Documentation of Patient/Client Management. American Physical Therapy Association Web site. http://www.apta.org/uploadedFiles/APTAorg/About_Us/Policies/BOD/Practice/DocumentationPatientClientMgmt.pdf#search=%22guidelines%20for%20physical%20therapy%20documentation%22. Accessed August 10, 2011.

9. Defensible Documentation Elements. American Physical Therapy Association Web site. http://www.apta.org/Documentation/DefensibleDocumentation/. Updated May 9, 2011. Accessed August 10, 2011.

10. Davis C. *Patient Practitioner Interaction*. Fourth Edition. Slack Inc. 2006.

11. Scott R: *Promoting Legal and Ethical Awareness: A Primer for Health Professionals and Patients*. Mosby. 2009.

12. Nosse L, Friberg D. *Managerial and Supervisory Principles for Physical Therapists*. Third Edition. Lippincott Williams & Wilkins. 2009.

13. Buchbinder S, Shanks N. *Introduction to Health Care Management*. Jones and Bartlett Publishers. 2007.

14. *Guide to Physical Therapist Practice*. Second Edition. Phys Ther. 2001; 81:583.

15. International Classification of Functioning, Disability and Health (ICF). World Health Organization Web site. http://www.who.int/classifications/icf/en/. Accessed August 10, 2011.

16. Direction and Supervision of the Physical Therapist Assistant. American Physical Therapy Association Web site. http://www.apta.org/uploadedFiles/APTAorg/About_Us/Policies/HOD/Practice/Direction.pdf. Updated December 14, 2009. Accessed August 10, 2011.

17. *Mosby's Dictionary of Medicine, Nursing and Health Professions*. Eighth Edition, Mosby. 2009.

18. Criteria for Standards of Practice for Physical Therapy. American Physical Therapy Association Web site. http://www.apta.org/uploadedFiles/APTAorg/About_Us/Policies/BOD/Practice/CriteriaforStandardsofPractice.pdf#search=%22criteria%20for%20standards%20of%20practice%22. Updated December 14, 2009. Accessed August 10, 2011.

19. Code of Ethics for the Physical Therapist. American Physical Therapy Association Web site. http://www.apta.org/uploadedFiles/APTAorg/About_Us/Policies/HOD/Ethics/CodeofEthics.pdf. Updated March 5, 2011. Accessed August 10, 2011.

20. Curtis K: *The Physical Therapist's Guide to Health Care*. Slack Inc. 1999.

21. Sandstrom R, Lohman H. *Health Services: Policy and Systems for Therapists*. Prentice Hall. 2003.

# Clinical Application Templates

Template 1: **Achilles Tendon Rupture** . . . . . . . . . . . . . . . . . . . . . . . . . . . . . . . . . . . . . . . . . . . . 568

Template 2: **Adhesive Capsulitis** . . . . . . . . . . . . . . . . . . . . . . . . . . . . . . . . . . . . . . . . . . . . . . . . . . 570

Template 3: **Alzheimer's Disease** . . . . . . . . . . . . . . . . . . . . . . . . . . . . . . . . . . . . . . . . . . . . . . . . . . 572

Template 4: **Amyotrophic Lateral Sclerosis** . . . . . . . . . . . . . . . . . . . . . . . . . . . . . . . . . . . . . . . . 574

Template 5: **Ankylosing Spondylitis** . . . . . . . . . . . . . . . . . . . . . . . . . . . . . . . . . . . . . . . . . . . . . . . . 576

Template 6: **Anterior Cruciate Ligament Sprain-Grade III** . . . . . . . . . . . . . . . . . . . . . . . . . . . 578

Template 7: **Bicipital Tendonitis** . . . . . . . . . . . . . . . . . . . . . . . . . . . . . . . . . . . . . . . . . . . . . . . . . . . 580

Template 8: **Breast Cancer** . . . . . . . . . . . . . . . . . . . . . . . . . . . . . . . . . . . . . . . . . . . . . . . . . . . . . . . . 582

Template 9: **Carpal Tunnel Syndrome** . . . . . . . . . . . . . . . . . . . . . . . . . . . . . . . . . . . . . . . . . . . . . . 584

Template 10: **Central Cord Syndrome** . . . . . . . . . . . . . . . . . . . . . . . . . . . . . . . . . . . . . . . . . . . . . . 586

Template 11: **Cerebral Palsy** . . . . . . . . . . . . . . . . . . . . . . . . . . . . . . . . . . . . . . . . . . . . . . . . . . . . . . . 588

Template 12: **Cerebrovascular Accident** . . . . . . . . . . . . . . . . . . . . . . . . . . . . . . . . . . . . . . . . . . . . 590

Template 13: **Congenital Torticollis** . . . . . . . . . . . . . . . . . . . . . . . . . . . . . . . . . . . . . . . . . . . . . . . . 592

Template 14: **Congestive Heart Failure** . . . . . . . . . . . . . . . . . . . . . . . . . . . . . . . . . . . . . . . . . . . . 594

Template 15: **Cystic Fibrosis** . . . . . . . . . . . . . . . . . . . . . . . . . . . . . . . . . . . . . . . . . . . . . . . . . . . . . . . 596

Template 16: **Degenerative Spondylolisthesis** . . . . . . . . . . . . . . . . . . . . . . . . . . . . . . . . . . . . . . 598

Template 17: **Diabetes Mellitus (Type 1)** . . . . . . . . . . . . . . . . . . . . . . . . . . . . . . . . . . . . . . . . . . . . 600

Template 18: **Down Syndrome** . . . . . . . . . . . . . . . . . . . . . . . . . . . . . . . . . . . . . . . . . . . . . . . . . . . . . 602

Template 19: **Duchenne Muscular Dystrophy** . . . . . . . . . . . . . . . . . . . . . . . . . . . . . . . . . . . . . . . 604

Template 20: **Emphysema** . . . . . . . . . . . . . . . . . . . . . . . . . . . . . . . . . . . . . . . . . . . . . . . . . . . . . . . . . 606

Template 21: **Erb's Palsy** . . . . . . . . . . . . . . . . . . . . . . . . . . . . . . . . . . . . . . . . . . . . . . . . . . . . . . . . . . 608

Template 22: **Fibromyalgia Syndrome** . . . . . . . . . . . . . . . . . . . . . . . . . . . . . . . . . . . . . . . . . . . . . . 610

Template 23: **Full-Thickness Burn** . . . . . . . . . . . . . . . . . . . . . . . . . . . . . . . . . . . . . . . . . . . . . . . . . . 612

SCOREBUILDERS

# Clinical Application Templates

The clinical application template allows candidates to explore many of the elements of patient/client management for a wide variety of medical conditions. Although candidates have been exposed to a variety of medical conditions during their clinical education experiences it is unlikely they have been exposed to the vast number of medical conditions commonly encountered on the examination. By utilizing clinical application templates students can broaden their experience base and as a result be better prepared to answer examination questions.

This section contains an executive summary of selected information associated with 60 different clinical application templates followed by an expansive two page summary of each medical condition. Candidates are encouraged to review the templates and carefully reflect on the presented information. Candidates should attempt to make this activity an active learning exercise and resist the urge to simply read each of the templates. For example, let's assume that a candidate was reviewing a clinical application template on an anterior cruciate ligament sprain. In each category of the clinical application template, candidates should assess their knowledge by asking specific questions. Two specific examples for the tests and measures section are listed below:

When reviewing range of motion, candidates should ask themselves the following:
- What is normal range of motion at the knee?
- Which type of end-feel would be considered normal for knee flexion and extension?
- Where should the axis, moving arm, and stationary arm of the goniometer be aligned when measuring range of motion?
- Where should the therapist stabilize when conducting the measurement?

When reviewing joint integrity and mobility, candidates should ask themselves the following:
- Which special test or tests would be the most appropriate to assess the ligamentous integrity of the anterior cruciate ligament?
- Describe the process for administering the special test?
- What finding would be indicative of a positive test?

By engaging in this type of active learning exercise, candidates are able to further assess their level of preparedness for the examination. Although some candidates may be quite comfortable reviewing selected clinical application templates, many candidates learn that they lack necessary content in many others. For example, do you feel adequately prepared to discuss the patient/client management of each of the following diagnoses: amyotrophic lateral sclerosis, cystic fibrosis, cerebrovascular accident, and rotator cuff tendonitis? Prior to taking the actual examination candidates should have some reasonable level of comfort discussing each of the 60 clinical application templates included in this unit.

Candidates should not rely solely on the presented clinical application templates and instead should utilize the template format to review a variety of other medical conditions. This type of active learning is best performed by a small group of candidates with a given candidate acting as the facilitator. In this manner students can share their individual clinical experience with the group and at the same time benefit from the knowledge of their classmates.

*The clinical application template was adapted from a document by the Academy of Specialty Boards entitled "Preparing Items that Measure More than Recall." The document was originally designed to help item writers develop sample questions for the Physical Therapy Specialty Examinations.

# 10

# CLINICAL APPLICATION TEMPLATES

**Scott Giles**
**Therese Giles**

555 Introduction

556 Index of Templates

559 Executive Summary

568 Clinical Application Templates

# Safety & Protection; Responsibilities; Research References

22.  Sadock B, Sadock V. *Kaplan & Sadock's Comprehensive Textbook of Psychiatry*. Eighth Edition. Lippincott Williams & Wilkins. 2005

23.  Edelman C, Mandle C. *Health Promotion Throughout the Lifespan*. Fifth Edition. Mosby. 2002

24.  Purtilo R, Haddad A. *Health Professional and Patient Interaction*. Seventh Edition. WB Saunders Company. 2007.

25.  Falvo DR. *Effective Patient Education*. Third Edition, Jones and Bartlett Publishers. 2004.

26.  Haggard A. *Handbook of Patient Education*. Aspen Publishers. 1989.

27.  Arends R. *Learning to Teach*. Third Edition, McGraw-Hill Inc. 2005.

28.  Scott R. *Foundations of Physical Therapy: A 21st Century-Focused View of the Profession*. McGraw-Hill Inc. 2002.

29.  Sackett DL, Straus SE, Richardson WS, Rosenburg W, Haynes RB. *Evidence-Based Medicine. How to Practice and Teach EBM*. 2nd ed. Edinburgh, Scotland; Churchill Livingstone; 2000.

30.  Asking focused questions. Centre for Evidence-Based Medicine Web site. http://www.cebm.net/index.aspx?o=1036. Updated April 7, 2009. Accessed October 7, 2010.

31.  Critical appraisal. Centre for Evidence-Based Medicine Web site. http://www.cebm.net/index.aspx?o=1157 Updated December 16, 2010. Accessed October 7, 2010.

32.  Practice Guidelines. *Physical Therapy* Web site. http://ptjournal.apta.org/cgi/collection/practice_guidelines Accessed October 3, 2010.

33.  Guidelines by Topic. National Guideline Clearinghouse Web site. http://www.guideline.gov/. Accessed October 3, 2010.

34.  Levels of evidence. Centre for Evidence-Based Medicine Web site. http://www.cebm.net/index.aspx?o=1025. Updated September 16, 2010. Accessed October 3, 2010.

35.  Portney LG, Watkins MP. *Foundations of Clinical Research: Applications to Practice*. 3rd ed. Upper Saddle River, NJ; Prentice Hall; 2009.

36.  Glossary of Statistical Terms. National Cancer Institute Web site. http://www.cancer.gov/statistics/glossary. Accessed October 3, 2010.

37.  Code of Federal Regulation Title 45. Public Welfare. Part 46. Protection of Human Subjects. US Department of Health and Human Services Web site. http://www.hhs.gov/ohrp/humansubjects/guidance/45cfr46.htm. Accessed October 3, 2010.

38.  Triola MF. *Elementary Statistics*. 9th ed. Boston, MA: Pearson Addison Wesley; 2004.

39.  Rothstein JM, Echternach JL. *Primer on Measurement: An Introductory Guide to Measurement Issues*. Alexandria, VA; American Physical Therapy Association; 1993.

40.  Iverson C, Christiansen S, Flanagin A, et al. *AMA Manual of Style: A Guide for Authors and Editors*. 10th ed. New York, NY: Oxford University Press; 2007.

41.  Code of Ethics for the Physical Therapist. American Physical Therapy Association Web site. http://www.apta.org/AM/Template.cfm?Section=Policies_and_Bylaws1&TEMPLATE=/CM/ContentDisplay.cfm&CONTENTID=73012. Accessed October 3, 2010

## Clinical Application Templates (continued)

Template 24: **Guillain-Barre Syndrome** . . . . . . . . . . . . . . . . . . . . . . . . . . . . . . . . . . . . **614**

Template 25: **Human Immunodeficiency Virus** . . . . . . . . . . . . . . . . . . . . . . . . . . . . . . **616**

Template 26: **Huntington's Disease** . . . . . . . . . . . . . . . . . . . . . . . . . . . . . . . . . . . . . . . **618**

Template 27: **Juvenile Rheumatoid Arthritis** . . . . . . . . . . . . . . . . . . . . . . . . . . . . . . . **620**

Template 28: **Lateral Epicondylitis** . . . . . . . . . . . . . . . . . . . . . . . . . . . . . . . . . . . . . . . . **622**

Template 29: **Lymphedema Post-Mastectomy** . . . . . . . . . . . . . . . . . . . . . . . . . . . . . . **624**

Template 30: **Medial Collateral Ligament Sprain-Grade II** . . . . . . . . . . . . . . . . . . . **626**

Template 31: **Multiple Sclerosis** . . . . . . . . . . . . . . . . . . . . . . . . . . . . . . . . . . . . . . . . . . **628**

Template 32: **Myocardial Infarction** . . . . . . . . . . . . . . . . . . . . . . . . . . . . . . . . . . . . . . . **630**

Template 33: **Osteoarthritis** . . . . . . . . . . . . . . . . . . . . . . . . . . . . . . . . . . . . . . . . . . . . . **632**

Template 34: **Osteogenesis Imperfecta** . . . . . . . . . . . . . . . . . . . . . . . . . . . . . . . . . . . **634**

Template 35: **Osteoporosis** . . . . . . . . . . . . . . . . . . . . . . . . . . . . . . . . . . . . . . . . . . . . . . **636**

Template 36: **Parkinson's Disease** . . . . . . . . . . . . . . . . . . . . . . . . . . . . . . . . . . . . . . . . **638**

Template 37: **Patellofemoral Syndrome** . . . . . . . . . . . . . . . . . . . . . . . . . . . . . . . . . . . **640**

Template 38: **Peripheral Vascular Disease** . . . . . . . . . . . . . . . . . . . . . . . . . . . . . . . . . **642**

Template 39: **Plantar Fasciitis** . . . . . . . . . . . . . . . . . . . . . . . . . . . . . . . . . . . . . . . . . . . . **644**

Template 40: **Pressure Ulcer** . . . . . . . . . . . . . . . . . . . . . . . . . . . . . . . . . . . . . . . . . . . . . **646**

Template 41: **Reflex Sympathetic Dystrophy** . . . . . . . . . . . . . . . . . . . . . . . . . . . . . . **648**

Template 42: **Restrictive Lung Disease** . . . . . . . . . . . . . . . . . . . . . . . . . . . . . . . . . . . . **650**

Template 43: **Rheumatoid Arthritis** . . . . . . . . . . . . . . . . . . . . . . . . . . . . . . . . . . . . . . . **652**

Template 44: **Rotator Cuff Tendonitis** . . . . . . . . . . . . . . . . . . . . . . . . . . . . . . . . . . . . **654**

Template 45: **Sciatica Secondary to a Herniated Disk** . . . . . . . . . . . . . . . . . . . . . . . **656**

Template 46: **Scoliosis** . . . . . . . . . . . . . . . . . . . . . . . . . . . . . . . . . . . . . . . . . . . . . . . . . . **658**

## Clinical Application Templates (continued)

Template 47: **Spina Bifida-Myelomeningocele** . . . . . . . . . . . . . . . . . . . . . . . . . . . . . . . . . . . . . .660

Template 48: **Spinal Cord Injury-Complete C7 Tetraplegia** . . . . . . . . . . . . . . . . . . . . . . . . . . .662

Template 49: **Spinal Cord Injury-Complete L3 Paraplegia** . . . . . . . . . . . . . . . . . . . . . . . . . . .664

Template 50: **Spondylolisthesis** . . . . . . . . . . . . . . . . . . . . . . . . . . . . . . . . . . . . . . . . . . . . . . . .666

Template 51: **Systemic Lupus Erythematosus** . . . . . . . . . . . . . . . . . . . . . . . . . . . . . . . . . . . . .668

Template 52: **Temporomandibular Joint Dysfunction** . . . . . . . . . . . . . . . . . . . . . . . . . . . . . .670

Template 53: **Thoracic Outlet Syndrome** . . . . . . . . . . . . . . . . . . . . . . . . . . . . . . . . . . . . . . . . .672

Template 54: **Total Hip Arthroplasty** . . . . . . . . . . . . . . . . . . . . . . . . . . . . . . . . . . . . . . . . . . . .674

Template 55: **Total Knee Arthroplasty** . . . . . . . . . . . . . . . . . . . . . . . . . . . . . . . . . . . . . . . . . . .676

Template 56: **Total Shoulder Arthroplasty** . . . . . . . . . . . . . . . . . . . . . . . . . . . . . . . . . . . . . . . .678

Template 57: **Transfemoral Amputation due to Osteosarcoma** . . . . . . . . . . . . . . . . . . . . . .680

Template 58: **Transtibial Amputation due to Arteriosclerosis Obliterans** . . . . . . . . . . . . . . .682

Template 59: **Traumatic Brain Injury** . . . . . . . . . . . . . . . . . . . . . . . . . . . . . . . . . . . . . . . . . . . .684

Template 60: **Urinary Stress Incontinence** . . . . . . . . . . . . . . . . . . . . . . . . . . . . . . . . . . . . . . . .686

## Clinical Application Template Executive Summary

### Achilles Tendon Rupture
- Typically occurs within one to two inches above the tendinous insertion on the calcaneus
- Incidence is greatest between 30-50 years of age without history of calf or heel pain
- Patients with an Achilles tendon rupture will typically be unable to stand on their toes and tend to exhibit a positive Thompson test

### Adhesive Capsulitis
- Occurs more in the middle-aged population with females having a greater incidence than males
- Arthrogram can assist with diagnosis by detecting decreased volume of fluid within the joint capsule
- Range of motion restriction typically in a capsular pattern (lateral rotation, abduction, medial rotation)

### Alzheimer's Disease
- Progressive neurological disorder that results in deterioration and irreversible damage within the cerebral cortex and subcortical areas of the brain
- Disease is initially noted by a change in higher cortical functions characterized by subtle changes in memory, impaired concentration, and difficulty with new learning
- Typical course of the disease averages between 7-11 years with death resulting from infection or dehydration

### Amyotrophic Lateral Sclerosis
- Risk is higher in males than females and usually occurs between 40-70 years of age
- Clinical presentation may include both upper and lower motor neuron involvement with weakness occurring in a distal to proximal progression
- Average course of the diagnosis is two to five years with 20-30% of patients surviving longer than five years

### Ankylosing Spondylitis
- Systemic condition characterized by inflammation of the spine and the larger peripheral joints
- Males are at two to three times greater risk than females with peak onset observed between 20-40 years of age
- Clinical presentation initially includes recurrent and insidious onset of back pain, morning stiffness, and impaired spinal extension

### Anterior Cruciate Ligament Sprain - Grade III
- Injury most commonly occurs during hyperflexion, rapid deceleration, hyperextension or landing in an unbalanced position
- Females involved in selected athletic activities have significantly higher ligament injury rates compared to males
- Approximately two-thirds of complete anterior cruciate ligament tears have an associated meniscal tear

### Bicipital Tendonitis
- Increased incidence of injury is associated with selected athletic activities such as baseball pitching, swimming, rowing, gymnastics, and tennis
- Characterized by subjective reports of a deep ache directly in front and on top of the shoulder made worse with overhead activities or lifting
- Examination may reveal a positive Speed's test or Yergason's test

## Clinical Application Template Executive Summary

### Breast Cancer
- May spread to the lymphatic system and commonly metastasizes to the brain, lungs, bones, adrenals, and liver
- Breast cancer makes up 30% of all female cancers and is the second leading cause of death for females in the United States
- Prognosis and ten-year survival rates for women are over 85% for stage I; 66% for stage II; 36% for stage III; and 7% for stage IV disease

### Carpal Tunnel Syndrome
- Incidence is higher in females than males with the most common age being from 35-55 years of age
- Muscle atrophy is often noted in the abductor pollicis brevis muscle and later in the thenar muscles
- Electromyography studies, Tinel's sign, and Phalen's test can be used to assist with confirming the diagnosis

### Central Cord Syndrome
- An incomplete spinal cord lesion that most often results from a cervical hyperextension injury
- Clinical presentation involves motor loss that is greater in the upper extremities than the lower extremities
- Most common incomplete spinal cord lesion accounting for approximately 30% of all incomplete forms of tetraplegia

### Cerebral Palsy
- Spastic cerebral palsy involves upper motor neuron damage; athetoid cerebral palsy involves damage to the cerebellum, cerebellar pathways or both
- Clinical presentation includes motor delays, abnormal muscle tone and motor control, reflex abnormalities, poor postural control, and balance impairments
- Mental retardation and epilepsy are present in 50-60% of children diagnosed with cerebral palsy

### Cerebrovascular Accident (CVA)
- Types of CVA include ischemic stroke (thrombus, embolus, lacunar) and hemorrhagic stroke (intracerebral, subdural, subarachnoid)
- Left CVA may present with weakness or paralysis to the right side, impaired processing, heightened frustration, aphasia, dysphagia, and motor apraxia
- Right CVA may present with weakness or paralysis to the left side, poor attention span, impaired awareness and judgment, spatial deficits, memory deficits, emotional lability, and impulsive behavior

### Congenital Torticollis
- Causes the neck to involuntarily contract to one side secondary to contraction of the sternocleidomastoid muscle
- The head is laterally flexed toward the contracted muscle, the chin faces the opposite direction, and there may be facial asymmetries
- Studies indicate that between 85-90% of patients with congenital torticollis respond to conservative treatment and passive stretching within the first year of life

### Congestive Heart Failure (CHF)
- Common etiologies contributing to CHF include arrhythmia, pulmonary embolism, hypertension, valvular heart disease, myocarditis, unstable angina, renal failure, and severe anemia
- Left-sided heart failure is generally associated with signs of pulmonary venous congestion; right-sided heart failure is associated with signs of systemic venous congestion
- Diminished cardiac output causes compensatory changes including an increase in blood volume, cardiac filling pressure, heart rate, and cardiac muscle mass

# Clinical Application Template Executive Summary

## Cystic Fibrosis

- Causes the exocrine glands to overproduce thick mucus which causes subsequent obstruction
- Autosomal recessive genetic disorder (both parents are carriers of the defective gene) located on the long arm of chromosome seven
- A terminal disease, however, the median age of death has increased to 35 years of age due to early detection and comprehensive management

## Degenerative Spondylolisthesis

- Caused by the weakening of joints that allows for forward slippage of one vertebral segment on the one below due to degenerative changes
- Most common site of degenerative spondylolisthesis is the L4-L5 level
- William's flexion exercises may be indicated to strengthen the abdominals and reduce lumbar lordosis

## Diabetes Mellitus (Type 1)

- Insulin is functionally absent due to the destruction of the beta cells of the pancreas; where the insulin would normally be produced
- Starts in children ages four years or older, with the peak incidence of onset coinciding with early adolescence and puberty
- Common symptoms include polyuria, polydipsia, polyphagia, nausea, weight loss, fatigue, blurred vision, and dehydration

## Down Syndrome

- Clinical manifestations include hypotonia, flattened nasal bridge, Simian line (palmar crease), epicanthal folds, enlargement of the tongue, and developmental delay
- Detection occurs in approximately 60-70% of women tested that are carrying a baby with Down syndrome
- Exercise is essential for a child with Down syndrome in order to avoid inactivity and obesity

## Duchenne Muscular Dystrophy

- X-linked recessive trait manifesting in only male offspring while female offspring become carriers
- Clinical presentation includes waddling gait, proximal muscle weakness, toe walking, pseudohypertrophy of the calf, and difficulty climbing stairs
- There is usually rapid progression of this disease with the inability to ambulate by ten to twelve years of age with death occurring as a teenager or less frequently in the 20's

## Emphysema

- Results from a long history of chronic bronchitis, recurrent alveolar inflammation or from genetic predisposition of a congenital alpha 1-antitrypsin deficiency
- Clinical presentation may include barrel chest appearance, increased subcostal angle, rounded shoulders secondary to tight pectorals, and rosy skin coloring
- Symptoms of emphysema worsen with the progression of the disease and include a persistent cough, wheezing, difficulty breathing especially with expiration, and an increased respiration rate

## Erb's Palsy

- Muscles affected are supplied by cervical roots C5 and C6 which result in a loss of function of the rotator cuff, deltoid, brachialis, coracobrachialis, and biceps brachii
- Brachial plexus injury in a newborn usually occurs during a difficult delivery, due to a large baby, a breech presentation with a prolonged labor or with the use of forceps
- Results in flaccid paralysis nicknamed the "waiter's tip deformity" (characterized by a loss of shoulder function, loss of elbow flexion, loss of forearm supination, and the hand positioned in a pinch grip manner)

## Clinical Application Template Executive Summary

### Fibromyalgia Syndrome
- Nonarticular rheumatic condition with pain caused by tender points within muscles, tendons, and ligaments
- Greater incidence in females (almost 75% of the cases) potentially affecting any age
- Widespread history of pain that exists in all four quadrants of the body (above and below the waist), axial pain is present, and there is pain in at least 11 of 18 standardized "tender point" sites

### Full-Thickness Burn
- Burn causes immediate cellular and tissue death and subsequent vascular destruction
- Eschar forms from necrotic cells and creates a dry and hard layer that requires debridement
- Absent sensation and pain due to destruction of free nerve endings, however, there may be pain from adjacent areas that experience partial-thickness burns

### Guillain-Barre Syndrome
- Results in motor weakness in a distal to proximal progression, sensory impairment, and possible respiratory paralysis
- Etiology of the disease is unknown, however, it is hypothesized to be an autoimmune response to a previous respiratory infection, influenza, immunization or surgery
- Majority of patients experience full recovery, 20% have remaining neurologic deficits, and 3-5% of patients die from respiratory complications

### Human Immunodeficiency Virus (HIV)
- Primary risk factors for contracting HIV include unprotected sexual relations, intravenous drug use or mother to fetus transmission
- Patients may actually be "symptom free" for one to two years post infection or may exhibit flu-like symptoms including rash and fever
- Leading cause of death for patients with the virus is kidney failure secondary to the extended drug therapies

### Huntington's Disease
- Chronic progressive genetic disorder that is fatal within 15 to 20 years after clinical manifestation
- Characterized by degeneration and atrophy of the basal ganglia (specifically the striatum) and cerebral cortex within the brain
- Clinical presentation includes enlarged ventricles secondary to atrophy of the basal ganglia, mental deterioration, speech disturbances, and ataxic gait

### Juvenile Rheumatoid Arthritis (JRA)
- Autoimmune disorder found in children less than 16 years of age that occurs when the immune cells mistakenly begin to attack the joints and organs causing local and systemic effects throughout the body
- Girls have a higher incidence of JRA and are most commonly diagnosed as toddlers or in early adolescence
- Clinical symptoms include persistent joint swelling, pain, and stiffness

### Lateral Epicondylitis "Tennis Elbow"
- Characterized by inflammation or degenerative changes at the common extensor tendon that attaches to the lateral epicondyle of the elbow
- Repeated overuse of the wrist extensors, particularly the extensor carpi radialis brevis can produce tensile stress and result in microscopic tearing and damage to the extensor tendon
- Clinical symptoms include difficulty holding or gripping objects and insufficient forearm functional strength

# Clinical Application Template Executive Summary

## Lymphedema Post-Mastectomy

- Caused by an excess load of lymph fluid or inadequate transport capacity within the lymphatic system secondary to the loss of homeostasis
- Primary contributing factor in the development of lymphedema following a mastectomy is the damage and/or removal of the axillary lymph nodes and vessels
- Intervention should focus on manual lymph drainage, short stretch compression bandages, retrograde massage, exercise, compression therapy, and use of a mechanical pump

## Medial Collateral Ligament Sprain – Grade II

- Grade II injury is characterized by partial tearing of the ligament's fibers resulting in joint laxity when the ligament is stretched
- Mechanism of injury is usually a blow to the outside of the knee joint causing excess force to the medial side of the joint
- Return to previous functional level should occur within four to eight weeks following the injury if no other associated structures are involved

## Multiple Sclerosis

- Characterized by demyelination of the myelin sheaths that surround nerves within the brain and spinal cord resulting in plaque development, decreased nerve conduction velocity, and eventual failure of impulse transmission
- Clinical symptoms may include visual problems, paresthesias, sensory changes, clumsiness, weakness, ataxia, balance dysfunction, and fatigue
- Intervention includes regulation of activity level, relaxation and energy conservation techniques, normalization of tone, balance activities, gait training, and core stabilization

## Myocardial Infarction

- Myocardial infarction occurs when there is poor coronary artery perfusion, ischemia, and subsequent necrosis of the cardiac tissue usually due to thrombus, arterial blockage or atherosclerosis
- Risk factors include patient or family history of heart disease, smoking, physical inactivity, stress, hypertension, elevated cholesterol, diabetes mellitus, and obesity
- Clinical presentation may include deep pain or pressure in the substernal area with or without pain radiating to the jaw or into the left arm or the back

## Osteoarthritis

- Degenerative process primarily involving articular cartilage resulting from excessive loading of a healthy joint or normal loading of an abnormal joint
- Typically diagnosed based on the results of a clinical examination and x-ray findings
- Prevalence is higher among women than men later in life with approximately 80-90% of individuals older than 65 years of age demonstrating evidence of osteoarthritis

## Osteogenesis Imperfecta

- Classified into four types with a wide range of clinical presentations ranging from normal appearance with mild symptoms to severe involvement that can be fatal during infancy
- Bone densitometry may be used to measure bone mass and estimate the risk of fracture for specific sites within the body
- Children with osteogenesis imperfecta often have delayed developmental milestones secondary to ongoing fractures with immobilization, hypermobility of joints, and poorly developed muscles

## Clinical Application Template Executive Summary

### Osteoporosis
- Metabolic bone disorder where the rate of bone resorption accelerates while the rate of bone formation slows down
- Patients may complain of low thoracic or lumbar pain and experience compression fractures of the vertebrae
- Bone mineral density test accounts for 70% of bone strength and is the easiest way to determine osteoporosis

### Parkinson's Disease
- Degenerative disorder characterized by a decrease in production of dopamine (neurotransmitter) within the corpus striatum of the basal ganglia
- Clinical presentation may include hypokinesia, difficulty initiating and stopping movement, festinating and shuffling gait, bradykinesia, poor posture, and "cogwheel" or "lead pipe" rigidity
- Medical management includes dopamine replacement therapy (Levodopa, Sinemet, Madopar) which is designed to minimize bradykinesia, rigidity, and tremor

### Patellofemoral Syndrome
- Causes damage to the articular cartilage of the patella ranging from softening to complete cartilage destruction resulting in exposure of subchondral bone
- Etiology is unknown, however, it is extremely common during adolescence, is more prevalent in females than males, and has a direct association with activity level
- Management includes controlling edema, stretching, strengthening, improving range of motion, and activity modification

### Peripheral Vascular Disease
- Characterized by narrowing of the lumen of blood vessels causing a reduction in circulation usually secondary to atherosclerosis
- Risk factors include phlebitis, injury or surgery, autoimmune disease, diabetes mellitus, smoking, hyperlipidemia, inactivity, hypertension, positive family history, increased age, and obesity
- Patient education is paramount regarding the disease process, limb protection, foot and skin care, and risk factor reduction (smoking cessation, avoid cold exposure)

### Plantar Fasciitis
- Chronic overuse condition that develops secondary to repetitive stretching of the plantar fascia through excessive foot pronation during the loading phase of gait
- Characterized by severe pain in the heel when first standing up in the morning (when the fascia is contracted, stiff, and cold)
- Intervention consists of ice massage, deep friction massage, heel insert, orthotic prescription, activity modification, and gentle stretching program of the Achilles tendon and plantar fascia

### Pressure Ulcer
- Unrelieved pressure deprives the tissues of oxygen which causes ischemia, subsequent cell death, and tissue necrosis
- High risk areas for pressure ulcers include the occiput, heels, greater trochanters, ischial tuberosities, sacrum, and epicondyles of the elbow
- Impaired cognition, poor nutrition, altered sensation, incontinence, decreased lean body mass, and infection contribute to the development of a pressure ulcer

# Clinical Application Template Executive Summary

## Reflex Sympathetic Dystrophy
- Increase in sympathetic activity causes a release of norepinephrine in the periphery and subsequent vasoconstriction of blood vessels resulting in pain and an increase in sensitivity to peripheral stimulation
- Affects all age groups, but is most likely found in individuals 35-60 years of age with females being three times more likely to be affected than males
- Patients experience intense burning and chronic pain in the affected extremity that eventually spreads in a proximal direction

## Restrictive Lung Disease
- Classification of disorders caused by a pulmonary or extrapulmonary restriction that produces impairment in lung expansion and an abnormal reduction in pulmonary ventilation
- Pulmonary restriction of the lungs can be caused by tumor, interstitial pulmonary fibrosis, scarring within the lungs, pleural effusion, chest wall stiffness, structural abnormality, and respiratory muscle weakness
- Pathogenesis includes a decrease in lung and chest wall compliance, decrease in lung volumes, and an increase in the work of breathing

## Rheumatoid Arthritis
- Systemic autoimmune disorder of the connective tissue that is characterized by chronic inflammation within synovial membranes, tendon sheaths, and articular cartilage
- Incidence is three times greater in females than males and is diagnosed most frequently between 30-50 years of age
- Blood work assists with the diagnosis of rheumatoid arthritis through evaluation of the rheumatoid factor, white blood cell count, erythrocyte sedimentation rate, hemoglobin, and hematocrit values

## Rotator Cuff Tendonitis
- Caused by an inability of a weak supraspinatus muscle to adequately depress the head of the humerus in the glenoid fossa during elevation of the arm
- Participating in activities that require excessive overhead activity such as swimming, tennis, baseball, painting, and other manual labor activities increase the risk of rotator cuff tendonitis
- Patients may experience a feeling of weakness and identify the presence of a painful arc of motion most commonly occurring between 60 and 120 degrees of active abduction

## Sciatica Secondary to a Herniated Disk
- The sciatic nerve experiences an inflammatory response and subsequent damage secondary to compression from the herniated disk
- Sciatica is characterized by low back and gluteal pain that typically radiates down the back of the thigh along the sciatic nerve distribution
- Pain will increase in a sitting position or when lifting, forward bending or twisting

## Scoliosis
- Curvature is usually found in the thoracic or lumbar vertebrae and can be associated with kyphosis or lordosis
- A patient with scoliosis that ranges between 25 and 40 degrees requires a spinal orthosis and physical therapy intervention for posture, flexibility, strengthening, respiratory function, and proper utilization of the spinal orthosis
- Scoliosis does not usually progress significantly once bone growth is complete if the curvature remains below 40 degrees at the time of skeletal maturity

## Clinical Application Template Executive Summary

### Spina Bifida – Myelomeningocele

- Classifications include occulta (incomplete fusion of the posterior vertebral arch with no neural tissue protruding), meningocele (incomplete fusion of the posterior vertebral arch with neural tissue/meninges protruding outside the neural arch), and myelomeningocele (incomplete fusion of the posterior vertebral arch with both meninges and spinal cord protruding outside the neural arch)
- Approximately 75% of vertebral defects are found in the lumbar/sacral region most often at L5-S1
- Prenatal testing of alpha-fetoprotein (AFP) in the blood will show an elevation in levels that indicate a probable neural tube defect at approximately week 16 of gestation

### Spinal Cord Injury – Complete C7 Tetraplegia

- Clinical presentation includes impaired cough and ability to clear secretions, altered breathing pattern, and poor endurance
- Outcomes at this level include independence with feeding, grooming, dressing, self-range of motion, independent manual wheelchair mobility, independent transfers, and independent driving with an adapted automobile
- The triceps, extensor pollicis longus and brevis, extrinsic finger extensors, and flexor carpi radialis will remain the lowest innervated muscles

### Spinal Cord Injury – Complete L3 Paraplegia

- Patients possess at least partial innervation of the gracilis, iliopsoas, quadratus lumborum, rectus femoris, and sartorius with full upper extremity use
- Additional findings that can exist include sexual dysfunction, a nonreflexive bladder, the need for a bowel program, urinary tract infections, muscle contractures, and pressure sores
- Patients with L3 paraplegia should be able to live independently with education regarding the management of their disability

### Spondylolisthesis

- Characterized by forward slippage of one vertebral body with respect to the vertebral body below it
- Patients participating in gymnastics, wrestling, football, and weight lifting are at greater risk for spondylolisthesis
- X-ray oblique views can show the pars as having the appearance of a "Scottie dog with a collar" when a spondylolysis is present

### Systemic Lupus Erythematosus

- Connective tissue disorder caused by an autoimmune reaction in the body
- Females are at greater risk than males with the most common age group ranging from 15-40 years of age
- Clinical presentation includes a red butterfly rash across the cheeks and nose, a red rash over light exposed areas, arthralgias, alopecia, pleurisy, kidney involvement, seizures, and depression

### Temporomandibular Joint Dysfunction

- Females are at greater risk than males with the most common age ranging from 20-40 years of age
- Clinical presentation includes pain (persistent or recurring), muscle spasm, abnormal or limited jaw motion, headache, and tinnitus
- Intervention includes patient education, posture retraining, and modalities such as moist heat, ice, biofeedback, ultrasound, electrostimulation, TENS, and massage

### Thoracic Outlet Syndrome

- Results from compression and damage to the brachial plexus nerve trunks, subclavian vascular supply, and/or the axillary artery
- Contributing factors in the development of the condition include the presence of a cervical rib, an abnormal first rib, postural deviations, hypertrophy or spasms of the scalene muscles, and an elongated cervical transverse process
- Females are at two to three times greater risk than males, with the most common age ranging from 30-40 years of age

## Clinical Application Template Executive Summary

### Total Hip Arthroplasty

- Patients are typically over 55 years of age and have experienced consistent pain that is not relieved through conservative measures which serve to limit the patient's functional mobility
- Posterolateral approach allows the abductor muscles to remain intact, however, there may be a higher incidence of post-operative joint instability due to the interruption of the posterior capsule
- Cemented hip replacement usually allows for partial weight bearing initially, while a noncemented hip replacement requires toe touch weight bearing for up to six weeks

### Total Knee Arthroplasty

- Primary indication for total knee arthroplasty is the destruction of articular cartilage secondary to osteoarthritis
- Post-operative care may include a knee immobilizer, elevation of the limb, cryotherapy, intermittent range of motion using a continuous passive motion (CPM) machine, and initiation of knee protocol exercises
- Patient education may include items such as avoid excessive stress to the knee, squatting, quick pivoting, using pillows under the knee while in bed, and low seating

### Total Shoulder Arthroplasty

- Surgical candidates typically have irreparable damage, deterioration, and destruction to the humeral head and the glenoid fossa within the shoulder complex
- Surgical complications include mechanical loosening of the prosthesis, instability, rotator cuff tear, implant failure, heterotopic ossification, and intraoperative fracture
- Life expectancy is longer for the shoulder compared to the knee or hip since the shoulder is a non-weight bearing joint

### Transfemoral Amputation due to Osteosarcoma

- Osteosarcoma is a highly malignant cancer that begins in the medullary cavity of a bone and leads to the formation of a mass
- A patient status post transfemoral amputation may present with fatigue, loss of balance, phantom pain or sensation, hypersensitivity of the residual limb, and psychological issues regarding the loss of the limb
- Lying in a prone position is beneficial to decrease the incidence of a hip flexion contracture

### Transtibial Amputation due to Arteriosclerosis Obliterans

- Arteriosclerosis obliterans results in ischemia and subsequent ulceration of the affected tissues
- A patient status post transtibial amputation may have a decrease in cardiovascular status depending on the frequency of intermittent claudication experienced prior to the amputation
- Preprosthetic intervention should focus on strength, range of motion, functional mobility, use of assistive devices, desensitization, and patient education for care of the residual limb

### Traumatic Brain Injury

- Occurs due to an open head injury where there is penetration through the skull or closed head injury where the brain makes contact with the skull secondary to a sudden, violent acceleration or deceleration
- Brain injury may include swelling, axonal injury, hypoxia, hematoma, hemorrhage and changes in intracranial pressure
- High risk groups include ages 0-4, 15-19, and greater than 65 (males are at greater risk in each category)

### Urinary Stress Incontinence

- Occurs during activities where there is an increase in abdominal pressure through straining, sneezing, coughing or lifting
- Risk factors include pregnancy, vaginal delivery, episiotomy, prostate or pelvic surgery, aging, diabetes mellitus, central nervous system dysfunction, and recurrent urinary infection
- Accounts for 50-60% of all incontinence cases and is manifested solely by the involuntary loss of urine with any form of exertion or increased abdominal pressure

# Achilles Tendon Rupture

## Diagnosis

### What condition produces a patient's symptoms?

Rupture of the Achilles tendon normally occurs within one to two inches above its tendinous insertion on the calcaneus. A patient will present with symptoms secondary to the rupture and discontinuity of the Achilles tendon.

### An injury was most likely sustained to which structure?

The Achilles tendon is the largest and strongest tendon in the human body, and is formed from the tendinous portions of the gastrocnemius and soleus muscles coalescing above the insertion on the calcaneal tuberosity. Theories suggest that an Achilles tendon rupture usually occurs in an Achilles tendon that has undergone degenerative changes. The degenerative changes will begin with hypovascularity in the Achilles tendon area. The impaired blood flow in combination with repetitive microtrauma creates degenerative changes within the tendon and as a result makes the tendon more susceptible to injury.

## Inference

### What is the most likely contributing factor in the development of this condition?

An Achilles tendon rupture occurs most frequently when pushing off of a weight bearing extremity with an extended knee, through unexpected dorsiflexion while weight bearing or with a forceful eccentric contraction of the plantar flexors. Participation in sports that require quick-changing footwork such as softball, tennis, basketball, and football are high-risk activities. Other contributing factors include poor stretching routine, tight calf muscles, improper shoe wear during high risk activities, and altered biomechanics at the foot during activities (such as a flattened arch). A person over 30 years of age is at a higher risk for rupture secondary to the decrease in blood flow to the area of the tendon associated with aging. A person with a history of corticosteroid injections to the tendon may also have a predisposition for rupture. The highest incidence for rupture is in individuals between 30 and 50 years of age that usually have no history of calf or heel pain and commonly participate in recreational activities.

## Confirmation

### What is the most likely clinical presentation?

A patient with an Achilles tendon rupture will present with swelling over the distal tendon, a palpable defect in the tendon above the calcaneal tuberosity, and pain and weakness with plantar flexion. The patient may limp and will often complain that during the injury there was a snap or a pop that was associated with the severe pain. A patient will not be able to stand on their toes and in a prone position will not demonstrate any passive plantar flexion with squeezing of the affected calf muscle (the Thompson test). A complete rupture will result in a palpable gap in the tendon prior to the insertion.

### What laboratory or imaging studies would confirm the diagnosis?

Confirmation of an Achilles tendon rupture should utilize x-ray to rule out an avulsion fracture or bony injury. MRI can be used to locate the presence and severity of the tear or rupture.

### What additional information should be obtained to confirm the diagnosis?

Diagnosis of an Achilles tendon rupture relies on patient history of the event and a positive Thompson's test. Patient history usually reveals a popping sound and a release from the back of the ankle. Physical examination and palpation reveal a discontinuity within the tendon. The O'Brien needle test may be used by the physician to confirm the rupture.

## Examination

### What history should be documented?

Important areas to explore include mechanism of present injury, past medical history, medications, current health status, social history and habits, occupation, living environment, and social support system.

### What test/measures are most appropriate?

**Anthropometric characteristics:** circumferential measurements for edema, palpation to determine ankle effusion

**Arousal, attention, and cognition:** examine mental status, learning ability, memory, motivation

**Assistive and adaptive devices:** potential utilization of crutches

**Gait, locomotion, and balance:** safety with/without an assistive device during gait; biomechanics of gait

**Integumentary integrity:** assessment of sensation

**Joint integrity and mobility:** special tests such as Thompson's test

**Muscle performance:** strength assessment, characteristics of muscle contraction

**Pain:** pain perception assessment scale

**Range of motion:** active and passive range of motion

**Sensory integration:** proprioception and kinesthesia

**Self-care and home management:** assessment of functional capacity

# Achilles Tendon Rupture

## What additional findings are likely with this patient?

An Achilles tendon rupture is more common in men and in individuals that do not consistently exercise, but are the "weekend warriors." There are risks and benefits to both philosophies of treatment (non-operative and operative) and the physician usually determines the course of treatment on a patient-by-patient basis accounting for the patient's age, activity level, and co-morbidities.

## Management

### What is the most effective management of this patient?

Medical management of a ruptured Achilles tendon incorporates immobilization through casting or a surgical approach for repair or reconstruction. Pharmacological intervention is not necessary for this condition except to relieve pain through NSAIDs, acetaminophen or narcotics depending on physician preference, and patient profile. Non-surgical treatment includes serial casting for approximately ten weeks followed by the use of a heel lift to ensure maximal healing without stress on the tendon for three to six months. Physical therapy begins when the cast is removed. If a patient requires surgical intervention then a cast or a brace is required for six to eight weeks. Physical therapy intervention is primarily the same for surgical and non-surgical patients and includes range of motion, stretching, icing, assistive device training, endurance programming, gait training, strengthening, plyometrics, and skill specific training. Modalities, pool therapy, and other cardiovascular equipment may assist in the recovery of functional motion and endurance.

### What home care regimen should be recommended?

A home care regimen is vital to the success of a patient's recovery. A program must be based on a patient's post-operative impairments and follow the physician's post-surgical protocol. A home program generally incorporates icing and elevation early in the rehabilitation process. A patient is required to continue a home program throughout the six to seven months of rehabilitation. Other areas of focus include range of motion, strengthening, gait, endurance activities, and high-level skill and sport specific tasks.

## Outcome

### What is the likely outcome of a course in physical therapy?

Physical therapy should begin after surgical intervention or when the cast is removed from a non-surgical patient. Assuming an unremarkable recovery, a patient should return to their previous functional level within six to seven months.

## What are the long-term effects of the patient's condition?

A patient that manages the Achilles tendon rupture without surgery and allows the tendon to heal on its own has a higher rate of rerupture (40% rerupture the tendon) compared to a patient that has surgical repair of the tendon (0-5% rerupture the tendon). An advantage to non-surgical management is a reduced risk of infection from surgery. However, it may result in an incomplete return of functional performance. A patient that has surgical intervention has a decreased risk for reinjury and a higher rate of return to athletic activities.

## Comparison

### What are the distinguishing characteristics of a similar condition?

Achilles tendonitis can be an acute or chronic condition due to repetitive microtrauma that builds scar tissue in the area over time. A patient initially feels an aching sensation after activity and progresses to pain with walking. There may be localized tenderness and swelling in the area. In the acute stage a patient should utilize anti-inflammatory medications, rest for 2-3 weeks and use a heel lift. In the chronic stage, the symptoms and pain may last beyond six weeks. Examination often reveals a thickened and nodular Achilles tendon. Surgical intervention may be warranted at this stage.

## Clinical Scenarios

### Scenario One

A 32-year-old female is playing soccer in a recreational league. A therapist that assists the team observes her kick the ball and then fall to the ground. The therapist examines the patient in the training room and finds that the patient has some plantar flexion in a non-weight bearing position, but is unable to plantar flex the foot while weight bearing. The patient states that something popped while running and palpation indicates a separation in the Achilles tendon.

### Scenario Two

A 46-year-old male is referred to physical therapy status post surgical reconstruction of a left Achilles tendon rupture. The patient has been casted for one week and has been using axillary crutches for household mobility. The patient has no significant past medical history. He is employed as a truck driver and resides in a one-story home. The patient sustained the injury while playing tennis.

# Adhesive Capsulitis

## Diagnosis

### What condition produces a patient's symptoms?

Adhesive capsulitis (also known as "frozen shoulder") is an enigmatic shoulder disorder characterized by inflammation and fibrotic thickening of the anterior joint capsule of the shoulder. The inflamed capsule becomes adherent to the humeral head and undergoes contracture. This condition is characterized by the symptoms of limitation in glenohumeral motion and pain.

### An injury was most likely sustained to which structure?

Adhesive capsulitis is classified as primary or secondary. Primary adhesive capsulitis occurs spontaneously and secondary adhesive capsulitis results from an underlying condition. Inflammation within the joint capsule causes fibrous adhesions to form and the capsule to thicken. A decrease in space within the capsule leads to a decrease of synovial fluid and further irritation to the glenohumeral joint.

## Inference

### What is the most likely contributing factor in the development of this condition?

Primary adhesive capsulitis has no known etiology, however, it is associated with conditions such as diabetes mellitus, hypothyroidism or cardiopulmonary conditions. Secondary adhesive capsulitis can result from trauma, immobilization, reflex sympathetic dystrophy, rheumatoid arthritis, abdominal disorders, and psychogenic disorders. Orthopedic intrinsic disorders that may initiate this process include supraspinatus tendonitis, partial tear of the rotator cuff, and bicipital tendonitis. Adhesive capsulitis occurs more in the middle-aged population with females having a greater incidence than males.

## Confirmation

### What is the most likely clinical presentation?

Data regarding the prevalence and incidence of adhesive capsulitis is lacking. According to a published study adhesive capsulitis occurs in 2% of the population within the United States and in 11% of individuals that are diagnosed with diabetes mellitus. A small percentage of patients (10-15%) develop bilateral adhesive capsulitis. Adhesive capsulitis is characterized by restricted active and passive range of motion at the glenohumeral joint. Characteristics of the acute phase include pain that radiates below the elbow and awakens the patient at night. Passive range of the shoulder is limited during this phase due to pain and guarding. During the chronic phase pain is usually localized around the lateral brachial region, the patient is not awakened by pain, and passive range is limited due to capsular stiffness. Pain is present with a loss of glenohumeral motion, restricted elevation, and lateral rotation.

### What laboratory or imaging studies would confirm the diagnosis?

An arthrogram can assist with the diagnosis of adhesive capsulitis by detecting a decreased volume of fluid within the joint capsule. The glenohumeral joint normally holds approximately 16-20 ml of fluid, however, adhesive capsulitis decreases the size of the capsule so it holds only 5-10 ml of fluid. Other tests should only be performed for differential diagnosis.

### What additional information should be obtained to confirm the diagnosis?

The diagnosis of adhesive capsulitis is confirmed from clinical evaluation and past medical history. The patient may present with the greatest restriction of glenohumeral motion in abduction and lateral rotation, but all planes of motion are usually affected. There is tightness within the anteroinferior joint capsule, pain with stretching, and restriction with passive and active range of motion.

## Examination

### What history should be documented?

Important areas to explore include past medical and surgical history, medications, family history, current symptoms, current health status, social history and habits, occupation, leisure activities, and social support system.

### What test/measures are most appropriate?

**Anthropometric characteristics:** circumferential measurements of bilateral upper extremities
**Arousal, attention, and cognition:** examine mental status, learning ability, memory, motivation
**Community and work integration:** analysis of community, work, and leisure activities
**Cranial nerve integrity:** assessment of muscle innervation by the cranial nerves, dermatome assessment
**Environmental, home, and work barriers:** analysis of current and potential barriers or hazards
**Integumentary integrity:** skin assessment, assessment of sensation
**Joint integrity and mobility:** assessment of hyper- and hypomobility of a joint, soft tissue swelling and inflammation
**Muscle performance:** strength assessment, muscle tone assessment
**Pain:** pain perception assessment scale, visual analogue scale, assessment of muscle soreness
**Posture:** analysis of resting and dynamic posture
**Range of motion:** active and passive range of motion
**Self-care and home management:** assessment of functional capacity

# Adhesive Capsulitis

**What additional findings are likely with this patient?**

A patient with adhesive capsulitis may encounter muscle spasms around the shoulder secondary to muscle guarding. A loss of reciprocal arm swing may be seen and disuse muscle atrophy may occur over time. A thorough examination must be completed to rule out concomitant systemic, rheumatologic, inflammatory, metastatic or infectious disorders.

## Management

**What is the most effective management of this patient?**

Medical management varies with adhesive capsulitis. Adhesive capsulitis is a self-limiting process that can take over 12 months in its course. Pharmacological intervention should emphasize the control of pain through acetaminophen, longer acting analgesics, NSAIDs or narcotics. A physician may inject the shoulder with corticosteroids to assist with recovery of motion. Surgical intervention to break up adhesions or release muscles adhered to the capsule is a last resort if conservative management fails. Physical therapy intervention during the acute phase includes icing or superficial heat, gentle joint mobilization, progressive strengthening, pendulum exercises, and isometric strengthening. During the chronic phase physical therapy intervention and goals may also include ultrasound, grade III and IV mobilization, increasing the extensibility of the joint capsule, and techniques such as PNF to restore painless functional range of motion.

**What home care regimen should be recommended?**

A home care regimen during the acute phase should include some self-stretching, but avoid abduction secondary to the risk of damage to subacromial tissue. Once the patient enters the chronic phase, the program should emphasize self-stretching, progressive exercises, posture management, PNF and other exercises such as pendulum exercises and "wall climbing" to assist with improving range of motion.

## Outcome

**What is the likely outcome of a course in physical therapy?**

Physical therapy is usually prescribed on an outpatient basis for three to five months after diagnosis. Adhesive capsulitis usually follows a nonlinear pattern of recovery. Spontaneous recovery is said to take 12-24 months in duration.

**What are the long-term effects of the patient's condition?**

Most patients are able to fully recover over time, but an estimated 7-14% of patients experience some permanent loss of range of motion at the shoulder joint. This loss is frequently asymptomatic and may not impair a patient's functional ability.

## Comparison

**What are the distinguishing characteristics of a similar condition?**

Acute bursitis is characterized by pain that is intense and sometimes throbbing over the lateral brachial region. This condition may arise secondary to calcific tendonitis. Active and passive motion in all directions is limited by pain. Abduction greater than 60 degrees and flexion greater than 90 degrees usually produce severe pain. Acute bursitis lasts for only a few days and unlike adhesive capsulitis this condition will usually resolve itself within a few weeks.

## Clinical Scenarios

### Scenario One

A 29-year-old was diagnosed with primary adhesive capsulitis and referred to outpatient physical therapy. The patient is self-employed as an artist and enjoys outdoor activities. Past medical history includes diabetes mellitus since age six and a femur fracture 11 months ago. The patient noticed reduced range of motion and an increase in pain over the last few weeks.

### Scenario Two

A 53-year-old female fell off her bike six months ago while cycling in a road race and sustained an injury to her shoulder complex. The patient attempted to immobilize her arm in a sling for two weeks. The patient states that she was unable to regain functional motion in her shoulder once she stopped using the sling. She saw a physician who diagnosed her with "frozen shoulder." The patient is limited to 10 degrees lateral rotation and 95 degrees of shoulder flexion.

# Alzheimer's Disease

## Diagnosis

### What condition produces a patient's symptoms?

Alzheimer's disease is a progressive neurological disorder that results in deterioration and irreversible damage within the cerebral cortex and subcortical areas of the brain. The loss of neurons results from the breakdown of several processes that would normally sustain the brain cells.

### An injury was most likely sustained to which structure?

Neurons that are normally involved with acetylcholine transmission deteriorate within the cerebral cortex of the brain. Postmortem biopsy reveals neurofibrillary tangles within cytoplasm, amyloid plaques, and cerebral atrophy. Amyloid plaques contain fragmented axons, altered glial cells, and cellular waste that result in an inflammatory response that provides further damage to the nervous system. Amyloid can also cause atrophy of the smooth muscle of the arteries of the brain, predisposing them to rupture.

## Inference

### What is the most likely contributing factor in the development of this condition?

The exact etiology of Alzheimer's disease is unknown, however, hypothesized causes include lower levels of neurotransmitters, higher levels of aluminum within brain tissue, genetic inheritance, autoimmune disease, abnormal processing of the substance amyloid, and virus. Approximately 4.5 million individuals are living with Alzheimer's disease in the United States. The risk of developing Alzheimer's disease increases with age and there is a higher incidence in women. The prevalence of Alzheimer's disease is 6% of individuals over 65 and 20% of individuals over 80 years of age.

## Confirmation

### What is the most likely clinical presentation?

Alzheimer's disease is initially noted by a change in higher cortical functions characterized by subtle changes in memory, impaired concentration, and difficulty with new learning. These symptoms progress in the early stages and there is a loss of orientation, word finding difficulties, emotional lability, depression, poor judgment, and impaired ability to perform self-care skills. During the middle stages of Alzheimer's disease the patient will develop behavioral and motor problems characterized by neurological symptoms such as aphasia, apraxia, perseveration, agitation, and violent or socially unacceptable behavior that can include wandering. Eventually all ability to learn is lost and long-term memory also disappears. End-stage Alzheimer's disease is characterized by severe intellectual and physical destruction. Patients in this stage will present with vegetative symptoms including incontinence, functional dependence, the inability to speak, and seizure activity.

### What laboratory or imaging studies would confirm the diagnosis?

Alzheimer's disease presently cannot be confirmed until a postmortem biopsy reveals the neurofibrillary tangles and amyloid plaques. MRI can be used to assess any abnormalities or signs of atrophy within the brain that is associated with Alzheimer's disease or to rule out other medical conditions. Single photon emission computed tomography (SPECT) may be used to determine brain activity and predict potential for Alzheimer's disease. Blood work, urine, and spinal fluid may be required to rule out other diseases that may cause signs of dementia.

### What additional information should be obtained to confirm the diagnosis?

A physical examination, neurological examination, and neuropsychological testing are required for diagnosis of probable Alzheimer's disease. The patient must demonstrate at least two deficits of cognition, memory, and related cognitive functioning with the absence of all other brain disease or disturbances in consciousness that may contribute to the identified deficits. Family history and symptoms may provide insight into the expected speed of progression of the disease.

## Examination

### What history should be documented?

Important areas to explore include past medical history, family history, history of current symptoms, current health status, living environment, social history and habits, occupation, and social support system.

### What test/measures are most appropriate?

**Aerobic capacity and endurance:** assessment of vital signs at rest and with activity

**Arousal, attention, and cognition:** examine mental status, learning ability, memory, motivation, Mini-Mental State Examination, level of consciousness

**Assistive and adaptive devices:** analysis of components and safety of a device

**Environmental, home, and work barriers:** analysis of current and potential barriers or hazards

**Gait, locomotion, and balance:** static and dynamic balance in sitting and standing, safety during gait with/without an assistive device, Functional Ambulation Profile, Berg Balance Scale

**Motor function:** equilibrium and righting reactions, coordination, physical performance scales

**Muscle performance:** strength assessment

**Posture:** analysis of resting and dynamic posture

**Range of motion:** active and passive range of motion

# Alzheimer's Disease

**Reflex integrity:** assessment of deep tendon and pathological reflexes (e.g., Babinski, ATNR)

**Self-care and home management:** assessment of functional capacity, Functional Independence Measure (FIM), Barthel Index

## What additional findings are likely with this patient?

A patient with end-stage Alzheimer's disease is at high risk for infection and pneumonia. These patients may experience complications from a persistent vegetative state such as contractures, decubiti, fracture, and pulmonary compromise.

## Management

### What is the most effective management of this patient?

Medical management of Alzheimer's disease may include pharmacological intervention during the early stages of the disease process. Medications are administered to inhibit acetylcholinesterase, alleviate cognitive symptoms, and control behavioral changes. Drug therapies are usually short-term in effect lasting six to nine months. Tacrine (Cognex), donepezil (Aricept), and rivastigmine (Exelon) are common pharmacological agents used to treat Alzheimer's disease, however, the side effects can be substantial. Physical therapy management should focus on maximizing the patient's remaining function and providing family and caregiver education. The therapist should attempt to create an emotional and physical environment that provides the patient with the opportunity to experience success. Modifying the layout of the patient's living space in order for the patient to easily find items is one example of creating an environment that encourages success. Safety with functional mobility and gait training may be indicated in the early stages of the disease. Later stages may require ongoing caregiver education regarding assistance with mobility, range of motion, and positioning. Many patients require a long-term care facility that specializes in Alzheimer's disease secondary to personality changes, aggressive behavior, and end-stage complications.

### What home care regimen should be recommended?

During the early stages of Alzheimer's disease a patient should continue with activity as tolerated and utilize a memory book or other compensatory strategies at home. As the disease progresses, a patient will rely on caregiver support to assist with a daily exercise program. The patient should be encouraged to exercise, ambulate, and participate in everyday activities such as folding laundry, making beds, and assisting with dinner in order to avoid restlessness and wandering.

## Outcome

### What is the likely outcome of a course in physical therapy?

Physical therapy may be indicated intermittently throughout the course of the disease, however, the therapy will not alter or cease the progression of the disease process.

### What are the long-term effects of the patient's condition?

Alzheimer's disease is a chronic and progressive disorder and is the fourth leading cause of death in adults. The typical course of the disease averages between seven and eleven years. The leading cause of death of a patient with Alzheimer's disease is infection or dehydration.

## Comparison

### What are the distinguishing characteristics of a similar condition?

Multi-infarct dementia produces symptoms in a step-like manner secondary to ongoing cerebral infarcts. This form of dementia is usually found in patients that are over 70 years of age and is more common in males. Hypertension is a primary risk factor and depression is common. A patient may also experience neurological deficits such as hemiplegia and emotional lability.

## Clinical Scenarios

### Scenario One

A 65-year-old female is referred to physical therapy for gait disturbances. The patient resides alone and drives on a regular basis. During the examination the patient reveals that she is sometimes confused when driving. The patient complains that she has difficulty managing her time around the house and requires an extended amount of time to get ready in the morning.

### Scenario Two

A 79-year-old male is seen by a therapist in an Alzheimer's residential facility. The physician recommends gait training with a walker. The patient enjoys walking around the unit, however, has fallen several times within the last month.

# Amyotrophic Lateral Sclerosis

## Diagnosis

### What condition produces a patient's symptoms?

Amyotrophic lateral sclerosis (ALS) is a chronic degenerative disease that produces both upper and lower motor neuron impairments. Demyelination, axonal swelling, and atrophy within the cerebral cortex, premotor areas, sensory cortex, and temporal cortex cause the symptoms of ALS.

### An injury was most likely sustained to which structure?

Rapid degeneration and demyelination occur in the giant pyramidal cells of the cerebral cortex and affect areas of the corticospinal tracts, cell bodies of the lower motor neurons in the gray matter, anterior horn cells, and areas within the precentral gyrus of the cortex. The rapid degeneration causes denervation of muscle fibers, muscle atrophy, and weakness.

## Inference

### What is the most likely contributing factor in the development of this condition?

The exact etiology of ALS is unknown (90% of all cases), however, there are multiple theories of causative factors that include genetic inheritance as an autosomal dominant trait, a slow acting virus, metabolic disturbances, and theories of toxicity of lead and aluminum. Familial ALS occurs in 5-10% of all cases. Risk for ALS is higher in men and usually occurs between 40 to 70 years of age.

## Confirmation

### What is the most likely clinical presentation?

Early clinical presentation of ALS may include both upper and lower motor neuron involvement. Early lower motor neuron signs include asymmetric muscle weakness, cramping, and atrophy that are usually found within the hands. Muscle weakness due to denervation eventually causes significant fasciculations, atrophy and wasting of the muscles. The weakness spreads throughout the body over the course of the disease and generally follows a distal to proximal path. Upper motor neuron symptoms occur due to the loss of inhibition of the muscle. Incoordination of movement, spasticity, clonus, and a positive Babinski reflex are some of the indicators of upper motor neuron involvement. Bulbar involvement is characterized by dysarthria, dysphagia, and emotional lability. Initially a person may have either upper or lower motor neuron involvement, but eventually both categories are affected. A patient with ALS will exhibit fatigue, oral motor impairment, fasciculations, spasticity, motor paralysis, and eventual respiratory paralysis.

### What laboratory or imaging studies would confirm the diagnosis?

There are multiple tests used to assist with diagnosing ALS. Electromyography assesses fibrillation and muscle fasciculations. Muscle biopsy verifies lower motor neuron involvement rather than muscle disease and a spinal tap may reveal a higher protein content in some patients with ALS. CT scan will appear normal until late in the disease process.

### What additional information should be obtained to confirm the diagnosis?

Diagnosis relies heavily on symptoms that determine both upper and lower motor neuron involvement. A patient that presents with motor impairment without sensory impairment is a primary indicator of ALS. Definitive diagnosis also first requires a physician to rule out other neurological conditions such as multiple sclerosis, spinal cord tumors, progressive muscular dystrophy, Lyme disease, and syringomyelia.

## Examination

### What history should be documented?

Important areas include past medical history, family history, history of current symptoms, current health status, living environment, social history and habits, occupation, and social support system.

### What test/measures are most appropriate?

**Aerobic capacity and endurance:** assessment of vital signs at rest and with activity, perceived exertion scale

**Anthropometric characteristics:** weight and height

**Arousal, attention, and cognition:** examines mental status, learning ability, memory, motivation

**Assistive and adaptive devices:** analysis of components and safety of a device

**Environmental, home, and work barriers:** analysis of current and potential barriers or hazards

**Gait, locomotion, and balance:** static and dynamic balance in sitting and standing, safety during gait with/without an assistive device

**Motor function:** motor assessment scales, coordination, equilibrium and righting reactions

**Muscle Performance:** strength assessment, muscle endurance, muscle tone assessment, muscle atrophy

**Neuromotor development and sensory integration:** analysis of reflex movement patterns, assessment of involuntary movements, sensory integration tests, gross and fine motor skills

**Posture:** analysis of resting and dynamic posture

**Range of motion:** active and passive range of motion

# Amyotrophic Lateral Sclerosis

**Reflex integrity:** assessment of deep tendon and pathological reflexes (e.g., Babinski, ATNR)

**Self-care and home management:** Barthel Index

**Ventilation, respiration, and circulation:** respiratory muscle strength, accessory muscle utilization, assessment of cough

## What additional findings are likely with this patient?

During the initial stages of ALS there are various effects on the body. Progression of the disease allows for significant deterioration within the brain and spinal cord and a patient may exhibit paralysis of vocal cords, swallowing impairment, contractures, decubiti, and breathing difficulty that requires ventilatory support. Throughout the course of ALS, however, sensation, eye movement, and bowel and bladder function remain preserved.

## Management

### What is the most effective management of this patient?

Effective management of ALS is based on supportive care and symptomatic therapy. Pharmacological intervention may include riluzole (Rilutek). This drug appears to have an effect on the progression of the disease process, however, its long-term effects are unknown. Symptomatic therapy may include anticholinergic, antispasticity, and antidepressant medications. Physical, occupational, speech, respiratory, and nutritional therapies may be warranted. Physical therapy intervention should focus on the quality of life and should include a low-level exercise program, range of motion, mobility training, assistive/adaptive devices, wheelchair prescription, bronchial hygiene, and energy conservation techniques. Patient, family, and caregiver training are important as the disease continues to progress.

### What home-care regimen should be recommended?

A home care regimen for a patient with ALS must consider the rate of disease progression and level of respiratory involvement. Goals should focus on maximizing the patient's functional capacity. A low-level exercise program may be indicated as long as the patient does not exercise to fatigue and promote further weakness. Family involvement is encouraged to support the patient through the course of the disease and assist with mobility, pacing skills, energy conservation techniques, and overall safety. During the later part of the disease the family and caregivers must be competent with positioning, bronchial hygiene, range of motion, and assistance with mobility.

## Outcome

### What is the likely outcome of a course in physical therapy?

Physical therapy intervention may assist with current issues, however, therapy does not hinder progression of ALS. Therapeutic goals will consider disease progression and focus on teaching for the patient and caregivers.

### What are the long-term effects of the patient's condition?

ALS is usually a rapidly progressing neurological disease with an average course of two to five years with 20-30% of patients surviving longer than five years. Research indicates that although there is no structured course of this disease process, if a patient is diagnosed before 50 years of age the disease is usually longer in course. Death usually occurs from respiratory failure.

## Comparison

### What are the distinguishing characteristics of a similar condition?

Muscular dystrophy (MD) is the term for a group of inherited disorders that are progressive and exhibit degeneration of muscles without sensory or neural impairment. Progressive weakness occurs to the muscle fibers secondary to the absence of dystrophin within the skeletal muscles. This group of disorders presents early in life and usually shortens life expectancy. Disuse atrophy, muscle deterioration, contractures, and cardiac and respiratory weakness are common characteristics of this disease process. A patient with MD usually dies from respiratory/cardiac complications secondary to the primary disease process.

## Clinical Scenarios

### Scenario One

A 56-year-old male is diagnosed with ALS and presents with mild atrophy of the hand. The patient owns his own business as a painter and wants to continue working for as long as he can. The patient is referred to physical therapy for a home exercise program.

### Scenario Two

A 60-year-old female is referred to physical therapy secondary to a left CVA. The patient was also diagnosed with ALS two years ago, requires the use of a wheelchair for mobility, and occasionally chokes while eating. The patient has assistance at home from her husband who is in good health.

# Ankylosing Spondylitis

## Diagnosis

### What condition produces a patient's symptoms?

Ankylosing spondylitis (AS), also known as Marie-Strumpell disease, is a systemic condition that is characterized by inflammation of the spine and larger peripheral joints. The chronic inflammation causes destruction of the ligamentous-osseous junction with subsequent fibrosis and ossification of the area.

### An injury was most likely sustained to which structure?

AS primarily affects the sacroiliac joint, intervertebral disks, spine, costovertebral and apophyseal joints, connective tissue, and larger peripheral joints (hips, knees, and shoulders). Ossification can occur within all affected joints resulting in pain and deformity.

## Inference

### What is the most likely contributing factor in the development of this condition?

AS is a progressive systemic disorder with uncertain etiology. Research supports the possibility of genetic inheritance combined with environmental influence. Gender, race, age, and family history are all factors to consider regarding risk for developing AS. A person born with a histocompatibility antigen HLA-B27 has a high risk for the disease. Approximately 80-90% of patients with AS are HLA-B27 positive, but only 2% of individuals that are HLA-B27 positive develop AS. HLA-B27 is found in 8.5% of Caucasians and only 2.5% of African Americans. Men are at a two to three time greater risk than women and onset is typically seen between twenty and forty years of age.

## Confirmation

### What is the most likely clinical presentation?

A patient with early AS will present with recurrent and insidious episodes of low back pain, morning stiffness, impaired spinal extension, and limited range of motion in the affected joints for over a three-month period of time. As the disease progresses pain will become severe, consistent, and extending to the midback, and sometimes towards the neck. The natural lumbar curve will eventually flatten due to muscle spasms. Other manifestations include fixed flexion at the hips, spinal kyphosis, fatigue, weight loss, and peripheral joint involvement. If the costovertebral joints are affected a patient will present with impaired chest mobility, compromised breathing, and decreased vital capacity.

### What laboratory or imaging studies would confirm the diagnosis?

X-ray of the spine may be negative in the initial stage of AS but with progression will reveal areas of erosion, demineralization, calcification, and syndesmophyte formation (ossification of the outside of the intervertebral disks). In the later stages of the disease x-ray will reveal fusion of the sacroiliac joint, calcification of apophyseal joints and spinal ligaments, and a bamboo appearance of the spine. Blood work can be used to rule out other diseases and assists with the diagnosis since the majority of patients with AS possess the HLA- B27 antigen and approximately 40% have an elevated erythrocyte sedimentation rate.

### What additional information should be obtained to confirm the diagnosis?

Physical examination may reveal joint tenderness, pain, and/ or limitation of the sacroiliac joint and the spine. Family inheritance and a thorough history of a patient's symptoms assist with the diagnosis of AS.

## Examination

### What history should be documented?

Important areas to explore include past medical history, medications, current health status, family inheritance, living environment, occupation, leisure activities, social history and habits, and social support system.

### What test/measures are most appropriate?

**Anthropometric characteristics:** baseline height measurement, circumferential chest measurements during inspiration

**Arousal, attention, and cognition:** examine mental status, learning ability, memory, motivation

**Assistive and adaptive devices:** analysis of components and safety of a device

**Community and work integration:** analysis of community, work, and leisure activities

**Environmental, home, and work barriers:** analysis of current and potential barriers or hazards

**Ergonomics and body mechanics:** analysis of dexterity and coordination

**Gait, locomotion, and balance:** assessment of static and dynamic balance in sitting and standing, safety during gait, Functional Ambulation Profile, analysis of wheelchair management

**Joint integrity and mobility:** assess hypomobility and limitation of a joint, Wright-Schober test for spinal mobility

**Muscle performance:** strength assessment

**Pain:** pain perception assessment scale

**Posture:** analysis of resting and dynamic posture

**Range of motion:** active and passive range of motion

**Reflex integrity:** assessment of deep tendon and pathological reflexes (e.g., Babinski, ATNR)

**Self-care and home management:** assessment of functional capacity

**Sensory integrity:** assessment of sensation

**Ventilation, respiration, and circulation:** analysis of thoracolumbar movement and chest expansion during breathing, measurement of vital capacity

# Ankylosing Spondylitis

### What additional findings are likely with this patient?

Long-term AS will present with progressive symptoms and multiple complications. Iritis, uveitis, osteoporosis, fracture, atlantoaxial subluxation, and complete spinal fusion can occur in severe long-standing cases of AS. Pericarditis, cardiac pathology, pulmonary fibrosis, cardiac arrhythmias, amyloidosis, and aortic insufficiency have also been noted as potential complications.

## Management

### What is the most effective management of this patient?

The goals of medical management are to reduce inflammation, maintain functional mobility, and relieve pain. Pharmacological intervention may include NSAIDs, disease-modifying drugs such as methotrexate, analgesics, and specifically Indomethacin to relieve pain. Physical therapy intervention should include postural exercises emphasizing extension, general range of motion, pain management, and energy conservation techniques. Low-impact and aerobic exercise with emphasis on extension and rotation are appropriate for a patient with AS. High-impact and flexion exercises are contraindicated. Patient education should include posture retraining, positioning for sleeping, and lifting techniques. Excessive exercise should be avoided as it can increase the inflammatory response and injury. Swimming is a highly recommended activity. Surgical intervention is rarely indicated to correct or stabilize a musculoskeletal deformity.

### What home care regimen should be recommended?

A home care regimen for a patient with AS should include a daily low-impact therapeutic exercise program. Range of motion should focus on spinal movement in all directions. The patient requires a firm sleeping surface and competence with proper positioning and use of pillows to maintain optimal alignment. Ongoing breathing exercises and posture retraining will assist with overall level of function.

## Outcome

### What is the likely outcome of a course in physical therapy?

Physical therapy cannot modify the progression of AS, however, it may assist to alleviate pain and improve a patient's functional capacity. A patient may require physical therapy on an intermittent basis for secondary complications throughout the disease process.

### What are the long-term effects of the patient's condition?

AS progresses slowly over a fifteen to twenty-five year period and may remain isolated to the spine and sacroiliac joint or spread to larger peripheral joints. Stiffness and joint limitation are common long-term effects of AS that can negatively impact a patient's functional mobility. The extent of disability varies greatly with only 1% of patients experiencing complete remission. Normal course includes periods of exacerbations and remissions. Hip disease with AS is a marker for a severe form of AS and is more likely to occur in a patient that is diagnosed at a young age.

## Comparison

### What are the distinguishing characteristics of a similar condition?

Sjogren's syndrome, like AS, is classified as a spondylarthropathy. Sjogren's is a chronic arthritis and autoimmune disease that also can affect several organs. Lymphocytes attack healthy tissues and organs and are usually found in combination with RA or lupus. Postmenopausal women are affected most often with over two to four million individuals in the United States living with the disease. It does not have a cure, but can be managed through medications, exercise, and proper nutrition. Exercise should follow general guidelines for the treatment of RA.

## Clinical Scenarios

### Scenario One

A 28-year-old male is seen in physical therapy shortly after being diagnosed with AS. The patient complains of sacroiliac pain and tenderness. The patient has a negative family history and is currently employed as a high school maintenance technician.

### Scenario Two

A 60-year-old female is seen in physical therapy with advanced AS. The patient has bilateral hip flexion contractures and kyphosis. The patient resides alone and receives daily assistance from her two sisters who live locally. The patient has previously refused recommendations to utilize an assistive device for ambulation.

# Anterior Cruciate Ligament Sprain – Grade III

## Diagnosis

### What condition produces a patient's symptoms?

The anterior cruciate ligament (ACL) extends from the anterior intracondylar region of the tibia to the medial aspect of the lateral femoral condyle in the intracondylar notch. The ligament prevents anterior translation of the tibia on the fixed femur and posterior translation of the femur on the fixed tibia. The ACL is a broad cord that has long collagen strands that permits up to 500 pounds of pressure prior to rupture. The ligament has a poor blood supply and does not have the ability to heal a complete tear. Injuries to the ACL most commonly occur during hyperflexion, rapid deceleration, hyperextension or landing in an unbalanced position.

### An injury was most likely sustained to which structure?

A grade III ACL sprain refers to a complete tear of the ligament with excessive laxity. Tears of the anterior cruciate ligament most often occur in the midsubstance of the ligament and not at the ligament's attachment on the femur or tibia. Laxity rarely occurs solely in a straight plane and instead is often classified as anterolateral or anteromedial.

## Inference

### What is the most likely contributing factor in the development of this condition?

Participation in athletic activities requiring high levels of agility (soccer, basketball, volleyball) and contact sports increases the incidence of an ACL injury. Recent studies indicate that women involved in selected athletic activities experienced significantly higher ACL injury rates than their male counterparts. There are many hypothesized reasons for this finding, but to date a definitive answer has not been identified. Causative factors for ACL disruption include body movement and positioning, muscle strength, joint laxity, Q angle, and a narrow intercondylar notch.

## Confirmation

### What is the most likely clinical presentation?

The peak incidence of ACL injury occurs between 14 and 29 years of age. This age group corresponds to an overall higher activity level, which increases the risk of injury. A grade III ACL sprain is characterized by significant pain, effusion, and edema that significantly limits range of motion. The patient may be unable to bear weight on the involved extremity resulting in dependence on an assistive device. Ligamentous testing reveals visible laxity in the knee and may exacerbate the patient's pain level.

### What laboratory or imaging studies would confirm the diagnosis?

MRI is the preferred imaging tool to identify the presence of an ACL tear and possible disruption of other soft tissue structures such as ligaments and menisci. X-rays may be used to rule out a fracture.

### What additional information should be obtained to confirm the diagnosis?

Subjective reports such as hearing a loud pop or feeling as though the knee buckled is often associated with a complete tear of the ACL. Special tests such as the Lachman, anterior drawer, and pivot shift test can be used to confirm the diagnosis. It is important to perform all special tests bilaterally.

## Examination

### What history should be documented?

Important areas to explore include mechanism of present injury, current symptoms, past medical history, medications, living environment, social history and habits, and social support system.

### What test/measures are most appropriate?

**Anthropometric characteristics:** knee effusion and lower extremity circumferential measurements

**Arousal, attention, and cognition:** examine mental status, learning ability, memory, motivation

**Assistive and adaptive devices:** analysis of components and safety of a device, potential utilization of crutches

**Gait, locomotion, and balance:** safety during gait with an assistive device

**Integumentary integrity:** assessment of sensation (pain, temperature, tactile), skin assessment

**Joint integrity and mobility:** special tests for ligaments and menisci, Lachman and reverse Lachman test, anterior drawer test, palpation of structures, joint play, soft tissue restrictions, joint pain

**Muscle performance:** strength and active movement assessment, resisted isometrics, muscle contraction characteristics, muscle endurance

**Orthotic, protective, and supportive devices:** utilization of bracing, taping or wrapping, foot orthotic assessment

**Pain:** pain perception assessment scale

**Range of motion:** active and passive range of motion

**Self-care and home management:** assessment of functional capacity

**Sensory integrity:** proprioception and kinesthesia

# Anterior Cruciate Ligament Sprain – Grade III

## What additional findings are likely with this patient?

Approximately two-thirds of the time the ACL is torn there is an accompanying meniscal tear. The collateral ligaments can also be involved although not as commonly as the menisci. When all three structures (ACL, MCL, and medial meniscus) are damaged it is referred to as the "unhappy triad."

## Management

### What is the most effective management of this patient?

Management of a patient following a grade III ACL sprain includes controlling edema, increasing range of motion, strengthening, and improving the fluidity of gait. For patients electing to have surgery, the patellar tendon is the most commonly utilized graft for intra-articular reconstruction. Patients often initially present with a knee immobilizer and crutches to protect the reconstructed ligament. Specific parameters are difficult to identify since many orthopedic surgeons utilize very specific protocols.

Physical therapy management in the initial post-operative phase includes protecting the integrity of the graft, controlling edema, and improving range of motion. Specific intervention activities include pain modulation, patellar mobility, active range of motion exercises, gait activities, and quadriceps exercises. As patients progress in their rehabilitation program, treatment begins to focus on strengthening activities emphasizing closed-chain exercises and selected functional activities. Closed-chain exercises are considered more desirable than open-chain exercises since they minimize anterior translation of the tibia. Patients should be required to complete a functional progression prior to returning to unrestricted athletics. For patients opting for a conservative (non-operative) approach, it is necessary to begin an aggressive strengthening program once the acute phase of the injury has subsided.

### What home care regimen should be recommended?

The home care regimen should consist of range of motion, strengthening, palliative care, and functional activities as warranted based on the results of the patient examination and course (operative versus non-operative) of treatment.

## Outcome

### What is the likely outcome of a course in physical therapy?

It is possible that with an aggressive strengthening program and/or activity modification, patients may be able to participate in light to moderate athletic activities without formal surgical reconstruction. Patients electing to have surgery can expect to return to their previous functional level in four to six months.

## What are the long-term effects of the patient's condition?

Patients that sustain a complete tear of the ACL and elect not to have reconstructive surgery will likely be at increased risk for instability and subsequent deterioration of joint surfaces.

## Comparison

### What are the distinguishing characteristics of a similar condition?

A grade III posterior cruciate ligament (PCL) sprain is less common than an ACL sprain. The most common mechanism of injury for a PCL sprain is a "dashboard" injury or forced knee hyperflexion as the foot is plantar flexed. A grade III PCL injury will typically produce effusion, posterior tenderness, and a positive posterior drawer test. Knee extension is often limited due to the effusion and stretching of the posterior capsule and gastrocnemius. The rehabilitation program typically emphasizes strengthening of the quadriceps muscles. Individuals with an isolated PCL sprain may not exhibit any functional performance limitations and as a result, surgical intervention is far less common than with an ACL sprain. A PCL sprain alters the arthrokinematics of the knee joint and as a result a patient will be susceptible to degenerative changes such as arthritis.

## Clinical Scenarios

### Scenario One

A 16-year-old gymnast sustains a grade I ACL injury after landing awkwardly on her left leg during a vault. The patient is two days status post injury and has mild effusion in the involved knee. The patient is a competitive gymnast and needs to compete in a regional meet in slightly less than four weeks.

### Scenario Two

A 35-year-old male is referred to physical therapy after injuring his knee in a softball game. The patient reports tearing the ACL ten years ago in a skiing accident. The patient is active, however, reports more recent episodes of instability. The physician notes significant arthritic changes in the involved knee including diminished joint space.

# Bicipital Tendonitis

## Diagnosis

### What condition produces a patient's symptoms?

Bicipital tendonitis is an inflammatory process of the tendon of the long head of the biceps. Impingement or an inflammatory injury can result in symptoms of shoulder pain. Repeated full abduction and lateral rotation of the humeral head can lead to irritation that produces inflammation, edema, microscopic tears within the tendon, and degeneration of the tendon itself.

### An injury was most likely sustained to which structure?

Continuous or repetitive shoulder motions can cause overuse of the biceps tendon. Damaged cells within the tendon do not have time to heal, leading to tendonitis. This is common in sports or work activities that require frequent and repeated use of the upper extremities, especially when the motion is performed overhead. Athletes who throw, swim or swing a racquet or club are at greatest risk. Years of shoulder wear and tear can cause the biceps tendon to become inflamed. Degeneration in a tendon causes a loss of the normal arrangement of the collagen fibers that join together to form the tendon. Some of the individual strands of the tendon become intertwined due to the degeneration, while allowing other fibers to break and the tendon to lose strength.

## Inference

### What is the most likely contributing factor in the development of this condition?

Bicipital tendonitis is often caused through repetitive overhead activity and motion. There is usually direct trauma to the tendon as the shoulder motion approaches excessive abduction and lateral rotation. Examples of high risk athletes include baseball pitchers, tennis players, gymnasts, rowers, and swimmers. Bicipital tendonitis can also be caused secondary to other shoulder pathology including rotator cuff disease, impingement syndrome or intra-articular pathology such as labral tears.

## Confirmation

### What is the most likely clinical presentation?

Patients generally report the feeling of a deep ache directly in the front and on the top of the shoulder. The ache may spread down into the biceps muscle and is usually made worse with overhead activities or lifting heavy objects. Resting the shoulder typically reduces the pain. A catching or slipping sensation of the biceps muscle may indicate a tear of the transverse humeral ligament. Bicipital tendinopathy, pain to palpation over the anterior shoulder in the area of the bicipital groove, pain with the biceps resistance test (i.e., shoulder flexion against resistance with elbow extended and forearm supinated), and a positive Yergason's or Speed's test (i.e., pain with resisted supination of the forearm or with the elbow flexed at 90° and the arm adducted against the body) are positive indicators for bicipital tendonitis.

### What laboratory or imaging studies would confirm the diagnosis?

There are no laboratory tests to assist with the diagnosis of bicipital tendonitis. Plain x-rays do not diagnose bicipital tendonitis, but may show calcification in the groove or subacromial spurring. Other x-rays of the neck and elbow may be indicated to rule out referred shoulder pain. MRI can view the tendon, but is expensive and not usually used unless the patient is not responding to conservative treatment.

### What additional information should be obtained to confirm the diagnosis?

Testing such as the biceps resistance test, Speed's test, and Yergason's test may be performed in conjunction with a full physical examination.

## Examination

### What history should be documented?

Important areas to explore include past medical history, medications, current health status, nutritional status, social history and habits, occupation, living environment, and social support system.

### What test/measures are most appropriate?

**Arousal, attention, and cognition:** examine mental status, learning ability, memory, motivation

**Community and work integration:** analysis of community, work, and leisure activities

**Environmental, home, and work barriers:** analysis of current and potential barriers or hazards

**Ergonomics and body mechanics:** analysis of dexterity and coordination

**Joint integrity and mobility:** assessment of hyper- and hypomobility of a joint, soft tissue swelling and inflammation

**Muscle performance:** strength assessment, muscle tone assessment

**Pain:** pain perception assessment scale, visual analogue scale, assessment of muscle soreness

**Posture:** analysis of resting and dynamic posture

**Range of motion:** active and passive range of motion, Speed's test, Yergason's test

**Reflex integrity:** assessment of deep tendon reflexes

**Self-care and home management:** assessment of functional capacity

**Sensory integrity:** assessment of proprioception and kinesthesia

# Bicipital Tendonitis

## What additional findings are likely with this patient?

Patients with long-term chronic tendonitis may experience shoulder instability and subluxation secondary to biceps degeneration. Bicipital tendonitis will also frequently accompany impingement syndrome, rotator cuff tendonitis, and forms of glenohumeral instability.

## Management

### What is the most effective management of this patient?

The primary goal of medical management is to relieve pain, reduce inflammation, and regain full available range of motion. Rest and/or immobilization using a splint or a removable brace may be indicated initially for a brief period of time. Generally, the patient should avoid all overhead movement, reaching, and lifting of objects. Pharmacological intervention may include nonsteroidal anti-inflammatory medications (NSAIDs) which will reduce both pain and inflammation. Active physical therapy is not often initiated immediately, however, the patient may be referred for instruction in general education of the pathology, guidelines for restrictions, pendulum exercises, and the use of TENS. The application of heat or cold to the affected area can also assist with relief of pain. The patient may benefit from the use of iontophoresis or phonophoresis. As the patient progresses out of the acute phase, physical therapy should focus on an exercise program that stretches and strengthens the affected muscle groups. This can restore the tendon's ability to function properly, improve healing, and prevent future injury. Surgical intervention is only recommended for patients that have not progressed with conservative treatment over a six month period of time. The typical procedure includes arthroscopic decompression and acromioplasty with anterior acromionectomy.

### What home care regimen should be recommended?

Patients with bicipital tendonitis are recommended to always perform warm-up activities prior to vigorous exercises, consistently perform passive selective stretching and strengthening, use proper body mechanics, and avoid any painful activity. The ongoing focus of a home program should be on strengthening and endurance surrounding the tendon. Patients will have to consistently participate in an ongoing home exercise program to prevent the risk of recurrence.

## Outcome

### What is the likely outcome of a course in physical therapy?

The goal of physical therapy is to restore full available range of motion without pain. Once the patient does not experience pain or discomfort with activity, they may slowly return to their previous level of activity. Most patients are successful with conservative treatment and are able to return to their activities after an average of six to eight weeks of physical therapy and rehabilitation.

## What are the long-term effects of the patient's condition?

Although the overall prognosis depends on the level of involvement, most patients have a positive long-term outcome and are able to return to their previous level of functioning. Statistically, there are approximately 10% of patients that do not achieve a positive outcome and have further deterioration or a rupture of the tendon.

## Comparison

### What are the distinguishing characteristics of a similar condition?

The glenoid labrum is a fibrocartilage rim that surrounds the glenoid cavity, attaches to the glenoid cavity of the scapula to increase its depth, and protects the edge of the bone within the joint capsule. A labral tear is most susceptible with anterior damage or subluxation. A Bankart lesion is the name given to the avulsion of the labral ligamentous complex from the anteroinferior aspect of the glenoid. This is the most common lesion resulting in anterior joint instability. A CT scan can diagnose the tear and surgical intervention is normally successful for repair.

## Clinical Scenarios

### Scenario One

A 27-year-old male is referred to physical therapy by his primary care physician for "probable bicipital tendonitis." He went to see his doctor secondary to pain when performing overhead activities and lifting objects of varying weight. He works as an auto mechanic 50 hours per week. He was trying to "work through the pain," but it has worsened over the last month. He resides with his wife and twin girls in a ranch style home.

### Scenario Two

A 56-year-old tennis instructor has noticed an increase in pain through a particular arc of motion at her shoulder. She was diagnosed with impingement syndrome years ago, but has not had any recurrence or discomfort again until now. She states that her goal is to return to teaching tennis.

# Breast Cancer

## Diagnosis

### What condition produces a patient's symptoms?

Breast cancer's primary symptom is a painless mass within the breast tissue. This mass is composed of malignant altered cells that proliferate and spread without control. A malignancy can occur anywhere within the breast tissue, however, the lump is usually found directly behind the areola in men and is usually located behind the areola or in the outer upper quadrant of the breast in women. There may or may not be generalized discomfort in the area of the mass.

### An injury was most likely sustained to which structure?

Injury occurs initially at the cellular level within the breast tissue. Breast cancer either begins in the lobules which are the milk producing glands or in the ducts that bring the milk to the nipples. Breast cancer can spread into the lymphatic system and will commonly metastasize to the brain, lungs, bones, adrenals, and liver.

## Inference

### What is the most likely contributing factor in the development of this condition?

The etiology of breast cancer is unknown, however, estrogen is believed to have some relationship to the disease process. Risk factors include gender, age, young menarche, late menopause, family history of breast cancer, high alcohol intake, high fat diet, radiation exposure, and past history of cancer. Breast cancer can occur in both males and females, however, males account for less then 1% of all breast cancer cases.

## Confirmation

### What is the most likely clinical presentation?

Breast cancer makes up approximately 30% of all female cancers and is the second leading cause of death in female cancers within the United States. Approximately 70% of all breast cancer occurs in women over the age of 50. A patient with breast cancer will present with a lump in the breast that is noticed by a physician (10%) or by the patient through self-examination (90%). Breast cancer is initially otherwise asymptomatic. As the disease progresses the breast may become painful, change shape, bleed from the nipple, and dimple over the area of the mass. Symptoms associated with metastases may include bone pain, upper extremity edema, and weight loss.

### What laboratory or imaging studies would confirm the diagnosis?

Mammography is used to detect the location and growth of a mass, however, definitive diagnosis of breast cancer is made only after microscopic examination of a suspected mass by needle or excision biopsy. Ultrasound can also be used to detect if a lump is filled with fluid or a solid mass. Sentinel lymph node mapping is used upon diagnosis to identify exact lymph node involvement.

### What additional information should be obtained to confirm the diagnosis?

Additional information such as family history of cancer, past medical history, and history of self-examination is helpful in support of a definitive diagnosis. This information is usually obtained prior to mammography and biopsy.

## Examination

### What history should be documented?

Important areas to explore include past medical history, family history of cancer, medications, current health status, social history and habits, hand dominance, occupation, living environment, and social support system.

### What test/measures are most appropriate?

**Aerobic capacity and endurance:** assessment of vital signs at rest and with activity

**Anthropometric characteristics:** upper extremity circumferential measurements

**Arousal, attention, and cognition:** examine mental status, learning ability, memory, motivation

**Community and work integration:** analysis of community, work, and leisure activities

**Gait, locomotion, and balance:** assess static/dynamic balance in sitting and standing, safety during gait

**Integumentary integrity:** assessment for potential infection of surgical incision

**Muscle performance:** strength assessment

**Pain:** pain perception assessment scale, visual analogue scale

**Range of motion:** active and passive range of motion

**Self-care and home management:** assessment of self-care and home management skills, assessment of functional capacity, Barthel Index

**Sensory integrity:** assessment of superficial and combined sensations, proprioception, and kinesthesia

# Breast Cancer

### What additional findings are likely with this patient?

Additional findings are dependent on the stage of the cancer (I, II, III, IV) and course of treatment. If a patient has undergone surgical resection or mastectomy the patient may experience pain, edema, fatigue, and psychological issues. Patients that are diagnosed with advanced breast cancer may experience pleural effusion, pathological fractures, and spinal compression.

## Management

### What is the most effective management of this patient?

The medical management of breast cancer is based on the size and the stage of the mass and corresponding involvement of the lymph nodes. Surgical management may range from excision of the mass (lumpectomy) to total radical mastectomy with axillary dissection. Chemotherapy, radiation therapy, and hormone therapies may be used in isolation or after a surgical procedure. Physical therapy may be indicated to assist with lymphedema management, post-surgical breathing exercises, positioning, pain management, strengthening and endurance activities, range of motion exercises, massage, intermittent compression, and patient education.

### What home care regimen should be recommended?

A home care regimen should include education, positioning, and techniques to manage lymphedema. Range of motion exercises, energy conservation techniques, as well as general exercise and endurance activities should continue on a regular basis at home.

## Outcome

### What is the likely outcome of a course in physical therapy?

Physical therapy may be indicated for post-surgical management to assist with impairments and promote independence with self-care and functional skills.

### What are the long-term effects of the patient's condition?

The long-term effects of breast cancer are varied. The risk of recurrence is always present and should be monitored closely. Post-surgical lymphedema may persist and require ongoing home management. Overall prognosis and ten-year survival rates for women are over 85% for stage I disease; 66% for stage II; 36% for stage III; and 7% for stage IV disease. The survival rate decreases as the tumor progresses and lymph nodes become involved. Overall mortality has decreased 1-2% annually within the United States secondary to changes in lifestyle, improved self-examination, earlier diagnosis, and better treatment.

## Comparison

### What are the distinguishing characteristics of a similar condition?

Fibrocystic breast disease (mammary dysplasia) usually occurs in both breasts and is characterized by nodular lumps within the breast tissue. The cysts are benign and become tender immediately prior to menstruation. Fibrocystic breast disease is the most common breast disorder in women. Other symptoms include aching and burning within the breast. Symptoms normally disappear after menstruation is over. Although benign, fibrocystic breast disease increases a patient's risk for breast cancer later in life.

## Clinical Scenarios

### Scenario One

A 65-year-old female is seen by a therapist 24 hours after total mastectomy. The patient was active prior to the surgery and walked for exercise two miles everyday. The patient's past medical history is positive for fibrocystic breast disease, diabetes mellitus, and skin cancer. The patient reports pain with coughing. The patient resides alone in a retirement village and lost her husband to cancer last year. She has three supportive children that reside in the local area.

### Scenario Two

A 45-year-old female is referred to outpatient physical therapy with lymphedema secondary to stage III breast cancer and radical mastectomy three months ago. The patient is fatigued and anxious about the increased size of her arm and limitation in range of motion. The patient runs a daycare center out of her home and is active in her church. Past medical history includes endometriosis and pharmacological treatment for depression.

# Carpal Tunnel Syndrome

## Diagnosis

### What condition produces a patient's symptoms?

The carpal tunnel is created by the transverse carpal ligament, the scaphoid tuberosity and trapezium, the hook of the hamate and pisiform, and the volar radiocarpal ligament and volar ligamentous extensions between the carpal bones. The median nerve, four flexor digitorum profundus tendons, four flexor digitorum superficialis tendons, and the flexor pollicis longus tendon pass through the carpal tunnel. Carpal tunnel syndrome (CTS) occurs as a result of compression of the median nerve where it passes through the carpal tunnel.

### An injury was most likely sustained to which structure?

The median nerve is injured by compression within the carpal tunnel at the wrist. Normal tissue pressure within the tunnel is seven to eight mm Hg but CTS can result in pressure above 30 mm Hg, which further increases with flexion and extension of the wrist. The increase in pressure produces ischemia in the nerve. This results in sensory and motor disturbances in the median nerve distribution of the hand.

## Inference

### What is the most likely contributing factor in the development of this condition?

Any condition such as edema, inflammation, tumor or fibrosis may cause compression of the median nerve within the carpal tunnel and result in ischemia. The exact etiology of CTS is unclear, however, conditions that produce inflammation of the carpal tunnel that can contribute to CTS include repetitive use, rheumatoid arthritis, pregnancy, diabetes, trauma, tumor, hypothyroidism, and wrist sprain or fracture. Other etiologies include a congenital narrowing of the tunnel and vitamin B6 deficiency.

## Confirmation

### What is the most likely clinical presentation?

Approximately five million individuals in the United States are diagnosed with CTS. Most patients are diagnosed between 35 and 55 years of age with greater prevalence in women. A patient with CTS will initially present with sensory changes and paresthesia along the median nerve distribution in the hand. It may also radiate into the upper extremity, shoulder, and neck. Symptoms include night pain, weakness of the hand, muscle atrophy, decreased grip strength, clumsiness, and decreased wrist mobility. Initially, muscle atrophy is often noted in the abductor pollicis brevis muscle and progresses to the thenar muscles.

### What laboratory or imaging studies would confirm the diagnosis?

Electromyography and electroneurographic studies can be used to diagnose a motor conduction delay along the median nerve within the carpal tunnel. MRI is sometimes used to identify inflammation of the median nerve, altered tendon or nerve positioning within the tunnel or thickening of the tendon sheath.

### What additional information should be obtained to confirm the diagnosis?

Physical examination, history, and review of symptoms are extremely important when diagnosing CTS. Provocation testing such as a positive Tinel's sign, a positive Phalen's test, and a positive tethered median nerve stress test along with the other symptoms will assist to confirm the diagnosis.

## Examination

### What history should be documented?

Important areas to explore include past medical history, medications, history of symptoms, current health status, occupation, living environment, social history and habits, leisure activities, and social support system.

### What test/measures are most appropriate?

**Anthropometric characteristics:** wrist and hand circumferential measurements
**Arousal, attention, and cognition:** examine mental status, learning ability, memory, motivation
**Community and work integration:** analysis of community, work, and leisure activities
**Environmental, home, and work barriers:** analysis of current and potential barriers or hazards
**Ergonomics and body mechanics:** analysis of dexterity and coordination
**Integumentary integrity:** skin and nailbed assessment, assessment of sensation
**Joint integrity and mobility:** assessment of hypomobility of a joint, assessment of soft tissue swelling/inflammation, Tinel's sign, Phalen's test, tethered median nerve stress test
**Muscle performance:** strength assessment including hand musculature
**Orthotic, protective, and supportive devices:** potential utilization of bracing or splinting
**Pain:** pain perception assessment scale
**Range of motion:** active and passive range of motion
**Self-care and home management:** assessment of functional capacity

# Carpal Tunnel Syndrome

### What additional findings are likely with this patient?

Advanced CTS can present with muscle atrophy of the hand, radiating pain in the forearm and shoulder, and nerve damage with motor and sensory loss. Unrelieved compression creates initial neurapraxia with some demyelination of the axons. This results in eventual axonotmesis and wallerian degeneration within the nerve distribution. The patient may present with ape hand deformity caused by atrophy of the thenar musculature and first two lumbricals. Research indicates that approximately 50% of cases include bilateral involvement.

## Management

### What is the most effective management of this patient?

A patient with CTS will initially receive conservative management including local corticosteroid injections, splinting, and physical therapy management. Recent pharmacological intervention has included Methylprednisolone injected proximally to the tunnel. Physical therapy is one aspect of conservative management and includes splinting, carpal mobilization, and gentle stretching. Biomechanical analysis and adaptation of a patient's occupation, work place, leisure activities, and living environment may be necessary.

If conservative treatment fails the patient may require surgery to release the carpal ligament and decompress the median nerve. Newer surgical techniques allow for smaller incisions, less manipulation of the nerve, and are highly successful for long-term relief of symptoms. Post-surgical physical therapy intervention should include the use of moist heat with electrical stimulation, iontophoresis, cryotherapy, gentle massage, desensitization of the scar, tendon gliding exercises, and active range of motion. A patient should initially avoid wrist flexion and a forceful grasp. After four weeks, a patient can progress with active wrist flexion, gentle stretching, putty exercises, light progressive resistive exercise, and continued modification of body mechanics. Radial deviation against resistance should be avoided due to the tendency for irritation and inflammation. Post-surgical rehabilitation usually lasts six to eight weeks.

### What home care regimen should be recommended?

A home care regimen should consist of continued stretching and strengthening exercises. The patient must be competent and compliant regarding the use of a splint and follow all work and leisure modifications.

## Outcome

### What is the likely outcome of a course in physical therapy?

Physical therapy intervention should improve a patient's condition and decrease symptoms of CTS within four to six weeks. If conservative treatment fails and the patient requires surgical intervention, rehabilitation may last six to eight weeks.

### What are the long-term effects of the patient's condition?

CTS can have minor effects on some patients while having debilitating effects on others. The overall long-term effects are dependent on the degree of involvement, the amount of permanent damage, and the level of success with conservative or surgical management. It is possible to have no long-term effects from this condition if the patient responds positively to physical therapy and the rehabilitation process. Other patients may be left with permanent motor and sensory impairments along the median nerve distribution.

## Comparison

### What are the distinguishing characteristics of a similar condition?

Compression in the tunnel of Guyon occurs with inflammation to the ulnar nerve between the hook of the hamate and the pisiform. This condition occurs from tasks such as leaning during extended handwriting, leaning on bike handles while riding, repetitive gripping activities or trauma. The patient will present with paresthesias along the ulnar distribution, weakness and atrophy of the hypothenar musculature, decreased mobility of the pisiform, and impaired grip strength. This condition can be treated with conservative management or surgical intervention.

## Clinical Scenarios

### Scenario One

A 26-year-old female is seen in physical therapy with a diagnosis of bilateral CTS. The patient has not been treated previously for this syndrome and is employed as a telephone sales specialist. The patient complains of pain in her hands, numbness when sleeping and while performing at work, and muscle soreness in both hands.

### Scenario Two

A 45-year-old male with CTS is referred to physical therapy ten days after surgical decompression. The patient's post-operative routine includes resting the hand, using a splint, icing, and elevation. Minimal edema is noted at the wrist. The patient is anxious to return to work.

# Central Cord Syndrome

## Diagnosis

### What condition produces a patient's symptoms?

Central cord syndrome (CCS) is an incomplete spinal cord lesion that most often results from a cervical hyperextension injury. Symptoms are secondary to damage to the central aspect of the spinal cord. CCS usually occurs from a fall but can occur from other forms of trauma such as a motor vehicle accident.

### An injury was most likely sustained to which structure?

The spinal cord sustains bleeding into the central gray matter that causes damage to the centrally located cervical tracts. Injury is caused by a ligamentum flavum (hyperextension) injury or otherwise from anterior compression of the cord due to osteophyte formation. Studies often reveal axonal disruption in the lateral columns at the level of injury with preservation of the gray matter.

## Inference

### What is the most likely contributing factor in the development of this condition?

The most common mechanism of injury for CCS is a hyperextension injury of the cervical spine. Other potential contributing factors in the development of CCS include cervical spondylosis, narrowing or congenital defect of the spinal canal, tumor, rheumatoid arthritis or syringomyelia. CCS predominantly affects the population over 50 years of age with a greater incidence in men.

## Confirmation

### What is the most likely clinical presentation?

CCS presents with motor loss that is greater in the upper extremities than the lower extremities and is most severe distally in the upper extremities. This presentation is due to the damage that occurs within the central location of the spinal cord. Sensory loss found below the level of the lesion is usually limited, but can be variable. Lumbar, thoracic, and cervical components proceed medially in order towards the center of the spinal cord. Sacral segments are usually unaffected since they are located laterally within the spinal cord. Bowel and bladder functions resolve in 55-85% of patients with CCS after six months.

### What laboratory or imaging studies would confirm the diagnosis?

MRI is used to assess spinal cord impingement from bone or disk. CT scan of the spine will assess spinal canal compromise and the degree of impingement. X-rays can be utilized to assess potential fractures, dislocations, and degree of spondylolitic deterioration.

### What additional information should be obtained to confirm the diagnosis?

Diagnosis is made using results of MRI, CT scan, and X-ray findings. Information may be obtained from past medical history and mechanism of injury that usually supports the diagnosis of CCS.

## Examination

### What history should be documented?

Important areas to explore include past medical history, medications, family history, current symptoms, mechanism of injury, social history and habits, occupation, leisure activities, and social support system.

### What test/measures are most appropriate?

**Aerobic capacity and endurance:** autonomic responses to positional changes, assessment of vital signs at rest/activity

**Arousal, attention, and cognition:** examine mental status, learning ability, memory, motivation

**Assistive and adaptive devices:** analysis of components and safety of a device, wheelchair prescription

**Community and work integration:** analysis of community, work, and leisure activities

**Environmental, home, and work barriers:** analysis of current and potential barriers or hazards

**Gait, locomotion, and balance:** static and dynamic balance in sitting and standing, safety during gait with/without an assistive device, Berg Balance Scale, Tinetti Performance Oriented Mobility Assessment, wheelchair management

**Integumentary integrity:** skin assessment, American Spinal Injury Association (ASIA)-Standard Neurological Classification of Spinal Cord Injury Sensory Examination

**Motor function:** equilibrium and righting reactions, posture and balance in sitting

**Muscle performance:** ASIA-Standard Neurological Classification of Spinal Cord Injury Motor Examination, muscle tone examination

**Neuromotor development and sensory integration:** analysis of reflex movement patterns

**Pain:** assessment of neuropathic pain

**Posture:** analysis of resting and dynamic posture

**Range of motion:** active and passive range of motion

**Reflex integrity:** assessment of deep tendon and pathological reflexes (e.g., Babinski, ATNR)

**Self-care and home management:** assessment of functional capacity, Functional Independence Measure (FIM), Barthel Index

**Ventilation, respiration, and circulation:** breathing patterns, auscultation of the lungs and heart

# Central Cord Syndrome

### What additional findings are likely with this patient?

Each patient with CCS will present differently based on location and extent of injury to the spinal cord. Potential side effects and complications include autonomic dysreflexia, spasticity, neurogenic bladder and bowel, allodynia, and pressure ulcers.

## Management

### What is the most effective management of this patient?

Rehabilitation services are initiated once the patient is medically stable. Medical management should include physiatry, physical therapy, occupational therapy, vocational counseling, and social services. Methylprednisolone should be administered within eight hours of injury to assist with neurologic recovery. Other pharmacological intervention may include blood pressure medication to combat autonomic dysreflexia, antispasticity medication for treatment of spasticity, anticonvulsants for treatment of neurogenic pain, prophylactic anticoagulants, and antidepressants if warranted.

Physical therapy intervention should include patient and caregiver education, range of motion, strengthening, endurance activities, balance retraining, proximal stabilization exercises, and functional mobility based on the patient's current functional status. Adaptive devices may be required to assist with overall mobility. If a patient ambulates, a platform attachment walker may initially be indicated since hand function is usually poor for grasp. Surgical intervention is rare, but may be indicated if compression within the spinal cord persists or progress ceases without cause.

### What home care regimen should be recommended?

A home care regimen should include a continuation of exercise, endurance, and functional mobility training based on the patient's current functional abilities. Outpatient physical therapy may be warranted and should modify the home program as necessary.

## Outcome

### What is the likely outcome of a course in physical therapy?

Physical therapy can assist a patient with CCS to attain maximum functional outcome based on level and extent of injury. Overall outcome, however, is based on age, motivation, compliance, and extent of injury.

### What are the long-term effects of the patient's condition?

CCS is the most common incomplete spinal cord lesion and accounts for approximately 30% of overall incomplete tetraplegia. Statistics indicate 77% of patients with CCS will ambulate, 53% will gain bowel and bladder control, and 42% regain some hand function. Older patients do not tend to recover as well as younger ones. Favorable long-term prognostic factors for a good outcome include early hand function, improvement of strength in all extremities during the inpatient stay, and little to no lower extremity involvement.

## Comparison

### What are the distinguishing characteristics of a similar condition?

Anterior cord syndrome (ACS) normally affects two-thirds of the spinal cord and can occur from a cervical flexion injury or anterior spinal artery embolization. There is a complete loss of motor function as well as pain and temperature below the level of the lesion due to damage of the spinothalamic and corticospinal tracts. Preservation of the posterior columns allow for intact vibration and proprioception. ACS has the worst prognosis for all the spinal cord syndromes with only 10-15% of patients achieving functional recovery.

## Clinical Scenarios

### Scenario One

A 22-year-old female is admitted to the rehabilitation floor with CCS secondary to a MVA. She has some motion in her lower extremities, shoulders, and trace motion at the elbows. She only wants to practice walking and refuses therapy for any other treatment. She also is currently refusing any form of adaptive equipment for use during ambulation and with dressing. The patient is currently living with her friend and planned to move out of state in six weeks. She is employed as a teacher assistant at a local middle school.

### Scenario Two

A 79-year-old male is diagnosed with CCS after being admitted through the emergency room secondary to a fall down his basement steps. He complains of severe neck pain and currently is not able to initiate movement in all four extremities. He is anxious and wants to return home to his second floor apartment as soon as he can. He misses his wife of 60 years who he has cared for since her stroke three years ago.

# Cerebral Palsy

## Diagnosis

### What condition produces a patient's symptoms?

Cerebral palsy (CP) is an umbrella term used to describe a group of non-progressive movement disorders that result from brain damage. CP is the most common cause of permanent disability in children.

### An injury was most likely sustained to which structure?

There is a wide variety of neurological damage that can occur with injury. Autopsy reports have indicated lesions that include hemorrhage below the lining of the ventricles, damage to the central nervous system that caused neuropathy and anoxia, and hypoxia that caused encephalopathy. Hypoxic and ischemic injuries disrupt normal metabolism that results in global damage to the developing fetus. CP is classified by neurological dysfunction and extremity involvement. Spastic CP involves upper motor neuron damage; athetoid CP involves damage to the cerebellum, cerebellar pathways or both.

## Inference

### What is the most likely contributing factor in the development of this condition?

The etiology may be multifactorial and is sometimes unknown. Risk factors are categorized as prenatal (80%) or perinatal and postnatal (20%) cases. Prenatal risk factors include Rh incompatibility, maternal malnutrition, hypothyroidism, infection, diabetes, and chromosome abnormalities. Perinatal factors include multiple or premature births, breech delivery, low birth weight, prolapsed cord, placenta abruption, and asphyxia. Postnatal factors include CVA, head trauma, neonatal infection, and brain tumor. The most common causative factor of CP is prenatal cerebral hypoxia.

## Confirmation

### What is the most likely clinical presentation?

CP is the second most common neurological impairment seen in children (following mental retardation). CP is a neuromuscular disorder of posture and controlled movement, however, clinical presentation is highly variable based on the area and extent of CNS damage. A child may present with high tone, low tone or athetoid movement. CP is classified as monoplegia (one involved extremity), hemiplegia (unilateral involvement of the upper and lower extremities), and quadriplegia (involvement of all extremities). CP is also classified as mild, moderate, and severe. General characteristics include motor delays, abnormal muscle tone and motor control, reflex abnormalities, poor postural control, high risk for hip dislocations, and balance impairments. Intellect, vision, hearing, and perceptual skills are usually altered in conjunction with CP. All other characteristics of CP are classification dependent.

### What laboratory or imaging studies would confirm the diagnosis?

If CP is suspected through clinical findings, including seizures, an electroencephalography (EEG) may be performed. X-ray of the hip may rule out hip dislocation; blood and urine tests can be used to investigate a metabolic cause of CP. Observation usually will diagnose CP secondary to the observed outward characteristics.

### What additional information should be obtained to confirm the diagnosis?

Diagnosis of CP is regularly confirmed through an extensive neurological evaluation, patient observation, and patient history including developmental progress, and the presence of pathological reflexes. Differential diagnosis is performed to rule out other potential disorders.

## Examination

### What history should be documented?

Important areas to explore include past medical history, risk factors, maternal course of pregnancy, medications, family history, current characteristics, social history, and social support system.

### What test/measures are most appropriate?

**Aerobic capacity and endurance:** assessment of vital signs at rest and with activity, auscultation of the lungs

**Arousal, attention, and cognition:** examine mental status, learning ability, memory, motivation

**Assistive and adaptive devices:** analysis of components and safety of a device

**Environmental, home, and work barriers:** analysis of current and potential barriers or hazards

**Gait, locomotion, and balance:** static/dynamic balance

**Integumentary integrity:** skin assessment, assessment of sensation

**Joint integrity and mobility:** assessment of hyper- and hypomobility of a joint

**Motor function:** equilibrium and righting reactions, coordination, posture and balance, sensorimotor integration, Barthel Index, Bayley Scale of Infant Development, Bruininks-Oseretsky Test of Motor Proficiency, Alberta Infant Motor Scale, Pediatric Evaluation of Disability Inventory

**Muscle performance:** muscle tone assessment, strength assessment if appropriate

**Neuromotor development and sensory integration:** analysis of reflex movement patterns, assessment of involuntary movements, sensory integration tests, gross and fine motor skills, developmental milestones

**Orthotic, protective, and supportive devices:** analysis of components of a device

## Cerebral Palsy

**Pain:** adapted pain scale
**Posture:** analysis of resting and dynamic posture
**Range of motion:** active and passive range of motion, assessment of contractures
**Reflex integrity:** assessment of deep tendon and pathological reflexes (e.g., Babinski, ATNR, Moro)
**Sensory integrity:** proprioception and kinesthesia
**Ventilation, respiration, and circulation:** breathing patterns, respiratory strength, accessory muscle utilization

### What additional findings are likely with this patient?

Specific additional findings are dependent on the classification and extent of CP. Generally, complications can include aspiration, pneumonia, contractures, scoliosis, and constipation. Mental retardation and epilepsy are present in 50-60% of children diagnosed with CP. Common co-morbidities include learning disabilities, seizure disorders, vision and hearing impairments, bowel and bladder dysfunction, microcephalus, and hydrocephalus. Secondary impairments may include psychosocial issues for the patient and family members.

## Management

### What is the most effective management of this patient?

Effective medical management of CP requires a life-long team approach. Pharmacological intervention may require antianxiety, antispasticity, and anticonvulsant medications. Physical therapy for CP often uses neurodevelopmental treatment and sensory integration techniques. Treatment should include normalization of tone, patient and caregiver education, motor learning, developmental milestones, positioning, stretching, strengthening, balance, and mobility skills. Adaptive equipment, specialized wheelchair seating, and orthotic prescription may be indicated. Surgical management may be required and include hip correction, contracture release, motor point block, dorsal rhizotomy or correction of scoliosis.

### What home care regimen should be recommended?

A home care regimen for a patient with CP is also a life-long process that will require ongoing modification to meet the progression of goals. Family and caregiver involvement is vital for patients with moderate to severe CP. A home program may include patient and caregiver education, exercise, positioning, stretching, mobility training, and strengthening.

## Outcome

### What is the likely outcome of a course in physical therapy?

Physical therapy will attempt to maximize a patient's level of current function and prevent secondary loss. If a patient is going to ambulate, this will usually occur by the age of eight. The ability or inability to ambulate will have a large impact on the direction and goals of therapeutic intervention.

### What are the long-term effects of the patient's condition?

CP is a non-progressive, but permanent condition. The long-term effects and overall functional outcome depend on the extent of injury, associated impairments, and caregiver support. Prognosis for mild to moderate CP is a near normal lifespan. Fifty percent of children with severe CP die by the age of ten.

## Comparison

### What are the distinguishing characteristics of a similar condition?

Arthrogryposis multiplex congenita (AMC) occurs in utero and is also considered to be non-progressive. AMC is a neuromuscular syndrome classified into three forms. The infant is born with multiple contractures and may have fibrous bands that developed in place of muscle. A patient with AMC should have a normal life expectancy and is typically of normal intelligence. It is usually difficult for these individuals to live independently due to their level of physical disability.

## Clinical Scenarios

### Scenario One

A two-year-old female diagnosed with moderate spastic quadriplegia is seen in physical therapy. She is delayed in developmental milestones and beginning to acquire contractures. The parents are very supportive and the child appears happy and cooperative. The child's chart indicates normal intelligence.

### Scenario Two

A nine-year-old male is seen in physical therapy at the request of his parents. The patient is diagnosed with moderate low tone quadriplegia, has minimal impairments with intelligence, and has acquired a 30-degree left thoracic scoliosis. The parents requested the evaluation since the child remains nonambulatory.

# Cerebrovascular Accident

## Diagnosis

### What condition produces a patient's symptoms?

Cerebrovascular accident (CVA) occurs when there is an interruption of cerebral circulation that results in cerebral insufficiency, destruction of surrounding brain tissue, and subsequent neurological deficit. The ischemia occurs from either a stroke in evolution (the infarct slowly progresses over one to two days) or as a completed stroke (an abrupt infarct with immediate neurological deficits).

### An injury was most likely sustained to which structure?

CVA results from prolonged ischemia to an artery within the brain. This condition can cause subsequent neurological damage relative to the size and location of the infarct. Disruption of blood flow to a certain artery will lead to damage of a specific area of the brain and its functions. There are different types of CVA that include ischemic stroke (thrombus, embolus, lacunar) and hemorrhagic stroke (intracerebral, subdural, subarachnoid).

## Inference

### What is the most likely contributing factor in the development of this condition?

The primary risk factors for CVA are classified as modifiable and non-modifiable. Modifiable factors include hypertension, atherosclerosis, heart disease, diabetes, elevated cholesterol, smoking, and obesity. Hypertension is the most prevalent modifiable cause of CVA. Non-modifiable risk factors include age, race, family history, and sex. Age constitutes the greatest risk for CVA, in fact 73% of patients sustaining a stroke are greater than 65 years of age.

## Confirmation

### What is the most likely clinical presentation?

It is estimated there are four million stroke survivors living today. The clinical presentation of a CVA is determined by the location and extent of the infarct. Typical characteristics can include hemiplegia or hemiparesis, sensory, visual, and perceptual impairments, balance abnormalities, dysphagia, aphasia, cognitive deficits, incontinence, and emotional lability.

### What laboratory or imaging studies would confirm the diagnosis?

Computed tomography can confirm an area of infarct in the brain and its vascular origin, however, it can present as negative for up to a few days after the event. MRI allows for the diagnosis of ischemia within the brain almost immediately after onset. Positron emission tomography (PET) can provide information regarding cerebral perfusion and cell function. Ultrasonography identifies areas of diminished blood flow in vessels and angiography may identify a clot and determine if surgical intervention is necessary.

### What additional information should be obtained to confirm the diagnosis?

A chest x-ray may be warranted to rule out lung disease, while an electrocardiogram is used to examine potential cardiac abnormalities. Diagnosis is usually based upon patient history, physical and neurological examinations, symptoms, and diagnostic testing.

## Examination

### What history should be documented?

Important areas to explore include past medical history, medications, risk factor profile, current health status, social history and habits, occupation, living environment, and social support system.

### What test/measures are most appropriate?

**Arousal, attention, and cognition:** examine mental status, learning ability, memory, motivation, Mini-Mental State Exam, Boston Diagnostic Aphasia Examination

**Assistive and adaptive devices:** analysis of components and safety of a device

**Gait, locomotion, and balance:** static and dynamic balance in sitting and standing, safety during gait with an assistive device, Berg Balance Scale, Tinetti Performance Oriented Mobility Assessment, Functional Ambulation Profile

**Integumentary integrity:** skin and sensation assessment

**Motor function:** equilibrium and righting reactions, coordination, motor assessment scales

**Muscle performance:** muscle tone assessment, assessment of active movement, Stroke Rehabilitation Assessment of Movement (STREAM)

**Neuromotor development and sensory integration:** assess involuntary movements, sensory integration, gross and fine motor skills, reflex movement patterns

**Orthotic, protective, and supportive devices:** analysis of components of a device, analysis of movement while wearing a device

**Posture:** analysis of resting and dynamic posture

**Pain:** pain perception assessment scale

**Range of motion:** active and passive range of motion

**Reflexes:** assessment of pathological reflexes (e.g., Babinski, ATNR)

**Self-care and home management:** assessment of functional capacity, Rankin Scale, NIH Stroke Scale, Functional Independence Measure (FIM)

**Sensory integrity:** proprioception and kinesthesia

# Cerebrovascular Accident

## What additional findings are likely with this patient?

A patient with a left CVA may present with weakness or paralysis to the right side, impaired processing, heightened frustration, aphasia, dysphagia, motor apraxia, and right hemianopsia. A patient with a right CVA may present with weakness or paralysis to the left side, poor attention span, impaired awareness and judgment, spatial deficits, memory deficits, left inattention, emotional lability, impulsive behavior, and left hemianopsia. Coma and death are the most severe consequences of a CVA. It is common for patients post CVA to have residual complications and deficits that persist.

## Management

### What is the most effective management of this patient?

Medical management will initially include medically stabilizing the patient through medication and surgical intervention. Pharmacological intervention can include thrombolytic agents, anticoagulants (contraindicated for hemorrhagic CVA), diuretics, antihypertensives, and potential long-term use of aspirin. Respiratory care must also be a priority during acute rehabilitation. Physical therapy during the acute phase focuses on positioning, pressure relief, sensory awareness and integration, ROM, weight bearing, facilitation, muscle re-education, balance, and postural control. The therapist is responsible for implementing the most appropriate therapeutic strategies based on the degree of impairment. There are many approaches to neurological rehabilitation that include, but are not limited to Bobath's Neuromuscular Developmental Treatment (NDT), motor control, Brunnstrom's Movement Therapy in Hemiplegia, Rood, and Kabat, Knott, and Voss' Proprioceptive Neuromuscular Facilitation (PNF). Many therapists integrate facets from multiple approaches based on the patient's response to selected interventions.

### What home care regimen should be recommended?

Approximately 75% of patients that have experienced a CVA return home at various levels of functional mobility. The majority of patients require ongoing therapy services as part of their home care regimen. A therapeutic program should be designed for a patient to continue at home independently or with the required level of assistance. Fall prevention, control of spasticity, endurance training, and optimizing functional mobility are important components of a successful home program.

## Outcome

### What is the likely outcome of a course in physical therapy?

A patient that experiences neurological deficits due to a CVA may require physical therapy to assist with motor re-education, sensory stimulation, and functional mobility. The outcome is dependent on the patient's overall health, level of cognition and motivation, motor recovery, residual deficits, and family support.

### What are the long-term effects of the patient's condition?

The effects of a CVA can be quite diverse ranging from spontaneous recovery to permanent disability requiring compensatory strategies and techniques in order to function. The first three months of recovery typically reveals the most measurable neurologic recovery and is usually a good indicator of the long-term outcome. Long-term outcome is based on several factors including the site and extent of CVA, premorbid status, age, potential for plasticity of the nervous system, and motivation. Research indicates that a patient can continue to improve the control of movement and show progress for an average of two to three years post CVA.

## Comparison

### What are the distinguishing characteristics of a similar condition?

A transient ischemic attack (TIA) is also characterized by diminished blood supply to the brain, however, it is transient. Although the patient may present with similar symptoms of a CVA, the symptoms last for only a brief period of time. Unlike a CVA, the TIA does not cause permanent residual neurological deficits. A TIA is an indication, however, of future risk for a CVA.

## Clinical Scenarios

### Scenario One

A 43-year-old male is diagnosed with a left hemorrhagic CVA due to an aneurysm of the middle cerebral artery. The patient resides with his wife and two teenage sons.

### Scenario Two

A 79-year-old female is diagnosed with a right CVA involving the anterior cerebral artery. The patient was unconscious for two days and is functioning at a very low-level. The patient was residing in an independent living facility where she had meals provided for her in the dining area.

# Congenital Torticollis

## Diagnosis

### What condition produces a patient's symptoms?

Congenital torticollis is a condition that causes the neck to involuntarily unilaterally contract to one side secondary to contraction of the sternocleidomastoid muscle. The head is laterally flexed toward the contracted muscle, the chin faces the opposite direction, and there may be facial asymmetries. The word torticollis means twisted neck. It is a disease, but also a symptom of many conditions.

### An injury was most likely sustained to which structure?

Congenital torticollis is not usually seen immediately at birth. Muscle injury may be due to birth trauma, breech position in utero or other forms of intrauterine malpositioning. Infants born with torticollis appear healthy at delivery, however, over days or weeks they develop swelling over the injured sternocleidomastoid.

## Inference

### What is the most likely contributing factor in the development of this condition?

The exact etiology of congenital torticollis is unknown, however, congenital torticollis may be caused by local trauma to the soft tissues of the neck just before or during delivery. The most common hypothesis is that birth trauma with resultant hematoma formation results in muscular contracture. Typically children with congenital torticollis have had breech or difficult forceps delivery. The fibrosis that develops in the muscle may be due to venous occlusion and pressure on the neck in the birth canal secondary to skull and neck position. Another theory includes malpositioning in utero resulting in intrauterine compartment syndrome.

## Confirmation

### What is the most likely clinical presentation?

The patient's head is laterally flexed towards the shortened muscle's side and the chin is pointed toward the opposite shoulder. Intermittent painful spasms of the sternocleidomastoid, trapezius, and other neck muscles may occur. The neck movements vary from jerky to smooth. The first sign may be a firm nontender enlargement of the sternocleidomastoid muscle visible at birth or within the infant's first few weeks of life. This mass, which is usually localized near the clavicular attachment of the sternocleidomastoid muscle, enlarges during the first few weeks of life, and then gradually decreases in size. Usually, the mass disappears by the sixth month of life and the only remaining clinical finding is the contracture of the sternocleidomastoid muscle that creates the torticollis posturing.

## What laboratory or imaging studies would confirm the diagnosis?

Cervical spine x-rays are used to assess potential fracture or subluxation. A CT scan or MRI of the cervical spine can identify the presence of a potential neck mass. Electromyography (EMG) study may be useful in defining the degree of muscle or nerve involvement.

## What additional information should be obtained to confirm the diagnosis?

The presence of the mass over the sternocleidomastoid along with the classic posturing will confirm the presence of congenital torticollis.

## Examination

### What history should be documented?

Important areas to explore include history of labor and delivery, family history, medications, current health status, and social support system.

### What test/measures are most appropriate?

**Arousal, attention, and cognition:** examine level of consciousness and alertness
**Cranial nerve integrity:** assessment of muscle innervation by the cranial nerves, dermatome assessment
**Environmental, home, and work barriers:** analysis of current and potential barriers or hazards in the home
**Integumentary integrity:** skin assessment, assessment of sensation
**Joint integrity and mobility:** assessment of hyper- and hypomobility of a joint, soft tissue swelling and inflammation
**Motor function:** motor assessment scales, coordination, Barthel Index, Bayley Scale of Infant Development, Denver II Scale, Neonatal Behavioral Assessment, Alberta Infant Motor Scale
**Neuromotor development and sensory integration:** analysis of reflex movement patterns, assessment of involuntary movements, sensory integration tests
**Posture:** analysis of resting and dynamic posture
**Range of motion:** active and passive range of motion
**Reflex integrity:** assessment of deep tendon and pathological reflexes (e.g., Babinski, ATNR)

# Congenital Torticollis

## What additional findings are likely with this patient?

Up to 20% of children with congenital torticollis have congenital dysplasia of the hips. In many instances, these infants will also present with facial asymmetries and plagiocephaly or flattening of the skull.

## Management

### What is the most effective management of this patient?

Congenital torticollis is usually treated with non-operative intervention for 12-24 months before considering surgical intervention. Pharmacological intervention may include non-steroidal anti-inflammatory drugs (NSAIDs), benzodiazepines and other muscle relaxants, anticholinergics, and local intramuscular injections of botulinum toxin or phenol. Physical therapy includes family/caregiver education and teaching, passive stretching exercises to the sternocleidomastoid and upper trapezius muscles, massage, local heat, analgesics, sensory biofeedback, and transcutaneous electrical nerve stimulation (TENS). Active range of motion with subsequent strengthening is also indicated to correct the infant's positioning of their head. Family training is extremely beneficial if there is consistency with handling and proper positioning during feeding and sleeping in order to promote stretch and active motion of the sternocleidomastoid muscle. If conservative treatment fails, surgical intervention will consist of unipolar sternocleidomastoid release, bipolar sternocleidomastoid release or selective denervation. Physical therapy is indicated after surgery and should include manual stretching of the neck to maintain the overcorrected position. Manual stretching should be continued three times daily for 3-6 months. A cervical collar may be used for the first 6-12 weeks after surgery.

### What home care regimen should be recommended?

The family must continue with the stretching program and the correct handling techniques that are recommended by the therapist. The family will need to include proper positioning for the infant's sleep and alert times in order to maximize the benefits of the intervention.

## Outcome

### What is the likely outcome of a course in physical therapy?

Studies indicate that between 85-90% of patients with congenital torticollis respond to conservative treatment and passive stretching within the first year of life. The best results for conservative management require the child to have had conservative treatment prior to the age of one. If surgical intervention is required, physical therapy will be required after surgery with an expected positive outcome for the patient.

## What are the long-term effects of the patient's condition?

If a child is left untreated, congenital torticollis could have detrimental effects including the impairment of normal growth and development. The vast majority of children with congenital torticollis that receive conservative management are expected to fully recover and live a normal life.

## Comparison

### What are the distinguishing characteristics of a similar condition?

Torticollis can also be acquired at an older age and presents in different forms. Acute wryneck is a term to describe a common type of torticollis that develops overnight without provocation. It is a self-limiting process and usually the symptoms subside within one to two weeks. Infectious torticollis may occur when the surrounding tissues become infected such as with a retropharyngeal abscess, nasopharyngeal abscess, tonsillitis, and sinusitis.

## Clinical Scenarios

### Scenario One

A three-week-old infant is referred to outpatient physical therapy with a moderate right torticollis. There is a mass felt over the sternocleidomastoid muscle belly. The parents are concerned with this diagnosis and are very eager to assist with the infant's program. The mother is at home during the day and they have three other children at home.

### Scenario Two

A child is referred to physical therapy status post unipolar sternocleidomastoid release two weeks ago. The child is 18 months old and was unsuccessful with conservative treatment for a significant left torticollis. The child resides with his foster mother in a studio apartment. The mother works full-time and the child participates in full-time daycare.

## Congestive Heart Failure

### Diagnosis

#### What condition produces a patient's symptoms?

Congestive heart failure (CHF) occurs when the heart can no longer meet the metabolic demands of the body. The heart's inability to pump a sufficient amount of blood occurs when there is insufficient or defective cardiac filling and/or impaired contraction and emptying of the heart. The impairment in cardiac output causes the body to compensate for this deficit and this results in an increase in blood volume, cardiac filling pressure, heart rate, and cardiac muscle mass.

#### An injury was most likely sustained to which structure?

CHF is not an independent disease process but rather a symptom of pathology within the heart muscle itself or in the cardiac valves. Injury within the heart can be left-sided, right-sided or both. The abnormal retention of fluids and diminished blood flow causes further stress and injury to the cardiac system.

### Inference

#### What is the most likely contributing factor in the development of this condition?

There are many pathologies (reversible and irreversible) that can contribute to CHF. Common etiologies shown to contribute to CHF include arrhythmia (e.g., atrial fibrillation), pulmonary embolism, hypertension, valvular heart disease, myocarditis, unstable angina, renal failure, medication-induced problems, high salt intake, and severe anemia. CHF occurs when there is a decrease in cardiac output, abnormalities in skeletal muscle metabolism, impaired left ventricular function or all of the above.

### Confirmation

#### What is the most likely clinical presentation?

A patient with CHF will initially show signs of tachycardia. Other signs include venous congestion, high catecholamine levels, and finally impaired cardiac output. As the severity of CHF increases, signs of venous congestion usually become apparent. Left-sided heart failure is generally associated with signs of pulmonary venous congestion; right-sided heart failure is associated with signs of systemic venous congestion. Impairment to either ventricle can affect the other, leading to both systemic and pulmonary venous congestion. A patient may present with pulmonary edema, nocturnal dyspnea, orthopnea, S3 gallop, dry cough, exertional dyspnea with low level exercise, sudden weight gain, possible cyanotic extremities, cardiac hypertrophy, and shortness of breath.

#### What laboratory or imaging studies would confirm the diagnosis?

Lab tests including urinalysis and a CBC count that includes electrolyte, thyroid stimulating hormone, blood urea nitrogen (BUN), and serum creatinine levels should be performed. A chest x-ray, electrocardiogram, and echocardiogram are also recommended. A Doppler echocardiogram can determine systolic and diastolic performance, the cardiac output (ejection fraction), and pulmonary artery and ventricular filling pressures.

#### What additional information should be obtained to confirm the diagnosis?

A patient history and administration of cardiac questionnaires will assist with diagnosis of CHF. In the Framingham classification system, the diagnosis of CHF requires that either two major criteria or one major and two minor criteria be present concurrently. The New York Heart Association Functional Capacity Classification also classifies heart disease based on symptomology as it relates to physical activity.

### Examination

#### What history should be documented?

Important areas to explore include past medical history, medications, current health status, nutritional status, social history and habits, occupation, living environment, and social support system.

#### What test/measures are most appropriate?

**Aerobic capacity and endurance:** assessment of vital signs at rest and with activity, perceived exertion scale, pulse oximetry, auscultation of the lungs

**Anthropometric characteristics:** circumferential measurements

**Arousal, attention, and cognition:** examine mental status, learning ability, memory, motivation

**Community and work integration:** analysis of community, work, and leisure activities

**Environmental, home, and work barriers:** analysis of current and potential barriers or hazards

**Gait, locomotion, and balance:** static and dynamic balance in sitting and standing, safety during gait with/without an assistive device

**Integumentary integrity:** skin assessment

**Muscle performance:** strength assessment

**Pain:** pain perception assessment scale, VAS

**Range of motion:** active and passive range of motion

**Self-care and home management:** assessment of functional capacity, Functional Independence Measure

**Sensory integrity:** proprioception and kinesthesia

**Ventilation, respiration, and circulation:** assessment of cough and clearance of secretions, breathing patterns, vital capacity, perceived exertion scale, pulse oximetry, palpation of pulses, auscultation of the lungs and heart

# Congestive Heart Failure

## What additional findings are likely with this patient?

Diagnoses such as left ventricular infarction, aortic or mitral valve disease, and hypertension create pulmonary congestion that may result in left-sided CHF. Over time, however, fluid accumulation spreads and ankle edema, congestive hepatomegaly, ascites, and pleural effusion occur. This leads the patient to develop right-sided CHF as well. Later stages of CHF are characterized by symptoms of low cardiac output.

## Management

### What is the most effective management of this patient?

A patient with CHF will be treated based on the root cause of the heart failure. Medical management includes the use of diuretics, nitrates, analgesics, and angiotensin-converting enzyme inhibitor agents. Medications play a vital role in the optimal management of this disease process. Therapists must be aware of the potential side effects such as digitalis toxicity when treating this population. The patient may be referred to physical therapy for generalized conditioning and mobility. Primary goals include improving exercise tolerance and increasing knowledge of the disease process. Therapeutic intervention has to be individualized by each patient since the etiology, current medications, and overall health play a role in the plan of care. Walking is commonly used to initiate an exercise program with cardiac patients. Patients can progress their overall endurance following their own heart rate and perceived exertion guidelines. Caregiver education and instruction may also be appropriate. Psychosocial support, nutritional counseling (no salt diet and no alcohol), and caretaker education are also important components of the plan of care.

### What home care regimen should be recommended?

A patient will usually follow a similar program at home once they are discharged from the hospital or in addition to their outpatient therapy. The patient should continue energy conservation and pacing techniques with all activities. The family and patient must be fully educated as to the signs and symptoms of concern as well as potential medication toxicity.

## Outcome

### What is the likely outcome of a course in physical therapy?

A patient can live with CHF and should benefit from physical therapy in order to improve endurance and strength after a decline in function from hospitalization or bed rest. Physical therapy will improve skeletal muscle function, blood flow, metabolic capacity, and overall exercise tolerance. Physical therapy, however, will not cure CHF or its cause.

## What are the long-term effects of the patient's condition?

CHF is a common disorder. Approximately 4.6 million Americans are being treated for CHF, and over 500,000 new cases are diagnosed each year. The prevalence of CHF increases significantly with age, occurring in 1-2% of persons aged 50-59 years and in up to 10% of persons older than 75 years. Despite the heart's compensatory mechanisms, the ability of the heart to contract and relax progressively worsens and eventually fails. Thirty-year data from the Framingham heart study demonstrated a median survival of 3.2 years for males and 5.4 years for females after diagnosis.

## Comparison

### What are the distinguishing characteristics of a similar condition?

Cor pulmonale is a form of right-sided heart failure but is normally seen as a consequence of chronic obstructive pulmonary disease. Sustained hypoxia produces an increase in pulmonary artery pressure that leads to right ventricular hypertrophy and finally, right-sided heart failure. When the right side fails, the left side does not receive adequate amounts of blood and then cannot sustain a normal cardiac output. This is not congestive in nature, however, as there is no fluid build up within the lungs. The right-sided heart failure also does not present with an audible S3 gallop.

## Clinical Scenarios

### Scenario One

A 69-year-old male has been hospitalized for five days with congestive heart failure. He was diagnosed last year with the condition and has been doing well on medication. He started having shortness of breath and noted a six pound weight gain. His medications have been adjusted and he is motivated to get home to his wife. The physician requests a physical therapy consult for baseline data and a home exercise program.

### Scenario Two

An 82-year-old female resides in a nursing home since her husband who cared for her passed away last summer. She was diagnosed with a left CVA three years ago that resulted in moderate weakness of her right upper extremity and as a result she requires assistance for ADLs. She requires a quad cane and supervision for ambulation. She has been in bed for the last month due to pneumonia and she currently has been diagnosed with CHF.

# Cystic Fibrosis

## Diagnosis

### What condition produces a patient's symptoms?

Cystic fibrosis (CF) is an inherited disease that affects the ion transport of the exocrine glands resulting in impairment of the hepatic, digestive, respiratory, and reproductive systems. The disease causes the exocrine glands to overproduce thick mucus (that causes subsequent obstruction), overproduce normal secretions or overproduce sodium and chloride.

### An injury was most likely sustained to which structure?

CF affects multi-systems within the body, however, the respiratory and gastrointestinal systems are usually the most involved in the disease process. There is an underlying impermeability of epithelial cells to chloride that results in viscosity of mucous gland secretions within the lungs, sweat glands, pancreas, and intestines. CF creates an elevation of sodium chloride and pancreatic enzyme insufficiency.

## Inference

### What is the most likely contributing factor in the development of this condition?

CF is an autosomal recessive genetic disorder (both parents are carriers of the defective gene) and is located on the long arm of chromosome seven. This disorder creates an abnormality in the CF transmembrane conductance regulator (CFTR) protein. CFTR normally is involved with the process that allows for chloride to pass through the plasma membrane of epithelial cells. It is estimated that 5% of the population carry a recessive gene for CF.

## Confirmation

### What is the most likely clinical presentation?

CF is the most common lethal genetic disorder affecting Caucasian children in the United States. Incidence is estimated at 1:2,500 births for Caucasians compared to 1:17,000 births for African Americans. CF can be diagnosed shortly after birth, however, it is sometimes not diagnosed for years. The most consistent symptom is the finding of high concentrations of sodium and chloride in the sweat. Parents will notice a salty taste when kissing their child. Other symptoms vary depending on the systems that are affected by the disease and the course of progression. These systems include pulmonary, gastrointestinal, digestive (liver, intestinal, pancreatic), genitourinary, and musculoskeletal impairments. Early symptoms may include a persistent cough, salty skin, sputum production, wheezing, poor weight gain, and recurrent infections.

### What laboratory or imaging studies would confirm the diagnosis?

Neonates' meconium can be tested as a screening tool for increased albumin. The quantitative pilocarpine iontophoresis sweat test is the sole diagnostic tool in determining the presence of CF. Sodium and chloride amounts greater than 60 mEq/l (standard value is 40 mEq/l) is a positive diagnosis for CF. The sweat test should be performed twice to ensure accuracy.

### What additional information should be obtained to confirm the diagnosis?

Additional information in the diagnosis of CF is found through a positive family history, genetic screening of the parents, a previous diagnosis of failure to thrive, and in the manifestation of symptoms.

## Examination

### What history should be documented?

Important areas to explore include past medical history (if diagnosed after birth), medications, current health status, developmental milestones, living environment, and social support system.

### What test/measures are most appropriate?

**Aerobic capacity and endurance:** assessment of vital signs at rest and with activity, perceived exertion scale
**Arousal, attention, and cognition:** examine mental status, learning ability, memory, motivation
**Assistive and adaptive devices:** analysis of components and safety of a device
**Integumentary integrity:** skin assessment, sweat test findings, clubbing of the digits
**Muscle performance:** active motion, strength assessment
**Posture:** analysis of resting and dynamic posture, especially thorax and shoulder girdle
**Range of motion:** active and passive range of motion, chest wall mobility
**Self-care and home management:** functional capacity
**Ventilation, respiration, and circulation:** assess cough and clearance of secretions, pulmonary function testing (FEV$_1$ and FVC), pulse oximetry, auscultation of the lungs, accessory muscle utilization and vital capacity

# Cystic Fibrosis

## What additional findings are likely with this patient?

The most common complication of CF is an exacerbation of obstructive pulmonary disease. Pulmonary function testing results in a decreased forced expiratory volume ($FEV_1$) and forced vital capacity (FVC). The functional residual capacity (FRC) and residual volume (RV) become increased. Hypoxemia and hypercapnia develop due to the alteration in perfusion. Chronic pulmonary infections and poor absorption often lead to barrel chest, pectus carinatum, and kyphosis deformities. Approximately 90% of patients have pancreatic enzyme deficiency, degeneration, and eventual progressive fibrosis of the pancreas. This process interferes with digestion and absorption of nutrients. Airway obstruction can cause pulmonary hypertension, atelectasis, pneumonia, and lung abscess. Severe complications can include cirrhosis, diabetes mellitus, pneumothorax, cardiac pathology, pancreatitis, cor pulmonale, and intestinal obstruction.

## Management

### What is the most effective management of this patient?

Medical management of CF is a multidisciplinary approach that should focus on the quality of life, providing emotional and psychosocial support, and controlling symptoms. Nutritional support is necessary throughout the patient's life to ensure adequate nutrition. Pharmacological intervention is required to treat infections, thin mucus secretions, replace pancreatic enzymes, reduce inflammation, and assist with breathing. Psychological counseling is indicated as needed. Gene therapy is experimental and attempts to correct the defect in CF cells. Physical therapy intervention is essential for management of the disease. Chest physical therapy should be performed several times per day and includes bronchial drainage, percussion, vibration, breathing and assistive cough techniques, and ventilatory muscle training. Posture training, mobilization of the thorax, and breathing exercises must be incorporated into the overall program. A patient may also be trained to use autogenic drainage, a positive expiratory pressure (PEP) device or Flutter valve therapy to assist with independent bronchial drainage. General exercise and stretching are indicated to optimize overall function. Family and patient education are vital to the survival of the patient.

### What home care regimen should be recommended?

A home care regimen for a patient with CF requires an ongoing routine performing postural drainage and chest physical therapy several times each day. Family members are trained to provide this ongoing support at home. Mechanical percussors may be used to ease the time and energy spent on manual percussion by the care provider. Mechanical percussors also offer the patient control and independence with treatment. Physical conditioning including exercise and endurance training are indicated except with severe lung disease. Exercise programs may improve pulmonary function, increase maximal work capacity, improve mucus expectoration, and increase self-esteem.

## Outcome

### What is the likely outcome of a course in physical therapy?

A patient with CF will require intermittent physical therapy throughout his or her life. The goals of physical therapy are to maximize secretion clearance from the lungs, optimize pulmonary function, and maximize the patient's quality of life.

### What are the long-term effects of the patient's condition?

CF is a terminal disease, however, the median age of death has increased to 35 years of age due to early detection and comprehensive management. The most common cause of death for patients with CF remains respiratory failure. A child that initially presents with gastrointestinal symptoms generally has a good clinical course whereas a child that initially presents with pulmonary symptoms is more likely to clinically deteriorate at a faster pace. Males generally have a better prognosis than females.

## Comparison

### What are the distinguishing characteristics of a similar condition?

There is no other respiratory disease that is similar to the etiology of CF, however, chronic obstructive pulmonary disease (COPD) has similar lung characteristics. COPD is characterized by altered pulmonary function tests, difficulty with expiration, cough, sputum production, and physical damage to specific portions of the lungs. Chest physical therapy and pharmacological intervention are indicated for moderate to advanced COPD.

## Clinical Scenarios

### Scenario One

A four-week-old infant is referred to physical therapy after being diagnosed with CF. The infant has a pleasant disposition and does not have any observable discomfort, however, the parents are very anxious. The patient has three siblings that do not have CF.

### Scenario Two

A 26-year-old female with CF is referred to physical therapy with a severe respiratory infection. The patient recently moved into an apartment with her boyfriend and works 30 hours per week in a hair salon. Prior to the infection the patient was living at home and was able to manage the disease with occasional assistance from family members. The physical therapy referral is for chest physical therapy.

# Degenerative Spondylolisthesis

## Diagnosis

### What condition produces a patient's symptoms?

Spondylolisthesis is the forward slippage of one vertebra on the vertebra below. There are several types of spondylolisthesis classified by the actual cause for the slippage. Classifications include congenital, isthmic, degenerative, post-traumatic, and pathologic spondylolisthesis. Degenerative spondylolisthesis (DS) is caused by the weakening of joints that allows for forward slippage of one vertebral segment on the one below due to degenerative changes. These changes include segmental ligamentous instability and hypertrophic subluxating facet joints which can result in stenosis of the spinal canal.

### An injury was most likely sustained to which structure?

The most common site of DS is the L4-L5 level. The slippage causes cauda equina symptoms secondary to stenosis of the canal. It is theorized that ischemia and poor nourishment secondary to the stenosis deprives the associated spinal nerves and results in pain. The L5 nerve root is compressed in an L4-L5 olisthesis. Other structures that can be irritated include the intervertebral disk, posterior and anterior longitudinal ligaments, and vertebral periosteum and bone.

## Inference

### What is the most likely contributing factor in the development of this condition?

DS is caused by arthritis and degenerative changes in the spine. The intervertebral disk loses some of its ability to resist motion and as a result the vertebral facets increase in size and develop bone spurs to compensate. This condition can actually produce spinal stenosis and weaken the spine itself resulting in the slippage of a vertebrae. Since all structures of the spine remain intact the slippage is usually limited due to the secondary bony restraints of the spine.

## Confirmation

### What is the most likely clinical presentation?

DS usually affects individuals over 50 years of age. It is more common with African Americans and women also have a higher incidence of occurrence than men. Back pain is a primary symptom that is said to increase with exercise, lifting overhead, prolonged standing, getting out of bed or a car, walking up stairs or an incline, and positioning in extension. The pain may be severe and radiate depending on the area of stenosis secondary to the vertebral slippage. Sensory and motor loss may be significant and follow a myotomal and/or dermatomal distribution. Most patients do not have significant neurologic deficits, however, a few do experience severe changes.

### What laboratory or imaging studies would confirm the diagnosis?

Plain radiographs of the vertebral column are adequate to confirm the diagnosis of DS. CT scan or MRI may be indicated to rule out any other contributing conditions or to further assess nerve impingement.

### What additional information should be obtained to confirm the diagnosis?

Physical and neurological examinations in combination with a full medical history usually provide adequate information for probable diagnosis, however, X-rays are required for definitive diagnosis of DS.

## Examination

### What history should be documented?

Important areas to explore include past medical history and previous testing, medications, family history, current symptoms, current health status, social history and habits, occupation, leisure activities, and social support system.

### What test/measures are most appropriate?

**Arousal, attention, and cognition:** examine mental status, learning ability, memory, motivation

**Assistive and adaptive devices:** analysis of components and safety of a device

**Community and work integration:** analysis of community, work, and leisure activities

**Environmental, home, and work barriers:** analysis of current and potential barriers or hazards

**Ergonomics and body mechanics:** analysis of dexterity and coordination, evaluation of proper lifting techniques

**Gait, locomotion, and balance:** static and dynamic balance in sitting and standing, safety during gait with/without an assistive device, Functional Ambulation Profile

**Joint integrity and mobility:** assessment of hyper- and hypomobility of a joint, soft tissue swelling and inflammation

**Muscle performance:** strength assessment

**Pain:** pain perception assessment scale, visual analogue scale, assessment of muscle soreness

**Posture:** analysis of resting and dynamic posture

**Range of motion:** active and passive range of motion

**Reflex integrity:** assessment of deep tendon and pathological reflexes (e.g., Babinski, ATNR)

**Self-care and home management:** assessment of functional capacity

**Sensory integrity:** assessment of sensation

# Degenerative Spondylolisthesis

## What additional findings are likely with this patient?

A patient with DS may or may not have additional slippage of the vertebra over time. If the slippage of the vertebra worsens it does not necessarily correspond to an increase in symptoms. Symptoms may increase with or without marked degenerative changes and vice versa. A patient that does experience ongoing neurological deficits will require surgical intervention regardless of the amount of slippage.

## Management

### What is the most effective management of this patient?

Medical management of a patient diagnosed with DS should initially include education, medication, activity modification, and physical therapy intervention. Pharmacological intervention should include NSAIDs to decrease acute inflammation. Corticosteroids may be indicated for severe symptoms. Epidural steroid injections and selective nerve root injections are sometimes indicated if oral medications fail. Activity modification and rest should be instituted to further allow inflammation to subside and improve overall symptoms. Long-term bed rest, however, should be avoided. Once the acute phase has subsided physical therapy should begin. William's flexion exercises should be performed to strengthen the abdominals and reduce lumbar lordosis. Back school, modalities, postural education, and other exercises that provide core stabilization and increase flexibility should be included in the patient's program. External support such as bracing or wearing of a corset may relieve intradiscal pressure. Surgical intervention is only indicated if conservative treatment fails, the pain becomes disabling or significant neurological impairment exists. Surgical intervention usually involves decompression with or without spinal fusion.

### What home care regimen should be recommended?

A patient with DS should initially take NSAIDs and decrease overall activities to allow for a reduction in the acute symptoms. Once a patient is able to tolerate physical therapy the home care regimen should include prescribed exercises to improve abdominal strength and core stabilization, flexibility exercises, and proper positioning. Goals for the home program are to alleviate pain and improve function. A patient should only modify the home program per therapist instruction.

## Outcome

### What is the likely outcome of a course in physical therapy?

The majority of patients with DS are successful with conservative treatment that may include physical therapy, home program, bracing, and use of NSAIDs as needed.

### What are the long-term effects of the patient's condition?

The long-term effects of DS vary based on progression and advancement of the slipped vertebrae and/or progression of symptoms. Some patients may be able to manage pain and maintain function without any further associated pathology. If symptoms continue to progress, then surgical intervention may be required.

## Comparison

### What are the distinguishing characteristics of a similar condition?

Congenital spondylolisthesis is the slippage of one vertebra on the vertebra below due to an anomaly or defect in the fusion of the neural arch. This usually occurs in the upper sacral vertebral arches or at the L5 level. The condition is usually diagnosed during the growth spurts between 12 and 16 years of age. Patients are normally pain free prior to this point and begin to express complaints of back pain, "sciatica" pain, and other symptoms. There is a strong genetic association found in this type of spondylolisthesis.

## Clinical Scenarios

### Scenario One

A 65-year-old female is seen in physical therapy with a diagnosis of L5 degenerative spondylolisthesis. She complains of pain in her back that can occasionally radiate down her left leg. She resides with her husband in their two-story home and works part-time at a grocery store as a clerk. She also enjoys gardening, but has been having a difficult time with all activities in the last eight weeks secondary to pain.

### Scenario Two

A 74-year-old male two weeks status post spinal fusion is examined in a nursing home. The patient was diagnosed six months ago with DS, shortly after he began to exhibit neurological symptoms. The physician prescribes physical therapy daily to improve strength and functional independence.

# Diabetes Mellitus (Type 1)

## Diagnosis

### What condition produces a patient's symptoms?

Type 1 diabetes mellitus (DM) is a multi-system disease with both biochemical and anatomical consequences. There is persistent hyperglycemia due to diminished or absent production of insulin. In type 1 DM, insulin is functionally absent due to the destruction of the beta cells of the pancreas where the insulin would normally be produced.

### An injury was most likely sustained to which structure?

Type 1 DM is characterized as an autoimmune disease in which circulating insulin is very low or absent, plasma glucose is elevated, and the pancreatic beta cells fail to respond to all insulin producing stimuli. The pancreas shows lymphocytic infiltration and destruction of insulin-secreting cells of the islets of Langerhans, causing insulin deficiency. Patients need exogenous insulin to reverse this catabolic condition, prevent ketosis, decrease hyperglycemia, and normalize lipid and protein metabolism.

## Inference

### What is the most likely contributing factor in the development of this condition?

The exact etiology of type 1 DM is unknown, however, there are several theories. It is an autoimmune process with a strong genetic component. It is also believed that the genetic predisposition in combination with an unknown factor, potentially environmental, triggers the ongoing cycle of destruction of the beta cells of the pancreas.

## Confirmation

### What is the most likely clinical presentation?

Type 1 DM usually starts in children ages 4 years or older, with the peak incidence of onset at 11-13 years of age, coinciding with early adolescence and puberty. Also, a relatively high incidence exists in people in their late 30s and early 40s, when it tends to present in a less aggressive manner. The most common symptoms of type 1 DM are polyuria, polydipsia, and polyphagia, along with nausea, weight loss, fatigue, blurred vision, and dehydration. A fasting glucose reading of 126 mg/dl is also a sign of DM. The disease onset is usually sudden or within a short period of time. It is not unusual for type 1 DM to present with ketoacidosis.

### What laboratory or imaging studies would confirm the diagnosis?

A test of blood glucose levels will be necessary. In asymptomatic patients, physicians use the American Diabetes Association (ADA) recommendation of two different fasting plasma glucose levels of greater than 125 mg/dl. In symptomatic patients, a random glucose of 200 mg/dl suggests DM. Other testing includes urinalysis for glucose, ketones, and protein and a white blood cell count as well as blood and urine cultures to rule out infection.

### What additional information should be obtained to confirm the diagnosis?

A detailed history and exam should provide the physician with confirmation of the previously mentioned symptoms that present with type 1 DM. Diagnosis is based on one of the subsequent factors: fasting glucose levels, two-hour post-load glucose levels or symptoms of DM.

## Examination

### What history should be documented?

Important areas to explore include past medical history, medications, current health status, history of incontinence, recent polyuria, polydipsia, nocturia or weight loss, nutritional status, social history and habits, occupation, living environment, and social support system.

### What test/measures are most appropriate?

**Arousal, attention, and cognition:** examine mental status, learning ability, memory, motivation

**Community and work integration:** analysis of community, work, and leisure activities

**Environmental, home, and work barriers:** analysis of current and potential barriers or hazards

**Gait, locomotion, and balance:** static and dynamic balance in sitting and standing, safety during gait

**Integumentary integrity:** skin assessment, assessment of sensation

**Motor function:** equilibrium and righting reactions, coordination, posture and balance in sitting

**Muscle performance:** strength assessment, muscle tone assessment

**Posture:** analysis of resting and dynamic posture

**Range of motion:** active and passive range of motion

**Self-care and home management:** assessment of functional capacity, Functional Independence Measure

# Diabetes Mellitus (Type 1)

## What additional findings are likely with this patient?

Complications of type 1 DM include hypoglycemia and hyperglycemia, diabetic ketoacidosis, increased risk of infections, cardiovascular and peripheral vascular disease, retinopathy, nephropathy, impotence, and acceleration of atherosclerosis. DM is the major cause of blindness in adults aged 20-74 years, as well as the leading cause of non-traumatic lower extremity amputation and end-stage renal disease.

## Management

### What is the most effective management of this patient?

Patients with type 1 DM require insulin therapy to control initial hyperglycemia and maintain serum electrolytes and hydration. At times, the first incidence of ketoacidosis is followed by a symptom-free period where patients do not need treatment. Pharmacological intervention includes the use of exogenous insulin per physician orders. Type 1 DM typically requires insulin delivery subcutaneously via continuous pump or self-administered injection. Supplemental insulin may also be delivered by oral or nasal route. Medical management should also include regular self-monitoring of blood glucose levels through finger stick samples and urine testing. Patient education and counseling is appropriate for nutritional components, weight loss if obese, the disease process, complications, medications, and long-term effects. Physical therapy may be indicated for a home exercise program and the patient may be seen intermittently for change and update of their program. Exercise is an important aspect in management of DM. Patients should be taught general exercise and strengthening, stretching, and self-monitoring of their cardiac status. The therapist should coordinate exercise sessions around the patient's meal schedule in order to avoid hypoglycemia and optimize exercise tolerance. Patients should exercise at 50-60% of their predicted maximum heart rate unless directed by a physician otherwise.

### What home care regimen should be recommended?

A patient with type 1 DM requires a good nutritional program, regular self-monitoring of blood glucose levels, and adequate and consistent daily exercise.

## Outcome

### What is the likely outcome of a course in physical therapy?

Type 1 DM is the most common metabolic disease of childhood, with a yearly incidence of 15 cases per 100,000 people less than 18 years of age. Approximately one million Americans have type 1 DM, and physicians diagnose 10,000 new cases every year. Physical therapy may be indicated initially for a patient with goals of optimizing exercise endurance and implementing a home exercise program. Otherwise, patients are usually seen in physical therapy for co-morbidities or due to complications from DM. Physical therapy attempts to maximize patients' functional and health status, but cannot alter the disease process.

### What are the long-term effects of the patient's condition?

Type 1 DM is associated with a high morbidity and premature mortality due to complications. As a result of these complications, people with diabetes have an increased risk of developing ischemic heart disease, cerebral vascular disease, peripheral vascular disease (that sometimes leads to amputation), chronic renal disease, reduced visual acuity and blindness, and autonomic and peripheral neuropathy.

## Comparison

### What are the distinguishing characteristics of a similar condition?

Type 2 DM is more common in the United States than type 1. Type 2 usually involves a defect in the insulin release sites within the pancreas or a resistance to the insulin due to impairment of the receptor sites in the peripheral tissues. In contrast to type 1, type 2 is usually diagnosed in a patient older than 40 years of age. This form of DM is significantly linked to a person's lifestyle, weight, and age. A patient with type 2 can present with the symptoms of type 1, but can also include paresthesias, visual changes, recurrent infections, inadequate wound healing, and cold extremities. In most cases, oral hypoglycemics are used instead of insulin injections.

## Clinical Scenarios

### Scenario One

A three-year-old girl is seen in physical therapy that has just been diagnosed with type 1 DM. She also has a greenstick fracture of the left tibia secondary to an auto accident, but otherwise is in good health. Her mother has stated that her blood sugar levels were not yet regulated and it has been difficult for the physician to find the correct amount and timing of insulin.

### Scenario Two

A 35-year-old male was just diagnosed with type 1 DM after he visited his physician for a routine check-up. He did note polyuria, polydipsia, and visual changes over the last six months time. He is referred to physical therapy for a home exercise program. The physician also recommended a nutritional consult as the patient is approximately 40 pounds overweight.

# Down Syndrome

## Diagnosis

### What condition produces a patient's symptoms?

Down syndrome (trisomy 21) occurs when there is an error in cell division either through nondisjunction (95%), translocation (4%) or mosaicism (1%) and the cell nucleus results in 47 chromosomes. Nondisjunction occurs when faulty cell division results in three specific chromosomes instead of two and extra chromosomes are then replicated for every cell. Translocation occurs when part of a chromosome breaks off during cell division and attaches to another chromosome. The total number of chromosomes remains 46, but Down syndrome exists. Mosaicism occurs right after fertilization when nondisjunction occurs in the initial cell divisions. This results in a mixture of cells with 46 and 47 chromosomes.

### An injury was most likely sustained to which structure?

The pair of 21$^{st}$ chromosomes is responsible for Down syndrome when nondisjunction, translocation or mosaicism occurs during cell division.

## Inference

### What is the most likely contributing factor in the development of this condition?

The exact etiology of Down syndrome is currently unknown. Some theories suggest that an increase in maternal age (and age of the oocyte) may cause predisposition to errors in meiosis. Environmental factors such as virus, paternal age, medical exposure, reproductive medications, and intrinsic predispositions have been associated with Down syndrome.

## Confirmation

### What is the most likely clinical presentation?

Down syndrome occurs once in every 800-1,000 live births. In the United States there are approximately 350,000 individuals living with Down syndrome. Down syndrome is the most common cause of mental retardation. Other clinical manifestations include hypotonia, flattened nasal bridge, almond-shaped eyes, abnormally shaped ears, Simian line (palmar crease), epicanthal folds, enlargement of the tongue, congenital heart disease, developmental delay, and a variety of musculoskeletal disorders.

### What laboratory or imaging studies would confirm the diagnosis?

During pregnancy a female can be tested for Alpha-fetoprotein, human chorionic gonadotropin, and unconjugated estrogen levels (the triple screen). Three diagnostic studies include chorionic villus sampling, amniocentesis or percutaneous umbilical blood sampling. Detection of Down syndrome occurs in approximately 60-70% of the women tested that are carrying a baby with Down syndrome. After birth a chromosome analysis called a karyotype can be performed to confirm the suspected diagnosis.

### What additional information should be obtained to confirm the diagnosis?

In most cases, diagnosis of Down syndrome is made through the physical attributes that are present at birth. Chromosomal testing is used to determine the exact chromosomal pathogenesis.

## Examination

### What history should be documented?

Important areas to explore include past medical history including cardiac status, family history, history of seizures, current health status, physical attributes, developmental delay, and social support system.

### What test/measures are most appropriate?

**Arousal, attention, and cognition:** mental status, learning ability, memory, intelligence testing

**Environmental, home, and work barriers:** analysis of current and potential barriers or hazards

**Ergonomics and body mechanics:** analysis of dexterity and coordination

**Gait, locomotion, and balance:** static and dynamic balance in sitting and standing, safety during gait with/without an assistive device

**Integumentary integrity:** skin and sensation assessment

**Joint integrity and mobility:** assessment of hypermobility and hypomobility of a joint, ligamentous laxity

**Motor function:** equilibrium and righting reactions, motor assessment scales, coordination, posture and balance in sitting, assessment of sensorimotor integration, Peabody Developmental Motor Scales

**Muscle performance:** strength and tone assessment

**Neuromotor development and sensory integration:** analysis of reflex movement patterns, assessment of involuntary movements, sensory integration tests, gross and fine motor skills, Bayley Scales of Infant Development

**Posture:** analysis of resting and dynamic posture

**Range of motion:** active and passive range of motion

**Reflex integrity:** assessment of deep tendon and pathological reflexes (e.g., Babinski, ATNR)

**Self-care and home management:** assessment of functional capacity, WEE-FIM

**Ventilation, respiration, and circulation:** assessment of cough and clearance of secretions, breathing patterns, respiratory muscle strength, accessory muscle utilization and vital capacity, perceived exertion scale, pulse oximetry, palpation of pulses, pulmonary function testing, auscultation of the lungs and heart

# Down Syndrome

## What additional findings are likely with this patient?

There are many associated impairments that a child with Down syndrome may inherit. Potential manifestations and secondary complications that are associated with Down syndrome include atlantoaxial instability, sensory, hearing, and visual impairments, umbilical hernia, respiratory compromise, and Alzheimer's disease. Persons with Down syndrome also have an increased incidence of celiac disease, epilepsy, constipation, as well as blood, dermatologic, and musculoskeletal disorders.

## Management

### What is the most effective management of this patient?

Medical management of Down syndrome is a team approach that requires life long intervention and should be directed toward the specific medical and developmental goals. The overall goal of treatment is to achieve maximum potential and level of function. Pharmacological intervention is based on a particular characteristic or complication such as leukemia or a seizure disorder. Physical therapy intervention plays an important role in the treatment of Down syndrome. Developmental delay, hypotonia, laxity of the ligaments, and poor strength are key areas for the focus of physical therapy treatment. A child with Down syndrome will also require learning strategies based on his or her level of mental retardation. Children with Down syndrome regularly have significant verbal-motor impairments when they verbally respond to a stimulus. Physical therapy will not accelerate developmental milestones, but will help the patient avoid compensatory patterns with static positioning and mobility.

### What home care regimen should be recommended?

A home care regimen should be multifaceted with caregivers being proficient with all aspects of care. A routine of exercise is highly important for a child with Down syndrome in order to avoid inactivity and obesity. Positioning and handling are key components in order to maximize proper alignment and to minimize pathological reflexes, malalignment, and instability.

## Outcome

### What is the likely outcome of a course in physical therapy?

Physical therapy will assist a child by teaching optimal movement patterns during developmental activities and by improving strength. Physical therapy will be indicated on an intermittent basis based on level of function and secondary complications. Strengthening and endurance activities should be encouraged within a home program.

## What are the long-term effects of the patient's condition?

Individuals with Down syndrome today have a longer life expectancy secondary to advances in medical care, however, it is still less than standard life expectancy. Higher mortality results from issues such as congenital heart defects and gastrointestinal anomalies. Immune system dysfunction, repeated respiratory infections, onset of leukemia, pulmonary hypertension, and complications from Alzheimer's disease all contribute to a higher overall mortality rate compared to the general population. Approximately 80% of patients with Down syndrome reach the age of 55.

## Comparison

### What are the distinguishing characteristics of a similar condition?

Prader-Willi syndrome is a genetic disorder that occurs when there is a partial deletion of chromosome 15. Characteristics include hypotonia, difficulties with feeding during infancy, short stature, excessive appetite, and obesity through childhood. Learning disabilities also exist.

## Clinical Scenarios

### Scenario One

A six-month-old boy with Down syndrome is evaluated for outpatient physical therapy. Moderate hypotonia exists and the child does not roll or sit with support. The child's chart indicates atlantoaxial instability with minimal subluxation between C1 and C2. The boy's parents are supportive but both work full-time and are concerned about the competence of the daycare provider.

### Scenario Two

A 12-year-old-girl with Down syndrome is seen in physical therapy two times per week at her school. The child is status post right femur fracture and the cast was taken off two weeks ago. The physician orders strengthening and cardiovascular endurance activities. The child has mild scoliosis and minimal learning deficits. The child is moderately obese and complains of pain consistently during treatment.

# Duchenne Muscular Dystrophy

## Diagnosis

### What condition produces a patient's symptoms?

Duchenne muscular dystrophy (DMD) is a progressive neuromuscular degenerative disorder that manifests symptoms once fat and connective tissue begin to replace muscle that has been destroyed by the disease process. The mutation of the dystrophin gene causes the symptoms of DMD.

### An injury was most likely sustained to which structure?

A patient with DMD is born with a mutation in the dystrophin gene Xp21 that normally codes for the muscle membrane protein dystrophin. This gene is found on the X-chromosome and since it is a recessive trait, only males are affected while females are carriers. The lack of dystrophin allows for damage within the sarcolema with contraction of the muscle. The mutated gene causes weakening of cell membranes, destruction of myofibrils, and loss of muscle contractility. The destroyed muscle cells are replaced with fatty deposits.

## Inference

### What is the most likely contributing factor in the development of this condition?

The etiology of DMD is inheritance as an X-linked recessive trait. The mother is the silent carrier of this disorder. Since it is a recessive trait, only male offspring will manifest the disorder while female offspring become carriers.

## Confirmation

### What is the most likely clinical presentation?

The incidence of DMD in the United States is 20-35:100,000 live male births. Diagnosis of DMD usually occurs between two and five years of age. The first symptoms include a waddling gait, proximal muscle weakness, clumsiness, toe walking, excessive lordosis, pseudohypertrophy of the calf and other muscle groups, and difficulty climbing stairs. DMD primarily affects the shoulder girdle musculature, pectorals, deltoids, rectus abdominis, gluteals, hamstrings, and calf muscles, and is initially identified when a child begins to have difficulty getting off the floor, needing to use the Gowers' maneuver. During this technique a patient uses his hands to stabilize and walk up his legs in order to attain an upright posture. Approximately one-third of patients have some form of learning disability secondary to the dystrophin abnormalities. The disabilities usually present as subtle cognitive and/or behavioral deficits. There is usually rapid progression of this disease with the inability to ambulate by ten to twelve years of age.

### What laboratory or imaging studies would confirm the diagnosis?

Electromyography is used to examine the electrical activity within the muscles. A muscle biopsy can be performed to determine the absence of dystrophin and evaluate the muscle fiber size. DNA analysis and high serum creatinine kinase levels in the blood also assist with confirming the diagnosis.

### What additional information should be obtained to confirm the diagnosis?

Clinical examination, current symptoms, and family history are used to assist in the diagnosis, the type, and progression of the disease. Definitive diagnosis is made from clinical findings along with EMG and muscle biopsy results.

## Examination

### What history should be documented?

Important areas to explore include past medical history, family history, medications, current symptoms, current health status, living and school environment, and social support system.

### What test/measures are most appropriate?

**Anthropometric characteristics:** circumferential measurements to monitor muscle atrophy

**Aerobic capacity and endurance:** assessment of vital signs at rest and with activity

**Arousal, attention, and cognition:** examine mental status, learning ability, memory, motivation

**Assistive and adaptive devices:** analysis of components and safety of a device

**Environmental, home, and work barriers:** analysis of current and potential barriers or hazards

**Gait, locomotion, and balance:** static and dynamic balance in sitting and standing, safety during gait with/without an assistive device

**Joint integrity:** assessment of hypermobility and hypomobility of a joint, assessment of deformity

**Muscle performance:** assessment of active movement

**Orthotic, protective, and supportive devices:** analysis of components of a device, analysis of movement while wearing a device

**Pain:** pain perception assessment scale

**Posture:** analysis of resting and dynamic posture

**Range of motion:** active and passive range of motion, contracture assessment

**Ventilation, respiration, and circulation:** breathing patterns, respiratory muscle strength, accessory muscle utilization, pulmonary function testing

# Duchenne Muscular Dystrophy

**What additional findings are likely with this patient?**

Additional findings occur with progression of the disease. Disuse atrophy, contractures, scoliosis, inability to ambulate, weight gain/obesity, cardiac and respiratory impairments, musculoskeletal deformity, and gastrointestinal dysfunction are the most common findings. Respiratory problems and scoliosis progress once the child is utilizing a wheelchair.

## Management

**What is the most effective management of this patient?**

Medical management of DMD focuses on maintaining function of the unaffected musculature for as long as possible. Pharmacological intervention may include glucocorticoids and immunosuppressant medications. Physical therapy intervention is initially indicated to assist a young child with progression through the developmental milestones. Once a child presents with impairments, physical therapy should focus on maintaining available strength, encouraging mobility, adapting to the loss of function, and promoting family involvement in a home program. Manual muscle testing and range of motion should be evaluated on a consistent basis to determine the pattern and rate of disability. Orthotic prescription, adaptive devices, and wheelchair prescription are areas that will require attention during the course of the disease. Respiratory care will also become a vital part of the plan of care as the patient weakens and strength diminishes. As DMD progresses, treatment will include range of motion, prevention of contracture/deformity, positioning, pain management, breathing exercises and postural drainage, and the use of a wheelchair or adaptive equipment. Ongoing emotional support for the child/family is necessary.

**What home care regimen should be recommended?**

A home care regimen relies on family involvement for a successful home program. Proper positioning, range of motion, submaximal exercise, and breathing exercises are all important aspects that assist a child to maintain function for as long as possible.

## Outcome

**What is the likely outcome of a course in physical therapy?**

Physical therapy is an important aspect in the care of a child with DMD, however, it will not alter the degenerative process of the disease. The goals of physical therapy throughout the course of the disease are to maintain present function, adapt to the progressive loss of mobility skills, and educate the patient and family. It is the role of the therapist to ensure that full and proper training has been completed on all aspects of a patient's care to ensure the highest level of function.

**What are the long-term effects of the patient's condition?**

DMD is a progressive disorder that occurs early in childhood and progresses rapidly. DMD usually affects cardiac muscle in the later stages of the disease. Death occurs primarily from cardiopulmonary complications due to cardiac muscle involvement or respiratory muscle dysfunction. Death usually takes place by the time a patient is a teenager or less frequently into their 20's.

## Comparison

**What are the distinguishing characteristics of a similar condition?**

Facioscapulohumeral dystrophy (FSHD), also known as Landouzy-Dejerine dystrophy, is a form of muscular dystrophy that is also inherited, but the exact genetic origin is unclear. This disease presents later in a child's life, usually between seven and twenty years of age. Characteristics include facial and shoulder girdle weakness, weakness lifting the arms over the head, and difficulty closing the eyes. This disease is more common in males than females. Females tend to be carriers of the disorder. Lifespan remains normal.

## Clinical Scenarios

**Scenario One**

A three-year-old male was recently diagnosed with DMD. The mother reports that the child can ambulate, but prefers to be carried. The child crawls up the stairs and has been falling more frequently. The patient has two sisters at home and resides in a two-story home. At present, both parents work full-time and the child is enrolled in a home daycare.

**Scenario Two**

A 12-year-old male diagnosed with DMD is referred to physical therapy secondary to increased weakness and frequent falls. The patient is currently ambulating with bilateral Lofstrand crutches. There is evidence of pseudohypertrophy and a mild plantar flexion contracture. The patient's mother is concerned that he is at risk for serious injury while ambulating at school.

# Emphysema

## Diagnosis

### What condition produces a patient's symptoms?

Emphysema refers to a pathologic accumulation of air in the lungs found with chronic obstructive pulmonary disease (COPD). There are three classifications of emphysema that include centrilobular emphysema, panlobular emphysema, and paraseptal emphysema. Emphysema results from a long history of chronic bronchitis, recurrent alveolar inflammation or from genetic predisposition of a congenital alpha 1-antitrypsin deficiency.

### An injury was most likely sustained to which structure?

Emphysema results from a non-reversible injury and destruction of elastin protein within the alveolar walls. This process causes permanent enlargement of the air spaces distal to the terminal bronchioles within the lungs. Anatomical changes include loss of elastic recoil, excessive airway collapse during exhalation, and chronic obstruction of airflow. Progression of the disease includes further destruction of the alveolar walls, collapse of the peripheral bronchioles, and impaired gas exchange. Emphysema causes pockets of air to form between the alveolar spaces, (known as blebs), and within the lung parenchyma (known as bullae). This results in an increase in dead space within the lungs that diminishes gas exchange.

## Inference

### What is the most likely contributing factor in the development of this condition?

The primary risk factors for the development of emphysema include chronic bronchitis, lower respiratory infections, cigarette smoking, and genetic predisposition. Environmental influence includes air pollution and other airborne toxins. The risk of acquiring emphysema increases with age.

## Confirmation

### What is the most likely clinical presentation?

COPD is the second leading cause of disability in individuals under 65 years of age worldwide. There are two million individuals in the United States diagnosed with emphysema (and another 14 million with some form of COPD). Emphysema can be asymptomatic until middle age and is most often diagnosed between 55 and 60 years of age. Centrilobular emphysema usually destroys the bronchioles in the upper lungs while the alveolar sacs usually remain intact. Panlobular emphysema destroys the air spaces of the acinus and is usually found in the lower lungs. Paraseptal emphysema destroys the alveoli in the lower lobes resulting in blebs along the lung periphery. Symptoms of emphysema worsen with the progression of the disease and include a persistent cough, wheezing, difficulty breathing especially with expiration, and an increased respiration rate. Advanced disease symptoms include increased use of accessory muscles, severe dyspnea, cor pulmonale, and cyanosis.

### What laboratory or imaging studies would confirm the diagnosis?

X-ray is utilized to visually evaluate the shape and spacing of the lungs. Other imaging studies include a planogram to detect bullae and a bronchogram to evaluate mucus ducts and detect possible enlargement of the bronchi. Arterial blood gases may indicate a decreased $PaO_2$.

### What additional information should be obtained to confirm the diagnosis?

A physical examination, thorough patient history (including cigarette smoking), and pulmonary function tests are required for diagnosis. Pulmonary function testing will result in impaired forced expiratory volume ($FEV_1$), vital capacity (VC), and forced vital capacity (FVC). Total lung capacity (TLC), residual volume (RV), and functional residual capacity (FRC) will be increased.

## Examination

### What history should be documented?

Important areas to explore include past medical history, history of smoking, medications, current health status, social history and habits, occupation, living environment, and social support system.

### What test/measures are most appropriate?

**Aerobic capacity and endurance:** assessment of vital signs at rest and with activity, perceived exertion scale, Six-Minute Walk Test, Three-Minute Step Test

**Arousal, attention, and cognition:** examine mental status, learning ability, memory, motivation

**Assistive and adaptive devices:** analysis of components and safety of a device

**Environmental, home, and work:** analysis of current and potential barriers or hazards

**Gait, locomotion, and balance:** static and dynamic balance in sitting and standing, safety during gait with/without an assistive device

**Muscle performance:** strength assessment, assessment of active movement, and muscle endurance

**Posture:** analysis of resting and dynamic posture

**Self-care and home management:** functional capacity

**Ventilation, respiration, and circulation:** assessment of thoracoabdominal movement, auscultation of vesicular sounds/potential rhonchi, pulse oximetry, pulmonary function testing, accessory muscle utilization

# Emphysema

## What additional findings are likely with this patient?

A patient with emphysema may present with a barrel chest appearance, an increased subcostal angle, rounded shoulders secondary to tight pectorals, rosy skin coloring, and may utilize pursed-lip breathing to assist with ventilation. Patients will also have high rates of anxiety associated with difficulty breathing and may present with claustrophobia, insomnia, and depression. Complications such as the formation and rupture of bullae and blebs can lead to pneumothorax. Cor pulmonale is a serious complication that can occur with advanced emphysema.

## Management

### What is the most effective management of this patient?

Medical management of a patient with emphysema includes pharmacological intervention, oxygen therapy, and physical therapy. Pharmacological intervention promotes bronchodilation, improved oxygenation, and ventilation. Drugs such as oral/inhaled bronchodilators, anti-inflammatory agents, mucolytic expectorants, mast cell membrane stabilizers, and antihistamines may be used in the treatment of emphysema. Preventative immunizations against influenza and pneumonia are also recommended. Physical therapy intervention is based on the severity of the disease process and can include general exercise and endurance training, breathing exercises including pursed-lip breathing, ventilatory muscle strengthening, chest wall exercises, and patient education on posture, airway secretion clearance, and energy conservation techniques. Pulse oximetry should be used to monitor a patient's oxygen saturation during activities and exercise. This will assist with patient education and deter the effects of hypoxemia. Chest physical therapy is required during advanced stages of emphysema.

### What home care regimen should be recommended?

The home care regimen should include breathing strategies and exercises, energy conservation, pacing techniques, and general strength and endurance training.

## Outcome

### What is the likely outcome of a course in physical therapy?

A patient with emphysema may require physical therapy intermittently as the disease progresses. The goals of physical therapy are to maximize the patient's functional abilities and optimize pulmonary function.

## What are the long-term effects of the patient's condition?

Emphysema is a chronic progressive disease process. Patients require ongoing medical care and intermittent physical therapy intervention. Life expectancy decreases to less than five years with severe expiratory slowing measured at a rate of <1L of air during forced expiratory volume ($FEV_1$).

## Comparison

### What are the distinguishing characteristics of a similar condition?

Bronchiectasis is inherited or acquired and is characterized by chronic inflammation and dilation of bronchi and destruction of the bronchial walls. This disease is associated with chronic bacterial infections and is an extreme form of bronchitis. Incidence within the United States is low. Bronchiectasis has a higher risk for development in patients with cystic fibrosis, sinusitis, Kartagener's syndrome, and endobronchial tumors. Characteristics include a chronic cough with sputum, hemoptysis, wheezing, dyspnea, and recurrent respiratory infections. Primary treatment includes physical therapy, bronchodilators, and antibiotics.

## Clinical Scenarios

### Scenario One

A 65-year-old male is referred to physical therapy after recently being diagnosed with emphysema. The patient works in an oil refinery part-time and manages a small dairy farm. The patient's past medical history is negative for smoking and consists of recurrent respiratory infections and chronic cough. The patient complains of shortness of breath with exertion, however, pulmonary function testing indicates only minimal impairment in lung volumes.

### Scenario Two

A 75-year-old female requires physical therapy for management of emphysema. The patient has a history of smoking cigarettes for over 40 years and continues to smoke approximately one pack per day. The patient has an oxygen saturation rate of 94% at rest and requires two liters of oxygen with exertion. The patient has moderate impairment in pulmonary function testing and a persistent cough. The patient presently resides in a two-story home and assists with the care of her disabled husband.

# Erb's Palsy

## Diagnosis

### What condition produces a patient's symptoms?

Erb's palsy is a term used to denote an upper brachial plexus injury or palsy that usually results from a difficult birth. This type of injury is the most common palsy related to the brachial plexus. It primarily affects the muscles of the shoulder and elbow.

### An injury was most likely sustained to which structure?

The brachial plexus is damaged with the most common avulsion located at Erb's point (which is an area in the anterolateral neck). This damages the nerves supplying the ipsilateral upper limb and shoulder. The muscles affected are those supplied by cervical roots C5 and C6; axillary, lateral pectoral, upper and lower subscapular, suprascapular and partial paralysis of the long thoracic and the musculocutaneous nerves. The result is loss of rotator cuff, deltoid, brachialis, coracobrachialis, and biceps brachii function.

## Inference

### What is the most likely contributing factor in the development of this condition?

A brachial plexus injury in a newborn usually occurs during a difficult delivery, due to a large baby, a breech presentation, with a prolonged labor or with the use of forceps. One side of the baby's neck is stretched which damages the nerves. If the upper nerves are affected the condition is termed Erb's palsy. One theory suggests that congenital chicken pox or amniotic bands may also produce this condition. When it occurs in adults, the cause typically is an injury that has caused stretching, tearing or other trauma to the upper brachial plexus network.

## Confirmation

### What is the most likely clinical presentation?

There are four types of brachial plexus injuries: avulsion, rupture, neuroma, and neurapraxia. The clinical presentation is a flaccid paralysis that is nicknamed the "Waiter's tip deformity," characterized by a loss of shoulder function, loss of elbow flexion, forearm pronation, and the hand positioned in a pinch grip manner.

### What laboratory or imaging studies would confirm the diagnosis?

An x-ray or magnetic resonance imaging (MRI) may be performed to see if there is any damage to the bones and joints of the neck and shoulder. The physician may also use an electromyogram (EMG) or nerve conduction studies (NCS) to see if any nerve signals are present in the upper extremity muscles. In complete injuries, motor and sensory nerve conduction studies of median, ulnar, and radial nerves may be conducted.

### What additional information should be obtained to confirm the diagnosis?

A complete history from the patient or parent should be taken regarding upper extremity weakness. Other testing that may assist with diagnosis include the active movement scale, Gilbert Shoulder Classification, and the Pediatric Outcomes Data Collection Instrument.

## Examination

### What history should be documented?

Important areas to explore include past medical history including labor and delivery (infant patients), mechanism of injury (adult patients), medications, current health status, nutritional status, social history, occupation, living environment, and support system.

### What test/measures are most appropriate?

**Anthropometric characteristics:** circumferential measurements of the extremities
**Cranial nerve integrity:** assessment of muscle innervation by the cranial nerves, dermatome assessment
**Environmental, home, and work barriers:** analysis of current and potential barriers or hazards (adult cases)
**Integumentary integrity:** assessment of sensation
**Joint integrity and mobility:** assessment of hypermobility and hypomobility of a joint
**Motor function:** equilibrium and righting reactions, motor assessment scales, coordination, posture and balance in sitting, assessment of sensorimotor integration, physical performance scales
**Muscle performance:** strength assessment, muscle tone assessment
**Neuromotor development and sensory integration:** analysis of reflex movement patterns, assessment of involuntary movements, sensory integration tests, gross and fine motor skills
**Posture:** analysis of resting and dynamic posture
**Range of motion:** active and passive range of motion
**Reflex integrity:** assessment of deep tendon and pathological reflexes (e.g., Babinski, ATNR)
**Self-care and home management:** assessment of functional capacity
**Sensory integrity:** proprioception and kinesthesia

# Erb's Palsy

## What additional findings are likely with this patient?

The child may exhibit characteristics such as an underdeveloped extremity or deformed area, if amniotic bands were the congenital cause for the brachial plexus injury. The patient may also experience glenohumeral subluxation or dislocation, skeletal deformity, poor bone growth, and a learned pattern of non-use of the upper extremity. Overall, the chance of a child having a brachial plexus palsy is equally distributed according to gender, gestational age, and race. It occurs frequently in normal and healthy infants. The reported incidence of brachial plexus palsies is approximately 1 in every 1,000 live births.

## Management

### What is the most effective management of this patient?

Physical therapy is recommended for a patient with Erb's palsy with the goal of developing a program that focuses on increasing active and passive movement and promoting use of the weak upper extremity for functional activities. Occupational and physical therapies are usually indicated immediately when the patient is diagnosed. The length of treatment will depend on the patient's recovery of active movements. If a patient has spontaneous recovery (full active movements) within three to four months, the caregivers are usually given a home program. However, if spontaneous recovery does not occur within that time frame, the patient may continue in therapy with close monitoring of progress. If conservative management fails, surgery may be indicated. Surgery will not restore normal function. After surgery, the infant will wear a splint for approximately three to four weeks. Caregiver education is very important regarding positioning to avoid any further traction during the child's daily activities. Other treatment techniques may include adaptation of developmental milestones and other functional activities, tapping, weight bearing activities, and other sensory techniques.

### What home care regimen should be recommended?

The patient's caregivers must be competent with all aspects of the home program and must perform the program in a consistent fashion. The program should include AROM, PROM, general strengthening, functional activities and integration of the weakened upper extremity into all functional activities.

## Outcome

### What is the likely outcome of a course in physical therapy?

The therapeutic management of a patient with Erb's palsy must begin in infancy (or immediately) in order to achieve optimal functional return. Nerve regeneration remains at a constant speed, however, physical therapy intervention can assist with overall strength and function during recovery. The chance of an infant having a brachial plexus palsy is equally distributed according to gender, gestational age, and race and occurs frequently in normal healthy infants.

## What are the long-term effects of the patient's condition?

Approximately nine out of ten infants with brachial plexus palsy can recover with conservative treatment. The final functional outcome will depend on the degree of damage to the nerves and the caregiver's ability to maintain their motion and their level of interest towards the affected upper extremity during the initial first few months of life. Since nerves grow at a rate of one inch per month, it may take several months or even years for nerves repaired at the cervical spine to reach the muscles of the hand.

## Comparison

### What are the distinguishing characteristics of a similar condition?

Klumpke palsy is the name for the brachial plexus palsy where there is an injury from childbirth affecting the spinal nerves C7, C8, and T1. It is uncommon and can be contrasted to Erb's palsy, which affects C5 and C6. Classically, it produces flexion and supination of the elbow, extension of the wrist, hyper-extension of the metacarpophalangeal joints, and flexion of the interphalangeal joints allowing for a "claw hand" posture. The mechanism of injury is traction of the upper extremity while in an abducted position.

## Clinical Scenarios

### Scenario One

A six-week-old infant is seen in outpatient physical therapy with a recent diagnosis of Erb's palsy. The mother has taken a leave of absence from her job in order to assist her infant. She also has a set of three-year-old twins and her husband has been deployed for 12 months for duty in Iraq.

### Scenario Two

A 56-year-old farmer was admitted to the hospital with a humeral fracture and traction injury to the upper brachial plexus. The injuries were sustained while the farmer was using a piece of faulty equipment. He cannot use the muscles in the C5-C6 distribution and is very anxious to return to work.

# Fibromyalgia Syndrome

## Diagnosis

### What condition produces a patient's symptoms?

Fibromyalgia syndrome (FMS) is classified as a rheumatology syndrome or a nonarticular rheumatic condition. Pain is the primary symptom caused by tender points within muscles, tendons, and ligaments.

### An injury was most likely sustained to which structure?

The exact etiology of FMS is unknown. Theories suggest potential biochemical, metabolic or immunologic pathology. Researchers believe it to be multifactorial in origin and suggest a link to a dysfunction within the stress system, autonomic nervous system, immune system and/or reproductive and hormone systems.

## Inference

### What is the most likely contributing factor in the development of this condition?

Since the exact etiology of FMS is unknown there is speculation linking many factors to the development of this condition. Factors include diet, sleep disorders, viral infections, psychological distress, occupational and environmental factors, hypothyroidism, trauma, and potential hereditary links. Many individuals diagnosed with FMS note multiple causative factors, however, there are individuals diagnosed with FMS that possess none of the theorized causative factors.

## Confirmation

### What is the most likely clinical presentation?

The American College of Rheumatology's data indicates that there are approximately six million individuals living with FMS, making it the most common musculoskeletal disorder in the United States. FMS has a greater incidence in females (almost 75% of the cases) and can affect any age, but most frequently is diagnosed between 14 and 68 years of age. FMS is diagnosed when a patient exhibits the criteria authored by the American College of Rheumatology. There is a widespread history of pain that exists in all four quadrants of the body (above and below the waist), axial pain is present, and there is pain in at least 11 of 18 standardized "tender point" sites. These sites include the occiput, low cervical area, trapezius, supraspinatus, second rib, lateral epicondyle, gluteal area, greater trochanter, and the knee. The patient may also complain of fatigue, memory and visual impairment, sleep disturbances, irritable bowel syndrome, headaches, and anxiety/depression.

### What laboratory or imaging studies would confirm the diagnosis?

FMS has been commonly misdiagnosed as myofascial pain, systemic lupus erythematosus, fibrocytis, and chronic fatigue syndrome. There are no specific tests used to diagnose FMS. Radiographs are negative and blood work often appears normal except for a possible alteration in the levels of substance P. This substance is a chemical involved with pain transmission. Image studies and other lab testing are performed only for differential diagnosis.

### What additional information should be obtained to confirm the diagnosis?

FMS is diagnosed according to the criteria from the American College of Rheumatology. A dolorimeter is used for reliability when testing the tender points by providing a consistent pressure (4 kg/cm$^2$). If the patient meets the criteria and has experienced symptoms for greater than three months, then a patient may be diagnosed with FMS. Diagnostic written tools that can assist with diagnosis include the Beck Depression Inventory and the Fibromyalgia Impact Questionnaire.

## Examination

### What history should be documented?

Important areas to explore include past medical history, medications, family history, current symptoms, current health status, social history and habits, occupation, leisure activities, and social support system.

### What test/measures are most appropriate?

**Aerobic capacity and endurance:** assessment of vital signs at rest and with activity, perceived exertion scale, pulse oximetry, auscultation of the lungs

**Arousal, attention, and cognition:** examine mental status, learning ability, memory, motivation

**Community and work integration:** analysis of community, work, and leisure activities

**Environmental, home, and work barriers:** analysis of current and potential barriers or hazards

**Ergonomics and body mechanics:** analysis of dexterity and coordination

**Gait, locomotion, and balance:** static and dynamic balance in sitting and standing, safety during gait

**Integumentary integrity:** skin assessment, assessment of sensation

**Joint integrity and mobility:** assessment of hypermobility and hypomobility of a joint, effusion, edema

**Muscle performance:** strength assessment, muscle tone assessment

**Neuromotor development and sensory integration:** analysis of reflex movement patterns, assessment of involuntary movements, sensory integration tests, gross and fine motor skills

**Pain:** pain perception assessment scale, visual analogue scale, assessment of muscle soreness and tender points

**Posture:** analysis of resting and dynamic posture

**Range of motion:** active and passive range of motion

**Self-care and home management:** assessment of functional capacity

# Fibromyalgia Syndrome

## What additional findings are likely with this patient?

The aforementioned symptoms can progress over time. Certain symptoms intensify and cause the patient to lose functional independence secondary to increased pain, decreased range of motion, and severe fatigue.

## Management

### What is the most effective management of this patient?

FMS is best treated with a multidisciplinary approach including education, medical management, and exercise. Medical management will attempt to normalize various dysfunctions of the autonomic nervous system, hormonal imbalances, and metabolic abnormalities. Physicians must address sleep disorders (which can be common) and pharmacological intervention based on symptoms. Psychotherapy may be warranted for anxiety or depression and must incorporate stress management and coping strategies into the plan of care. Physical therapy intervention may include relaxation techniques, energy conservation, gentle stretching, moist heat, ultrasound, posture and body mechanics, biofeedback, and exercise to tolerance. Aquatic therapy is recommended to improve a patient's fitness level and an ergonomic evaluation should be performed at the patient's work place. This population should not work through pain. They require short exercise sessions initially (three to five minutes) due to a low tolerance for exertion.

### What home care regimen should be recommended?

A home care regimen should include short duration exercise, aquatic therapy (if indicated), energy conservation strategies, the use of proper positioning, proper body mechanics, and gentle stretching. Patient education is the key to success. Exercises that strain muscles such as weight lifting should be avoided. A comprehensive plan should also include lifestyle management, nutritional support, and stress management.

## Outcome

### What is the likely outcome of a course in physical therapy?

A patient with FMS may benefit from multidisciplinary intervention. Patient compliance with a home program increases the overall success rate. In many cases, symptoms can remain unchanged even with intervention and patient compliance. Some patients will report improvement in areas of fatigue, sleep, and self-reported pain.

## What are the long-term effects of the patient's condition?

FMS is presently not "curable." Many patients that have mild symptoms do not require multidisciplinary intervention and have a good long-term outcome. The majority of patients diagnosed with FMS exhibit moderate levels of symptoms and usually continue to experience these symptoms for years or even their entire lifetime.

## Comparison

### What are the distinguishing characteristics of a similar condition?

Myofascial pain syndrome (MPS) is often misdiagnosed for FMS. MPS is characterized by trigger points rather than tender points and lacks associated symptoms. MPS is a localized musculoskeletal condition that is specific to a muscle. FMS, on the other hand, is a systemic condition. MPS is usually caused by overuse, reduced muscle activity or repetitive motions.

## Clinical Scenarios

### Scenario One

A 32-year-old female recently diagnosed with FMS is seen in physical therapy. Her chief complaints are fatigue, pain throughout her body, and difficulty with sleeping which has effected her employment as a mail carrier. She has been on disability for the last six months and under a physician's care for depression.

### Scenario Two

A 45-year-old construction worker is referred to physical therapy with diagnosis of FMS. His history reveals mild symptoms for the last year. He has seen specialists and was diagnosed last week by a rheumatologist. He is positive for 12 tender points and denies any sleep disturbances or other medical history. He is currently working and appears motivated for therapy.

# Full-Thickness Burn

## Diagnosis

### What condition produces a patient's symptoms?

Full-thickness burns can be caused by thermal (fire, hot fluids, steam), chemical (acid, alkalis, vesicants) or electrical (lightning, high voltage, faulty wiring) agents. This severe burn causes immediate cellular and tissue death and subsequent vascular destruction. The patient will experience primary and secondary symptoms secondary to the extent and area of injury.

### An injury was most likely sustained to which structure?

A full-thickness burn indicates complete destruction of the epidermis, dermis, hair follicle, and nerve endings within the dermis; and also affects the subcutaneous fat layer and underlying muscles, resulting in red blood cell destruction. There is irreversible damage sustained to all epithelial elements.

## Inference

### What is the most likely contributing factor in the development of this condition?

The National Burn Information Exchange indicates that 75% of burns are a direct result of the patient's actions. There are approximately two million individuals burned annually with 70,000 hospitalized and 6,000-7,000 deaths. There is higher risk for burns in children between one and five years of age as well as individuals over 70 years of age. Burns are currently the third leading cause of accidental death in all age categories with males having a higher overall frequency of injury.

## Confirmation

### What is the most likely clinical presentation?

A full-thickness burn is characterized by a variable appearance of deep red, black or white coloring. Eschar forms from necrotic cells and creates a dry and hard layer that requires debridement. Edema is present at the site of injury and in surrounding tissues. Hairs within the region of the burn are easily pulled from the follicle due to the destruction. An area of full-thickness burn does not have sensation or pain due to destruction of free nerve endings, however, there may be pain from adjacent areas that experience partial-thickness burns. During the initial stages the patient will experience thermoregulation impairment, shortness of breath, electrolyte disturbances, poor urine output, and variation in level of consciousness.

### What laboratory or imaging studies would confirm the diagnosis?

Blood work should include a complete blood count, electrolytes, blood urea nitrogen, creatinine, bilirubin, and arterial blood gases. This will indicate baseline data, systemic changes, level of shock, and metabolic complications.

Bronchoscopy and pulmonary function tests may be indicated to assess airway damage and pulmonary insufficiency.

### What additional information should be obtained to confirm the diagnosis?

Diagnosis is primarily based on observation and assessment regarding the extent and depth of the burn. The rule of nines and the Lund-Browder charts grossly approximate the percentage of the body affected by a burn.

## Examination

### What history should be documented?

Important areas to explore include past medical history, mechanism of injury, medications, family history, type and percentage of burn, current symptoms and health status, social history and habits, occupation, leisure activities, and social support system.

### What test/measures are most appropriate?

**Aerobic capacity and endurance:** assessment of vital signs, perceived exertion scale, pulse oximetry

**Anthropometric characteristics:** circumferential measurements of affected areas

**Arousal, attention, and cognition:** examine mental status, learning ability, memory, motivation

**Cranial nerve integrity:** dermatome assessment

**Gait, locomotion, and balance:** static and dynamic balance in sitting and standing

**Integumentary integrity:** sensation assessment, assessment of burn, size, color, eschar, hair follicle integrity, wound mapping

**Joint integrity and mobility:** assessment of contracture, hypomobility of joints, soft tissue swelling

**Muscle performance:** strength and tone assessment

**Pain:** pain perception assessment scale, visual analogue scale to the area of the burn and surrounding tissues

**Posture:** analysis of resting and dynamic posture

**Range of motion:** active and passive range of motion

**Reflex integrity:** assessment of deep tendon and pathological reflexes (e.g., Babinski, ATNR)

**Self-care and home management:** functional capacity, Functional Independence Measure (FIM)

**Ventilation, respiration, and circulation:** cough and clearance of secretions, auscultation of the lungs, breathing patterns, respiratory muscle strength, accessory muscle utilization, vital capacity, pulse oximetry and palpation, pulmonary function testing

# Full-Thickness Burn

### What additional findings are likely with this patient?

A patient with a full-thickness burn will present with multiple secondary effects based on the mechanism of the burn, size of the burn, and location of the burn. Infection, hypertrophic scarring, and contractures are the most common complications. Other secondary damage may include impairments of the cardiovascular system, renal system, gastrointestinal system, respiratory system and/or immune system. Damage to these vital areas can result in metabolic disorders, acidosis, sepsis, and dehydration.

## Management

### What is the most effective management of this patient?

The initial management includes medically stabilizing the patient followed by a full assessment of primary and secondary damage. This emergent phase lasts 48-72 hours and concludes with regaining capillary permeability and hemodynamic stability. An autograft procedure is usually required for full-thickness burns. The rehabilitation phase is a long-term commitment that includes all aspects of functional recovery. Physical therapy intervention begins immediately following skin grafting and includes wound care, pulmonary exercises, positioning, splinting, and immobilization for the first three to five days. A therapist will also provide education regarding skin care, positioning, and contracture prevention. Early ambulation and mobility activities should be incorporated as soon as possible in order to decrease complications such as atelectasis, pneumonia, and contracture. Continued physical therapy management will involve edema control, monitoring of any elastic garments, massage, stretching, hydrotherapy, ROM, debridement, relaxation techniques, progressive exercise, ambulation, and functional mobility training.

### What home care regimen should be recommended?

A patient must continue with the established splinting and positioning schedule at home. Physical therapy may initially be warranted for continued pulmonary management, stretching, and functional mobility. A home program is vital to the patient's continued success and should include strengthening exercises, massage, scar management, positioning, and stretching. As the patient progresses, participation in wound management, activities of daily living, and functional activities should be incorporated into the daily routine.

## Outcome

### What is the likely outcome of a course in physical therapy?

Patient outcome is dependent on location, extent, and secondary complications of the burn. Physical therapy will provide the patient with education for an ongoing therapeutic program. Therapeutic exercise, stretching, compression garments, and other modalities will enhance the probability of a positive outcome.

### What are the long-term effects of the patient's condition?

The mortality rate has decreased over the last two decades due to improvement in burn care, prevention of infection, and advances in grafting procedures. Mortality rates are highest for children under four and adults over 65 years of age. Overall prognosis is dependent on factors such as cardiac pathology, alcoholism, peripheral vascular disease, and obesity. Other factors that also require consideration are depression, social and emotional shock, and level of difficulty reintegrating into a daily routine (with employment, spouse, children, community). Long-term outcome is also based on the extent of secondary effects such as scarring and contractures. Garments may be worn up to two years after injury. Without significant complications a patient should achieve independence within a few months post injury.

## Comparison

### What are the distinguishing characteristics of a similar condition?

A superficial partial-thickness burn damages the epidermis and the papillary layer of the dermis (the dermis remains largely intact). This burn presents with blister formation, bright red coloring, intact blanching, moderate edema, and pain. The burn will heal without surgical intervention within 5-21 days with minimal to no scarring noted.

## Clinical Scenarios

### Scenario One

A 32-year-old female six weeks status post full-thickness burns to 50% of her right arm and 70% of her right leg is referred to physical therapy. She wears compression garments and has decreased range of motion. She resides alone in a two-story home and is employed as a cook.

### Scenario Two

A three-year-old boy is referred to physical therapy 48 hours after an autograft for a full-thickness burn on the left side of his thorax. The chart review notes the mechanism of injury as pulling a cup of coffee off a table. Other medical history includes developmental delay, seizures, and hydrocephaly.

# Guillain-Barre Syndrome

## Diagnosis

### What condition produces a patient's symptoms?

Guillain-Barre syndrome (GBS) or acute polyneuropathy is a temporary inflammation and demyelination of the peripheral nerves' myelin sheaths, potentially resulting in axonal degeneration. GBS results in motor weakness in a distal to proximal progression, sensory impairment, and possible respiratory paralysis.

### An injury was most likely sustained to which structure?

The autoantibodies of GBS attack segments of the myelin sheath of the peripheral nerves. The infecting organism is of similar structure to molecules found on the surface of myelin sheaths. The antibodies produced attack both the organism of infection as well as the Schwann cells due to the similar structure. This decreases nerve conduction velocity and results in weakness or paralysis of the involved muscles. The demyelination that is initiated at Ranvier's nodes occurs secondary to macrophage response and inflammation, and as a result, destruction of the myelin. The body responds to this process and attempts to repair the damage through Schwann cell division and myelinization of the damaged nerves. Motor fibers are predominantly affected.

## Inference

### What is the most likely contributing factor in the development of this condition?

The exact etiology of GBS is unknown, however, it is hypothesized to be an autoimmune response to a previous respiratory infection, influenza, immunization or surgery. Viral infections, Epstein-Barr syndrome, cytomegalovirus, bacterial infections, surgery, and vaccinations have been associated with the development of GBS.

## Confirmation

### What is the most likely clinical presentation?

GBS can occur at any age, however, there is a peak in frequency in the young adult population and again in adults that are between their fifth and eighth decades. Incidence is slightly greater in males than females and in Caucasians than African Americans. A patient with GBS will initially present with distal symmetrical motor weakness and will likely experience mild distal sensory impairments and transient paresthesias. The weakness will progress towards the upper extremities and head. The level of disability usually peaks within two to four weeks after onset. Muscle and respiratory paralysis, absence of deep tendon reflexes, and the inability to speak or swallow may also occur. GBS can be life threatening if there is respiratory involvement. There are multiple subtypes of GBS, but the classic type involves acute onset of symptoms with peak impairment within four weeks, followed by a two to four week static period and gradual recovery that can take months to years.

### What laboratory or imaging studies would confirm the diagnosis?

GBS can be diagnosed through a cerebrospinal fluid sample that contains high protein levels and little to no lymphocytes. Electromyography will result in abnormal and slowed nerve conduction.

### What additional information should be obtained to confirm the diagnosis?

A physical and neurological examination, strength testing, and a review of relevant medical history are all important in the diagnosis of GBS. The National Institute of Neurologic and Communicative Disorders and Stroke has established criteria to assist with the diagnosis of GBS.

## Examination

### What history should be documented?

Important areas to explore include past medical, family, and surgical history, recent illness, medications, immunizations, current symptoms and health status, social history and habits, occupation, living environment, and social support system.

### What test/measures are most appropriate?

**Aerobic capacity and endurance:** vital signs at rest/activity, responses to positional changes

**Arousal, attention, and cognition:** examine mental status, learning ability, memory, motivation

**Assistive and adaptive devices:** analysis of components and safety of a device

**Cranial nerve integrity:** assessment of muscles innervated by the cranial nerves, dermatome assessment

**Community and work integration:** analysis of community, work, and leisure activities

**Gait, locomotion, and balance:** static and dynamic balance in sitting and standing, safety during gait with/without an assistive device, Berg Balance Scale, Tinetti Performance Oriented Mobility Assessment, analysis of wheelchair management

**Integumentary integrity:** skin and sensation assessment

**Motor function:** equilibrium and righting reactions, coordination, motor assessment scales

**Muscle performance:** strength and tone assessment

**Orthotic, protective, and supportive devices:** potential utilization of bracing

**Pain:** pain perception assessment scale

**Range of motion:** active and passive range of motion

**Reflex integrity:** assessment of deep tendon and pathological reflexes

**Self-care and home management:** assessment of functional capacity

**Ventilation, respiration and circulation:** pulmonary function tests, assessment of cough and secretions

# Guillain-Barre Syndrome

## What additional findings are likely with this patient?

The extent of impairment for each patient depends on the clinical course of the GBS. The patient may also experience bladder weakness, deep muscle pain, and autonomic nervous system involvement including arrhythmia, tachycardia, postural hypotension, heart block, and absent reflexes. Up to 30% of patients require mechanical ventilation during the acute stage. Respiratory assistance can last as long as 50-60 days.

## Management

### What is the most effective management of this patient?

Medical management of a patient with GBS may require hospitalization for treatment of symptoms. Pharmacological intervention often includes immunosuppressive and analgesic/ narcotic medications. Corticosteroids are controversial and usually contraindicated. Cardiac monitoring, plasma exchange (through plasmapheresis), and mechanical ventilation may be required. A tracheostomy may be performed for ventilation. Physical, occupational, and speech therapies are indicated to facilitate neurological rehabilitation. Physical therapy should be initiated upon admission to the hospital with focus on passive range of motion, positioning, and light exercise. During the acute stage a therapist must limit overexertion and fatigue to avoid exacerbation of symptoms. As the patient progresses, intervention may include orthotic, wheelchair or assistive device prescription, exercise and endurance activities, family teaching, functional mobility and gait training, and progressive respiratory therapy. The therapeutic pool may be indicated to initiate movement without the effects of gravity.

### What home-care regimen should be recommended?

A home care regimen should include breathing exercises and incentive spirometry for respiratory involvement. A patient, along with the caregiver, must continue with therapeutic exercise, ongoing functional mobility training, and endurance activities as tolerated.

## Outcome

### What is the likely outcome of a course in physical therapy?

Physical therapy may assist with recovery, but it cannot alter the course of the disease. Physical therapy intervention may be required on an ongoing basis to assist with recovery that can last from 3-12 months.

## What are the long-term effects of the patient's condition?

GBS is an autoimmune response that varies in severity from person to person. Recovery is slow and can last up to two years after onset. Although most patients experience full recovery, statistics indicate that 20% have remaining neurologic deficits, and 3-5% of patients die from respiratory complications.

## Comparison

### What are the distinguishing characteristics of a similar condition?

Polyneuropathy is a progressive condition that affects the nerves. The most common etiology is metabolic conditions such as diabetes mellitus. Polyneuropathy develops slowly, bilaterally, and symmetrically. The first symptom is often sensory impairment of the distal lower extremities. Pain, diminished deep tendon reflexes, and motor loss are other symptoms of this condition that is marked by exacerbations and remissions. Medical management will focus on stabilizing the underlying metabolic condition.

## Clinical Scenarios

### Scenario One

A 25-year-old female has been hospitalized for one week with a diagnosis of GBS. The patient's strength assessment reports 3-/5 bilateral hip strength, 2+/5 bilateral knee strength, and 2-/5 bilateral ankle strength. The patient is anxious to improve and is eager to begin physical therapy. The patient resides alone in a second floor apartment and works as a bank teller.

### Scenario Two

A 43-year-old male was admitted to the hospital one month ago with GBS. The patient had significant paralysis and was ventilator dependent. The patient began to improve two weeks ago and was taken off the ventilator. The patient was in good health prior to admission and worked as an independent international sales representative. The patient is diabetic and has a history of alcoholism. He is divorced with no children.

# Human Immunodeficiency Virus

## Diagnosis

### What condition produces a patient's symptoms?

The human immunodeficiency virus (HIV) is a retrovirus that initially invades and destroys cells within the immune system; specifically CD4+ T-lymphocytes (T-cells). This virus also affects monocytes, macrophages, and B-cells. Once the T-cells decrease beyond a specific level a patient will begin to demonstrate symptoms of the HIV infection.

### An injury was most likely sustained to which structure?

HIV infects T-cells within the immune system. Other cells that eventually house HIV include monocytes, macrophages, microglia, cervical cells, and epithelial cells of the GI tract. HIV uses and destroys the cells that possess the antigen CD4 on their surface in order to replicate HIV, and as a result the immune system becomes weaker and unable to function.

## Inference

### What is the most likely contributing factor in the development of this condition?

HIV is transmitted through contact with blood, semen, vaginal secretions, and breast milk. Contact can be sexual, perinatal or through contact with blood or body fluids that carry infected cells. Risk factors for contracting HIV include unprotected sexual relations, intravenous drug use or mother to fetus transmission. The largest risk factors for contracting HIV are homosexual male sex (46%), intravenous drug use (25%), and heterosexual sex (11%).

## Confirmation

### What is the most likely clinical presentation?

The incidence of newly diagnosed cases of HIV is approximately 40,000 per year within the United States (decreased from 150,000 new cases yearly during the mid-1980s). A patient will not immediately present with symptoms after the initial transmission of the infection. A patient may actually be "symptom free" for one to two years post infection or may exhibit flu-like symptoms including rash and fever. HIV immediately begins a latent phase where replication of the virus is minimal. The three phases of this disease process include asymptomatic HIV, symptomatic HIV, and acquired immunodeficiency syndrome (AIDS). The T-cell count will begin to decrease during the "asymptomatic" phase, however, symptoms will not appear until the count decreases to a certain level. Manifestations of HIV may lead to other infections, malignancies, neurological dysfunction, dementia, and cardiac pathologies.

### What laboratory or imaging studies would confirm the diagnosis?

HIV is diagnosed through various blood tests such as the enzyme-linked immunosorbent test or Western blot test. Once diagnosed the lab results can also assist with classifying the stage of HIV infection.

### What additional information should be obtained to confirm the diagnosis?

Definitive diagnosis is made through blood tests, however, the physician should ascertain accurate medical and social history. Accurate drug use and sexual partner history will allow for appropriate patient education in order to cease the spread of the virus. A positive diagnosis will allow the patient to notify others at risk.

## Examination

### What history should be documented?

Important areas to explore include past medical history, medications, family history, current symptoms, current health status, social history and habits, occupation, leisure activities, and social support system.

### What test/measures are most appropriate?

**Aerobic capacity and endurance:** assessment of vital signs, perceived exertion scale, auscultation of the lungs

**Arousal, attention, and cognition:** examine mental status, learning ability, memory, and level of motivation

**Community and work integration:** analysis of community, work, and leisure activities

**Environmental, home, and work barriers:** analysis of current and potential barriers or hazards

**Gait, locomotion, and balance:** static and dynamic balance in sitting and standing, safety during gait with/without an assistive device, Tinetti Performance Oriented Mobility Assessment, analysis of wheelchair management

**Integumentary integrity:** skin assessment and sensation assessment

**Motor function:** equilibrium and righting reactions, motor assessment scales, coordination, posture and balance in sitting, assessment of sensorimotor integration, physical performance scales

**Muscle performance:** strength assessment, muscle tone assessment

**Pain:** pain perception assessment scale

**Range of motion:** active and passive range of motion

**Reflex integrity:** assessment of deep tendon and pathological reflexes (e.g., Babinski, ATNR)

**Self-care and home management:** assessment of functional capacity

**Ventilation, respiration, and circulation:** pulmonary function testing, breathing patterns, perceived exertion scale, assessment of cough

# Human Immunodeficiency Virus

## What additional findings are likely with this patient?

The Centers for Disease Control classifies HIV into three categories based on the T-cell count. Symptoms and secondary illnesses occur as the T-cell count decreases. The onset of AIDS occurs when the T-cell count falls below 200 cells per mm$^3$ (normal ranges 650-1,200 cells) or when one of 26 specific AIDS defining disorders is present or both. A patient may experience musculoskeletal, neuromuscular, cardiopulmonary, integumentary, and other impairments secondary to HIV.

## Management

### What is the most effective management of this patient?

Early detection is important so that pharmacological intervention can be initiated and slow the progression of the virus. There is no cure for HIV, however, proper medical intervention can allow the virus to remain a manageable chronic condition. Medical management will institute antiretroviral therapy (HAART) when T-cells drop below 500 mm$^3$. The goal of drug therapy is to significantly decrease the virus' ability to replicate, and therefore, decrease the progression of the disease. Drugs may include nucleoside analogs, protease inhibitors, and non-nucleoside reverse transcriptase inhibitors. Physical therapy intervention may be indicated during the course of HIV/AIDS due to secondary impairments. Physical therapy goals and intervention include the promotion of optimal fitness, flexibility, energy conservation, stress management, ADL equipment, relaxation, aquatic therapy, modalities, positioning, pain management, breathing exercises, and neurological rehabilitation.

### What home care regimen should be recommended?

A patient with HIV must follow a home regimen including medication, proper nutrition and sleep, and fitness in order to remain as healthy as possible. A physical therapy home program can also minimize the negative effects on functional ability and improve the overall independence and quality of life.

## Outcome

### What is the likely outcome of a course in physical therapy?

Physical therapy may be warranted for periods of time throughout the progression of HIV/AIDS. Physical therapy cannot alter the progression of the virus, but can foster improvement in functional mobility, conditioning, and overall independence.

## What are the long-term effects of the patient's condition?

There are currently 42 million individuals around the world living with HIV/AIDS. There is presently no cure for HIV/AIDS, however, with early combination therapies patients are surviving longer and living more productive lives. Studies indicate that psychosocial factors influence progression of the virus as well as survival. Presently, the leading cause of death is kidney failure secondary to the extended drug therapies.

## Comparison

### What are the distinguishing characteristics of a similar condition?

Hepatitis B (HBV) is a form of viral hepatitis that produces inflammation and damage to the liver. Like HIV, hepatitis B is transmitted parenterally through intravenous drug use, sexual relations, blood transfusions, perinatal transmission or dialysis. A vaccine is available for prevention and blood tests are used for diagnosis. Approximately 95% of those infected with HBV fully recover, however, 10% of these individuals become carriers. Some of the carriers develop chronic liver disease and may die prematurely.

## Clinical Scenarios

### Scenario One

A 19-year-old female is seen in outpatient physical therapy secondary to weakness and balance impairments. She was diagnosed with HIV two years ago, but the physician believes that she was infected at least one to two years prior to diagnosis by IV drug use. Her T-cell count is 404 mm$^3$ using HIV drug therapies.

### Scenario Two

A 58-year-old male was diagnosed with AIDS one year ago and has lost significant weight. He presents with general muscle atrophy and is having difficulty with ambulation and ADLs. The patient is referred to physical therapy for adaptive and assistive devices. He lives with his partner in a ranch style home and is on medical disability.

# Huntington's Disease

## Diagnosis

### What condition produces a patient's symptoms?

Huntington's disease (HD), also known as Huntington's chorea, is a neurological disorder of the CNS and is characterized by degeneration and atrophy of the basal ganglia (specifically the striatum) and cerebral cortex within the brain.

### An injury was most likely sustained to which structure?

HD affects the basal ganglia and cerebral cortex of the brain. The ventricles of the brain become enlarged secondary to atrophy of the basal ganglia and there is extensive loss of small and medium sized neurons. There appears to be an overall decrease in the quantity and activity of gamma-aminobutyric acid (GABA) and acetylcholine neurons that are produced in these areas. The identified neurotransmitters become deficient and are unable to modulate movement. Loss of neurons creates dysfunction in inhibition that results in the symptoms of chorea, bradykinesia, and rigidity. The thalamus is also believed to contribute to the movement disorders associated with the disease process.

## Inference

### What is the most likely contributing factor in the development of this condition?

HD is genetically transmitted as an autosomal dominant trait with the defect linked to chromosome four and to the gene identified as IT-15. The disease is usually perpetuated by a person that has children prior to the normal onset of symptoms and without knowledge that he/she possesses the defective gene. Genetic testing is able to identify the defective gene for HD prior to the onset of symptoms.

## Confirmation

### What is the most likely clinical presentation?

The prevalence of HD is approximately 4-8:100,000 in North America with 25,000 individuals diagnosed with HD in the United States. The average age for developing symptoms ranges between 35 and 55 years, however, symptoms can develop at any age. HD is a disease that produces a movement disorder, affective dysfunction, and cognitive impairment. The patient will initially present with involuntary choreic movements and a mild alteration in personality. Unintentional facial expressions such as a grimace, protrusion of the tongue, and elevation of the eyebrows are common. As the disease progresses gait will become ataxic and a patient experiences choreoathetoid movement of the extremities and the trunk. Speech disturbances and mental deterioration are common. Late stage HD is characterized by a decrease in IQ, dementia, depression, dysphagia, incontinence, inability to ambulate or transfer, and progression from choreiform movements to rigidity.

### What laboratory or imaging studies would confirm the diagnosis?

Magnetic resonance imaging (MRI) or computed tomography (CT scan) may indicate atrophy or abnormalities within the cerebral cortex as well as the basal ganglia. Positron-emission tomography (PET) may be used to augment other testing and obtain information regarding blood flow, oxygen uptake, and metabolism of the brain. A DNA marker study may be administered to determine if the autosomal dominant trait is present for HD.

### What additional information should be obtained to confirm the diagnosis?

A physical examination, review of symptoms, and family history are important components in the diagnosis of HD.

## Examination

### What history should be documented?

Important areas to explore include past medical history, medications, family history, current symptoms, health status, social history/habits, occupation, living environment, and social support system.

### What test/measures are most appropriate?

**Aerobic capacity and endurance:** assessment of vital signs at rest and with activity

**Arousal, attention, and cognition:** examine mental status, learning ability, memory, motivation

**Gait, locomotion, and balance:** static/dynamic balance in sitting/standing, safety during gait, Functional Reach Test, Tinetti Performance Oriented Mobility Assessment, Functional Ambulation Profile

**Motor function:** equilibrium/righting reactions, coordination

**Muscle performance:** strength and tone assessment, tremor assessment, testing for dysdiadochokinesia

**Neuromotor development and sensory integration:** analysis of reflex movement patterns, assessment of involuntary movements

**Posture:** analysis of resting and dynamic posture

**Range of motion:** active and passive range of motion

**Self-care and home management:** assessment of functional capacity, Functional Independence Measure (FIM), Barthel Index

# Huntington's Disease

## What additional findings are likely with this patient?

Dementia and other psychological changes usually occur after neurological symptoms appear. The emotional disorder worsens with progression and may require admission to a psychiatric facility for severe depression and/or suicidal attempts. Secondary complications that can occur from symptoms of HD include loss of range of motion, deformity, pain, communication breakdown, aspiration and choking, fatigue, and weakness from weight loss.

## Management

### What is the most effective management of this patient?

Medical management of HD requires a team approach including genetic, psychological, and social counseling for the patient and family. Education regarding disease process, coping strategies, and genetic consequences should initiate immediately following diagnosis. Medical treatment will focus on symptoms and pharmacological management. Drug classes such as anticonvulsants and antipsychotics may assist as these block dopamine transmission, however, have very serious side effects. Commonly utilized drugs include Perphenazine, Haloperidol (Haldol), and Reserpine. Physical, occupational, and speech therapy interventions may be warranted intermittently throughout the course of the disease and should focus on current problems with mobility and self-care skills. Physical therapy should maximize endurance, strength, balance, postural control, and functional mobility. Intervention should focus on motor control and utilize techniques including coactivation of muscles, trunk stabilization, the use of biofeedback, and relaxation in an attempt to maintain a patient's functional status. Patient education should include prone lying, stretching, prevention of deformity and contracture, and safety with mobility. As the disease progresses, the degree of dementia will influence treatment and goals. The therapist must continue to emphasize family involvement and caregiver teaching. As the patient continues to lose function the caregiver will require education regarding posture, seating, assistance with transfers, mobility, and the use of adaptive equipment.

### What home care regimen should be recommended?

A home care regimen should include an exercise routine, functional mobility skills, relaxation techniques, range of motion, stretching exercises, and endurance activities. Participation in a home care regimen can assist to maintain the optimal quality of life during the progression of the disease process.

## Outcome

### What is the likely outcome of a course in physical therapy?

Physical therapy is recommended on an intermittent basis throughout the course of the disease. Physical therapy will not prevent further degeneration, however, it will maximize the patient's functional potential and safety. The goal of physical therapy is to attain an optimal functional outcome within the limitations of the disease process.

### What are the long-term effects of the patient's condition?

HD is a chronic progressive genetic disorder that is fatal within 15 to 20 years after clinical manifestation. Late stages of the disease result in total physical and mental incapacitation. The patient usually requires an extended care facility due to the burden of care and physical, cognitive, and emotional dysfunction.

## Comparison

### What are the distinguishing characteristics of a similar condition?

Athetoid (dyskinetic) cerebral palsy is a non-progressive motor disorder caused by central nervous system damage specifically to the basal ganglia. Clinical manifestations include slow and involuntary movements, choreiform movements, severe dysarthria, and an increased risk of aspiration pneumonia. The involuntary movements will increase with stress and fatigue and subside with sleep. Physical therapy intervention should focus on motor control and mobility deficits in order to attain the highest level of functioning.

## Clinical Scenarios

### Scenario One

A 48-year-old attorney is referred for physical therapy home services. The patient was diagnosed with HD two years ago and resides in a two-story home. The patient has a significant other and they reside together. The patient's primary complaint is a loss of balance while ambulating. The patient refuses to utilize an assistive device.

### Scenario Two

A 45-year-old female is referred to physical therapy. She was diagnosed with HD seven years ago and has recently fallen multiple times. According to family members the patient is short-tempered, irritable, and occasionally demonstrates poor judgment. The physician requests physical therapy for an evaluation and home program.

# Juvenile Rheumatoid Arthritis

## Diagnosis

### What condition produces a patient's symptoms?

Juvenile rheumatoid arthritis (JRA) is a form of arthritis found in children less than 16 years of age. JRA causes inflammation and stiffness to multiple joints for a period of greater than six weeks. The inflammatory process affects the tissues surrounding the affected synovial joints causing symptoms of JRA.

### An injury was most likely sustained to which structure?

JRA, like adult rheumatoid arthritis, is an autoimmune disorder that occurs when the immune cells mistakenly begin to attack the joints and organs causing local and systemic effects throughout the body. The severity of ongoing injury is based on the specific classification and subtype of the disease.

## Inference

### What is the most likely contributing factor in the development of this condition?

The etiology for JRA is currently unknown. Research postulates that JRA develops in children with a genetic predisposition for the disease. The predisposition may be triggered by environmental factors or a viral or bacterial infection. Girls have a higher incidence of JRA and it is found to begin most commonly in the toddler or adolescent.

## Confirmation

### What is the most likely clinical presentation?

JRA is an umbrella term for three specific classifications and subtypes of childhood arthritis. Classification is based on the number of joints involved, symptoms, presence of the rheumatoid factor (RF) or antinuclear antibody (ANA), and systemic involvement. General symptoms include persistent joint swelling, pain, and stiffness. Pauciarticular JRA involves four or less joints, is asymmetric, and is usually a mild form of JRA. This is the most common form of JRA and accounts for 50% of the cases, with girls under eight most likely to develop this subtype. ANA can also be found in 20-30% of patients and correlates with eye disease. Polyarticular JRA involves more than four joints, is usually symmetrical, involves the joints of the hands and feet as well as larger joints, and has potential for severe destruction. This subtype accounts for 30-40% of the cases and children may have the IgM rheumatoid factor (RF) similar to adult RA. Systemic JRA accounts for 10-20% of the cases and is otherwise known as Still's disease. Onset includes a high fever, chills, and a rash that may last for weeks, followed by severe myalgia and polyarthritis. This form presents with severe extraarticular manifestations including anemia, hepatosplenomegaly, lymphadenopathy, pericarditis, and myocarditis. Most children in this subtype are negative for RF or ANA antibodies. About 25% experience severe and unremitting arthritis.

### What laboratory or imaging studies would confirm the diagnosis?

There is not a single test to identify the presence of JRA. Blood tests may include serum evaluation to measure inflammation and detect RF, ANA or HLAB27 (human leukocyte antigen). Only a small percentage of patients with JRA possess RF or ANA. An erythrocyte sedimentation rate (ESR or "sed rate") may also indicate rheumatic disease. Other tests or procedures may be used to rule out other conditions such as Lyme disease, lupus, infection, and cancers.

### What additional information should be obtained to confirm the diagnosis?

Diagnosis is made largely through physical examination, a patient's past and present medical status, and meeting the criteria set forth by the American Rheumatoid Association regarding the diagnosis and classification of JRA.

## Examination

### What history should be documented?

Important areas to explore include past medical history, medications, family history, current symptoms, current health status, social history and habits, leisure activities, and social support system.

### What test/measures are most appropriate?

**Aerobic capacity and endurance:** vital signs at rest and with activity, timed walk, aerobic endurance, $VO_2$ max

**Anthropometric characteristics:** circumferential measurements of all affected joints

**Arousal, attention, and cognition:** examine mental status, learning ability, memory, motivation

**Assistive and adaptive devices:** analysis of components and safety of a device

**Environmental and home barriers:** analysis of current and potential barriers or hazards

**Ergonomics and body mechanics:** analysis of dexterity and coordination

**Gait, locomotion, and balance:** static/dynamic balance in sitting and standing, visual inspection of gait with and without shoes, timed walk, gait over level and unlevel surfaces, gait analysis with videography

**Integumentary integrity:** skin and sensation assessment

**Joint integrity and mobility:** active joint count, joint effusion, articular tenderness

**Motor function:** equilibrium and coordination

**Muscle performance:** break testing of isometric contractions, manometer method of strength testing, dynamic muscle strength using repetition maximum (only if pain free)

# Juvenile Rheumatoid Arthritis

**Neuromotor development and sensory integration:** analysis of reflex movement patterns, assessment of involuntary movements, sensory integration tests, gross and fine motor skills

**Orthotic, protective, and supportive devices:** analysis of components and movement using a device

**Pain:** Pediatric Pain Questionnaire (PPQ), visual analogue scale

**Posture:** analysis of resting and dynamic posture, scoliosis screening

**Range of motion:** active/passive range of motion for extremities, active motion only for cervical spine, angular deformities and joint play assessments

**Self-care and home management:** Pediatric Evaluation of Disability Inventory (PEDI), Child Health Assessment Questionnaire (CHAQ), Juvenile Arthritis Functional Status Index (JASI)

## What additional findings are likely with this patient?

Potential complications are dependent on the subtype of JRA and the presence (or absence) of RF or ANA. Joint swelling, stiffness, and pain are the most common symptoms. Eye inflammation and development of iritis/uveitis can be a significant complication. Some patients have periods of exacerbations and remissions while other patient's symptoms will persist.

## Management

### What is the most effective management of this patient?

A pediatric rheumatologist is ideal to direct a multidisciplinary team in the complex care of JRA. Primary goals of treatment are to maintain a high level of physical functioning and quality of life. Pharmacological intervention may include NSAIDS, immunosuppressive medications, disease-modifying antirheumatic drugs, and corticosteroids. Physical therapy intervention is a key component and should include range of motion, exercise, and pain control. Functional mobility, strengthening, endurance, and aerobic training will assist a patient in overall function. Range of motion exercises, modalities, splints and orthotics, patient/family education, and the integration of recreational activities should optimize the quality of life. Surgical intervention is sometimes warranted for severe contractures or irreversible joint destruction. Soft tissue release, supracondylar osteotomy, and arthroplasty are the most common surgical procedures.

## What home care regimen should be recommended?

A home care regimen should provide an individualized exercise program. The program should be simple and take no more than 20 minutes to complete in order to optimize compliance. Swimming is also a beneficial activity for a child with JRA.

## Outcome

### What is the likely outcome of a course in physical therapy?

Physical therapy may be indicated periodically throughout a patient's childhood based on symptoms and complications. Ongoing education and revision of a home program is vital to promote patient compliance. Physical therapy outcome is variable depending on the severity of the patient's symptoms.

### What are the long-term effects of the patient's condition?

Long-term effects of JRA are dependent on subtype, symptoms, and any complications encountered. Some patients "outgrow" JRA and are not affected as adults while others experience pain and other manifestations of the disease on a consistent and long-term basis.

## Comparison

### What are the distinguishing characteristics of a similar condition?

Infectious bacterial arthritis most often develops within a joint secondary to systemic corticosteroid use, trauma, HIV or alcohol/drug abuse. If treated immediately, long-term prognosis is good. If left uncontrolled, toxemia and septicemia can be fatal. Inflammation and pannus within the synovium erodes articular cartilage. There is an acute onset of swelling, tenderness, and loss of range of motion. A child will usually not bear weight through the involved joint.

## Clinical Scenarios

### Scenario One

A 12-year-old boy diagnosed with systemic JRA is seen in physical therapy two days status post soft tissue release of the bilateral heel cords. The patient primarily uses a wheelchair for mobility.

### Scenario Two

A six-year-old girl is seen in physical therapy shortly after diagnosis of pauciarticular JRA two months ago. The patient's primary complaint is pain in the right ankle with any weight bearing activity. The patient enjoys playing outside and participates in soccer in the fall.

# Lateral Epicondylitis

## Diagnosis

### What condition produces a patient's symptoms?

Lateral epicondylitis (tennis elbow) is characterized by inflammation or degenerative changes at the common extensor tendon that attaches to the lateral epicondyle of the elbow. The primary symptom of this condition is pain.

### An injury was most likely sustained to which structure?

Repeated overuse of the wrist extensors, particularly the extensor carpi radialis brevis can produce tensile stress and result in microscopic tearing and damage to the extensor tendon. Other muscles that can be affected include the extensor digitorum, extensor carpi radialis longus, and extensor carpi ulnaris.

## Inference

### What is the most likely contributing factor in the development of this condition?

The exact etiology is uncertain, however, repetitive wrist action against resistance during extension and supination appear to produce this condition. Over time inflammation of the periosteum may develop with formation of adhesions. The continued microtrauma does not allow for proper healing and will continue to injure the tissues. This pattern is best seen while hitting a backhand in tennis, however, overuse with painting, hand tools, gardening, and any repeated activity that involves forceful wrist extension can result in lateral epicondylitis. Men are more likely to develop lateral epicondylitis and it is also more common for individuals in their late 30's and 40's secondary to the normal loss of the extensibility of connective tissue with age.

## Confirmation

### What is the most likely clinical presentation?

A typical patient with lateral epicondylitis is usually between the third and fifth decades of life and has unilateral involvement of the elbow. Lateral epicondylitis presents with pain along the lateral aspect of the elbow especially over the lateral epicondyle that sometimes radiates into the dorsum of the hand. The pain will increase with wrist flexion with elbow extension, resisted wrist extension, and resisted radial deviation. The patient may also have difficulty holding or gripping objects and insufficient forearm functional strength. Range of motion of the elbow usually remains normal, however, may be limited in severe cases. The patient will have localized tenderness over the lateral epicondyle and may present with localized swelling. The pain usually increases with activity and is noted at night.

### What laboratory or imaging studies would confirm the diagnosis?

No lab or imaging studies are required to diagnose lateral epicondylitis. X-ray or MRI may be used to rule out other conditions. Electrodiagnostic tests are only beneficial if there is radial nerve involvement.

### What additional information should be obtained to confirm the diagnosis?

Lateral epicondylitis is usually diagnosed based on history, physical examination of the extremity, and several manual maneuvers that specifically identify the presence of lateral epicondylitis. An increase in pain at the lateral epicondyle with resisted wrist extension implies extensor carpi radialis brevis involvement.

## Examination

### What history should be documented?

Important areas to explore include past medical history, medications, family history, current symptoms, current health status, social history and habits, occupation, leisure and sport activities, and social support system.

### What test/measures are most appropriate?

**Anthropometric characteristics:** circumferential measurements of the forearm

**Arousal, attention, and cognition:** examine mental status, learning ability, memory, motivation

**Community and work integration:** analysis of community, work, and leisure activities

**Environmental, home, and work barriers:** analysis of current and potential barriers or hazards

**Integumentary integrity:** skin assessment, assessment of sensation

**Joint integrity and mobility:** assessment of hypermobility and hypomobility of a joint, soft tissue swelling and inflammation, quality of movement of the elbow complex, provocative tests for lateral epicondylitis including Cozen's test, Mill's test, and lateral epicondylitis test

**Muscle performance:** strength assessment, muscle tone assessment, grip test dynamometer

**Orthotic, protective, and supportive devices:** potential utilization of bracing, splinting

**Pain:** pain perception assessment scale, visual analogue scale, assessment of muscle soreness

**Posture:** analysis of resting and dynamic posture

**Range of motion:** active and passive range of motion of bilateral upper extremities

**Reflex integrity:** assessment of deep tendon reflexes

**Self-care and home management:** assessment of functional capacity

# Lateral Epicondylitis

## What additional findings are likely with this patient?

If the patient is involved in tennis or some other potential overuse activity, there should be remediation and modification in training, technique, and equipment to minimize the chance of recurrence.

## Management

### What is the most effective management of this patient?

Medical management initially treats the pain and inflammation through protection, rest, ice, compression, and elevation. During the initial phase the patient should avoid all activities that aggravate the injury. Pharmacological intervention should include NSAIDs to alleviate pain and inflammation. Modalities may also be used such as phonophoresis with hydrocortisone or iontophoresis with dexamethasone. On occasion, resting splints may be used during the acute stage to relieve tension of the involved muscles. Physical therapy intervention should initiate stretching and strengthening to improve flexibility and increase functional activities. All exercise must remain pain free. Other modalities including electrical stimulation and cryotherapy may be beneficial. Strengthening should include elbow, wrist, and hand exercises. As a patient progresses resistive, isokinetic, and sport-specific exercises should be introduced. Counter-force bracing in the form of a forearm band may be indicated to reduce the degree of tension in the region of the muscular attachment. A patient should wean from the brace, prior to the completion of rehabilitation so the patient does not depend on it or use it as a replacement for rehabilitation.

### What home care regimen should be recommended?

A home care regimen should include the same therapeutic program the patient performs during physical therapy. Patient education should include modification of all activities that exacerbate the symptoms. It is imperative that the patient not rush or advance beyond the parameters of the home program as it will exacerbate the condition. A patient must avoid all activities that produce pain and use ice, elevation, and rest as needed.

## Outcome

### What is the likely outcome of a course in physical therapy?

Physical therapy may be indicated with goals of regaining appropriate strength, flexibility, and endurance while reducing inflammation and pain of the involved muscles. Overall outcome is favorable and a patient should be able to return to all previous functional activities without restrictions.

## What are the long-term effects of the patient's condition?

Lateral epicondylitis will commonly recur, however, continued stretching and exercise will decrease the risk of future recurrence. If conservative treatment does not improve symptoms after two to three months, surgical intervention may be indicated.

## Comparison

### What are the distinguishing characteristics of a similar condition?

Medial epicondylitis (golfer's or swimmer's elbow) results from repeated microtrauma to the flexor carpi radialis and/ or the humeral head of the pronator teres during pronation and wrist flexion. There is pain with resisted wrist flexion and resisted pronation and point tenderness over the medial epicondyle. Treatment is similar in protocol to lateral epicondylitis, however, is directed at the appropriate location. Complete immobilization is never recommended, however, counter-force bracing or splinting may be indicated.

## Clinical Scenarios

### Scenario One

A 27-year-old tennis player is seen in physical therapy diagnosed with right lateral epicondylitis. The patient plays in a competitive league and recently changed his instructor and increased the number of games played per week. He complains of pain and point tenderness over the lateral epicondyle. He is very frustrated, as this pain has had a large impact on his ability to win games.

### Scenario Two

A 42-year-old female diagnosed with right lateral epicondylitis has been seen in physical therapy for four weeks. She has a past medical history that includes reflex sympathetic dystrophy two years ago in the right upper extremity and is status post hysterectomy three months ago. She has not had any relief of pain and states that she cannot hold anything in her right hand. She enjoys gardening and works at a vegetable farm.

# Lymphedema Post-Mastectomy

## Diagnosis

### What condition produces a patient's symptoms?

Lymphedema following a mastectomy is termed secondary lymphedema and is the result of damage to the lymphatic nodes and vessels during surgery. Excessive accumulation of lymph fluid within the soft tissues is caused by an excess load of lymph fluid or inadequate transport capacity within the lymphatic system secondary to the loss of homeostasis.

### An injury was most likely sustained to which structure?

The lymphatic system is damaged as a result of the mastectomy, the surgical removal of the breast, whereby the lymphatic nodes and vessels are removed or damaged. The lymph system is unable to compensate, the lymph vessels dilate, and the valve flaps are not able to fully stop lymph flow. This allows for backflow of lymph into the tissues. This chain reaction causes further injury, chronic inflammation and progression including fibrosis, hypoxia within the tissues, and an increase risk of infection.

## Inference

### What is the most likely contributing factor in the development of this condition?

The most likely contributing factor in the development of lymphedema following a mastectomy is the damage and/or removal of the axillary lymph nodes and vessels in an attempt to prevent the spread of breast cancer. If the lymphatic nodes have not been removed, but have received radiation they may stop functioning due to chronic inflammation, fibrosis, and scarring. Globally, the parasitic infection called filariasis is the most common cause of secondary lymphedema. The virus is carried by mosquitoes in regions such as Africa, India, and Malaysia. Other causes include severe infection, crush injuries, burns or repeated pregnancies. There are an estimated three million new cases of secondary lymphedema each year with approximately 30% of breast cancer survivors affected by this condition. Primary lymphedema statistics indicate 15% of the cases are present at birth and 75% of the cases are acquired from adolescence through midlife years. Females are affected more than males with a 4:1 ratio.

## Confirmation

### What is the most likely clinical presentation?

The clinical presentation of lymphedema includes edema in an affected area/extremity that increases with dependent positioning. The patient usually does not experience pain, but rather a tight or heavy sensation. Lymphedema is classified into three stages that present differently based on the severity of the condition. Stage I is characterized by pitting edema that reduces with elevation overnight and does not exhibit any fibrotic changes. Stage II is identified by some fibrotic changes that begin to occur and increase in non-pitting edema that does not reduce with elevation. Stage III is characterized by

skin changes, frequent infections, and severe edema that is non-pitting and fibrotic.

### What laboratory or imaging studies would confirm the diagnosis?

Diagnosis is confirmed through history, observation, and several diagnostic tools to rule out other potential disorders. A Doppler study of the affected area is able to rule out a deep vein thrombosis. A CT scan or MRI may be performed before treatment of lymphedema is initiated to rule out malignancy. A lymphoscintigram is a nuclear medicine procedure that tests the function of the lymphatic system.

### What additional information should be obtained to confirm the diagnosis?

A medical evaluation should include a thorough history including all illnesses, hospitalizations, and surgeries. History should be noted regarding the current edema and its course. Date of onset, progression, and symptoms associated with the edema are important to attain and note in the patient's record.

## Examination

### What history should be documented?

Important areas to explore include past medical history and surgical history, medications, history of swelling, family history, current symptoms, current health status, living environment, social history and habits, occupation, and social support system.

### What test/measures are most appropriate?

**Aerobic capacity and endurance:** assessment of vital signs at rest and with activity, perceived exertion scale, pulse oximetry, auscultation of the lungs

**Anthropometric characteristics:** circumferential and volumetric measurements of involved areas, skinfold measurements

**Arousal, attention, and cognition:** examine mental status, learning ability, memory, motivation

**Community and work integration:** analysis of community, work, and leisure activities

**Environmental, home, and work barriers:** analysis of current and potential barriers or hazards

**Gait, locomotion, and balance:** static and dynamic balance in sitting and standing, safety during gait with/without an assistive device

**Integumentary integrity:** skin assessment, assessment of sensation, nailbed assessment

**Joint integrity and mobility:** soft tissue swelling and inflammation

**Muscle performance:** strength and tone assessment

# Lymphedema Post-Mastectomy

**Pain:** pain perception assessment scale
**Range of motion:** active and passive range of motion
**Self-care and home management:** assessment of functional capacity
**Ventilation, respiration, and circulation:** assessment of brachial and radial pulses, capillary refill assessment

## What additional findings are likely with this patient?

Additional findings are based on the etiology, stage, and progression of the lymphedema. Complications can include ulcer formation, increased risk for fungal and bacterial infections, loss of range, fatigue, and fibrotic edema with atrophic skin changes. If left untreated a patient could progress to stage III "lymphostatic elephantiasis."

## Management

### What is the most effective management of this patient?

Effective medical management of secondary lymphedema may involve pharmacological intervention or natural substances that increase proteolysis and macrophage activity, however, there is no particular class of drugs that can "cure" lymphedema. Surgery is used in the treatment of severe lymphedema, but only achieves limited results since the cause remains unchanged. Physical therapy intervention usually follows a treatment approach termed combined decongestive physiotherapy (CDP). The philosophy of lymphatic management includes patient education in skin care, hygiene, bandaging, self-massage, and exercise. Therapeutic intervention should focus on manual lymph drainage, short stretch compression bandages, retrograde massage, exercise, compression therapy, and use of a mechanical pump. Care must be taken, however, not to exceed 45 mm Hg during compression therapy since a greater pressure can damage or collapse the lymphatic walls.

### What home care regimen should be recommended?

A home care regimen is vital to the success of the CDP treatment of lymphedema. A patient must understand and comply with skin care, bandaging, self-massage, lymphatic drainage techniques, compression therapy, and an exercise program. Each patient must also understand the lifetime precautions that can increase lymphedema such as sunburn, air travel, excessive exercise, poor nutrition, and obesity.

## Outcome

### What is the likely outcome of a course in physical therapy?

Comprehensive lymphedema intervention such as CDP has shown significant reduction in lymphedema during treatment and continued reduction with an ongoing home program over time.

## What are the long-term effects of the patient's condition?

Lymphedema is progressive if left untreated, but can be managed through intervention and education. Patients must comply with a home program and must remain aware of all activities that place the patient at an increased risk for lymphedema.

## Comparison

### What are the distinguishing characteristics of a similar condition?

Lipedema is a condition where there appears to be swelling throughout the bilateral lower extremities from the hips to the ankle joints. This swelling is actually subcutaneous adipose tissue. This condition is sometimes confused with lymphedema, but does not affect the lymphatic system. It most often occurs in women with hormonal disorders and is believed to have a family history in approximately 20% of the cases. Medical management treats the hormonal imbalance and assists with nutritional guidance to allow for effective weight management.

## Clinical Scenarios

### Scenario One

A 39-year-old female status post right mastectomy secondary to malignancy develops lymphedema in her right arm four months after surgery. She resides alone and is employed as a web design consultant. She complains of heaviness in the arm, but denies pain. She was referred by her oncologist for outpatient physical therapy.

### Scenario Two

A 68-year-old male is seen in physical therapy with stage II lymphedema in his right lower extremity. He underwent total hip arthroplasty two months ago and experienced immediate swelling and discomfort. His history includes multiple abdominal surgeries with edema present after each surgery. He presents with non-pitting edema that does not reduce with elevation.

# Medial Collateral Ligament Sprain – Grade II

## Diagnosis

### What condition produces a patient's symptoms?

The medial collateral ligament (MCL) connects the medial epicondyle of the femur to the medial tibia and as a result resists medially directed force at the knee. The MCL is the primary stabilizer of the medial side of the knee against valgus force and lateral rotation of the tibia (especially during knee flexion). This extra-articular ligament is a thick and flat band which attaches proximally on the medial femoral condyle and extends to the medial surface of the tibia approximately six centimeters below the joint line. A common mechanism of injury is a direct blow against the lateral surface of the knee causing valgus stress and subsequent damage to the medial aspect of the knee.

### An injury was most likely sustained to which structure?

The medial collateral ligament is comprised of two parts. A deep part of the ligament attaches to the meniscus and the superficial part attaches further down the joint. A grade II injury of the MCL is characterized by partial tearing of the ligament's fibers resulting in joint laxity when the ligament is stretched. Often the medial capsular ligament is involved in a grade II sprain of the MCL.

## Inference

### What is the most likely contributing factor in the development of this condition?

Individuals participating in contact activities requiring a high level of agility are particularly susceptible to a MCL injury. Mechanism of injury is usually a blow to the outside of the knee joint causing excess force to the medial side of the joint. The MCL can also be injured by a twisting of the knee. Muscle weakness resulting in poor dynamic stabilization may also increase the incidence of this type of injury.

## Confirmation

### What is the most likely clinical presentation?

A patient with a grade II MCL injury will likely present with an inability to fully extend and flex the knee, pain and significant tenderness along the medial aspect of the knee, possible decrease in strength, potential loss of proprioception, and an antalgic gait. There is typically discernable laxity with valgus testing, instability of the joint, and slight to moderate swelling around the knee. More severe swelling may be indicative of meniscus or cruciate ligament involvement.

### What laboratory or imaging studies would confirm the diagnosis?

MRI is a non-invasive imaging technique that can be utilized to view soft tissue structures such as ligaments. The imaging technique is extremely expensive and therefore may not be commonly employed on an individual with a suspected MCL injury without other extenuating circumstances.

### What additional information should be obtained to confirm the diagnosis?

A valgus stress test is a technique designed to detect medial instability in a single plane. The examiner applies a valgus stress at the knee while stabilizing the ankle in slight lateral rotation. The test is often performed initially in full extension and then in 30 degrees of flexion. A patient with a grade II MCL sprain may exhibit 5-15 degrees of laxity with valgus stress at 30 degrees of flexion.

## Examination

### What history should be documented?

Important areas to explore include mechanism of present injury, current symptoms, past medical history, medications, living environment, occupation, social history and habits, and social support system.

### What test/measures are most appropriate?

**Anthropometric characteristics:** palpation to determine knee effusion, lower extremity circumferential measurements

**Arousal, attention, and cognition:** examine mental status, learning ability, memory, motivation

**Assistive and adaptive devices:** analysis of components and safety of a device, potential utilization of crutches

**Community and work integration:** analysis of community, work, and leisure activities

**Environmental, home, and work barriers:** analysis of current and potential barriers or hazards

**Gait, locomotion, and balance:** safety during gait with an assistive device

**Integumentary integrity:** assessment of sensation (pain, temperature, tactile), skin assessment

**Joint integrity and mobility:** special tests for ligaments and menisci, valgus stress test, palpation of structures, joint play, soft tissue restrictions, joint pain

**Muscle performance:** strength assessment, assessment of active movement, resisted isometrics, muscle contraction characteristics, muscle endurance

**Orthotic, protective, and supportive devices:** potential utilization of bracing, taping or wrapping

**Pain:** pain perception assessment scale, visual analogue scale

**Range of motion:** active and passive range of motion

**Self-care and home management:** assessment of functional capacity

**Sensory integrity:** assessment of proprioception and kinesthesia

# Medial Collateral Ligament Sprain – Grade II

## What additional findings are likely with this patient?

Anterior cruciate ligament and/or meniscal damage often accompanies a grade II MCL injury. As a result it is often prudent to perform special tests directed at these particular structures. The MCL normally has a good secondary support system with weight bearing forces compressing the medial side of the joint and adding to the overall stability of the joint. This allows the structures to be protected after injury along with use of a brace.

## Management

### What is the most effective management of this patient?

Medical management for a grade II MCL sprain usually involves conservative management including R.I.C.E. (rest, icing, compression, and elevation). Pharmacological intervention is directed towards pain management through acetaminophen or NSAIDs. The patient may utilize a full-length knee immobilizer or a hinge brace and crutches to limit weight bearing through the involved lower extremity for initial rehabilitation. Physical therapy intervention should be directed towards increasing range of motion in the involved extremity and beginning light resistive exercises. Range of motion exercises may include heel slides or stationary cycling without resistance. Resistive exercises should be directed towards the quadriceps and may include isometrics and closed kinetic chain exercises. Functional activities such as gait and stair climbing should be incorporated into the treatment program. Superficial modalities and electrical stimulation may be utilized to combat pain and inflammation. Transverse friction massage may be applied to the healing ligament so it does not adhere to surrounding and adjacent structures. Care must be taken not to massage the proximal attachment of the MCL due to potential bony periosteal disruption. A patient should be required to complete a functional progression prior to returning to unrestricted activity.

### What home care regimen should be recommended?

The home care regimen should consist of range of motion, strengthening, palliative care, and functional activities as warranted based on the results of the patient examination. The use of crutches should continue until the patient can adequately extend the knee joint.

## Outcome

### What is the likely outcome of a course in physical therapy?

A grade II MCL sprain should progress fairly quickly if no other structures (ACL or meniscus) are involved. A patient should be able to return to their previous functional level within four to eight weeks following the injury.

### What are the long-term effects of the patient's condition?

Proper healing time and rehabilitation management should allow the patient to return to all forms of activity once the patient demonstrates full range of motion, ambulation without a limp, no visual swelling, and competence with all agility testing. If the patient has residual laxity from the injury the patient may be susceptible to reinjury.

## Comparison

### What are the distinguishing characteristics of a similar condition?

A grade II lateral collateral ligament injury differs from a MCL injury in several ways. The lateral collateral ligament attaches proximally on the lateral femoral condyle and runs distally and posteriorly to insert on the head of the fibula. Lateral collateral ligament injuries are far less common than MCL injuries. Management should focus on the same general goals (range of motion, strengthening, palliative care, and functional activities) as those outlined for the MCL injury.

## Clinical Scenarios

### Scenario One

A 17-year-old male is diagnosed with a left grade III MCL sprain and a small tear in the medial meniscus. The patient was playing football when he was injured. The patient has no significant past medical history and plans to participate in football at the collegiate level.

### Scenario Two

A 20-year-old college field hockey player complains of knee pain after being diagnosed with a grade I MCL sprain. The patient is mildly tender to palpation over the medial joint line and exhibits trace effusion. The patient has no significant past medical history and would like to return to athletic competition as soon as possible.

# Multiple Sclerosis

## Diagnosis

### What condition produces a patient's symptoms?

Multiple sclerosis (MS) produces patches of demyelination that decreases the efficiency of nerve impulse transmission. Symptoms vary based on the location and the extent of demyelination.

### An injury was most likely sustained to which structure?

Multiple sclerosis is characterized by demyelination of the myelin sheaths that surround the nerves within the brain and spinal cord. Myelin breakdown results in plaque development, decreased nerve conduction velocity, and eventual failure of impulse transmission. Lesions are scattered throughout the central nervous system and do not follow a particular pattern.

## Inference

### What is the most likely contributing factor in the development of this condition?

The exact etiology of MS is unknown. Genetics, viral infections, and environment all have a role in the development of MS. It is theorized that a slow acting virus initiates the autoimmune response in individuals that have environmental and genetic factors for the disease. The incidence of MS is higher in Caucasians between the ages of 20 and 35 years and is nearly twice as common in women as in men. There is also a higher incidence of MS in temperate climates.

## Confirmation

### What is the most likely clinical presentation?

The prevalence of MS differs by geographic area, sex, and race. In the United States the prevalence is 30-80:100,000 with 250,000-350,000 current cases. The highest incidence is 20-35 years of age, however, MS can occur at any age. MS can be classified as relapsing-remitting MS (85%), secondary-progressive MS, primary-progressive MS or progressive-relapsing MS. The clinical presentation varies based on the type of disease, the location, extent of demyelination, and degree of sclerosis. Initial symptoms can include visual problems, paresthesias and sensory changes, clumsiness, weakness, ataxia, balance dysfunction, and fatigue. The clinical course usually consists of periods of exacerbations and remissions, however, the degree of neurologic dysfunction and subsequent recovery will follow typical patterns of the specific type of MS. The frequency and intensity of exacerbations may indicate the speed/course of the disease process.

### What laboratory or imaging studies would confirm the diagnosis?

There is not a single testing procedure to diagnose MS early in the disease. MRI may assist with observation and establishing a baseline for lesions, evoked potentials may demonstrate slowed nerve conduction, and cerebrospinal fluid can be analyzed for an elevated concentration of gamma globulin and protein levels.

### What additional information should be obtained to confirm the diagnosis?

Clinical presentation and reliable patient history of symptoms are vital in the diagnosis of MS. Guidelines indicate that a clinically definitive diagnosis of MS can be made if a person experiences two separate attacks and shows evidence of two separate lesions. Other diagnoses (having specific criteria) include laboratory-supported definite MS, clinically probable MS, and laboratory-supported probable MS.

## Examination

### What history should be documented?

Important areas to explore include past medical history, history of symptoms, medications, current health status, social history, occupation, living environment, and social support system.

### What test/measures are most appropriate?

**Aerobic capacity and endurance:** assessment of vital signs at rest and with activity

**Arousal, attention and cognition:** examine mental status, learning ability, memory, and motivation, Mini-Mental State Examination

**Assistive and adaptive devices:** analysis of components and safety of a device

**Community and work integration:** analysis of community, work, and leisure activities

**Gait, locomotion, and balance:** static/dynamic balance in sitting/standing, Tinetti Performance Oriented Mobility Assessment, Berg Balance Scale

**Motor function:** assessment of dexterity and coordination; assessment of postural, equilibrium, and righting reactions; gross and fine motor skills

**Muscle performance:** strength and tone assessment, tremor assessment, muscle endurance, Modified Fatigue Impact Scale

**Neuromotor development and sensory integration:** analysis of reflex movement patterns

**Pain:** pain perception assessment scale

**Posture:** resting/dynamic posture, potential contracture

**Range of motion:** active and passive range of motion

**Self-care and home management:** Barthel Index, assessment of functional capacity and safety, Kurtzke Expanded Disability Status Scale

# Multiple Sclerosis

## What additional findings are likely with this patient?

A low percentage of patients experience benign MS and have little to no long-term disability. The majority experience progressive degeneration through periods of exacerbations and remissions. As the disease advances exacerbations leave greater ongoing disability and the length of remissions decrease. Ongoing symptoms can include emotional lability, depression, dementia, psychological problems, spasticity, tremor, weakness, paralysis, sexual dysfunction, and loss of bowel and bladder control.

## Management

### What is the most effective management of this patient?

Management of MS includes pharmacological, medical, and therapeutic intervention. The goal of medical treatment of MS is to lessen the length of exacerbations and maximize the health of the patient. Pharmacological intervention is quite complex and can include ABC drugs (approved in the treatment of MS) that are classified as immunomodulatory medications. Physical, occupational, and speech therapies are indicated throughout the clinical course of the disease and well as nutritional and psychological counseling. Physical therapy intervention includes regulation of activity level, relaxation and energy conservation techniques, normalization of tone, balance activities, gait training, core stabilization and control, and adaptive/assistive device training. Patient and caregiver education regarding safety, energy conservation, patterns of fatigue, and the use of adaptive devices is vital to the quality of life.

### What home care regimen should be recommended?

A home care regimen should include a submaximal exercise/endurance program. Exercise in the morning when the patient is rested is advisable to avoid fatigue. The patient may need frequent rest periods throughout the day and may benefit from breaking a task into smaller steps to avoid fatigue. Ongoing ambulation and mobility activities are important to maintain endurance and prevent disuse atrophy. Aquatic therapy may also be beneficial to this population.

## Outcome

### What is the likely outcome of a course in physical therapy?

Physical therapy is indicated intermittently throughout the clinical course of MS with the goal of maximizing functional capacity and the quality of life. Physical therapy will not alter the progression of the disease process, but rather treat the current symptoms and assist the patient to attain the highest level of function. Factors that influence exacerbations include heat, stress, infection, trauma, and pregnancy.

## What are the long-term effects of the patient's condition?

MS is generally a progressive degenerative disease process that creates permanent damage and disability. Factors that influence exacerbations include heat, stress, and trauma. Most patients live with MS for many years and die from secondary complications such as disuse atrophy, pressure sores, contractures, pathological fractures, renal infection, and pneumonia. If left untreated 50% of patients will require a wheelchair within 15 years post diagnosis. Overall mortality rate and long-term outcome correlates to age at diagnosis, number of attacks and exacerbations, frequency and duration of remissions, and type of MS. Suicide is also seven times greater when compared to the same age control group without MS.

## Comparison

### What are the distinguishing characteristics of a similar condition?

Dystonia is a neurologic syndrome that presents with involuntary and sustained muscle contractions that cause repetitive movements. Idiopathic dystonia has a genetic basis and accounts for two-thirds of all cases. Secondary dystonia usually results from brain damage or CNS damage. There are no definitive tests to diagnose dystonia. Treatment is based on current symptoms and includes pharmacological intervention, physical therapy, and occasional surgical intervention. Prognosis is based on age of onset and spontaneous remission occurs in 25-30% of the cases.

## Clinical Scenarios

### Scenario One

A 28-year-old female has recently had visual difficulty, urinary urgency, tingling, and upper extremity weakness on two separate occasions. The patient has an aunt with MS, however, has no other significant medical history. The patient was referred to physical therapy by her primary physician.

### Scenario Two

A 42-year-old male with MS is referred to physical therapy. The patient has experienced several exacerbations and remissions with full recovery in the past. The patient presently appears to have an exacerbation of symptoms including excessive fatigue. He lives alone and works in a library.

# Myocardial Infarction

## Diagnosis

### What condition produces a patient's symptoms?

Myocardial infarction (MI) occurs when there is poor coronary artery perfusion, ischemia, and subsequent necrosis of the cardiac tissue usually due to thrombus, arterial blockage or atherosclerosis. The location and severity of the infarct will determine symptoms and the overall acute clinical picture.

### An injury was most likely sustained to which structure?

A MI produces ischemia and subsequent necrosis to a portion of the myocardium. The extent of the damage to the myocardium is dependent on the duration of ischemia and on the thickness of the tissue involved. A transmural MI involves the full-thickness of the myocardium while a nontransmural MI involves the subendocardial area (inner third of the myocardium). The myocardium has three zones that form concentric circles around the point of infarct termed zone of infarct, zone of hypoxic injury, and zone of ischemia. Thrombosis of the anterior descending branch of the left coronary artery is the most common location of infarct and affects the left ventricle. A right coronary artery thrombosis can result in an infarct of the posteroinferior portion of the left ventricle and can potentially affect the right ventricular myocardium.

## Inference

### What is the most likely contributing factor in the development of this condition?

The primary risk factors for MI include patient or family history of heart disease, smoking, physical inactivity, stress, hypertension, elevated cholesterol, diabetes mellitus, and obesity. The use of cocaine and aortic stenosis may also cause a MI. It has been documented that a MI will occur more frequently in the morning hours and during the November to December holiday season.

## Confirmation

### What is the most likely clinical presentation?

MI occurs in 1.5 million individuals each year within the United States with a mortality rate of 500,000 deaths annually. Approximately two-thirds of patients experience prodromal symptoms days to weeks before the event, including unstable angina, shortness of breath, and fatigue. A patient that is experiencing a MI will initially present with deep pain or pressure in the substernal area. The pain may or may not radiate to the jaw and down the left arm or to the back. The patient cannot alleviate the pain with rest or nitroglycerin and the pain may last for hours. The patient is usually anxious, pale, sweating, fatigued, and may present with nausea and vomiting. Symptoms of a MI frequently do not follow a typical pattern, especially in females. There are also instances of a silent MI where no symptoms are noted.

## What laboratory or imaging studies would confirm the diagnosis?

The primarily tool to detect a MI is a 12-lead electrocardiogram. An inverted T wave indicates myocardial ischemia, elevated ST segment indicates acute infarction, and a depressed ST segment indicates a pending subendocardial or transmural infarction. A blood serum analysis can be utilized to determine the level of selected cardiac enzymes. The level of selected enzymes such as creatine phosphokinase (CPK), aspartate transferase (AST), and lactic dehydrogenase (LDH) can be dramatically altered during and after a MI. A complete blood count (CBC), chest radiograph, radionuclide imaging, and amylase level may be ordered to assist with the diagnosis.

## What additional information should be obtained to confirm the diagnosis?

Additional information in the diagnosis of a MI is found through the manifestation of symptoms and clinical examination including a thorough past medical history and history of current symptoms.

## Examination

### What history should be documented?

Important areas to explore include past medical history, family history, medications, current health status, living environment, social history and habits, occupation, and social support system.

### What test/measures are most appropriate?

**Aerobic capacity and endurance:** vital signs at rest and during activity, palpation of pulses, perceived exertion scale, electrocardiogram analysis, auscultation of the heart and lungs, pulse oximetry

**Arousal, attention, and cognition:** examine mental status, learning ability, memory, motivation

**Assistive and adaptive devices:** analysis of components and safety of a device

**Environmental, home, and work:** analysis of current and potential barriers or hazards

**Gait, locomotion, and balance:** assessment of static and dynamic balance in sitting and standing, safety during gait with/without an assistive device

**Muscle performance:** strength assessment through active movement only (no manual muscle testing)

**Pain:** pain perception scale, visual analogue scale

**Posture:** analysis of resting and dynamic posture

**Self-care and home management:** assessment of functional capacity, Barthel Index

**Ventilation, respiration, and circulation:** ventilation, respiration, and circulation; assessment of pulses

# Myocardial Infarction

## What additional findings are likely with this patient?

A patient status post MI is at risk for complications that include arrhythmias, hypotension, pericarditis, impaired cardiac output, pulmonary edema, congestive heart failure, pericarditis, cardiogenic shock, recurrent infarction and sudden death. Arrhythmias occur in 90% of patients post MI and are caused by ischemia, ANS impairment, electrolyte imbalances, conduction defects, and other chemical imbalances.

## Management

### What is the most effective management of this patient?

Initial medical management of a MI is to stabilize the patient and initiate pharmacological intervention to hinder the evolution of the MI. Anticoagulants, beta-blockers, thrombolytic agents, angiotensin-converting enzyme inhibitors, vasodilators, and estrogen (in women) may be used. Once stable, the patient is managed through a cardiac rehabilitation program. Surgical intervention including angioplasty, stenting, endarterectomy, and bypass grafting may be indicated based on the underlying cause of the MI. Exercise testing is performed within three days of the MI in order to establish baseline guidelines for patients that are cleared to exercise and do not exhibit any arrhythmias or angina. Physical therapy intervention usually follows a multi-phase cardiac rehabilitation program and continues in an outpatient setting once the patient is discharged from the hospital. Low-level therapeutic exercise, functional activities, relaxation, breathing techniques, endurance training, and continuous monitoring of vital signs are key components of this program. Patient education regarding reduction of risk factors, return to activity, and commitment to fitness and health are also important to the success of physical therapy intervention.

### What home care regimen should be recommended?

A home care regimen should follow the guidelines indicated for each phase of cardiac rehabilitation. A patient must continue with safe exercise and integration of risk factor reduction. Symptom recognition and nutritional strategies are also important in a daily routine.

## Outcome

### What is the likely outcome of a course in physical therapy?

Cardiac rehabilitation is recommended status post MI. The patient should start in the coronary care unit (CCU) and progress through each of the phases of cardiac rehabilitation. The goal is successful completion of a cardiac rehabilitation program allowing the patient to resume all activities of daily living and recreational pursuits. Upon completion, the patient should possess self-management skills associated with symptoms/risk factors of heart disease.

## What are the long-term effects of the patient's condition?

A patient that has experienced a MI may be able to return to all previous activities after successful completion of a cardiac rehabilitation program. A patient must continue to reduce the modifiable risk factors and maintain an appropriate level of exercise in order to limit a possible subsequent MI. Long-term outcome is dependent on prior functional ability, the extent and damage to the heart, and factors that negatively affect prognosis such as age, cardiovascular disease, hypotension, the presence of co-morbidities, and an abnormal treadmill exercise test.

## Comparison

### What are the distinguishing characteristics of a similar condition?

Angina pectoris is a myocardial ischemic disorder that occurs when there is an oxygen deficit to the coronary arteries. Coronary artery disease accounts for 90% of all cases of angina. Angina is classified as stable, post-infarction, Prinzmetal's, resting, unstable, nocturnal or variant. Symptoms often occur during exertion and include chest pain that may radiate. Rest or nitroglycerin normally provides relief of the symptoms. Treatment of the underlying cause is essential to prevent further damage to the heart.

## Clinical Scenarios

### Scenario One

A 51-year-old male is referred to a phase I cardiac rehabilitation program after a transmural MI two days ago. The patient has hypertension, high cholesterol, smokes, and is obese. The patient currently supervises a local automobile dealership. The patient is divorced and lives in a two-story home.

### Scenario Two

A 78-year-old female is status post nontransmural MI. The patient is very active and plays golf. The patient's past medical history includes treatment for a cardiac arrhythmia, obesity, and diabetes mellitus. The physician referred the patient for cardiac rehabilitation.

# Osteoarthritis

## Diagnosis

### What condition produces a patient's symptoms?

Osteoarthritis (OA) is a heterogeneous group of conditions resulting in common physiological changes. The most common type of joint disease, OA is a degenerative chronic disorder resulting from the biochemical breakdown of articular cartilage in the synovial joints. Although theories indicate that OA is due to excessive wear and tear, secondary inflammatory changes may also affect the involved joints. OA has been divided into primary and secondary forms.

### An injury was most likely sustained to which structure?

The progression of OA begins with degenerative alterations primarily in the articular cartilage. This degenerative process is usually a result of excessive loading of a healthy joint or normal loading of an abnormal joint. External forces create the breakdown of the chondrocytes and cause disruption of the cartilaginous matrix. Loss of cartilage results in the loss of the joint space. Through this process, reactive new bone forms, usually at the margins and subchondral areas of the joint.

## Inference

### What is the most likely contributing factor in the development of this condition?

The etiology of primary OA is idiopathic occurring within intact joints with no history that supports the initiation of this condition. Primary OA is related to the aging process and typically occurs in older individuals. Secondary OA refers to degenerative disease of the synovial joints that results from some predisposing condition (i.e., trauma) that has adversely altered the articular cartilage and/or subchondral bone of the affected joints. Secondary OA often occurs in relatively young individuals. General risk factors include age, obesity, trauma, infection, repetitive microtrauma, genetic factors, inflammatory arthritis, neuromuscular and metabolic disorders.

## Confirmation

### What is the most likely clinical presentation?

Potential sites for primary OA include joints of the hands specifically the distal interphalangeal joints (DIP) and proximal interphalangeal joints (PIP), knees, hips, and the spine. Bilateral symmetry is often seen in cases of primary OA, particularly when the hands are affected. A patient with OA may experience a decrease in range of motion accompanied by crepitus within the affected joints. The patient will frequently complain of deep and aching joint pain exacerbated by prolonged activity and use. Heberden's nodes consist of palpable osteophytes in the DIP joints and are usually seen in women, but not men. Pain is the main reason patients seek medical attention. Initially, patients have pain during activity that is alleviated by rest and usually respond to analgesics.

Morning stiffness in the affected joints usually occurs with progression of the disease, resulting in an increased pain level even at rest that may not respond to analgesics. Erythema or warmth over the joints is not usually present, but effusion may exist. Malalignment and limitation of the joint may occur as the disease progresses in severity. The patient may also present with a deviated gait pattern, atypical movement patterns, and muscle atrophy.

### What laboratory or imaging studies would confirm the diagnosis?

OA is typically diagnosed on the basis of clinical examination and x-ray findings. Laboratory tests will not diagnose OA.

### What additional information should be obtained to confirm the diagnosis?

Visual inspection of the affected joints, a thorough examination, and a history of the condition will normally support the diagnosis.

## Examination

### What history should be documented?

Important areas to explore include past medical history, medications, current health status, nutritional status, social history and habits, occupation, living environment, and social support system.

### What test/measures are most appropriate?

**Aerobic capacity and endurance:** assessment of vital signs at rest and with activity, perceived exertion scale, pulse oximetry, auscultation of the lungs

**Anthropometric characteristics:** circumferential measurements

**Arousal, attention, and cognition:** mental status exam

**Assistive and adaptive devices:** analysis of components and safety of a device

**Community and work integration:** analysis of community, work, and leisure activities

**Environmental, home, and work barriers:** analysis of current and potential barriers or hazards

**Ergonomics and body mechanics:** analysis of dexterity and coordination

**Gait, locomotion, and balance:** static and dynamic balance in sitting and standing, safety during gait with/without an assistive device, Berg Functional Balance Scale, Functional Ambulation Profile

**Integumentary integrity:** assessment of sensation

**Joint integrity and mobility:** hypermobility and hypomobility of a joint, soft tissue swelling and inflammation

# Osteoarthritis

**Motor function:** equilibrium and righting reactions, motor assessment scales, coordination

**Muscle performance:** strength assessment

**Pain:** pain perception assessment scale, VAS

**Posture:** analysis of resting and dynamic posture

**Range of motion:** active and passive range of motion

**Self-care and home management:** assessment of functional capacity, Functional Independence Measure

**Sensory integrity:** proprioception and kinesthesia

## What additional findings are likely with this patient?

In patients greater than 55 years old, the prevalence of OA is higher among women than men. DIP and PIP joint involvement resulting in Heberden's and Bouchard's nodes is also more common in women. Disease progression characteristically is slow, occurring over several years or decades. Pain is usually the initial and principal source of morbidity in OA. The patient can become progressively inactive leading to additional co-morbidities including weight gain. There is also an increased incidence of strains and sprains around joints affected with OA.

## Management

### What is the most effective management of this patient?

Medical management of a patient with OA is usually multi-faceted based on symptoms and the specific affected joints. Long-term management would include pharmacological intervention using acetaminophen or other NSAIDs to alleviate the pain. Glucocorticoid intra-articular injections may also be prescribed to improve a patient's symptoms, however, must be used sparingly due to the long-term negative effects. Nutritional education and weight reduction may be indicated to reduce the stress on the affected joints. Physical therapy may be indicated intermittently in order to preserve joint motion and flexibility. Other treatment may include posture retraining, work site evaluation, general strengthening, relaxation and endurance activities, icing or heat for pain management, hydrotherapy, modalities, patient education, aquatic therapy, and functional activities. If conservative treatment fails, a patient may be a candidate for joint replacement surgery with the goal of pain relief.

### What home care regimen should be recommended?

A home care regimen for OA should include general strengthening to tolerance, AROM exercises, endurance activities, continued use of relaxation techniques, and supportive or assistive devices that would decrease pain and improve functional ability. It is very important that the patient avoid overexertion and fatigue.

## Outcome

### What is the likely outcome of a course in physical therapy?

Physical therapy can assist the patient during periods of exacerbation of the disease process, however, cannot change the ultimate outcome of the condition. OA is a progressive and chronic condition. Physical therapy can assist in minimizing the effects of the process and allow for as much independence as allowed by patient tolerance during functional activities.

### What are the long-term effects of the patient's condition?

Approximately 80-90% of individuals older than 65 years have evidence of primary OA. The degree of disability also depends on the site(s) of involvement and rate of progression. Usually, the pain slowly worsens over time, but it may stabilize. OA of the knee is a leading cause of disability in elderly persons.

## Comparison

### What are the distinguishing characteristics of a similar condition?

Psoriatic arthritis is a rheumatic condition characterized by inflammatory arthritis and is often seen in combination with psoriatic skin lesions. Symptoms include silver or grey scaly spots on the scalp, elbows, knees and spine, pitting of fingernails and toenails, pain and swelling in one or more joints, and swelling of the fingers and toes. Psoriatic arthritis affects men and women of all races and usually occurs between the ages of 20 and 50, but can occur at any age. The etiology is unknown, but theories suggest a relationship to genetic inheritance, psoriasis, and environmental factors.

## Clinical Scenarios

### Scenario One

A 71-year-old female is referred to physical therapy with significant OA in her hands, knees, and hips. She is approximately 35 pounds overweight and has lost mobility. She rates her pain as an eight out of ten and wants to have surgery to "fix" her legs. She resides in a two-story home with her husband.

### Scenario Two

A 39-year-old male has developed secondary OA as a result of a 15-year career in semi-professional football. The patient lives a very active lifestyle, however, has a significant amount of pain in both knee joints. The patient is currently married and working full-time.

# Osteogenesis Imperfecta

## Diagnosis

### What condition produces a patient's symptoms?

Osteogenesis Imperfecta (OI) is a rare congenital disorder of collagen synthesis that affects all connective tissue in the body. The genetic defect affects collagen-producing genes and reduces production of collagen from 20-50%. There are many mutations identified and various underlying causes that combine to produce the phenotypic expression of OI in a patient.

### An injury was most likely sustained to which structure?

The genes for type I collagen production (COL1A1 and COL1A2) have been identified as the genes that become mutated and result in OI. Since collagen production is vital throughout the body, bones and all forms of connective tissue are compromised. OI can also compromise growth, hearing, cardiopulmonary function, and joint integrity.

## Inference

### What is the most likely contributing factor in the development of this condition?

Most children inherit OI from parents as either an autosomal dominant or autosomal recessive trait. Twenty-five percent of the time the genetic defect occurs by spontaneous mutation of the genes. Statistics estimate that 30 to 50 thousand individuals are living with OI in the United States.

## Confirmation

### What is the most likely clinical presentation?

OI is classified into four types and has a wide range of clinical presentations ranging from normal appearance with mild symptoms to severe involvement that is fatal during infancy. Type I is the mildest form where a child has near normal growth and appearance with frequency of fractures usually ceasing after puberty. The patient experiences mild or moderate fragility, but most times without deformity. This patient will usually present with blue sclera, easy bruising, triangular face, and possible hearing loss. Type II is the most severe form where a child dies in utero or by early childhood. This child has significant fragility of connective tissue, experiences multiple fractures with extreme deformities, and has a soft skull. Type III is severe, but these children present with greater ossification of the skull. Type III characteristics include significant growth, retardation, progressive deformities, ongoing fractures, severe osteoporosis, triangular face, blue sclera, and significant limitations with functional mobility. Type IV is usually a milder course that involves mild to moderate fragility and osteoporosis (but greater than type I). The patient will experience fractures easily prior to puberty, but some children improve at that time. Type IV may or may not have a shorter stature, will have bowing of long bones, a barrel shape of their rib cage, possible hearing loss, brittle

teeth, and will present with near normal sclera. These children have a near normal life expectancy.

### What laboratory or imaging studies would confirm the diagnosis?

A skin biopsy is used to examine the collagen and determine what type of OI is present. X-rays and bone scans may be used for evidence of deformities and old fractures. Bone densitometry may also be used to measure bone mass and estimate the risk of fracture for specific sites within the body. The diagnosis is made through these tests and in combination with the examination and history.

### What additional information should be obtained to confirm the diagnosis?

Diagnosis should be determined based on physical examination, family and personal medical history, and formal testing.

## Examination

### What history should be documented?

Important areas to explore include past medical history including falls, medications, family history, current symptoms and health status, and social support system.

### What test/measures are most appropriate?

**Arousal, attention, and cognition:** examine mental status, learning ability, memory, motivation

**Environmental, home, and work barriers:** analysis of current and potential barriers or hazards

**Ergonomics and body mechanics:** analysis of dexterity and coordination

**Gait, locomotion, and balance:** static/dynamic balance in sitting/standing, safety during gait with/without an assistive device, analysis of wheelchair management

**Integumentary integrity:** skin and sensation assessment

**Joint integrity and mobility:** assessment of hypermobility and hypomobility of a joint

**Muscle performance:** strength assessment of active motion, muscle tone assessment

**Neuromotor development and sensory integration:** reflex movement patterns and involuntary movements, sensory integration tests, gross/fine motor skills

**Orthotic, protective, and supportive devices:** analysis of components of a device, analysis of movement while wearing a device

**Pain:** pain perception assessment scale, visual analog scale, assessment of muscle soreness

**Posture:** analysis of resting and dynamic posture, scoliosis assessment

**Range of motion:** active range of motion only

**Self-care and home management:** assessment of functional capacity

# Osteogenesis Imperfecta

## What additional findings are likely with this patient?

Children with OI often have delayed developmental milestones secondary to ongoing fractures with immobilization, hypermobility and laxity of joints, and poorly developed muscles. Most Type I children are community ambulators, approximately 57% of Type IV are household ambulators and 26% are community ambulators, and only 26% of Type III become household ambulators.

## Management

### What is the most effective management of this patient?

Medical management is directed at controlling the symptoms of OI. General goals include maximizing independence with mobility, improving optimal bone mass and muscle strength, and prevention of fractures and deformities. Pharmacological interventions have been studied, but have not shown any strong effect. Children should not be given steroids since it may deplete bone and increase fragility. Nutritional counseling and strong dental care are important in the management of OI. Lightweight orthotics may be indicated early to support the extremities, assist with ambulation, encourage weight bearing, and prevent fractures. Physical therapy intervention initially focuses on parent handling techniques, recognition of fractures, positioning, and activities that facilitate safe movement. Treatment of a child with OI should incorporate developmental activities, strengthening, positioning, weight bearing, and the use of mobility aids (scooters, riding toys or wheelchair). Swimming is also a good alternative for strengthening and exercise. All strengthening exercises should avoid rotational forces, placing weights/resistance near a joint, and using long lever arms. Surgical procedures known as "rodding" may also be indicated if a child has more than two fractures to the same bone within six months or if the angle of the long bone would not allow for stable ambulation.

### What home care regimen should be recommended?

A home care regimen will be successful if parents are competent with many of the relevant aspects of care. Handling techniques, recognition of fractures, precautions and contraindications, standing program, and exercise through activities are all key components of a home program for a child with OI. A child needs to continue to move and exercise in a safe fashion in order to optimize strength and bone mass.

## Outcome

### What is the likely outcome of a course in physical therapy?

Physical therapy may be required intermittently over the course of the patient's childhood depending on the severity of OI and the secondary complications. A home program must be established for optimal therapeutic results. Physical therapy may be in an outpatient setting or through the school

system. The therapist should work closely with the physician and caregivers for comprehensive care.

### What are the long-term effects of the patient's condition?

A patient with OI has outcome potential based on the type of disorder, symptoms, and secondary complications encountered. A strong predictor of a child's ability to ambulate in the future also lies in the child's ability to sit by ten months of age. Some children live normal lives with minimal involvement while others use power wheelchairs for mobility and experience multiple secondary complications.

## Comparison

### What are the distinguishing characteristics of a similar condition?

Arthrogryposis multiplex congenita (AMC) is a non-progressive neuromuscular disorder that results from multiple conditions that ultimately limit fetal movement in an intact skeleton and cause multiple congenital contractures at birth. Children are also born with muscle atrophy and weakness, and articular rigidity. Primary forms of AMC include contracture syndromes, amyoplasia, and distal arthrogryposis. Some children will ambulate and others will require wheelchairs for mobility.

## Clinical Scenarios

### Scenario One

A nine-month-old boy is seen in physical therapy with Type IV OI. He currently has a cast on his left lower extremity due to a femur fracture. His mother wants to learn activities in sitting and handling techniques that would help her son.

### Scenario Two

A 12-year-old female is seen by a school therapist. She underwent intramedullary rod placement in her right femur six weeks ago. She has type III OI and uses a wheelchair. She also presents with a 45 degree thoracic scoliosis and bowing in her upper extremities.

## Osteoporosis

### Diagnosis

#### What condition produces a patient's symptoms?

Osteoporosis is a metabolic bone disorder where the rate of bone resorption accelerates while the rate of bone formation slows down; osteoclast activity exceeds osteoblast activity. This reduction of bone mass decreases the overall bone density and strength. Primary osteoporosis includes classifications such as idiopathic osteoporosis, involutional (senile) osteoporosis, and postmenopausal osteoporosis. Secondary osteoporosis occurs due to a primary disease process or as a result of taking certain medications.

#### An injury was most likely sustained to which structure?

Osteoporosis primarily affects trabecular bone in a postmenopausal patient, however, is primarily seen in both trabecular and cortical bone in the geriatric population. Impaired bone formation due to declining osteoblast function in addition to the loss of calcium and phosphate salts within the bone structure cause brittle and porous bones that easily fracture. All bones can be affected with fractures of the vertebrae, distal radius/ulna, and femoral neck being the most common.

### Inference

#### What is the most likely contributing factor in the development of this condition?

The exact cause of primary osteoporosis is unknown, however, risk factors include inadequate dietary calcium, smoking, excessive caffeine, high intake of alcohol or salt, small stature, Caucasian race, inactive lifestyle, family history or history of chronic disease. Secondary osteoporosis may be caused by prolonged drug therapies of heparin or corticosteroid use, endocrine disorders, malnutrition, and other disease processes. Postmenopausal osteoporosis targets women approximately 50-60 years of age. Involutional (senile) osteoporosis usually targets men and women >70 years of age. Idiopathic osteoporosis can occur in both genders at all ages.

### Confirmation

#### What is the most likely clinical presentation?

Osteoporosis is the most frequently seen metabolic bone disease that affects approximately 10 million individuals within the United States. The prevalence is expected to increase with the increase in the aging population. A patient diagnosed with osteoporosis may complain of low thoracic or lumbar pain, experience compression fractures of the vertebrae, and complain of back pain. Vertebral and other crush fractures may occur with little to no trauma. Pain is acute and increases with weight bearing and palpation. A patient may also present with deformities such as kyphosis, Dowager's hump, a decrease in height, and other postural changes.

#### What laboratory or imaging studies would confirm the diagnosis?

There is not an accurate measure of overall bone strength or standards for routine screening that have been established, however, X-rays are taken to investigate the amount of degeneration and the decrease in density of a particular area. A bone mineral density test accounts for 70% of bone strength and is the easiest way to determine osteoporosis. Photon absorptiometry is used to measure bone mass particularly of the vertebrae, hips, and extremities. Quantitative CT scans may be used to aid diagnosis by examining the bone density of the spine.

#### What additional information should be obtained to confirm the diagnosis?

Differential diagnosis including lab testing and urinalysis must exclude other disease processes through examination and testing. A patient's past medical history, current symptoms, and location of pain all play a role in diagnosing osteoporosis.

### Examination

#### What history should be documented?

Important areas to explore include past medical history, medications, family history, current symptoms, current health status, social history and habits, occupation, leisure activities, and social support system.

#### What test/measures are most appropriate?

**Aerobic capacity and endurance:** assessment of vital signs at rest and with activity, perceived exertion scale

**Arousal, attention, and cognition:** examine mental status, learning ability, memory, motivation

**Assistive and adaptive devices:** analysis of components and safety of a device

**Environmental, home, and work barriers:** analysis of current and potential barriers or hazards

**Ergonomics and body mechanics:** analysis of dexterity and coordination

**Gait, locomotion, and balance:** static and dynamic balance in sitting and standing, safety during gait with/without an assistive device, Berg Balance Scale, functional capacity evaluation

**Integumentary integrity:** skin and sensation assessment

**Motor function:** coordination, posture/balance in sitting

**Muscle performance:** strength of active range of motion only

**Pain:** pain perception scale, visual analog scale

**Posture:** analysis of resting and dynamic posture

**Range of motion:** active range of motion

**Self-care and home management:** assessment of functional capacity

# Osteoporosis

## What additional findings are likely with this patient?

Once osteoporosis progresses in severity it can affect areas other than weight bearing bones such as the skull, long bones, and ribs. Spontaneous fractures and skeletal deformities may increase due to the continuing bone loss. A single fracture significantly increases the risk for subsequent fractures and skeletal deformities such as kyphosis.

## Management

### What is the most effective management of this patient?

Effective management of osteoporosis includes vitamin and pharmaceutical supplements, proper nutrition, education and physical therapy intervention. Hormone replacement therapy is recommended for postmenopausal patients. Calcium supplements, vitamin D, Raloxifene, and Fosamax (prevents bone resorption) may be recommended in the treatment of osteoporosis. Physical therapy intervention should include patient education regarding exercise, positioning, pain management, nutrition, and fall prevention. Physical therapy should include an exercise program that emphasizes weight bearing activities as tolerated. A patient may require a corset or lumbar support if at risk for vertebral fractures and many patients will require training with an assistive device. Aquatic therapy will assist with conditioning, however, should not replace weight bearing activities. Surgical intervention may be indicated for a patient requiring fracture stabilization.

### What home care regimen should be recommended?

The home care regimen for osteoporosis includes a consistent home exercise program that combines exercise, walking, and other activities within a patient's tolerance. Exercise is crucial to slow the bone resorption process and increase bone development. Patients should be educated to avoid heavy resistive exercise, excessive flexion during exercise or household activities, and the use of ballistic movements. Light resistance such as small dumbbells or Theraband can be used with caution after consulting with the physician.

## Outcome

### What is the likely outcome of a course in physical therapy?

Physical therapy should prescribe an exercise program that the patient can follow independently. Patient education should allow for independent decision making regarding proper nutrition and activities that incorporate precautions and fall prevention techniques. This level of patient competency should assist in decreasing the risk of fractures and other complications. Physical therapy cannot cease the process, but can empower the patient to effectively manage this bone disorder.

## What are the long-term effects of the patient's condition?

Osteoporosis will create thin and porous bones that will fracture easily and result in direct and indirect complications. Deformity and pain can become long-term effects of osteoporosis. Early detection and management of osteoporosis is important to limit the long-term effects of the disease.

## Comparison

### What are the distinguishing characteristics of a similar condition?

Paget's disease (osteitis deformans) is a chronic bone disease of unknown etiology where there is thickened, spongy, and abnormal bone formation. Large multinucleated osteoblasts, fibrous tissue, and thickened lamellae and trabeculae form and create weak and brittle bones. Bone pain, headache, hearing loss, fatigue, and stiffness are some early characteristics of Paget's disease. Progression of the disease includes bowing of long bones, an increase in skull size, bone deformities, and fractures (especially of the vertebrae).

## Clinical Scenarios

### Scenario One

A 63-year-old female is seen in outpatient physical therapy for a home exercise program. She is postmenopausal and does not take hormone replacement therapy. She has been recently diagnosed with osteoporosis and X-rays revealed three old vertebral fractures. The patient's major complaints are pain and stiffness.

### Scenario Two

A 92-year-old male was admitted to the hospital for internal fixation of a femoral neck fracture. The patient's history reveals osteoporosis, diabetes, and anxiety. He wants to be discharged home to care for his cat. The physician orders are for physical therapy two times per week with the goal of returning home alone.

# Parkinson's Disease

## Diagnosis

### What condition produces a patient's symptoms?

Parkinsonism syndrome is used to describe a group of disorders within subcortical gray matter of the basal ganglia that produces a similar disturbance of balance and voluntary movements. This syndrome occurs as a secondary effect or disorder from another disease process. Parkinson's disease is a primary degenerative disorder and is characterized by a decrease in production of dopamine (neurotransmitter) within the corpus striatum portion of the basal ganglia. The degeneration of the dopaminergic pathways creates an imbalance between dopamine and acetylcholine. This process produces the symptoms of Parkinson's disease.

### An injury was most likely sustained to which structure?

Injury occurs to the subcortical gray matter within the basal ganglia, specifically the substantia nigra and the corpus striatum. The basal ganglia stores the majority of dopamine and is responsible for modulation and control of voluntary movement. A patient with Parkinson's disease exhibits degeneration of dopaminergic neurons that results in depletion of dopamine production within the basal ganglia. Change in the neurochemical production damages the complex loop between the basal ganglia and the cerebrum.

## Inference

### What is the most likely contributing factor in the development of this condition?

Primary Parkinson's disease has an unknown etiology and accounts for the majority of patients with Parkinsonism. Contributing factors that can produce symptoms of Parkinson's disease include genetic defect, toxicity from carbon monoxide, excessive manganese or copper, carbon disulfide, vascular impairment of the striatum, encephalitis, and other neurodegenerative diseases such as Huntington's disease or Alzheimer's disease.

## Confirmation

### What is the most likely clinical presentation?

There are approximately 500,000 individuals affected by Parkinsonism and about 42% of these are diagnosed specifically with Parkinson's disease. The risk for developing Parkinson's disease increases with age and 1:100 are affected over the age of 75. The majority of patients are between 50 and 79 years of age and approximately 10% are diagnosed before 40 years. The majority of patients with Parkinson's disease will initially notice a resting tremor in the hands (sometimes called a pill-rolling tremor) or feet that increases with stress and disappears with movement or sleep. Early in the disease process a patient may attribute symptoms to "old age" such as balance disturbances, difficulty rolling over and rising from bed, and impairment with fine manipulative movements seen in writing, bathing and dressing. A patient's symptoms slowly progress and often include hypokinesia, sluggish movement, difficulty with initiating (akinesia) and stopping movement, festinating and shuffling gait, bradykinesia, poor posture, dysphagia, and "cogwheel" or "lead pipe" rigidity of skeletal muscles. Patients may also experience "freezing" during ambulation, speech, blinking, and movements of the arms. A patient with Parkinson's disease will also have a mask-like appearance with no facial expression.

### What laboratory or imaging studies would confirm the diagnosis?

There are no laboratory or imaging studies that initially diagnose Parkinson's disease. CT scan or MRI may be used to rule out other neurodegenerative diseases and obtain a baseline for future comparison.

### What additional information should be obtained to confirm the diagnosis?

Definitive diagnosis is difficult during the early stages of the disease. Parkinson's disease is believed to progress slowly over 25 to 30 years prior to the onset of pharmacological intervention. Diagnosis is made from patient history, history of symptoms, and differential diagnosis to rule out other potential disorders. There are evaluation tools that are utilized to classify a patient by stage of the disease process.

## Examination

### What history should be documented?

Important areas to explore include past medical history, medications, current symptoms, current health status, social history and habits, occupation, living environment, and social support system.

### What test/measures are most appropriate?

**Aerobic capacity and endurance:** assessment of vital signs at rest and with activity

**Arousal, attention, and cognition:** examine mental status, learning ability, memory, motivation, and Mini-Mental State Examination

**Environmental, home, and work barriers:** analysis of current and potential barriers or hazards

**Gait, locomotion, and balance:** static and dynamic balance in sitting and standing, Functional Reach Test, Tinetti Performance Oriented Mobility Assessment, Berg Balance Scale, outcome measurement tools, safety with/without an assistive device during gait

**Joint integrity and mobility:** analysis of quality of movement, examine joint hypermobility and hypomobility

**Motor function:** assessment of dexterity, coordination and agility, assessment of postural, equilibrium, and righting reactions

**Muscle performance:** strength assessment, muscle tone assessment, and tremor assessment

# Parkinson's Disease

**Posture:** analysis of resting and dynamic posture
**Range of motion:** active and passive range of motion
**Self-care and home management:** functional capacity, Barthel Index, safety assessments, Parkinson's disease Questionnaire (PDQ-39)
**Sensory integration:** assessment of combined sensation, assessment of proprioception and kinesthesia
**Ventilation, respiratory, and circulation:** assessment of chest wall mobility, expansion, and excursion

## What additional findings are likely with this patient?

Since Parkinson's disease is a progressive condition there are ongoing physical and cognitive impairments. A patient may develop a stooped posture and an increased risk for falling. Progression of the disease may result in dysphagia, difficulty with speech, and pulmonary impairment. Greater attention is required for skin care once nutrition and mobility are further compromised. Many patients with Parkinson's disease die from complications of bronchopneumonia.

## Management

### What is the most effective management of this patient?

The medical management of Parkinson's disease relies heavily on pharmacological intervention. Dopamine replacement therapy, (Levodopa, Sinemet, Madopar) is the most effective treatment in reducing the symptoms of Parkinson's disease such as movement disorders, bradykinesia, rigidity, and tremor. Antihistamines, anticholinergics, and antidepressants are also utilized. Physical, occupational, and speech therapies may be warranted intermittently throughout the course of the disease. Physical therapy intervention should include maximizing endurance, strength, and functional mobility. Verbal cueing and oral/visual feedback are effective tools to use with this population. Family teaching, balance activities, gait training, stretching, trunk rotation activities, assistive device training, relaxation techniques, and respiratory therapy are all important components in the treatment of Parkinson's disease. Psychological and nutritional counseling are recommended.

### What home care regimen should be recommended?

A home care regimen should include an exercise routine, functional mobility skills, the use of relaxation techniques, range of motion and stretching exercises, and endurance activities. A competent caretaker is vital to the success of the home program and must continuously motivate the patient to continue with mobility and endurance activities in order to avoid deleterious effects of the disease process.

## Outcome

### What is the likely outcome of a course in physical therapy?

Physical therapy is recommended on an intermittent basis throughout the course of the disease and will focus on current symptoms that arise. Physical therapy will not prevent further degeneration or cure the movement disorder, however, it will assist the patient to maximize their level of function and quality of life.

### What are the long-term effects of the patient's condition?

Parkinson's disease does not significantly alter a patient's lifespan if the patient is diagnosed with a generalized form between 50 and 60 years of age. As the disease progresses, however, there will be an exacerbation of all symptoms and significant loss of mobility. The inactivity and deconditioning allows for complications and eventual death.

## Comparison

### What are the distinguishing characteristics of a similar condition?

Wilson's disease is inherited as an autosomal recessive trait and causes a defect in the metabolism of copper. The accumulation of copper within the erythrocytes, liver, brain, and kidneys produces the associated degenerative changes. The patient presents with hepatic insufficiency, tremor, choreoathetoid movements, dysarthria, and progressive rigidity.

## Clinical Scenarios

### Scenario One

A 35-year-old female is sent to physical therapy shortly after being diagnosed with Parkinson's disease. She is presently having difficulty maintaining a grasp on items from an assembly line at work and complains of frequently tripping.

### Scenario Two

A 42-year-old male was diagnosed with Parkinson's disease four years ago. The patient requires physical therapy to reassess gait and prescribe an assistive device. The son states that the patient sits a great deal at home and lacks motivation to engage in exercise.

# Patellofemoral Syndrome

## Diagnosis

### What condition produces a patient's symptoms?

Patellofemoral syndrome is caused by an abnormal tracking of the patella between the femoral condyles. The tracking problem places increased and misdirected forces between the patella and femur. This most commonly occurs when the patella is pulled too far laterally during knee extension.

### An injury was most likely sustained to which structure?

Patellofemoral syndrome causes damage to the articular cartilage of the patella. The damage can range from softening of the cartilage to complete cartilage destruction resulting in exposure of subchondral bone.

## Inference

### What is the most likely contributing factor in the development of this condition?

The exact etiology of patellofemoral syndrome is unknown, however, it is extremely common during adolescence, is more prevalent in females than males, and has a direct association with the activity level of the patient. In an older population patellofemoral syndrome is often associated with osteoarthritis. Additional factors associated with patellofemoral syndrome include patella alta, insufficient lateral femoral condyle, weak vastus medialis obliquus, excessive pronation, excessive knee valgus, and tightness in lower extremity muscles (iliopsoas, hamstrings, gastrocnemius, and vastus lateralis).

## Confirmation

### What is the most likely clinical presentation?

A patient with patellofemoral syndrome often describes a gradual onset of anterior knee pain following an increase in physical activity. The pain is characteristically located behind the patella (retropatellar pain) and may be exacerbated with activities that increase patellofemoral compressive forces (stair climbing, jumping) and also with prolonged static positioning (sitting with the knee flexed at 90 degrees as in a car, plane, theatre). Point tenderness is common over the lateral border of the patella and crepitus may be elicited when the patella is manually compressed into the trochlear groove. Visible quadriceps atrophy may be noted in the involved lower extremity particularly along the vastus medialis obliquus. The patient may also complain of burning pain when sitting for prolonged periods of time or when ascending stairs.

### What laboratory or imaging studies would confirm the diagnosis?

Laboratory or imaging studies are not commonly used to diagnose patellofemoral syndrome. X-rays are often used to rule out a fracture, examine the configuration of the patellofemoral joint, and identify potential osteophytes, joint space narrowing, patella alta, and arthritic changes. Arthrogram and arthroscopy can be used to examine the articular cartilage.

### What additional information should be obtained to confirm the diagnosis?

Special tests such as Clarke's sign can be useful when attempting to confirm the diagnosis. The test is performed by applying pressure immediately proximal to the upper pole of the patient's patella. The physician/therapist then asks the patient to isometrically contract the quadriceps. A positive test is indicated by a failure to fully contract the quadriceps or by the presence of retropatellar pain. The test should be performed at varying degrees of flexion and extension. It is helpful to determine the patient's Q angle and examine the alignment of the patient's feet, as these factors can contribute to the causative factors.

## Examination

### What history should be documented?

Important areas to explore include past medical history, medications, current symptoms and health status, social history, occupation/recreational activities, living environment, and social support system.

### What test/measures are most appropriate?

**Anthropometric characteristics:** knee effusion, lower extremity circumferential measurements

**Arousal, attention, and cognition:** examine mental status, learning ability, memory, motivation

**Assistive and adaptive devices:** components and safety of a device, potential utilization of crutches

**Environmental, home, and work barriers:** analysis of current and potential barriers or hazards

**Gait, locomotion, and balance:** safety during gait with an assistive device

**Integumentary integrity:** assessment of sensation (pain, temperature, tactile), skin assessment

**Joint integrity and mobility:** Clarke's sign, patella grind test (active and passive), dynamic patella tracking, patella glide test, palpation of structures, joint play, soft tissue restrictions, joint pain

**Muscle performance:** strength assessment, assessment of active movement, resisted isometrics, muscle contraction characteristics, muscle endurance

**Orthotic, protective, and supportive devices:** potential utilization of bracing, taping or wrapping

**Pain:** pain perception assessment scale

**Range of motion:** active and passive range of motion

**Self-care and home management:** functional capacity

**Sensory integrity:** proprioception and kinesthesia

# Patellofemoral Syndrome

### What additional findings are likely with this patient?

Patients diagnosed with patellofemoral syndrome often have an increased Q angle. The normal Q angle is 13 degrees in males and 18 degrees in females. The Q angle is measured using the anterior superior iliac spine, the midpoint of the patella, and the tibial tubercle. Differential diagnosis should rule out other problems such as referred pain from the hip, Osgood-Schlatter syndrome, neuroma, patellar tendonitis, plica syndrome, and infection of the knee joint.

## Management

### What is the most effective management of this patient?

Medical management of patellofemoral syndrome is usually successful with conservative measures, surgical intervention is rare. Pharmacological intervention may include acetaminophen, NSAIDs, and steroid injections into the joint. Physical therapy management includes controlling edema, stretching, strengthening, improving range of motion, and activity modification. Mobilization activities to increase medial glide can be beneficial to increase the flexibility of the lateral fascia. Strengthening activities emphasizing the vastus medialis obliquus in non-weight bearing and weight bearing positions are recommended. Biofeedback can be a useful tool in order to selectively train the muscle. Stretching activities should emphasize the hamstrings, iliotibial band, tensor fasciae latae, and rectus femoris. Strengthening activities may include quadriceps setting exercises, straight leg raising and mini-squats incorporating the hip adductors. Exercises such as deep squats should be avoided since they will tend to aggravate the patient's condition. Patellar taping to improve the position and tracking of the patella during dynamic activities can be useful to limit irritation.

### What home care regimen should be recommended?

The home care regimen should consist of range of motion, strengthening, stretching, palliative care, and functional activities. An active patient must decrease their level of activities to relieve the additional stress placed on the patellofemoral joint. A patient must also comply with recommendations for proper footwear and orthotics to improve alignment and lessen aggravation of symptoms, specifically knee pain.

## Outcome

### What is the likely outcome of a course in physical therapy?

A patient with patellofemoral syndrome that undergoes conservative management may be able to return to their previous functioning within four to six weeks.

### What are the long-term effects of the patient's condition?

Prognosis for a full recovery is good with successful conservative management, however, failure to adequately address the cause of the patellofemoral syndrome will likely result in a patient's condition further deteriorating. The patient may experience increased irritation of the patellofemoral joint that further impacts their ability to participate in activities of daily living. Periodic exacerbations of the condition most commonly due to an increased activity level may require further physical therapy intervention.

## Comparison

### What are the distinguishing characteristics of a similar condition?

Patellar tendonitis is an overuse condition characterized by inflammatory changes of the patellar tendon. The condition is most prevalent in athletes who participate in activities requiring repetitive jumping skills. The primary complaint is often pain over the anterior portion of the superior tibia with activities such as jumping or ascending/descending stairs. Patients may also experience pain after prolonged sitting and often exhibit point tenderness at the superior pole of the patella tendon. Management of patellar tendonitis incorporates many of the same interventions as patellofemoral syndrome such as range of motion, stretching, and palliative care.

## Clinical Scenarios

### Scenario One

A 14-year-old female is referred to physical therapy with patellofemoral syndrome. The patient has mild edema and is sensitive to light touch over the anterior surface of the knee. The patient reports gaining ten pounds and expresses that she is willing to do "anything" to improve her present condition.

### Scenario Two

A 45-year-old male is referred to physical therapy after experiencing anterior knee pain for the last week. The patient is 19 weeks status post ACL reconstruction and has recently returned to a softball league. The patient reports an insidious onset of pain and insists that he has been faithful to his home program. A note from the referring physician confirms that the integrity of the graft is fine and he suspects patellofemoral syndrome.

# Peripheral Vascular Disease

## Diagnosis

### What condition produces a patient's symptoms?

Peripheral vascular disease (PVD) is a condition where there has been narrowing of the lumen of blood vessels causing a reduction in circulation usually secondary to atherosclerosis. This can be compounded by either emboli or thrombi.

### An injury was most likely sustained to which structure?

PVD, also known as arteriosclerosis obliterans, is primarily the result of atherosclerosis. Damage can occur to the walls of both arteries and veins from fatty plaque buildup that creates hard and narrow vessels. The atherosclerotic process will gradually progress to significant or complete occlusion of medium and large arteries.

## Inference

### What is the most likely contributing factor in the development of this condition?

The primary factor for developing PVD is atherosclerosis. Other etiologies and risk factors that have been associated with the development of PVD may include phlebitis, injury or surgery, autoimmune disease, diabetes mellitus, smoking, hyperlipidemia, inactivity, hypertension, positive family history, increased age, and obesity.

## Confirmation

### What is the most likely clinical presentation?

Symptoms and clinical presentation will differ depending on which vessel or blood flow has been compromised. During the early stages of PVD intermittent claudication may be the only manifestation. Symptoms are precipitated by walking a predictable distance and are normally relieved by rest. Claudication also may present as buckling or "giving out" of the lower extremity after a certain period of exertion and may not demonstrate the typical symptom of pain on exertion. Other symptoms may include tingling and numbness of the affected extremities, pain at rest and during sleep, slowed healing, changes in skin coloring, a decrease in skin temperature, absence of hair on the extremity, and a weak or absent pulse.

### What laboratory or imaging studies would confirm the diagnosis?

Routine blood tests generally are indicated and include CBC, BUN, creatinine, and electrolytes studies. Doppler ultrasound studies are used to determine flow status. MRI, angiogram or arteriogram can also be used to assist with the diagnosis.

### What additional information should be obtained to confirm the diagnosis?

The ankle-brachial index (ABI) can be used to provide a ratio of systolic blood pressure of the lower extremity compared to the upper extremity. An ABI above 0.90 is normal; 0.70-0.90 indicates mild peripheral vascular disease; 0.50-0.70 indicates moderate disease; and less than 0.50 indicates severe peripheral vascular disease. A rubor of dependency test, transcutaneous oximetry, and treadmill exercise test may also assist with baseline information and diagnosis of insufficiency.

## Examination

### What history should be documented?

Important areas to explore include past medical history, medications, current health status, nutritional status, social history and habits, occupation, living environment, and social support system.

### What test/measures are most appropriate?

**Aerobic capacity and endurance:** assessment of vital signs at rest and with activity, perceived exertion scale, pulse oximetry, auscultation of the lungs

**Arousal, attention, and cognition:** examine mental status, memory, motivation

**Assistive and adaptive devices:** analysis of components and safety of a device

**Community and work integration:** analysis of community, work, and leisure activities

**Environmental, home, and work barriers:** analysis of current and potential barriers or hazards

**Gait, locomotion, and balance:** static and dynamic balance in sitting and standing, safety during gait with/without an assistive device, Functional Ambulation Profile

**Integumentary integrity:** skin assessment, assessment of sensation

**Muscle performance:** strength assessment

**Pain:** pain perception assessment scale, visual analogue scale, assessment of muscle soreness

**Posture:** analysis of resting and dynamic posture

**Range of motion:** active and passive range of motion

**Self-care and home management:** assessment of functional capacity, Functional Independence Measure

**Sensory integrity:** proprioception and kinesthesia

**Ventilation, respiration, and circulation:** palpation of pulses, pulse oximetry, ABI, capillary refilling test

### What additional findings are likely with this patient?

Ischemic rest pain can occur from the combination of PVD and inadequate perfusion. It is fairly common for a patient with PVD to be diagnosed with coronary artery disease or diabetes mellitus. There is a higher risk for complications such as deep vein thrombosis, insufficiency ulcers, gangrene, and amputation.

# Peripheral Vascular Disease

## Management

### What is the most effective management of this patient?

The medical management of a patient with PVD should include a physician, psychiatrist or psychologist, nurse, nutritionist, occupational therapist, physical therapist, vocational therapist, and case manager. Pharmacological intervention may be utilized to reduce morbidity and prevent complications. Anticoagulants such as heparin, antiplatelet agents and thrombolytics may be indicated. Patient education is paramount regarding the disease process, limb protection, foot and skin care, and risk factor reduction (smoking cessation, avoid cold exposure). Physical therapy is an important component in the treatment of PVD. A walking program will initially have the patient walk until near maximal pain and then rest until the pain is relieved. The goal is to have the patient achieve longer walking periods with less rest, eventually walking for 30 minutes continuously. Non-weight bearing exercises such as swimming or stationary cycling can supplement the program. After 4-6 weeks of therapy including isometric and active range exercises, the patient should tolerate the implementation of resistive exercise. Physical rehabilitation, involving dynamic aerobic exercise and resistance training improves cardiovascular endurance and demonstrates a positive impact on patient function and independence. In more severe cases, surgical intervention may be required. Common procedures include balloon angioplasty, endarterectomy, stent implantation or bypass surgery.

### What home care regimen should be recommended?

A patient must continue with their walking program and a generalized exercise program to tolerance. They should perform skin and foot inspections daily and continue with smoking cessation and a low cholesterol diet. For patients with pain at rest, particularly at night, the head of the bed should be elevated 4-6 inches, which should improve lower extremity perfusion by the effects of gravity on blood flow.

## Outcome

### What is the likely outcome of a course in physical therapy?

Physical therapy can be instrumental in managing PVD through education of the disease process, implementing a walking program that allows for the development of collateral circulation, and designing an exercise program that allows the patient to gain strength and endurance for activities. The patient must have the desire, discipline, and motivation to continue with habit modification and maintain their exercise regimen in order to be successful.

### What are the long-term effects of the patient's condition?

PVD can be controllable with pharmacological treatment, risk factor reduction, and in some cases, surgical intervention. Patients with PVD are at a higher risk overall for complications such as permanent numbness, tingling or weakness in lower extremities and/or feet, permanent sensory changes such as burning or aching pain, gangrene, and amputation of the affected body part. Patients with PVD are also at higher risk of heart attack and stroke. Symptomatic PVD has at least a 30% risk of death within five years and approximately 50% in ten years, secondary to MI or cerebrovascular disease.

## Comparison

### What are the distinguishing characteristics of a similar condition?

Coronary artery disease (CAD) is the narrowing or blockage due to fatty build up (cholesterol) within the artery walls reducing the overall blood flow to the cardiac muscle. Patient symptoms will vary based on the location and severity of blockage. Patients range from asymptomatic to symptoms at rest. These symptoms can include nausea, vomiting, heartburn, shortness of breath, and profuse sweating. Risk factors include hypertension, smoking, obesity, stress, elevated cholesterol, and sedentary lifestyle. Electrocardiograms and angiograms are typically used to diagnose CAD.

## Clinical Scenarios

### Scenario One

A 66-year-old male is seen in physical therapy with a new diagnosis of PVD. The patient's past medical history consists of L5 disc herniation with surgical stabilization and type 2 diabetes mellitus. The patient complains of increasing lower extremity pain with ambulation while at his job as a surveyor. The patient lives alone and has two dogs.

### Scenario Two

An 82-year-old female is seen in physical therapy in an acute care hospital with orders for whirlpool secondary to an ulcer on her right lower extremity. The patient has moderate to severe PVD affecting both lower extremities. She presents with sensory loss and significant pain with ambulation greater than 20 feet. She also complains of pain at night. She resides with her husband in a first floor apartment.

# Plantar Fasciitis

## Diagnosis

### What condition produces a patient's symptoms?

The plantar fascia is a thin layer of tough connective tissue that supports the arch of the foot. Plantar fasciitis is an inflammatory process of the plantar fascia (or aponeurosis) at its origin on the calcaneus. Plantar fasciitis is a chronic overuse condition that develops secondary to repetitive stretching of the plantar fascia through excessive foot pronation during the loading phase of gait. This results in stress at the calcaneal origin of the plantar fascia.

### An injury was most likely sustained to which structure?

Injury can occur to the plantar fascia itself and cause microtearing, inflammation, and pain. The abductor hallucis, flexor digitorum brevis, and quadratus plantae muscles share the same origin on the medial tubercle of the calcaneus and may also become inflamed and irritated.

## Inference

### What is the most likely contributing factor in the development of this condition?

Factors that contribute to the development of plantar fasciitis include excessive pronation during gait, tightness of the foot and calf musculature, obesity, and possessing a high arch. A person participating in endurance sports such as running and dancing or a person with an occupation that requires prolonged walking or standing has an increased risk for plantar fasciitis. It is believed that development of plantar fasciitis results from a combination of predisposing factors. Although it is more common in the middle-age population, it also occurs in younger individuals, but usually in combination with calcaneal apophysitis.

## Confirmation

### What is the most likely clinical presentation?

A patient with plantar fasciitis presents with severe pain in the heel when first standing up in the morning (when the fascia is contracted, stiff, and cold). This pain has also been reported to radiate proximally up the calf and/or distally to the toes. This is the most common symptom that relates directly to the diagnosis of plantar fasciitis and in one study was expressed in over 84% of cases. Pain typically subsides for a few hours during the day, but increases with prolonged activity or when the patient has been non-weight bearing and resumes a weight bearing posture. Pain has also been described by patients as "pain that moves around." A patient will typically experience point tenderness and pain with palpation over the calcaneal insertion of the plantar fascia. There may be bony growths in the plantar fascia near its insertion. Plantar fasciitis is usually unilateral and tightness in the Achilles tendon is found in the majority of the patients.

### What laboratory or imaging studies would confirm the diagnosis?

Plantar fasciitis is initially treated based on symptoms and physical examination. If pain persists after six to eight weeks of physical therapy intervention, MRI may be used to confirm the diagnosis. Other diagnostic tools may include x-ray and bone scan to rule out a stress fracture, rheumatology work up to rule out systemic etiology, and EMG testing to rule out nerve entrapment.

### What additional information should be obtained to confirm the diagnosis?

A thorough history and biomechanical assessment of the foot, observation of the fat pad, examination for Achilles tendon tightness, analysis of footwear, and gait disturbances all assist in diagnosing plantar fasciitis.

## Examination

### What history should be documented?

Important areas to explore include mechanism of current injury, training routine, past medical history, medications, social history and habits, occupation, living environment, and social support system.

### What test/measures are most appropriate?

**Anthropometric characteristics:** circumferential measurements of affected area or extremity
**Arousal, attention, and cognition:** examine mental status, learning ability, memory, motivation
**Community and work integration:** analysis of community, work, and leisure activities
**Environmental, home, and work barriers:** analysis of current and potential barriers or hazards
**Gait, locomotion, and balance:** biomechanical analysis of gait during walking and running (if appropriate), footprint analysis, dynamic plantar pressure distribution
**Integumentary inspection:** assessment of sensation, skin assessment
**Joint integrity and mobility:** assessment of swelling, inflammation, and joint restriction
**Muscle performance:** strength assessment, muscle endurance
**Pain:** pain perception scale, visual analogue scale
**Orthotic, protective, and supportive devices:** potential utilization of taping or use of cushions
**Posture:** analysis of resting and dynamic posture
**Range of motion:** active and passive range of motion
**Sensory integrity:** assessment of proprioception and kinesthesia
**Self-care and home management:** assessment of functional capacity

# Plantar Fasciitis

## What additional findings are likely with this patient?

Bony hypertrophy can occur at the origin of the plantar fascia resulting in a heel spur. Plantar fasciitis is a relative of heel spur syndrome, but is not the same condition. Heel spurs develop initially as calcium deposits that form due to the repetitive stress and inflammation in the plantar fascia.

## Management

### What is the most effective management of this patient?

Medical and pharmacological management of a patient with plantar fasciitis usually requires local corticosteroid injections or anti-inflammatory medications to reduce inflammation within the plantar fascia. Physical therapy intervention consists of ice massage, deep friction massage, shoe modification, heel insert application, foot orthotic prescription, modification of activities to include non-weight bearing endurance activities, and a gentle stretching program of the Achilles tendon and plantar fascia. Muscle strengthening exercises for the intrinsic and extrinsic muscles should be implemented once the acute symptoms have subsided. During the acute phase the patient must also modify activities and rest the affected foot. Heel cup prescription and casting may also be indicated.

### What home care regimen should be recommended?

A home care regimen for a patient with plantar fasciitis should include ongoing strengthening and stretching exercises (especially stretching of the gastrocnemius and plantar fascia in the morning and prior to and after exercise), maintenance of a fitness program, the use of proper footwear, and the use of foot orthotics and heel inserts if warranted. Night tension splints may be indicated if symptoms persist.

## Outcome

### What is the likely outcome of a course in physical therapy?

Conservative physical therapy intervention on an outpatient basis in combination with a consistent home program should allow the patient to return to a more functional level within eight weeks. Total resolution of symptoms can take up to twelve months. Physical therapy, orthotic prescription, splinting, pharmacological injections, and physician follow-up are all components of the treatment program that may be required for a positive outcome.

### What are the long-term effects of the patient's condition?

A patient previously diagnosed with plantar fasciitis is at an increased risk for recurrence, however, successful conservative management, compliance with a home program, and proper footwear will decrease the incidence of any negative long-term effects. If conservative management fails the patient may require surgical intervention, however, this option is relatively rare. Approximately 10% of patients can develop persistent, chronic, and disabling symptoms.

## Comparison

### What are the distinguishing characteristics of a similar condition?

The tarsal tunnel is the region where the tibial nerve passes between the medial malleolus and the calcaneus. The tibial nerve splits into the medial and lateral plantar nerves while still traversing in the tunnel along with other nerves in this region. Tarsal tunnel syndrome is characterized by pain that is experienced with weight bearing, but not with direct palpation to the plantar fascia. Characteristics of tarsal tunnel syndrome include complaints of numbness, burning pain, tingling, and paresthesias at the heel. Etiology consists of entrapment and compression of the posterior tibial nerve or plantar nerves within the tarsal tunnel due to inflammation or thickening of the flexor retinaculum.

## Clinical Scenarios

### Scenario One

A 19-year-old male athlete is referred to physical therapy with bilateral heel pain. The physician has ruled out systemic disorders and diagnosed bilateral mechanical plantar fasciitis. The athlete is a swimmer and began running cross-country last fall. The patient is otherwise healthy, but wants to return to athletic activities as soon as possible.

### Scenario Two

A 56-year-old female is referred to physical therapy with left plantar fasciitis. The patient is mildly obese and works the night shift at a paper mill. She stands at her station throughout the shift and is required to walk between the two buildings every hour. The patient has a history of mild asthma and a cardiac murmur. She is anxious to obtain relief from her symptoms since she feels that her employment may be jeopardized.

# Pressure Ulcer

## Diagnosis

### What condition produces a patient's symptoms?

A pressure ulcer is a type of ulcer or wound caused by unrelieved pressure to a specific area that results in damage to the underlying tissues. The unrelieved pressure deprives the tissues of oxygen, which causes ischemia to the site, subsequent cell death, and tissue necrosis. A definition of unrelieved pressure is >32 mm Hg of pressure to an area for more than two hours.

### An injury was most likely sustained to which structure?

A pressure ulcer can affect different structures based on the degree or staging of the ulcer. Damage can be contained to only the epidermis in stage I ulcers, while stage IV ulcers will include damage to the epidermis, dermis, the fascia and deeper, potentially damaging muscles, ligaments, tendons and/or bones. The most high risk areas for pressure ulcers include the occiput, heels, greater trochanters, ischial tuberosities, sacrum, and epicondyles of the elbow.

## Inference

### What is the most likely contributing factor in the development of this condition?

A pressure ulcer can occur at any time secondary to unrelieved pressure, but there are certain populations and risk factors that are associated with its development. Immobility is a leading factor and is seen with populations such as spinal cord injury, other paralysis, and hemiplegia. Impaired cognition, poor nutrition, altered sensation, incontinence, decreased lean body mass, and infection are other contributing factors in the development of a pressure ulcer. At the cellular level, the interface pressure, shear and/or friction are the contributing factors in the development of a pressure ulcer.

## Confirmation

### What is the most likely clinical presentation?

A patient will usually develop a pressure ulcer over a bony prominence with common sites including the greater trochanter, ischium, sacrum, and heel. A stage I pressure ulcer is classified as an area of nonblanchable erythema of intact skin. There may also be an increase in warmth to the site or altered coloration. Stage II is classified as a partial thickness wound involving the epidermis, dermis or both. This ulcer does not extend through the entire dermis. Stage III is classified as an ulcer that has extended into subcutaneous tissue, but not through fascia. Stage IV is classified as an ulcer that extends through the fascia and deeper. It is a full thickness wound that may damage muscles, bones, ligaments and/or tendons. Pressure ulcers will vary in color, odor, drainage, and volume.

### What laboratory or imaging studies would confirm the diagnosis?

A diagnosis is made from visual inspection, however, blood studies such as a CBC, electrolyte, and protein levels, as well as tests for bacteremia or sepsis may be indicated. Urinalysis and stool samples may be indicated to determine contributing factors in the development of the ulcer. Coagulation studies and tissue sampling may also be indicated.

### What additional information should be obtained to confirm the diagnosis?

Extensive examination and photography of the site are necessary for accurate baseline data. A patient's history and current status are also important factors in designing the plan of care. Diagnosis of staging of the ulcer requires the use of the Braden Scale, Gosnell Scale or Norton Scale along with baseline measurements of size and depth of the ulcer.

## Examination

### What history should be documented?

Important areas to explore include past medical history, medications, current health status, history of incontinence, nutritional status, social history, living environment, occupation, and social support system.

### What test/measures are most appropriate?

**Aerobic capacity and endurance:** assessment of vital signs at rest and with activity

**Arousal, attention, and cognition:** examine mental status, learning ability, memory and motivation

**Environmental, home, and work barriers:** analysis of current and potential barriers or hazards

**Gait, locomotion, and balance:** static and dynamic balance in sitting and standing, safety during gait with/without an assistive device

**Integumentary integrity:** skin assessment, assessment of sensation, Braden Scale, Norton Scale, photography of ulcer, eschar, granulation formation, Gosnell Scale

**Joint integrity and mobility:** assessment of hypermobility and hypomobility of a joint, soft tissue swelling and inflammation

**Muscle performance:** strength assessment

**Pain:** pain perception assessment scale, visual analogue scale

**Posture:** analysis of resting and dynamic posture

**Range of motion:** active and passive range of motion

**Sensory integrity:** proprioception and kinesthesia

# Pressure Ulcer

## What additional findings are likely with this patient?

Complications that may prevent healing of the ulcer include infection, osteomyelitis, sepsis, pain, spasticity, malnutrition, incontinence, and depression. Patients at high risk may also develop multiple ulcers at once.

## Management

### What is the most effective management of this patient?

Patient and caregiver education for the prevention of subsequent pressure ulcers is very important and should include skin inspection, positioning, and pressure relief techniques. The use of pressure reducing devices such as seat cushions, multipodus boots or specialized mattresses is also an important aspect to the overall care of ulcers. Pharmacological intervention may include antimicrobials and antibiotics to fight infection and allow for proper healing. Dressings for the ulcer may include nonocclusive or occlusive types of dressings. Nonocclusive dressings include dry to dry, wet to wet, wet to dry or composite dressings. Occlusive dressings include semipermeable films, hydrocolloids, hydrogels, semipermeable foams, and alginates. The ulcer may require cleansing agents, and/or debridement (enzymatic, mechanical non-selective or sharp). Mobility training and proper positioning for the patient will also be vital in order to decrease forces of shear and friction upon the site of the ulcer. A general exercise program should be initiated as well as mobility training to tolerance. Skin inspection should be provided daily and photography should be documented regularly to track the progress of healing. Patients should avoid the use of hot water and the use of massage surrounding the site. The therapist should promote proper positioning techniques (such as positioning of the bed at less than a 45 degree angle) in order to decrease friction and shear forces.

### What home care regimen should be recommended?

The home care regimen is dependent on the size and staging of the pressure sore. The patient should continue with the appropriate schedule for dressings and follow physician orders. The patient should maintain an appropriate activity level, use correct positioning, and receive adequate protein and calorie intake to assist with the healing process. The patient should use a mild cleansing agent, dry and wrinkle free sheets for their bed, and appropriate moisturizers.

## Outcome

### What is the likely outcome of a course in physical therapy?

The care of ulcers is estimated to cost $6 billion dollars annually which makes this diagnosis the most costly preventable injury. Approximately 60,000 patients die annually due to secondary complications from ulcers. However, many people that develop a pressure ulcer completely recover with no residual impairments.

## What are the long-term effects of the patient's condition?

Treatment of a pressure ulcer should provide a normal path of recovery without any residual deficits. If there is infection or complications to healing, the patient may have to undergo additional treatment such as further pharmacological intervention or surgical procedures. If the patient is in a high risk group for skin breakdown the patient may require the ongoing use of a pressure relief seating system or air mattress for the bed.

## Comparison

### What are the distinguishing characteristics of a similar condition?

A neuropathic ulcer is an ulcer that develops due to the lack of neural function, which occurs commonly in patients with diabetes mellitus. Other high risk groups include spinal cord injury, stroke, spina bifida, sensory neuropathies, and tumors. The feet are the prime region for neuropathic ulcers in the diabetic patient. These ulcers occur in areas of weight bearing where there are mechanical shear forces such as under the metatarsal heads. These ulcers are usually round in shape and are not painful. It is believed that these ulcers occur not only due to motor neuropathy, but also impairment of the sensory and autonomic systems. Approximately 15% of patients with diabetes mellitus will develop a foot ulcer. Treatment is usually the same as with a pressure ulcer, but care must be taken to continually assess progress since there is usually motor and sensory damage surrounding the ulcer site.

## Clinical Scenarios

### Scenario One

A 31-year-old male has been in the hospital for four weeks secondary to a motor vehicle accident. He was in a coma for ten days and was required to stay in bed due to multiple fractures for three of the four weeks. He developed a stage two pressure ulcer on his right heel and has orders for whirlpool treatment. He is being discharged home alone in two weeks to his two-story home and is currently NWB on the right lower extremity and WBAT on the left lower extremity.

### Scenario Two

An 85-year-old female is admitted to the hospital due to a stage four pressure ulcer on her sacrum. She had been cared for at home by her husband since her stroke four months ago. The husband states that the wife remained in bed most of the time, has lost over 30 pounds, and presents with some mild cognitive deficits.

# Reflex Sympathetic Dystrophy

## Diagnosis

### What condition produces a patient's symptoms?

Reflex sympathetic dystrophy (RSD), also known as complex regional pain syndrome type I (occurring subsequent to trauma) or complex regional pain syndrome type II (associated with peripheral nerve injury) is usually found in an extremity that has experienced some form of trauma. Symptoms result from a disturbance in the functioning of the sympathetic nervous system. The increase in sympathetic activity causes a release of norepinephrine in the periphery and subsequent vasoconstriction of blood vessels. This results in pain and an increase in sensitivity to peripheral stimulation.

### An injury was most likely sustained to which structure?

RSD results from injured sensory nerve fibers at one somatic level that initiates sympathetic efferent activity that affects many segmental levels. The extremity of origin sustains injury as well as areas adjacent to the extremity.

## Inference

### What is the most likely contributing factor in the development of this condition?

The exact etiology of RSD is unknown, however, predisposing factors include trauma, surgery, CVA, TBI, repetitive motion disorders, and lower motor neuron and peripheral nerve injuries. RSD is reported to occur following 5% of all injuries. While many cases of RSD resolve, others progress and become a disabling disorder. RSD can affect all age groups but is most likely found in the age group of 35-60 years with females three times more likely to be affected by RSD than males.

## Confirmation

### What is the most likely clinical presentation?

A patient with RSD will experience intense, burning, and chronic pain in the affected extremity that will eventually spread proximally. Early in the syndrome the degree of pain is greater than expected based on the amount of trauma that the tissue sustained. Edema, thermal changes, discoloration, stiffness, and dryness are seen during stage I (acute stage) of RSD. Progression to stage II (dystrophic stage) is characterized by worsening and constant pain, continued edema, and trophic skin changes. X-rays may reveal bone loss, osteoporosis, and subchondral bone erosion in the affected extremity. Stage III (atrophic stage) is characterized by pain that continues to spread, hardened edema, decreased limb temperature, and atrophic changes to fingertips or toes. X-rays at this stage may reveal demineralization and ankylosis. Motor disorders such as tremor, spasms, and atrophy may also be present throughout each stage of RSD.

### What laboratory or imaging studies would confirm the diagnosis?

Imaging studies that can assist with the diagnosis of RSD include X-rays, thermographic studies, a three-phase bone scan, and laser Doppler flowmetry.

### What additional information should be obtained to confirm the diagnosis?

RSD is diagnosed primarily through a complete physical examination and a patient's complete medical history including a history and course of illness.

## Examination

### What history should be documented?

Important areas to explore include past medical history, medications, family history, current symptoms, current health status, social history and habits, occupation, leisure activities, and social support system.

### What test/measures are most appropriate?

**Anthropometric characteristics:** circumferential measurements of affected area or extremity

**Arousal, attention, and cognition:** examine mental status, learning ability, memory, motivation

**Environmental, home, and work barriers:** analysis of current and potential barriers or hazards

**Gait, locomotion, and balance:** static and dynamic balance in sitting and standing, safety during gait

**Integumentary integrity:** skin assessment, assessment of sensation, skin temperature changes

**Joint integrity and mobility:** assessment of hypermobility and hypomobility of a joint, soft tissue swelling

**Motor function:** motor assessment scales, assessment of sensorimotor integration, physical performance scales

**Muscle performance:** strength assessment, muscle tone assessment

**Pain:** pain perception scale, visual analogue scale, assessment of muscle soreness, McGill Pain Questionnaire

**Reflex integrity:** assessment of deep tendon and pathological reflexes

**Posture:** analysis of resting and dynamic posture

**Range of motion:** active and passive range of motion

**Sensory integrity:** assessment of proprioception and kinesthesia

**Self-care and home management:** assessment of functional capacity

# Reflex Sympathetic Dystrophy

## What additional findings are likely with this patient?

RSD will affect a patient's function throughout the progression of this neurovascular syndrome. RSD may progress to the point of bone demineralization and joint ankylosis (seen in stage III). Muscle atrophy, contractures, spasms, and incoordination will also contribute to functional decline. Depression and anxiety are also frequently seen and require medical attention. Malingering for secondary gain has been documented in some cases and should be monitored by the rehabilitation team.

## Management

### What is the most effective management of this patient?

RSD requires prolonged medical management. Treatment is based on identifying the underlying cause and stage of RSD at the time of diagnosis. Pharmacological intervention may include NSAIDs and corticosteroids for pain relief in early stages. Amitriptyline may be used for sleep and calcium channel blockers used for increasing peripheral circulation. Baclofen has been used as a long-term intervention to assist motor function. Bisphosphonate administration is warranted in later stages to combat bone loss. Surgical interventions such as sympathetic blocks or a sympathectomy are used to alleviate pain. Physical therapy intervention is a key component in the management of RSD. Pain control, patient education, skin care, joint mobilization, desensitization, and functional activity training are vital to the program. Modalities, pool therapy, relaxation training, and a home program all assist a patient with management of this syndrome.

### What home care regimen should be recommended?

A home program is vital to the management of RSD. Stretching and ROM, light weight bearing activities, ice and/or heat, TENS, and light exercise for conditioning are all key components of a home program. The patient must be educated and encouraged to use the involved extremity as tolerated. Edema management using a pump or compression garments may be indicated. Functional activities must also be encouraged.

## Outcome

### What is the likely outcome of a course in physical therapy?

Overall prognosis is better for a patient that begins treatment early in the cycle of the disease process. Physical therapy attempts to break the pain cycle and allows for a patient to continue with functional activities. Outcome is also dependent on a patient's motivation to maintain all aspects of a home program.

## What are the long-term effects of the patient's condition?

RSD can spontaneously resolve, continue with ongoing symptoms that can last for years or follow a pattern of remissions and recurring symptoms that develop from subsequent injuries. A patient's long-term outcome is dependent on how early the RSD was detected and treated. Research indicates a better prognosis if treatment is initiated within the first six months of the disease process.

## Comparison

### What are the distinguishing characteristics of a similar condition?

Sympathetically maintained pain (SMP) is a pain syndrome that is maintained by sympathetic efferent activity and is caused by a partial peripheral nerve lesion. SMP occurs less than RSD and is characterized by pain that is produced by a non-painful stimulus, vasomotor disturbances, and trophic changes. These symptoms remain localized to the affected nerve and the pain can usually be temporarily alleviated by sympathetic nerve block. Physical therapy intervention is warranted to assist with pain control through the use of modalities.

## Clinical Scenarios

### Scenario One

A 39-year-old female is seen in physical therapy with stage I (acute) RSD. The patient complains of burning pain in her left arm and presents with mild edema. The patient injured her shoulder two months ago. Past medical history includes being diagnosed with fibromyalgia two years ago. She is a team manager for a photography company and works approximately 50 hours per week.

### Scenario Two

A 62-year-old female is evaluated in physical therapy. She was diagnosed with RSD 13 months ago. She complains of significant pain in her right lower extremity and cannot walk without a walker. She has both hip and knee flexion contractures and significant swelling of the affected lower extremity.

# Restrictive Lung Disease

## Diagnosis

### What condition produces a patient's symptoms?

Restrictive lung disease (RLD) is a classification of disorders caused by a pulmonary or extrapulmonary restriction that produces impairment in lung expansion and an abnormal reduction in pulmonary ventilation. There are multiple conditions that can cause restrictive lung disease. Many symptoms are common regardless of the underlying etiology and other symptoms are disease-specific.

### An injury was most likely sustained to which structure?

Pulmonary restriction of the lungs can be caused by tumor, interstitial pulmonary fibrosis, scarring within the lungs, and pneumonia. Extrapulmonary restrictions of the lungs include pleural effusion, chest wall stiffness, structural abnormality, postural deformity, respiratory muscle weakness, and central nervous system injury.

## Inference

### What is the most likely contributing factor in the development of this condition?

There are varying etiologies for the group of disorders that cause restrictive lung disease. Musculoskeletal etiology includes scoliosis, pectus excavatum or other chest wall deformity, rib fractures, ankylosing spondylitis, and kyphosis. Pulmonary etiology includes idiopathic pulmonary fibrosis, pneumonia, pleural effusion, sarcoidosis, hyaline membrane disease, and tumor within the lungs. Other etiologies include inhalation of toxic fumes, drug therapy, asbestos, rheumatoid arthritis, systemic lupus erythematosus, muscular dystrophy, spinal cord injury, obesity, and other neurologic and neuromuscular diseases.

## Confirmation

### What is the most likely clinical presentation?

The clinical presentation varies based on the underlying cause or disease process. The pathogenesis of RLD includes a decrease in lung and chest wall compliance, decrease in lung volumes and an increase in the work of breathing. Generally, restrictive lung disease is characterized by a reduction of lung volumes (total lung capacity, vital capacity, inspiratory reserve volume, tidal volume, expiratory reserve volume, and inspiratory capacity) due to impaired lung expansion. A patient with restrictive lung disease will present with decreased chest mobility, decreased breath sounds, shortness of breath, hypoxemia, a rapid and shallow respiratory pattern (tachypnea), respiratory muscle weakness, ineffective cough, and increased use of accessory muscles.

### What laboratory or imaging studies would confirm the diagnosis?

A chest radiograph is utilized to evaluate lung structure and evidence of fibrosis, infiltrates, tumor, and deformity. Arterial blood gas analysis may indicate a decrease in $PaO_2$.

### What additional information should be obtained to confirm the diagnosis?

Pulmonary function testing will result in impaired vital capacity (VC), forced vital capacity (FVC), and total lung capacity (TLC). The patient will usually present with normal residual volume (RV) and expiration flow rates. Expiratory reserve volume (ERV) and functional residual capacity (FRC) are often decreased. Arterial blood gas analysis examines the presence of hypoxemia and hypocapnia.

## Examination

### What history should be documented?

Important areas to explore include past medical history, medications, current health status, social history and habits, occupation, living environment, and social support system.

### What test/measures are most appropriate?

**Aerobic capacity and endurance:** assessment of vital signs at rest and with activity, perceived exertion scale, pulse oximetry, auscultation of the lungs

**Arousal, attention, and cognition:** examine mental status, learning ability, memory, motivation

**Assistive and adaptive devices:** analysis of components and safety of a device

**Environmental, home, and work barriers:** analysis of current and potential barriers or hazards

**Gait, locomotion, and balance:** static and dynamic balance in sitting and standing, safety during gait with/without an assistive device, Berg Balance Scale, Tinetti Performance Oriented Mobility Assessment, Functional Ambulation Profile

**Motor function:** assessment of dexterity, coordination and agility, assessment of postural, equilibrium, and righting reactions

**Muscle performance:** strength assessment, active movement

**Posture:** analysis of resting and dynamic posture

**Range of motion:** active and passive range of motion

**Self-care and home management:** assessment of functional capacity

**Ventilation, respiration, and circulation:** auscultation of breath sounds, thoracoabdominal movement, pulmonary function testing, perceived exertion scale, assessment of cough and clearance of secretions

## Restrictive Lung Disease

### What additional findings are likely with this patient?

A patient with restrictive lung disease may become incapable of deep inspiration due to poor lung expansion. As restrictive lung disease progresses, respiratory muscle fatigue will lead to impaired alveolar ventilation and carbon dioxide retention. A patient will initially present with exertional dyspnea and progress to dyspnea at rest if the restriction progresses. Hypoxemia, pulmonary hypertension, cor pulmonale, severe decrease in oxygenation, and ventilatory failure are complications and outcomes of advanced restrictive lung disease.

## Management

### What is the most effective management of this patient?

Medical management of restrictive lung disease includes treatment of the underlying cause through pharmacological intervention, physical therapy, and potential surgical intervention. Physical therapy intervention is based on the severity of the condition, but is consistently oriented toward the goals of maximizing gas exchange and obtaining maximal functional capacity. Physical therapy intervention may include body mechanics, posture training, diaphragm and ventilatory muscle strengthening, relaxation and energy conservation techniques, and the use of these techniques during functional mobility. Breathing exercises, coughing techniques, and airway secretion clearance are often components of a comprehensive care plan.

### What home care regimen should be recommended?

A home care regimen should include breathing strategies and exercises, proper positioning, energy conservation and pacing techniques, general strengthening and endurance activities, and postural awareness with mobility. Low-level general strengthening and endurance training are indicated as tolerated.

## Outcome

### What is the likely outcome of a course in physical therapy?

Physical therapy intervention is specific to the underlying cause of the restrictive lung disease. Outcome is based on the etiology of the restrictive lung disease and patient response to physical therapy intervention. Treatment goals should include improving oxygenation and obtaining the maximal level of functioning.

### What are the long-term effects of the patient's condition?

Long-term effects from restrictive lung disease are also specific to the underlying cause. Some disorders require surgical intervention that alleviates the condition while other conditions are progressive and irreversible. Some patients with end-stage disease may be candidates for lung transplantation, however, most eventually progress to ventilatory failure.

Idiopathic pulmonary fibrosis is a restrictive lung disease that has a high mortality rate within four to six years of diagnosis whereas many conditions that cause restrictive lung disease are alleviated through appropriate management.

## Comparison

### What are the distinguishing characteristics of a similar condition?

Tuberculosis is an infectious and inflammatory systemic disease that can result in restrictive lung disease. The condition is a chronic pulmonary and extrapulmonary disease that causes fibrosis within the lungs. It is caused by the mycobacterium tuberculosis (tubercle bacillus) and transmitted through infected airborne droplets that are inhaled. Pulmonary symptoms include fatigue, weakness, an initial non-productive cough, and dyspnea with exertion. The disease also can affect other systems within the body including the lymph nodes and organs. Pharmacological intervention is the primary means of treating a patient with tuberculosis.

## Clinical Scenarios

### Scenario One

A 32-year-old male shows signs of restrictive lung disease. The patient is slightly short of breath with activity, has difficulty with deep inspiration, and complains of a non-productive cough. The patient had prolonged exposure to asbestos at his last place of employment and is under a physician's care. The physician referred the patient to physical therapy to improve the patient's general pulmonary status.

### Scenario Two

A 65-year-old female is seen in physical therapy for restrictive lung disease secondary to the removal of a benign tumor from the left lung. The patient reports having difficulty breathing, limited inhalation capability, and a productive cough. The patient has not been able to perform self-care and home activities secondary to breathing difficulties and relies solely on her 72-year-old husband.

# Rheumatoid Arthritis

## Diagnosis

### What condition produces a patient's symptoms?

Rheumatoid arthritis (RA) is a systemic autoimmune disorder of the connective tissue that is characterized by chronic inflammation within synovial membranes, tendon sheaths, and articular cartilage. The acute and chronic inflammatory changes produce the symptoms of this condition.

### An injury was most likely sustained to which structure?

Smaller peripheral joints are usually the first to be affected by RA, however, all connective tissue may become involved. Inflammation is present within the synovial membrane and granulation tissue forms as a result of the synovitis. The granulation tissue and protein degrading enzymes erode articular cartilage resulting in destruction, adhesions, and fibrosis within the joint.

## Inference

### What is the most likely contributing factor in the development of this condition?

The etiology of RA is unknown, however, there appears to be evidence of genetic predisposition with viral or bacterial triggers. Approximately 80% of individuals diagnosed with RA possess a positive rheumatoid factor (RF). RF represents the presence of autoantibodies that conflict with immunoglobulin antibodies found in the blood. The incidence of RA in women is three times greater than the incidence in men.

## Confirmation

### What is the most likely clinical presentation?

RA affects approximately 1-2% of the population within the United States or two million individuals (1.5 million women, 600,000 men). This condition is characterized by periods of exacerbations and is diagnosed most frequently between 30 and 50 years of age. RA will vary in onset and progression from patient to patient. Onset of RA may be sudden or develop over a period of weeks. Early characteristics include fatigue, bilateral involvement, tenderness of smaller joints, and low-grade fever. Patients often experience pain with motion, stiffness including prolonged morning stiffness, and progression of symptoms to larger synovial joints. In late stages of the disease the heart can become affected and deformities, subluxations, and contractures can occur.

### What laboratory or imaging studies would confirm the diagnosis?

Blood work assists with the diagnosis of RA through evaluation of the rheumatoid factor (RF), white blood cell count, erythrocyte sedimentation rate, hemoglobin, and hematocrit values. A synovial fluid analysis evaluates the content of synovial fluid within a joint. X-rays can be used to evaluate the joint space and the extent of decalcification.

### What additional information should be obtained to confirm the diagnosis?

Physical examination and patient history of symptoms are required to confirm the diagnosis. The American Rheumatoid Association has designed diagnostic criteria for RA that can be used as a guide to determine a definite, possible, probable or classic diagnosis.

## Examination

### What history should be documented?

Important areas to explore include past medical history, family history, medications, current symptoms and health status, living environment, social history and habits, occupation, and social support system.

### What test/measures are most appropriate?

**Aerobic capacity and endurance:** assessment of vital signs at rest and with activity, timed walk, $VO_2$ max

**Anthropometric characteristics:** circumferential measurements of all affected joints

**Arousal, attention, and cognition:** examine mental status, learning ability, memory, motivation

**Community and work integration:** analysis of community, work, and leisure activities

**Ergonomics and body mechanics:** analysis of dexterity and coordination

**Environmental, home, and work barriers:** analysis of current and potential barriers or hazards

**Gait, locomotion, and balance:** safety during gait with/without an assistive device, Functional Ambulation Profile, gait over level/unlevel surfaces, visual inspection of gait with and without shoes

**Integumentary integrity:** skin and sensation assessment

**Joint integrity and mobility:** assessment of joint hypomobility, soft tissue inflammation, presence of deformity, active joint count, articular tenderness

**Motor function:** equilibrium and righting reactions, motor assessment scales, coordination, posture and balance in sitting, physical performance scales

**Muscle performance:** break testing of isometric contractions, manometer method of strength testing

**Orthotic, protective, and supportive devices:** potential utilization of bracing, analysis of movement while wearing a device

**Pain:** pain perception assessment scale

**Range of motion:** active and passive range of motion

**Self-care and home management:** assessment of functional capacity

**Sensory integrity:** assessment of sensation, kinesthesia, and proprioception

# Rheumatoid Arthritis

### What additional findings are likely with this patient?

Extraarticular manifestations with RA can include pericarditis, anemia, tearing of tendons and musculature, osteoporosis, swan neck and/or boutonniere deformities, compression neuropathies, peripheral neuropathies, depression, pleurisy, skin changes, and anorexia.

## Management

### What is the most effective management of this patient?

Early medical management of a patient with RA is critical to improve the long-term outcomes of the disease. Medical treatment will focus on pain relief, reduction of edema, and preservation of joint integrity. Pharmacological intervention is required to decrease inflammation and retard the progression of the disease. NSAIDs, corticosteroids, and disease-modifying medications such as methotrexate are indicated. Physical therapy management during the acute stage or exacerbation includes patient education regarding regular rest, pain relief, relaxation, positioning, joint protection techniques, splinting, energy conservation, and body mechanics. Treatment may include gentle massage, hydrotherapy, hot pack, paraffin or cold modalities, gentle isometrics, and instruction in the use of assistive devices. Treatment during the acute stage should avoid resistive exercise, deep heating modalities, and any form of active stretching since these activities will further exacerbate the arthritis. Physical therapy management during the chronic stage or remission focuses on improving overall functional capacity, endurance, and strength. Treatment consists of low-impact conditioning through swimming or the stationary bicycle. Gentle stretching may be indicated to maintain available range of motion, however, aggressive stretching is contraindicated.

### What home care regimen should be recommended?

A home care regimen for a patient with RA must maintain a delicate balance between activity and rest. The patient should perform low-level exercise, utilize relaxation and energy conservation techniques, and use splints as needed. The patient should recognize when total rest is indicated due to an acute exacerbation.

## Outcome

### What is the likely outcome of a course in physical therapy?

Physical therapy cannot halt the progression of RA, however, it can improve a patient's ability to function. Physical therapy may be indicated intermittently throughout the disease process with goals that focus on pain relief, relaxation, improving motion, and preventing deformity.

### What are the long-term effects of the patient's condition?

RA is a chronic disease process that currently does not have a known cure, progresses at a varied rate, creates irreversible damage and deformity, and results in disability. As the disease progresses there is bilateral and symmetrical involvement of joints. Systemic effects include insomnia, fatigue, and organ involvement including the heart and lungs.

## Comparison

### What are the distinguishing characteristics of a similar condition?

Osteoarthritis is a chronic degenerative condition that usually develops secondary to repetitive trauma, disease or obesity. The hyaline cartilage in the joint softens and breaks apart allowing bone-to-bone contact that results in joint deformity, crepitus, impaired range of motion, and pain. Pain typically increases with prolonged activity. Joints become swollen and tender and joint deformity develops. Women have a slightly greater risk for OA than men. Surgical procedures including osteotomy and joint replacement may be indicated if conservative treatment is unsuccessful.

## Clinical Scenarios

### Scenario One

A 38-year-old female diagnosed with RA is seen in an outpatient clinic. The patient history reveals fatigue and malaise for two to three weeks and pain in the fingers and wrists. The patient has difficulty caring for herself at home and is on medical leave from her job. The patient does not have any other significant past medical history and resides alone.

### Scenario Two

A 74-year-old male diagnosed with RA is treated by a therapist. The patient presents with multi-joint involvement, deformities of the hands and feet, poor endurance, stiffness, and pain. The patient is ambulatory, however, is currently in a wheelchair secondary to pain from an exacerbation. The patient is oriented and has a history of COPD.

## Rotator Cuff Tendonitis

### Diagnosis

#### What condition produces a patient's symptoms?

Repetitive overhead activities can produce impingement of the supraspinatus tendon immediately proximal to the greater tubercle of the humerus. The impingement is caused by an inability of a weak supraspinatus muscle to adequately depress the head of the humerus in the glenoid fossa during elevation of the arm. As a result the humerus translates superiorly due to the disproportionate action of the deltoid muscle. Primary impingement occurs from intrinsic or extrinsic factors within the subacromial space. Secondary impingement describes symptoms that occur from poor mechanics or instability at the shoulder joint.

#### An injury was most likely sustained to which structure?

The supraspinatus muscle has the most commonly involved tendon in rotator cuff tendonitis. The muscle originates on the supraspinatus fossa of the scapula and inserts on the greater tubercle of the humerus. Bicipital and infraspinatus tendonitis as well as bursitis may also coexist as other contributing factors.

### Inference

#### What is the most likely contributing factor in the development of this condition?

Individuals participating in activities that require excessive overhead activity such as swimming, tennis, baseball, painting, and other manual labor activities are at increased risk for rotator cuff tendonitis. Excessive use of the upper extremity following a prolonged period of inactivity also can produce this condition. Statistically, individuals from 25-40 years of age are the most likely to develop this condition.

### Confirmation

#### What is the most likely clinical presentation?

A patient with rotator cuff tendonitis often reports difficulty with overhead activities and a dull ache following periods of activity. The patient may experience a feeling of weakness and identify the presence of a painful arc of motion most commonly occurring between 60 and 120 degrees of active abduction. The patient usually presents with pain with palpation of the musculotendinous junction of the involved muscle and/or with stretching or resisted contraction of the muscle. Pain often increases at night resulting in difficulty sleeping on the affected side. The patient will often have difficulty with dressing and repetitive shoulder motions such as lifting, reaching, throwing, swinging or pushing and pulling with the involved upper extremity.

#### What laboratory or imaging studies would confirm the diagnosis?

Magnetic resonance imaging can be used to identify the presence of rotator cuff tendonitis, however, due to the high cost it is not commonly employed prior to the initiation of formal treatment. X-rays with the shoulder laterally rotated can be used to identify the presence of calcific deposits or other bony abnormalities.

#### What additional information should be obtained to confirm the diagnosis?

A number of specific special tests including the empty can test, Jobe test, Neer impingement test, and Hawkins-Kennedy impingement test can be used to confirm the presence of rotator cuff tendonitis or impingement.

### Examination

#### What history should be documented?

Important areas to explore include past medical history, family history, medications, history of symptoms, current health status, living environment, social history and habits, occupation, and social support system.

#### What test/measures are most appropriate?

**Anthropometric characteristics:** upper extremity circumferential measurements

**Arousal, attention, and cognition:** examine mental status, learning ability, memory, motivation

**Assistive and adaptive devices:** analysis of components and safety of a device

**Community and work integration:** analysis of community, work, and leisure activities

**Integumentary integrity:** skin assessment, assessment of sensation

**Joint integrity and mobility:** soft tissue swelling and inflammation, assessment of joint play, palpation of the joint, empty can test, Neer impingement test, Hawkins-Kennedy impingement test

**Motor function:** posture and balance

**Muscle performance:** strength assessment

**Pain:** pain perception assessment scale

**Posture:** analysis of resting and dynamic posture

**Range of motion:** active and passive range of motion

**Reflex integrity:** assessment of deep tendon reflexes

**Self-care and home management:** assessment of functional capacity

# Rotator Cuff Tendonitis

### What additional findings are likely with this patient?

Rotator cuff tendonitis often presents in association with impingement syndrome. Impingement syndrome typically involves the supraspinatus tendon, glenoid labrum, long head of the biceps, and subacromial bursa. It is extremely difficult to determine through examination the exact level of involvement of each of the identified structures.

## Management

### What is the most effective management of this patient?

Medical management of acute rotator cuff tendonitis usually includes pharmacological intervention and physical therapy. Pharmacological intervention will focus on pain relief through analgesics and NSAIDs. Acute physical therapy intervention guidelines should include cryotherapy, activity modification, range of motion, and rest. As the acute phase subsides the patient is often instructed in strengthening exercises. Since the rotator cuff muscles are dependent on adequate blood supply and oxygen, it is essential that all range of motion and strengthening exercises are pain free. Range of motion exercises using a pulley system or a cane can serve as an effective intervention. Strengthening exercises are initiated with the arm at the patient's side in order to prevent the possibility of impingement. Elastic tubing or handheld weights are often the preferred equipment of choice. It is important for the entire rotator cuff to be strong prior to initiating overhead activities. Shoulder shrugs and push-ups with the arms abducted to 90 degrees can effectively be used to strengthen the upper trapezius and serratus anterior. This type of activity promotes elevation of the acromion without direct contact with the rotator cuff.

### What home care regimen should be recommended?

The home care regimen should consist of range of motion, strengthening, palliative care, and functional activities as warranted based on the results of the patient examination.

## Outcome

### What is the likely outcome of a course in physical therapy?

A patient with rotator cuff tendonitis should be able to return to their previous level of functioning with conservative management within four to six weeks. Outcome can be dependent, however, on the patient's classification of stage I, II or III impingement syndrome. Stage I is usually found in the population less than 25 years of age and consists of localized inflammation, edema, and minimal bleeding around the rotator cuff. Stage II represents progressive deterioration of the tissues surrounding the rotator cuff and is common in 25 to 40-year-old patients. Stage III represents the end-stage and is usually found in patients over 40 years of age. There is usually disruption and/or rupture of numerous soft tissue structures.

### What are the long-term effects of the patient's condition?

Failure to adequately treat rotator cuff tendonitis may necessitate significant activity modification or more aggressive surgical management such as subacromial decompression. Prolonged inflammation of the rotator cuff tendon may facilitate eventual tearing of the rotator cuff musculature.

## Comparison

### What are the distinguishing characteristics of a similar condition?

A rotator cuff tear is usually the result of repetitive microtrauma but can also result suddenly from a single traumatic event. Partial tears often occur in a younger population while complete tears more commonly occur in older individuals. The mechanism of injury is often a fall on an outstretched arm or a sudden strain applied to the shoulder during pushing or pulling activities. Diagnosis is made through MRI to identify the tear. Surgical repair of the rotator cuff is often required and may be done with arthroscopy or through a traditional open technique. The shoulder is usually protected by a sling and small abduction pillow for the first six weeks post surgery. Rehabilitation and return to full function can take upwards of six months, heavy lifting may be restricted for six to twelve months following surgery.

## Clinical Scenarios

### Scenario One

A 23-year-old female diagnosed with rotator cuff tendonitis is referred to physical therapy after experiencing pain while swimming the breaststroke in a competitive swim meet one week ago. The patient participates on a school swim team and a private club and practices four to six times per week. A few days after experiencing shoulder pain the patient was back in the pool, however, was unable to return to her previous training regimen.

### Scenario Two

A 45-year-old male employed as a pipe fitter is referred to physical therapy after subacromial decompression. The patient is one week status post surgery and is anxious to "test" his involved shoulder. Prior to surgery the patient was placed on "light duty." It has been six months since the patient was able to perform his job without restrictions. The patient presently denies any pain in the involved shoulder.

# Sciatica Secondary to a Herniated Disk

## Diagnosis

### What condition produces a patient's symptoms?

A herniated disk is an intervertebral disk that bulges and protrudes posterolaterally against a nerve root. Sciatica is the diagnosis of compression of the sciatic nerve (L4, L5, S1, S2, S3) secondary to a herniated disk causing a patient's symptoms. Other causes for sciatica include tumor, infection, spondylolisthesis, narrowing of the canal, and blood clots.

### An injury was most likely sustained to which structure?

As a patient gets older there are natural and significant alterations in the composition of the intervertebral disks and supporting structures. In a herniated disk the nucleus pulposus has bulged posterolaterally secondary to a weakening of the outer annulus fibrosis and posterior longitudinal ligament. The sciatic nerve experiences an inflammatory response and subsequent damage secondary to the compression from the herniated disk.

## Inference

### What is the most likely contributing factor in the development of this condition?

The most common contributing factor for this condition is the natural aging process. Each decade the composition of the annulus fibrosus and nucleus pulposus is altered and decreases in overall stability. Once there is adequate structural breakdown within the disk, a patient becomes a high risk for injury. A "normal mechanical load on a normal disk" is now an "excessive load on a compromised disk." As expected, sciatica secondary to a herniated disk is most often seen in patients between 40 and 60 years of age.

## Confirmation

### What is the most likely clinical presentation?

Sciatica is characterized by low back and gluteal pain that typically radiates down the back of the thigh along the sciatic nerve distribution. Sciatic pain occurs from nerve root compression and can be dull, aching or sharp. Pain may have a sudden onset or develop gradually over time. Early sciatica may involve discomfort or pain limited to the low back and gluteal region. Leg pain can become greater than the back pain and can radiate the entire length of the nerve to the toes. The patient may also experience intermittent numbness and tingling localized to the dermatomal distribution, limited thoracolumbar range of motion in all planes, tenderness to palpation at the segment of herniation, and muscle guarding.

### What laboratory or imaging studies would confirm the diagnosis?

Radiologic testing of the spine and electrophysiologic studies are initially performed to assist with diagnosis. Other imaging may include myelogram, discography, CT scan or MRI. Blood work may assist with differential diagnosis.

### What additional information should be obtained to confirm the diagnosis?

A full examination should be performed that includes history (trauma, osteoporosis, corticosteroid use), functional assessment, inspection, palpation, and special tests. The straight leg raise test will reproduce symptoms in the case of a herniated disk. The exam should also include testing for non-organic back pain to rule out psychological factors.

## Examination

### What history should be documented?

Important areas to explore include past medical history and treatment, history of trauma and accidents, medications, family history, current symptoms, current health status, social history and habits, occupation, leisure activities, and social support system.

### What test/measures are most appropriate?

**Arousal, attention, and cognition:** examine mental status, learning ability, memory, motivation

**Assistive and adaptive devices:** analysis of components and safety of a device

**Community and work integration:** analysis of community, work, and leisure activities

**Environmental, home, and work barriers:** analysis of current and potential barriers or hazards

**Ergonomics and body mechanics:** analysis of dexterity and coordination

**Gait, locomotion, and balance:** static and dynamic balance in sitting and standing, Functional Ambulation Profile

**Integumentary integrity:** skin assessment, assessment of sensation, dermatome testing of the lower extremities

**Joint integrity and mobility:** assessment of hypermobility and hypomobility of a joint, soft tissue swelling and inflammation

**Muscle performance:** strength assessment, resisted isometrics, straight leg raise testing

**Pain:** Oswestry Function Test, McGill Pain Questionnaire, visual analogue scale

**Posture:** analysis of resting and dynamic posture

**Range of motion:** active and passive movement of the spine, combined movements, segmental mobility testing

**Reflex integrity:** assessment of deep tendon and pathological reflexes (clonus)

**Self-care and home management:** assessment of functional capacity, Functional Independence Measure

# Sciatica Secondary to a Herniated Disk

### What additional findings are likely with this patient?

Sciatica will produce pain that increases with certain positions due to an increase in intradiskal pressure. Pain will increase in a sitting position or when lifting, forward bending or twisting. Sneezing and coughing can also exacerbate the pain. Although a patient may want to stop all activity to relieve pain, prolonged bed rest is contraindicated and will not relieve pain on a long-term basis.

## Management

### What is the most effective management of this patient?

Medical management of sciatica due to a herniated disk includes short-term bed rest, overall reduction of intradiskal pressure, patient education, physical therapy, medications, and in rare instances surgical intervention. Pharmacological intervention will incorporate NSAIDs initially to relieve pain followed by epidural injections of cortisone and local anesthetics that may be indicated for temporary relief, however, do not alter the root of the problem. Physical therapy intervention should include patient education on positioning and biomechanics, pain management, traction, heat, lumbar stabilization exercises, McKenzie exercises, stretching, and endurance activities. Swimming, stationary bicycling and walking are indicated within tolerance. Lifting, squatting, and climbing are contraindicated due to the significant increase in intradiskal pressure. Most herniations will spontaneously decrease in size with conservative treatment. Research indicates that the majority of patients improve with two to four months of conservative treatment, however, approximately 2% of patients undergo surgery. Common surgical intervention may include laminectomy, discectomy, chemonucleolysis, laser discectomy or laminotomy.

### What home care regimen should be recommended?

A home care regimen should include ongoing caution regarding positioning and constant effort to decrease intradiskal pressure. A home exercise program including stabilization exercises is indicated as well as other aerobic/endurance activities to tolerance.

## Outcome

### What is the likely outcome of a course in physical therapy?

Most patients improve with conservative treatment over a two to four month period. Physical therapy intervention combined with a consistent home program will provide the patient with the necessary tools to relieve pain and improve function.

### What are the long-term effects of the patient's condition?

Sciatica secondary to a herniated disk can be corrected through rest and physical therapy intervention. Healing of the disk can also occur and scarring can reinforce the posterior aspect and annular fibers so that it is protected from further protrusion. Restoration of functional mobility is plausible, however, surgical intervention may be required if neurological symptoms increase or no progress is made with conservative measures.

## Comparison

### What are the distinguishing characteristics of a similar condition?

Spinal stenosis is another condition that can be a causative factor of sciatica. Symptoms that would indicate spinal stenosis include lower extremity weakness with or without sciatica, back and leg pain after ambulating a short distance, increasing symptoms with continued ambulation, and relief of symptoms through flexion. Radiologic results reveal disk narrowing and degenerative spondylolisthesis. Surgery is only recommended as a last resort when conservative treatment fails.

## Clinical Scenarios

### Scenario One

A 42-year-old female is referred to physical therapy with an L5 herniated disk and sciatica. The patient injured her back skiing three months ago. She presently works 50 hours per week at a daycare facility. Current symptoms include radiating pain down the left leg, a "feeling of weakness," and an inability to sleep at night due to pain.

### Scenario Two

A 65-year-old male has been seen in physical therapy for three months with sciatica secondary to a L4 herniated disk. The patient states that he experiences constant pain. The therapist questions the patient's overall compliance with his established home exercise program. The physician orders are prescribed as physical therapy three times per week.

# Scoliosis

## Diagnosis

### What condition produces a patient's symptoms?

A patient with scoliosis presents with a lateral curvature of the spine. The curvature is usually found in the thoracic or lumbar vertebrae and can be associated with kyphosis or lordosis. The curvature of the spine may be towards the right or towards the left and rotation of the spine may or may not occur. Typically, the rotation will occur towards the convex side of the major curve.

### An injury was most likely sustained to which structure?

The injury or deformity begins when the vertebrae of the spine deviate from the normal vertical position. The curvature disrupts normal alignment of the ribs and muscles and can create compensatory curves that attempt to keep the body in proper alignment. The vertebral column, rib cage, supporting ligaments, and muscles are all affected by a scoliosis of the spine.

## Inference

### What is the most likely contributing factor in the development of this condition?

Idiopathic scoliosis, termed for its unknown etiology, accounts for approximately 80% of all cases. Upwards of 1:10 children are affected by some form of scoliosis with 1:4 requiring treatment for the curvature. The age of onset determines the subset of classification as infantile (0 to 3), juvenile (four to puberty), adolescent (12 for girls and 14 for boys) or adult (skeletal maturation) scoliosis. Non-structural scoliosis is a reversible curve that can change with repositioning. This type of curve is non-progressive and is usually caused by poor posture or leg length discrepancy. Structural scoliosis cannot be corrected with movement and can be caused by congenital, musculoskeletal, and neuromuscular reasons. Contributing factors of a structural curve include altered development of the spine in utero, association with neuromuscular diseases (cerebral palsy, muscular dystrophy, congenital defect of the vertebrae), and inheritance as an autosomal dominant trait. Research indicates a predisposition for scoliosis with a multifactorial etiology.

## Confirmation

### What is the most likely clinical presentation?

A patient with a structural curve will present with asymmetries of the shoulders, scapulae, pelvis, and skinfolds. Juvenile idiopathic scoliosis is characterized by a thoracic curve with convexity towards the right. This curve may progress quickly and develop compensatory curves above and below. As the curve progresses there will be a rib hump posteriorly over the thoracic region on the convex side of the curve. The patient does not typically experience pain or other subjective symptoms until the curve has progressed. Adolescent scoliosis

of greater than 30 degrees is seen more in females than males (10:1). Adult scoliosis affects approximately 500,000 adults in the United States. Curves that are less than 20 degrees rarely cause a person to experience significant problems or impairments.

### What laboratory or imaging studies would confirm the diagnosis?

X-rays should be taken in an anterior and lateral view with the patient standing and with the patient bending over. A device called a scoliometer can be used to measure the angle of trunk rotation. The Cobb method can be used to determine the angle of curvature. A bone scan or MRI can be used to determine and rule out conditions such as infections, neoplasms, spondylolysis, disk herniations or compression fractures.

### What additional information should be obtained to confirm the diagnosis?

Physical examination allows visual inspection of the curvature and physical asymmetries. A scoliometer can assist with measurement and the examiner can determine if the curve is non-structural or structural.

## Examination

### What history should be documented?

Important areas to explore include past medical history, family history, medications, current health status, living environment, school activities, and social support system.

### What test/measures are most appropriate?

**Aerobic capacity and endurance:** assessment of vital signs at rest and with activity, perceived exertion scale

**Arousal, attention, and cognition:** examine mental status, learning ability, memory, motivation

**Ergonomics and body mechanics:** analysis of dexterity and coordination

**Integumentary integrity:** skin and sensation assessment

**Gait, locomotion, and balance:** static and dynamic balance in sitting and standing, safety during gait with/without an assistive device, analysis of wheelchair management

**Joint integrity and mobility:** assessment of hypermobility and hypomobility of a joint

**Muscle performance:** strength assessment

**Orthotic, protective, and supportive devices:** analysis of components of a device, analysis of movement while wearing a device

**Pain:** assessment of muscle soreness

**Posture:** analysis of resting and dynamic posture

**Range of motion:** active and passive range of motion

**Self-care and home management:** assessment of functional capacity

# Scoliosis

## What additional findings are likely with this patient?

Common postural findings with scoliosis include increased spacing between the elbow and trunk during standing, leg length discrepancy, uneven shoulder and hip heights, and prominence on one side of the pelvis or breast (due to rotation of the curve). If a progressive scoliosis is untreated, the deformity can increase to an angle in excess of 60 degrees and cause pulmonary insufficiency, significant pain, impairment in lung capacity, and degenerative changes including arthritis and disk pathology. Early screening, detection, and treatment are necessary to control the curvature and avoid surgical intervention.

## Management

### What is the most effective management of this patient?

Medical management of scoliosis is based on the type and severity of the curve, patient age, and previous management. Patients with scoliosis may utilize electrical stimulation to alleviate pain and biofeedback for education with proper posture and positioning. A patient with scoliosis that is less than 25 degrees should be monitored every three months. Breathing exercises and a strengthening program for the trunk and pelvic muscles are indicated. A patient with scoliosis that ranges between 25 and 40 degrees requires a spinal orthosis and physical therapy intervention for posture, flexibility, strengthening, respiratory function, and proper utilization of the spinal orthosis. A patient with scoliosis that is greater than 40 degrees usually requires surgical spinal stabilization. One method to surgically correct scoliosis is through posterior spinal fusion and stabilization with a Harrington rod. Physical therapy intervention after surgical fusion is indicated for breathing exercises, posture, flexibility, general strengthening, and respiratory muscle strengthening.

### What home care regimen should be recommended?

A home care regimen is based on the type and severity of the curve. Exercise, stretching, posture, and flexibility are important components of an exercise program.

## Outcome

### What is the likely outcome of a course in physical therapy?

Physical therapy intervention should improve a patient's condition through patient education and therapeutic exercise. Physical therapy may be indicated for implementation of a home program, pain management, posture retraining, orthotic training or following surgical stabilization.

## What are the long-term effects of the patient's condition?

Prognosis for structural scoliosis is based on the age of onset and the severity of the curve. Early intervention results in the best possible outcome. Scoliosis does not usually progress significantly once bone growth is complete if the curvature remains below 40 degrees at the time of skeletal maturity. If the curvature is over 50 degrees there likely will be ongoing progression of the curve each year of life.

## Comparison

### What are the distinguishing characteristics of a similar condition?

Torticollis is a deformity of the neck that is caused by shortened or spastic sternocleidomastoid muscles. The patient presents with a bending of the neck towards the affected side and rotation of the head towards the unaffected side. Causative factors include damage to the sternocleidomastoid muscle, malpositioning in utero, spasms secondary to central nervous system impairment or psychogenic origin. Conservative treatment for acquired torticollis includes heat, traction, massage, stretching, positioning, and bracing. Surgical intervention may be indicated if conservative management fails.

## Clinical Scenarios

### Scenario One

An 11-year-old female is seen in physical therapy with diagnosis of a 30-degree right thoracic scoliosis. The physician has prescribed a spinal orthosis and physical therapy. The patient denies any pain, but states that she has soreness in her back. The patient is in the marching band and plays basketball. There is no past medical history and her parents are very supportive.

### Scenario Two

A seven-year-old boy is referred to physical therapy with a 12-degree right thoracic scoliosis. The physical therapy prescription requests evaluation for a home exercise program. The patient has type 1 diabetes mellitus and a low I.Q. The mother is present for the evaluation and appears to be supportive.

# Spina Bifida – Myelomeningocele

## Diagnosis

### What condition produces a patient's symptoms?

Spina bifida is a congenital neural tube defect that generally occurs in the lumbar spine but can also occur at the sacral, cervical, and thoracic levels. Spina bifida has three classifications that include spina bifida - occulta (incomplete fusion of the posterior vertebral arch with no neural tissue protruding), spina bifida - meningocele (incomplete fusion of the posterior vertebral arch with neural tissue/meninges protruding outside the neural arch), and spina bifida - myelomeningocele (incomplete fusion of the posterior vertebral arch with both meninges and spinal cord protruding outside the neural arch).

### An injury was most likely sustained to which structure?

Spina bifida - myelomeningocele is characterized by a sac or cyst that protrudes outside the spine and contains a herniation of meninges, cerebrospinal fluid, and the spinal cord through the defect in the vertebrae. The cyst may or may not be covered by skin. Spina bifida results from failure of neural tube closure by day 28 of gestation when the spinal cord is expected to form. Approximately 75% of vertebral defects are found in the lumbar/sacral region, typically L5-S1 with injury to the structures at that level and below. Defects can also occur in the cervical or thoracic spine, however, this is rare.

## Inference

### What is the most likely contributing factor in the development of this condition?

The Centers for Disease Control estimates the incidence for neural tube defects to be five per 10,000 live births within the United States. The incidence varies by socioeconomic status, geographic area, and ethnic background. The overall incidence is declining due to improved prenatal care. The exact etiology for spina bifida - myelomeningocele has not been identified, however, causative and risk factors include genetic predisposition, environmental influence (certain solvents, lead, herbicides, glycol ethers), insulin-dependent diabetes, low-levels of maternal folic acid, alcohol, maternal hyperthermia, and certain classifications of drugs (teratogenic exposure and vitamin A toxicity). Theories suggest that the cause is multifactorial rather than a single source of etiology. Prenatal care including recommended amounts of folic acid, especially in the first six weeks of pregnancy, appears to be the most effective way to prevent neural tube defects.

## Confirmation

### What is the most likely clinical presentation?

Myelomeningocele is a severe condition that is characterized by a sac that is seen on an infant's back protruding from a specific area of the spinal cord. Impairments associated with myelomeningocele include motor and sensory loss below the vertebral defect, hydrocephalus, Arnold-Chiari type II malformation, clubfoot, scoliosis, bowel and bladder dysfunction, and learning disabilities. The higher the neural lesion the worse the prognosis is for survival. The infant will require surgical intervention to close the lesion and in 90% of the cases a shunt is required for hydrocephalus. Approximately two-thirds of children with myelomeningocele and shunted hydrocephalus have normal intelligence and the other third demonstrate only mild retardation. Regardless of intelligence, children with myelomeningocele exhibit difficulties with perceptual abilities, attention, problem solving, and memory.

### What laboratory or imaging studies would confirm the diagnosis?

Prior to birth a fetal ultrasound may identify the myelomeningocele defect in the spine. Prenatal testing of alpha-fetoprotein (AFP) in the blood will show an elevation in levels that indicate a probable neural tube defect at approximately week 16 of gestation. At birth an obvious sac will be present over the spinal defect. Spinal films and CT scan can evaluate for the presence of defects and hydrocephalus.

### What additional information should be obtained to confirm the diagnosis?

Diagnosis is confirmed through prenatal testing or upon visual observation at birth. Past medical history of the mother, history of the pregnancy, and family history of neural tube defects may be noted.

## Examination

### What history should be documented?

Important areas to explore with the parents include past medical history, current symptoms and health status, medications, past surgical procedures, living environment, and social support system.

### What test/measures are most appropriate?

**Aerobic capacity and endurance:** assessment of vital signs at rest and with activity

**Arousal, attention, and cognition:** examine mental status, learning ability, memory, motivation

**Assistive and adaptive devices:** use of appropriate devices, analysis of components/safety of a device

**Ergonomics and body mechanics:** analysis of dexterity and coordination

**Gait, locomotion, and balance:** developmental milestones assessment, static/dynamic balance in prone and sitting, analysis of wheelchair management, standing with frame, gait with assistive device

**Integumentary integrity:** skin and sensation assessment

**Motor function:** equilibrium and righting reactions, motor assessment scales, balance in sitting

## Spina Bifida – Myelomeningocele

**Muscle performance:** assessment of active movement, muscle tone assessment
**Orthotic, protective, and supportive devices:** analysis of components of a device, analysis of movement while wearing a device
**Range of motion:** active and passive range of motion
**Reflex integrity:** assessment of deep tendon and pathological reflexes (e.g., Babinski, ATNR)

### What additional findings are likely with this patient?

Immediately after birth, an infant with myelomeningocele has an increased risk of meningitis, hemorrhage, and hypoxia, however, surgical intervention may significantly reduce the risks. Ongoing additional findings with myelomeningocele include hydrocephalus, clubfoot, neuropathic fracture, visual problems, osteoporosis, kyphosis, hip dislocations, and latex allergy.

## Management

### What is the most effective management of this patient?

Medical management of a patient with myelomeningocele begins with immediate surgical intervention to repair and close the defect and for placement of a shunt to alleviate hydrocephalus. Orthopedic surgical intervention may be warranted throughout a patient's life to correct deformities such as clubfoot, hip dysplasia, and scoliosis. Pharmacological intervention may include medications that assist in the management of bowel and bladder dysfunction. Physical and occupational therapies are important components in the management of myelomeningocele. Physical therapy is initiated immediately and focuses on family education regarding positioning, handling techniques, range of motion, and therapeutic play. Long-term physical therapy attempts to maximize functional capacity and may include range of motion, facilitation of developmental milestones, therapeutic exercise, skin care, strengthening, balance, and mobility training. Physical therapy will also assist with wheelchair prescription, assistive and adaptive device selection, and the use of orthotics and splinting.

### What home care regimen should be recommended?

A home care regimen should include a formal exercise program, range of motion, and mobility training. Family and caregiver involvement are important in assisting a patient through their exercise program. The home program will require modification as the child matures and goals change.

## Outcome

### What is the likely outcome of a course in physical therapy?

Physical therapy initially evaluates and documents the baseline information regarding the patient's motor and sensory function and level of ability. Physical therapy is ongoing through adolescence and is based on the severity of impairments and the needs of the child. Physical therapy is usually initiated based on symptoms, functional problems, and disability.

### What are the long-term effects of the patient's condition?

A patient with myelomeningocele has a near normal life expectancy as long as the patient receives consistent and thorough health care. Functional outcome of the patient depends on the level of injury, the amount of associated impairments, and the caregiver support that is provided.

## Comparison

### What are the distinguishing characteristics of a similar condition?

Anencephaly is a condition that is characterized by failed closure of the cranial end of the neural tube. The cerebral hemispheres do not form and some neural tissue may protrude through the defect. This type of neural tube defect cannot be repaired. Many infants with this condition are stillborn, while others only survive a short time after birth.

## Clinical Scenarios

### Scenario One

A six-month-old boy is seen in physical therapy after revision of a ventriculoperitoneal shunt. The parents state that the child has been responsive at home and has been doing well. The child can position himself in prone on elbows and is able to sit with support.

### Scenario Two

An 11-year-old girl with a T12 spinal cord lesion is seen in outpatient physical therapy. The patient presently uses a wheelchair for mobility, however, indicates that her goal is to walk in her home. The patient's upper body strength is good and intellect is normal.

# Spinal Cord Injury – Complete C7 Tetraplegia

## Diagnosis

### What condition produces a patient's symptoms?

The majority of traumatic spinal cord injuries result from compression, flexion or extension of the spine with or without rotation. Spinal cord injuries are classified as a concussion, contusion or laceration, and injury results in primary and secondary neural destruction. Traumatic injury to the spinal cord produces a physiological and biochemical chain of events that results in vascular impairment and permanent tissue and nerve damage.

### An injury was most likely sustained to which structure?

A patient sustains primary damage to the spinal cord and surrounding tissues at the C7 level through disruption of the membrane, displacement or compression of the spinal cord, and subsequent hemorrhage and vascular damage. Secondary damage occurs beyond the level of injury due to biochemicals that are released as a result of the initial damage. This process destroys adjacent cells and neural tracts due to the acute inflammation and can last for days or even weeks. After injury, C7 is the most distal segment of the spinal cord that both the motor and sensory components remain intact.

## Inference

### What is the most likely contributing factor in the development of this condition?

There is an estimated 250,000 persons living with SCI within the United States. Statistics from the National Spinal Cord Injury Database (NSCID) indicate that motor vehicle accidents, violence, and falls are the top causes of traumatic spinal cord injury. Statistics also indicate a higher ratio of injury in men (approximately 80%) and Caucasians. The highest incidence of age of injury (over 50%) occurs between 15 to 30 years of age.

## Confirmation

### What is the most likely clinical presentation?

Spinal shock, which is the total depression of all nervous system function below the level of lesion, occurs immediately following injury and may last for days. Presentation includes total flaccid paralysis and loss of all reflexes and sensation. Surgical intervention may be required after injury in order to stabilize the spinal cord through decompression and fusion at the site of injury. A Halo device is commonly used with cervical injuries to stabilize the spine. As spinal shock subsides, a patient will experience an increase in muscle tone below the level of lesion and neurologic reflexes reappear. Spasticity will evolve and may become problematic. Autonomic dysreflexia and loss of thermoregulation are other impairments that occur secondary to autonomic nervous system dysfunction. A patient with C7 tetraplegia will also present with impaired cough and ability to clear secretions, altered breathing pattern, and poor endurance. The patient is at high risk for contractures and impaired skin integrity.

### What laboratory or imaging studies would confirm the diagnosis?

X-rays of the cervical spine observe the positioning and damage of the involved vertebrae. The results of imaging determine subsequent medical intervention including stabilization of the spine. A myelogram or tomogram may be useful to confirm the extent of surrounding damage at the level of the injury.

### What additional information should be obtained to confirm the diagnosis?

Other information commonly obtained in order to support the diagnosis includes physician conducted interviews regarding the mechanism of injury as well as a full neurological examination.

## Examination

### What history should be documented?

Important areas to explore include past medical history, medications, mechanism of injury, precautions, current health status, social history and habits, occupation or school responsibilities, living environment, and social support system.

### What test/measures are most appropriate?

**Aerobic capacity and endurance:** autonomic responses to positional changes, vital signs at rest/activity

**Arousal, attention, and cognition:** examine mental status, learning ability, memory, motivation

**Assistive and adaptive devices:** analysis of components and safety of a device, wheelchair prescription, adaptive devices, environmental controls

**Integumentary integrity:** skin assessment, American Spinal Injury Association (ASIA) - Standard Neurological Classification of Spinal Cord Injury Sensory Examination

**Motor function:** posture and balance in sitting

**Muscle performance:** ASIA - Standard Neurological Classification of Spinal Cord Injury Motor Examination, muscle tone assessment

**Neuromotor development and sensory integration:** analysis of reflex movement patterns

**Pain:** dysesthetic pain (deafferentation pain), nerve root pain, musculoskeletal pain

**Posture:** positioning, resting and dynamic posture

**Range of motion:** active and passive range of motion

**Reflex integrity:** assessment of deep tendon reflexes and pathological reflexes

**Sensory integrity:** proprioception and kinesthesia

**Ventilation, respiration, and circulation:** assessment of cough and clearance of secretions, breathing patterns, respiratory muscle strength, accessory muscle utilization, pulmonary function tests

# Spinal Cord Injury – Complete C7 Tetraplegia

## What additional findings are likely with this patient?

There are many additional findings that can exist with a C7 injury, but the most common complications include orthostatic hypotension, pressure sores, spasticity, heterotopic ossification, and autonomic dysreflexia. Autonomic dysreflexia is considered a medical emergency and requires immediate attention to remove the noxious stimuli and lower the blood pressure or the patient will be at risk for subarachnoid hemorrhage. Other findings that require management include sexual dysfunction, respiratory complications, and pain management (neurogenic, central cord, peripheral nerve or musculoskeletal pain).

## Management

### What is the most effective management of this patient?

Medical management of a SCI injury has both an acute and rehabilitation phase. The acute phase begins at injury and includes medically stabilizing the patient. Pharmacological intervention is started immediately using methylprednisolone (corticosteroid), lipid peroxidation inhibitors, and drugs that block opiate receptors. These drugs appear to control the amount of secondary damage and improve neurological outcome. Once a patient is medically stable, inpatient rehabilitation, which is typically six to eight weeks, should initially focus on range of motion, positioning in bed, and respiratory management such as cough, clearance of secretions, bronchial drainage, and incentive spirometry. Compensatory techniques, strengthening, muscle substitution, the use of momentum, and the head-hips relationship should be utilized during all activities. Ongoing intervention should include mat and endurance activities, pressure relief training, wheelchair skills, self-range of motion, transfer skills, and community reintegration.

### What home care regimen should be recommended?

A home care regimen should include breathing exercises, incentive spirometry, stretching, and mobility skills. Physical therapy intervention may be indicated for continuation of community skills and furthering the patient's independence within the boundaries of the physical limitations.

## Outcome

### What is the likely outcome of a course in physical therapy?

A patient diagnosed with C7 tetraplegia will require extensive physical therapy with projected outcomes based upon the C7 level of motor and sensory innervation. Typical outcomes at this level include independence with feeding, grooming, and dressing, self-range of motion, independent manual wheelchair mobility, independent transfers, and independent driving with an adapted automobile. Independent living with adaptive equipment is possible.

## What are the long-term effects of the patient's condition?

At this time there is no cure for a complete spinal cord injury, therefore a patient with a complete C7 injury will not regain innervation below this level. The triceps, extensor pollicis longus and brevis, extrinsic finger extensors, and flexor carpi radialis will remain the lowest innervated muscles. There will be ongoing musculoskeletal and cardiopulmonary deficits that can increase the risk for other health issues. The latest research suggests, however, that approximately 40% of the spinal cord injured population have a life expectancy over 45 years of age.

## Comparison

### What are the distinguishing characteristics of a similar condition?

Brown-Sequard's syndrome is a condition that results from injury to one side of the spinal cord. Motor function, proprioception, and vibration are lost ipsilateral to the lesion and vibration, pain, and temperature are absent contralateral to the lesion.

## Clinical Scenarios

### Scenario One

A patient is diagnosed with T12 paraplegia after a motor vehicle accident. Neurological examination reveals no active movement or sensation below T12. The patient is a chemistry teacher and coaches basketball. He is otherwise in good health.

### Scenario Two

A 25-year-old male was injured when he was hit from behind. The blow produced cervical hyperextension and bleeding within the central gray matter of the spinal cord. The patient was diagnosed with central cord syndrome and referred to physical therapy. The patient resides alone in a second floor apartment and is a full-time graduate student.

# Spinal Cord Injury – Complete L3 Paraplegia

## Diagnosis

### What condition produces a patient's symptoms?

The majority of traumatic spinal cord injuries result from compression, flexion or extension of the spine with or without rotation. Spinal cord injuries are classified as a concussion, contusion or laceration, and injury results in primary and secondary neural destruction. Traumatic injury to the spinal cord produces a physiological and biochemical chain of events that results in vascular impairment and permanent tissue and nerve damage.

### An injury was most likely sustained to which structure?

The forces responsible for spinal fractures are compression, flexion, extension, rotation, shear or distraction forces or a combination of these. A patient sustains primary damage to the spinal cord and surrounding tissues at the L3 level through the disruption of the membrane, displacement or compression of the spinal cord, and subsequent hemorrhage and vascular damage. Secondary damage occurs beyond the level of injury due to biochemicals that are released as a result of the initial damage. This process destroys adjacent cells and neural tracts due to the acute inflammation that can last for days or even weeks. After a complete injury at this level, L3 is the most distal segment of the spinal cord that both the motor and sensory components remain intact.

## Inference

### What is the most likely contributing factor in the development of this condition?

There is an estimated 190,000 to 230,000 persons living with SCI within the United States. Statistics from the National Spinal Cord Injury Database (NSCID) indicate that motor vehicle accidents, violence, and falls are the top causes of traumatic spinal cord injury. Statistics also indicate a higher ratio of injury in men (approximately 80%) and Caucasians. The highest incidence of age of injury (over 50%) occurs between 15 to 30 years of age. It is also reported that 40% of spinal injuries are caused by motor vehicle accidents.

## Confirmation

### What is the most likely clinical presentation?

Spinal shock occurs immediately after the injury and can last for days. Surgical intervention may be required for stabilization of the spine. The patient is usually required to wear a spinal orthosis to maintain stability. As spinal shock subsides, a patient will experience an increase in muscle tone below the level of lesion and neurologic reflexes reappear. Spasticity will evolve and may become problematic. Patients specifically with a complete lesion at the L3 level typically have at least partial innervation of the gracilis, iliopsoas, quadratus lumborum, rectus femoris, and sartorius. Patients have full use of their upper extremities and have hip flexion, adduction, and knee extension.

### What laboratory or imaging studies would confirm the diagnosis?

The evaluation of a patient with an acute lumbar spine fracture should include routine laboratory tests, such as CBC, and electrolytes. X-rays, CT scan, and MRI allows for bony and ligamentous injury diagnosis.

### What additional information should be obtained to confirm the diagnosis?

A detailed neurological evaluation should include evaluation of sensory level, posterior column function, normal and abnormal reflexes, and examination of rectal tone and perianal sensation. The cutaneous abdominal reflex, bulbocavernosus reflex, and the presence of the Babinski sign also should be examined.

## Examination

### What history should be documented?

Important areas to explore include past medical history, medications, mechanism of injury, precautions, current health status, nutritional status, social history, living environment occupation, and social support system.

### What test/measures are most appropriate?

**Aerobic capacity and endurance:** autonomic responses to positional changes, vital signs at rest/activity

**Arousal, attention, and cognition:** examine mental status, memory, motivation, level of consciousness

**Assistive and adaptive devices:** analysis of components and safety of a device, wheelchair prescription, adaptive devices, environmental controls

**Community and work integration:** analysis of community, work, and leisure activities

**Environmental, home, and work barriers:** analysis of current and potential barriers or hazards

**Gait, locomotion, and balance:** static and dynamic balance in sitting, analysis of wheelchair management

**Integumentary integrity:** skin assessment, American Spinal Injury Association (ASIA) – Standard Neurological Classification of Spinal Cord Injury Sensory Examination

**Motor function:** equilibrium and righting reactions, posture and balance in sitting

**Muscle performance:** ASIA – Standard Neurological Classification of Spinal Cord Injury Motor Examination, muscle tone assessment

**Neuromotor development and sensory integration:** analysis of reflex movement patterns

**Orthotic, protective, and supportive devices:** analysis of components of a device and movement with a device

**Pain:** dysesthetic pain (deafferentation pain), nerve root pain, musculoskeletal pain

## Spinal Cord Injury – Complete L3 Paraplegia

**Range of motion:** active and passive range of motion
**Reflex integrity:** assessment of deep tendon and pathological reflexes
**Self-care and home management:** assessment of functional capacity, Functional Independence Measure
**Sensory integrity:** proprioception and kinesthesia

### What additional findings are likely with this patient?

There are many additional findings that can exist with a L3 injury including sexual dysfunction, a nonreflexive bladder, and the need for a bowel program. These patients usually present with flaccid paralysis below the level of lesion and are at risk for pain, urinary tract infections, muscle contractures, and pressure sores.

## Management

### What is the most effective management of this patient?

Medical emergency management of a patient with a L3 SCI is initiated by stabilization of the patient's airway in order to secure adequate oxygenation. As soon as the patient is stabilized all patients with spinal cord injuries should immediately receive intravenous methylprednisolone since it has proven to control the amount of secondary damage and improve the neurological outcome. The patient may be placed in a thoracolumbar orthosis (TLSO) with restriction of activities or undergo stabilization surgery followed by the use of a TLSO. Once the patient's spine is stable, rehabilitation should be initiated on an inpatient basis for approximately four to eight weeks. Rehabilitation management may include physical, occupational, vocational therapies, physiatry, nutritional consult, counseling services, and case management. Physical therapy should initially focus on mobility including transfers, bed mobility, and wheelchair mobility. Range of motion and selective strengthening programs, endurance activities, and balance activities should be performed on an ongoing basis in order to optimize functional outcomes. Orthotic prescription (KAFOs or AFOs) is recommended once the patient has gained strength to assist with ambulation using crutches. Community reintegration must be a component of the overall rehabilitation program.

### What home care regimen should be recommended?

A home care regimen for a patient with L3 SCI should include continued selective strengthening, selective stretching, endurance activities, balance and postural control training, and continued use of all orthotics and assistive/adaptive devices. The patient must continue with a home program in order to attain and maintain the highest level of functioning and endurance.

## Outcome

### What is the likely outcome of a course in physical therapy?

A patient with L3 SCI will usually participate in four to eight weeks of inpatient rehabilitation immediately after injury and stabilization. The patient should be able to function independently from a wheelchair level and ambulation level. Outcome is based on the degree of injury, the patient's mental capacity, outside support, emotional stability, motivation, and co-morbidities.

### What are the long-term effects of the patient's condition?

There are approximately 12,000 persons that sustain a spinal cord injury each year and nearly 5,000 of these cases are diagnosed with paraplegia. Patients with SCI are always at a greater risk for osteoporosis, pressure ulcers, hypertension, and heterotopic ossification. The leading cause of death at present is pneumonia, followed by nonischemic heart disease and sepsis. Patients with L3 paraplegia should be able to live independently with education regarding the management of their disability.

## Comparison

### What are the distinguishing characteristics of a similar condition?

There are various outcomes from spinal cord injuries that occur in the lumbosacral region. Fractures of the thoracolumbar junction can produce a mixture of cord and root syndromes caused by lesions of the conus medullaris and lumbar nerve roots. Complete damage of the conus medullaris presents with no motor function or sensation below L1. Patients with complete damage to the sacral portion of the cord have no control of bowel and bladder function and sacral motor paralysis.

## Clinical Scenarios

### Scenario One

A 16-year-old male involved in a MVA sustained a complete L4 injury that required surgery to stabilize his spine. He has just been transferred to rehabilitation and has a TLSO for support. His parents are divorced and he lives between their two homes.

### Scenario Two

A 23-year-old male sustained a conus medullaris injury in a MVA. He was admitted to the acute care hospital and has been having complications regulating his blood glucose level. The patient was diagnosed with type 1 diabetes mellitus when he was seven years old. The patient resides in a two-story condominium.

# Spondylolisthesis

## Diagnosis

### What condition produces a patient's symptoms?

Spondylolisthesis is a descriptive term referring to forward slippage of one vertebral body with respect to the vertebral body below it. The patient's symptoms will vary based on the type and degree of the slippage.

### An injury was most likely sustained to which structure?

Spondylolisthesis may not produce collateral injury to other structures, but in many cases there can be symptoms that range from localized or radiating pain to significant nerve compression, radiculopathy or neurogenic claudication.

## Inference

### What is the most likely contributing factor in the development of this condition?

Spondylolysis is a term used to describe a defect in the pars interarticularis that may produce the forward slippage of a vertebrae as found with spondylolisthesis. There are several etiologies (all are multifactorial) that can produce a spondylolisthesis. All categories ultimately lead to a loss in stability of the locking mechanism of the articular processes with subsequent slippage. The etiologies can be classified as congenital (a defect at birth in the upper sacrum or sacral facet joints); isthmic (results from a defect in the pars interarticularis which allows for increased stress and subsequent fracture); degenerative (usually found later in life as a result of degenerative changes primarily through facet arthropathy or discopathy); traumatic (can occur at any age from acute fracture of the pars or facets that results in listhesis); and pathologic (results secondary to bone disease that compromises the joint). High risk activities include gymnastics, wrestling, football, and weight lifting.

## Confirmation

### What is the most likely clinical presentation?

The presentation of spondylolisthesis is dependent on the causative factors and age of the patient. Pain is the most common symptom of spondylolysis and spondylolisthesis. Pain may originate in the area of lysis or may arise from other structures that have been affected by secondary changes of lysis or spondylolisthesis. These include degenerative changes in the disk, facet arthropathy, and ligamentous sprain or strain. If the patient is young, pain is usually confined to the area of slippage and may occasionally radiate. Progression involves neurological, motor, sensory and reflex changes. Pain is usually provoked with activity especially when it involves extension of the spine. The patient may also present with a palpable step-off over the spine, hamstrings tightness, lumbar spasm, trunk shortening, and gait abnormalities due to a shortened stride length. The most common location of isthmic spondylolisthesis is at L5-S1, while degenerative spondylolisthesis most commonly occurs at L4-L5.

### What laboratory or imaging studies would confirm the diagnosis?

Lateral and anteroposterior plain x-rays of the lumbar spine should be obtained. The oblique view can show the pars as having the appearance of a "Scottie dog with a collar" when a spondylolysis is present. Other studies may include a bone scan, CT scan and myelogram. Laboratory studies will not assist with diagnosis.

### What additional information should be obtained to confirm the diagnosis?

Once a spondylolisthesis is diagnosed, it should also be graded. Meyerding's scale is used frequently and measures the degree of slippage as Grade 1 through 5. The slippage is measured as the percentage of distance that the vertebral body has moved anteriorly over the superior end plate of the vertebral body below it. Grade 1=1-25%; grade 2= 26-50%; grade 3= 51-75%; grade 4= 76-100%; and grade 5= greater than 100%.

## Examination

### What history should be documented?

Important areas to explore include past medical history, medications, current health status, history of illness, nutritional status, social history and habits, occupation, living environment, and social support system.

### What test/measures are most appropriate?

**Assistive and adaptive devices:** analysis of components and safety of a device
**Community and work integration:** analysis of community, work, and leisure activities
**Cranial nerve integrity:** dermatome assessment, assessment of muscle innervation by the cranial nerves
**Environmental, home, and work barriers:** analysis of current and potential barriers or hazards
**Ergonomics and body mechanics:** analysis of dexterity and coordination
**Gait, locomotion, and balance:** static and dynamic balance in sitting and standing, safety during gait with/without an assistive device
**Integumentary integrity:** assessment of sensation
**Joint integrity and mobility:** assessment of hypermobility and hypomobility of a joint, assessment of sprain
**Muscle performance:** strength assessment, muscle tone assessment
**Orthotic, protective, and supportive devices:** analysis of components of a device, analysis of movement while wearing a device
**Pain:** pain perception assessment scale, visual analogue scale, assessment of muscle soreness
**Posture:** analysis of resting and dynamic posture
**Range of motion:** active and passive range of motion
**Reflex integrity:** assessment of deep tendon reflexes
**Self-care and home management:** assessment of functional capacity, Functional Independence Measure

# Spondylolisthesis

## What additional findings are likely with this patient?

Spondylolysis has a 2:1 male-to-female predominance compared to all forms of spondylolisthesis, which indicate a female-to-male predominance of 2:1 (congenital) and 5:1 (degenerative). Overall, females tend to be more prone to progressive spondylolisthesis and require surgery more often than males. Most patients are diagnosed with isthmic type by the age of 15 with a significant increase in symptoms during puberty whereas patients diagnosed with degenerative type are usually over 40 when diagnosed.

## Management

### What is the most effective management of this patient?

Patients with spondylolisthesis are initially treated conservatively regardless of the type or causative factors. Medical management may initially include rest if the spondylolisthesis is acute in nature. Pharmacological intervention may include NSAIDs, acetaminophen, hydrocodone, and/or vicodin. Steroid injections may be used to assist with radicular pain or neurogenic claudication. Physical therapy is indicated with emphasis on activity modification, patient education regarding disease process, bracing, and therapeutic stretching and strengthening. Exercise protocols should include exercise and activity that reduces stress with spinal extension. Bracing (typically a thoracolumbosacral spinal orthosis) may be prescribed to increase spinal stability and reduce symptoms. Conservative treatment is very successful especially with the younger patient, however, surgery may be indicated for unsuccessful patients or patients that present with neurological deficits secondary to the spondylolisthesis. Goals of surgery would include decompression of neural impingement and stabilization of the unstable segments of the spinal cord.

### What home care regimen should be recommended?

A home care regimen should include a stretching program, posture exercises, and compliance with a wearing schedule if bracing is indicated.

## Outcome

### What is the likely outcome of a course in physical therapy?

Physical therapy can play a vital role in the rehabilitation process, however, outcome is also based on the type and amount of slippage present, age, and comorbidities. Generally, the higher the grade of the slippage, the more variable the outcome becomes.

## What are the long-term effects of the patient's condition?

Spondylolisthesis can be asymptomatic or can cause significant neurological deficits due to compression of the neural components surrounding the slippage. Conservative management is effective for many people, especially those with an isthmic type of spondylolisthesis. The degenerative type may continue with some persistent low back pain. Surgical intervention is warranted for patients with significant pain, failed conservative treatment, and/or neurological involvement. Surgery provides most patients with a relief of symptoms and improvement in function.

## Comparison

### What are the distinguishing characteristics of a similar condition?

Retrolisthesis is a slippage in the posterior direction (opposite of anterolisthesis) or the relative posterior displacement of a vertebra on the one below it that usually results from degenerative factors. Initially treatment incorporates activity modification and pharmacological intervention for pain control. If the pain worsens or a progressive neurologic deficit develops despite treatment, surgery may be indicated.

## Clinical Scenarios

### Scenario One

A 14-year-old gymnast is seen in physical therapy shortly after she was diagnosed with a grade 2 spondylolisthesis. She is highly motivated to return to her physical activity, but has pain in the low back that will frequently go down her leg. She resides with her parents and younger sister in a two-story home.

### Scenario Two

A 50-year-old male that works construction is seen in physical therapy after two months on medical leave for back pain. The patient just underwent surgical fusion of L4-L5 due to degenerative spondylolisthesis. He needs to work to provide for his family and wants to get back to his activity as soon as possible. He still complains of back pain and has some residual neurological deficits. He resides in a three-story townhouse with his wife and four children.

# Systemic Lupus Erythematosus

## Diagnosis

### What condition produces a patient's symptoms?

Systemic lupus erythematosus (SLE) is a connective tissue disorder caused by an autoimmune reaction in the body. The primary manifestation of the condition is the production of destructive antibodies that are directed at the individual's own body. The chronic inflammatory disorder produces a variety of symptoms depending on the severity and extent of involvement.

### An injury was most likely sustained to which structure?

SLE is an autoimmune disorder that creates high levels of autoantibodies (antinuclear antibodies) that attack various cells and tissues within the body. The autoantibodies form immune complexes that produce an inflammatory response and cause further tissue destruction. Proliferation of immune complexes precipitates inflammation responses that in turn destroy cells, tissues, and organs. Specific injury is organ or system dependent depending on which areas of the body are affected by SLE.

## Inference

### What is the most likely contributing factor in the development of this condition?

The exact etiology of SLE is unknown, however, it is described as an immunoregulatory disturbance from genetic, environmental, viral, and hormonal contributing factors. Environmental factors associated with SLE include ultraviolet light exposure, infection, antibiotics (specifically penicillin and sulfa drugs), extreme stress, immunization, and pregnancy. SLE can occur at any age, but the most common age group is 15 to 40 years of age. The disorder is 10-15 times more common in women.

## Confirmation

### What is the most likely clinical presentation?

There are an estimated 1.4 million individuals diagnosed with SLE in the United States. A patient with SLE will have diverse symptoms based on the involvement of the connective tissue throughout the body. Symptoms will appear with exacerbations and disappear with remissions throughout the course of the disease. Symptoms such as arthralgias, malaise, and fatigue may persist even during a remission period. A patient may initially see a physician for symptoms that include fever, malaise, rash, arthralgias, headache, and weight loss. Common clinical presentation throughout the course of SLE includes a red butterfly rash across the cheeks and nose, a red rash over light exposed areas, arthralgias, alopecia, pleurisy, kidney involvement, seizures, depression, fibromyalgia, and cardiac involvement. SLE can affect the skin, joints, kidneys, lungs, heart, and other organs and tissues within the body. Patients can also have CNS involvement that can lead to

neuropsychiatric manifestations that present with depression, irritability, emotional instability, and seizures.

### What laboratory or imaging studies would confirm the diagnosis?

Microscopic fluorescent techniques are indicated to detect the presence of the antinuclear antibody (ANA) within the blood. A positive ANA test warrants an additional test for antideoxyribonucleic acid antibodies. These two tests in combination with the physical presentation support the presence of SLE. Other testing including erythrocyte sedimentation rate, complete blood count, and urinalysis.

### What additional information should be obtained to confirm the diagnosis?

The American Rheumatism Association has designated criteria to confirm the diagnosis of SLE. A patient requires at least four of fourteen characteristics that occur during the same period of time. A patient evaluation including a thorough history and current symptoms assists with confirming a diagnosis of SLE.

## Examination

### What history should be documented?

Important areas to explore include past medical and family history, medications, current symptoms and health status, living environment, social history and habits, occupation, and social support system.

### What test/measures are most appropriate?

**Aerobic capacity and endurance:** assessment of vital signs at rest/activity, auscultation of the lungs/heart

**Arousal, attention, and cognition:** examine mental status, learning ability, memory, motivation

**Assistive and adaptive devices:** analysis of components and safety of a device

**Community and work integration:** analysis of community, work, and leisure activities

**Environmental, home, and work barriers:** analysis of current and potential barriers or hazards

**Ergonomics and body mechanics:** analysis of dexterity and coordination

**Gait, locomotion, and balance:** static/dynamic balance in sitting and standing, safety during gait, Tinetti Performance Oriented Mobility Assessment, Berg Balance Scale, Functional Ambulation Profile

**Integumentary integrity:** skin assessment, assessment of sensation, presence and assessment of rash

**Joint integrity and mobility:** soft tissue swelling and inflammation, presence of deformity

**Motor function:** posture and balance

**Muscle performance:** strength assessment

**Neuromotor development and sensory integration:** analysis of reflex movement patterns, sensory integration tests, gross and fine motor skills

# Systemic Lupus Erythematosus

**Orthotic, protective, and supportive devices:** potential utilization of bracing
**Pain:** pain perception assessment scale
**Range of motion:** active and passive range of motion
**Self-care and home management:** assessment of functional capacity

## What additional findings are likely with this patient?

SLE can produce skeletal deformities such as ulnar deviation and subluxed interphalangeal joints. Kidney involvement and cardiovascular impairments such as endocarditis, myocarditis, and pericarditis can occur during an exacerbation. Patients that experience nephritis, myocarditis or neurological implications have a poor prognosis. Modifiable risk factors for exacerbation include high stress, limited emotional and social support, and psychological distress.

## Management

### What is the most effective management of this patient?

Medical management of SLE focuses on reversing the autoimmune response in order to avoid complications and exacerbations of symptoms. Pharmacological intervention for a patient with mild SLE will include salicylates, Indomethacin or NSAIDs. Antimalarial medications, corticosteroids, and immunosuppressive therapy may be used. General management of SLE includes good nutrition, ongoing medical supervision, and avoidance of ultraviolet exposure. Physical therapy intervention is usually indicated after a period of exacerbation and includes a slow resumption of physical activity, energy conservation techniques, gradual endurance activities and significant patient education regarding skin care, pacing, exercise, and strengthening to tolerance.

### What home care regimen should be recommended?

A home care regimen during an acute exacerbation of SLE should include relaxation and energy conservation techniques, stress reduction strategies, therapeutic exercise as tolerated, and pain management.

## Outcome

### What is the likely outcome of a course in physical therapy?

Physical therapy cannot cease or alter the clinical course of SLE, however, it may assist in controlling the debilitating effects during an acute phase/exacerbation of the disease. Goals include focus on pain relief, relaxation, strengthening, and preventing deformity.

## What are the long-term effects of the patient's condition?

The clinical course of SLE is highly unpredictable. A patient may only exhibit symptoms for skin and joint involvement or may exhibit multi-system involvement. Periods of remission may last years and the prognosis depends on the severity and the extent of the disease process. The overall prognosis for SLE is good, although in rare cases the disease process can remain acute and become fatal within a short period of time. There is a high ten-year survival rate with SLE. Death is usually attributed to kidney failure or secondary infections.

## Comparison

### What are the distinguishing characteristics of a similar condition?

Scleroderma, also termed progressive systemic sclerosis, is a chronic disease that primarily affects the skin, but can involve articular structures and internal organs. There is long-term hardening and shrinking of the affected connective tissues. The two subtypes of this disease are systemic scleroderma and localized scleroderma. Etiology is unknown and the disease varies in course (months, years or a lifetime) and progression.

## Clinical Scenarios

### Scenario One

A 25-year-old female is referred to physical therapy for a therapeutic exercise program. The patient was diagnosed last year with SLE and has not exercised since that time. The patient is currently taking corticosteroids and antimalarial medications to manage a recent exacerbation.

### Scenario Two

A 43-year-old female was seen in outpatient physical therapy to assist with pain management. The patient was diagnosed five years ago with SLE and has recently experienced increased difficulty using her hands secondary to deformity and pain. The patient's goal is to reduce the pain in her hands.

# Temporomandibular Joint Dysfunction

## Diagnosis

### What condition produces a patient's symptoms?

The temporomandibular joint (TMJ) is a complex joint that is classified as a condylar, hinge, and synovial joint. The TMJ contains fibrocartilaginous surfaces and articular discs. Temporomandibular joint dysfunction (TMD) occurs due to a change in the joint structure that can cause multiple symptoms and a limitation in function. In many instances inflammation and muscle spasm surrounding the joint produces symptoms for the patient with TMD.

### An injury was most likely sustained to which structure?

TMD results from injury, derangement or incongruence of the TMJ itself, intra-articular disks, and/or supporting surrounding structures. Over time the meniscus of the TMJ becomes compressed and torn allowing for the bony portion of the joint (the ball and socket) to deteriorate secondary to the grinding of bone on bone.

## Inference

### What is the most likely contributing factor in the development of this condition?

TMD can be classified by three primary etiological factors: predisposing factors, triggering factors, and perpetuating/sustaining factors. TMD can occur secondary to multiple causative factors including injury or trauma to the joint, congenital abnormalities, internal derangement of joint structure, arthritis, dislocation, disk degeneration, metabolic conditions or stress. Risk factors include chewing on one side, eating tough food, clenching, and grinding of teeth. Habits of gum chewing and nail biting may increase the incidence of injury to the TMJ. Patients are typically between 20 to 40 years of age with a greater incidence in women. Research indicates a possible link between gender-specific hormones and the risk for TMD.

## Confirmation

### What is the most likely clinical presentation?

The National Institute of Dental and Craniofacial Research indicates that approximately 10.8 million individuals have TMD within the United States and 90% of the individuals that are seeking treatment are women in their childbearing years. A patient with TMD will present with symptoms that include pain (persistent or recurring), muscle spasm, abnormal or limited jaw motion, headache, and tinnitus. These symptoms can be unilateral or bilateral. The patient will often complain of feeling and hearing a "clicking or popping" sound with motion at the TMJ. Clinical manifestation of symptoms relates to the actual cause of the TMD.

### What laboratory or imaging studies would confirm the diagnosis?

Procedures used in diagnosing TMD and its origin may include X-ray, MRI, mandibular kinesiography, CT scan, and a dental examination.

### What additional information should be obtained to confirm the diagnosis?

A physical examination, upper quarter screening, TMJ loading, condyle-meniscus relationship, review of symptoms, and past medical history are all important components in the diagnosis of TMD. An occlusion examination may be indicated to evaluate a patient's bite.

## Examination

### What history should be documented?

Important areas to explore include past medical history, medications, family history, current symptoms, current health status, diet, social history and habits, occupation, leisure activities, and social support system.

### What test/measures are most appropriate?

**Arousal, attention, and cognition:** examine mental status, learning ability, memory, motivation

**Community and work integration:** analysis of community, work, and leisure activities

**Cranial nerve integrity:** assessment of muscle innervation by the cranial nerves, dermatome assessment

**Integumentary integrity:** skin assessment, assessment of sensation

**Joint integrity and mobility:** assessment of hypermobility and hypomobility of a joint, soft tissue swelling and inflammation, joint play

**Muscle performance:** strength assessment including mastication, tongue, and lips; upper quarter screening

**Pain:** pain perception assessment scale, visual analogue scale, assessment of muscle soreness

**Posture:** analysis of resting and dynamic posture

**Range of motion:** active and passive range of motion

**Self-care and home management:** assessment of functional capacity

**Ventilation, respiration, and circulation:** breathing patterns, respiratory muscle strength, accessory muscle utilization

# Temporomandibular Joint Dysfunction

## What additional findings are likely with this patient?

TMD produces a general clinical presentation that includes pain, headache, muscle spasms, and tinnitus. Specific findings result from the specific cause of the TMD. Other findings can include popping and clicking when opening the mandible, locking of the TMJ, restriction of movement of the unaffected side, and/or pulling of the mandible towards the affected side. Common underlying causes include arthritis, fracture, congenital abnormalities, dislocations, and tension-relieving habits (chewing gum, bruxism, clenching or grinding the teeth).

## Management

### What is the most effective management of this patient?

Medical management of TMD may include pharmacological intervention, the use of splinting, physical therapy treatment, and possible surgical intervention. Pharmacological treatment of TMD may include analgesics, NSAIDs, muscle relaxants, and antianxiety medications. A patient may also benefit from a splint to assist with realignment of the joint and a guard or bite plate to maintain proper positioning and avoid grinding of the teeth throughout the night. Specific physical therapy intervention is based on the exact etiology of the TMD. Generally, physical therapy intervention includes patient education regarding habits such as nail biting, posture retraining, the use of modalities such as moist heat, ice, biofeedback, ultrasound, electrostimulation, TENS, and massage. Soft tissue manipulation, joint mobilization, ROM, stretching, occlusal appliance prescription, and relaxation techniques are also appropriate. If conservative treatment fails or the exact etiology warrants surgical intervention, (approximately 5% of cases) the patient may require a condylectomy, osteotomy, arthrotomy, arthroscopy, reduction of subluxation or joint debridement.

### What home care regimen should be recommended?

A home care regimen for a patient with TMD should include relaxation techniques, self-stretching, posture retraining exercises, and progressive ROM. A patient should avoid all foods and activities (such as gum chewing) that aggravate and stress the TMJ. The patient should continue with the proper use of an occlusal appliance if indicated. In order to maintain progress the patient must have ongoing consistency with the home program.

## Outcome

### What is the likely outcome of a course in physical therapy?

Physical therapy intervention should improve a patient's condition and decrease the symptoms of the TMD. Physical therapy is usually conducted on an outpatient basis with focus on maximizing function and alleviating pain.

## What are the long-term effects of the patient's condition?

A patient previously diagnosed with TMD is at an increased risk of recurrence, however, with successful management, ongoing compliance with the home program, and use of an indicated appliance, the patient may not have any long-term effects. If conservative management fails the patient may require surgical intervention for the underlying cause in order to alleviate the TMD.

## Comparison

### What are the distinguishing characteristics of a similar condition?

Myofascial pain dysfunction (MPD) syndrome is a nonarticular disorder that affects the area surrounding the TMJ, however, symptoms are produced secondary to muscle spasm. MPD occurs more in females and can be of psychophysiologic origin. Habits such as grinding and jaw clenching increase tension in the muscles of mastication and create spasm. MPD can mimic the symptoms of TMD, however, differential diagnosis will rule out true TMJ involvement.

## Clinical Scenarios

### Scenario One

A 12-year-old female is referred to physical therapy with a diagnosis of TMD secondary to condylar hyperplasia. The patient required a condylectomy with post-operative orders for physical therapy. The female is motivated and she has very supportive parents.

### Scenario Two

A 30-year-old male is referred to physical therapy with a diagnosis of TMD. The physician referral notes inflammation, muscle spasm, and poor posture. The patient states that he will feel clicking when he eats certain foods. The patient has a history of childhood scoliosis that was controlled with exercise and short-term bracing. The patient is a stockbroker and spends a great deal of time talking on the phone.

# Thoracic Outlet Syndrome

## Diagnosis

### What condition produces a patient's symptoms?

Thoracic outlet syndrome is a term used to describe a group of disorders that presents with symptoms secondary to neurovascular compression of fibers of the brachial plexus. This usually occurs between the points of the interscalene triangle and the inferior border of the axilla. Compression of the nerves and blood supply can also occur as they pass over the first rib.

### An injury was most likely sustained to which structure?

Thoracic outlet syndrome results from compression and damage to the brachial plexus nerve trunks, subclavian vascular supply, and/or the axillary artery. Nerve injury can result in neurapraxia with segmental degeneration and progress to axonotmesis due to continued and unrelieved compression.

## Inference

### What is the most likely contributing factor in the development of this condition?

Contributing factors in the development of thoracic outlet syndrome include the presence of a cervical rib, an abnormal first rib, postural deviations or changes, body composition, chronic hyperabduction of the arm, hypertrophy or spasms of the scalene muscles, degenerative disorders, and an elongated cervical transverse process.

## Confirmation

### What is the most likely clinical presentation?

A patient with thoracic outlet syndrome will present with symptoms based on nerve and/or vascular compression. Typical symptoms include diffuse pain in the arm most often at night, paresthesias in the fingers and through the upper extremities, weakness and muscle wasting, poor posture, edema, and discoloration. If the upper plexus is involved, pain will be reported in the neck that may radiate to the face and may follow the lateral aspect of the forearm into the hand. If the lower plexus is involved, pain is reported in the back of the neck and shoulder, which will radiate over the ulnar distribution to the hand. A patient's symptoms are usually enhanced with behaviors that aggravate the symptoms such as poor posture, lifting activities, and movements overhead.

### What laboratory or imaging studies would confirm the diagnosis?

X-ray will confirm the presence of a cervical rib or other bony abnormality. Nerve conduction velocity testing may be valuable if a neuropathy exists. Otherwise, diagnosis relies solely on a thorough history of patient symptoms, provocative testing, and a physical examination. Other testing should be used for differential diagnosis to rule out cervical radiculopathy, RSD, myofascial pain syndrome, tumor, carpal tunnel syndrome, brachial plexus injury, ulnar never compression, and angina.

### What additional information should be obtained to confirm the diagnosis?

A patient can be diagnosed with thoracic outlet syndrome following a thorough history of symptoms, physical examination, and provocative testing that includes Adson maneuver, Wright test, Roo's test, Halstead maneuver, Allen test, and the costoclavicular and hyperabduction tests.

## Examination

### What history should be documented?

Important areas to explore include past medical history, family history, medications, history of symptoms, current health status, living environment, social history and habits, occupation, and social support system.

### What test/measures are most appropriate?

**Anthropometric characteristics:** upper extremity circumferential measurements
**Arousal, attention, and cognition:** examine mental status, learning ability, memory, motivation
**Community and work integration:** analysis of community, work, and leisure activities
**Cranial nerve integrity:** assessment of muscles innervation by the cranial nerves, dermatome assessment
**Environmental, home, and work barriers:** analysis of current and potential barriers or hazards
**Ergonomics and body mechanics:** analysis of dexterity and coordination
**Integumentary integrity:** skin assessment, assessment of sensation
**Joint integrity and mobility:** soft tissue swelling and inflammation, assessment of joint play, palpation of the joint
**Motor function:** posture and balance; upper quarter screening
**Muscle performance:** strength assessment
**Pain:** pain perception assessment scale, assessment of interscalene triangle point tenderness
**Posture:** analysis of resting and dynamic posture
**Range of motion:** active and passive range of motion
**Reflex integrity:** assessment of deep tendon and pathological reflexes (e.g., Babinski, ATNR)
**Self-care and home management:** assessment of functional capacity

# Thoracic Outlet Syndrome

## What additional findings are likely with this patient?

A patient with thoracic outlet syndrome may have difficulty sleeping due to excessive pillows or malpositioning of the arm. The patient may have difficulty at work with carrying items on the affected side or with driving a car. Thoracic outlet most commonly affects the population between 30 and 40 years of age with women being affected two to three times more than men.

## Management

### What is the most effective management of this patient?

Initial medical management of thoracic outlet syndrome takes a conservative approach. If conservative management fails, it is followed by surgical intervention. A patient with thoracic outlet syndrome requires physical therapy intervention to assist with modification of posture, breathing patterns, positioning in bed and at the work site, and gentle stretching. Physical therapy should focus on pain management, strengthening (especially the trapezius, levator scapulae, and rhomboids), joint mobilization, body mechanics, flexibility, and postural awareness. A therapist may utilize modalities such as transcutaneous nerve stimulation, ultrasound, and biofeedback to attain goals. Work site analysis and subsequent activity modification may be necessary to relieve the pain and other symptoms. A patient may benefit from anti-inflammatory agents in combination with physical therapy. If physical therapy management fails, the patient may require surgical decompression of bony or fibrotic abnormalities. The exact type of surgical intervention and approach is chosen by the surgeon based on symptoms and current damage.

### What home care regimen should be recommended?

A home care regimen for a patient with thoracic outlet syndrome should include stretching, strengthening, and postural awareness. The patient should utilize these strategies on an ongoing basis at work and with recreational activities in order to promote pain free movement and limit undesirable symptoms associated with the condition.

## Outcome

### What is the likely outcome of a course in physical therapy?

Most patients with thoracic outlet syndrome have positive results from physical therapy intervention and are able to return to their previous level of function within four to eight weeks.

## What are the long-term effects of the patient's condition?

If a patient has positive results from physical therapy intervention, there will not be any long-term impairments, however, if the patient's symptoms persist for three to four months, surgical intervention may be warranted. Approximately 75% of patients post surgery have a positive response, however, complications from surgery can include winging of the scapula, pneumothorax, and nerve compression. Research indicates no significant long-term difference between surgical resection of the first rib and successful conservative management.

## Comparison

### What are the distinguishing characteristics of a similar condition?

A radial nerve lesion may be caused by direct trauma, excessive traction, entrapment or compression. A patient presents with an inability to extend the wrist, thumb, and fingers. The patient will also present with impaired grip strength and coordination. Splinting is recommended to maintain proper positioning. Passive range of motion is necessary to prevent secondary impairments such as contractures within the hand.

## Clinical Scenarios

### Scenario One

A 35-year-old female is seen in physical therapy secondary to pain and paresthesias throughout the left upper extremity. The patient's work history reveals that she is employed as a telemarketer and is required to hold the phone between her ear and shoulder throughout her shift. The patient carries a five-pound brief case with a shoulder strap as she walks one-half mile to work. The patient has a one-year-old child.

### Scenario Two

A 45-year-old female is referred to physical therapy secondary to pain when reaching overhead and carrying objects. The patient recently complains of waking up during the night with pain and paresthesias in the involved arm. The patient is very anxious and concerned because she is required to carry items and place them above her head as part of her job at a local production mill.

# Total Hip Arthroplasty

## Diagnosis

### What condition produces a patient's symptoms?

A total hip arthroplasty (THA) may be warranted secondary to progressive and severe osteoarthritis or rheumatoid arthritis in the hip joint, developmental dysplasia of the hip, tumors, failed reconstruction of the hip or other hip conditions that produce incapacitating pain and disability. A THA may also be required secondary to trauma, avascular necrosis or a nonunion fracture.

### An injury was most likely sustained to which structure?

Arthritis causes the hip joint to undergo a degenerative process including destruction of articular cartilage that results in bone-to-bone contact. Degenerative changes are usually apparent in both the acetabulum and the femoral head requiring a THA, however, if the acetabulum does not exhibit degenerative changes then only the femoral head will be replaced in a hemiarthroplasty procedure.

## Inference

### What is the most likely contributing factor in the development of this condition?

Intra-articular disease or the destruction of articular cartilage may come from arthritis, repetitive microtrauma, obesity, nutritional imbalances, falls or abnormal joint mechanics. Indications for THA include osteoarthritis, rheumatoid arthritis, avascular necrosis, developmental dysplasia, osteomyelitis, failed fixation of a fracture, ankylosing spondylitis, and failed conservative management.

## Confirmation

### What is the most likely clinical presentation?

A patient that requires a THA will present with decreased range of motion, impaired mobility skills, and persistent pain that increases with motion and weight bearing. The patient is usually over 55 years of age and has experienced consistent pain that is not relieved through conservative measures and limits the patient's functional mobility on a consistent basis.

### What laboratory or imaging studies would confirm the diagnosis?

X-ray, computed tomography, and magnetic resonance imaging procedures may be used to view the integrity of the joint. These procedures are also used to rule out a fracture or a tumor.

## What additional information should be obtained to confirm the diagnosis?

Patient history, current functional status, and level of pain and disability are important factors in determining the need for surgical intervention. A standardized pain assessment scale and the Arthritis Impact Measurement tool may be used to establish an objective baseline. Relative or absolute contraindications must be considered prior to the recommendation for a THA. Contraindications may include but are not limited to active infection, severe obesity, arterial insufficiency, neuromuscular disease, and certain mental illness.

## Examination

### What history should be documented?

Important areas to explore include past medical history, family history, medications, current symptoms, current health status, living environment, social history and habits, occupation, and social support system.

### What test/measures are most appropriate?

**Aerobic capacity and endurance:** assessment of vital signs at rest and with activity, perceived exertion scale

**Anthropometric characteristics:** hip circumferential measurements, leg length measurements

**Arousal, attention, and cognition:** examine mental status, learning ability, memory, motivation

**Assistive and adaptive devices:** analysis of components and safety of a device

**Environmental, home, and work barriers:** analysis of current and potential barriers or hazards

**Gait, locomotion, and balance:** safety during gait with/without an assistive device, Functional Ambulation Profile

**Joint integrity and mobility:** soft tissue swelling and inflammation

**Muscle performance:** strength assessment, assessment of active movement

**Pain:** pain perception assessment scale

**Range of motion:** active and passive range of motion

**Self-care and home assessment:** assessment of functional capacity, Barthel Index

**Sensory integrity:** assessment of sensation

# Total Hip Arthroplasty

## What additional findings are likely with this patient?

A patient that requires a THA may also have arthritis in other areas of the body. The patient may present with low endurance and may be deconditioned secondary to inactivity from the effects of arthritis. Post-surgical complications may include nerve injury, vascular damage, dislocation, pulmonary embolism, myocardial infarction, and CVA. The prosthesis is also at risk for loosening, infection, heterotopic ossification, and fracture.

## Management

### What is the most effective management of this patient?

Medical management includes choosing a surgical approach that meets the patient's needs and level of activity. A THA that utilizes a posterolateral approach allows the abductor muscles to remain intact, however, there may be a higher incidence of post-operative joint instability due to the interruption of the posterior capsule. This type of surgical approach requires a patient to avoid excessive hip flexion greater than 90 degrees, hip adduction, and hip medial rotation. A patient with a THA that utilizes an anterolateral approach should avoid hip flexion and lateral rotation. A direct lateral approach leaves the posterior portion of the gluteus medius attached to the greater trochanter and the posterior capsule left intact. This method is preferred for patients that may be noncompliant in order to avoid posterior dislocation. Pharmacological intervention status post THA will include anticoagulant therapy and pain medication. The patient's post-operative care includes hip precautions, use of an abduction pillow (with posterolateral approach), initiation of hip protocol exercises, and physical therapy intervention. The hip protocol exercises usually include ankle pumps, quadriceps sets, gluteal sets, heel slides, and isometric abduction. Physical therapy should emphasize patient education regarding hip precautions and weight bearing status, scar management, and soft tissue mobilization. At the time of hospital discharge the patient should be able to extend the hip to neutral and flex the hip to 90 degrees. A cemented hip replacement usually allows for partial weight bearing initially and a noncemented hip replacement requires toe touch weight bearing for up to six weeks. Physical therapy encourages early ambulation training in order to avoid deconditioning and the risk of deep vein thrombosis. A patient must practice all mobility skills using the proper hip precautions. Outpatient physical therapy may be indicated to assist with progression to a cane.

### What home care regimen should be recommended?

The patient should be instructed in a home care regimen that includes range of motion, strengthening, and progressive ambulation. The patient must adhere to the hip precaution guidelines for a minimum of three months or until a physician determines that the hip demonstrates adequate stability.

## Outcome

### What is the likely outcome of a course in physical therapy?

A patient status post THA will benefit from physical therapy and should attain an improved functional outcome. The patient should have diminished to no pain, increased strength and endurance, and improved mobility within six to eight weeks after surgery.

### What are the long-term effects of the patient's condition?

A THA is a highly successful surgical procedure. The current lifespan of the prosthesis is less than 20 years and as a result some patients may require a subsequent replacement. Studies indicate pain relief and improved function with good to excellent results in 85-95% of the patients at 15 to 20 years post THA. Validated scoring systems such as the Harris Hip Scoring System or the Special Surgery Rating system are measures used to determine the quality of life after the THA.

## Comparison

### What are the distinguishing characteristics of a similar condition?

A hemiarthroplasty of the hip is a replacement of the femoral head due to a subcapital fracture of the femur or degeneration of the femoral head. This type of surgical intervention is sometimes used as an alternative to a THA for elderly patients that sustain a hip fracture or patients that have a shortened expected lifespan.

## Clinical Scenarios

### Scenario One

A patient is seen in physical therapy after THA surgery. The surgeon performed an anterolateral approach and used a noncemented prosthesis. The patient is mildly obese and has a lengthy cardiac history. The patient has osteoarthritis and had progressive pain and difficulty with mobility prior to surgery. The patient complains of soreness in the hip and is anxious to get home.

### Scenario Two

A 75-year-old male is seen in physical therapy status post reduction of a dislocated right hip prosthesis. The patient had a THA three weeks ago and dislocated the hip two days ago while bending over to tie his shoes. The patient is currently using a walker for mobility and is toe touch weight bearing. The patient resides alone in a garden apartment and does not have any family in the area.

# Total Knee Arthroplasty

## Diagnosis

### What condition produces a patient's symptoms?

A total knee arthroplasty (TKA) may be warranted secondary to progressive and disabling pain within the knee joint. The pain is most often due to severe degenerative osteoarthritic destruction and deformity that can occur within the knee.

### An injury was most likely sustained to which structure?

Arthritis causes the knee joint to undergo a degenerative process that includes destruction of articular cartilage and resultant bone-to-bone contact within the joint. The knee presents with decreased joint space and osteophyte formation. Injury occurs to the femoral condyles, tibial articulating surface, and the dorsal side of the patella.

## Inference

### What is the most likely contributing factor in the development of this condition?

The destruction of articular cartilage secondary to osteoarthritis is the most common indication for a TKA. A patient with a history of participation in high-impact sports or has experienced trauma to the knee is at a higher risk for arthritis and subsequent TKA. Obesity, varus/valgus deformity, previous mechanical derangement, infection, rheumatoid arthritis, hemophilia, crystal deposition diseases, avascular necrosis or bone dysplasia at the knee are some other contributing factors that may warrant a TKA.

## Confirmation

### What is the most likely clinical presentation?

Approximately 130,000 TKAs are performed each year within the United States. A patient that requires a TKA will present with severe knee pain that worsens with motion and weight bearing, impaired range of motion, possible deformity of the knee, and impaired mobility skills. Night pain is common and may include localized or diffuse pain. Other symptoms may include stiffness, swelling, locking, and giving way of the affected knee. Patients often attempt conservative treatment measures to address the condition with only limited success.

### What laboratory or imaging studies would confirm the diagnosis?

X-ray, computed tomography, and magnetic resonance imaging are used to determine the extent of deterioration and bony abnormalities within the knee joint. Radiographic images can be utilized post-operatively to ensure proper fit and obtain baseline information.

### What additional information should be obtained to confirm the diagnosis?

Patient history, current functional status, and level of pain and disability are important factors in determining the need for surgical intervention. A pain assessment scale and the Arthritis Impact Measurement tool may be used to establish an objective baseline.

## Examination

### What history should be documented?

Important areas to explore include past medical history, family history, medications, current symptoms, living environment, social history and habits, occupation, current functional status, and social support system.

### What test/measures are most appropriate?

**Aerobic capacity and endurance:** assessment of vital signs at rest and with activity, perceived exertion scale
**Anthropometric characteristics:** knee circumferential measurements
**Arousal, attention, and cognition:** examine mental status, learning ability, memory, motivation
**Assistive and adaptive devices:** analysis of components and safety of a device
**Environmental, home, and work barriers:** analysis of current and potential barriers or hazards
**Gait, locomotion, and balance:** safety during gait/stairs with device, Functional Ambulation Profile
**Joint integrity and mobility:** soft tissue swelling and inflammation
**Muscle performance:** strength/active movement assessment
**Pain:** pain perception assessment scale
**Range of motion:** active and passive range of motion
**Self-care and home assessment:** assessment of functional capacity, Barthel Index
**Sensory integrity:** assessment of sensation

### What additional findings are likely with this patient?

A patient that requires TKA may have arthritis in other joints, previous replacement surgeries or previous trauma to the knee joint. Patients with significant osteoarthritis and severe pain may exhibit sleep disorders or depression due to the disease process. Relative or absolute contraindications must be considered prior to the recommendation for a TKA. Contraindications may include but are not limited to active infection of the knee, severe obesity, significant genu recurvatum, arterial insufficiency, neuropathic joint, and certain mental illnesses. Post-surgical complications after a TKA include infection, vascular damage, patellofemoral instability, fracture surrounding the prosthesis, pulmonary embolism, nerve damage, loosening of the prosthesis, and arthrofibrosis.

# Total Knee Arthroplasty

## Management

### What is the most effective management of this patient?

Medical management of a patient requiring a TKA includes choosing of the appropriate surgical procedure based on the patient's symptoms and level of activity. Pharmacological intervention status post TKA will require anticoagulant therapy and pain medications. The patient's post-operative care includes a knee immobilizer, elevation of the limb, cryotherapy, intermittent range of motion using a continuous passive motion (CPM) machine, and initiation of knee protocol exercises. A cemented knee prosthesis allows for either partial weight bearing or weight bearing as tolerated post surgery based on the individual physician's discretion. A noncemented knee prosthesis requires toe touch weight bearing for up to six weeks to allow for the bone to grow and affix to the prosthesis. Physical therapy should focus on mobility training with the proper weight bearing status using an appropriate assistive device. Early ambulation training is encouraged in order to avoid deconditioning and the risk of deep vein thrombosis. Physical therapy intervention should emphasize ankle pumps, quad sets, and hamstrings sets as well as range of motion and stretching. A goal of 90 degrees of knee flexion and 0 degrees knee extension is often established prior to discharge from the hospital or rehabilitation facility. The following precautions should be used for several months after surgery to avoid excessive stress to the knee: avoid squatting, avoid quick pivoting, do not use pillows under the knee while in bed, and avoid low seating. Outpatient therapy may be recommended to progress the patient from an assistive device. Once the physician progresses the patient to weight bearing as tolerated, physical therapy intervention should include strengthening with closed-chain exercises and functional activities.

### What home care regimen should be recommended?

A home care regimen would typically include range of motion, strengthening, and progressive ambulation exercises. The patient must adhere to precautions, use of an immobilizer, and proper weight bearing status until a physician determines that the knee joint demonstrates adequate stability.

## Outcome

### What is the likely outcome of a course in physical therapy?

A patient status post TKA will benefit from physical therapy and should attain an improved functional capacity. The patient should experience relief of pain that will allow for a full return to previous functional activities within eight to twelve weeks after surgery depending on a cemented or noncemented prosthesis and potential complications that were encountered.

### What are the long-term effects of the patient's condition?

A TKA is a highly successful surgical procedure that should significantly reduce pain and increase function. After finishing a rehabilitation protocol, a patient may have only minor limitations in knee range of motion. A knee replacement may loosen over time and require revision, however, the life expectancy of the knee prosthesis is between 15 and 20 years.

## Comparison

### What are the distinguishing characteristics of a similar condition?

A patellectomy (surgical removal of the patella) is a surgical procedure that is indicated for a comminuted facture of the patella that cannot be repaired with internal fixation. A patellectomy can include the entire patella or just the inferior or superior pole of the patella. The retinaculum and extensor mechanism are repaired with the surgical procedure and the patient is immobilized for six to eight weeks. Once rehabilitation is initiated the patient starts with range of motion and closed-chain exercises.

## Clinical Scenarios

### Scenario One

An 80-year-old female in an acute care hospital is two days status post left TKA. The patient presents with partial hearing loss and moderate dementia. The patient's past medical history includes a right CVA with no residual impairment and hypertension that is controlled by medication. The patient resides with her sister in a ranch style home with three steps to enter.

### Scenario Two

A 49-year-old male is referred to outpatient physical therapy seven weeks after surgery. The patient received a noncemented knee prosthesis and has recently advanced to weight bearing as tolerated. The patient's range of motion in the involved knee is 10-85 degrees. The patient is otherwise independent with axillary crutches. No significant past medical history is noted.

# Total Shoulder Arthroplasty

## Diagnosis

### What condition produces a patient's symptoms?

A patient that is a candidate for a total shoulder arthroplasty (TSA) will have severe pain and impaired shoulder motion due to deterioration of the glenohumeral joint. These candidates have undergone conservative treatment measures that have failed to improve their condition.

### An injury was most likely sustained to which structure?

TSA candidates will have irreparable damage, deterioration, and destruction to the humeral head and the glenoid fossa within the shoulder complex. The joint surfaces are severely damaged or destroyed by wear and tear, inflammation, injury or previous surgery.

## Inference

### What is the most likely contributing factor in the development of this condition?

Indications for a TSA include severe glenohumeral degenerative joint disease, pain and limited range of motion secondary to osteoarthritis, rheumatoid arthritis, avascular necrosis, fracture or rotator cuff arthropathy. Other patients that may require a TSA would include a patient with a bone tumor, Paget's disease or with recurrent dislocations. A patient will be considered for TSA if conservative treatment of the underlying cause fails.

## Confirmation

### What is the most likely clinical presentation?

A patient will exhibit impaired range of motion at the shoulder, may lack independence with functional mobility and ADLs, and will experience severe pain. It is this unremitting pain (with failed conservative treatment) that is the primary indication for the TSA. A TSA performed secondary to arthritis is usually performed on patients between 55 and 70 years of age while TSA performed secondary to irreparable damage from dislocation or avascular necrosis is usually performed on patients between 40 and 50 years of age.

### What laboratory or imaging studies would confirm the diagnosis?

X-ray will reveal the level of degeneration within the shoulder complex. MRI or CT scan will allow the physician to assess the integrity of the rotator cuff and deltoid muscles surrounding the joint as well as the overall integrity of the shoulder complex.

### What additional information should be obtained to confirm the diagnosis?

A full medical history along with a physical examination is a key component that is required in determining if a patient is a candidate for a TSA. The patient must possess motivation, realistic expectations, and appropriate goals regarding outcome.

## Examination

### What history should be documented?

Important areas to explore include past medical and family history, medication, current symptoms, surgical precautions/contraindications, rehabilitation protocol, social history and habits, occupation, leisure activities, and social support system.

### What test/measures are most appropriate?

**Aerobic capacity and endurance:** assessment of vital signs at rest and with activity

**Anthropometric characteristics:** circumferential measurements of the affected upper extremity

**Arousal, attention, and cognition:** examine mental status, learning ability, memory, motivation

**Community and work integration:** analysis of community, work, and leisure activities

**Environmental, home, and work barriers:** analysis of current and potential barriers or hazards

**Integumentary integrity:** skin assessment, assessment of sensation

**Joint integrity and mobility:** assessment of hypermobility and hypomobility of a joint, soft tissue swelling and inflammation

**Muscle performance:** strength assessment except for surgical extremity

**Pain:** pain perception assessment scale, visual analogue scale, assessment of muscle soreness

**Range of motion:** passive range of motion within limits of physician protocol for involved shoulder, active and passive range of motion for all other extremities

**Self-care and home management:** assessment of functional capacity, Functional Independence Measure (FIM)

**Sensory integrity:** assessment of proprioception and kinesthesia

### What additional findings are likely with this patient?

Surgical complications post TSA include mechanical loosening of the prosthesis, instability, rotator cuff tear, implant failure, heterotopic ossification and intraoperative fracture. Risk for complication is dependent on the type of prosthesis (unconstrained, semiconstrained, constrained), surgical skill in reproducing proper alignment, use of cemented prosthesis versus press-fit prosthesis, and integrity of rotator cuff musculature.

# Total Shoulder Arthroplasty

## Management

### What is the most effective management of this patient?

A patient status post TSA will remain hospitalized for an average of two to five days. Medical management of the patient will rely on a team approach including nursing, physician services, and rehabilitation therapies. The success of the TSA will rely on the style of the implant, the quality of the soft tissue, bone, and the rehabilitation program. A CPM may be prescribed by the surgeon for use during the patient's hospitalization. Pharmacological intervention includes anticoagulation and pain medications. Physical therapy is initiated the day after surgery and should follow the shoulder rehabilitation protocol designed by the surgeon. The shoulder usually remains immobilized using a sling during initial rehabilitation. The Neer shoulder protocol advocates initiating isometric shoulder exercises approximately three weeks after surgery and active shoulder exercises approximately six weeks after surgery. PROM and AAROM are indicated but AROM at the shoulder is contraindicated during the first phase of rehabilitation. Physical therapy intervention includes pain management, prevention of adhesions, functional activities, PROM/AAROM/ AROM, therapeutic exercise, edema management, patient education in self-ROM and wand/pendulum exercises, and the use of modalities.

### What home care regimen should be recommended?

The home care regimen should include a range of motion and therapeutic exercise program that follows the surgeon's shoulder rehabilitation protocol. During initial recovery, pendulum and wand exercises are appropriate as well as self-ROM. A patient must not perform any form of medial rotation or lateral rotation beyond 35 to 40 degrees during the first two to three weeks post surgery. Controlled motion and return to functional activity are incorporated into the home program as directed by the physician protocol. A patient must also continue to manage edema and follow other physician orders regarding precautions.

## Outcome

### What is the likely outcome of a course in physical therapy?

The goal of a TSA is to relieve pain and regain functional motion. Physical therapy should assist the patient to meet these goals unless hindered by post-surgical or other complications.

### What are the long-term effects of the patient's condition?

Since the shoulder is a non-weight bearing joint there is a longer life expectancy for the prosthesis than for the knee or hip. There is a high success rate for long-term results with a TSA. Patients should avoid activities such as heavy lifting, chopping wood or contact sports since these can increase the risk of fracture, loosening or rotator cuff tear.

## Comparison

### What are the distinguishing characteristics of a similar condition?

A shoulder hemiarthroplasty is a similar surgery that involves the replacement of the head and neck of the humerus leaving the glenoid fossa of the scapula intact. This surgery is indicated when the humeral head has deteriorated or fractured without healing. This procedure may also be performed if the patient does not have enough bone density to support the glenoid component or when there are significant rotator cuff deficiencies that exist.

## Clinical Scenarios

### Scenario One

A 60-year-old female is 14 days status post left TSA and is currently attending outpatient therapy three days per week. The patient's rehabilitation is complicated by right upper extremity paralysis secondary to a CVA two years ago. The patient is motivated, cooperative, and does not have any residual cognitive deficits.

### Scenario Two

A 58-year-old male is one-month status post TSA and has been attending outpatient therapy three days per week. His wife states that he complains of significant pain during his home exercise program. He appears to be progressing otherwise. He has no significant medical history other than the rheumatoid arthritis that created the need for the TSA.

## Transfemoral Amputation due to Osteosarcoma

### Diagnosis

#### What condition produces a patient's symptoms?

Osteosarcoma (osteogenic sarcoma) is the second most common primary bone tumor and accounts for 15-20% of bone tumors. Osteosarcoma is a highly malignant cancer that begins in the medullary cavity of a bone and leads to the formation of a mass. It usually affects bones with an active growth phase such as the femur or tibia and is often located in the metaphysis. Amputation may be necessary to remove the tumor and surrounding tissues to avoid metastatic disease.

#### An injury was most likely sustained to which structure?

The cancer cells are found in osteoblasts within the primitive mesenchymal cells of the medullary cavity of a bone. The cancer rapidly proliferates, replaces normal bone, and causes tissue destruction. Osteosarcoma will also metastasize to the lungs very early in the disease process.

### Inference

#### What is the most likely contributing factor in the development of this condition?

Osteosarcomas can occur as a primary or secondary cancer and the etiology remains unknown. This form of tumor primarily affects young children (especially males), adolescents, and young adults under 30 years of age. A peak time for incidence is during a growth spurt as an adolescent. Risk factors associated with secondary osteosarcoma include Paget's disease, osteoblastoma, giant cell tumor or chronic osteomyelitis. Environmental and genetic factors have been associated with the disease. In many instances amputation is required to cease the disease process.

### Confirmation

#### What is the most likely clinical presentation?

Osteosarcoma can be found most often in the long bones especially at the site of the most active epiphyseal growth plate, the distal femur, proximal tibia, proximal humerus and pelvis. The knee region accounts for approximately 50% of osteosarcomas. Patients that require amputation secondary to an osteosarcoma will present with a mass often found in the tibia or femur. The most common symptoms of osteosarcoma are pain and swelling within the extremity. Pain may worsen at night or with exercise and a lump may develop in the extremity sometime after the onset of pain. The osteosarcoma may weaken the involved extremity leading to a fracture. In some cases, a fracture may be the first sign of the osteosarcoma. Metastases appear in the lungs early in 90% of the cases.

#### What laboratory or imaging studies would confirm the diagnosis?

X-ray, MRI, and scintigraphy allow the physician to determine the presence, location, and size of a tumor. The "Codman's triangle" can be seen on x-ray indicating reactive bone at the site where the periosteum has been elevated by the neoplasm. Definitive diagnosis for an osteosarcoma is made through tissue biopsy of the tumor.

#### What additional information should be obtained to confirm the diagnosis?

Diagnosis of osteosarcoma is confirmed solely through biopsy. The course of treatment and the need for surgical amputation is determined by the size, location of the tumor, and progression of the malignancy.

### Examination

#### What history should be documented?

Important areas to explore include past medical history, medications, family history, current symptoms and health status, social history and habits, occupation, leisure activities, and social support system.

#### What test/measures are most appropriate?

**Aerobic capacity and endurance:** assessment of vital signs at rest and with activity, auscultation of the lungs, palpation of pulses

**Anthropometric characteristics:** residual limb circumferential measurements, length of limb

**Arousal, attention, and cognition:** examine mental status, learning ability, memory, motivation

**Assistive and adaptive devices:** analysis of components and safety of a device

**Community and work integration:** analysis of community, work, and leisure activities

**Gait, locomotion, and balance:** analysis of wheelchair mobility, static and dynamic balance in sitting and standing, safety during gait with an assistive device

**Integumentary integrity:** skin assessment, assessment of sensation, temperature of limb

**Muscle performance:** strength and tone assessment

**Pain:** phantom pain, pain perception assessment scale

**Prosthetic requirements:** analysis and safety of the prosthesis; alignment, efficiency, and fit of the prosthesis with the residual limb

**Range of motion:** active and passive range of motion

**Self-care and home management:** assessment of functional capacity, Barthel Index, Functional Independence Measure (FIM)

**Sensory integrity:** proprioception and kinesthesia

# Transfemoral Amputation due to Osteosarcoma

## What additional findings are likely with this patient?

A patient status post transfemoral amputation secondary to an osteosarcoma may present with fatigue, loss of balance, phantom pain or sensation, hypersensitivity of the residual limb, and psychological issues regarding the loss of the limb. The patient may also have associated symptoms from chemotherapy that can include anemia, abnormal bleeding, infection, and kidney impairment. The presence of these findings can have a negative influence on a patient's ability to utilize a prosthesis.

## Management

### What is the most effective management of this patient?

Medical management will focus on adjunctive therapies to treat the osteosarcoma. Pharmacological intervention may include pain medication and other medication to deter effects from cancer treatment. Physical and occupational therapies should begin immediately after the transfemoral amputation. Preprosthetic intervention should focus on range of motion, positioning, strengthening, desensitization, residual limb wrapping, functional mobility, gait training, and patient education for care of the residual limb. Patients with a transfemoral amputation should lie prone for a period of time each day to prevent a hip flexion contracture. Modalities may be used to improve range of motion and decrease pain. Serial casting may be indicated if a contracture develops. Without complication the patient should be able to return home with support and receive short-term physical therapy for prosthetic training.

### What home care regimen should be recommended?

A home care regimen for a patient status post transfemoral amputation should include limb desensitization, stretching, proper positioning, and prone lying. The patient must be independent with residual limb care, skin inspection, and proper wrapping. Endurance activities, strengthening, and mobility with an assistive device are necessary as a precursor to prosthetic training.

## Outcome

### What is the likely outcome of a course in physical therapy?

Physical therapy is necessary for both preprosthetic and prosthetic training. A patient should be able to achieve the established goals and function with a prosthesis for all mobility including ambulation, balance, transfers, and stair activities. The general health, cognition, motivation, and social support system of the patient will influence the patient's functional outcome.

## What are the long-term effects of the patient's condition?

The survival rate for a patient status post osteosarcoma has increased in recent years to a five-year cure rate of 70-80% with treatment that may include amputation, radiation, and chemotherapy. The transfemoral amputation should not permanently impair the patient's independence with mobility, self-care or ambulation using a prosthesis. The patient's long-term outcome is dependent on the status of the cancer.

## Comparison

### What are the distinguishing characteristics of a similar condition?

Ewing's sarcoma is a malignant nonosteogenic primary bone tumor that infiltrates the bone marrow and usually affects children and adolescents under 20 years of age. A patient will present with pain of increasing severity, swelling, and fever. This tumor is not found consistently in a specific location within the bone and is extremely malignant with a high frequency of metastases. Ewing's sarcoma requires aggressive treatment that may include amputation and adjunctive chemotherapy. The five-year survival rate is approximately 70%.

## Clinical Scenarios

### Scenario One

A 10-year-old female is seen in physical therapy after a right transfemoral amputation. The patient was diagnosed with osteosarcoma four months ago. The patient is in good spirits and is anxious to receive "a new leg" and begin walking. Her parents are supportive and are eager to assist her during rehabilitation.

### Scenario Two

A 16-year-old male is seen for the first time in physical therapy since a left transfemoral amputation. The boy states that his leg had bothered him for a few weeks and the pain got worse everyday. He also stated that he was told that the cancer was now also found in his lungs. He wants to start an exercise program so that he will be ready for his prosthesis when his residual limb heals.

# Transtibial Amputation due to Arteriosclerosis Obliterans

## Diagnosis

### What condition produces a patient's symptoms?

Arteriosclerosis obliterans, also known as peripheral arterial disease (PAD), is a form of peripheral vascular disease that produces thickening, hardening, and eventual narrowing and occlusion of the arteries. Arteriosclerosis obliterans results in ischemia and subsequent ulceration of the affected tissues. The affected area may become necrotic, gangrenous, and require amputation.

### An injury was most likely sustained to which structure?

Injury will occur to all structures that receive blood supply from vessels that have become occluded. Prolonged ischemia results in tissue death and infection. Arteriosclerosis obliterans is the most common arterial occlusive disease and accounts for approximately 95% of the cases of vascular disease.

## Inference

### What is the most likely contributing factor in the development of this condition?

Risk factors associated with arteriosclerosis obliterans include age, diabetes, sex, hypertension, high serum cholesterol and low-density lipid levels, smoking, impaired glucose tolerance, obesity, and sedentary lifestyle. Unsuccessful management of peripheral vascular disease may ultimately lead to uncontrolled infection, gangrene, necrosis, and amputation. Males have an overall higher incidence of arteriosclerosis than female counterparts.

## Confirmation

### What is the most likely clinical presentation?

The patient that requires a transtibial amputation secondary to arteriosclerosis obliterans is typically an individual over 45 years that smokes (75-90%) and will present with intermittent claudication that produces cramps and pain in the affected areas. Intermittent claudication will typically present in the gastrocnemius-soleus complex, secondary to its high oxygen demand. Other characteristics include resting pain, decreased pulses, ischemia, pallor skin, and decreased skin temperature.

### What laboratory or imaging studies would confirm the diagnosis?

Arteriosclerosis obliterans can be diagnosed using Doppler ultrasonography, MRI or arteriography. These diagnostic tests examine the degree of blood flow throughout the extremities. A patient with arteriosclerosis obliterans would typically demonstrate poor results including blockage, tissue damage, and tissue death.

### What additional information should be obtained to confirm the diagnosis?

The physician should examine the limb for temperature, skin condition, the presence of hair, sensation, and palpable pulses when determining the need for amputation. The physician may perform a selected non-invasive test such as a claudication test that examines the presence of intermittent claudication that can occur with prolonged ambulation. The ankle-brachial index, segmental limb pressures or pulse volume recordings may also be used to assist with the diagnosis.

## Examination

### What history should be documented?

Important areas to explore include past medical history, medications, current health status, social history and habits, occupation, living environment, and social support system.

### What test/measures are most appropriate?

**Aerobic capacity and endurance:** palpation of pulses, pulse oximetry, assessment of vital signs at rest and with activity

**Anthropometric characteristics:** residual limb circumferential measurements, length of limb

**Arousal, attention, and cognition:** examine mental status, learning ability, memory, motivation

**Assistive and adaptive devices:** analysis of components and safety of a device

**Gait, locomotion, and balance:** analysis of wheelchair mobility, static and dynamic balance in sitting and standing, safety during gait with an assistive device

**Integumentary integrity:** examine presence of hair growth, color, temperature, assessment of sensation

**Muscle performance:** strength assessment, muscle tone assessment

**Pain:** phantom pain, pain perception assessment scale

**Prosthetic requirements:** (when appropriate) analysis and safety of the prosthesis; assessment of alignment, efficiency, and fit of the prosthesis; assessment of residual limb with the prosthesis

**Range of motion:** active and passive range of motion

**Self-care and home management:** assessment of functional capacity, Barthel Index, Functional Independence Measure (FIM)

**Sensory integrity:** assessment of proprioception and kinesthesia

# Transtibial Amputation due to Arteriosclerosis Obliterans

## What additional findings are likely with this patient?

A patient status post transtibial amputation may have a decrease in cardiovascular status depending on the frequency of intermittent claudication the patient experienced prior to the amputation. The patient may initially experience diminished balance secondary to the loss of the limb. Other issues that directly affect the residual limb include phantom pain, decreased range of motion, poor skin integrity, and hypersensitivity. The presence of any of these findings can have a negative influence on a patient's ability to utilize a prosthesis.

## Management

### What is the most effective management of this patient?

A patient should be a candidate for inpatient physical therapy services immediately after the transtibial amputation. Preprosthetic intervention should focus on strength, range of motion, functional mobility, use of assistive devices, desensitization, and patient education for care of the residual limb. Intervention should focus on proper positioning in order to avoid the risk of contractures, especially a knee flexion contracture. If the patient does not experience complications they should be able to return home either independently or with support. The patient may receive continued short-term physical therapy for prosthetic intervention once the residual limb has fully healed.

### What home care regimen should be recommended?

A home care regimen for a patient status post transtibial amputation should include exercises, limb desensitization, proper positioning, and stretching. Since ambulation with a prosthesis increases the energy cost, the patient should be encouraged to perform cardiovascular activities on a frequent basis. In order to be successful, the patient will need to consistently monitor the residual limb and wrap the limb to ensure proper shaping until the prosthesis is tolerated.

## Outcome

### What is the likely outcome of a course in physical therapy?

Physical therapy for both preprosthetic and prosthetic intervention is typically necessary. A patient should be able to achieve the established goals and function with a prosthesis and an assistive device if warranted. The general health, cognition, motivation, and social support system of the patient will influence the patient's functional outcome.

## What are the long-term effects of the patient's condition?

Arteriosclerosis obliterans is a chronic disease that a patient should continue to manage. The current transtibial amputation should not permanently alter a patient's level of functional mobility. The patient should be able to manage all aspects of self-care and functional mobility after prosthetic training with the permanent prosthesis unless hindered by other ailments. Approximately 20% of all individuals with arteriosclerosis obliterans have a myocardial infarction or CVA at some point after diagnosis.

## Comparison

### What are the distinguishing characteristics of a similar condition?

Any amputation would be considered a similar condition, with each level of amputation possessing distinguishing characteristics. Regardless, physical therapy intervention will include desensitization, phantom pain education, proper compression and shaping, strengthening, self-care, and mobility. In most instances, patients status post amputation share the common goal of functional prosthetic use.

## Clinical Scenarios

### Scenario One

A two-year-old female born with congenital malformation of the ankle joint and without a foot is referred to physical therapy for a pre-operative evaluation. The child is in good health, active, and has no other past medical history. The child has become increasingly frustrated with her alternate means of mobility. Her parents are supportive and carry her for community mobility. She prefers to scoot and crawl around the house since she cannot bear weight through the affected lower extremity. She is scheduled for a Syme's amputation in one week.

### Scenario Two

An 83-year-old male, status post right transtibial amputation secondary to insulin-dependent diabetes mellitus, is admitted to a skilled nursing facility for rehabilitation. The patient is obese and presents with cardiopulmonary insufficiency. The patient previously resided alone with intermittent home health care and requires two liters of oxygen with activity.

# Traumatic Brain Injury

## Diagnosis

### What condition produces a patient's symptoms?

Traumatic brain injury (TBI) occurs due to an open head injury where there is penetration through the skull or closed head injury where the brain makes contact with the skull secondary to a sudden, violent acceleration or deceleration impact. Traumatic brain injury can also occur secondary to anoxia as with cardiac arrest or near drowning.

### An injury was most likely sustained to which structure?

Any structure within the brain is vulnerable to injury; however, primary damage will occur at the site of impact. Secondary damage occurs as a result of metabolic and physiologic reactions to the trauma. Brain injury may include swelling, axonal injury, hypoxia, hematoma, hemorrhage and changes in intracranial pressure (ICP).

## Inference

### What is the most likely contributing factor in the development of this condition?

Statistics from the Centers for Disease Control indicate that falls (32.5%) and motor vehicle accidents (17.3%) are the two leading causes of TBI. Pediatric TBI occurs 50% of the time as a result of a fall. Motor vehicle accidents account for 31.8% of deaths from TBI. High risk groups include ages 0-4, 15-19, and greater than 65. Males are at greater risk in each demographic category.

## Confirmation

### What is the most likely clinical presentation?

The incidence of head injury is close to two million individuals per year with an estimated five million individuals living with a brain injury. The clinical presentation of a TBI varies due to the type, area, extent of injury, and secondary damage within the brain. Characteristics of a TBI may include altered consciousness (coma, obtundity, delirium), cognitive and behavioral deficits, changes in personality, motor impairments, alterations in tone, and speech and swallowing issues.

### What laboratory or imaging studies would confirm the diagnosis?

Diagnostic imaging such as CT scan or MRI should be performed immediately in order to rule out hemorrhage, infarction, and swelling. X-rays taken of the cervical spine can be used to rule out fracture and potential for subluxation. An electroencephalogram (EEG), positron emission tomography (PET), and cerebral blood flow mapping (CBF) may also be utilized for diagnosis and baseline data.

### What additional information should be obtained to confirm the diagnosis?

A full neurological evaluation by a physician should include a mental examination, cranial nerve assessment, tonal assessment and papillary reactivity assessment. The physician will classify the patient using the Glasgow Coma Scale and indicate severe (coma), moderate or mild brain injury. The Rancho Los Amigos Levels of Cognitive Functioning can also be used to classify injury and assist with developing an appropriate plan of care.

## Examination

### What history should be documented?

Important areas to explore include past medical history, medications, family history, current symptoms, level of cognitive functioning, social history and habits, occupation, leisure activities, and social support system.

### What test/measures are most appropriate?

**Aerobic capacity and endurance:** vital signs at rest/activity, pulse oximetry, auscultation of lungs

**Arousal, attention, and cognition:** using Rancho Los Amigos Levels of Cognitive Functioning

**Assistive and adaptive devices:** analysis of components and safety of a device

**Cranial nerve integrity:** muscle innervation by the cranial nerves, dermatome assessment

**Environmental, home, and work barriers:** analysis of current and potential barriers or hazards

**Gait, locomotion, and balance:** static and dynamic balance in sitting and standing, safety during gait with/without an assistive device, Berg Balance Scale, Tinetti Performance Oriented Mobility Assessment, analysis of wheelchair management

**Integumentary integrity:** skin and sensation assessment

**Joint integrity and mobility:** assessment of hypermobility and hypomobility of a joint

**Motor function:** equilibrium and righting reactions, motor assessment scales, coordination, posture and balance in sitting, assessment of sensorimotor integration, physical performance scales

**Muscle performance:** strength assessment, muscle tone assessment

**Neuromotor development and sensory integration:** analysis of reflex movement patterns, assessment of involuntary movements, sensory integration tests, gross and fine motor skills

**Orthotic, protective, and supportive devices:** analysis of components and movement while wearing a device

**Pain:** pain perception assessment scale, visual analogue scale, assessment of muscle soreness

## Traumatic Brain Injury

**Posture:** analysis of resting and dynamic posture
**Range of motion:** active and passive range of motion
**Reflex integrity:** assessment of deep tendon and pathological reflexes (e.g., Babinski, ATNR)
**Self-care and home management:** assessment of functional capacity, Functional Independence Measure (FIM), Barthel Index, Rankin Scale, Rivermead Motor Assessment

### What additional findings are likely with this patient?

There are multiple impairments that can develop secondary to TBI. Intracranial pressure must be monitored initially since it is at risk to increase or develop hemorrhage. A patient can develop heterotopic ossification, contractures, skin breakdown, seizures, and deep vein thrombosis. A patient with a severe TBI may remain in a persistent vegetative state.

## Management

### What is the most effective management of this patient?

Medical management is initiated at the site of injury or in the emergency room for life preserving measures. The initial goal is to stabilize the patient, control intracranial pressure, and prevent secondary complications. Surgical intervention may be required in attempt to regain homeostasis within the brain secondary to hemorrhage or fracture. Once a patient is medically stable, physical therapy rehabilitation is initiated. Treatment of a patient with TBI usually includes a team approach with goals based on the patient's level of injury. Pharmacological intervention may include cerebral vasoconstrictive agents, psychotropic agents, hypertensive agents, antispasticity agents, and medication to assist with cognition and attention. Physical therapy will focus on sensory stimulation and PROM for a comatose patient or pathfinding and high-level balance activities for a patient with a mild injury. Physical therapy may include functional mobility training, behavior modification, serial casting, compensatory strategies, vestibular rehabilitation, task specific activities, wheelchair seating, and pulmonary intervention.

### What home care regimen should be recommended?

A home care regimen should include ongoing therapeutic activities that focus on goals associated with the patient's current Rancho Los Amigos level. Consistency is vital to the success of a home program. The patient may also participate in a community re-entry based program for the TBI population if warranted by their level of current function.

## Outcome

### What is the likely outcome of a course in physical therapy?

A patient diagnosed with TBI does not have a specific projected outcome. Outcome is based on the degree of primary and secondary damage and the extent of cognitive and behavioral impairments. Physical therapy should continue in all settings until the patient has attained all realistic goals.

### What are the long-term effects of the patient's condition?

TBI affects approximately 1.7 million Americans each year. Approximately 52,000 individuals die each year as a result of TBI. Long-term effects are determined by the extent of injury and impairments resulting from the TBI. Many patients experience life long deficits that do not allow them to return to their pre-injury lifestyle.

## Comparison

### What are the distinguishing characteristics of a similar condition?

Meningitis is a bacterial or viral infection that spreads through the cerebrospinal fluid to the brain. The meninges of the brain become inflamed as well as the meningeal membranes. The patient will have a headache and may complain of stiffness in the neck. The patient may also show symptoms of confusion, fatigue, and irritability. As the virus progresses the patient may experience seizures and may progress into a coma. Medical treatment varies based on the causative strain of the virus/bacteria. Mortality ranges from 5-25% and approximately 30% have some degree of permanent neurological impairment.

## Clinical Scenarios

### Scenario One

A 22-year-old male with TBI is admitted to an inpatient rehabilitation hospital. The patient is presently classified as Rancho Los Amigos Level IV. The patient required surgical decompression after the TBI. The patient's parents are with the patient almost constantly.

### Scenario Two

A 42-year-old female sustained a severe TBI in a motor vehicle accident and is presently classified as Rancho Los Amigos Level II. The accident was two weeks ago. Prior to admission the patient was healthy and worked full-time. She has a supportive husband.

## Urinary Stress Incontinence

### Diagnosis

**What condition produces a patient's symptoms?**

Urinary incontinence is the involuntary loss of urine. There are five classifications that include functional incontinence, stress incontinence, urge incontinence, mixed incontinence, and overflow incontinence. Urinary stress incontinence may occur during activities when there is an increase in abdominal pressure through straining, sneezing, coughing or lifting.

**An injury was most likely sustained to which structure?**

Urinary stress incontinence usually occurs from loss of strength and/or integrity of the contractile and noncontractile tissues that maintain bladder control. Urinary stress incontinence is caused by weakness of the pelvic floor musculature (urogenital diaphragm, levator ani muscle group), damage of the pudendal nerve, malposition of the urethra, and/or urethral sphincter incompetence.

### Inference

**What is the most likely contributing factor in the development of this condition?**

Risk factors for the development of urinary stress incontinence include pregnancy, vaginal delivery, episiotomy, prostate or pelvic surgery, aging, diabetes mellitus, central nervous system and peripheral system dysfunction, and recurrent urinary tract infections. A prolapsed bladder, uterus or bowel may contribute to leakage and is seen in women that have had multiple vaginal deliveries. Medications that treat other illnesses can sometimes contribute to incontinence especially with the older population. Obesity is another risk factor that is believed to increase the risk of stress incontinence due to increased intra-abdominal pressure and the effect of obesity on the neuromuscular function of the genitourinary tract.

### Confirmation

**What is the most likely clinical presentation?**

It is estimated that approximately 10 million adults experience some form of urinary incontinence. Urinary stress incontinence accounts for 50-60% of all incontinence cases and is manifested solely by the involuntary loss of urine with any form of exertion or increased abdominal pressure. The amount of urine that leaks is typically less than 50 milliliters with coughing, sneezing or straining. Physical activity or exercise can also produce leakage due to exertion with these activities. Other manifestations may include dribbling of urine, urgency, frequency, nocturia, and a weak stream while voiding.

**What laboratory or imaging studies would confirm the diagnosis?**

Cystometry is used to evaluate bladder capacity, control, contractility, and sensation. During this procedure provocative stress testing will be performed when stress incontinence is suspected. Urodynamic testing observes the stability of the bladder and electromyography observes bladder contractions. Urinalysis is used for differential diagnosis to rule out infection, diabetes, and other conditions.

**What additional information should be obtained to confirm the diagnosis?**

Urinary stress incontinence can be determined through history, pelvic examination, and noted loss of urine with straining activities. The Marshall-Marchetti test utilizes finger elevation of the paraurethral vaginal tissues at the neck of the bladder in order to stop the leakage of urine during coughing, sneezing or straining. Baseline exam should include the amount of time that a patient can hold urine, repetitions performed of a holding contraction, and the amount of pelvic floor contractions a patient can perform.

### Examination

**What history should be documented?**

Important areas to explore include past medical history, childbirth history, medications, current health status, fluid intake, social history, occupation, living environment, and social support system.

**What test/measures are most appropriate?**

**Aerobic capacity and endurance:** assessment of vital signs at rest and with activity, perceived exertion scale

**Arousal, attention, and cognition:** examine mental status, learning ability, memory, motivation, Urge Impact scale

**Community and work integration:** analysis of community, work, and leisure activities

**Environmental, home, and work barriers:** analysis of current and potential barriers or hazards

**Ergonomics and body mechanics:** analysis of dexterity and coordination, assessment of lifting techniques (intra-abdominal pressure)

**Integumentary integrity:** skin assessment, examination of the pelvic floor

**Muscle performance:** strength assessment of the pelvic floor and abdominal muscles, muscle tone assessment

**Pain:** pain perception assessment scale

**Posture:** analysis of resting and dynamic posture

**Range of motion:** active and passive range of motion

**Self-care and home management:** assessment of functional capacity, bladder diary, fluid intake

## Urinary Stress Incontinence

### What additional findings are likely with this patient?

A patient with urinary stress incontinence may be at increased risk for a urinary tract infection with subsequent skin breakdown. Pelvic floor weakness, uterine prolapse, and kidney infection may all relate to urinary stress incontinence. A patient that has poor diet and nutrition, constipation, inadequate hydration, and urinary frequency will further promote incontinence.

## Management

### What is the most effective management of this patient?

Medical management of urinary incontinence usually consists of conservative measures (physical therapy) as a first line of defense followed by pharmacological and surgical interventions depending on the underlying cause and response to conservative treatment. Physical therapy intervention for pelvic floor muscle weakness that is tested as 0/5 – 2/5 includes biofeedback, electrical stimulation, bladder retraining, and therapeutic exercise. Pelvic floor muscle strengthening at this level includes facilitation and tapping of the pelvic floor muscles, overflow exercises using the buttocks, adductors, and lower abdominals, and implementation of Kegel exercises. Physical therapy intervention for pelvic floor muscle weakness that is tested as 3/5 – 5/5 includes continued biofeedback and bladder retraining, weighted vaginal cones for resistance training, and implementation of pelvic floor muscle exercise during activities.

### What home care regimen should be recommended?

A home care regimen for a patient with urinary stress incontinence should emphasize an active exercise program that includes pelvic floor strengthening in order to regain control of the flow of urine. Patients are encouraged to perform the recommended exercises throughout the day and integrate the pelvic exercises during activities that may trigger an increase in abdominal pressure within their daily routine. In addition to exercise, patients are advised to make behavioral and dietary modifications based on their personal bladder diary.

## Outcome

### What is the likely outcome of a course in physical therapy?

Outpatient physical therapy for urinary stress incontinence should alleviate pelvic floor weakness and involuntary leakage of urine within eight to twelve weeks. If a patient requires surgical intervention or presents with multiple impairments then physical therapy may be warranted for a longer period of time to assist with gaining bladder control.

### What are the long-term effects of the patient's condition?

The long-term effects of urinary stress incontinence depend on the exact cause for the incontinence and the responsiveness to therapeutic intervention. Some patients do not have any long-term effects upon successful completion of physical therapy while other patients do not benefit from physical therapy intervention and require surgical intervention for the underlying cause. Compliance with the home exercise program is required when the underlying cause is weakness of the pelvic floor musculature. Research indicates that in an older population approximately 50% of all admissions to skilled nursing facilities have a direct relationship to unresolved urinary incontinence and impairments.

## Comparison

### What are the distinguishing characteristics of a similar condition?

Bowel incontinence can occur from birth defects, trauma to the rectum, spinal cord injuries, fecal impaction, and tumor. Conservative treatment is preferred and includes diet, pharmacological agents, and strengthening of the sphincter muscles through exercise, electrical stimulation, and biofeedback. Surgical intervention may be warranted.

## Clinical Scenarios

### Scenario One

A 32-year-old female is referred to physical therapy with a diagnosis of incontinence. The patient gave birth to her fourth child six weeks ago. The patient reports involuntary leakage of urine with exertion. The patient has no significant past medical history; however, reports that she is very anxious about participating in physical therapy.

### Scenario Two

A 68-year-old female complains to her doctor during her annual examination that she has difficulty controlling her bladder since a kidney infection six months ago. The patient states that she is unable to hold her urine if she sneezes or coughs and cannot perform any activity of exertion without wearing feminine pads due to leakage. The physician referred the patient to physical therapy for Kegel exercises.

# 11

## PHYSICAL THERAPY EXAM ONE

### Scott Giles

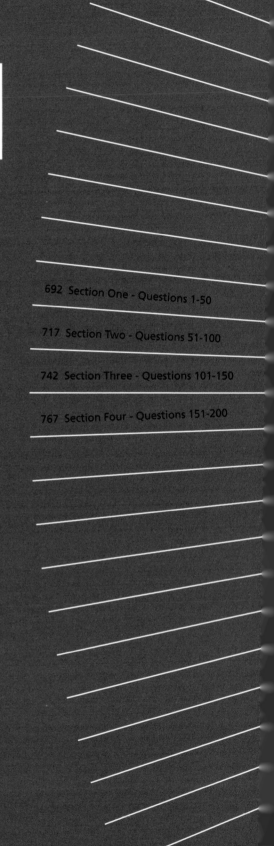

692 Section One - Questions 1-50

717 Section Two - Questions 51-100

742 Section Three - Questions 101-150

767 Section Four - Questions 151-200

# Computer-Based Examinations
# Answer Key

The unit contains the answer key for the three, 200 question sample examinations located on a CD-ROM attached to the inside of the back cover of the text. Candidates should take the examinations on the CD-ROM and then consult the answer key. Candidates who are exposed to sample examinations have several distinct opportunities that otherwise may not be available.

- Candidates have the opportunity to refine their test taking skills with sample questions that are similar in design and format to actual examination questions.

- Candidates have the opportunity to assess their current level of preparedness prior to the actual examination.

The sample examinations on the CD-ROM include questions representative of each of the categories and subcategories of the current content outline of the National Physical Therapy Examination. A sophisticated performance analysis section offers candidates detailed feedback on their examination performance according to six system specific areas and six content outline areas.

**System Specific Summary**

> Musculoskeletal System
>
> Neuromuscular & Nervous Systems
>
> Cardiovascular/Pulmonary and Lymphatic Systems
>
> Other Systems
>
> Non-Systems

**Content Outline Summary**

> Physical Therapy Examination
>
> Foundations for Evaluation, Differential Diagnosis, and Prognosis
>
> Interventions
>
> Equipment & Devices; Therapeutic Modalities
>
> Safety & Protection; Professional Responsibilities; Research

The answer key includes the correct answer, explanations supporting the correct answer and each of the incorrect answers, a cited resource with page number, and the system specific and content outline area classification. A complete index for the sample examinations begins on page 1,000. The index allows candidates to identify the location of specific subject matter within each of the sample examinations.

There are a number of indicators that must be closely examined after completing each sample examination in order to assess a candidate's performance. Perhaps the most obvious indicator is the number of questions a candidate answers correctly. Candidates should attempt to answer 75% or more of the questions correctly. Although this is a relatively lofty goal 75% was selected since the score is safely above a typical criterion-referenced score and therefore would likely be considered a passing score.

There are a number of less obvious indicators that can offer candidates feedback as they prepare for the National Physical Therapy Examination. These indicators often are best examined by answering several specific questions.

- Were you able to maintain the same level of concentration throughout the entire examination?

- Did you have adequate time to complete the examination?

- Did you effectively incorporate test taking strategies?

- Did you misinterpret or fail to identify what selected questions were asking?

- Did the questions that were answered incorrectly exhibit any similar characteristics?

- Did you make any careless mistakes?

- Candidates should attempt to integrate this information in conjunction with the performance analysis summary to accurately identify current strengths and weaknesses and develop appropriate remedial strategies. The computer-based examinations include a number of helpful tools to assist candidates to integrate this information. Candidates should avoid becoming overly excited or depressed based on the results of a given sample examination and use the number of questions answered correctly only as a general indicator of their current level of preparedness. Studying for the examination is much closer to running a marathon than running a sprint. By engaging in meaningful self-assessment activities candidates can gather valuable information to improve future examination performance.

# PHYSICAL THERAPY
# EXAM ONE

# STRATEGY

**"Good fortune is what happens when opportunity meets preparation."**

— Thomas Edison

Candidates need to have a strategy or plan to prepare for the National Physical
Therapy Examination. An important component of any comprehensive study plan
involves answering multiple-choice questions and carefully analyzing the results.
Identifying strengths and weaknesses in the various system specific and content
outline areas can be a useful activity to direct remedial activities.

## Exam One: Question 1

A physical therapist using an electrical stimulation device attempts to quantify several characteristics of a monophasic waveform. When measuring phase charge, the standard unit of measure is the:

1. coulomb
2. ampere
3. ohm
4. second

**Correct Answer: 1** (Prentice - Therapeutic Modalities p. 98)

Physical therapists should possess an understanding of the basic principles associated with electricity. As part of this knowledge, therapists should be aware of the standard units associated with commonly utilized electrical terminology.

1. **A coulomb is a term used to describe electrical charge. One coulomb equals 6.25 X $10^{18}$ electrons per second.**

2. An ampere is a unit of measure used to describe the rate of current. One ampere equals the delivery of one coulomb of electrical charge per second. Flow

3. An ohm is a unit used to describe resistance or electrical impedance. An electrical circuit with high resistance (ohms) will have less flow (amperes) than a circuit with less resistance and the same voltage.

4. A second is a unit used to measure time. There are 60 seconds in a minute. Common terms used with electrical current include microseconds and milliseconds.

System Specific: Non-Systems
Content Outline: Equipment & Devices; Therapeutic Modalities

## Exam One: Question 2

A physical therapist assesses the functional strength of a patient's hip extensors while observing the patient move from standing to sitting. What type of contraction occurs in the hip extensors during this activity?

1. concentric
2. **eccentric**
3. isometric
4. isokinetic

**Correct Answer: 2** (Levangie p. 376)

The gluteus maximus and the hamstrings muscles function as primary hip extensors. These muscles contract in an eccentric fashion when moving from standing to sitting.

1. Concentric contractions require a shortening of the involved muscle. The hip extensors would lengthen when moving from standing to sitting and therefore the contraction would not be labeled concentric.

2. **Eccentric contractions require a lengthening of the involved muscle. The contraction generally occurs when there is a need to decelerate a body part. The hip extensors would lengthen when moving from standing to sitting.**

3. Isometric contractions do not change the length of a muscle or produce movement. As a result, the hip extensors cannot contract isometrically when moving from standing to sitting.

4. Isokinetic contractions occur when a muscle contracts and shortens at a constant speed. This can occur only when a muscle's maximal force of contraction exceeds the total load on the muscle. The hip extensors would not lengthen at a constant speed when moving from standing to sitting.

System Specific: Musculoskeletal System
Content Outline: Physical Therapy Examination

## Exam One: Question 3

A patient referred to physical therapy with chronic low back pain has failed to make any progress toward meeting established goals in over three weeks of treatment. The physical therapist has employed a variety of treatment techniques, but has yet to observe any sign of subjective or objective improvement in the patient's condition. The MOST appropriate action would be to:

1. transfer the patient to another therapist's schedule
2. re-examine the patient and establish new goals
3. continue to modify the patient's treatment plan
4. **alert the referring physician to the patient's status**

**Correct Answer: 4** (Criteria for Standards of Practice)
Physical therapists must be willing to consult with a referring physician when there is ample evidence suggesting that the patient is not benefitting from physical therapy services.

1. There is no supporting evidence to suggest that the patient's failure to make progress is influenced by the patient-therapist relationship or the therapist's level of competence.

2. Re-examining the patient and establishing new goals is a viable option, however, failing to make progress during a relatively long period of time (i.e., three weeks) necessitates formal communication with the physician.

3. Modifying an established treatment plan is desirable when progress has not been made or the rate of progress is not satisfactory. Although a desirable option, the length of time the patient has failed to make progress would necessitate formal communication with the physician.

4. **Formal communication should occur with the referring physician when a patient fails to make progress in physical therapy. This is particularly relevant in the described scenario since the physical therapist has employed a variety of treatment techniques and has not observed any sign of subjective or objective improvement.**

System Specific: Musculoskeletal System
Content Outline: Interventions

## Exam One: Question 4

A patient recently admitted to an acute care hospital is referred to physical therapy. The physical therapist documents the following clinical signs: pallor, cyanosis, and cool skin. These clinical signs are MOST consistent with:

1. cor pulmonale
2. **anemia**
3. hypertension
4. diaphoresis

**Correct Answer: 2** (Paz p. 405)
Anemia refers to a reduction in the number of circulating red blood cells or a reduction in hemoglobin. Anemia is the most common disorder of the blood. The three main categories of anemia include excessive blood loss (i.e., hemorrhage), excessive blood cell destruction (i.e., hemolysis), and deficient red blood cell production (i.e., hematopoiesis).

1. Cor pulmonale is right-sided heart failure arising from disease of the lungs. Signs of right ventricular failure are elevated central venous pressure with distension of the neck veins. Ascites (accumulation of fluid in the peritoneal cavity) and peripheral edema of the feet and ankles are common. Individuals with heart failure often experience fatigue and exercise intolerance.

2. **A decrease in the number of red blood cells that carry oxygen in the blood results in a variety of symptoms including pallor, cyanosis, cool skin, vertigo, weakness, headache, and malaise.**

3. Hypertension, or increased blood pressure, is diagnosed when diastolic blood pressure equals or exceeds 90 mm Hg or when systolic blood pressure equals or exceeds 140 mm Hg. Hypertension often goes unrecognized as mild to moderate elevations in blood pressure usually are not symptomatic.

4. Diaphoresis refers to profuse perspiration and is often associated with shock or other emergent medical conditions.

System Specific: Cardiovascular/Pulmonary and Lymphatic Systems
Content Outline: Foundations for Evaluation, Differential Diagnosis, & Prognosis

## Exam One: Question 5

A physical therapist instructs a patient in a home stretching program that includes the pictured stretch. The MOST likely structure targeted is the:

1. gluteus medius
2. iliotibial band
3. **piriformis**
4. rectus femoris

**Correct Answer: 3** (Hall p. 494)
The picture shows a patient stretching the right piriformis. The patient uses the left leg to assist with lateral rotation of the right hip. The patient will perceive tension in the right buttock when performing the stretch.

1. The gluteus medius originates on the ilium and inserts on the greater trochanter. The primary action of the muscle is abduction of the hip. As a result, the hip would not be abducted when stretching the gluteus medius.

2. The iliotibial band is a thick tendon like reinforcement of the tensor fasciae latae that runs from the iliac crest to the lateral condyle of the tibia. The iliotibial band acts to flex and abduct the hip. As a result, the hip would not be in a flexed and laterally rotated position when stretching the iliotibial band.

3. **The piriformis muscle originates on the sacrum and inserts on the greater trochanter. The muscle acts to laterally rotate the femur, however, with the hip flexed more than 60 degrees, the piriformis medially rotates the femur.**

4. The rectus femoris originates on the anterior inferior iliac spine and inserts into the patellar tendon. The muscle acts to flex the hip and extend the knee. As a result, the hip would not be in a flexed position when stretching the rectus femoris.

System Specific: Musculoskeletal System
Content Outline: Interventions

## Exam One: Question 6

A physical therapist receives a referral for a two-month-old infant diagnosed with osteogenesis imperfecta. After completing the examination, the therapist discusses the physical therapy plan of care with the infant's parents. The PRIMARY goal of therapy should be:

1. improve muscle strength and diminish tone
2. facilitate protected weight bearing
3. **promote safe handling and positioning**
4. diminish pulmonary secretions

**Correct Answer: 3** (Ratliffe p. 254)
Osteogenesis imperfecta is an autosomal disorder of collagen synthesis that affects bone metabolism. Children with osteogenesis imperfecta often have delayed developmental milestones secondary to ongoing fractures with immobilization, hypermobility of joints, and poorly developed muscles. The disorder is classified into four types with diverse clinical presentations ranging from normal appearance with mild symptoms to severe involvement that can be fatal during infancy.

1. The patient would likely have diminished muscle strength due to atrophy, hypermobility of joints, and multiple fractures. Improving strength is therefore desirable, however, would not be the primary goal of therapy for the patient. In addition, tone is not typically altered with osteogenesis imperfecta.

2. Protected weight bearing is desirable in order to reduce the risks associated with fracture and prevent disuse atrophy. Given the patient's age this goal would not be the primary focus of therapy.

3. **A patient with osteogenesis imperfecta is extremely susceptible to fractures during even basic activities such as being carried or bathing. As a result, safe handling and positioning would be the primary goal. This information would be critical to convey to all caregivers, perhaps most notably, the infant's parents.**

4. Osteogenesis imperfecta is a disorder of collagen synthesis that affects bone metabolism. The disorder would not directly influence pulmonary secretions.

System Specific: Musculoskeletal System
Content Outline: Foundations for Evaluation, Differential Diagnosis, & Prognosis

## Exam One: Question 7

A physical therapist elects to utilize the Six-Minute Walk Test as a means of quantifying endurance for a patient rehabilitating from a lengthy illness. Which variable would be the MOST appropriate to measure when determining the patient's endurance level with this objective test?

1. perceived exertion
2. heart rate response
3. elapsed time
4. **distance walked**

**Correct Answer: 4** (Paz p. 915)

The Six-Minute Walk Test is used to determine a patient's functional exercise capacity. The test is commonly used upon admission, discharge, and to monitor progress or decline throughout physical therapy. This tool is administered to various populations including those with cardiac impairments, pulmonary disease, chronic conditions, and patients recovering from orthopedic surgical procedures.

1. The patient is instructed to walk as quickly as they can and attempt to cover as much ground as possible within the six minute period. The therapist does not attempt to record the patient's perceived exertion, however, the patient must let the therapist know if they experience chest pain or dizziness.
2. The heart rate response will likely increase as the intensity and duration of the test increases, however, the test is not designed to examine the heart rate response. Heart rate, blood pressure, oxygen saturation, and a dyspnea score are typically assessed prior to and after the administration of the test.
3. The elapsed time for the Six-Minute Walk Test is six minutes, as the name implies, and therefore does not vary during the administration of the test.
4. **The test requires the therapist to measure the distance the patient walks within a six minute period with rest periods permitted as necessary.**

System Specific: Cardiovascular/Pulmonary and Lymphatic Systems
Content Outline: Physical Therapy Examination

## Exam One: Question 8

A physician orders an electrocardiogram (ECG) for a patient diagnosed with congestive heart failure. The medical record indicates the patient is currently taking digitalis. What effect would you expect digitalis to have on the patient's ECG?

1. sinus tachycardia
2. **lengthened PR interval**
3. lengthened QT interval
4. elevated ST segment

**Correct Answer: 2** (Brannon p. 227)

Digitalis is a medication given to increase the force of myocontractility and is often prescribed for patients with heart failure. Increased contractility increases cardiac output and decreases preload, cardiac workload, and myocardial oxygen demand, thus reducing the clinical effects of congestive heart failure.

1. Sinus tachycardia is a fast heart rate (greater than 100 bpm) that has its origin in the SA node.
2. **By increasing conduction time through the AV node, digitalis prolongs the PR interval on the ECG.**
3. The QT interval measures the depolarization and repolarization time of the ventricles and extends from the beginning of the QRS complex to the end of the T wave. Digitalis may produce shortening of the QT interval.
4. The ST segment represents the beginning of ventricular repolarization and is generally isoelectric. In healthy African American men it can be elevated as much as 2 mm. The ST segment is also elevated in an acute myocardial infarction. Digitalis may produce sagging in the ST segment.

System Specific: Cardiovascular/Pulmonary and Lymphatic Systems
Content Outline: Foundations for Evaluation, Differential Diagnosis, & Prognosis

## Exam One: Question 9

A physical therapist completes an examination on a five-year-old boy diagnosed with Duchenne muscular dystrophy. The referral indicates that the boy was diagnosed with the disease less than one year ago. Assuming a normal progression, which of the following findings would be the FIRST to occur?

1. distal muscle weakness
2. **proximal muscle weakness**
3. impaired respiratory function
4. inability to perform activities of daily living

**Correct Answer: 2** (Ratliffe p. 241)
Duchenne muscular dystrophy is an inherited disorder, characterized by rapidly worsening muscle weakness that starts in the proximal muscles of the lower extremities and pelvis, and later affects all voluntary muscles.

1. Distal muscles are affected later in the course of the disease process.
2. **Muscle weakness and atrophy begin in the proximal muscles of the lower extremities and pelvis, then progresses to the muscles of the shoulders and neck, followed by loss of upper extremity muscles and respiratory muscles.**
3. The muscles of respiration are not initially affected in patients with Duchenne muscular dystrophy.
4. As the condition progresses, weakness begins to interfere with activities of daily living.

System Specific: Musculoskeletal System
Content Outline: Foundations for Evaluation, Differential Diagnosis, & Prognosis

## Exam One: Question 10

A physical therapist obtains an x-ray of a 14-year-old female recently referred to physical therapy after experiencing an increase in back pain following activity. The patient previously participated in competitive gymnastics, however, states that her back was unable to tolerate the intensity of training. Based on the presented x-ray, the therapist would expect the patient's medical diagnosis to be:

1. spondylitis
2. spondylolysis
3. **spondylolisthesis**
4. spondyloptosis

**Correct Answer: 3** (Magee p. 515)
There are a variety of commonly encountered medical conditions that significantly impact the lumbar spine. Physical therapists should be familiar with the clinical presentation and management of these medical conditions.

1. Spondylitis refers to inflammation of a vertebra.
2. Spondylolysis refers to a defect in the pars interarticularis or the arch of the vertebra. This is most common in the L5 vertebra, but can also occur in other lumbar or thoracic vertebra.
3. **Spondylolisthesis refers to the forward displacement of one vertebra over another. The x-ray involves spondylolisthesis at the L5-S1 level. Individuals involved in physical activities such as weight lifting, gymnastics or football are particularly susceptible to this condition. The severity of the spondylolisthesis is classified on a scale of 1-5 based on how much a given vertebral body has slipped forward over the vertebral body beneath it.**
4. Spondyloptosis refers to the condition where a vertebral body is completely off of the adjacent vertebral body (grade 5).

System Specific: Musculoskeletal System
Content Outline: Foundations for Evaluation, Differential Diagnosis, & Prognosis

## Exam One: Question 11

A physical therapist completes a developmental assessment on a five-month-old infant. If the therapist elects to examine the infant's palmar grasp reflex, which of the following stimuli is the MOST appropriate?

1. contact to the ball of the foot in upright standing
2. **maintained pressure to the palm of the hand**
3. noxious stimulus to the palm of the hand
4. sudden change in the position of the head

> **Correct Answer: 2** (O'Sullivan p. 240)
>
> Primitive reflexes are reflexes which begin during gestation or in early infancy. Most of these reflexes become integrated as the infant ages. Integration indicates that the reflex is no longer present when the stimulus is provided. Failure to integrate primitive reflexes can lead to impaired movement and function.
>
> 1. Contact to the ball of the foot in an upright position will elicit the plantar grasp reflex, resulting in curling of the toes. The reflex begins at 28 weeks of gestation and is fully integrated by 9 months of age.
>
> 2. **The palmar grasp reflex is elicited through maintained pressure to the palm of the hand resulting in finger flexion. The reflex begins at birth and is integrated at approximately four to six months of age.**
>
> 3. The palmar grasp reflex is stimulated by maintained pressure to the palm of the hand and not via noxious stimuli.
>
> 4. A sudden change in the position of the head will stimulate the Moro reflex and will cause extension, abduction of the upper extremities, hand opening and crying; followed by flexion and adduction of the upper extremities across the chest. The reflex begins at 28 weeks of gestation and is fully integrated by 5-6 months of age.
>
> System Specific: Neuromuscular & Nervous Systems
> Content Outline: Physical Therapy Examination

## Exam One: Question 12

A physical therapist treats a nine-year-old child diagnosed with cystic fibrosis. As part of the treatment session the therapist attempts to improve the efficiency of the patient's breathing. The MOST appropriate technique to encourage full expansion at the base of the lungs is:

1. manual percussion over the posterior portion of the ribs with the patient in prone
2. **manual contacts with pressure over the lateral borders of the ribs with the patient in supine**
3. manual vibration over the lateral portion of the ribs with the patient in sidelying
4. manual cues over the epigastric area with the patient in supine

> **Correct Answer: 2** (Frownfelter p. 369)
>
> Applying direct pressure with the hands on the lateral borders of the ribs with the patient in supine can promote a more efficient breathing pattern. Physical therapy management for a child with cystic fibrosis may include bronchial drainage techniques, chest percussion, vibration, and suctioning.
>
> 1. Manual percussion over the posterior ribs with the patient in prone describes the postural drainage position and technique used for airway clearance, not lung expansion, of the posterior basal lung segments
>
> 2. **Direct pressure of the hands over the lateral ribs can facilitate expansion of the basal lobes of the lungs.**
>
> 3. Manual vibration over the lateral portion of the ribs in sidelying describes the postural drainage position and technique used for airway clearance, not expansion, of the lateral basal lung segments.
>
> 4. The epigastric area refers to the upper central region of the abdomen. Manual cues on this area would not encourage expansion at the base of the lungs.
>
> System Specific: Cardiovascular/Pulmonary and Lymphatic Systems
> Content Outline: Interventions

## Exam One: Question 13

A physician discusses a patient's plan of care with a physical therapist. The patient is a 29-year-old male that sustained deep partial-thickness burns to the anterior surface of his lower extremities. The physician discusses the possibility of discontinuing use of the topical antibiotic silver sulfadiazine after identifying an irregularity in the patient's laboratory results. Which finding could be MOST related to the use of silver sulfadiazine?

1. **leukopenia**
2. peripheral edema
3. hypokalemia
4. altered pH balance

**Correct Answer: 1** (Paz p. 357)

Silver sulfadiazine is a topical antibiotic that works by interfering with bacterial nucleic acid production by disrupting folic acid synthesis in susceptible bacteria. The antibiotic is a broad spectrum agent that can be applied directly to the skin. Additional problems encountered with sulfa drugs include gastrointestinal distress and allergic reactions.

1. **Silver sulfadiazine is a sulfa drug that can produce a decrease in the number of circulating white blood cells (leukopenia), usually below 5,000 mm³.**

2. Peripheral edema refers to the swelling of tissues in the lower limbs due to the accumulation of fluid. Peripheral edema frequently is associated with heart failure, venous insufficiency, pregnancy, kidney disease, and selected pharmacological agents.

3. Hypokalemia refers to an abnormally low potassium concentration in the blood. The condition can be caused by vomiting, diarrhea, burns, uncontrolled diabetes mellitus, diuretic therapy, and steroid therapy.

4. The pH is a measure of the degree to which a solution is acidic or alkaline. A pH of 7.0 indicates neutrality, a pH of less than 7.0 indicates acidity, a pH of more than 7.0 indicates alkalinity. The body's fluids are usually between 7.35-7.45. Topical agents such as mafenide acetate would be more likely to alter pH.

System Specific: Other Systems
Content Outline: Interventions

## Exam One: Question 14

A patient recently admitted to the hospital with an acute illness is referred to physical therapy. During a scheduled treatment session the patient asks what effect anemia will have on his ability to complete a formal exercise program. The MOST appropriate therapist response is:

1. you may feel as though your muscles are weak
2. you may experience frequent nausea
3. your aerobic capacity may be reduced
4. **you may have a tendency to become fatigued**

**Correct Answer: 4** (Goodman - Pathology p. 685)

Anemia refers to a reduction in the number of circulating red blood cells or reduction in hemoglobin. Symptoms of anemia include pallor of the skin, vertigo, and general malaise.

1. Although a patient may sense that their muscles are weak, fatigue will have a greater impact on the patient's ability to complete a formal exercise program.

2. Nausea refers to the sensation of unease and discomfort in the stomach with an urge to vomit. Nausea is a common side effect of many medications and is commonly associated with chemotherapy, pregnancy, and general anesthesia. Nausea is not typically associated with anemia.

3. Anemia may adversely affect aerobic capacity. However, this is not a term that most patients would readily understand.

4. **Anemia is a common cause of fatigue. Fatigue often results since there are an inadequate number of red blood cells available to transport oxygen to the tissues of the body.**

System Specific: Cardiovascular/Pulmonary and Lymphatic Systems
Content Outline: Foundations for Evaluation, Differential Diagnosis, and Prognosis

## Exam One: Question 15

When performing range of motion exercises with a patient that sustained a head injury, a physical therapist notes that the patient lacks full elbow extension and classifies the end-feel as hard. The MOST likely cause is:

1. **heterotopic ossification**
2. spasticity of the biceps
3. anterior capsular tightness
4. triceps weakness

**Correct Answer: 1** (Goodman - Pathology p. 1237)
Heterotopic ossification refers to abnormal bone growth in tissue and is relatively common in patients following head injury. Signs and symptoms include decreased range of motion, local swelling, and warmth.

1. **The presence of abnormal bone growth in tissue (i.e., heterotopic ossification) could result in an end-feel that is classified as hard due to the bony contact.**
2. Spasticity of the biceps would tend to produce a firm end-feel due to the presence of increased muscle tone.
3. Anterior capsular tightness would tend to produce a firm end-feel. Other common examples of a firm end-feel include muscular, ligamentous, and fascial shortening.
4. Muscle weakness would not be associated with an end-feel of any type since by definition end-feel is a passive assessment.

System Specific: Musculoskeletal System
Content Outline: Foundations for Evaluation, Differential Diagnosis, & Prognosis

## Exam One: Question 16

A physical therapist develops a problem list after examining a patient with a transtibial amputation. Which of the following would be the MOST appropriate entry in the patient problem list?

1. donning and doffing prosthesis requires verbal cues
2. donning and doffing prosthesis requires verbal cues and minimal assist of one
3. **dependence with donning and doffing prosthesis**
4. independent donning and doffing prosthesis in one week

**Correct Answer: 3** (Quinn p. 34)
The problem list, located in the assessment portion of a S.O.A.P. note, should summarize the significant findings from the examination. Since the problem list relates back to the subjective and objective portion of the note, each entry should be described in broad terms. Items in the problem list should be capable of being influenced or changed by physical therapy intervention.

1. The entry describes the patient's current difficulty, but should be expressed in a more general manner without qualifiers (i.e., requires verbal cues).
2. The entry is similar to option 1 with an additional qualifier (i.e., minimal assist of one).
3. **The entry summarizes the patient's problem without providing unnecessary specificity which would already be included in the objective section of the S.O.A.P. note.**
4. The entry more closely approximates a goal since it describes a hypothesized future level of performance.

System Specific: Musculoskeletal System
Content Outline: Interventions

## Exam One: Question 17

A physical therapist monitors a 6 foot 3 inch, 275 pound male's blood pressure using the brachial artery. Which of the following is MOST important when selecting an appropriate size blood pressure cuff for the patient?

1. patient age
2. percent body fat
3. somatotype
4. **extremity circumference**

**Correct Answer: 4** (Pierson p. 58)

If the bladder of the blood pressure cuff is too narrow in relation to the circumference of the patient's arm, the reading will be erroneously high. Conversely, if the bladder is too wide, the reading will be erroneously low.

1. The patient's age is relevant to differentiate whether the patient is an infant, child or adult, however, age becomes a poor predictor of extremity circumference once an individual becomes an adult.

2. A patient with a high percent body fat may need a larger cuff, however, the measure is not nearly as sensitive as extremity circumference.

3. Somatotype is a term used to classify a system of body typing. The most common classifications of somatotype include endomorph, mesomorph, and ectomorph. This information may be useful, however, would not be nearly as specific as a more direct measure such as extremity circumference.

4. **The width of a bladder should be approximately 40% of the circumference of the midpoint of the limb. Bladder width for an average size adult is 5-6 inches.**

System Specific: Cardiovascular/Pulmonary and Lymphatic Systems
Content Outline: Physical Therapy Examination

## Exam One: Question 18

A physical therapist works with a patient with a moderate disk protrusion on an extension progression. Which position would have immediately preceded the pictured position?

1. prone press-up
2. prone lying with a pillow under the waist
3. standing extension
4. **prone lying**

**Correct Answer: 4** (Dutton p. 1556)

The patient in the picture is demonstrating prone on elbows. A patient assumes the position by lying in prone with their elbows directly under their shoulders. The patient then moves their sternum away from the surface as the spine moves up and away from the shoulder blades. The extension progression sequence from least provocative to most provocative is: 1. prone with a pillow under the waist; 2. prone; 3. prone on elbows; 4. prone press-up; 5. standing extension.

1. A patient performing a prone press-up lies in prone with their palms on the surface. The patient performs a press-up by straightening their arms as much as possible while keeping the pelvis flat on the surface.

2. Prone with a pillow under the waist is often the most comfortable position for a patient since the pillow allows the spine to assume a more flexed position.

3. Standing extension occurs with the patient in standing with their feet slightly separated. The patient places their hands on the small of the back with the fingers pointing downward and the thumbs pointing anteriorly. The patient then bends backwards at the waist.

4. **A prone position refers to a patient lying on their stomach. This position requires the spine to be in a slightly extended position.**

System Specific: Musculoskeletal System
Content Outline: Interventions

## Exam One: Question 19

A physical therapist works with a patient status post stroke on a mat program. The therapist assists the patient in lateral weight shifting activities while positioned in prone on elbows. Which therapeutic exercise technique would allow the patient to improve dynamic stability with this activity?

1. alternating isometrics
2. **approximation**
3. rhythmic initiation
4. timing for emphasis

**Correct Answer: 2** (Sullivan p. 27)

Facilitation techniques are designed to reduce the effects of impairments and disabilities while promoting motor recovery and improved function. It is important to select a facilitation technique whose purpose is consistent with the established therapeutic objectives.

1. Alternating isometrics are designed to facilitate isometric holding first in agonists acting on one side of the joint, followed by holding of the antagonist muscle groups. This technique is indicated when there is instability in weight bearing, poor static postural control, and/or weakness.

2. **Approximation is a therapeutic exercise technique designed to facilitate contraction and stability through joint compression. The compression force is most often applied to joints through gravity acting on body weight, manual contacts or weight belts.**

3. Rhythmic initiation is a facilitation technique that begins with voluntary relaxation followed by passive movement through increments in range. This is followed by active-assistive movements progressing to resisted movements. The technique is indicated when there is a need to relax, hypertonicity, inability to initiate movement, motor learning deficits, and communication deficits.

4. Timing for emphasis is a facilitation technique that uses maximum resistance to elicit a sequence of contractions from major muscle components of a pattern of motion. This technique allows overflow to occur from strong to weak muscles. The technique is indicated when there is weakness and/or incoordination and is commonly used in conjunction with repeated contractions.

System Specific: Neuromuscular & Nervous Systems
Content Outline: Interventions

## Exam One: Question 20

A patient informs a physical therapist how frustrated she feels after being examined by her physician. The patient explains that she becomes so nervous, she cannot ask any questions during scheduled office visits. The therapist's MOST appropriate response is to:

1. offer to go with the patient to her next scheduled physician visit
2. offer to call the physician and ask any relevant questions
3. **suggest that the patient write down questions for the physician and bring them with her to the next scheduled visit**
4. tell the patient it is a very normal response to be nervous in the presence of a physician

**Correct Answer: 3** (Davis p. 95)

The physical therapist should attempt to identify a strategy or strategies that the patient can use to take a more active role during visits with the physician.

1. It is probably not realistic for the physical therapist to go with the patient to her next scheduled visit. In addition, the action places the burden on the therapist and does not promote a long-term change in the patient's current behavior.

2. Offering to call the physician and ask any relevant questions is similar to the previous option, however, may be slightly more practical. The action, however, does not require the patient to take a more active role and instead uses the physical therapist as an intermediary.

3. **Writing down questions allows the patient to reflect on the information she would like to gather in advance and provides the structure necessary to reduce the influence of the patient's anxiety during office visits.**

4. Acknowledging that many people are nervous in the presence of a physician may make the patient momentarily feel better, however, it does not provide the patient with a viable method to change her current behavior.

System Specific: Non-Systems
Content Outline: Safety and Protection; Professional Responsibilities; Research

## Exam One: Question 21

A physical therapist observes an electrocardiogram of a patient on beta-blockers. Which of the following electrocardiogram changes could be facilitated by beta-blockers?

1. **sinus bradycardia**
2. sinus tachycardia
3. premature ventricular contractions
4. ST segment sagging

**Correct Answer: 1** (Brannon p. 134)

Beta-adrenergic blocking agents (beta-blockers) decrease heart rate, blood pressure, and myocardial contractility.

1. **Sinus bradycardia is a slow sinus rhythm of less than 60 beats per minute. It may occur from beta-blocker medication, during sleep, in physically fit individuals, acute myocardial infarction, carotid sinus pressure, and in response to increased vagal tone due to pain.**

2. Sinus tachycardia is a rapid sinus rhythm of greater than 100 beats per minute. It is usually caused by something that increases sympathetic activity, such as excitement, pain, fever, hypoxia, exercise, and stimulants. Beta-blockers have the opposite effect on heart rate.

3. A premature ventricular contraction (PVC) is a premature beat arising from an ectopic focus in the ventricle. PVCs may be precipitated by anxiety, tobacco, alcohol, caffeine, and any condition causing myocardial ischemia. PVCs are not caused by beta-blockers.

4. ST segment sagging or depression is indicative of myocardial ischemia and is not caused by beta-blockers.

System Specific: Cardiovascular/Pulmonary and Lymphatic Systems
Content Outline: Foundations for Evaluation, Differential Diagnosis, and Prognosis

## Exam One: Question 22

An athlete is forced to contemplate knee surgery after spraining the anterior cruciate ligament (ACL) while playing soccer. Which situation would provide the MOST direct support for an anterior cruciate ligament reconstruction?

1. grade III ACL sprain with a grade I posterior cruciate ligament (PCL) sprain
2. grade III ACL sprain with a lateral meniscus tear
3. grade II ACL sprain with a medial meniscus tear
4. **functional instability**

**Correct Answer: 4** (Kisner p. 726)

Surgical intervention is based on the amount of functional instability, however, is also influenced by a number of other variables including skeletal maturity, previous ligament injury, activity level, and age.

1. A grade III ACL sprain refers to a complete tear of the ACL. A grade I PCL sprain refers to a mild injury to the PCL without discernable laxity.

2. A grade III ACL sprain refers to a complete tear of the ACL. The addition of a lateral meniscus tear would likely enhance the instability already caused by the complete tear of the ACL.

3. A grade II ACL sprain refers to a moderate tear of the ACL with discernable laxity with the presence of an endpoint. The amount of laxity would be compounded by the presence of the medial meniscus tear. Meniscal tears contribute to knee instability since the meniscus, when healthy, contribute to the stability of the knee.

4. **Many individuals are able to continue to function at high levels despite a variety of ligamentous and meniscal injuries, therefore functional instability provides the most direct support for an anterior cruciate ligament reconstruction.**

System Specific: Musculoskeletal System
Content Outline: Foundations for Evaluation, Differential Diagnosis, & Prognosis

## Exam One: Question 23

A physical therapist employed in a long-term care setting attempts to identify a screening tool that examines a patient's ability to perform a variety of activities of daily living independently. The therapist would like to readminister the tool to assess patient progress. The MOST appropriate screening tool is the:

1. **Barthel Index**
2. Berg Balance Scale
3. Functional Reach Test
4. Tinetti Performance Oriented Mobility Assessment

---

**Correct Answer: 1** (Physical Therapist's Clinical Companion p. 104)

There are a vast number of available screening tools utilized in physical therapy. A selected screening tool must be both valid and reliable and the individuals administering the tool must be qualified and capable in order to obtain meaningful results.

1. **The Barthel Index consists of ten activities of daily living and is often used as a screening tool in rehabilitation, long-term care settings, and home care. Scoring ranges from 0-100 in increments of 5. A score of 100 indicates that the patient is independent.**

2. The Berg Balance Scale consists of 14 tasks of everyday life activities that are scored according to a 0-4 scale. The maximum total score possible is 56, with a score of less than 45 indicating the patient is at risk for multiple falls.

3. The Functional Reach Test was developed to assess standing balance and the risk for falls. A person is required to stand upright against a wall with a static base of support. The patient is asked to make a fist and raise the arm nearest the wall to 90 degrees of shoulder flexion. The patient is then asked to lean forward as far as possible. The beginning position is subtracted from the ending position in order to obtain the final value.

4. The Tinetti Performance Oriented Mobility Assessment measures balance and gait using an ordinal scale of 0-2. The test has a total possible score of 28. Patients scoring less than 19 are considered to be at high risk for falling.

System Specific: Neuromuscular and Nervous Systems
Content Outline: Physical Therapy Examination

## Exam One: Question 24

A patient rehabilitating from a lower extremity injury is referred to physical therapy for hydrotherapy treatments. The physical therapist would like the patient to fully extend the involved lower extremity while sitting in the hydrotherapy tank. Which type of whirlpool would NOT allow the patient to extend the involved lower extremity?

1. Hubbard tank
2. **highboy tank**
3. lowboy tank
4. walk tank

---

**Correct Answer: 2** (Michlovitz p. 122)

Whirlpools consist of a tank that holds water and a turbine that produces movement of the water. Whirlpools are available in a variety of shapes and sizes. The type of whirlpool selected is primarily influenced by the size and shape of the body part to be treated and the established therapeutic objectives.

1. A Hubbard tank is used for full-body immersion. Approximate dimensions for the Hubbard tank are a depth of four feet, a length of eight feet, and a width of six feet.

2. **A highboy tank is designed for immersion of larger body parts. The length of a highboy tank does not permit a patient to fully extend the lower extremities in sitting, however, its depth permits immersion to the midthoracic region.**

3. A lowboy tank is also designed for immersion of larger body parts. The length of a lowboy tank permits a patient to fully extend the lower extremities in sitting, however, its depth is significantly less than the highboy.

4. A walk tank would allow for near full body immersion with the patient in an upright posture. The patient would have the ability to bear weight through the lower extremities and simulate selected functional activities.

System Specific: Non-Systems
Content Outline: Equipment & Devices; Therapeutic Modalities

## Exam One: Question 25

While examining a patient diagnosed with Achilles tendonitis, a physical therapist notes that the foot and ankle appear to be pronated. Which motions combine to create pronation in a non-weight bearing foot?

1. abduction, dorsiflexion, eversion
2. adduction, dorsiflexion, inversion
3. abduction, plantar flexion, eversion
4. adduction, plantar flexion, inversion

**Correct Answer: 1** (Magee p. 854)

Pronation and supination are triplanar multi-joint motions that occur between the hindfoot, the midfoot, and the forefoot. A non-weight bearing foot is synonymous with the term open-chain.

1. Pronation of the foot consists of abduction of the forefoot, dorsiflexion of the subtalar and midtarsal joints, and eversion and inward rotation of the heel.

2. Pronation requires abduction of the forefoot and eversion of the heel, instead of adduction of the forefoot and inversion of the heel.

3. Pronation requires dorsiflexion and not plantar flexion of the subtalar and midtarsal joints.

4. Supination of the foot consists of adduction of the forefoot, plantar flexion of the subtalar and midtarsal joints, and inversion and outward rotation of the heel.

System Specific: Musculoskeletal System
Content Outline: Physical Therapy Examination

## Exam One: Question 26

A physical therapist performs goniometric measurements on a patient rehabilitating from injuries sustained in a motor vehicle accident. When measuring rotation of the cervical spine, which of the following landmarks would be the MOST appropriate for the axis of the goniometer?

1. centered over the external auditory meatus
2. centered over the center of the cranial aspect of the head
3. centered over the C7 spinous process
4. centered over the midline of the occiput

**Correct Answer: 2** (Norkin p. 341)

Cervical rotation occurs in the transverse plane around a vertical axis. The patient should be positioned sitting in a chair with back support. The cervical spine should be positioned in neutral.

1. Centering the axis of the goniometer over the external auditory meatus would be appropriate when measuring the range of motion for cervical flexion and extension. The stationary arm should be either perpendicular or parallel to the ground, while the moving arm should be aligned with the base of the nares.

2. The axis of the goniometer should be positioned over the center of the cranial aspect of the head when measuring rotation of the cervical spine. The stationary arm should be parallel to an imaginary line between the two acromial processes, while the moving arm should be aligned with the tip of the nose.

3. Centering the axis of the goniometer over the C7 spinous process would be appropriate when measuring the range of motion for cervical sidebending. The stationary arm should be aligned with the spinous processes of the thoracic vertebrae (perpendicular to the ground), while the moving arm is aligned with the dorsal midline of the head, using the occipital protuberance for reference.

4. Centering the axis of the goniometer over the midline of the occiput is not a commonly used landmark for cervical spine range of motion.

System Specific: Musculoskeletal System
Content Outline: Physical Therapy Examination

## Exam One: Question 27

A physical therapist performs girth measurements on a patient rehabilitating from knee surgery. The therapist takes the measurements 5 cm and 10 cm above the superior pole of the patella with the patient in supine. The girth measurements are recorded as 32 cm and 37 cm on the right and 34 cm and 40 cm on the left. Which of the following conclusions can be made regarding the strength of the patient's quadriceps?

1. The right quadriceps will be capable of producing a greater force than the left.
2. The left quadriceps will be capable of producing a greater force than the right.
3. The right and left quadriceps will be capable of producing equal force.
4. **Not enough information is given to form a conclusion.**

**Correct Answer: 4** (Magee p. 805)

Girth (circumferential) measurements using a flexible tape measure are commonly used to obtain a gross estimate of muscle atrophy or edema.

1. The circumference of the right quadriceps at the two identified measurement sites is less than the circumference of the equivalent sites on the left quadriceps. The obtained measurements would not likely support the statement that the right quadriceps are stronger than the left.

2. The circumference of the left quadriceps at the two identified measurement sites is greater than the circumference of the equivalent sites on the right quadriceps. The therapist may therefore hypothesize that the right quadriceps are stronger than the left, however, girth measurements are not used to determine strength.

3. The right and left quadriceps could be capable of producing equal force despite different circumferences, however, this is impossible to prove or disprove using girth measurements.

4. **The physical therapist cannot rely on girth measurements to determine strength and would instead need to utilize a formal test and measure for strength such as manual muscle testing or isokinetic testing.**

System Specific: Musculoskeletal System
Content Outline: Foundations for Evaluation, Differential Diagnosis, & Prognosis

## Exam One: Question 28

A physical therapist instructs a patient to expire maximally after taking a maximal inspiration. The therapist can use these instructions to measure the patient's:

1. expiratory reserve volume
2. inspiratory reserve volume
3. total lung capacity
4. **vital capacity**

**Correct Answer: 4** (Brannon p. 293)

Vital capacity is the maximum volume of gas that can be exhaled after a maximum inhalation.

1. Expiratory reserve volume (ERV) is the additional volume of air that can be exhaled beyond the normal tidal exhalation. ERV is one component of vital capacity.

2. Inspiratory reserve volume (IRV) is the additional volume of air that can be inhaled beyond the normal tidal inhalation. IRV is one component of vital capacity.

3. Total lung capacity is the maximum volume to which the lungs can be expanded. It is the sum of vital capacity and residual volume: TLC = VC + RV.

4. **Vital capacity is the maximum volume of gas that can be exhaled after a maximum inhalation. It is equal to the sum of inspiratory reserve volume, tidal volume, and expiratory reserve volume: VC = IRV + TV + ERV.**

System Specific: Cardiovascular/Pulmonary and Lymphatic Systems
Content Outline: Physical Therapy Examination

## Exam One: Question 29

A physical therapist participating in a research project decides it will be necessary to utilize a relatively large sample. By including a large number of subjects, the researcher hopes to increase:

1. the effect size
2. **the likelihood of rejecting the null hypothesis**
3. the validity of the outcome measurements
4. the reliability of the outcome measurements

**Correct Answer: 2** (Portney p. 423)
Sample size is critical to the probability that a statistical test will lead to rejection of the null hypothesis (i.e., statistical power). Besides sample size, statistical power is a function of the significance criterion (alpha), the variance in the data, and the effect size.

1. Effect size is a statistical expression of the magnitude of the difference between different treatments or the magnitude of the relationship between variables. Sample size has no specific effect on the effect size.

2. **The larger the sample, the greater the probability that a statistical test will lead to rejection of the null hypothesis. Small samples are less likely to represent the population of interest. Therefore, true differences or relationships (whatever is being tested) are more likely to be detected in large samples.**

3. Validity of measurement refers to the degree to which an instrument measures what it is intended to measure. Sample size has no specific effect on the validity of measurements.

4. Reliability of measurement refers to the consistency with which an instrument or rater measures a variable. Sample size has no specific effect on the reliability of measurements.

System Specific: Non-Systems
Content Outline: Safety and Protection; Professional Responsibilities; Research

## Exam One: Question 30

A physical therapist monitors a patient's vital signs while exercising in a phase I cardiac rehabilitation program. The patient is status post myocardial infarction and has progressed without difficulty while involved in the program. Which of the following vital sign recordings would exceed the typical limits of a phase I program?

1. heart rate elevated 18 beats per minute above resting level
2. respiration rate of 18 breaths per minute
3. **systolic blood pressure decreased by 25 mm Hg from resting level**
4. diastolic blood pressure less than 100 mm Hg

**Correct Answer: 3** (Brannon p. 4)
Physical therapists should closely monitor the response to exercise of patients in a phase I cardiac rehabilitation program. A drop in the systolic blood pressure of 20 mm Hg or greater is indicative of exercise hypotension and is an indication to stop exercise.

1. An increase in heart rate of 18 beats per minute above resting heart rate is acceptable. Most guidelines for phase I cardiac rehabilitation recommend that heart rate not exceed 130 beats per minute or a heart rate more than 20 beats above resting for post myocardial infarction patients or a heart rate more than 30 beats above resting for post-surgical patients.

2. Dyspnea is a reason to terminate exercise during phase I exercise. However, a respiration rate of 18 breaths per minute is at the upper limit of the normal range and would not typically cause a patient to report a sense of dyspnea.

3. **A decrease in systolic pressure of 25 mm Hg exceeds the 10 mm Hg limit allowed during exercise in a phase I cardiac rehabilitation program.**

4. A diastolic blood pressure of 110 mm Hg is considered the upper limit for exercise in phase I cardiac rehabilitation. A diastolic pressure less than 110 mm Hg is acceptable.

System Specific: Cardiovascular/Pulmonary and Lymphatic Systems
Content Outline: Interventions

## Exam One: Question 31

A physical therapist establishes the following short-term goal for a patient rehabilitating from total knee arthroplasty surgery: Patient will ambulate with a walker 50% weight bearing and moderate assist of 1 for 20 feet within one week. Three days later, the patient successfully achieves the established goal. Which of the following would be the MOST appropriate revision of the short-term goal?

1. ambulate with walker 75% weight bearing and moderate assist of 1 for 30 feet within one week
2. ambulate with walker 50% weight bearing and moderate assist of 2 for 30 feet within one week
3. **ambulate with walker 50% weight bearing and minimal assist of 1 for 30 feet within one week**
4. ambulate with walker 75% weight bearing and minimal assist of 1 for 10 feet within one week

**Correct Answer: 3** (Guide for Professional Conduct)
Physical therapists must frequently revise short-term goals to facilitate the achievement of an established long-term goal.

1. The physician would be the health care professional responsible for modifying the patient's weight bearing status. The physical therapist would typically modify parameters associated with level of assistance, frequency, and duration.

2. The goal maintains the patient's present weight bearing status while it increases the assistance from 1 to 2 and increases the ambulation distance by 10 feet. The item does not provide adequate justification to increase the level of assistance based solely on an increase in ambulation distance of 10 feet.

3. **The goal maintains the patient's present weight bearing status while it decreases the level of assistance from moderate to minimal and increases the ambulation distance by 10 feet. This would appear to be a reasonable modification based on the previously achieved goal and the surgical procedure.**

4. Increasing the patient's weight bearing status from 50% to 75% would be inappropriate without physician approval.

System Specific: Musculoskeletal System
Content Outline: Interventions

## Exam One: Question 32

A physician orders a nasogastric tube for a patient on an acute rehabilitation unit. Which of the following does NOT accurately describe a potential use of the nasogastric tube?

1. administer medications directly into the gastrointestinal tract
2. obtain gastric specimens
3. remove fluid or gas from the stomach
4. **obtain venous blood samples from the stomach**

**Correct Answer: 4** (Pierson p. 281)
A nasogastric tube is a plastic tube that enters the body through a nostril and terminates in a patient's stomach. As a result, the tube is not used for obtaining venous samples.

1. A nasogastric tube can administer medications directly into the gastrointestinal tract. The patient can also be fed nutrients directly through the nasogastric tube if they are unable to take in adequate nutrition orally. Oral feeding or drinking is contraindicated when the nasogastric tube is in place, but exercise is permitted with caution. Head and neck movements should be closely monitored.

2. A nasogastric tube can be used to obtain gastric specimens. The tube is best taped to the patient's face so that it does not easily become dislodged.

3. A nasogastric tube can be used to remove fluid or gas from the stomach and may be utilized to keep the stomach empty after surgery. This would also allow the bowels to rest if needed.

4. **An intravenous line can be used to obtain venous blood samples (but not from the stomach). Intravenous lines also infuse fluids, nutrients, medications, and electrolytes. A nasogastric tube does not obtain venous samples.**

System Specific: Other Systems
Content Outline: Interventions

## Exam One: Question 33

When observing a patient ambulating, a physical therapist notes that the patient's gait has the following characteristics: narrow base of support, short bilateral step length, and decreased trunk rotation. This gait pattern is often observed in patients with a diagnosis of:

1. CVA
2. **Parkinson's disease**
3. post-polio syndrome
4. multiple sclerosis

**Correct Answer: 2** (Paz p. 190)

Patients with Parkinson's disease often exhibit gait abnormalities due to difficulty initiating movement, rigidity, absence of equilibrium responses, and diminished associated reactions.

1. A patient that has experienced a CVA may present with a wide range of diverse impairments, however, a common finding is hemiplegia or hemiparesis. Other characteristics may include gait deviations secondary to weakness and tonal influence. Patients often present with foot drop and decreased stability at the ankle, knee, and hip.
2. **The gait of a patient with Parkinson's disease is characterized by a decrease in stride length and velocity. As the disease progresses, the patient appears to be attempting to catch up with their center of gravity as the step length becomes smaller; this is termed festination. Festination places the patient at higher risk for a fall.**
3. The gait of a patient with post-polio syndrome is characterized by asymmetrical gait patterns secondary to weakness, fatigue, and pain.
4. The gait of a patient with multiple sclerosis is characterized by impaired trunk control and balance. There is often circumduction to assist with foot clearance and ataxia due to weakness and tonal influence.

System Specific: Neuromuscular & Nervous Systems
Content Outline: Foundations for Evaluation, Differential Diagnosis, & Prognosis

## Exam One: Question 34

A physical therapist prepares to complete an assisted standing pivot transfer with a patient that requires moderate assistance. In order to increase a patient's independence with the transfer, which of the following instructions would be the MOST appropriate?

1. I want you to help me perform the transfer.
2. **Try to utilize your own strength to complete the transfer.**
3. Only grab onto me if it is absolutely necessary.
4. Pretend you were home alone and needed to complete the transfer.

**Correct Answer: 2** (Purtilo p. 168)

When treating a patient there must be clear and specific instructions given prior to the initiation of any task. Failure to offer clear and specific instructions increases the probability of an unwanted action. Requesting that the patient utilize their own strength to complete the transfer is the most appropriate instruction for the patient.

1. The statement, "I want you to help me perform the transfer," states that the therapist wants the patient to assist, but does not give the patient exact expectations on how to perform during the transfer.
2. **The statement, "Try to utilize your own strength to complete the transfer," is a direct statement that explains the exact expectations of the patient during the transfer.**
3. The statement, "Only grab onto me if it is absolutely necessary," does not encourage any kind of active participation on the patient's behalf and allows for a "high risk" behavior of grabbing onto the therapist at the patient's discretion.
4. The statement, "Pretend you were home alone and needed to complete the transfer," would not be appropriate since the patient currently requires moderate assistance and if they were "pretending to be alone" they would not follow the correct and safe method for transferring independently.

System Specific: Musculoskeletal System
Content Outline: Interventions

## Exam One: Question 35

A physical therapist instructs a patient with a lower extremity amputation to wrap her residual limb. The patient has mildly impaired sensation on several localized areas of the residual limb. Which of the following would be the LEAST acceptable method of securing the bandage?

1. clips
2. safety pins
3. tape
4. Velcro

**Correct Answer: 1** (Seymour p. 132)

Bandaging of the residual limb is an important aspect of care in rehabilitation following amputation. Goals include shaping, stabilizing the volume, and desensitization of the residual limb. Patients should avoid the use of clips for securing the bandage due to the potential risk for damage to the skin of the residual limb.

1. **Clips should not be used to secure bandages, especially for patients that exhibit impaired sensation. Failure of the patient to recognize that a clip is causing damage to the residual limb could lead to a wound that would significantly delay rehabilitation progress.**

2. Safety pins should not be used on a patient with impaired sensation. If the pin opens, there is risk for damage to the patient's residual limb. Although safety pins are not desirable, they are not as dangerous as clips.

3. Tape would be one of the most acceptable methods for securing the bandage since the tape does not pose any risk to the residual limb.

4. Velcro is an acceptable method to secure the bandage, however, it is not as feasible and affordable as tape.

System Specific: Other Systems
Content Outline: Interventions

## Exam One: Question 36

A physical therapist attempts to identify a patient's risk factors for coronary artery disease as part of a health screening. The patient's heart rate is recorded as 78 beats per minute and blood pressure as 110/70 mm Hg. A recent laboratory report indicates a total cholesterol level of 170 mg/dL with high-density lipoproteins reported as 20 mg/dL and low-density lipoproteins as 110 mg/dL. Which of the following values would be considered atypical?

1. heart rate
2. blood pressure
3. **high-density lipoproteins (HDL)**
4. low-density lipoproteins (LDL)

**Correct Answer: 3** (American Heart Association)

A value less than 40 mg/dL is considered low for HDL cholesterol. Values of 60 mg/dL or greater are considered high. A low HDL value is strongly associated with an increased risk for coronary artery disease.

1. 78 beats per minute is a normal resting heart rate. The range of normal is 60–100 beats per minute.

2. A systolic blood pressure of 110 mm Hg and a diastolic blood pressure of 70 mm Hg are considered within normal limits for blood pressures.

3. **A HDL cholesterol level of 20 mg/dL is very low and is associated with an increased risk of coronary artery disease. The patient would likely be treated by their physician with pharmacological and non-pharmacological therapies to raise the HDL cholesterol level.**

4. The optimal level of low-density lipoprotein cholesterol is less than 100. A value of 110 mg/dL is considered near optimal. High levels of LDL cholesterol increase the risk of coronary artery disease.

System Specific: Cardiovascular/Pulmonary and Lymphatic Systems
Content Outline: Foundations for Evaluation, Differential Diagnosis, & Prognosis

## Exam One: Question 37

A physical therapist performs palpation with a patient positioned in standing as part of a respiratory assessment. Which structure would be the MOST appropriate to assess with the therapist positioned behind the patient?

1. mediastinum
2. upper chest wall motion
3. middle chest wall motion
4. **lower chest wall motion**

---

**Correct Answer: 4** (Frownfelter p. 210)

Palpation of chest wall motion is performed segmentally to compare the motion over the upper, middle, and lower lobes while the patient is breathing quietly and while breathing deeply.

1. The physical therapist palpates the mediastinum to evaluate for deviation of the trachea by inserting the tip of the index finger in the suprasternal notch. This is done facing the patient.

2. The physical therapist evaluates upper chest wall expansion by placing the palms of the hands anteriorly over the chest wall from the fourth rib upward. The therapist's fingers are stretched over the trapezius and the thumbs placed together along the midline of the chest. The therapist faces the patient.

3. The physical therapist evaluates middle chest wall expansion by placing the fingers laterally over the posterior axillary folds with the thumbs together along the midline of the chest. The therapist faces the patient.

4. **The lower chest wall expansion is evaluated with the patient's back to the therapist and the therapist's fingers wrapped around the anterior axillary folds with the tips of the thumbs together at the vertebral spines.**

System Specific: Cardiovascular/Pulmonary and Lymphatic Systems
Content Outline: Physical Therapy Examination

---

## Exam One: Question 38

A physical therapist prepares a whirlpool treatment for a scheduled patient. Which treatment area would place the patient at the GREATEST risk for hyperthermia?

1. wrist and hand
2. **thigh**
3. elbow
4. foot and ankle

---

**Correct Answer: 2** (Cameron p. 264)

Whirlpool treatments stress the body's ability to dissipate heat and therefore can result in hyperthermia or other forms of heat illness. The larger the portion of the body immersed in the whirlpool the greater the level of heat stress.

1. Whirlpool treatment to the wrist and hand would require only a small portion of the upper extremity to be immersed.

2. **Whirlpool treatment to the thigh would require the patient to be immersed up to the waist, possibly including a portion of the torso, depending on the configuration of the whirlpool tank. This level of immersion would place the patient at the greatest risk for hyperthermia.**

3. Whirlpool treatment to the elbow would require the majority of the upper extremity to be immersed. This is greater than the level of immersion for the wrist and hand, but it still represents a relatively small percentage of the total body surface.

4. Whirlpool treatment to the foot and ankle would require the lower extremity to be immersed only to the midcalf.

System Specific: Other Systems
Content Outline: Interventions

## Exam One: Question 39

A group of physical therapists conducts scoliosis screenings on adolescents as part of physical therapy week. The MOST appropriate action after identifying an adolescent with a moderate scoliotic curve is to:

1. refer the adolescent for further orthopedic assessment
2. educate the adolescent as to the cause of the scoliosis
3. devise an exercise program for the adolescent
4. instruct the adolescent in the importance of proper posture

**Correct Answer: 1** (Goodman - Pathology p. 1113)
A patient with moderate scoliosis should be referred to an orthopedic physician since treatment for moderate curves requires a spinal orthosis and physical therapy intervention for posture, flexibility, strengthening, respiratory function, and proper utilization of the spinal orthosis.

1. **Scoliosis is a condition that will respond to treatment best when detected early. Common postural findings with scoliosis include increased spacing between the elbow and trunk during standing, leg length discrepancy, uneven shoulder and hip heights, and prominence on one side of the pelvis or breast (due to rotation of the curve).**
2. Although education regarding scoliosis is important, the most appropriate action when identifying a moderate curve is to refer the patient to a physician for further assessment and treatment. The physician will educate the patient based on their findings regarding the scoliosis.
3. A physician should always evaluate a patient with moderate scoliosis prior to the development and implementation of an exercise program.
4. Postural training will not rectify or maintain a moderate scoliotic curve. Moderate curves require multifaceted treatment and physician involvement.

System Specific: Musculoskeletal System
Content Outline: Interventions

## Exam One: Question 40

A physical therapist checks the water temperature of the hot pack machine after several patients report the heat being very strong. Which of the following temperatures would be acceptable?

1. 64 degrees Celsius (147 degrees Fahrenheit)
2. **71 degrees Celsius (160 degrees Fahrenheit)**
3. 83 degrees Celsius (181 degrees Fahrenheit)
4. 94 degrees Celsius (201 degrees Fahrenheit)

**Correct Answer: 2** (Cameron p. 161)
A hot pack must be stored in hot water between 158 to 167 degrees Fahrenheit (70 to 75 degrees Celsius). Six to eight towel layers should be applied between the hot pack and the treatment surface. The size and shape of the hot pack varies depending on the size and contour of the treatment area.

1. 64 degrees Celsius (147 degrees Fahrenheit) would be less than the recommend water temperature in the hot pack unit. As a result, the hot pack would not possess the necessary thermal energy with the traditional number of towel layers.
2. **71 degrees Celsius (160 degrees Fahrenheit) is consistent with the recommended range of water temperature and therefore the hot pack will possess the requisite amount of thermal energy.**
3. 83 degrees Celsius (181 degrees Fahrenheit) would be greater than the recommended water temperature and therefore may create a potential safety risk for the patient without adding additional towel layers.
4. 94 degrees Celsius (201 degrees Fahrenheit) would be significantly greater than the recommended water temperature and would place the patient at significant risk for a superficial burn.

System Specific: Non-Systems
Content Outline: Equipment & Devices; Therapeutic Modalities

## Exam One: Question 41

A physical therapist employed in an outpatient physical therapy clinic attempts to obtain informed consent from a 17-year-old male prior to initiating a formal exercise test. The patient signs the informed consent form, however, the patient's parents dropped him off at the clinic and are now unavailable to sign the form. The MOST appropriate therapist action is:

1. complete the exercise test
2. secure another physical therapist to witness the exercise test
3. contact the referring physician and request approval to complete the exercise test
4. **reschedule the exercise test**

**Correct Answer: 4** (Scott - Promoting Legal and Ethical Awareness p. 222)
Obtaining informed consent from patients before exercise testing is an important ethical and legal consideration. Physical therapists have an obligation to obtain informed consent from patients prior to initiating intervention activities. If a patient is under the age of 18 the therapist is required to obtain informed consent from the patient and a parent or legal guardian.

1. The physical therapist should have a valid consent form before performing the exercise test.

2. Having another physical therapist witness the test is not a substitute for legal informed consent.

3. Having the physician approve the test is not a substitute for legal informed consent.

4. **A patient's status as a minor makes it necessary that a parent or legal guardian sign the consent form. The physical therapist should reschedule the test to a time when a parent can sign the consent form.**

System Specific: Cardiovascular/Pulmonary and Lymphatic Systems
Content Outline: Interventions

## Exam One: Question 42

A physical therapist attempts to obtain a general assessment of a patient's cognitive status. The patient is a 62-year-old female three days status post total hip arthroplasty. The MOST appropriate action is:

1. review the patient's medical record
2. **conduct a patient interview**
3. conduct a physical examination
4. consult with family members

**Correct Answer: 2** (Bickley p. 55)
A patient interview provides a physical therapist with an opportunity to assess patient cognition. This approach is often more appropriate than relying on a previous entry in the medical record, particularly with a patient status post surgery.

1. It is important to review a patient's medical record prior to the initial examination so that the therapist has an understanding of past medical history, current medical status, physician orders, and any precautions or contraindications, however, this is not the optimal choice for assessment of the patient's cognitive status.

2. **Conducting a patient interview allows the therapist to evaluate the patient's cognitive status through a routine screening of person, place, and time or through more extensive testing such as the Mini Mental State Examination.**

3. A physical examination would focus on a patient's physical attributes and impairments. Items such as muscle strength, range of motion, and anthropometric measurements are examples of common components of a physical examination.

4. Consultation with family members may assist in certain scenarios, however, cannot replace direct screening of the patient when assessing cognition.

System Specific: Other Systems
Content Outline: Physical Therapy Examination

## Exam One: Question 43

A physical therapist attempts to secure a wheelchair for a patient with an incomplete spinal cord injury. The patient is a 28-year-old female that is very active and relies on a wheelchair as her primary mode of transportation. Which type of wheelchair design would be the MOST appropriate for the patient?

1. standard chair with a rigid frame
2. **lightweight chair with a rigid frame**
3. standard chair with a folding frame
4. lightweight chair with a folding frame

**Correct Answer: 2** (Physical Therapist's Clinical Companion p. 324)
A lightweight wheelchair will be significantly easier for the patient to propel and maneuver, while a rigid frame provides the necessary durability and strength required for an active individual.

1. A standard chair would not be optimal secondary to the increased weight of the chair and the patient's decreased strength due to the incomplete spinal cord injury.

2. **A lightweight wheelchair is easier to propel and maneuver. The chair is made from stainless steel or aluminum which also enhances durability. The rigid frame allows for strength and a smoother ride for the patient.**

3. A standard wheelchair with a folding frame would not be optimal secondary to the increased weight of the chair which would necessitate greater effort for mobility and transportation. The folding frame would not possess the durability required for an active individual.

4. The lightweight wheelchair is a better choice for the patient, however, the folding frame is not an optimal choice based on the patient's activity level.

System Specific: Neuromuscular and Nervous Systems
Content Outline: Interventions

## Exam One: Question 44

A physical therapist attempts to select an assistive device for a patient rehabilitating from a traumatic brain injury. The patient is occasionally impulsive, however, has fair standing balance and good upper and lower extremity strength. Which of the following would be the MOST appropriate assistive device?

1. cane
2. axillary crutches
3. Lofstrand crutches
4. **walker**

**Correct Answer: 4** (Pierson p. 219)
A walker would be the most appropriate assistive device to use since the patient can stand without support, however, has only fair standing balance and is impulsive at times. A walker does not require a great deal of coordination.

1. A cane is appropriate to assist with balance and stability, however, it does not provide a large amount of assistance due to the small base of support. A cane would not be appropriate for a patient that presents with impulsivity and only fair standing balance.

2. Axillary crutches are appropriate for patients of all weight bearing levels, however, require a higher level of coordination. Injury can occur to axillary vessels and nerves if used improperly. The device would not be appropriate for the patient based on their present balance and the medical diagnosis.

3. Lofstrand crutches are an option for patients that need more support than a cane. The crutches provide minimal stability and require functional standing balance and coordination for use. Lofstrand crutches would not be appropriate for a patient with fair balance and impulsivity.

4. **A walker is appropriate for patients of varying weight bearing levels. The device offers the greatest amount of stability due to its large base of support. The stability offered by the walker is necessary due to the patient's fair standing balance and impulsivity. Proper supervision would be necessary based on the patient's diagnosis.**

System Specific: Neuromuscular and Nervous Systems
Content Outline: Interventions

## Exam One: Question 45

A physical therapist examines a 16-year-old male diagnosed with left knee anterior cruciate ligament insufficiency. During the examination a Lachman test is performed. Ideally, the therapist should perform the test with the knee in:

1. **20-30 degrees flexion**
2. 30-40 degrees flexion
3. 40-50 degrees flexion
4. 80-90 degrees flexion

**Correct Answer: 1** (Magee p. 767)

The Lachman test is perhaps the most common ligamentous instability test designed to assess the integrity of the anterior cruciate ligament. It is typically performed with the patient in a supine position and the knee flexed 20-30 degrees. The therapist applies an anterior directed force to the tibia on the femur. A positive test is indicated by excessive anterior translation of the tibia on the femur with a diminished or absent end-point and may be indicative of an anterior cruciate ligament injury.

1. **20-30 degrees of knee flexion is generally accepted as the amount of knee flexion used for the Lachman test. The position approximates a functional position and all parts of the anterior cruciate ligament are relatively taut.**

2. 30-40 degree of knee flexion is slightly greater than the recommended amount of knee flexion for the Lachman test.

3. 40-50 degrees is significantly greater than the recommended amount of knee flexion for the Lachman test.

4. 80-90 degrees of knee flexion more closely approximates the position of the knee when performing the anterior drawer test.

System Specific: Musculoskeletal System
Content Outline: Physical Therapy Examination

## Exam One: Question 46

A patient with cerebellar dysfunction exhibits signs of dysmetria. Which of the following activities would be the MOST difficult for the patient?

1. rapid alternating pronation and supination of the forearms
2. **placing feet on floor markers while walking**
3. walking at varying speeds
4. marching in place

**Correct Answer: 2** (Umphred p. 840)

Dysmetria refers to an inability to modulate movement where patients will either overestimate or underestimate their targets. The cerebellum is normally responsible for the timing, force, extent, and direction of the limb movement in order to correctly reach a target.

1. Dysdiadochokinesia refers to the inability to perform rapid alternating movements such as pronation and supination of the forearms. As speed increases there is typically a rapid loss of range of movement and rhythm of movement. This condition is a result of damage to the cerebellum.

2. **Dysmetria occurs with cerebellar lesions and is defined as the inability to appropriately reach a target. An example of dysmetria would be the inability of a patient to place their feet on floor markers successfully while walking.**

3. Difficulty walking at varying speeds is common with cerebellar pathology, however, the activity is not associated with dysmetria.

4. Patients with cerebellar lesions often have difficulty modulating movement. As a result, irregular stepping patterns and poor upright stance make activities such as marching in place difficult.

System Specific: Neuromuscular & Nervous Systems
Content Outline: Interventions

# Exam One: Question 47

A physical therapist examines a patient referred to physical therapy diagnosed with a medial collateral ligament sprain. During the examination the patient appears to be relaxed and comfortable, however, is extremely withdrawn. Which of the following questions would be the MOST appropriate to further engage the patient?

1. Is this the first time you have injured your knee?
2. Have you ever been to physical therapy before?
3. How long after your injury did you see a physician?
4. **What do you hope to achieve in physical therapy?**

**Correct Answer: 4** (Goodman – Differential Diagnosis p. 36)
Physical therapists often use a variety of strategies to increase the level of patient participation in treatment sessions. Open-ended questions allow patients to answer with a myriad of responses, while closed-ended questions can often be answered with a yes or no response.

1. The question can be answered with a simple "yes or no" and therefore would be unlikely to increase patient participation.
2. The question would also require a simple "yes or no" response.
3. The question requires the patient to respond with an amount of time. The response, although not a "yes or no," would be equally unlikely to further engage the patient.
4. **The question requires the patient to provide some level of insight towards their physical therapy goals and may provide a foundation for a meaningful exchange between the patient and therapist. The information obtained by the therapist can be valuable when designing an appropriate plan of care.**

System Specific: Musculoskeletal System
Content Outline: Physical Therapy Examination

# Exam One: Question 48

A physical therapist conducts a pre-operative training session for a patient scheduled for surgery to repair a large rotator cuff tear. The patient is a 54-year-old male who is employed as an insurance agent. During the pre-operative training session the patient inquires as to the amount of time before he is able to return to recreational activities such as tennis and golf. The MOST appropriate time frame is typically:

1. 6-8 weeks
2. 12-14 weeks
3. **24-28 weeks**
4. 36-40 weeks

**Correct Answer: 3** (Brotzman p. 159)
The majority of rotator cuff tears occur in individuals greater than 40 years of age with a history of recurrent shoulder symptoms. A large tear is most often considered to be between 3-5 centimeters in diameter.

1. At 6-8 weeks following surgery the patient may be ready to begin to focus on strength, endurance, and neuromuscular control while continuing to attain or maintain range of motion. Since the tear was classified as "large" in some cases the patient may not be permitted to perform strengthening exercises until 10-12 weeks.
2. At 12-14 weeks following surgery the patient focuses on task specific strengthening activities. The activities occur in a controlled environment and the patient is closely monitored.
3. **At 24-28 weeks the patient is typically allowed to return to recreational activities such as tennis and golf. Strengthening activities may continue during this period since studies have shown that on average patients regain approximately 80% of their strength in the involved shoulder compared to the uninvolved shoulder in the first six months following surgery. The actual rate of recovery is influenced significantly by the size of the tear.**
4. At 36-40 weeks the patient typically has returned to their previous lifestyle and continues to gain strength in the involved shoulder. Studies have shown that even after one year only 90% of the strength in the shoulder has been achieved compared to the uninvolved shoulder.

System Specific: Musculoskeletal System
Content Outline: Foundations for Evaluation, Differential Diagnosis, & Prognosis

## Exam One: Question 49

A physical therapist determines a patient's heart rate by counting the number of QRS complexes in a six second electrocardiogram strip. Assuming the therapist identifies eight QRS complexes in the strip, the patient's heart rate should be recorded as:

1. 40 beats per minute
2. 60 beats per minute
3. **80 beats per minute**
4. 100 beats per minute

**Correct Answer: 3** (Brannon p. 193)

The QRS complex reflects the depolarization of the ventricles during the cardiac cycle. If the heart rhythm is regular, the minute heart rate can be determined by counting the number of QRS complexes in 6 seconds on the electrocardiogram paper, then multiply this number by 10 to get the heart rate for one minute.

1. For a heart rate of 40 beats per minute, there would be four QRS complexes in six seconds.
2. For a heart rate of 60 beats per minute, there would be six QRS complexes in six seconds.
3. **Eight QRS complexes per six second interval x 10 (six second intervals per minute) = 80 QRS complexes per minute.**
4. For a heart rate of 100 beats per minute, there would be 10 QRS complexes in six seconds.

System Specific: Cardiovascular/Pulmonary and Lymphatic Systems
Content Outline: Physical Therapy Examination

## Exam One: Question 50

A physical therapist prepares to apply a sterile dressing to a wound after debridement. The therapist begins the process by drying the wound using a towel. The therapist applies medication to the wound using a gauze pad and then applies a series of dressings that are secured using a bandage. Which step would NOT warrant the use of sterile technique?

1. **bandage**
2. dressings
3. medication
4. towel

**Correct Answer: 1** (Pierson p. 303)

Application of a bandage does not require sterile technique since the bandage does not come in direct contact with the wound. All other aspects of the scenario require sterile technique to protect the wound and surrounding area, the patient, and the caregiver from contamination.

1. **A bandage is applied over a dressing. The function of a bandage is to keep the dressing in position, provide a barrier between the dressing and the environment, provide pressure, and protect the wound. Since the bandage does not come in direct contact with the area surrounding the wound, sterile technique is not required.**
2. A dressing for a wound is usually comprised of several layers. The function of a dressing is to prevent contamination to the wound, keep microorganisms within the wound from infecting other areas, assist with healing, apply pressure, absorb drainage, and prevent further injury to the wound. Application of all layers of a dressing requires sterile technique.
3. The application of medication is part of the dressing in this scenario and should be applied using sterile technique.
4. If the patient is using the towel directly on the area of the wound, the towel must be sterile and the therapist must use sterile technique to avoid contamination.

System Specific: Other Systems
Content Outline: Interventions

## Exam One: Question 51

A physical therapist inspects a wound over the sacrum of a 58-year-old female. The therapist would MOST accurately classify the presented wound as:

1. stage I
2. stage II
3. **stage III**
4. stage IV

**Correct Answer: 3** (Sussman p. 78)
The National Pressure Ulcer Advisory Panel pressure ulcer staging criteria was developed for use with pressure ulcers. The staging criteria range from I - IV.

1. A stage I ulcer is characterized by an observable pressure related alteration of intact skin whose indicators, as compared to an adjacent or opposite area on the body, may include changes in skin color, skin temperature, skin stiffness or sensation.
2. A stage II ulcer is characterized by partial-thickness skin loss that involves the epidermis and/or dermis. The ulcer is superficial and presents clinically as an abrasion, a blister or a shallow crater.
3. **A stage III ulcer is characterized by full-thickness skin loss that involves damage or necrosis of subcutaneous tissue that may extend down to, but not through, underlying fascia. The ulcer presents clinically as a deep crater with or without undermining adjacent tissue.**
4. A stage IV ulcer is characterized by full-thickness skin loss with extensive destruction, tissue necrosis or damage to muscle, bone or supporting structures (e.g., tendon, joint capsule).

System Specific: Other Systems
Content Outline: Physical Therapy Examination

## Exam One: Question 52

A physical therapist observes a patient's breathing as part of a respiratory assessment. Which muscle of respiration is MOST active during forced expiration?

1. diaphragm
2. external intercostals
3. **internal intercostals**
4. upper trapezius

**Correct Answer: 3** (Frownfelter p. 50)
Unlike quiet expiration, which is mainly a passive process primarily dependent on the elastic properties of lung tissue, forced expiration is an active process. In addition to the rectus abdominis, external and internal obliques, and transverse abdominis contracting to compress the abdominal viscera, the ribs are pulled downward by action of the internal intercostals and quadratus lumborum.

1. The diaphragm is the principal inspiratory muscle.
2. The external intercostals act to lift the ribs during deep inspiration.
3. **The internal intercostals assist to pull the ribs downward during forced expiration.**
4. The upper trapezius acts as an accessory muscle of inspiration by assisting to elevate and stabilize the scapulae.

System Specific: Cardiovascular/Pulmonary and Lymphatic Systems
Content Outline: Physical Therapy Examination

## Exam One: Question 53

A physical therapist treats a patient who sustained a right lateral ankle sprain less than six hours ago. The therapist contemplates the use of cold water immersion as a cryotherapeutic agent. What would be the primary limitation of this type of intervention?

1. decreased cell metabolism
2. excessive vasoconstriction of blood vessels
3. the involved extremity cannot be elevated
4. decreased nerve conduction velocity

**Correct Answer: 3** (Cameron p. 267)

There are a wide range of cryotherapeutic agents commonly used in physical therapy including cold whirlpool, ice packs, ice massage, cold sprays, and contrast baths. Physical therapists should be aware of the advantages and limitations of each of the identified cryotherapeutic agents.

1. Cryotherapy decreases metabolic reactions including those involved in the inflammatory process.
2. Cryotherapy initially causes local vasoconstriction of smooth muscles in an attempt to conserve heat. Vasoconstriction is responsible for decreasing the formation and accumulation of edema.
3. Cold water immersion is an acceptable form of cryotherapy, however, is not ideal when treating an acute lower extremity injury since the injured limb cannot be elevated. Inflammation is most effectively controlled if the cryotherapeutic agent is applied in conjunction with elevation and compression. Several other cryotherapeutic agents such as ice packs or Cryocuff may be more desirable interventions.
4. Cryotherapy decreases the nerve conduction velocity of both sensory and motor nerves. Cryotherapy has the greatest effect on the conduction velocity of myelinated and small fibers, and the least effect on the conduction velocity of unmyelinated and large fibers.

System Specific: Musculoskeletal System
Content Outline: Interventions

## Exam One: Question 54

A physical therapist reviews the results of a pulmonary function test for a 58-year-old male patient recently admitted to the hospital. The therapist notes that the patient's total lung capacity is significantly increased when compared to established norms. Which medical condition would MOST likely produce this type of result?

1. chronic bronchitis
2. emphysema
3. spinal cord injury
4. pulmonary fibrosis

**Correct Answer: 2** (Frownfelter p. 86)

Emphysema is a chronic obstructive pulmonary disease characterized by an abnormal and permanent enlargement of the air spaces distal to the terminal bronchiole, accompanied by destructive changes in their walls. Changes in lung tissue resulting from these anatomic changes include loss of elastic recoil, collapse of airways during exhalation, and airflow obstruction.

1. In chronic bronchitis there is hypertrophy of the submucosal glands in the large and small bronchi and trachea with hypersecretion of mucus sufficient to cause a productive cough. Pulmonary function tests demonstrate a forced expiratory volume in one second ($FEV_1$) of < 65% of the predicted value. Total lung capacity is not increased in true chronic bronchitis.
2. As a result of the pathologic changes to the lung tissue in emphysema, the lungs become hyperinflated. Due to the loss of elastic recoil, obstruction to airflow is seen as an increase in total lung capacity, residual volume, and functional residual capacity.
3. Spinal cord injury is a neuromuscular cause of restrictive lung dysfunction. Characteristic changes in pulmonary function tests may include decreases in total lung capacity, vital capacity, and inspiratory capacity.
4. Pulmonary fibrosis is an inflammatory process affecting the alveoli that grossly distorts the architecture of the lung. These changes cause a decrease in lung compliance and a decrease in lung volumes including total lung capacity, vital capacity, functional residual capacity, and residual volume.

System Specific: Cardiovascular/Pulmonary and Lymphatic Systems
Content Outline: Foundations for Evaluation, Differential Diagnosis, & Prognosis

## Exam One: Question 55

A patient rehabilitating from an upper extremity injury affecting the left shoulder performs a resistive exercise as shown. Which muscle would be primarily emphasized when performing the pictured exercise?

1. pectoralis major
2. **supraspinatus**
3. teres major
4. teres minor

**Correct Answer: 2** (Magee p. 262)
The image shows a patient performing an isometric shoulder exercise emphasizing shoulder abduction. An isometric exercise utilizes isometric contractions that occur when tension develops, but there is no change in the length of the muscle.

1. The clavicular head of the pectoralis major originates on the anterior surface of the medial half of the clavicle. The sternocostal head originates on the anterior surface of the sternum and six costal cartilages and the aponeurosis of the external oblique muscle. The muscles insert on the lateral lip of the intertubercular groove of the humerus. The clavicular head acts to flex the humerus while the sternocostal head extends the humerus. Collectively, the muscle adducts and medially rotates the humerus.

2. **The supraspinatus originates on the middle two-thirds of the supraspinous fossa of the scapula and inserts on the greater tubercle of the humerus. The muscle acts to abduct the shoulder and stabilize the head of the humerus in the glenoid fossa.**

3. The teres major originates on the dorsal surface of the inferior angle of the scapula and lower third of the border of the scapula. The muscle inserts on the lesser tubercle of the humerus. The muscle acts to medially rotate, adduct, and extend the shoulder.

4. The teres minor originates on the upper two-thirds of the dorsal surface of the lateral border of the scapula and inserts on the greater tubercle of the humerus. The muscle acts to laterally rotate the shoulder.

System Specific: Musculoskeletal System
Content Outline: Interventions

## Exam One: Question 56

A physical therapist prepares a patient status post CVA with global aphasia for discharge from a rehabilitation hospital. The patient will be returning home with her husband and daughter. The MOST appropriate form of education to facilitate a safe discharge is to:

1. **perform hands-on training sessions with the patient and family members**
2. videotape the patient performing transfers and activities of daily living
3. provide written instructions on all activities of daily living and functional tasks
4. meet with family members to discuss the patient's present status and abilities

**Correct Answer: 1** (O'Sullivan p. 761)
In order to facilitate a safe discharge, it is imperative that the physical therapist is certain that the patient and family are aware of and can perform the necessary activities of daily living (ADLs) and functional tasks that will be required. The most effective manner in which to ascertain the family's readiness is to have them perform the required tasks and observe their competence.

1. **Hands-on training sessions provide unique opportunities for the therapist to assess the competence of family members in a structured environment.**

2. Videotaping the necessary transfers and ADLs will provide the family with a visual aid, however, it does not ensure that they are able to safely perform the tasks with the patient.

3. Providing written instructions on all ADLs and functional tasks is an important part of a home exercise program and should be included in all discharge plans. This action, however, does not ensure that family members are able to perform the tasks safely with the patient.

4. Meeting with the family member to discuss the patient's present status and abilities is an important part of any discharge planning, however, it will not provide the therapist with enough information on the family's competence with the required tasks.

System Specific: Neuromuscular and Nervous Systems
Content Outline: Interventions

## Exam One: Question 57

A physical therapist treats a 36-year-old male status post knee surgery. The therapist performs goniometric measurements to quantify the extent of the patient's extension lag. Which of the following would NOT provide a plausible rationale for the extension lag?

1. muscle weakness
2. **bony obstruction**
3. inhibition by pain
4. patient apprehension

---

**Correct Answer: 2** (Kisner p. 891)

Patients that demonstrate an extension lag have greater passive extension than active extension. The difference in the passive and active extension range of motion is used to quantify the amount of the lag.

1. Muscle weakness would provide a plausible rationale for an extension lag since force production is necessary to produce active motion. Inability to produce adequate force to move the tibia on the femur while performing active extension would produce the lag.

2. **A bony obstruction would not produce an extension lag since passive range of motion and active range of motion would be equal. In essence, the obstruction would interfere with the ability to perform both passive and active knee extension.**

3. Inhibition by pain would provide a plausible rationale for an extension lag. The amount of pain produced during an active muscle contraction may make it impossible for the muscle to generate the required amount of force to actively extend the tibia on the femur. The difference in the passive extension versus the active extension would determine the amount of the extension lag.

4. Patient apprehension would provide a plausible rationale for an extension lag since the patient may be unwilling to actively move the knee through the available active range of motion due to fear or anxiety.

System Specific: Musculoskeletal System
Content Outline: Physical Therapy Examination

---

## Exam One: Question 58

A patient successfully completes ten anterior lunges. The physical therapist would like to modify the activity to maximally challenge the patient in the sagittal plane. Which of the following modifications would be the MOST appropriate?

1. anterior lunge with concurrent bilateral elbow flexion to 45 degrees with five pound weights
2. **anterior lunge with concurrent bilateral shoulder flexion to 90 degrees with five pound weights**
3. anterior lunge with concurrent unilateral shoulder flexion to 90 degrees with a five pound weight
4. anterior lunge with concurrent bilateral shoulder abduction to 45 degrees with five pound weights

---

**Correct Answer: 2** (Norkin p. 5)

The sagittal plane divides the body into left and right halves. Motions in the sagittal plane include flexion and extension. In order to maximally challenge the patient in this plane, therapists should choose the option that moves the patient's center of gravity furthest outside the base of support in the sagittal plane.

1. Bilateral elbow flexion would challenge the patient in the sagittal plane, however, the movement would not significantly change the center of gravity since the upper extremities would be held close to the body.

2. **Bilateral shoulder flexion would create the largest forward movement and would therefore provide the greatest challenge for the patient due to the center of gravity moving forward outside the base of support.**

3. Unilateral shoulder flexion would challenge the patient in the sagittal plane, however, it would not provide as much of a challenge as the bilateral shoulder flexion due to the decreased amount of mass moving outside the base of support (one upper extremity versus two upper extremities).

4. Bilateral shoulder abduction would challenge the patient in the frontal plane.

System Specific: Musculoskeletal System
Content Outline: Interventions

# Exam One: Question 59

A physical therapist teaches a patient positioned in supine to posteriorly rotate her pelvis. The patient has full active and passive range of motion in the upper extremities, but is unable to achieve full shoulder flexion while maintaining a posterior pelvic tilt. Which of the following could BEST explain these findings?

1. capsular tightness
2. **latissimus dorsi tightness**
3. pectoralis minor tightness
4. quadratus lumborum tightness

**Correct Answer: 2** (Kendall p. 325)

A posterior pelvic tilt results in the posterior superior iliac spines of the pelvis moving posteriorly and inferiorly. This motion results in hip extension and lumbar spine flexion.

1. The capsular pattern at the glenohumeral joint is lateral rotation, abduction, and medial rotation. A capsular pattern of restriction at the glenohumeral joint would limit range of motion, however, would not be influenced by the position of the pelvis.

2. **Shortening of the latissimus dorsi often results in a limitation of shoulder flexion or abduction due to the muscle's origin on the external lip of the iliac crest and its insertion on the intertubercular groove of the humerus.**

3. Pectoralis minor tightness may have a direct effect on shoulder range of motion, however, would not be influenced by the position of the pelvis. Pectoralis minor tightness is often best identified by positioning a patient in supine with the arms at their side and the palms facing upward. The relative tightness of the muscle is determined by the extent to which the shoulder is raised from the table and the amount of resistance felt to downward pressure on the shoulder.

4. Quadratus lumborum tightness may affect the ability of the pelvis to achieve the posterior pelvic tilt position required in the question, however, would not affect shoulder range of motion since the muscle does not directly attach to the shoulder joint.

System Specific: Musculoskeletal System
Content Outline: Interventions

# Exam One: Question 60

A physical therapist observes a burn on the dorsal surface of a patient's arm. The wound area is mottled red with a number of blisters. The therapist informs the patient that healing should take place in less than three weeks. This description is MOST indicative of a:

1. superficial burn
2. **superficial partial-thickness burn**
3. deep partial-thickness burn
4. full-thickness burn

**Correct Answer: 2** (Goodman - Pathology p. 436)

The burn classification system most commonly utilized uses the terms superficial, partial-thickness (superficial and deep), and full-thickness. The system provides a general description of the most common clinical findings associated with each type of burn.

1. A superficial burn involves only the outer epidermis. The involved area may be red with slight edema. Healing occurs without evidence of scarring in 2-5 days.

2. **A superficial partial-thickness burn involves the epidermis and the upper portion of the dermis. The involved area may be extremely painful and exhibit blisters. Healing occurs with minimal to no scarring in 5-21 days.**

3. A deep partial-thickness burn involves complete destruction of the epidermis and the majority of the dermis. The involved area may appear to be discolored with broken blisters and edema. Damage to nerve endings may result in only moderate levels of pain. Healing occurs with the potential for hypertrophic scars and keloids in 21-35 days.

4. A full-thickness burn involves complete destruction of the epidermis and dermis along with partial damage of the subcutaneous fat layer. The involved area often presents with eschar formation and minimal to no pain. Patients with full-thickness burns require grafts and may be susceptible to infection.

System Specific: Other Systems
Content Outline: Foundations for Evaluation, Differential Diagnosis, & Prognosis

## Exam One: Question 61

A group of physical therapists develops a research project that examines the effect of increased abdominal muscle strength on forced vital capacity and forced expiratory volume. In order to conduct the study, the therapists are required to have the approval of the hospital Institutional Review Board. The PRIMARY purpose of the committee is to:

1. protect the hospital from unnecessary litigation
2. **ensure the rights of research subjects are protected**
3. examine the design of the research project
4. assess the financial ramifications of the research project

**Correct Answer: 2** (Portney p. 52)
Federal regulations require an Institutional Review Board (IRB) review all research proposals prior to implementation to ensure that the rights of research subjects are protected.

1. By ensuring the rights of research subjects, the IRB may protect the hospital from litigation, however, protection from litigation is not the primary purpose of the committee.

2. **Ensuring the rights of research subjects is the primary purpose of the IRB. To do this, the IRB evaluates the scientific merit of the project, the competence of the investigators, the risk to subjects, and the feasibility of the project based on available resources.**

3. In evaluating the scientific merit of the project, the IRB will examine the research design. This is done to ensure that the rights of research subjects are protected since if the project is not scientifically sound, there can be no benefit.

4. In evaluating the research proposal, the IRB will consider the feasibility of the project based on the identified resources.

System Specific: Non-Systems
Content Outline: Safety and Protection; Professional Responsibilities; Research

## Exam One: Question 62

Members of a community health task force evaluate a proposal for a new adolescent screening program. Several members of the task force raise questions as to the validity of the screening instrument. Which measure of validity examines the instrument's ability to identify diseased persons by comparing true positives?

1. adaptability
2. selectivity
3. **sensitivity**
4. specificity

**Correct Answer: 3** (Portney p. 620)
The validity of a diagnostic test is evaluated by its ability to accurately assess the presence or absence of the target condition. A diagnostic test can have four possible outcomes: true positive, true negative, false positive, and false negative.

1. Adaptability is not a measure of the accuracy or validity of a diagnostic or screening test.

2. Selectivity is not a measure of the accuracy or validity of a diagnostic or screening test.

3. **Sensitivity is a measure of the validity of a screening test, based on the probability that the screening test will be positive in someone with the disease or target condition (i.e., true positive).**

4. Specificity is a measure of the validity of a screening test, based on the probability that the screening test will be negative in someone who does not have the disease or target condition (i.e., true negative).

System Specific: Non-Systems
Content Outline: Safety and Protection; Professional Responsibilities; Research

## Exam One: Question 63

A physical therapist attempts to quantify a patient's endurance level by administering a maximal exercise test. What is the PRIMARY limitation of a maximal exercise test?

1. Maximal exercise testing requires participants to exercise to the point of volitional fatigue.
2. Maximal exercise testing does not typically allow a steady state heart rate at each work rate.
3. Maximal exercise testing is not useful in diagnosing coronary artery disease.
4. Maximal exercise testing requires progressive stages of increasing work intensities without rest intervals.

**Correct Answer: 1** (American College of Sports Medicine p. 352)

The decision to use a maximal or submaximal exercise test depends largely on the reasons for the test and the availability of the appropriate equipment and personnel. Maximal exercise testing offers increased sensitivity for diagnosing coronary artery disease in asymptomatic individuals and provides a better estimate of maximum oxygen uptake than a submaximal test.

1. **The primary limitation of a maximal exercise test is that it requires the individual to exercise to the point of volitional fatigue. Some subjects terminate the exercise test due to fatigue or exercise intolerance before reaching their physiological maximum. This reduces the sensitivity of the estimate of maximum oxygen uptake.**
2. Most standardized exercise test protocols have the individual exercise at two or three minute intervals before increasing to a higher workload. This type of design allows the subject to come to a steady state heart rate for each workload before increasing the workload.
3. Maximal exercise testing is used to help diagnose coronary artery disease and offers better sensitivity than submaximal exercise testing.
4. Most standard exercise test protocols are continuous and do not allow formal rest intervals, however, this is not considered the primary limitation of the test.

System Specific: Cardiovascular/Pulmonary and Lymphatic Systems
Content Outline: Physical Therapy Examination

## Exam One: Question 64

A physical therapist prepares to complete a sensory examination on a patient rehabilitating from a lower extremity burn. Which of the following would serve as the BEST predictor of altered sensation?

1. presence of a skin graft
2. **depth of burn injury**
3. percentage of body surface affected
4. extent of hypertrophic scarring

**Correct Answer: 2** (Rothstein p. 960)

Patients with burns often experience a number of sensory changes. These changes can include impaired sensation or increased sensitivity. Although many factors contribute to sensory alteration, the depth of the burn appears to be the best predictor.

1. Skin grafts are typically used with full-thickness burns and although there is a predictable pattern of sensory alteration with full-thickness burns, the absence of a skin graft would not be useful to predict sensory changes in less severe burns (i.e., superficial and partial-thickness).
2. **It is possible to predict the relative extent of sensory alteration based on the depth of the burn. For example, a superficial partial-thickness burn is characterized by extreme pain and significant sensitivity to temperature change, while a full-thickness burn is characterized by an absence of pain and inability to identify temperature change.**
3. The percentage of body surface affected provides information on the size or extent of the burn, but does not provide information on other important variables such as the depth or severity of the burn.
4. Hypertrophic scarring refers to an overgrowth of dermal constituents that remain within the boundaries of the wound. This occurs as a result of scar formation when the burn extends into the dermis. Hypertrophic scarring results in poor cosmesis and the development of contractures that may limit function. The presence of hypertrophic scarring provides only limited information regarding the extent of altered sensation.

System Specific: Other Systems
Content Outline: Foundations for Evaluation, Differential Diagnosis, & Prognosis

## Exam One: Question 65

In a randomized control trial, the best way for a researcher to protect against the biases associated with the patient's and investigator's knowledge of the treatment the patient is receiving is to:

1. randomly assign patients to the intervention group
2. perform an intent-to-treat analysis of the data
3. **use a double-blind research design**
4. use a single-blind research design

**Correct Answer: 3** (Portney p. 170)

Blinding is a form of experimental control implemented to protect against bias since both the patients' knowledge of their treatment and the investigator's expectations can influence performance or the recording and reporting of the outcomes under study.

1. Random assignment of patients to groups is recommended to ensure that each individual has an equal chance of being assigned to any group so that no systematic bias exists with respect to the attributes that might differentially affect the outcomes. Random assignment does not protect against the biases associated with the patient's and investigator's knowledge of the treatment the patient is receiving.

2. In an intent-to-treat analysis, the data is analyzed according to the original random assignments, according to the way subjects were intended to be treated, regardless of the treatment they actually received. An intent-to-treat analysis does not protect against the biases associated with the patient's and investigator's knowledge of the treatment the patient is receiving.

3. **Protection against bias associated with the patient's and investigator's knowledge of the treatment is best achieved by a double-blind research design. In a double-blind study, neither the subject nor the investigator is aware of the identity of the treatment group to which the subject was assigned until after the data is collected and the subject has completed the study.**

4. In a single-blind study, only the subject is kept unaware of the identity of the treatment group to which the subject was assigned. The potential for bias from the investigator remains uncontrolled.

System Specific: Non-Systems
Content Outline: Safety and Protection; Professional Responsibilities; Research

## Exam One: Question 66

A physician orders compression garments for an ambulatory patient who has significant difficulty with lower extremity edema. How much pressure would typically be necessary to control lower extremity edema?

1. 10 mm Hg
2. 18 mm Hg
3. 25 mm Hg
4. **35 mm Hg**

**Correct Answer: 4** (Cameron p. 331)

Compression garments are available in different thicknesses and different levels of pretension. The garments offer varying levels of pressure ranging from 10 mm Hg to 50 mm Hg. The amount of pressure selected must be determined based on the intended goals of the therapeutic intervention.

1. A pressure of 10 mm Hg would not be adequate to control lower extremity edema in an ambulatory patient.

2. A pressure of 16-18 mm Hg is characteristic of off the shelf stockings used to prevent deep vein thrombosis in patients who are in bed.

3. A pressure of 20-30 mm Hg is used to control scar tissue formation.

4. **A pressure of 30-40 mm Hg is used to control edema in ambulatory patients.**

System Specific: Cardiovascular/Pulmonary and Lymphatic Systems
Content Outline: Interventions

## Exam One: Question 67

A physical therapist monitors the vital signs of a 52-year-old male during a graded exercise test. The patient was prompted to seek medical assistance two weeks ago after becoming short of breath on two separate occasions. When interpreting the data collected during the exercise test, which finding would serve as the BEST indicator that the patient had exerted a maximal effort?

1. **failure of the heart rate to increase with further increases in intensity**
2. rise in systolic blood pressure of 50 mm Hg when compared to the resting value
3. rating of 12 on a perceived exertion scale
4. rating of 2/4 on the dyspnea scale

**Correct Answer: 1** (American College of Sports Medicine p. 352)
Failure of the heart rate to increase with further increases in intensity occurs when the patient can no longer meet the demands imposed by the exercise, signifying the patient has produced a maximal effort.

1. **Failure of the heart rate to increase with further increases in exercise intensity is an objective indicator that the patient made a maximal effort during graded exercise testing.**
2. The normal response to exercise is a progressive increase in systolic blood pressure, typically 10 mm Hg per MET, with a possible plateau at peak exercise. A rise in systolic blood pressure of 50 mm Hg over the resting rate is common during graded exercise testing, however, is not necessarily an indication of a maximal effort.
3. A rating of 12 on the 6-20 perceived exertion scale corresponds only to a perception of "fairly light" to "somewhat hard." A rating of > 17 ("very hard") is an indicator of a maximal effort.
4. A rating of 2 out of 4 on the dyspnea scale corresponds to a perception of "moderate, bothersome" degree of breathlessness. This level does not indicate a maximal effort.

System Specific: Cardiovascular/Pulmonary and Lymphatic Systems
Content Outline: Interventions

## Exam One: Question 68

A physical therapist performs an examination on a patient with hip-knee-ankle-foot orthoses. The patient can ambulate independently with the orthoses and Lofstrand crutches, however, due to the high energy expenditure often becomes fatigued very rapidly. Which disorder would be MOST consistent with this scenario?

1. amyotrophic lateral sclerosis
2. peripheral neuritis
3. neurogenic arthropathy
4. **spina bifida**

**Correct Answer: 4** (Physical Therapist's Clinical Companion p. 314)
A hip-knee-ankle foot orthosis (HKAFO) consists of bilateral knee-ankle-foot orthoses with an extension to the hip joints with use of a pelvic band. The orthosis can control rotation at the hip and abduction/adduction. The orthosis is heavy and restricts patients to a swing-to or swing-through gait pattern. The HKAFO is indicated for patients with hip, knee, ankle, and foot weakness.

1. Amyotrophic lateral sclerosis is a chronic degenerative disease that produces both upper and lower motor neuron impairments. Motor weakness typically presents in a distal to proximal progression. The weakness combined with fatigue make it unlikely the patient would be able to ambulate with HKAFOs.
2. Peripheral neuritis refers to the inflammation of the nerves and is synonymous with the term peripheral neuropathy. Since every peripheral nerve has a highly specialized function, a wide array of symptoms can occur when nerves are damaged. Symptoms may include numbness, tingling, paresthesia, sensitivity to touch, and muscle weakness. As a result, it is difficult to determine the type of orthoses that would be appropriate based on the diagnosis alone.
3. Neurogenic arthropathy is a rapidly destructive arthropathy due to impaired pain perception and position sense, which can result from various underlying disorders, most commonly diabetes and stroke. Symptoms may include joint swelling, effusion, deformity, and instability. Treatment most often consists of joint immobilization which slows the disease progression.
4. **Spina bifida is a neural tube defect characterized by defective closure of the vertebral column. Although the exact clinical presentation of spina bifida can vary considerably, HKAFOs are often employed to assist pediatric patients with ambulation activities. The high energy cost of ambulating with the orthosis often makes community ambulation difficult.**

System Specific: Neuromuscular & Nervous Systems
Content Outline: Foundations for Evaluation, Differential Diagnosis, & Prognosis

## Exam One: Question 69

A physician orders electromyography for a patient with a brachial plexus injury to objectively determine the extent of pathology. Which of the following responses is MOST indicative of a normal muscle at rest?

1. electrical silence
2. spontaneous potentials
3. polyphasic potentials
4. occasional motor unit potentials

**Correct Answer: 1** (Cameron p. 81)

Electromyography is a test that assesses the health of the muscles and the nerves controlling the muscles. A needle electrode is inserted through the skin into the muscle. The electrical activity detected by this electrode is displayed on an oscilloscope, and may be heard through a speaker. The presence, size, and shape of the wave form (i.e., the action potential) produced on the oscilloscope provides information about the ability of the muscle to respond when the nerves are stimulated.

1. A normally innervated muscle is electrically silent at rest. Once the insertion activity (caused by the trauma of needle insertion) resolves, there should be no action potential on the oscilloscope.

2. Spontaneous electrical potentials, like fibrillations and positive sharp waves, are seen in an acutely denervated muscle. Fibrillation and positive sharp waves are the result of spontaneous discharge of a single muscle fiber.

3. Polyphasic potentials are the electrical potentials from a denervated motor unit. A motor unit that exhibits five or more phases is referred to as polyphasic.

4. Occasional motor unit potentials occurring during minimal effort muscle contractions two to three weeks after injury suggest neurapraxia (a temporary failure of nerve conduction in the absence of structural nerve changes due to blunt injury, compression or ischemia).

System Specific: Other Systems
Content Outline: Foundations for Evaluation, Differential Diagnosis, & Prognosis

## Exam One: Question 70

A physical therapist completes a quantitative gait analysis on a patient rehabilitating from a lower extremity injury. As part of the examination the therapist measures the number of steps taken by the patient in a 30 second period. This measurement technique can be used to measure:

1. acceleration
2. cadence
3. velocity
4. speed

**Correct Answer: 2** (Levangie p. 528)

Time and distance parameters are often used to provide a basic description of gait. Commonly used temporal variables include stance time, single limb and double support time, cadence, and speed. Commonly used distance variables include stride length, step length, width of base of support, and degrees of toe-out.

1. Acceleration is the rate of change of velocity with respect to time.

2. Cadence is defined as the number of steps taken by a person per unit of time. Walking with increased cadence decreases the duration of double support time. A cadence of 110 steps per minute is typical in a male, while 116 steps per minute is typical in a female.

3. Velocity is the rate of linear forward motion of the body which is measured most often in centimeters per second, meters per second or miles per hour. Walking velocity equals distance walked divided by time.

4. Speed is usually classified as slow, free or fast. Free speed of gait refers to a person's normal walking speed.

System Specific: Musculoskeletal System
Content Outline: Physical Therapy Examination

# Exam One: Question 71

Members of a health promotion task force design a program that annually will screen individuals in selected retirement communities for osteoporosis. Which screening tool would be the MOST cost effective and reliable to incorporate as part of the program?

1. physical activity survey
2. dietary analysis
3. **measuring height**
4. urinalysis screening

**Correct Answer: 3** (Goodman – Differential Diagnosis p. 439)
Osteoporosis is a metabolic bone disorder where the rate of bone resorption accelerates while the rate of bone formation slows down. This reduction of bone mass decreases the overall bone density and strength. The disease is more common in women and in particular postmenopausal women who are not taking hormone replacement therapy.

1. Physical activity is critical throughout the lifespan to maintain and possibly increase peak bone mass. The effect of exercise on slowing the decline of bone mineral density later in life has been found to be only modest. Regular activity has been found to decrease the incidence of hip fractures in individuals greater than 65 years of age.

2. A dietary analysis is an important component of a comprehensive plan of care for a patient with osteoporosis. This is important at all ages and in particular with postmenopausal women who require more than 1,500 mg of calcium daily. Adequate levels of Vitamin D are also necessary to assist in the absorption of dietary calcium. A dietary analysis would be expensive to implement and analyze and would be heavily influenced by a variety of other factors other than the presence or absence of osteoporosis.

3. **Measuring a person's height is an inexpensive and relatively reliable method to screen for osteoporosis. Patients with osteoporosis often lose height due to a reduction in bone mass, postural changes (e.g., kyphosis, Dowager's hump), and vertebral compression fractures.**

4. A urinalysis screening would be of minimal benefit since osteoporosis is a metabolic bone disorder and the primary affect of the condition is on the musculoskeletal system.

System Specific: Other Systems
Content Outline: Physical Therapy Examination

# Exam One: Question 72

A physical therapist treats a patient diagnosed with lateral epicondylitis using iontophoresis. The therapist uses dexamethasone with a current intensity of 3 mA for 20 minutes. How often during the treatment session should the therapist check the skin?

1. every minute
2. **every three to five minutes**
3. every ten minutes
4. at the conclusion of the treatment session

**Correct Answer: 2** (Prentice - Therapeutic Modalities p. 180)
Iontophoresis is the process by which medications are induced through the skin into the body by means of continuous direct current electrical stimulation. Sensitivity reactions most often occur due to the use of direct current, and in some cases, due to a particular therapeutic ion. A physical therapist should frequently check the patient's skin for a sensitivity reaction during iontophoresis treatment.

1. Checking the skin every minute would be both impractical and unnecessary since the time period is too short.

2. **An interval of three to five minutes provides the necessary frequency to detect an adverse reaction and take the necessary corrective action.**

3. An interval of ten minutes would be too long especially given the duration of the iontophoresis treatment (i.e., 20 minutes). Checking the skin at ten minute intervals would make it difficult for the physical therapist to detect a sensitivity reaction in a timely manner.

4. Checking the skin at the conclusion of treatment is common, however, additional skin checks need to occur at regular intervals throughout the duration of the 20 minute session.

System Specific: Non-Systems
Content Outline: Equipment & Devices; Therapeutic Modalities

## Exam One: Question 73

A physical therapist strongly suspects a patient is intoxicated after arriving for his treatment session. When asked if he has been drinking, the patient indicates he consumed six or seven alcoholic beverages before driving to therapy. The therapist's MOST appropriate action is to:

1. continue to treat the patient, assuming he can remain inoffensive to other patients
2. modify the patient's present treatment program to minimize the effects of alcohol
3. **contact a member of the patient's family to take the patient home**
4. instruct the patient to leave the clinic

**Correct Answer: 3** (Guide for Professional Conduct)

A physical therapist should never treat a patient under the influence of alcohol. Therapists should be aware of signs and symptoms associated with intoxication and be willing to take necessary action to avoid harm to the patient and others when this situation is identified.

1. The amount of alcohol consumed would make it unsafe for the patient to participate in physical therapy. Effects of alcohol include impaired judgment, delayed reactions, impaired memory, and poor coordination.

2. Modifying the program to minimize the effects of alcohol condones the patient's behavior and makes it likely the same behavior would occur in the future.

3. **Contacting a member of the patient's family allows the physical therapist to discontinue the session and at the same time provides the patient with a safe method to return home.**

4. Instructing the patient to leave the clinic could create a safety issue for the patient and possibly others, particularly if the patient is driving a motor vehicle.

System Specific: Non-Systems
Content Outline: Safety and Protection; Professional Responsibilities; Research

## Exam One: Question 74

A physical therapist observes a patient's postural strategies following a series of perturbations. Which strategy is BEST illustrated in the image?

1. ankle strategy
2. **hip strategy**
3. suspensory strategy
4. stepping strategy

**Correct Answer: 2** (O'Sullivan p. 253)

Automatic postural strategies are automatic motor responses that are used to maintain the center of gravity over the base of support. These responses occur in a predictable pattern based on the magnitude of the perturbation.

1. The ankle strategy is the first strategy to be elicited by a small range and slow velocity perturbation when the feet are on the ground. Muscle groups contract in a distal to proximal progression to control postural sway from the ankle joint.

2. **The presented image is an example of the hip strategy which is elicited by a greater force, challenge or perturbation. The hips will move (in the opposite direction from the head) in order to maintain balance. Muscle groups contract in a proximal to distal progression in order to counteract the loss of balance.**

3. The suspensory strategy is used to lower the center of gravity during standing or ambulation in order to better control the center of gravity. Examples of this strategy include knee flexion, crouching or squatting. This strategy is often used when both mobility and stability are required during a task (e.g., surfing).

4. The stepping strategy is elicited through unexpected challenges or perturbations during static standing or when the perturbation produces a movement that displaces the center of gravity beyond the base of support. The lower extremities step and/or upper extremities reach to regain a new base of support.

System Specific: Neuromuscular and Nervous Systems
Content Outline: Physical Therapy Examination

## Exam One: Question 75

A patient rehabilitating from cardiac surgery is monitored using an arterial line. The PRIMARY purpose of an arterial line is to:

1. measure right atrial pressure
2. measure heart rate and oxygen saturation
3. measure pulmonary artery pressure
4. **measure blood pressure**

**Correct Answer: 4** (Pierson p. 276)

An arterial line is inserted directly into an artery and is used to continuously monitor blood pressure or to obtain blood samples.

1. Right atrial pressure, (i.e., blood pressure in the right atrium) is measured by a balloon tipped catheter which is advanced from the femoral, brachial or internal jugular vein into the pulmonary artery. A common version is the Swan-Ganz catheter.

2. In addition to the primary purpose of measuring blood pressure, an arterial line can be used as an access point for sampling arterial blood. Oxygen saturation can be determined by the analysis of blood gases, however, an arterial line does not monitor heart rate.

3. Like right atrial pressure, pulmonary artery pressure is measured by a Swan-Ganz catheter or another form of pulmonary artery catheter.

4. **An arterial line is a monitoring device consisting of a catheter that is inserted into an artery and attached to an electronic monitoring system. The device is considered to be more accurate than traditional measures of blood pressure and does not require repeated needle punctures.**

System Specific: Cardiovascular/Pulmonary and Lymphatic Systems
Content Outline: Interventions

## Exam One: Question 76

A physical therapist listens to the lung sounds of a 56-year-old male with chronic bronchitis. The patient was admitted to the hospital two days ago after complaining of shortness of breath and difficulty breathing. While performing auscultation the therapist identifies distinct lung sounds with a high constant pitch during exhalation. This type of sound is MOST consistent with:

1. crackles
2. rales
3. rhonchi
4. **wheezes**

**Correct Answer: 4** (Frownfelter p. 206)

Wheezes are described as high-pitched, musical sounds made by air passing through narrowed tracheobronchial airways.

1. Crackles are discontinuous, adventitious breath sounds heard during auscultation of the lungs due to fluid accumulation in the distal airways or when collapsed alveoli reopen during inspiration.

2. Rales are synonymous with crackles.

3. Rhonchi are lower-pitched, continuous, adventitious breath sounds occurring during inspiration or expiration and are caused by the turbulence of air passing through secretions in large and mid-sized bronchi.

4. **Wheezes are continuous, high-pitched, adventitious breath sounds that are most frequently heard on exhalation and are associated with airway obstruction or bronchospasm. There can also be inspiratory wheezing caused by movement of air through secretions. Wheezes are commonly associated with asthma and bronchitis.**

System Specific: Cardiovascular/Pulmonary and Lymphatic Systems
Content Outline: Physical Therapy Examination

## Exam One: Question 77

A physical therapist administers iontophoresis to a patient with a lower extremity ulceration in an attempt to promote tissue healing. Which ion would BEST meet the stated objective?

1. acetate
2. magnesium
3. lidocaine
4. **zinc**

**Correct Answer: 4** (Prentice - Therapeutic Modalities p. 185)

Iontophoresis refers to the transcutaneous delivery of ions into the body for therapeutic purposes using an electrical current. Physical therapists must possess an in-depth awareness of the most appropriate ions to treat specific conditions.

1. Acetate, from acetic acid, is a negatively charged ion used to treat calcific deposits.
2. Magnesium, from magnesium sulfate, is a positively charged ion used as a muscle relaxant and vasodilator.
3. Lidocaine, from xylocaine, is a positively charged ion used to treat pain and inflammation associated with acute inflammatory conditions.
4. **Zinc, from zinc oxide, is a positively charged ion used to promote healing, most often with open lesions and ulcerations.**

System Specific: Non-Systems
Content Outline: Equipment & Devices; Therapeutic Modalities

## Exam One: Question 78

A twelve-month-old child with cerebral palsy demonstrates an abnormal persistence of the positive support reflex. During therapy this would MOST likely interfere with:

1. sitting activities
2. **standing activities**
3. prone on elbows activities
4. supine activities

**Correct Answer: 2** (Ratliffe p. 27)

The positive support reflex promotes extension of the lower extremities and trunk with weight bearing through the balls of the feet. If this reflex persists, it can interfere with standing, ambulation, balance reactions and weight shifting in standing, and can lead to plantar flexion contractures.

1. Sitting activities would not be influenced by the positive support reflex since there would not be stimulation to the ball of the foot. An infant is usually able to sit unsupported at six to seven months.
2. **The positive support reflex is elicited by contact of the ball of the foot with the floor surface when placed into a standing position. The reflex causes rigid extension of the lower extremities and trunk with weight bearing. This reflex is typically integrated at two to four months of age.**
3. Prone on elbows activities would not be influenced by the positive support reflex since there would not be stimulation to the ball of the foot. An infant is usually able to maintain the prone on elbows position at three to four months.
4. Supine activities would not be influenced by the positive support reflex since there would not be stimulation to the ball of the foot while in supine.

System Specific: Neuromuscular & Nervous Systems
Content Outline: Interventions

## Exam One: Question 79

A physical therapist treats a patient with limited shoulder range of motion. The therapist hypothesizes that the patient's range of motion limitation is due to pain and not a specific tissue restriction. Which graded oscillation techniques would be the MOST appropriate to treat this patient?

1. grades I, II
2. grades II, III
3. grades III, IV
4. grades IV, V

**Correct Answer: 1** (Kisner p. 116)
Graded oscillation techniques include grade I, II, III, IV, and V. The type of grade selected is dependent on the intended treatment objective.

1. **Grade I refers to small amplitude oscillations at the beginning of the range. Grade II refers to large amplitude oscillations performed within the range, but not reaching the limit of range. Grade I and II are primarily used to treat pain by stimulating mechanoreceptors.**

2. Grade II was previously defined. Grade III refers to large amplitude oscillations performed to the limit of available range and stressed into tissue resistance.

3. Grade III was previously defined. Grade IV refers to small amplitude oscillations performed at the limit of available range and stressed into the tissue resistance. Grade III and IV are primarily used as stretching maneuvers.

4. Grade IV was previously defined. Grade V refers to small amplitude, high velocity thrust techniques used to break up adhesions.

System Specific: Musculoskeletal System
Content Outline: Interventions

## Exam One: Question 80

A patient diagnosed with lateral epicondylitis is referred to physical therapy. The therapist elects to use iontophoresis over the lateral epicondyle. Which type of current would the physical therapist use to administer the treatment?

1. direct
2. alternating
3. pulsatile
4. interferential

**Correct Answer: 1** (Cameron p. 223)
Iontophoresis refers to the transcutaneous delivery of ions into the body for therapeutic purposes using an electrical current.

1. **Direct current is characterized by an uninterrupted flow of electrons toward the positive pole. This type of current is necessary to move the charged ions across the dermal barrier. Polarity remains constant and is determined by the physical therapist based on treatment goals and the polarity of the chosen ion.**

2. Alternating current is characterized by the bidirectional (constantly changing) continuous flow of electrons. Electrons flowing in an alternating current move from the negative to positive pole, reversing direction when the polarity is reversed.

3. Pulsatile current is characterized by three or more pulses grouped together and may be unidirectional or bidirectional. A series of unidirectional pulses is known as monophasic pulsed current and a series of bidirectional pulses is known as biphasic pulsed current.

4. Interferential current combines two high frequency alternating waveforms that are biphasic. The two waveforms are delivered through two sets of electrodes through separate channels in the same stimulator.

System Specific: Non-Systems
Content Outline: Equipment & Devices; Therapeutic Modalities

## Exam One: Question 81

A physical therapist sets up a patient for mechanical traction to the lumbar spine. The therapist's objective is to provide soft tissue stretch to surrounding muscles. Assuming the therapist uses a force equivalent to 25% of the patient's body weight and the patient has tolerated treatment without difficulty on several other occasions, the MOST appropriate duration of treatment is:

1. 5 minutes
2. 10 minutes
3. **25 minutes**
4. 40 minutes

**Correct Answer: 3** (Cameron p. 299)

Physical therapists must carefully select the parameters associated with mechanical traction (i.e., force, hold/relax times, duration) based on the desired outcomes.

1. A duration of five minutes would be appropriate for a brief trial of traction. This may be warranted if the patient's initial symptoms are severe. Shorter treatment times are generally recommended for the initial session or in the acute phase of rehabilitation.

2. A duration of 10 minutes would be appropriate for an initial session if the patient's symptoms are mild or moderate.

3. **A duration of 25 minutes would be appropriate when attempting to stretch soft tissue in a patient who has previously tolerated traction without difficulty. A duration of 20-30 minutes is most often recommended for stretching soft tissue or reducing muscle spasm. This amount of time allows for a prolonged stretch without compromising the integrity of other structures.**

4. A duration of 40 minutes or more using spinal traction is not necessary since the literature has shown that treatment of this duration generally provides no additional benefit.

System Specific: Non-Systems
Content Outline: Equipment & Devices; Therapeutic Modalities

## Exam One: Question 82

A physical therapist designs an exercise program for a patient rehabilitating from cardiac surgery. During the treatment session the therapist monitors the patient's oxygen saturation rate. Which of the following would be MOST representative of a normal oxygen saturation rate?

1. 82%
2. 87%
3. 92%
4. **97%**

**Correct Answer: 4** (Brannon p. 296)

Oxygen saturation ($SaO_2$) measures the percentage of hemoglobin saturated with oxygen. The normal range for oxygen saturation is between 95-98% in healthy individuals.

1. A value of 82% $SaO_2$ demonstrates significant hypoxemia resulting in the patient requiring continuous use of supplemental oxygen. Exercise would be contraindicated at this level.

2. A value of 87% $SaO_2$ is below the range for acceptable oxygen saturation. The patient would likely use supplemental oxygen at rest and with exercise. The patient should maintain 90% $SaO_2$ or better with supplemental oxygen use.

3. A value of 92% $SaO_2$ is not within normal limits for oxygen saturation. In most cases, the patient would be monitored to ensure that $SaO_2$ does not fall below 90% during exertion or exercise.

4. **A value of 97% $SaO_2$ is within the specified range of 95-98% for normal arterial oxygen saturation.**

System Specific: Cardiovascular/Pulmonary and Lymphatic Systems
Content Outline: Physical Therapy Examination

## Exam One: Question 83

A physical therapist attempts to assess the integrity of the L4 spinal level. Which deep tendon reflex would provide the therapist with the MOST useful information?

1. lateral hamstrings
2. medial hamstrings
3. **patellar reflex**
4. Achilles reflex

**Correct Answer: 3** (Magee p. 805)
Deep tendon reflexes are assessed to examine the integrity of the afferent and efferent peripheral nervous systems and the ability of the central nervous system to inhibit the reflex. The physical therapist should attempt to assess the reflex by striking the tendon with the reflex hammer after placing the tendon on slight stretch.

1. The lateral hamstrings reflex is innervated at the S1-S2 spinal level.
2. The medial hamstrings reflex is innervated at the L5-S1 spinal level.
3. **The patellar reflex is innervated at the L3-L4 spinal level.**
4. The Achilles reflex is innervated at the S1-S2 spinal level.

System Specific: Neuromuscular & Nervous Systems
Content Outline: Physical Therapy Examination

## Exam One: Question 84

A physical therapist examines a patient diagnosed with rotator cuff tendonitis in physical therapy. The physician referral indicates the patient should be seen three times a week, however, after examining the patient the therapist feels once a week is adequate. The MOST appropriate therapist action is to:

1. **schedule the patient once a week and notify the referring physician of your rationale**
2. schedule the patient as indicated on the physician referral
3. ask the patient how often they would like to be seen in physical therapy
4. attempt to determine if the patient's insurance will cover physical therapy visits three times a week

**Correct Answer: 1** (Guide for Professional Conduct)
The *Guide for Professional Conduct* published by the American Physical Therapy Association states that a physical therapist shall avoid overutilization of physical therapy services.

1. **The physical therapist should determine the frequency of physical therapy sessions based solely on the needs of the patient. The therapist should communicate the rationale for the change in the frequency of the physical therapy sessions to the physician.**
2. Scheduling the patient three times a week when it is not necessary would result in overutilization of physical therapy services. The Code of Ethics published by the American Physical Therapy Association states that a physical therapist shall seek only such remuneration as is deserved and reasonable for physical therapy services.
3. The patient's wishes should always be considered, however, only the physical therapist can determine the actual frequency of physical therapy visits necessary.
4. If the additional visits are not necessary it does not matter if the services will be reimbursed by the patient's insurance.

System Specific: Musculoskeletal System
Content Outline: Interventions

## Exam One: Question 85

A patient receiving physical therapy services in an outpatient clinic explains that he has felt nauseous since having his methotrexate medication level altered. The MOST appropriate physical therapist action is to:

1. explain to the patient that nausea is very common when altering medication levels
2. ask the patient to stop taking the prescribed medication
3. request that the patient make an appointment with the physician
4. **request that the patient contact the physician's office**

**Correct Answer: 4** (Ciccone p. 226)

Methotrexate is used as a disease-modifying agent in the treatment of rheumatoid arthritis. Adverse effects include nausea, gastrointestinal distress, hemorrhage, cough, shortness of breath, and lower extremity edema. Nausea refers to the sensation of unease and discomfort in the stomach with an urge to vomit. Although nausea is not a medical emergency, it is appropriate for the patient to inform the physician of any persistent side effects as soon as possible.

1. A physical therapist may inform a patient about common side effects of medications, however, the patient's acknowledgement of feeling nauseous after having their medication level altered would still require contact with the physician.
2. A physical therapist is not able to ask a patient to discontinue the use of a prescribed medication. This action is the sole responsibility of the physician.
3. A recommendation to make an appointment with the physician is appropriate, however, would not typically be as timely as contacting the physician's office. Given the patient's present status (i.e., feeling nauseous), it is necessary to advocate for an immediate resolution to the problem.
4. **A patient should contact the physician's office whenever they experience side effects that may be associated with prescribed medication. Direct contact with the physician is an immediate response which makes the physician aware of the patient's present status and allows them to potentially modify or discontinue medication.**

System Specific: Other Systems
Content Outline: Foundations for Evaluation, Differential Diagnosis, and Prognosis

## Exam One: Question 86

A physical therapist completes a fitness screening on a 34-year-old male prior to prescribing an aerobic exercise program. Which value is MOST representative of the patient's age-predicted maximal heart rate?

1. 168
2. 174
3. **186**
4. 196

**Correct Answer: 3** (Minor p. 124)

Age-predicted maximal heart rate can be determined as follows: 220-age.

1. Based on the formula of 220-age, the rate of 168 is too low for this patient's age-predicted maximal heart rate.
2. Based on the formula of 220-age, the rate of 174 is too low for this patient's age-predicted maximal heart rate.
3. **Based on the formula of 220-age, the rate of 186 is equal to this patient's age-predicted maximal heart rate.**
4. Based on the formula of 220-age, the rate of 196 is too high for this patient's age-predicted maximal heart rate. This would be an unsafe rate for exercise.

System Specific: Cardiovascular/Pulmonary and Lymphatic Systems
Content Outline: Physical Therapy Examination

## Exam One: Question 87

A physical therapist observes a patient ambulating in the clinic. The therapist notes that the patient's pelvis drops on the left during left swing phase. This deviation is usually caused by weakness of the:

1. left gluteus medius
2. **right gluteus medius**
3. left gluteus minimus
4. right gluteus minimus

**Correct Answer: 2** (Magee p. 966)

A Trendelenburg gait pattern is characterized by excessive lateral trunk flexion and weight shifting over the stance leg. The gait pattern is often seen with lesions of the superior gluteal nerve, L5 radiculopathy, and poliomyelitis.

1. The gluteus medius acts to abduct the hip joint. The anterior fibers medially rotate and may assist in flexion of the hip joint. The posterior fibers laterally rotate and may assist in extension. Weakness of the left gluteus medius would be characterized by the pelvis dropping on the right during right swing phase.

2. **Weakness of the right gluteus medius would be characterized by the pelvis dropping on the left during left swing phase.**

3. The gluteus minimus acts to abduct and medially rotate the hip and may assist in hip flexion. Weakness of the left gluteus minimus would be identified by diminished strength in medial rotation and abduction of the left hip.

4. Weakness of the right gluteus minimus would be identified by diminished strength in medial rotation and abduction of the right hip.

System Specific: Musculoskeletal System
Content Outline: Physical Therapy Examination

## Exam One: Question 88

A physical therapist examines a patient diagnosed with cerebellar degeneration. Which of the following clinical findings is NOT typically associated with this condition?

1. **athetosis**
2. dysmetria
3. nystagmus
4. dysdiadochokinesia

**Correct Answer: 1** (O'Sullivan p. 201)

Athetosis is a term used to describe slow, writhing, and involuntary movements that may occur with damage to the basal ganglia.

1. **Athetosis is characterized by extraneous and involuntary movements, slowness of movement, and alterations in muscle tone. Athetoid movements may look "wormlike" with a rotatory component evident.**

2. Dysmetria occurs with cerebellar lesions and is defined as the inability to appropriately reach a target. The cerebellum is normally responsible for the timing, force, extent, and direction of the limb movement in order to correctly reach the target.

3. Nystagmus can occur with cerebellar lesions and is usually classified as gaze-evoked nystagmus. The patient will attempt to look toward an object in the periphery, but the eyes will drift involuntarily back to neutral. This may occur unilaterally or bilaterally depending on the cause of cerebellar dysfunction.

4. Dysdiadochokinesia occurs with cerebellar lesions and is defined as the inability to perform rapid alternating movements.

System Specific: Neuromuscular & Nervous Systems
Content Outline: Foundations for Evaluation, Differential Diagnosis, & Prognosis

## Exam One: Question 89

A physical therapist examines a 36-year-old female referred to physical therapy after experiencing back pain two weeks ago. The patient identifies the majority of pain in the buttock and lateral thigh and denies any referred pain down the posterior leg. Presently she rates the pain as a "3" on a 0-10 scale, however, indicates that the pain is a "6" or a "7" during activity or at night. This description MOST closely resembles:

1. sacroilitis
2. iliolumbar syndrome
3. piriformis syndrome
4. **trochanteric bursitis**

**Correct Answer: 4** (Goodman – Differential Diagnosis p. 654)

There are a multitude of medical diagnoses that are associated with low back pain. Physical therapists should be familiar with the typical clinical presentation of these diagnoses and be able to identify a given diagnosis after completing a thorough examination.

1. Sacroilitis refers to inflammation of one or both of the sacroiliac joints. The patient is typically tender to palpation directly over the sacroiliac joint.

2. Iliolumbar syndrome, also known as iliac crest pain syndrome, is caused by inflammation or a tear of the iliolumbar ligament. The condition often leads to referred pain in the pelvis or groin. The patient is often tender to palpation over the iliac crest and pain tends to be exacerbated with sidebending.

3. Piriformis syndrome refers to a condition in which the piriformis muscle irritates the sciatic nerve causing pain in the buttocks and referred pain along the course of the sciatic nerve. The primary patient complaint is buttock pain that is made worse by sitting, stair climbing or squatting.

4. **Trochanteric bursitis refers to inflammation of the trochanteric bursa, which is a pad-like sac that protects the soft tissue structures that cross the posterior portion of the greater trochanter. The patient is often extremely sensitive to palpation over the bursa and may experience lateral thigh pain that is exacerbated by activity or periods of prolonged rest.**

System Specific: Musculoskeletal System
Content Outline: Foundations for Evaluation, Differential Diagnosis, & Prognosis

## Exam One: Question 90

A physical therapist completes a sensory assessment on a 61-year-old female diagnosed with multiple sclerosis. As part of the assessment the therapist examines stereognosis, vibration, and two-point discrimination. What type of receptor is primarily responsible for generating the necessary information?

1. deep sensory receptors
2. **mechanoreceptors**
3. nociceptors
4. thermoreceptors

**Correct Answer: 2** (O'Sullivan p. 134)

Mechanoreceptors generate information related to discriminative sensations. The information is then mediated through the dorsal column-medial lemniscal system. Examples of mechanoreceptors include free nerve endings, Merkel's disks, Ruffini endings, hair follicle endings, Meissner's corpuscles, and Pacinian corpuscles.

1. Deep sensory receptors are sensory receptors that are located in the muscles, tendons, and joints. Muscle and joint receptors are both classified as deep sensory receptors and include Golgi tendon organs, Pacinian corpuscles, muscle spindle, Ruffini endings, free nerve endings, and joint receptors. They evaluate position sense, proprioception, muscle tone, and movement.

2. **Mechanoreceptors are sensory receptors that respond to mechanical deformation of the area surrounding a receptor. They are responsible for sensations of touch, pressure, itch, tickle, vibration, and discriminative touch.**

3. Nociceptors are specialized peripheral free nerve endings that are found throughout different tissues within the body that respond to noxious stimuli and result in the perception of pain. A painful stimulus will ascend through the spinal cord via the lateral spinothalamic tract. Several areas of the brain provide specific responses to the painful stimulus.

4. Thermoreceptors are sensory receptors that respond to changes in temperature. Stimulation of the cold or warm receptors will ascend through the spinal cord via the lateral spinothalamic tract.

System Specific: Neuromuscular & Nervous Systems
Content Outline: Physical Therapy Examination

## Exam One: Question 91

A physical therapist is employed at a physician owned physical therapy clinic that charges by the modality. One of the physicians, who is an owner of the practice, requests that all of his patients receive a minimum of heat, ultrasound, and electrical stimulation during each session. The therapist feels that the majority of patients receive little benefit from the treatment regimen. The MOST appropriate IMMEDIATE action is:

1. ignore the physician's request and treat each patient as you feel is indicated
2. **discuss with the physician the rationale for requesting modalities on each patient**
3. report the physician's conduct to the American Medical Association
4. inform the physician that he is abusing the health care system

**Correct Answer: 2** (Guide for Professional Conduct)
The *Guide for Professional Conduct* states that physical therapists seek remuneration for their services that is deserved and reasonable.

1. The physical therapist must treat each patient as they feel is indicated, however, it would be inappropriate to ignore the physician's request without addressing the issue directly.

2. **The physical therapist should have a candid conversation with the physician and attempt to understand the rationale for the physician's current approach. The physical therapist can use the opportunity to educate the physician on appropriate utilization of physical therapy services.**

3. The physical therapist should address the issue directly with the physician prior to considering a formal complaint with an external licensing agency.

4. Informing a physician that he is abusing the health care system would likely place the physician in a defensive posture and negate any opportunity to have a meaningful conversation. In addition, the action could be considered slanderous.

System Specific: Non-Systems
Content Outline: Safety and Protection; Professional Responsibilities; Research

## Exam One: Question 92

A physical therapist completes a developmental assessment on an infant. At what age should an infant begin to sit with hand support for an extended period of time?

1. **6-7 months**
2. 8-9 months
3. 10-11 months
4. 12-15 months

**Correct Answer: 1** (Ratliffe p. 46)
Infants typically develop the stability to sit with hand support in the sixth to seventh month.

1. **Sitting for a prolonged period of time with upper extremity support usually occurs at 6-7 months of age. The infant will also bring objects to midline, hold a bottle with two hands, and roll to prone.**

2. When an infant is 8-9 months of age, they will typically manipulate toys in sitting, raise themselves from supine to sit, pull to stand with support, and transfer objects with a controlled release.

3. When an infant is 10-11 months of age, they will typically stand briefly without support, transition from supine to sitting or quadruped, pull to stand through half kneel, and use a pincer grasp.

4. When an infant is 12 months of age, they will typically stand up through quadruped, use a wide array of sitting positions, walk without support, creep up stairs, throw a ball in sitting, and mark paper with crayons.

System Specific: Neuromuscular and Nervous Systems
Content Outline: Physical Therapy Examination

## Exam One: Question 93

A physical therapist collects data as part of a preseason athletic screening program designed to identify individuals susceptible to heat illness. Which of the following measures would be the MOST valuable to collect?

1. height
2. weight
3. **percent body fat**
4. vital capacity

**Correct Answer: 3** (American College of Sports Medicine p. 551)

A variety of factors can increase a patient's susceptibility to heat illness. Some of the more common risk factors include age extremes (i.e., children, elderly), excessive muscle mass or obese individuals, previous history of heat illness, salt or water depletion, and acute or chronic illness.

1. Height without additional information such as weight would provide little benefit to identify individuals susceptible to heat illness.

2. Weight without additional information such as height would provide little benefit to identify individuals susceptible to heat illness.

3. **Patients with a higher percent body fat are more susceptible to heat illness since the larger the person is, the more difficult it will be to dissipate excess heat since the body's cooling system cannot work quickly enough. In addition, research has revealed that overweight individuals may generate up to 18% greater heat production than underweight individuals.**

4. Vital capacity is defined as the maximal volume forcefully expired after a maximal inspiration. The pulmonary function test measure would not be useful in isolation to identify individuals susceptible to heat illness.

System Specific: Other Systems
Content Outline: Foundations for Evaluation, Differential Diagnosis, & Prognosis

## Exam One: Question 94

A physical therapist employed in an acute care hospital works with a patient on bed mobility activities. The therapist would like to incorporate a strengthening activity for the hip extensors that will improve the patient's ability to independently reposition in bed, however, the patient does not have adequate strength to perform bridging. The MOST appropriate exercise activity is:

1. anterior pelvic tilts
2. heel slides
3. straight leg raises
4. **isometric gluteal sets**

**Correct Answer: 4** (O'Sullivan p. 525)

Bridging occurs when a patient positioned in hooklying lifts their buttocks and low back from a fixed surface. The activity can be used to facilitate pelvic motion and for strengthening the hip extensors.

1. An anterior pelvic tilt requires the anterior superior iliac spines of the pelvis to move anteriorly and inferiorly. Anterior pelvic tilts result in hip flexion and increased lumbar spine extension. The hip flexors and back extensors are the primary muscles active during the exercise.

2. Heel slides require the patient to lie on their back with the hips and knees flexed and the feet flat on the floor. The patient attempts to straighten the leg by sliding the heel on the floor while maintaining the low back in a flattened position. The patient then returns the leg to the upright starting position. The exercise is most often used as an active stretching technique to promote knee flexion.

3. Straight leg raises combine dynamic hip flexion with an isometric contraction of the quadriceps. The rectus femoris is the primary muscle active during the exercise.

4. **Isometric gluteal sets are an appropriate precursor to bridging since the activity incorporates the hip extensors.**

System Specific: Musculoskeletal System
Content Outline: Interventions

# Exam One: Question 95

A patient on supplemental oxygen participates in a series of active exercises. During the exercise session the patient's oxygen saturation falls to the lower limit of her established acceptable range of 92-95%. When asked by the physical therapist how she is feeling the patient reports that she feels fine. The MOST appropriate therapist action is:

1. **continue the exercise session**
2. increase the amount of oxygen
3. discontinue the exercise session
4. contact the patient's physician

**Correct Answer: 1** (Paz p. 441)

Supplemental oxygen is most commonly administered by a nasal cannula at flow rates between one and six liters per minute.

1. **Since the oxygen saturation rate has not fallen below the patient's established acceptable range and the patient reports feeling fine it is reasonable to continue with the exercise session.**

2. Physical therapists should not routinely increase the amount of oxygen even if the patient's oxygen saturation level falls below their acceptable range as the increased levels of oxygen may depress the hypoxic drive in patients with chronically high $PaCO_2$ (partial pressure of carbon dioxide).

3. Since the oxygen saturation level did not fall below the acceptable range, it is not necessary to discontinue the exercise session.

4. The acceptable oxygen saturation level for exercise should be established by the patient's physician. Since the oxygen saturation level did not fall below the acceptable range, contacting the physician is not necessary.

System Specific: Cardiovascular/Pulmonary and Lymphatic Systems
Content Outline: Interventions

# Exam One: Question 96

A physical therapist performs segmental breathing exercises with a patient following atelectasis. Which manual contact would be the MOST appropriate to emphasize lingula expansion?

1. **place the hands on the left side of the chest below the axilla**
2. place the hands below the clavicle on the anterior chest wall
3. place the hands over the posterior aspect of the lower ribs
4. place the hands on the right side of the chest below the axilla

**Correct Answer: 1** (Tan p. 735)

Segmental breathing, also known as localized breathing or thoracic expansion exercise, is intended to improve regional ventilation in patients with pulmonary disease and to prevent and treat pulmonary complications after surgery. The technique combines positioning with tactile and verbal cueing and resistance to enhance expansion of a specific lung segment to facilitate chest wall motion and increase ventilation.

1. **The lingula is a segment of the left upper lobe. Placing the hands on the left side of the chest below the axilla would provide tactile stimulation to facilitate expansion of the chest wall to improve ventilation of the left upper lobe.**

2. Placing the hands below the clavicle on the anterior chest wall would provide tactile stimulation to the anterior segments of the upper lobes, but not the lingula.

3. Placing the hands over the posterior aspect of the lower ribs would provide tactile stimulus over the lateral basal segments of the right and left lower lobes, not the lingula.

4. Placing the hands on the right side of the chest below the axilla would be overlying the right middle lobe, not the lingula.

System Specific: Cardiovascular/Pulmonary and Lymphatic Systems
Content Outline: Interventions

## Exam One: Question 97

A patient with C5 tetraplegia exercises on a mat table. Suddenly, the patient begins to demonstrate signs and symptoms of autonomic dysreflexia including headache and sweating above the level of the lesion. The MOST appropriate assessment to validate the presence of autonomic dysreflexia is:

1. pulse rate
2. **blood pressure**
3. respiratory rate
4. oxygen saturation

**Correct Answer: 2** (Umphred p. 622)

Autonomic dysreflexia occurs when a noxious stimulus below the level of the lesion triggers the autonomic nervous system causing a sudden elevation in blood pressure. The condition is common in patients with spinal cord lesions above the T6 level. Symptoms include profuse sweating, goose bumps below the level of the lesion, and vasodilation (flushing) above the level of injury. This condition should be treated as a medical emergency.

1. Pulse rate can be somewhat variable with autonomic dysreflexia and therefore it is not particularly useful when attempting to validate the presence of the condition.

2. **A significant increase in the patient's blood pressure is associated with autonomic dysreflexia. As a result, the measure should be assessed when attempting to confirm the presence of the condition. Management of autonomic dysreflexia includes placing the patient in an upright position in an attempt to control the rising blood pressure.**

3. Respiration rate may increase slightly with autonomic dysreflexia, but the measurement would not be useful to validate the presence of the condition.

4. Oxygen saturation rate measures the oxygen saturation of blood. This measure would not be immediately impacted by the presence of autonomic dysreflexia.

System Specific: Neuromuscular & Nervous Systems
Content Outline: Physical Therapy Examination

## Exam One: Question 98

A patient rehabilitating from a spinal cord injury informs a therapist that he will walk again. Which type of injury would make functional ambulation the MOST unrealistic?

1. **complete T9 paraplegia**
2. posterior cord syndrome
3. Brown-Sequard's syndrome
4. cauda equina injury

**Correct Answer: 1** (Umphred p. 647)

The ability to functionally ambulate following a spinal cord injury is primarily dependent on the patient's available motor and sensory innervation and the associated energy requirements.

1. **A patient with complete T9 paraplegia would possess full upper extremity innervation and would be able to utilize the lower abdominals and intercostals. The patient would not possess any lower extremity innervation and therefore, functional ambulation would be unrealistic.**

2. Posterior cord syndrome refers to a relatively rare incomplete lesion caused by compression of the posterior spinal artery. The condition is characterized by loss of pain perception, proprioception, two-point discrimination, and stereognosis. Motor function is preserved.

3. Brown-Sequard's syndrome refers to an incomplete lesion usually caused by a stab wound, which produces hemisection of the spinal cord. The condition is characterized by paralysis and loss of vibratory and position sense on the same side as the lesion and loss of pain and temperature sense on the opposite side of the lesion.

4. Cauda equina injury occurs below the L1 spinal level where the long nerve roots transcend. Cauda equina injuries can be complete, however, are frequently incomplete due to the large number of nerve roots in the area. The condition is characterized by flaccidity, areflexia, and impairment of bowel and bladder function. Full recovery is not typical due to the distance needed for axonal regeneration.

System Specific: Neuromuscular & Nervous Systems
Content Outline: Foundations for Evaluation, Differential Diagnosis, & Prognosis

## Exam One: Question 99

A physical therapist monitors a 29-year-old male with a C6 spinal cord injury positioned on a tilt table. After elevating the tilt table to 30 degrees, the patient begins to complain of nausea and dizziness. The patient's blood pressure is measured as 70/35 mm Hg. The patient's signs and symptoms are MOST indicative of:

1. spinal shock
2. postural hypertension
3. autonomic dysreflexia
4. **orthostatic hypotension**

**Correct Answer: 4** (Umphred p. 621)

Patients status post spinal cord injury are particularly susceptible to several potentially emergent conditions. Physical therapists must closely monitor patients for signs and symptoms associated with these conditions and, if necessary, provide appropriate and immediate medical management.

1. Spinal shock refers to a physiologic response that occurs between 30 and 60 minutes after trauma to the spinal cord and can last up to several weeks. The patient presents with total flaccid paralysis and loss of all reflexes below the level of injury.

2. Postural hypertension is a term used to describe dizziness caused by a change in position in the presence of high blood pressure (systolic blood pressure greater than 140 mm Hg and diastolic greater than 90 mm Hg). A far more common term is postural hypotension which is synonymous with orthostatic hypotension.

3. Autonomic dysreflexia occurs when a noxious stimulus below the level of the lesion triggers the autonomic nervous system causing a sudden elevation in blood pressure. If not treated, this condition can lead to convulsions, hemorrhage, and death. The condition frequently occurs in patients with lesions at or above T6.

4. **Orthostatic hypotension or postural hypotension occurs due to a loss of sympathetic control of vasoconstriction in combination with absent or severely reduced muscle tone. A decrease in systolic blood pressure greater than 20 mm Hg after moving from supine to sitting is typically indicative of orthostatic hypotension.**

System Specific: Cardiovascular/Pulmonary and Lymphatic Systems
Content Outline: Foundations for Evaluation, Differential Diagnosis, & Prognosis

## Exam One: Question 100

A physical therapist attempts to examine the relationship between scores on a functional independence measure and another measurement whose validity is known. This type of example BEST describes:

1. face validity
2. predictive validity
3. **concurrent validity**
4. content validity

**Correct Answer: 3** (Portney p. 103)

Concurrent validity refers to the relationship between test scores and either criterion states or measurements whose validity is known.

1. Face validity refers to whether the test "looks valid" to those who take and administer it. It refers, not to what the test actually measures, but to what it appears superficially to measure.

2. Predictive validity is a form of validity that is demonstrated when a score is helpful in predicting a specific future outcome. Examples of tests with predictive validity are career or aptitude tests, which are helpful in determining who is likely to succeed or fail in certain subjects or occupations.

3. **Concurrent validity is demonstrated when a test score correlates well with a measure that has previously been validated. This is the circumstance in the example, where the functional balance measure would have concurrent validity if a strong relationship can be shown between its scores and scores on a previously validated measurement.**

4. Content validity refers to the extent to which a measure represents all facets of a given concept or construct.

System Specific: Non-Systems
Content Outline: Safety and Protection; Professional Responsibilities; Research

## Exam One: Question 101

A physical therapist develops a chart detailing expected functional outcomes for a variety of spinal cord injuries. Which is the highest spinal cord injury level at which independent transfers with a sliding board would be feasible?

1. C4
2. C6
3. T1
4. T3

**Correct Answer: 2** (Rothstein p. 404)

The ability to independently transfer with a sliding board following a spinal cord injury is primarily dependent on the patient's available motor and sensory innervation. In addition to performing independent sliding board transfers, a patient with a C6 spinal cord injury should be able to perform independent bed mobility, coughing, skin inspection, and pressure relief with equipment and adaptations.

1. A patient with a C4 spinal cord injury would not have adequate upper extremity movement to be capable of completing the transfer. Primary muscles innervated include the diaphragm and trapezius.
2. A patient with a C6 spinal cord injury would possess the requisite upper extremity strength to make the transfer feasible. Primary muscles innervated include the extensor carpi radialis, infraspinatus, latissimus dorsi, pectoralis major, pronator teres, serratus anterior, and teres minor.
3. A patient with a T1 spinal cord injury would possess full upper extremity innervation and should be able to complete the transfer. The option is not the correct response since the item asks the highest spinal cord injury level where the transfer is feasible.
4. A patient with a T3 spinal cord injury should also be able to complete the transfer. The patient's clinical presentation would be consistent with the patient at the T1 level.

System Specific: Neuromuscular & Nervous Systems
Content Outline: Foundations for Evaluation, Differential Diagnosis, & Prognosis

## Exam One: Question 102

A patient rehabilitating from a spinal cord injury has significant lower extremity spasticity which often results in the patient's feet becoming dislodged from the wheelchair footrests. The MOST appropriate modification to address this problem is:

1. hydraulic reclining unit
2. elevating legrests
3. **heel loops and/or toe loops**
4. detachable swing-away legrests

**Correct Answer: 3** (O'Sullivan p. 976)

There are a variety of wheelchair components that can assist patients to achieve maximum function, comfort, stability, and protection. The specific components selected are based on the unique needs of each patient.

1. A hydraulic reclining unit would allow the patient to recline in the actual chair. Semireclining chairs recline to approximately 30 degrees from the vertical and fully reclining chairs recline to a horizontal position.
2. Elevating legrests allow the entire front rigging to be elevated and maintained at varying heights. Patients with inadequate knee flexion, a long leg cast or circulatory compromise may use this type of adaptation.
3. Heel loops and/or toe loops can maintain the foot on the footrest. This is often necessary in the presence of spasticity.
4. Detachable swing-away legrests allow the front rigging to be pivoted outward away from the wheelchair frame. This adaptation allows the wheelchair to be positioned closer to objects and provides more unobstructed space to transfer.

System Specific: Non-Systems
Content Outline: Equipment & Devices; Therapeutic Modalities

## Exam One: Question 103

A physical therapist utilizes a manual assisted cough technique on a patient with a mid-thoracic spinal cord injury. When completing this technique with the patient in supine, the MOST appropriate location for the therapist's hand placement is:

1. manubrium
2. **epigastric area**
3. xiphoid process
4. umbilical region

**Correct Answer: 2** (O'Sullivan p. 959)

The degree of respiratory impairment is related to the level of the spinal cord injury, residual muscle function, trauma at the time of injury, and premorbid respiratory status. Weakness or paralysis of the external oblique muscles compromises the patient's ability to cough and expel secretions.

1. The manubrium is the broad, quadrangular shaped upper part of the sternum. This region is too high to provide effective pressure support for coughing.
2. **The epigastric area is the upper central region of the abdomen, located between the costal margins and the subcostal plane. Applying manual hand pressure inwards and upwards over the epigastric area can assist the patient to cough and promote airway clearance.**
3. The xiphoid process is a small cartilaginous extension to the lower part of the sternum that is usually ossified in the adult. Pressure over this region should be avoided.
4. The umbilical region is the area surrounding the umbilicus (i.e., belly button). This region is too low to provide effective pressure support for coughing.

System Specific: Cardiovascular/Pulmonary and Lymphatic Systems
Content Outline: Interventions

## Exam One: Question 104

A patient 72 hours status post stroke is referred to physical therapy. As part of the patient care program, the physical therapist makes positioning recommendations to the nursing staff. How often should turning occur?

1. every thirty minutes
2. **every two hours**
3. every four hours
4. every six hours

**Correct Answer: 2** (Pierson p. 86)

During the initial stages of rehabilitation a patient status post stroke should be repositioned in bed on a regular basis. Failure to reposition could result in contractures or excessive pressure to the skin and associated structures. The greatest pressure typically occurs to tissues that cover bony prominences.

1. Turning a patient on a 30 minute interval would be desirable to reduce the risk of tissue damage, however, the time frame would place an unrealistic burden on the nursing staff without adequate clinical justification.
2. **Turning a patient on a two hour interval is the most widely accepted positioning rule. This interval is sufficient to reduce the risk of tissue damage and is realistic for the nursing staff.**
3. Turning a patient every four hours is inadequate and would place the patient at significant risk for tissue damage.
4. Turning a patient every six hours is also inadequate. The greater the interval beyond two hours, the greater the probability that the patient will experience tissue damage.

System Specific: Other Systems
Content Outline: Interventions

## Exam One: Question 105

A physical therapist prepares to use soft tissue massage as part of a treatment plan for a patient with an adductor strain. The MOST appropriate therapist action prior to initiating treatment is:

1. utilize proper draping
2. **explain the treatment procedure and obtain patient consent**
3. ask another therapist to be present during the treatment session
4. describe the benefits of soft tissue massage on muscle strains

**Correct Answer: 2** (Scott - Promoting Legal and Ethical Awareness p. 224)

The *Criteria for Standards of Practice for Physical Therapy* published by the American Physical Therapy Association state that "Within the patient/client management process, the physical therapist and the patient/client establish and maintain an ongoing collaborative process of decision making that exists throughout the provision of services."

1. Proper draping is essential given the location of the adductors, however, explaining the treatment procedure and obtaining consent would be the prerequisite activity.
2. Explaining the treatment procedure and obtaining patient consent provides the patient with a broad understanding of the intervention and permits them with the opportunity to refuse. Failure to take this action may result in the therapist assuming unnecessary legal risk.
3. Asking another physical therapist to be present provides the therapist with a witness who could verify that the intervention was applied in a professional manner. Although this is a commonly used risk management strategy, it ignores the patient's right to be involved in decision making.
4. A patient should be aware of the benefits associated with a specific intervention, however, this would likely be a component of explaining the treatment procedure and obtaining patient consent.

System Specific: Musculoskeletal System
Content Outline: Interventions

## Exam One: Question 106

A physical therapist moves a patient from sidelying to supine after the patient was unable to maintain the manual muscle test position for the hip abductors. Assuming the patient is able to complete full range of motion in the horizontal plane, the MOST appropriate muscle grade is:

1. fair
2. fair minus
3. **poor**
4. poor minus

**Correct Answer: 3** (Kendall p. 20)

Physical therapists are required to modify the traditional manual muscle testing position when a patient is unable to complete range of motion against gravity. The primary hip abductors are the gluteus minimus and gluteus medius.

1. A grade of fair is characterized by the patient completing range of motion against gravity without manual resistance.
2. A grade of fair minus is characterized by the patient being unable to complete the range of motion against gravity, but does complete more than half of the range.
3. A grade of poor is characterized by the patient completing range of motion with gravity eliminated.
4. A grade of poor minus is characterized by the patient being unable to complete range of motion in a gravity eliminated position.

System Specific: Musculoskeletal System
Content Outline: Physical Therapy Examination

## Exam One: Question 107

A physical therapist completes a lower quarter screening examination on a patient diagnosed with trochanteric bursitis. Assuming a normal end-feel, which of the following classifications would be MOST consistent with hip extension?

1. soft
2. firm
3. hard
4. empty

**Correct Answer: 2** (Norkin p. 202)
End-feel is the type of resistance that is felt when passively moving a joint through the end range of motion.

1. A soft end-feel results in a yielding compression that halts further movement. An example of a soft end-feel would be associated with knee flexion secondary to compression of soft tissue.
2. The end-feel most often associated with hip extension is firm due to tension in the anterior joint capsule and the iliofemoral ligament.
3. A hard or bony end-feel results in an unyielding sensation most often caused by bone to bone contact. An example of a hard or bony end-feel would be elbow extension.
4. An empty end-feel results when pain prevents reaching the end of range of motion. Resistance is not felt, although protective muscle splinting or muscle spasm may be detected. An empty end-feel is always considered abnormal.

System Specific: Musculoskeletal System
Content Outline: Physical Therapy Examination

## Exam One: Question 108

A physician utilizes diagnostic imaging to show motion within a joint through x-ray. This type of imaging is BEST termed:

1. computed tomography
2. fluoroscopy
3. discography
4. radionuclide scanning

**Correct Answer: 2** (Magee p. 64)
Knowledge of diagnostic imaging techniques allows therapists to better understand the rationale associated with physician orders for imaging and the interpretation of the obtained results.

1. Computed tomography is a non-invasive imaging technique that uses cross-sectional images based on x-ray attenuation. Computer enhancement allows the imaging to have significantly better contrast resolution when compared to conventional x-rays.
2. Fluoroscopy refers to examination by means of the fluoroscope. A fluoroscope allows an examiner to observe the actions of joints, organs or entire systems of the body. The instrument requires a specific body segment to be placed between a fluorescent screen and an x-ray tube. X-rays from the tube pass through the body and project images on the screen.
3. Discography is an invasive imaging technique that involves injecting a radiopaque dye into the nucleus pulposus of an intervertebral disc using radiographic guidance. The technique can be used to identify disruptions of the nucleus pulposus or the annulus fibrosus.
4. Radionuclide scanning is an invasive imaging technique that can be used in conjunction with bone scans to identify areas where there is a high level of bone turnover relative to the rest of the bone. The technique requires the intravenous injection of chemicals labeled with isotopes.

System Specific: Musculoskeletal System
Content Outline: Foundations for Evaluation, Differential Diagnosis, & Prognosis

## Exam One: Question 109

A physical therapist reviews the medical record of a patient recently admitted to the intensive care unit. A note from the patient's physician indicates an order for arterial blood gas analysis six times daily. Which type of indwelling line would be used to collect the necessary samples?

1. intravenous line
2. **arterial line**
3. central venous line
4. pulmonary artery line

**Correct Answer: 2** (Pierson p. 278)

Samples for blood gas analysis may be obtained from different regions of the vascular bed. Arterial samples are taken from either a needle puncture or indwelling catheter in a peripheral artery.

1. An intravenous line consists of a short catheter inserted through the skin into a peripheral vein. Intravenous lines are used as a route to administer medications or fluids.

2. **An arterial line consists of a catheter inserted through the skin into an artery connected to pressure tubing, a transducer, and a monitor. The device can be used for continuous direct blood pressure readings and to sample arterial blood for arterial blood gas analysis. The radial and brachial arteries are the most common sites for an arterial line.**

3. A central venous line consists of a catheter inserted through the skin into a large vein, usually the superior vena cava or inferior vena cava, or within the right atrium of the heart to measure right atrial pressure. The catheter also may be used as a route for medication or fluid administration, blood sampling, and emergency placement of a pacemaker.

4. A pulmonary artery line is a balloon-tipped catheter introduced via the internal jugular vein or subclavian vein passing through the right atrium, tricuspid valve, right ventricle, pulmonary valve, and into the pulmonary artery. It is used to monitor cardiovascular pressures and to sample mixed venous blood for gas analysis.

System Specific: Cardiovascular/Pulmonary and Lymphatic Systems
Content Outline: Foundations for Evaluation, Differential Diagnosis, & Prognosis

## Exam One: Question 110

A physical therapist completes a family training session with a patient rehabilitating from a spinal cord injury. During the training the patient asks a question regarding their functional ability following rehabilitation. The MOST appropriate therapist response is to:

1. explain that it is difficult to predict since all patients progress differently
2. **provide information on the expected prognosis based on the nature and severity of the injury**
3. refer the patient to the director of rehabilitation
4. refer the patient to the physiatrist

**Correct Answer: 2** (Purtilo p. 33)

Patients often ask physical therapists questions about their functional abilities following rehabilitation. It is reasonable for the therapist to provide the patient with information on this topic given the patient's level of motor and sensory innervation.

1. The statement, although accurate, does not directly address the patient's question. Physical therapists should attempt to answer questions posed by patients in a direct and forthcoming manner whenever possible.

2. **Physical therapists can share information with patients related to projected functional outcomes following rehabilitation. Physical therapists should be careful to make sure that the topics addressed fall within their scope of practice.**

3. The director of rehabilitation is typically responsible for oversight of the therapy services provided by the various health care disciplines. The position is primarily administrative and therefore the director would not typically be well suited to respond to questions regarding expected patient outcome.

4. Referring the patient to the physiatrist, although appropriate, would be a more attractive option if the question posed by the patient was directly related to their medical management or another similar topic that would fall under the scope of practice of the physiatrist.

System Specific: Neuromuscular & Nervous Systems
Content Outline: Foundations for Evaluation, Differential Diagnosis, & Prognosis

## Exam One: Question 111

A patient is referred to physical therapy following a modified radical mastectomy for treatment of associated soft tissue restrictions and pain. During the examination, the physical therapist becomes concerned since the surgical site is extremely warm to touch, tender, and discolored. Given the patient's recent history, the MOST likely etiology is:

1. dermatitis
2. **cellulitis**
3. mastitis
4. erysipelas

**Correct Answer: 2** (Goodman–Pathology p. 673)
A modified radical mastectomy includes removal of all tissues of the affected breast including the areola, nipple, and most of the axillary lymph nodes. The local lymphatic disruption and resultant impairment of local immune responses increases the likelihood of post-operative cellulitis.

1. Dermatitis presents in numerous forms (e.g., contact, seborrheic, atopic), all of which involve some degree of general skin irritation. Although contact dermatitis may have a visible presentation similar to cellulitis, it would not typically be warm to touch nor is it consistent with the described clinical scenario.

2. **Cellulitis tends to develop in areas where the skin's protective barrier (e.g., surgical site, wound) and lymphatic flow (e.g., lymph node removal, excessive soft tissue, edema) have been disrupted. Cellulitis is a common post-operative complication of surgical breast cancer treatment.**

3. Mastitis is an infection of the fatty breast tissue typically associated with postpartum breast feeding. The infection may present with a superficial appearance similar to cellulitis, but is further characterized by painful lumps within the breast tissue.

4. Erysipelas is a specific form of cellulitis caused by streptococcal bacteria. Like cellulitis, the skin is typically warm and tender to the touch, however, it is much more defined in its appearance. Erysipelas is characterized by a raised, sharp demarcation of borders with an unmistakable bright red discoloration.

System Specific: Other Systems
Content Outline: Foundations for Evaluation, Differential Diagnosis, and Prognosis

## Exam One: Question 112

A physical therapist uses a self-care assessment to examine change over time in rehabilitation programs. The assessment uses a seven-point scale to examine 18 items. The collected information is based on observations of patient performance. This type of assessment MOST closely describes:

1. **Functional Independence Measure**
2. Functional Status Index
3. Physical Self-Maintenance Scale
4. Katz Index of Activities of Daily Living

**Correct Answer: 1** (Van Deusen p. 425)
There are a variety of outcome measures which examine self-care and activities of daily living. Physical therapists should have general knowledge of the more commonly used measures and consider the conceptual and measurement model, reliability, validity, responsiveness, and interpretability inherent to each measure.

1. **The Functional Independence Measure (FIM) tests a subject in multiple areas to determine the overall degree of disability experienced by an adult rehabilitation patient. A seven-point scale is utilized to examine 18 areas, which include self-care, sphincter control, transfers, locomotion, communication, and social cognitive activities. The FIM is commonly used to examine changes in disability status that occur over time.**

2. The Functional Status Index was developed as a comprehensive ADL assessment for adults living in the community. The 18 items include the following domains: gross mobility, personal care, social/role activities, hand activities and home chores. Scores are generated in three areas: dependence, difficulty, and pain.

3. The Physical Self-Maintenance Scale (PSMS) is a Guttman scale containing six items of self-care. The PSMS was designed as a disability measure for use in planning and evaluating treatment in elderly people living in the community or within institutions.

4. The Katz Index of Activities of Daily Living uses a nominal scale index to identify self-care problems and the level of assistance required within six areas: bathing, dressing, toileting, transfers, continence, and feeding.

System Specific: Neuromuscular and Nervous Systems
Content Outline: Physical Therapy Examination

## Exam One: Question 113

A physical therapist working on a pulmonary rehabilitation unit works with a patient on therapeutic positioning. The patient has experienced a lengthy inpatient hospitalization and was only recently referred to physical therapy. The patient has significant weakness of the diaphragm and is hypertensive. The MOST appropriate patient position to initiate treatment is:

1. prone
2. supine
3. Trendelenburg
4. **reverse Trendelenburg**

---

**Correct Answer: 4** (Hillegass p. 578)

The reverse Trendelenburg position refers to a position in which the patient's head is elevated on an inclined plane in relation to the feet.

1. The prone position would be a difficult position in which to teach the patient diaphragmatic breathing since the weight of the abdominal contents on the diaphragm makes it more difficult for a weakened diaphragm to contract.

2. In supine, the weight of the abdominal contents on the diaphragm makes it more difficult for a weakened diaphragm to contract. Also, the supine position can reduce the functional residual volume of the lungs by as much as fifty percent.

3. In the Trendelenburg position the patient's head is lower than their feet. The position is used to facilitate drainage from the lower lobes of the lungs and to increase blood pressure in hypotensive patients. The position would tend to increase the blood pressure of a patient that is already hypertensive.

4. **The reverse Trendelenburg position is recommended to reduce hypertension and facilitate movement of the diaphragm by using gravity to reduce the weight of the abdominal contents on the diaphragm.**

System Specific: Cardiovascular/Pulmonary and Lymphatic Systems
Content Outline: Interventions

---

## Exam One: Question 114

A physical therapist works with a patient who is HIV positive and has been admitted to an acute care hospital for a course of intravenous antibiotics. The patient's medical record states that he has had a persistent cough producing bloody sputum for four weeks and that airborne precautions should be observed. The most likely rationale for this level of precaution is:

1. decrease the risk of exposing the immunocompromised patient to pneumonia
2. decrease the risk of exposing the immunocompromised patient to active tuberculosis
3. decrease the risk of staff and visitor exposure to pneumonia
4. **decrease the risk of staff and visitor exposure to active tuberculosis**

---

**Correct Answer: 4** (Pierson p. 34)

Standard precautions should be observed with all patients regardless of their reported medical history. Physical therapists must also be aware of additional precautions which may be associated with more specific forms of infections. Airborne precautions typically include protection of respiratory pathways (e.g., wearing a mask or face shield) in order to prevent the risk of airborne transmission of infectious agents through evaporated droplets in air or dust particles containing infectious agents.

1. Although it is important to protect a patient from exposure to potential sources of infection, airborne precautions are typically designated with the intent of preventing transmission of disease from the patient to others. Pneumonia is contracted via droplet transmission.

2. Neutropenic precautions may be instituted in addition to standard precautions for patients who are so immunocompromised that even a mild infection may be lethal. However, the patient's clinical presentation is consistent with active tuberculosis making it much more likely that the precautions have been instituted to protect others.

3. Pneumonia may produce symptoms similar to those described, however, the infection responsible is contracted via droplet transmission of an infectious virus, bacteria or fungi.

4. **Airborne precautions are typically instituted to protect staff and visitors from contracting an infection spread through airborne transmission. There is a significant prevalence of tuberculosis among patients who are HIV positive and the reported persistent cough and bloody sputum are consistent with the clinical presentation of the disease.**

System Specific: Non-Systems
Content Outline: Safety and Protection; Professional Responsibilities; Research

## Exam One: Question 115

A physical therapist observes an intravenous line that is tangled around a patient's bed rail. What type of medical asepsis is indicated prior to coming in contact with the intravenous line?

1. gloves
2. gloves, gown
3. gloves, gown, mask
4. **none**

---

**Correct Answer: 4** (Pierson p. 282)

An intravenous (I.V.) system can be used to infuse fluids, electrolytes, nutrients, and medication. The I.V. line most commonly consists of plastic tubing and is considered a non-sterile object.

1. Gloves offer protection to the physical therapist's hands to reduce the likelihood of becoming infected with microorganisms from a patient and reduce the risk of the patient receiving microorganisms from the physical therapist. Gloves would not be necessary when handling an I.V. line.

2. A gown is used to protect the physical therapist's clothing from being contaminated or soiled by a contaminant. The gown also reduces the probability of the physical therapist transmitting a microorganism from their clothing to the patient. Gloves and gown would not be necessary when handling an I.V. line.

3. A mask is designed to reduce the spread of microorganisms that are transmitted through the air. The mask protects the physical therapist from inhalation of particles or droplets that may contain pathogens and also reduces the transmission of pathogens from the physical therapist to the patient. Gloves, gown, and mask would not be necessary when handling an I.V. line.

4. **The tubing is a non-sterile object that would not require the use of protective clothing. The physical therapist can reposition the I.V. line through direct hand contact.**

System Specific: Non-Systems
Content Outline: Safety and Protection; Professional Responsibilities; Research

---

## Exam One: Question 116

A physical therapist presents an inservice to the rehabilitation staff that compares traditional gait terminology with Rancho Los Amigos terminology. Which pair of descriptive terms describes the same general point in the gait cycle?

1. midstance to heel off and initial swing
2. **heel strike and initial contact**
3. foot flat to midstance and loading response
4. toe off and midswing

---

**Correct Answer: 2** (Rothstein p. 678)

Traditional gait terminology and Rancho Los Amigos terminology can be used to describe the various components of gait. There are a fair number of similarities between the two classification systems, however, there are also a number of differences. Rancho Los Amigos terminology tends to be more descriptive since it describes intervals of gait, usually with a well defined beginning and end point.

1. Midstance to heel off occurs during stance phase. Initial swing begins when the stance foot lifts from the floor and ends with maximal knee flexion during swing (i.e., swing phase).

2. **Heel strike and initial contact are both terms that describe the moment that the heel contacts the ground and stance phase begins.**

3. The loading response corresponds to the amount of time between initial contact and the beginning of the swing phase for the other leg. This is not the same point in the gait cycle as foot flat to midstance since the loading response does not include the period of time when the other foot is off the floor until the body is directly over the stance limb (i.e., midstance).

4. Toe off is the point in which only the toe of the stance limb remains on the ground, however, midswing occurs during swing phase.

System Specific: Musculoskeletal System
Content Outline: Physical Therapy Examination

## Exam One: Question 117

A physical therapist selects a therapeutic ultrasound generator with a frequency of 3.0 MHz. Which condition would MOST warrant the use of this frequency?

1. lumbar paravertebral muscle spasm
2. hip flexion contracture
3. quadriceps strain
4. **anterior talofibular ligament sprain**

> **Correct Answer: 4** (Cameron p. 192)
> A higher frequency results in greater attenuation of energy in superficial structures. As a result, an ultrasound generator with a frequency of 3.0 MHz may be more desirable than a generator with a frequency of 1.0 MHz when treating a superficial structure.
>
> 1. The lumbar paravertebral muscles refer to a relatively diverse group of muscles next to the spine. The muscles collectively support the spine and produce movement. The relative depth of the muscles would make it necessary to utilize a frequency of 1.0 MHz to reach the target area.
> 2. A hip flexion contracture typically results from shortening of the iliopsoas muscle. The iliopsoas is formed by the iliacus and psoas major muscles and is considered to be the most powerful flexor of the hip. Ultrasound in this area would require a frequency of 1.0 MHz due to the depth of the muscle.
> 3. The quadriceps muscles are a large muscle group consisting of the rectus femoris, vastus lateralis, vastus medialis, and vastus intermedius. A strain in this area would require a frequency of 1.0 MHz due to the depth of the structures.
> 4. **The anterior talofibular ligament is a thickening of the anterior joint capsule that extends from the anterior surface of the lateral malleolus to the lateral facet of the talus and the lateral surface of the talar neck. The ligament is only two to five millimeters thick and therefore a frequency of 3.0 MHz would be adequate.**
>
> System Specific: Non-Systems
> Content Outline: Equipment & Devices; Therapeutic Modalities

## Exam One: Question 118

A physical therapist employed in a rehabilitation hospital utilizes a variety of transfer techniques to move patients of various functional abilities. Which type of transfer would NOT be classified as dependent?

1. sliding transfer
2. hydraulic lift
3. **sliding board transfer**
4. two-person lift

> **Correct Answer: 3** (Minor p. 190)
> Physical therapists should select transfers for patients based on their unique abilities and limitations. Types of transfers range from completely dependent to independent.
>
> 1. The sliding transfer is considered a dependent transfer most often used when transferring a patient in supine from a treatment table or bed to a similar surface. When performing the transfer therapists often use a "draw" sheet to move the patient from one surface to the other.
> 2. The hydraulic lift is a device required for dependent transfers when a patient is obese, there is only one therapist available to assist with the transfer or the patient is totally dependent.
> 3. **The sliding board transfer is used for a patient that possesses sitting balance, upper extremity strength, and can adequately follow directions. The transfer is used when patients can assist or are independent.**
> 4. The two-person lift is considered a dependent transfer used to transfer a patient between two surfaces of different heights or when transferring a patient to the floor.
>
> System Specific: Non-Systems
> Content Outline: Equipment & Devices; Therapeutic Modalities

## Exam One: Question 119

A 28-year-old male referred to physical therapy by his primary physician complains of recurrent ankle pain. As part of the treatment program, the therapist uses ultrasound over the peroneus longus and brevis tendons. The MOST appropriate location for ultrasound application is:

1. inferior to the sustentaculum tali
2. over the sinus tarsi
3. **posterior to the lateral malleolus**
4. anterior to the lateral malleolus

**Correct Answer: 3** (Kendall p. 412)

The peroneus longus and brevis are innervated by the superficial peroneal nerve (L4, L5, S1) and act to evert the foot and assist in plantar flexion of the ankle joint. The peroneus longus also acts to depress the head of the first metatarsal.

1. The sustentaculum tali is a horizontal eminence arising from the medial surface of the calcaneus. The bony prominence serves as the attachment for several ligaments including the plantar calcaneonavicular ligament, also known as the spring ligament.

2. The sinus tarsi is a small osseous canal which runs into the ankle under the talus bone. The structure is at the same approximate level as the lateral malleolus.

3. **The peroneus longus and brevis tendons pass posterior to the lateral malleolus. The peroneus longus inserts on the lateral side of the base of the first metatarsal and first cuneiform, while the peroneus brevis inserts on the tuberosity of the fifth metatarsal.**

4. The tendon of the extensor digitorum longus can be palpated slightly anterior to the lateral malleolus.

System Specific: Musculoskeletal System
Content Outline: Interventions

## Exam One: Question 120

A physical therapist treats a patient rehabilitating from an Achilles tendon repair using cryotherapy. Which cryotherapeutic agent would provide the GREATEST magnitude of tissue cooling?

1. frozen gel packs
2. **ice massage**
3. Fluori-Methane spray
4. cold water bath

**Correct Answer: 2** (Cameron p. 145)

Cryotherapy is a commonly used therapeutic intervention in rehabilitation. Primary uses of cryotherapy include reducing inflammation, pain control, and spasticity management. Physical therapists must be aware of contraindications and precautions of cryotherapy as well as signs or symptoms of cold intolerance.

1. Frozen gel packs contain silica gel and are available in a variety of shapes and sizes. The packs are stored in a refrigeration unit and are usually applied with a moist towel. Cold packs may not maintain uniform contact with the treatment surface and require a treatment time of approximately 20 minutes.

2. **Ice massage is typically performed by freezing water in paper cups and applying the ice directly to the treatment area. Ice massage tends to create a more intense cooling since the ice is applied directly to a localized target area. The treatment time is 5-10 minutes using ice massage due to the intensity of the cooling.**

3. Fluori-Methane is a commonly used vapocoolant spray. Vapocoolant sprays allow for a brief cooling to a very localized area of application. The vapocoolant spray is applied in parallel strokes along the skin in the area of trigger points. Stretching immediately follows the application of the vapocoolant spray.

4. A cold water bath is commonly used for immersion of the distal extremities. A basin or whirlpool is most often used to hold the cold water. A cold bath requires water temperature ranging from 55 to 64 degrees Fahrenheit (13 to 18 degrees Celsius). The body part typically requires a treatment time of 15-20 minutes to attain the desired therapeutic effects.

System Specific: Non-Systems
Content Outline: Equipment & Devices; Therapeutic Modalities

## Exam One: Question 121

A physical therapist treats a 32-year-old female rehabilitating from a closed head injury presently functioning at Rancho Los Amigos level IV. The therapist treats the patient in her home for 60 minute sessions, three times per week. Recently the therapist has noticed that the patient becomes increasingly combative as the session progresses and believes the deterioration in behavior is linked to the patient becoming fatigued. The MOST appropriate treatment modification is:

1. reduce the treatment sessions to 30 minutes, three times per week
2. reduce the frequency of the treatment sessions to two times per week
3. **increase the rest periods during existing treatment sessions**
4. increase the treatment sessions to 90 minutes, two times per week

**Correct Answer: 3** (O' Sullivan p. 913)

The Rancho Los Amigos Levels of Cognitive Functioning Scale is used to describe cognitive and behavioral recovery in individuals following traumatic brain injury. A patient at level IV is labeled "Confused-Agitated."

1. Reducing the treatment sessions to 30 minutes in length would result in a fifty percent decrease in therapy time. It is possible that this may be necessary, however, the therapist should attempt to modify other parameters of treatment prior to implementing such a drastic reduction in therapy time.

2. Reducing the frequency of the sessions to two times per week would likely have minimal impact on the patient's behavior without reducing the length of the sessions or incorporating more frequent rest periods.

3. **A patient functioning at level IV may be particularly susceptible to changes in behavior based on fatigue. Ideally, the physical therapist should attempt to maintain the integrity of the current treatment regimen, however, if increased rest periods do not produce an observable change in the patient's behavior it may be appropriate to modify other parameters such as the frequency or length of treatment.**

4. It is likely that the length of the session, currently 60 minutes, may be more challenging for the patient than the frequency of the sessions. As a result, increasing the duration of the treatment sessions to 90 minutes would likely exacerbate the current situation.

System Specific: Neuromuscular & Nervous Systems
Content Outline: Interventions

## Exam One: Question 122

A physical therapist positions a patient in supine in preparation for goniometric measurements. When measuring medial rotation of the shoulder, the therapist should position the fulcrum:

1. on the lateral midline of the humerus using the lateral epicondyle as a reference
2. perpendicular to the floor
3. along the midaxillary line of the thorax
4. **over the olecranon process**

**Correct Answer: 4** (Norkin p. 76)

According to the American Academy of Orthopaedic Surgeons normal shoulder medial rotation is 0-70 degrees.

1. The lateral midline of the humerus using the lateral epicondyle as a reference should be used to align the moveable arm of the goniometer when measuring shoulder flexion and extension.

2. The stationary arm of the goniometer should be aligned parallel or perpendicular to the floor when measuring medial rotation of the shoulder.

3. The midaxillary line of the thorax should be used to align the stationary arm of the goniometer when measuring shoulder flexion and extension.

4. **The fulcrum of the goniometer should be aligned over the olecranon process. The moveable arm of the goniometer should be aligned with the ulna, using the olecranon and ulnar styloid as a reference when measuring medial rotation of the shoulder.**

System Specific: Musculoskeletal System
Content Outline: Physical Therapy Examination

## Exam One: Question 123

A physical therapist examines a patient diagnosed with left-sided heart failure. Which finding is NOT typically associated with this condition?

1. pulmonary edema
2. persistent cough
3. **dependent edema**
4. muscular weakness

**Correct Answer: 3** (Hillegass p. 93)
Heart failure refers to the heart's inability to maintain a cardiac output that is adequate to meet the demands of the tissues due to an abnormality in the pumping ability of the heart muscle. Left-sided heart failure means it is the left side of the heart that is failing which causes fluid to build up behind the left ventricle. Left-sided failure is frequently caused by myocardial infarction, hypertension or aortic valve disease.

1. Pulmonary edema is the abnormal accumulation of fluid in the alveolar spaces of the lungs. This is the "congestion" of congestive heart failure. It is often caused by increased pulmonary hydrostatic pressure from left-sided heart failure.
2. Patients with left-sided failure may be in respiratory distress and have a cough that produces pink, frothy (blood-tinged) sputum.
3. **Dependent edema is associated with right-sided heart failure. Fluid backs up behind the right ventricle and produces the accumulation of fluid in the liver, abdomen, and ankles.**
4. Muscle weakness, fatigue, and decreased exercise tolerance are universal among patients with left-sided heart failure due to the decreased blood flow to the extremities.

System Specific: Cardiovascular/Pulmonary and Lymphatic Systems
Content Outline: Foundations for Evaluation, Differential Diagnosis, & Prognosis

## Exam One: Question 124

A physical therapist monitors a patient with a single lead electrocardiogram. After carefully examining the obtained data, the therapist classifies the rhythm as sinus bradycardia. Which description is MOST indicative of this condition?

1. R-R interval is irregular with a rate between 100 and 200 beats per minute
2. R-R interval is irregular with a rate between 40 and 100 beats per minute
3. R-R interval is regular with a rate greater than 100 beats per minute
4. **R-R interval is regular with a rate less than 60 beats per minute**

**Correct Answer: 4** (Brannon p. 195)
The electrocardiogram is composed of a number of different waves – P, R, T, sometimes U – and the terms "irregular" and "regular" usually refer to the rhythm of the heart rate (i.e., the distance between similar waves). A sinus rhythm indicates that the cardiac impulse originates in the sinoatrial node. Sinus bradycardia is a sinus rhythm with a heart rate of less than 60 beats per minute.

1. Irregular R-R intervals with a heart rate between 100 and 200 beats per minute is characteristic of atrial tachycardia. Atrial tachycardia is defined as three or more consecutive premature atrial complexes, where an ectopic focus in either atria initiates an impulse before the SA node.
2. Irregular R-R intervals with a heart rate between 40 and 100 beats per minute is characteristic of sinus arrhythmia. Sinus arrhythmia is an irregularity in rhythm where the cardiac impulse is initiated at the SA node, but with a variable quickening and slowing of the impulse formation.
3. Regular R-R intervals with a heart rate greater than 100 beats per minute is sinus tachycardia.
4. **Regular R-R intervals with a heart rate of less than 60 beats per minute is sinus bradycardia.**

System Specific: Cardiovascular/Pulmonary and Lymphatic Systems
Content Outline: Foundations for Evaluation, Differential Diagnosis, and Prognosis

## Exam One: Question 125

A physical therapist washes his hands thoroughly after treating a patient with a suspected infection. Which statement regarding hand washing is NOT accurate?

1. **wash all hand and wrist jewelry**
2. wash your hands, wrists, and two to three inches of your distal forearms
3. wash for at least 30 seconds
4. select warm water to allow soap to lather easily

**Correct Answer: 1** (Pierson p. 32)

Hand washing is one of the most effective methods to reduce and prevent the spread of microorganisms.

1. **All hand and wrist jewelry should be removed prior to hand washing. Washing the hands without removing jewelry will increase the likelihood of microorganism transmission.**

2. Hand washing should include the wrist and a portion of the distal forearm. Washing of the wrist and the distal forearm should include both friction and rotary motions.

3. Hand washing should occur for a minimum of 30 seconds and longer in instances where a physical therapist has treated a patient known to have an infection.

4. Warm water allows the soap to lather more easily and causes minimum irritation to the skin.

System Specific: Non-Systems
Content Outline: Safety and Protection; Professional Responsibilities; Research

## Exam One: Question 126

A physical therapist uses a 3.0 MHz ultrasound beam at 1.5 W/cm² to treat a patient diagnosed with carpal tunnel syndrome. The MAJORITY of ultrasound energy will be absorbed within a depth of:

1. 1-2 centimeters
2. 2-3 centimeters
3. 4-5 centimeters
4. 5-6 centimeters

**Correct Answer: 1** (Cameron p. 192)

Frequency should be selected according to the depth of tissues to be treated. The most common frequency settings are 1 MHz and 3 MHz. A frequency setting of 1 MHz is used for heating of deeper tissues (up to five centimeters) where a setting of 3 MHz is used for heating superficial tissues with a depth of penetration of less than two centimeters.

1. **Tissues 1-2 centimeters in depth can be effectively treated with ultrasound using a frequency of 3 MHz.**

2. Tissues 2-3 centimeters in depth require ultrasound using a frequency of 1 MHz since a frequency of 3 MHz would not provide sufficient depth.

3. Tissues up to 5 centimeters in depth can be treated with ultrasound using a frequency of 1 MHz.

4. Tissues greater than 5 centimeters in depth are not effectively treated with ultrasound.

System Specific: Non-Systems
Content Outline: Equipment & Devices; Therapeutic Modalities

## Exam One: Question 127

A physical therapist serves as an accessibility consultant for a local retail store. What is the MINIMUM width required for a patient using a wheelchair to safely traverse through a doorway?

1. 24 inches
2. 30 inches
3. **32 inches**
4. 36 inches

**Correct Answer: 3** (Minor p. 4)

The Americans with Disabilities Act was designed to provide a clear and comprehensive national mandate for the elimination of discrimination. Title III provides information on public accommodations including minimum accessibility standards.

1. The seat width in an average adult size wheelchair is 18 inches. As a result, 24 inches would not be nearly sufficient to accommodate the remainder of the wheelchair and still have adequate space available to propel the wheelchair through the doorway.
2. A wheelchair would likely be able to traverse through a doorway that was 30 inches wide, however, it would not meet the minimum width required by the Americans with Disabilities Act.
3. **The Americans with Disabilities Act requires that the minimum width of a doorway is 32 inches.**
4. The Americans with Disabilities Act requires that the minimum width of a corridor (hallway) is 36 inches. This width allows the patient to change the direction of the wheelchair within the corridor.

System Specific: Non-Systems
Content Outline: Safety and Protection; Professional Responsibilities; Research

## Exam One: Question 128

A physical therapist reviews the medical record of a 52-year-old male status post myocardial infarction. The patient is currently in the coronary care unit and is scheduled to begin cardiac rehabilitation tomorrow. Which potential complication of a myocardial infarction is the patient MOST susceptible to?

1. heart failure
2. **arrhythmias**
3. thrombus formation
4. heart structural damage

**Correct Answer: 2** (Brannon p. 102)

Myocardial infarction has four major complications: arrhythmias, heart failure, thrombolytic complications, and damage to the heart structures.

1. Heart failure is a syndrome that reflects an inability of the heart to maintain a cardiac output sufficient to meet the oxygen and nutritional needs of the tissues. Heart failure is not as common as arrhythmias.
2. **Arrhythmias are caused by abnormalities in cardiac impulse generation, conduction, or both and occur in 90% of individuals who have experienced a myocardial infarction.**
3. Venous or mural thrombi can occur due to venous stasis after myocardial infarction. Thrombus formation is not as common as arrhythmias.
4. Damage to the papillary muscle, ventricle wall, and intraventricular septum can occur after a myocardial infarction. Heart structural damage is not as common as arrhythmias.

System Specific: Cardiovascular/Pulmonary and Lymphatic Systems
Content Outline: Foundations for Evaluation, Differential Diagnosis, & Prognosis

## Exam One: Question 129

A physical therapist positions a patient in prone on a treatment plinth in preparation for a hot pack. When preparing the hot pack for the low back, the therapist should utilize:

1. 2-4 towel layers
2. 4-6 towel layers
3. **6-8 towel layers**
4. 8-10 towel layers

---

**Correct Answer: 3** (Cameron p. 162)

A hot pack must be stored in hot water between 158 to 167 degrees Fahrenheit (70 to 75 degrees Celsius). As a result, it is necessary to use a barrier between the hot packs' canvas or nylon covered case and the body part to be treated. Most often towels or hot pack covers are used. Hot pack covers count for two towel layers because of their thickness.

1. Two to four towel layers would be inadequate and would result in the patient being at risk for excessive heat.

2. Four to six towel layers may be inadequate to properly protect the patient from excessive heat. It is possible to use only four to six towel layers in instances where the patient complains of not feeling enough heat or the therapist is aware that the hot pack may not possess its typical amount of heat. Therapist's must be cautious, however, to avoid removing towels during the session since increased skin temperature may diminish the patient's thermal sensitivity and their ability to accurately assess heat tolerance.

3. **Six to eight towel layers placed between a hot pack and the treatment surface is generally adequate to allow for the necessary transmission of heat without jeopardizing patient safety.**

4. Eight to ten towel layers may be excessive and as a result would significantly diminish the transmission of heat.

System Specific: Non-Systems
Content Outline: Equipment & Devices; Therapeutic Modalities

---

**Test Taking Tip:** When an option provides a range of answers, it is essential that candidates are satisfied with both the lower and upper limit of the range. For example, in option 2 a candidate may be satisfied with six towel layers, however, may feel that four towel layers would be inadequate. As a result, a candidate should not select option 2.

## Exam One: Question 130

A physical therapist attempts to determine if a wheelchair is the appropriate size for a patient recently admitted to a rehabilitation program. As part of the assessment, the therapist examines the distance from the front edge of the seat to the posterior aspect of the lower leg. If the seat depth is appropriate, how much space should exist between these two landmarks?

1. 1 inch
2. **2 inches**
3. 4 inches
4. 6 inches

---

**Correct Answer: 2** (Pierson p. 136)

Seat depth is determined by measuring from the patient's posterior buttock, along the lateral thigh to the popliteal fold; then subtracting approximately 2 inches to avoid pressure from the front edge of the seat against the popliteal space. Normal seat depth in an adult size wheelchair is 16 inches.

1. One inch of space may result in the patient experiencing increased pressure in the popliteal area or even potentially compromised circulation since the amount of space between the front edge of the seat and the popliteal space is less than the recommended amount of two inches.

2. **Two inches of space between the front edge of the seat and the popliteal space is the recommended amount of space. This distance corresponds to the width of three or four fingers.**

3. Four inches of space may result in the patient experiencing decreased trunk stability, increased weight bearing on the ischial tuberosities due to the body weight being shifted posteriorly secondary to the lack of support to the thighs, and poor balance since the base of support has been reduced.

4. Six inches of space would serve to exacerbate the difficulties discussed in option 3.

System Specific: Non-Systems
Content Outline: Equipment & Devices; Therapeutic Modalities

## Exam One: Question 131

A patient using a wheelchair arranges for a local contractor to build a ramp that will allow entry into the patient's house. What is the MAXIMUM recommended grade for the ramp?

1. 6.2%
2. **8.3%**
3. 9.5%
4. 10.4%

**Correct Answer: 2** (O'Sullivan p. 409)

Percent grade reflects the angle of inclination. The percent grade is determined by taking the rise and dividing the value by the run and then multiplying the number by 100 to convert the value to a percentage. A percent grade of 100% would be completely vertical and a percent grade of 0% would be completely horizontal.

1. A grade of 6.2% would be acceptable for the ramp, however, the item asks for the maximum recommended grade.

2. **A grade of 8.3% would result from a ramp that had one inch of rise for every 12 inches of run. This value represents the maximum percent grade of a ramp according to the Americans with Disabilities Act.**

3. A grade of 9.5% exceeds the maximum percent grade of a ramp allowable according to the Americans with Disabilities act by 1.2%.

4. A grade of 10.4% exceeds the maximum percent grade of a ramp allowable according to the Americans with Disabilities act by 2.1%.

System Specific: Non-Systems

Content Outline: Safety and Protection; Professional Responsibilities; Research

## Exam One: Question 132

A 16-year-old female accompanied by her mother receives exercise instructions. During the treatment session the mother makes several comments to her daughter that appear to be extremely upsetting and result in the daughter losing concentration. The MOST appropriate physical therapist action is:

1. document the mother's comments in the medical record
2. ask the patient if her mother is verbally abusive
3. **ask the mother to return to the waiting area**
4. discontinue the treatment session

**Correct Answer: 3** (Purtilo p. 344)

The physical therapist's primary concern should be to establish an environment that is conducive to instructing the patient in the exercise program. Failure to address the negative interaction between the mother and daughter may limit the effectiveness of the session.

1. Documentation may be an appropriate option, however, it does not address the primary objective which is to allow the patient to receive exercise instructions in an appropriate learning environment.

2. It would be inappropriate to ask the child a question about this topic, particularly in the presence of the mother.

3. **The therapist increases the likelihood that the child will be able to concentrate on the exercise instructions by asking the mother to return to the waiting area. The question provides ample information to hypothesize that the mother's actions may be the reason the child is upset.**

4. The child appears to be upset and is losing concentration, however, there is no indication that the session is hopeless and therefore the decision to discontinue the treatment session would be premature without first trying to modify the current learning environment.

System Specific: Non-Systems

Content Outline: Safety and Protection; Professional Responsibilities; Research

## Exam One: Question 133

A physical therapist working on a medical/surgical rotation returns from a morning inservice and finds a number of items that require her attention. Which of the following items should be given the highest priority?

1. **a patient requiring pre-operative instruction**
2. an incomplete exercise flow sheet
3. an unfinished wheelchair order form
4. a written note from a staff dietician

---

**Correct Answer: 1** (Code of Ethics)

Physical therapists routinely have to multi-task, however, as part of this process therapists need to be able to prioritize the importance of selected activities.

1. **Pre-operative instruction most often occurs in close proximity to a scheduled surgical procedure. As a result, delaying the pre-operative instruction may result in the patient not receiving the necessary instruction or the surgery being delayed or cancelled.**

2. It is important to document exercise activities using a flow sheet or other suitable tracking form, however, the activity can be deferred without immediate consequence.

3. It is important to submit all order forms for equipment or other devices in a timely manner. This need is particularly important in today's health care environment due to the reduced length of stay. Despite the importance, this would not supersede the need to complete the pre-operative instruction.

4. The physical therapist should read and, if necessary, respond to the note from the staff dietician, however, this would not supersede the need for the direct patient care activity.

System Specific: Musculoskeletal System
Content Outline: Interventions

---

## Exam One: Question 134

A physical therapist employed in a busy outpatient orthopedic clinic attempts to determine a schedule for calibration and maintenance of an ultrasound unit. The MOST important factor for the therapist to consider when determining an appropriate schedule is:

1. beam nonuniformity ratio
2. **frequency of use**
3. cost associated with calibration and maintenance
4. availability of qualified personnel to inspect the unit

---

**Correct Answer: 2** (Belanger p. 237)

Electrical equipment must be calibrated and maintained by qualified personnel on a regular schedule consistent with the manufacturer's recommendations. The regular schedule, once established, can be modified based on variables such as increased frequency of use or reports of faulty performance.

1. Beam nonuniformity ratio (BNR) refers to the ratio of intensity of the highest peak to the average intensity of all peaks. The BNR is determined by the intrinsic biophysical properties of the piezoelectric transducer. The BNR of an ultrasound device would not be a factor in determining a calibration and maintenance schedule.

2. **The frequency of use of an ultrasound device is extremely important when determining a schedule for calibration and maintenance. Ultrasound units used frequently may be calibrated several times a year, while a unit used sparingly would likely warrant a longer interval.**

3. The cost associated with calibration and maintenance of the ultrasound unit should not be a factor in establishing a calibration and maintenance schedule. Relying on a variable such as cost implies that when there are ample resources available calibration and maintenance take place and when resources are not available calibration and maintenance can be deferred.

4. The availability of qualified personnel to inspect the ultrasound unit would not be a factor in determining a calibration and maintenance schedule. If appropriate personnel are not available within the health care organization, there are a variety of external companies who can provide the necessary service.

System Specific: Non-Systems
Content Outline: Equipment & Devices; Therapeutic Modalities

## Exam One: Question 135

A patient rehabilitating from a fractured acetabulum is referred to physical therapy for ambulation activities. The patient has been on bed rest for three weeks and appears to be somewhat apprehensive about weight bearing. The MOST appropriate device to use when initiating ambulation activities is:

1. **parallel bars**
2. walker
3. axillary crutches
4. straight cane

**Correct Answer: 1** (Pierson p. 215)

A physical therapist must carefully assess a patient's needs prior to initiating ambulation activities. The question provides ample evidence that the patient will need a secure and stable environment to initiate ambulation.

1. **The magnitude of the injury (i.e., fractured acetabulum), the length of time the patient has been on bed rest, and the degree of patient apprehension make it imperative that the therapist initiate ambulation in a controlled and stable environment (i.e., parallel bars).**

2. A walker is a relatively stable assistive device, however, the parallel bars provide a safer environment to initiate ambulation. It is likely that the patient will quickly transition to the walker in subsequent sessions.

3. Axillary crutches allow altered weight bearing levels, but would not likely provide the level of stability required given the presented information.

4. A straight cane does not permit partial weight bearing, if desired, and offers significantly less stability than any of the other presented options.

System Specific: Musculoskeletal System
Content Outline: Interventions

## Exam One: Question 136

A seven-year-old boy sitting in the physical therapy waiting area suddenly grasps his throat and appears to be in distress. The boy slowly stands, but is obviously unable to breathe. The physical therapist recognizing the signs of an airway obstruction should administer:

1. **abdominal thrusts**
2. chest thrusts
3. rescue breathing
4. finger sweep

**Correct Answer: 1** (American Heart Association)

An airway obstruction in a child or an adult is best treated by using abdominal thrusts.

1. **Abdominal thrusts (Heimlich maneuver) can be used on a child until the object is expelled or the victim becomes unresponsive. The American Red Cross recommends back blows in combination with abdominal thrusts. Abdominal thrusts are not recommended for infants (less than one year of age) because of an increased risk of injury.**

2. If abdominal thrusts are ineffective, the health care provider may consider using chest thrusts. Research has demonstrated that approximately 50% of the episodes of airway obstruction were not relieved by a single technique. As a result, the likelihood of success may be increased when using combinations of back blows, abdominal thrusts, and chest thrusts.

3. Rescue breathing is recommended for an unresponsive patient who has a palpable pulse, but is not breathing. This would not be an immediate reaction for an airway obstruction since the priority should focus on clearing the airway.

4. A finger sweep is recommended if the health care provider can see solid material obstructing the airway of an unresponsive patient. In the question, the boy is conscious.

System Specific: Non-Systems
Content Outline: Safety and Protection; Professional Responsibilities; Research

## Exam One: Question 137

A physical therapist assesses a patient's upper extremity deep tendon reflexes as part of a screening examination. The MOST appropriate location to elicit the brachioradialis reflex is the:

1. radial tuberosity
2. antecubital fossa
3. biceps tendon
4. **styloid process of the radius**

---

**Correct Answer: 4** (Magee p. 52)

The brachioradialis muscle is innervated by the radial nerve via the C5-C6 nerve root, however, the reflex is largely a function of C6. The brachioradialis muscle is the only muscle in the body that extends from the distal end of one bone to the distal end of another.

1. The radial tuberosity is an oval projection from the medial surface of the radius, immediately distal to the neck. The biceps brachii tendon inserts on the radial tuberosity.

2. The antecubital fossa is a triangular cavity of the elbow that contains the tendon of the biceps, the median nerve, and the brachial artery.

3. The biceps reflex (C5-C6) is tested by tapping over the biceps tendon or the thumb of the therapist placed directly over the biceps tendon in the antecubital fossa.

4. **The brachioradialis reflex is tested by tapping the brachioradialis tendon at the distal end of the radius with the flat edge of the reflex hammer.**

System Specific: Neuromuscular & Nervous Systems
Content Outline: Physical Therapy Examination

---

## Exam One: Question 138

A physical therapist prepares to assist a patient with a sliding board transfer from a wheelchair to a mat table. Which of the following would be the MOST appropriate INITIAL instruction to the patient?

1. place the sliding board under your buttocks
2. move your buttocks onto the mat table
3. complete a series of push-ups
4. **secure the wheelchair brakes**

---

**Correct Answer: 4** (Minor p. 136)

Securing the wheelchair brakes is the most appropriate action when initiating a transfer from a wheelchair.

1. Placing the sliding board under the buttocks occurs after the wheelchair is positioned, after the wheelchair brakes are secure, and after the armrests are removed.

2. Moving the buttocks onto the mat table is performed after the patient has actually slid out of the wheelchair, onto and across the sliding board, and is ready to complete the transfer.

3. Completing a series of push ups is performed after the sliding board is placed under the buttocks in order to move across the sliding board.

4. **Securing the wheelchair brakes is always the most appropriate action when initiating a transfer from a wheelchair. It is a safety concern that must be addressed in order for the patient to safely complete the transfer.**

System Specific: Non-Systems
Content Outline: Equipment & Devices; Therapeutic Modalities

## Exam One: Question 139

A physical therapist completes a respiratory assessment on a patient in an acute care hospital. The examination reveals decreased breath sounds and decreased fremitus. This finding is MOST indicative of:

1. **pleural effusion**
2. pulmonary edema
3. consolidation
4. atelectasis

**Correct Answer: 1** (Hillegass p. 554)

Decreased breath sounds and decreased fremitus are most likely caused by pleural effusion or pneumothorax. Pulmonary edema, consolidation, and atelectasis are often associated with decreased breath sounds and increased fremitus.

1. **Pleural effusion is an accumulation of fluid between the layers of the membrane that lines the lungs and chest cavity. Abnormal lung pressures secondary to congestive heart failure often cause transudative pleural effusion. Exudative effusion results from inflammation of the pleura caused by lung disease.**
2. Pulmonary edema is an accumulation of fluid in the alveolar spaces. The condition is most often associated with decreased breath sounds and increased fremitus.
3. Consolidation refers to an area of the lung that is filled with fluid. The fluid may be edema, inflammatory exudate, pus, water or blood. The condition is most often associated with decreased breath sounds and increased fremitus on the side of the consolidation.
4. Atelectasis is the absence of gas in part or all of a lung due to a collapse of the lung tissue. The condition is most often associated with decreased breath sounds and increased fremitus.

System Specific: Cardiovascular/Pulmonary and Lymphatic Systems
Content Outline: Foundations for Evaluation, Differential Diagnosis, & Prognosis

## Exam One: Question 140

A physical therapist records the parameters of an electrical stimulation treatment in a patient's medical record. The standard unit of measure when recording alternating current frequency is:

1. volt
2. **hertz**
3. coulomb
4. pulses per second

**Correct Answer: 2** (Cameron p. 236)

Frequency controls, often labeled rate, determine the type of response or muscle contraction that electrical stimulation will produce. As the frequency of any waveform is increased, the amplitude tends to increase and decrease more rapidly.

1. Voltage refers to the electrical force capable of moving charged particles through a conductor between two regions or points.
2. **Hertz is a unit of measure which describes the number of cycles per second when using alternating current.**
3. A coulomb is the amount of electrical charge transported in one second by a steady current of one ampere.
4. Pulses per second is utilized to describe the frequency of pulsed current.

System Specific: Non-Systems
Content Outline: Equipment & Devices; Therapeutic Modalities

## Exam One: Question 141

A physical therapist working in cardiac rehabilitation progresses a patient involved in a phase II program through an established exercise protocol. The patient weighs 70 kg and has progressed without difficulty through the rehabilitation program. The protocol indicates the patient should be performing activities requiring 3-4 METs. An example of an appropriate activity would be:

1. level walking at 1 mph
2. jogging at 5 mph
3. cycling at 10 mph
4. **walking on a treadmill at 3 mph**

**Correct Answer: 4** (Brannon p. 317)
One metabolic equivalent is the amount of oxygen consumed at rest and is equal to approximately 3.5 milliliters of oxygen per kilogram of body weight per minute.

1. Level walking at 1 mph is approximately 1-2 METs.

2. Jogging at 5 mph is approximately 7-8 METs.

3. Cycling at 10 mph is approximately 5-6 METs.

4. **Walking on a treadmill at 3 mph is approximately 3-4 METs.**

System Specific: Cardiovascular/Pulmonary and Lymphatic Systems
Content Outline: Interventions

## Exam One: Question 142

A physical therapist utilizes continuous ultrasound to supply thermal effects to a patient rehabilitating from a lower extremity injury. During the treatment session, the patient suddenly becomes startled and reports feeling an electrical shock from the ultrasound machine. The MOST appropriate therapist action is to:

1. decrease the intensity of the ultrasound
2. modify the duty cycle
3. discontinue ultrasound treatment
4. **unplug the machine and label – "defective, do not use"**

**Correct Answer: 4** (Prentice – Therapeutic Modalities p. 398)
Any equipment that is potentially defective should be formally inspected prior to being used to treat patients.

1. Decreasing the intensity of the ultrasound will diminish the total amount of sound energy delivered to tissues, however, it does not significantly protect the patient from the potential harm of a malfunctioning ultrasound unit.

2. Modifying the duty cycle would be used to increase or decrease the amount of sound energy delivered to tissues or to emphasize to a greater or lesser extent the thermal or non-thermal effects, however, the option does not offer adequate protection for the patient.

3. Discontinuing ultrasound treatment, although appropriate, places other patients at risk by exposing them to potential harm from a malfunctioning ultrasound unit. It is an appropriate therapist response to discontinue any physical agent when the patient reports an abnormal response to treatment such as "feeling an electrical shock."

4. **By unplugging the machine and labeling it – "defective, do not use," the therapist not only guarantees that the current treatment is stopped, but also eliminates any potential risk from using the ultrasound unit with other patients. The unit requires a formal inspection from a qualified individual prior to being used again.**

System Specific: Non-Systems
Content Outline: Equipment & Devices; Therapeutic Modalities

## Exam One: Question 143

A physical therapy department embarks on a quality improvement program. Results from a random sample of patient charts reveal that 40% of the charts do not include a discharge summary. A logical next step to the quality improvement program would be:

1. dismiss the findings because discharge summaries are not directly related to the quality of patient care
2. discipline the staff members who did not complete the discharge summaries and continue to monitor the situation
3. dismiss the findings because a random sample does not provide accurate information
4. **notify the staff that discharge summaries are to be completed on all patients and continue to monitor the situation**

**Correct Answer: 4** (Nosse p. 295)

Quality improvement refers to activities or programs designed to achieve a desired degree or grade of care. Findings from quality improvement initiatives should be communicated directly to staff in a manner that is constructive, instead of punitive.

1. Discharge summaries are an essential component of physical therapy documentation and offer important information that can be used as part of a quality improvement program.

2. Disciplining staff members based on the identification of a significant finding from a quality improvement program would be considered a punitive action, especially given the fact that the problem had not been previously addressed.

3. A random sample of patient charts is a commonly used form of sampling that allows individuals to draw inferences without having to examine every patient chart. Given the significance of the findings (i.e., 40% of patient charts did not include a discharge summary), it would be inappropriate to dismiss the findings.

4. **The identified finding is unacceptable and therefore compels the therapist to act. By notifying staff of the findings the therapist has emphasized the importance of completing discharge summaries. Continued monitoring is necessary to determine if the staffs' performance improves. Failure to improve may warrant disciplinary action.**

System Specific: Non-Systems
Content Outline: Safety and Protection; Professional Responsibilities; Research

## Exam One: Question 144

A physical therapist employed in a rehabilitation hospital examines a patient that exhibits several signs and symptoms of anemia. Which question would be the MOST useful to gather additional information related to anemia?

1. Does it hurt to take a deep breath?
2. **Do you experience heart palpitations or shortness of breath at rest or with mild exertion?**
3. Do you frequently experience dizziness, headaches or blurred vision?
4. Are you susceptible to bruising?

**Correct Answer: 2** (Goodman - Differential Diagnosis p. 230)

Anemia is a condition in which the number of red blood cells is reduced. Due to the reduction of red blood cells, delivery of oxygen to the tissues is impaired. Symptoms of anemia include pallor, cyanosis, cool skin, weakness, and malaise.

1. Pain with deep breathing may be from pleurisy, pneumothorax or from an injury to the muscles, ribs, cartilage or nerves of the chest.

2. **Heart palpitations and shortness of breath are symptoms of anemia.**

3. Dizziness, headaches or blurred vision are signs and symptoms commonly associated with hypertension.

4. Susceptibility to bruising is a sign of a coagulation disorder, possibly from recent use of thrombolytic agents after a myocardial infarction or hemophilia.

System Specific: Cardiovascular/Pulmonary and Lymphatic Systems
Content Outline: Physical Therapy Examination

## Exam One: Question 145

A physical therapist performs postural drainage to the anterior basal segments of the lower lobes. During the treatment session the patient suddenly complains of dizziness and mild dyspnea. The MOST appropriate therapist action is:

1. reassure the patient that the response is normal
2. assess the patient's vital signs
3. **elevate the patient's head**
4. call for assistance

**Correct Answer: 3** (Hillegass p. 570)

Postural drainage is the assumption of one or more body positions that allow gravity to drain secretions from each of the patient's lung segments. In each position, the segmental bronchus of the area to be drained is positioned perpendicular to the floor. Postural drainage to the anterior basal segment of the lower lobes would require the bottom of the bed to be elevated 18 inches.

1. A subjective complaint of dizziness and mild dyspnea would exceed a "normal" patient response. The physical therapist must act based on the patient's comment even though it would not be entirely unexpected given the necessary patient position for postural drainage of the anterior basal segment of the lower lobes.

2. Assessing the patient's vital signs is a desirable option, however, only after the patient is repositioned with the head elevated.

3. **Dizziness and dyspnea are signs of intolerance to the head down postural drainage position required to drain the anterior basal segments of the lower lobes. Elevating the patient's head will likely relieve the symptoms.**

4. Calling for assistance is not necessary since the patient's symptoms should subside once the head is elevated.

System Specific: Cardiovascular/Pulmonary and Lymphatic Systems
Content Outline: Interventions

## Exam One: Question 146

A terminally ill patient completes a formal document that names his daughter as the individual to make health care decisions in the event that he is unable. This type of advanced directive is termed:

1. living will
2. physician's directive
3. **durable power of attorney**
4. euthanasia

**Correct Answer: 3** (Scott – Promoting Legal and Ethical Awareness p. 194)

Durable power of attorney for health care decisions refers to a legal document that delegates decision making to a specified individual in the event another individual is found to be incompetent to make a medical decision.

1. A living will is a legal document that a person uses to make known his or her wishes regarding life prolonging medical treatments. It can also be referred to as an advance directive, health care directive or a physician's directive.

2. The term "physician's directive" is synonymous with a living will.

3. **The power associated with the durable power of attorney becomes operative when and if the patient becomes legally incompetent to make decisions. The patient often designates a spouse, relative, friend or attorney to act on their behalf.**

4. Euthanasia is the act of ending a person's life and usually pertains to patients in either vegetative states or that are terminally ill. Passive euthanasia is the practice of withholding or withdrawing life sustaining devices and measures. Active euthanasia involves the deliberate intervention in order to facilitate a person's death.

System Specific: Non-Systems
Content Outline: Safety and Protection; Professional Responsibilities; Research

## Exam One: Question 147

A patient recently diagnosed with a deep venous thrombophlebitis is placed on heparin. The PRIMARY side effect associated with heparin is:

1. hypotension
2. depression
3. **excessive anticoagulation**
4. thrombocytopenia

**Correct Answer: 3** (Ciccone p. 352)

Anticoagulant agents delay or prevent blood coagulation (clotting). Heparin is an anticoagulant used to prevent and treat disorders such as pulmonary embolism, which result from vascular thrombosis. Heparin inhibits coagulation by preventing the conversion of prothrombin to thrombin and by preventing the release of thromboplastin from platelets.

1. Hypotension, a lower than normal systolic or diastolic blood pressure, is not a side effect of heparin.
2. Depression, a mood disorder characterized by loss of interest or pleasure in living, is not a side effect associated with heparin.
3. **The most common side effect of heparin is abnormal bleeding. A physical therapist should be careful to avoid excessive contact or bumping of the limbs of a patient on heparin since this may cause bruising or bleeding.**
4. Thrombocytopenia, or an abnormal decrease in the number of blood platelets, has been associated with heparin use, but is not the primary side effect.

System Specific: Cardiovascular/Pulmonary and Lymphatic Systems
Content Outline: Foundations for Evaluation, Differential Diagnosis, and Prognosis

## Exam One: Question 148

A patient is asked to complete a pain questionnaire. The patient selects words such as cramping, dull, and aching to describe the pain. What related structure is MOST consistent with the pain description?

1. nerve root
2. **muscle**
3. bone
4. vascular

**Correct Answer: 2** (Magee p. 7)

The patient interview provides a physical therapist with an opportunity to identify specific characteristics of pain. Subjective pain descriptors can provide valuable information related to a patient's condition. Characteristics to explore may include location, intensity, description, duration, and pattern.

1. Nerve root pain is often characterized as sharp, shooting, and burning. The pain tends to travel in the distribution of the specific nerve root.
2. **Muscle pain is often characterized as cramping, dull, and aching. The pain tends to worsen when the involved muscle contracts or is lengthened.**
3. Bone pain is often characterized as deep, intolerable, boring, and highly localized.
4. Vascular pain is often characterized as diffuse, throbbing, aching, and poorly localized. The pain is often referred to other parts of the body.

System Specific: Other Systems
Content Outline: Foundations for Evaluation, Differential Diagnosis, & Prognosis

## Exam One: Question 149

A physical therapist examines a patient with suspected vascular compression in the shoulder region. Which special test would be LEAST beneficial to confirm the therapist's suspicions?

1. Adson maneuver
2. Halstead maneuver
3. **Froment's sign**
4. Wright Test

**Correct Answer: 3** (Magee p. 442)

There are a variety of special tests designed to identify vascular compression in the shoulder. When performing the tests, a positive sign is often indicated by diminution or disappearance of a pulse or reproduction of neurological signs or symptoms.

1. Adson maneuver is performed with the patient in sitting or standing. The therapist monitors the radial pulse and asks the patient to rotate their head to face the test shoulder. The patient is then asked to extend their head while the therapist laterally rotates and extends the patient's shoulder. A positive test is indicated by an absent or diminished radial pulse.

2. The Halstead maneuver is performed with the patient sitting over the edge of a table. The therapist palpates the radial pulse and applies a downward traction on the symptomatic side. The patient is then asked to extend the head and turn away from the tested side. A positive test is indicated by an absent or diminished pulse.

3. **Froment's sign requires a patient to grasp a piece of paper between the thumb and index finger. A positive test is indicated by flexion of the terminal phalanx of the thumb caused by paralysis of the adductor pollicis longus. The test is used to assess the integrity of the ulnar nerve.**

4. The Wright test or hyperabduction test is performed with the patient in sitting or supine. The therapist moves the patient's arm overhead in the frontal plane while monitoring the patient's radial pulse. A positive test is indicated by an absent or diminished radial pulse and may be indicative of compression in the costoclavicular space.

System Specific: Musculoskeletal System
Content Outline: Physical Therapy Examination

## Exam One: Question 150

A physical therapist asks a patient to complete a visual analogue scale designed to assess pain intensity. The scale consists of a 10 centimeter line with descriptive labels at each end. Which terminology would be the MOST appropriate for the FIRST label?

1. **no pain**
2. mild pain
3. weak pain
4. faint pain

**Correct Answer: 1** (Magee p. 9)

A visual analogue scale is a tool used to assess pain intensity using a 10-15 cm line with the left anchor indicating "no pain" and the right anchor indicating "the worst pain you can have." The level of perceived pain is indicated on the line and is reassessed frequently over the course of physical therapy to qualify changes in the pain level and to assess progress.

1. **The left anchor of a visual analogue pain scale is often described as no pain, pain free or the absence of pain.**

2. Mild pain is defined as not acute or serious. The term mild pain would be more appropriately used on a verbal descriptor scale where a patient may be asked to point to a term that best matches their pain (e.g., slight pain, mild pain, moderate pain, severe pain).

3. Weak pain is characterized as not strong or lacking force. This would correspond to a rating on the lower portion of the visual analogue scale, but would not be used as an anchor definition.

4. Faint pain is characterized as lacking strength or vividness. This would correspond to a rating slightly above the visual analogue scale's left anchor.

System Specific: Other Systems
Content Outline: Physical Therapy Examination

## Exam One: Question 151

A physical therapist prepares to treat a patient with continuous ultrasound. Which general rule BEST determines the length of treatment when using ultrasound?

1.  two minutes for an area that is two times the size of the transducer face
2.  **five minutes for an area that is two times the size of the transducer face**
3.  five minutes is the maximum treatment time regardless of the treatment area
4.  ten minutes is the maximum treatment time regardless of the treatment area

**Correct Answer: 2** (Prentice - Therapeutic Modalities p. 378)
The duration of ultrasound treatment is based on a number of variables including the treatment goal, the size of the area to be treated, and the effective radiating area of the transducer face.

1.  Two minutes would not be enough time to use ultrasound in an area that was two times the size of the transducer face.
2.  **An accepted recommendation is that ultrasound can be administered to an area two to three times the size of the effective radiating area of the transducer face in a five minute period. This recommendation equates to roughly twice the size of the transducer face.**
3.  There is not a specified maximum amount of time when using ultrasound. Most often ultrasound is used for periods ranging from five to eight minutes in duration.
4.  Ten minutes is a relatively long duration for treatment with ultrasound, however, this could be plausible in situations where the size of the area to be treated is large.

System Specific: Non-Systems
Content Outline: Equipment & Devices; Therapeutic Modalities

## Exam One: Question 152

A physical therapist attempts to prevent alveolar collapse in a patient following thoracic surgery. Which breathing technique would be the MOST beneficial to achieve the established goal?

1.  inspiratory muscle trainer
2.  mechanical percussors
3.  **incentive spirometer**
4.  flutter valve

**Correct Answer: 3** (Hillegass p. 583)
An incentive spirometer provides visual or in some cases auditory feedback as the patient takes a maximum inspiration. Incentive spirometry increases the amount of air that is inspired and as a result, can be used as a treatment to prevent alveolar collapse after thoracic surgery.

1.  Inspiratory muscle trainers are handheld breathing training devices used primarily to increase the strength and endurance of the muscles of inspiration. They are not used to prevent alveolar collapse after thoracic surgery.
2.  Mechanical percussors are electronically or pneumatically powered devices employed as a substitute for manual percussion with the hands. They can be used to help mobilize bronchial secretions after thoracic surgery, but only if the patient was retaining secretions.
3.  **Incentive spirometers are devices that provide visual or other feedback while the patient performs sustained maximal inspirations. The device is most often used following upper abdominal or thoracic surgery. Indications may include chest wall pain, loss of mobility, weakness of the muscles of inspiration, and to prevent or treat atelectasis.**
4.  Flutter valves are mucus clearance devices that combine positive expiratory pressure with high frequency oscillations at the airway opening during exhalation.

System Specific: Cardiovascular/Pulmonary and Lymphatic Systems
Content Outline: Interventions

## Exam One: Question 153

A physical therapist reviews the surface anatomy of the hand in preparation for a patient status post wrist arthrodesis. Which bony structure does NOT articulate with the lunate?

1. **trapezium**
2. radius
3. capitate
4. scaphoid

**Correct Answer: 1** (Hoppenfeld p. 66)

The lunate is located in the center of the proximal row between the scaphoid and the triquetrum. The lunate is distinguished by its crescent-like outline. The proximal row of carpal bones from lateral to medial consists of the scaphoid, lunate, triquetrum, and pisiform. The distal row of carpal bones from lateral to medial consists of the trapezium, trapezoid, capitate, and hamate.

1. **The trapezium is located on the lateral side of the carpus between the scaphoid and the first metacarpal. It is distinguished by a deep groove on its palmar surface. The proximal portion of the trapezium articulates with the scaphoid. The distal portion articulates with the base of the second metacarpal.**

2. The radius articulates with the wrist at the radiocarpal joint. The concave surface of the distal end of the radius articulates with the scaphoid and lunate of the proximal row of carpals.

3. The capitate is the most central and largest of the carpal bones. The proximal portion of the capitate articulates with the lunate and scaphoid. The distal portion articulates with the base of the third metacarpal.

4. The scaphoid links the proximal and distal carpal rows and helps provide stability to the wrist. Patients who fracture the proximal aspect of the scaphoid are susceptible to avascular necrosis due to disrupted blood supply. The proximal portion of the scaphoid articulates with the radius. The distal portion articulates with the trapezium and trapezoid. The medial surface articulates with the lunate and capitate.

System Specific: Musculoskeletal System
Content Outline: Physical Therapy Examination

## Exam One: Question 154

A physical therapist conducts a sensory assessment on numerous areas of a patient's face. The cranial nerve MOST likely assessed using this type of testing procedure is:

1. facial nerve
2. oculomotor nerve
3. **trigeminal nerve**
4. trochlear nerve

**Correct Answer: 3** (Magee p. 74)

The cranial nerves refer to twelve pairs of nerves that have their origin in the brain. The majority of cranial nerves contain both sensory and motor fibers, however, there are several exceptions including the oculomotor and trochlear nerves.

1. The afferent component of the facial nerve (cranial nerve VII) can be assessed by examining a patient's ability to accurately identify sweet and salty substances. The efferent component is tested by performing a manual muscle test of selected muscles involved in facial expression.

2. The efferent component of the oculomotor nerve (cranial nerve III) can be assessed by asking a patient positioned in sitting to follow an object such as a writing utensil with their eyes as it is moved vertically, horizontally, and diagonally. The therapist should make sure the patient does not rotate their head during the testing and should inspect the patient's eyes for asymmetry or ptosis.

3. **The afferent component of the trigeminal nerve (cranial nerve V) can be assessed by examining sensation of the face and jaw. The efferent component is assessed by examining the muscles of mastication.**

4. The efferent component of the trochlear nerve (cranial nerve IV) can be assessed by asking a patient positioned in sitting to follow an object such as a writing utensil with their eyes as it is moved in an inferior direction. The therapist should make sure the patient does not move their head downward.

System Specific: Neuromuscular & Nervous Systems
Content Outline: Physical Therapy Examination

## Exam One: Question 155

A physical therapist treats a patient in a medical intensive care unit. The therapist notices that intravenous solution appears to be infusing into the tissues surrounding the dorsum of the patient's hand. The MOST appropriate therapist action is:

1. **contact nursing**
2. reposition the intravenous line
3. remove the intravenous line
4. document the incident in the medical record

**Correct Answer: 1** (Pierson p. 282)

An intravenous system consists of a sterile fluid source, a pump, a clamp, and a catheter to insert into a vein. An intravenous system can be used to infuse fluids, electrolytes, nutrients, and medication. The described scenario suggests that the catheter has become dislodged from the superficial vein. Nursing should be immediately alerted to any problems with the intravenous system.

1. **Nurses have the requisite training necessary to adjust, modify or discontinue the use of an intravenous system. In some instances, other health care providers are permitted to make selected modifications, however, only after being adequately instructed and trained.**

2. Repositioning the intravenous line for the purpose of straightening the tubing or removing an object that is occluding the tubing is an appropriate activity for a physical therapist. The action would not be useful to address the primary issue which is the intravenous solution infusing into the tissues of the hand.

3. Removing the intravenous line is a skilled activity that should be performed by a nurse.

4. Documenting the incident is appropriate, however, addressing the patient care issue would remain the priority.

System Specific: Cardiovascular/Pulmonary and Lymphatic Systems
Content Outline: Foundations for Evaluation, Differential Diagnosis, and Prognosis

## Exam One: Question 156

A physical therapist completes a cognitive function test on a patient status post stroke. As part of the test, the therapist examines the patient's abstract ability. Which of the following tasks would be the MOST appropriate?

1. orientation to time, person, and place
2. copy drawn figures of varying size and shape
3. **discuss how two objects are similar**
4. identify letters or numbers traced on the skin

**Correct Answer: 3** (O'Sullivan p. 232)

A patient with impaired abstract thinking may have involvement of the frontal lobe, diffuse encephalopathy or psychiatric illness.

1. Orientation can be assessed by asking a person to identify time (e.g., day, month, season), person (e.g., name), and place (e.g., city, state). Disorientation is most commonly associated with traumatic brain injury, delirium, and advanced dementia.

2. Copying drawn figures of varying size and shape assesses constructional ability. Impairments in constructional ability are often associated with damage to the parietal lobe or stroke.

3. **Abstract ability is commonly tested using two specific methods. The first method is by asking a patient to describe how two items such as a cat and a mouse are similar. The other method is by asking a patient to interpret the meaning of a proverb such as "a rolling stone gathers no moss." Patients with difficulty in abstract thinking may provide answers that tend to be literal or concrete.**

4. The ability to recognize symbols, letters or numbers traced on the skin refers to graphesthesia. Patients with language or speech disorders secondary to stroke can identify the correct figure by pointing at an image located in a table instead of through verbal identification.

System Specific: Neuromuscular & Nervous Systems
Content Outline: Physical Therapy Examination

## Exam One: Question 157

A patient fails to attain established physical therapy goals within the number of visits approved by the patient's third party payer. The patient has made progress in therapy, however, has been slowed somewhat by an adverse reaction to medication. The MOST appropriate physical therapist action is:

1. request additional visits from the referring physician
2. **request additional visits from the third party payer**
3. inform the patient that physical therapy services may not be fully covered by the third party payer
4. discharge the patient from physical therapy with a home exercise program

**Correct Answer: 2** (Criteria for Standards of Practice)

According to the *Criteria for Standards of Practice for Physical Therapy* published by the American Physical Therapy Association, "The physical therapist discharges the patient/client from physical therapy when the anticipated goals or expected outcomes for the patient/client have been achieved. The physical therapist discontinues intervention when the patient/client is unable to continue to progress toward goals or when the physical therapist determines that the patient/client will no longer benefit from physical therapy."

1. The question does not provide any evidence suggesting that the physician has limited the patient's number of physical therapy visits or that an established limit has been reached.

2. **A physical therapist should attempt to secure approval for additional physical therapy visits when there is ample evidence that the patient is progressing towards the established goals.**

3. It is reasonable for the physical therapist to provide information to the patient regarding reimbursement when possible, however, the greater priority would be to have the additional visits approved by the third party payer.

4. It would not be in the best interest of the patient to be discharged from physical therapy since they have made progress, however, have yet to attain the established goals.

System Specific: Non-Systems
Content Outline: Safety and Protection; Professional Responsibilities; Research

## Exam One: Question 158

A physical therapist documents in the medical record that a patient has moved from stage 5 to stage 6 of Brunnstrom's Stages of Recovery. This type of transition is characterized by:

1. absence of associated reactions
2. **disappearance of spasticity**
3. voluntary movement begins outside of synergy patterns
4. normal motor function

**Correct Answer: 2** (Brunnstrom p. 47)

Brunnstrom separates neurological recovery into seven separate stages based on progression through abnormal tone and spasticity. The seven stages of recovery describe tone, reflex activity, and volitional movement.

1. In stage 2, movement occurs primarily in the form of associated reactions and spasticity begins to develop. In stage 3 voluntary movement begins within basic limb synergies.

2. **In stage 5, spasticity is still present although it continues to decrease. Stage 6 is characterized by the disappearance of spasticity and the ability to complete isolated joint movements in a coordinated fashion.**

3. In stage 4, movement patterns are not dictated solely by limb synergies and voluntary movement patterns begin outside of limb synergies.

4. In stage 7, normal motor function is restored.

System Specific: Neuromuscular & Nervous Systems
Content Outline: Physical Therapy Examination

## Exam One: Question 159

A physical therapist preparing a hot pack notices the water in the hot pack unit is cloudy. The MOST probable explanation is:

1. power failure
2. **seepage from a hot pack**
3. ineffective heating element
4. thermostat set too low

**Correct Answer: 2** (Cameron p. 161)

A hot pack consists of a canvas or nylon covered pack filled with hydrophilic silicate gel that provides a moist heat. The size and shape of the hot pack varies depending on the size and contour of the treatment area.

1. A power failure would result in the water temperature being low. As a result, the hot packs would not possess the necessary amount of heat to transfer to the target area.

2. **A disruption in the canvas case may cause small quantities of the silicate to be released into the water which often results in the water appearing cloudy.**

3. An ineffective heating element would fail to heat the water or would heat it to less than the desired temperature. A change in water temperature would not significantly influence the clarity of the water.

4. A thermostat that is set too low would not heat the water within the hot pack unit to the desired temperature.

System Specific: Non-Systems
Content Outline: Equipment & Devices; Therapeutic Modalities

**Test Taking Tip:** A power failure, ineffective heating element, and a thermostat set too low would all result in insufficient heating. Since the options would result in the same objective finding it would be unlikely that one of the options would be correct and the others would be incorrect. In essence, the options mutually exclude each other from being correct.

## Exam One: Question 160

A physical therapist designs a home exercise program for a patient rehabilitating from a lower extremity injury. Which step would be the MOST appropriate to maximize patient compliance?

1. limit the exercise program to 10 minutes
2. select a maximum of five different exercises
3. **select exercises consistent with the patient's rehabilitation goals**
4. avoid physically demanding exercises

**Correct Answer: 3** (Kisner p. 20)

Many factors can influence patient compliance with a home exercise program, however, regardless of the construction of the program it is essential that the program is designed to be consistent with the patient's rehabilitation goals.

1. An exercise program that can be completed in a relatively short period of time is more likely to be completed since patients have a better opportunity to fit the program into their existing schedule.

2. Limiting the number of exercises tends to promote compliance since it is easier for the patient to focus and complete each exercise.

3. **Patients are typically highly motivated to complete home exercise programs when they believe the exercises will help them to achieve their personal rehabilitation goals. Options such as limiting the length of the exercise program and limiting the number of exercises are helpful strategies to promote compliance, however, they would not be as critical as aligning the exercises with the patient's rehabilitation goals.**

4. There is no information presented which implies the patient is averse to physically demanding activities.

System Specific: Musculoskeletal System
Content Outline: Interventions

**Test Taking Tip:** Many items on the National Physical Therapy Examination require candidates to differentiate between good, better, and best options. Candidates must therefore carefully assess the relative value of each of the presented options. In this particular item, candidates must differentiate between several options that are plausible and attractive. Candidates must remain open minded when examining each of the options and avoid the tendency to select the first viable option that they encounter since in many cases there is an additional option that may be better.

## Exam One: Question 161

A physical therapist performs gait training activities with an eight-year-old child who utilizes a reciprocating gait orthosis. Which medical diagnosis is MOST often associated with the use of this type of orthotic device?

1. cerebral palsy
2. Down syndrome
3. Legg-Calve-Perthes disease
4. **spina bifida**

**Correct Answer: 4** (Tecklin p. 256)

A reciprocating gait orthosis is a type of hip-knee-ankle-foot orthosis that incorporates a cable connecting the two hip joint mechanisms. The device assists the child to advance the lower extremities during ambulation.

1. Cerebral palsy is an umbrella term used to describe a group of non-progressive movement disorders that result from brain damage. Clinical presentation includes motor delays, abnormal muscle tone and motor control, reflex abnormalities, poor postural control, and balance impairments.

2. Down syndrome (trisomy 21) occurs when there is an error in cell division. Clinical manifestations include hypotonia, flattened nasal bridge, Simian line (palmar crease), epicanthal folds, enlargement of the tongue, and developmental delay.

3. Legg-Calve-Perthes disease is the name given to idiopathic osteonecrosis of the capital femoral epiphysis of the femoral head. Clinical presentation includes short limb, high greater trochanter, quadriceps atrophy, and adductor spasm. Bracing using a Scottish-Rite brace may be used in an attempt to contain the femoral head in the acetabulum.

4. **Spina bifida is a congenital neural tube defect that generally occurs in the lumbar spine, but can also occur at the sacral, thoracic, and cervical levels. Classifications include occulta, meningocele, and myelomeningocele. Since the impairments associated with some of the classifications of spina bifida can include motor and sensory loss below the vertebral defect a reciprocating gait orthosis is often used.**

System Specific: Neuromuscular and Nervous Systems
Content Outline: Interventions

## Exam One: Question 162

A physical therapist instructs a patient rehabilitating from thoracic surgery how to produce an effective cough. Which patient position would be the MOST appropriate to initiate treatment?

1. standing
2. **sitting**
3. sidelying
4. hooklying

**Correct Answer: 2** (Kisner p. 868)

An effective cough requires an inspiration greater than tidal volume, followed by closure of the glottis, abdominal muscle contraction, and sudden opening of the glottis for the forceful expulsion of the inspired air.

1. Although it is possible to perform a maximal inhalation needed for an effective cough, the standing position would not be the MOST appropriate position to initiate treatment after thoracic surgery.

2. **Sitting upright will maximize all of the steps needed to produce an effective cough.**

3. The sidelying position does not promote the maximal inhalation needed for an effective cough.

4. The hooklying position does not promote the maximal inhalation needed for an effective cough. Hooklying refers to a position where the patient is lying in supine with their hips and knees bent and the feet flat on the floor with the arms positioned at the their side.

System Specific: Cardiovascular/Pulmonary and Lymphatic Systems
Content Outline: Interventions

## Exam One: Question 163

A physical therapist provides pre-operative instructions for a patient scheduled for hip arthroplasty surgery. As part of the session, the therapist discusses the importance of preventing deep vein thrombosis following surgery. Which finding is the BEST indicator that the patient is at minimal risk of acquiring a deep vein thrombosis?

1. ability to perform ankle pumps and muscle setting exercises
2. **ability to ambulate on a frequent schedule**
3. ability to achieve full hip range of motion within the allowable limits
4. ability to utilize pneumatic compression devices and elastic stockings

**Correct Answer: 2** (Kisner p. 833)

Deep vein thrombosis results from the formation of a blood clot that becomes dislodged and is termed an embolus. This is a serious medical condition since the embolus may obstruct a selected artery. Patients are often at risk for acquiring a deep vein thrombosis after surgery. Other risk factors include advanced age, obesity, infection, tobacco, and air travel.

1. Ankle pumps and muscle setting exercises are beneficial, but would not produce the magnitude of muscle pumping action compared to an activity such as ambulation since the exercises tend to involve muscles working in relative isolation.

2. **The ability to ambulate on a frequent schedule requires a significant amount of muscle pumping action generated from contraction of the lower extremity muscles. The initiation of this activity signifies that the patient is progressing toward a more dynamic state which significantly decreases the risk of acquiring deep vein thrombosis.**

3. Range of motion is a desirable activity following surgery since it requires muscle activity and promotes circulation, however, the intensity of the activity is relatively low when compared to ambulation.

4. Pneumatic compression devices and elastic stockings are often utilized following surgery since they can help to prevent coagulation and the formation of a thrombus. The interventions are less desirable than an activity like ambulation, however, can be successfully integrated into a comprehensive program to prevent deep vein thrombosis.

System Specific: Other Systems
Content Outline: Interventions

## Exam One: Question 164

A physical therapist performs an examination on an 84-year-old female in the physical therapy gym. The patient answers the therapist's questions in a very soft voice and appears to be intimidated by the bustling environment. The MOST appropriate therapist action is:

1. ask the patient if she understands why she was referred to physical therapy
2. tell the patient to relax and speak louder
3. **complete the examination in a private treatment room**
4. ask the patient about her rehabilitation goals

**Correct Answer: 3** (Purtilo p. 344)

A physical therapist should make every attempt to ensure that the patient is comfortable with the environment. The fact that the patient is speaking with a very soft voice and appears to be intimidated by the bustling environment provides adequate justification that the environment is less than ideal.

1. Asking the patient if she understands why she was referred to physical therapy may provide insight toward the patient's awareness of her current abilities and limitations, however, it ignores the fact that the patient appears to be uncomfortable with the existing environment.

2. Telling the patient to relax and speak louder forces the patient to adapt to the existing environment without attempting to modify it.

3. **Completing the examination in a private treatment room attempts to create a more desirable environment for the initial session. A private treatment room offers a secure, quiet location that can be much less intimidating than a physical therapy gym.**

4. Asking the patient about her rehabilitation goals may provide the therapist with important information on how to design an appropriate plan of care, however, it does not address the immediate need which is to modify the existing environment.

System Specific: Non-Systems
Content Outline: Safety and Protection; Professional Responsibilities; Research

## Exam One: Question 165

A group of physical therapists design a research study which examines the reliability of the Functional Independence Measure. To measure reliability the therapists utilize a test-retest design. What is the MOST significant source of error with this type of research design?

1. sampling error
2. tendency to rate too strictly or leniently
3. change in test forms due to sampling of items
4. **change in subject situation over time**

**Correct Answer: 4** (Portney p. 85)

The repeatability of scores on the Functional Independence Measure (FIM) from one test administration to another provides evidence of test-retest reliability.

1. Sampling error refers to the differences between samples drawn from the same population due to chance. This is not an issue in test-retest design for reliability because the same individuals are tested each time.

2. In a test-retest design for reliability, the therapists rating the patients use the same scoring rules on each occasion.

3. In a test-retest design for reliability, the FIM would be administered both times, therefore the form of the test would not change.

4. **Because test-retest design necessitates an interval of time between test administrations, a real change in the patient's function during this time would adversely affect the reliability score.**

System Specific: Non-Systems
Content Outline: Safety and Protection; Professional Responsibilities; Research

## Exam One: Question 166

A patient status post knee surgery receives instructions on the use of a continuous passive motion machine. Which of the following would be the MOST essential to ensure patient safety?

1. instructions on progression of range of motion
2. utilization of proximal and distal stabilization straps
3. recommendations for cryotherapy following treatment sessions
4. **orientation to remote on/off switch**

**Correct Answer: 4** (Kisner p. 62)

The continuous passive motion machine (CPM) is a mechanical device designed to provide continuous motion at a particular joint using a predetermined range and speed. The primary indication for CPM use is to improve range of motion that may have been impaired secondary to a surgical procedure.

1. The physical therapist would likely provide the patient with a description of the anticipated range of motion progression, however, this does not ensure patient safety.

2. The CPM includes proximal and distal stabilization straps which serve to stabilize the upper and lower leg and ensure the knee joint is aligned with the axis of the CPM. Utilization of the straps is a standard procedure when using the CPM.

3. Cryotherapy could be used following the treatment session with the CPM, however, this action would do little to protect the patient while using the CPM.

4. **Physical therapists must orient patients to the CPM's remote on/off switch since the device allows patients to terminate the treatment immediately without direct assistance from a health care provider.**

System Specific: Musculoskeletal System
Content Outline: Interventions

## Exam One: Question 167

A physical therapist instructs a patient rehabilitating from a rotator cuff repair in a home exercise program. The patient is a 27-year-old male who is illiterate. The MOST appropriate action to promote compliance with the exercise program is:

1. ask the patient to memorize the exercises
2. use short sentences consisting of simple words
3. **draw pictures to describe the exercises**
4. do not utilize a home exercise program

**Correct Answer: 3** (Kisner p. 22)

Illiterate refers to the inability to read or write simple sentences. Functional illiteracy refers to the inability of an individual to use reading, writing, and computational skills efficiently in everyday life situations. It is estimated that seven million individuals in the United States are illiterate and 27 million individuals are unable to read well enough to complete a job application.

1. Memorizing the exercises would be a formidable challenge for many patients. The absence of a handout for the patient to refer to would likely decrease compliance and may increase the probability of the exercises being performed incorrectly.
2. Physical therapists should try to keep exercise instructions as simple as possible, however, given the patient's illiteracy this modification may still be inadequate to meet the patient's needs.
3. **Pictures provide the patient with an image of the exercises without relying solely on formal written instructions or memorization.**
4. Home exercise programs are a critical component of almost any patient care plan and can be effective with patients that are illiterate. Physical therapists should use alternate forms of educational media (e.g., pictures) whenever possible since it is an erroneous assumption to believe that the vast majority of patients possess basic reading and writing skills.

System Specific: Musculoskeletal System
Content Outline: Interventions

## Exam One: Question 168

A physical therapist treats a patient status post femur fracture with external fixation. While monitoring the patient during an exercise session, the therapist observes clear drainage from a distal pin site. The MOST appropriate therapist action is:

1. discontinue the exercise session and contact the referring physician
2. use a gauze pad to absorb the drainage and notify nursing
3. **use a gauze pad to absorb the drainage and continue with the exercise session**
4. document the finding and discontinue the exercise session

**Correct Answer: 3** (Pierson p. 288)

External fixation devices provide stabilization to fracture sites through the use of pins that are inserted into bone fragments. Clear drainage from a pin site is not uncommon and should not be viewed as a sign of infection or any other serious medical complication.

1. Clear drainage from a distal pin site would not warrant discontinuing the exercise session or contacting the referring physician. If the scenario offered compelling data suggestive of infection, it would be appropriate to notify the referring physician and/or the nurse.
2. The gauze pad is an acceptable method to absorb the drainage. The observation of clear drainage from a distal pin site is relatively common and therefore would not require consultation with nursing.
3. **The exercise session can continue after the drainage has been absorbed.**
4. Documenting the observation would be acceptable, however, the presented scenario does not provide adequate justification for discontinuing the exercise session.

System Specific: Other Systems
Content Outline: Interventions

## Exam One: Question 169

A physical therapist reviews the medical record of a patient with a suspected head injury. During testing using the Glasgow Coma Scale, the patient exhibited spontaneous eye opening, was able to follow selected motor commands, and was considered to be "oriented" based on verbal responses. The MOST likely score assigned to the patient would be:

1. 6
2. 12
**3. 15**
4. 18

**Correct Answer: 3** (O'Sullivan p. 900)

The Glasgow Coma Scale is a neurological assessment tool used initially after injury to determine arousal and cerebral cortex function. The assessment tool utilizes an ordinal scale ranging from 3-15 with a higher score representing a greater level of consciousness. The Glasgow Coma Scale examines eye opening, motor response, and verbal response. The scale was initially used to assess level of consciousness after head injury and is often used on selected patients in acute care or following trauma.

1. A score of 8 or less is indicative of a severe head injury.

2. A score of 9-12 is indicative of a moderate head injury.

**3. A score of 15 is the highest attainable score on the Glasgow Coma Scale. A score of 13-15 is indicative of a mild head injury.**

4. A score of 18 is not possible on the Glasgow Coma Scale since the maximum score is 15.

System Specific: Neuromuscular & Nervous Systems
Content Outline: Physical Therapy Examination

## Exam One: Question 170

A physical therapist uses a subjective pain scale to assess pain intensity in a patient with multiple sclerosis. The pain scale consists of a 10 cm line with each end anchored by one extreme of perceived pain intensity. The patient is asked to mark on the line the point that best describes their present pain level. This type of scale is BEST termed:

1. Descriptor Differential Scale
2. Verbal Rating Scale
**3. Visual Analogue Scale**
4. Numerical Rating Scale

**Correct Answer: 3** (Van Deusen p. 127)

There are a variety of commonly used pain scales in physical therapy. Physical therapists should have familiarity with the various scales and be able to select an appropriate scale based on the breadth and depth of information they are hoping to collect.

1. The Descriptor Differential Scale consists of 12 descriptor items each centered over 21 horizontal dashes. At the extreme left dash is a minus sign and at the extreme right dash is a plus sign. Patients are asked to rate the magnitude of their pain in terms of each descriptor.

2. A Verbal Rating Scale is most often used to assess pain affect. The scale typically consists of a series of adjectives describing increasing levels of unpleasantness such as "distracting," "oppressive" or "agonizing."

**3. A Visual Analogue Scale is a tool used to assess pain intensity using a 10-15 centimeter line with the left anchor indicating "no pain" and the right anchor indicating "the worst pain you can have." The level of perceived pain is indicated on the line and is reassessed frequently over the course of physical therapy to qualify changes in the pain level and to assess progress.**

4. A Numerical Rating Scale asks patients to rate their perceived level of pain intensity on a numerical scale from 0-10 or 0-100. The 0 represents "no pain" and the 10 or 100 represents "pain as bad as it could be."

System Specific: Other Systems
Content Outline: Physical Therapy Examination

## Exam One: Question 171

A physical therapist assesses end-feel while completing passive plantar flexion range of motion. The therapist classifies the end-feel as firm. Which of the following structures does NOT contribute to the firm end-feel?

1. tension in the anterior joint capsule
2. tension in the tibialis anterior
3. tension in the anterior talofibular ligament
4. **tension in the calcaneofibular ligament**

---

**Correct Answer: 4** (Norkin p. 274)
End-feel refers to the type of resistance that is felt when passively moving a joint through the end range of motion.

1. The anterior joint capsule experiences increased tension with passive plantar flexion range of motion which contributes to a firm end-feel.

2. The tibialis anterior acts to dorsiflex the ankle joint and invert the foot. As a result, the muscle would experience increased tension while lengthening during passive plantar flexion range of motion.

3. The anterior talofibular ligament resists movement into plantar flexion and inversion. The ligament would therefore experience increased tension during passive plantar flexion range of motion.

4. **Tension in the calcaneofibular ligament is often associated with the normal end-feel of dorsiflexion (i.e., firm). Other structures contributing to an end-feel associated with dorsiflexion include the posterior joint capsule, soleus, Achilles tendon, posterior portion of the deltoid ligament, and the posterior talofibular ligament.**

System Specific: Musculoskeletal System
Content Outline: Physical Therapy Examination

---

## Exam One: Question 172

A physical therapist prepares to use phonophoresis as a component of a patient's plan of care, but is concerned about the potential of the ultrasound to exacerbate the patient's current inflammation. The MOST effective method to address the therapist's concern is:

1. utilize ultrasound with a frequency of 1 MHz
2. limit treatment time to five minutes
3. **incorporate a pulsed 20% duty cycle**
4. select an ultrasound intensity less than 1.5 W/cm$^2$

---

**Correct Answer: 3** (Cameron p. 192)
Physical therapists must select ultrasound treatment parameters that are consistent with the desired therapeutic outcome. Failure to select appropriate parameters can lead to poor outcomes and potentially jeopardize patient safety.

1. The frequency of ultrasound selected primarily determines the depth of penetration. A frequency setting of 1 MHz is used for heating of deeper tissues (up to five centimeters).

2. Limiting the treatment time to five minutes does effectively control the duration of ultrasound, but it does not address several other critical factors that significantly influence changes in tissue temperature (e.g., duty cycle, intensity).

3. **When ultrasound is used in a pulsed mode with a 20% or lower duty cycle, the heat produced during the on time of the cycle is dispersed during the off time and as a result there is no measurable net increase in temperature. Ultrasound using a 20% or lower duty cycle would typically be used for nonthermal effects.**

4. Limiting the intensity of ultrasound to less than 1.5 W/cm$^2$ is helpful to avoid exacerbating the patient's current inflammation, however, the patient's condition could still be exacerbated at many intensity levels below 1.5 W/cm$^2$.

System Specific: Non-Systems
Content Outline: Equipment & Devices; Therapeutic Modalities

## Exam One: Question 173

A physical therapist attempts to assess the integrity of the first cranial nerve. Which test would provide the therapist with the desired information?

1. the patient protrudes the tongue while an examiner checks lateral deviation
2. the patient completes a vision examination
3. the patient performs a shoulder shrug against resistance
4. **the patient is asked to identify familiar odors with the eyes closed**

**Correct Answer: 4** (Tan p. 14)

Lesions affecting the cranial nerves often produce specific and predictable alterations. As a result, it is often desirable to perform cranial nerve testing.

1. The hypoglossal nerve (cranial nerve XII) is assessed by asking the patient to protrude the tongue. A positive test may be indicated by an inability to fully protrude the tongue or the tongue deviating to one side during protrusion.

2. The optic nerve (cranial nerve II) is assessed by asking the patient to identify objects or read selected items from a chart or diagram. A positive test may be indicated by an inability to identify objects at a reasonable distance.

3. The accessory nerve (cranial nerve XI) is assessed by asking a patient, positioned in sitting with the arms at their side, to shrug their shoulders and maintain the position while the therapist applies resistance through the shoulders in the direction of shoulder depression. A positive test may be indicated by an inability to maintain the test position against resistance.

4. **The olfactory nerve (cranial nerve I) is assessed by placing an item with a familiar odor under the patient's nostril and the patient is then asked to identify the odor. A positive test may be indicated by an inability to identify familiar odors.**

System Specific: Neuromuscular & Nervous Systems
Content Outline: Physical Therapy Examination

## Exam One: Question 174

A patient eight days status post anterior cruciate ligament reconstruction using a patellar tendon autograft is examined in physical therapy. Which of the following exercises would be the MOST appropriate based on the patient's post-operative status?

1. limited range isokinetics at 30 degrees per second
2. unilateral leg press
3. **mini-squats in standing**
4. active knee extension in short sitting

**Correct Answer: 3** (Kisner p. 732)

Anterior cruciate ligament reconstruction refers to the use of a graft to replace a damaged anterior cruciate ligament. The graft is placed through drilled holes in the femoral and tibial tunnels and then anchored with a fixation device. The focus of the early post-operative period is to protect the healing graft and donor site, and at the same time avoid post-operative complications such as adhesions, contractures, and articular degeneration.

1. Performing isokinetics at 30 degrees per second on a patient eight days status post anterior cruciate ligament reconstruction could potentially jeopardize the integrity of the graft.

2. A unilateral leg press is similar to a squat, however, it is usually performed in a supine position. The exercise is not as desirable as the mini-squat given the patient's post-operative status since the leg press activity is unilateral and therefore the patient would not have the benefit of using the uninvolved lower extremity to assist, if necessary. In addition, the mini-squat implies limited range where the unilateral leg press does not.

3. **A mini-squat is a closed chain exercise typically performed in standing that enables the patient to vary the force through the involved extremity by simply shifting their weight. This exercise significantly limits the amount of knee flexion and as a result does not place a great deal of stress through the reconstructed knee. When completing mini-squats in standing it is important that the knees do not move anterior to the toes as the hips descend since this will increase the shear forces of the tibia and could unnecessarily stress the graft.**

4. Active knee extension in short sitting is an open kinetic chain activity that places a significant amount of force on the anterior surface of the knee and in particular, the patellar tendon donor area.

System Specific: Musculoskeletal System
Content Outline: Interventions

## Exam One: Question 175

A physical therapy department in an acute care hospital utilizes physical therapy aides to perform a variety of patient care services. What health care professional is directly responsible for the actions of the physical therapy aide?

1. **the physical therapist of record**
2. the physical therapist assistant of record
3. the director of physical therapy
4. the director of rehabilitation

**Correct Answer: 1** (Guide to Physical Therapist Practice)
The physical therapy aide is a non-licensed worker who is specifically trained under the direction and supervision of a physical therapist. Activities performed by the aide are limited to those tasks that do not require clinical decision making by the physical therapist.

1. **The determination of what tasks are appropriately directed to the aide must be made by the physical therapist. As a result, the physical therapist would be responsible for the actions of the aide.**

2. The physical therapist assistant can direct and supervise the aide in selected jurisdictions, however, the physical therapist is able to function in this capacity in all jurisdictions. The availability of an option that includes the physical therapist makes the physical therapist assistant option less desirable.

3. The director of physical therapy is an administrative position that would typically be responsible for the daily operations of the physical therapy department.

4. The director of rehabilitation is an administrative position within the health care organization. The position would typically be responsible for the oversight of a number of different departments including physical therapy, occupational therapy, and speech-language pathology.

System Specific: Non-Systems
Content Outline: Safety and Protection; Professional Responsibilities; Research

## Exam One: Question 176

A physical therapist is scheduled to treat a patient requiring droplet precautions. What type of protective equipment would be necessary prior to entering the patient's room?

1. gloves
2. **mask**
3. gloves and mask
4. gloves, gown, and mask

**Correct Answer: 2** (Pierson p. 30)
Droplet precautions are designed to prevent transmission of infectious agents through close respiratory or mucous membrane contact. Droplets are most often deposited on the host's nasal mucosa, conjunctivae or mouth. Examples of diseases requiring droplet precautions include pertussis, influenza, and diphtheria.

1. Gloves would be required for contact precautions, but would not be required for droplet precautions.

2. **Droplet precautions require individuals coming within three feet of the patient to wear a mask, however, it is prudent to wear the mask upon entering the room of a patient on droplet precautions to avoid any inadvertent exposure.**

3. A mask is required when working with a patient with droplet precautions, however, gloves are not.

4. Only a mask is required when treating a patient with droplet precautions. Gloves, gown, and mask are typically required with direct contact with a patient with contact precautions.

System Specific: Non-Systems
Content Outline: Safety and Protection; Professional Responsibilities; Research

## Exam One: Question 177

A physical therapist collects data as part of a research project that requires direct observation of children performing selected gross motor activities. The therapist is concerned about the influence of an observer on the children's performance. The MOST effective strategy to control for this source of error is to:

1. provide initial and refresher observer training
2. increase observer awareness of the influence of their background
3. **have an observer spend time with the children before direct observation**
4. ask the children to ignore the presence of the observer

> **Correct Answer: 3** (Portney p. 310)
> A research project should be designed to eliminate as many extraneous variables as possible. Failure to eliminate or at least reduce the potential impact of an observer on the children's performance would be a significant limitation of the study.
>
> 1. Observer training would be beneficial in order to provide the observers with a better sense of their purpose, role, and actions. This action would be desirable, but would not address the nuance of the observer for the children.
> 2. An individual's background can influence their observations particularly when the data collected is open for interpretation. This option also focuses on the observer and not the children.
> 3. **Spending time with the children prior to direct observation will allow the children to feel more at ease and as a result their performance may be more reflective of their current abilities.**
> 4. Asking the children to ignore the presence of the observer would likely serve to bring additional attention to the observer and therefore influence behavior.
>
> System Specific: Musculoskeletal System
> Content Outline: Physical Therapy Examination

## Exam One: Question 178

A patient reports to a physical therapist that she completely tore one of the ligaments in her ankle. If the patient's comment is accurate, the injury to the ligament is MOST likely classified as a:

1. grade I sprain
2. **grade III sprain**
3. grade I strain
4. grade III strain

> **Correct Answer: 2** (Dutton p. 1128)
> Ligamentous injuries are termed sprains and are graded based on the amount of tissue damage that the ligament has sustained. A strain refers specifically to an injury involving a muscle or tendon.
>
> 1. A first degree sprain involves a stretch of the ligament where there is no discontinuity of the ligament. The injury usually results in minimal if any joint hypermobility.
> 2. **A third degree sprain involves a complete rupture or break in the continuity of a ligament. The injury usually results in gross instability and laxity.**
> 3. A first degree strain involves minimal disruption in the continuity of a muscle or tendon. The question asks specifically about a ligament tear or sprain.
> 4. A third degree strain involves a complete rupture or break in the continuity of a muscle or tendon. The question is asking about a ligament tear or a sprain.
>
> System Specific: Musculoskeletal System
> Content Outline: Foundations for Evaluation, Differential Diagnosis, and Prognosis

## Exam One: Question 179

A physical therapist prepares to treat a patient diagnosed with impingement syndrome with iontophoresis directly over the insertion of the supraspinatus muscle. What bony landmark BEST corresponds to this site?

1. lesser tubercle of the humerus
2. **greater tubercle of the humerus**
3. supraspinous fossa of the scapula
4. deltoid tuberosity of the humerus

**Correct Answer: 2** (Kendall p. 314)

Impingement syndrome is a commonly used term describing mechanical impingement of the rotator cuff tendon beneath the anteroinferior portion of the acromion. Symptoms of impingement syndrome include difficulty reaching up behind the back, pain with overhead use of the arm, and weakness of the shoulder muscles.

1. The subscapularis muscle originates on the subscapular fossa of the scapula and inserts on the lesser tubercle of the humerus. The muscle is innervated by the subscapular nerve.

2. **The supraspinatus muscle inserts on the greater tubercle of the humerus. The muscle is innervated by the suprascapular nerve.**

3. The supraspinatus muscle originates on the supraspinous fossa of the scapula. The question asks about the insertion of the muscle.

4. The deltoid tuberosity is the insertion point for the three heads of the deltoid. The anterior deltoid originates on the lateral third of the clavicle, the middle deltoid originates on the acromion process, and the posterior deltoid originates on the spine of the scapula. The deltoid is innervated by the axillary nerve.

System Specific: Musculoskeletal Systems
Content Outline: Interventions

## Exam One: Question 180

A patient status post motor vehicle accident is referred to physical therapy. The patient has multiple injury sites including the hand, wrist, elbow, and knee. As part of the patient care plan, the physical therapist attempts to increase tissue temperature at each of the involved sites. The MOST appropriate thermal agent is:

1. diathermy
2. ultrasound
3. **hydrotherapy**
4. hot packs

**Correct Answer: 3** (Michlovitz p. 122)

There are a large number of thermal agents that are used in physical therapy. When selecting the most appropriate thermal agent, physical therapists must consider a number of variables including the location and size of the area or areas to be treated.

1. Diathermy refers to the application of shortwave or microwave electromagnetic energy to produce heat within tissues. Diathermy relies on inductive coil applicators or capacitive plates which provide energy to a localized area.

2. Ultrasound uses inaudible acoustic mechanical vibrations of high frequency to produce thermal and nonthermal effects. Ultrasound is most often performed by placing a transducer in direct contact with a body surface or through a medium such as water. The size of the ultrasound transducer would significantly limit the surface area treated with ultrasound.

3. **Hydrotherapy transfers heat through conduction or convection and is administered in tanks of varying size ranging from extremity whirlpools to Olympic size pools. The ability to select the size of the tank makes hydrotherapy an attractive option considering the multiple injury sites.**

4. A hot pack consists of a canvas or nylon covered pack filled with a hydrophilic silicate gel that provides a moist heat. The size and shape of the hot pack varies depending on the size and contour of the treatment area, however, the number of different injury sites makes the use of hot packs impractical.

System Specific: Non-Systems
Content Outline: Equipment & Devices; Therapeutic Modalities

## Exam One: Question 181

A physical therapist presents an inservice on graded oscillation techniques. Which grades of oscillation are the MOST appropriate for stretching maneuvers?

1. I, II
2. I, III
3. II, III
4. **III, IV**

**Correct Answer: 4** (Kisner p. 116)

Physical therapists must select the appropriate rate, rhythm, and intensity of mobilization techniques. Graded oscillation techniques range from grades I-V. Grades I and II oscillations are used primarily to treat joints limited by pain, while grades III and IV oscillations are used as stretching maneuvers. Grade V oscillations are thrust techniques used to snap adhesions at the limit of available motion.

1. Grade I oscillations refer to small amplitude rhythmic oscillations performed at the beginning of the range. Grade II oscillations refer to large amplitude rhythmic oscillations performed within the range, but not reaching the limit of the range and not returning to the beginning of the range. Grade I and II oscillations are used to treat joints limited by pain. The oscillations inhibit pain by stimulating mechanoreceptors that block nociceptive pathways at the spinal cord or brain stem.

2. Grade I oscillations were previously defined. Grade III oscillations refer to large amplitude rhythmic oscillations performed up to the limit of the available motion and are stressed into the tissue resistance. Grade I oscillations are used primarily to treat joints limited by pain, while grade III oscillations are used as stretching maneuvers.

3. Grade II and III oscillations were previously defined. Grade II oscillations are used primarily to treat joints limited by pain, while grade III oscillations are used as stretching maneuvers.

4. **Grades III oscillations were previously defined. Grade IV oscillations refer to small amplitude rhythmic oscillations performed at the limit of the available motion and are stressed into the tissue resistance. Grades III and IV oscillations are used as stretching maneuvers.**

System Specific: Musculoskeletal System
Content Outline: Interventions

## Exam One: Question 182

A physical therapist examines the breath sounds of a 55-year-old male diagnosed with pulmonary disease. The therapist identifies rales during both inspiration and expiration. This finding is MOST representative of:

1. pleural effusion
2. pulmonary fibrosis
3. **impaired secretion clearance**
4. localized stenosis

**Correct Answer: 3** (Hillegass p. 551)

Auscultation of the lungs with a stethoscope is an examination procedure physical therapists use to identify abnormalities in lung sounds. Abnormal lung sounds may suggest problems with ventilation or airway clearance.

1. Pleural effusion is the accumulation of fluid in the pleural space. Lung sounds are usually decreased, but a pleural friction rub may be heard if the pleural surfaces are inflammed.

2. Pulmonary fibrosis is a type of restrictive lung dysfunction characterized by changes to the alveoli and lung architecture from an inflammatory process. The inflammatory changes cause scarring and fibrotic lesions in the lungs which result in decreased lung compliance, lung volumes, diffusing capacity, increased pulmonary arterial pressure, and work of breathing. Auscultation often reveals decreased breath sounds.

3. **Crackles or rales are abnormal breath sounds heard during auscultation of the lungs with a stethoscope. Crackles are extra sounds caused by the "popping open" of small airways blocked by secretions or fluid and may be heard during both the inspiratory and expiratory phases of the breathing cycle.**

4. Localized stenosis is not a term associated with breath sounds.

System Specific: Cardiovascular/Pulmonary and Lymphatic Systems
Content Outline: Foundations for Evaluation, Differential Diagnosis, & Prognosis

## Exam One: Question 183

The components of a clinical question posed in order to search the literature for information about the effectiveness of a therapy include:

1. subjective, objective, assessment, plan (S.O.A.P.)
2. **patient or problem, intervention, comparison, outcome (P-I-C-O)**
3. validity, reliability, applicability
4. diagnosis, prognosis, intervention

**Correct Answer: 2** (Portney p. 10)
Asking a patient-centered clinical question is the first step in searching the literature for information about the effectiveness of a therapy.

1. Subjective, objective, assessment, and plan (S.O.A.P.) refer to the elements commonly used for recording daily notes of a patient's physical therapy sessions.

2. **The acronym P-I-C-O helps to focus on the appropriate pieces of information needed to search the literature for information about the effectiveness of a therapy. The P refers to the target population or characteristics of the patient or problem of interest. The I refers to the intervention being considered. The C refers to the comparison or control condition that may be considered along with the intervention and is most appropriate when the need is to compare the effectiveness of two or more interventions. The O refers to the outcomes or measurements that will be relevant to understanding the effect of the interventions.**

3. Validity, reliability, and applicability are properties of measurements.

4. Diagnosis, prognosis, and intervention are elements of the patient/client management model as described in the Guide to Physical Therapist Practice, along with examination, and evaluation.

System Specific: Non-Systems
Content Outline: Safety and Protection; Professional Responsibilities; Research

## Exam One: Question 184

A physical therapist completes a study which examines the effect of goniometer size on the reliability of passive shoulder joint measurements. The therapist concludes that goniometric measurements of passive shoulder range of motion can be highly reliable when taken by a single therapist, regardless of the size of the goniometer. This study demonstrates the use of:

1. interrater reliability
2. **intrarater reliability**
3. internal validity
4. external validity

**Correct Answer: 2** (Norkin p. 41)
Reliability, or the extent to which a measurement is consistent and free from error, is a prerequisite of any measurement. There are a number of types of reliability that may be estimated: test-retest, rater (intrarater and interrater), alternate forms, and internal consistency.

1. Interrater reliability refers to the reproducibility of measurements made by two or more raters who measure the same group of subjects.

2. **Intrarater reliability refers to the reproducibility of measurements made by one individual across two or more trials.**

3. Internal validity focuses on cause and effect relationships. Specifically, is there evidence that, given a statistical relationship between the independent variable and dependent variable in an experiment, one causes the other.

4. External validity refers to the extent to which the results of a study can be generalized beyond the study sample to persons, settings, and times that are different from those employed in the experimental situation. External validity is concerned with the usefulness of the information outside the experimental situation.

System Specific: Musculoskeletal System
Content Outline: Physical Therapy Examination

## Exam One: Question 185

A physical therapist employed in an acute care hospital examines a patient rehabilitating from surgery. The patient has diabetes, however, has no other significant past medical history. Which of the following situations would MOST warrant IMMEDIATE medical attention?

1. **signs of confusion and lethargy**
2. systolic blood pressure increase of 20 mm Hg during exercise
3. lack of significant clinical findings following the examination
4. discovery of significant past medical history unknown to the physician

**Correct Answer: 1** (Goodman - Differential Diagnosis p. 431)
Confusion and lethargy in a patient with diabetes are signs of hypoglycemia or low blood glucose. If untreated, hypoglycemia can rapidly progress towards a life-threatening situation.

1. **It is important to treat hypoglycemia immediately using glucose tablets or sugar in order to raise blood glucose levels.**
2. An increase in systolic blood pressure of 20 mm Hg is a normal response to exercise.
3. The lack of significant findings in the examination does not warrant immediate medical attention.
4. Discovery of significant unknown medical history warrants referral to the physician for possible future examination and follow-up, but does not warrant immediate medical attention.

System Specific: Other Systems
Content Outline: Interventions

## Exam One: Question 186

A patient with a peripheral nerve injury is examined in physical therapy. The patient's primary symptoms result from an injury to the superficial peroneal nerve. The MOST likely area of sensory alteration is:

1. sole of the foot
2. plantar surface of the toes
3. **lateral aspect of the leg and dorsum of the foot**
4. triangular area between the first and second toes

**Correct Answer: 3** (Kendall p. 369)
The superficial peroneal nerve innervates the peroneus longus and brevis. It is a branch of the sciatic nerve.

1. The sole of the foot receives cutaneous innervation from the medial and lateral plantar nerves, which are branches of the tibial nerve. The tibial nerve is a branch of the sciatic nerve.
2. The plantar surface of the toes are innervated by the medial and lateral plantar nerves, which are branches of the tibial nerve. The tibial nerve is a branch of the sciatic nerve.
3. **A peripheral nerve injury affecting the superficial peroneal nerve often results in sensory alterations along the lateral aspect of the leg and dorsum of the foot.**
4. The triangular area between the first and second toes is innervated by the deep peroneal nerve. It is a branch of the sciatic nerve.

System Specific: Neuromuscular & Nervous Systems
Content Outline: Physical Therapy Examination

## Exam One: Question 187

A physical therapist reviews a physician examination which indicates diminished sensation in the L3 dermatome. The MOST appropriate location to confirm the physician's findings is:

1. dorsum of the foot
2. **anterior thigh**
3. groin
4. lateral calf

**Correct Answer: 2** (Magee p. 22)

A dermatome refers to an area of skin supplied by a dorsal root of a spinal nerve.

1. Sensation in the dorsum of the foot is supplied by the L5 and S1 spinal nerves. The L5 dermatome corresponds to the medial portion of the dorsum of the foot and the S1 dermatome corresponds to the lateral portion of the dorsum of the foot.

2. **Sensation in the anterior thigh is supplied by the L2 and L3 spinal nerves.**

3. Sensation in the groin is supplied by the S3 and S4 spinal nerves. The S3 dermatome corresponds to the groin and medial thigh and the S4 dermatome corresponds to the perineum, genitals, and lower sacrum.

4. Sensation in the lateral calf is supplied by the L5 spinal nerve.

System Specific: Neuromuscular & Nervous Systems
Content Outline: Physical Therapy Examination

## Exam One: Question 188

A physical therapist attempts to obtain a history from a patient that recently immigrated to the United States. The patient does not speak English and seems to be intimidated by the hospital environment. The MOST appropriate action is to:

1. ask the patient to communicate in writing
2. ask another physical therapist to complete the examination
3. move the patient to a private treatment room
4. **request an interpreter**

**Correct Answer: 4** (Haggard p. 39)

A physical therapist must utilize available resources to ensure that all patients receive quality health care. Title VI, of the Civil Rights Act of 1964 prohibits exclusion from services and discrimination on grounds of race, color or national origin. This extends to people with non-English or limited English proficiency. Failure to request an interpreter given the patient's obvious need would be a violation of the patient's rights.

1. Communicating in writing is not desirable in this situation since it is unlikely that the patient would be able to communicate in a written form that would be understood by the physical therapist. In addition, writing alone does not provide the patient with an effective method of communication especially in the hospital environment.

2. This option may be more desirable if it was clear that the other physical therapist possessed the necessary language skills to communicate effectively with the patient.

3. Moving the patient to a private treatment room may address the patient's intimidation with the hospital environment, however, it does not address the more critical communication element.

4. **An interpreter would provide the patient and physical therapist with an effective method to communicate with each other. This action would ensure that the patient can actively participate in their care and that the physical therapist can appropriately direct future sessions.**

System Specific: Non-Systems
Content Outline: Safety and Protection; Professional Responsibilities; Research

## Exam One: Question 189

A physical therapist prepares to perform volumetric measurements as a means of quantifying edema. Which patient would appear to be the MOST appropriate candidate for this type of objective measure?

1. **a 38-year-old female with a Colles' fracture**
2. a 27-year-old male with bicipital tendonitis
3. a 48-year-old male with a rotator cuff tear
4. a 57-year-old male with pulmonary edema

> **Correct Answer: 1** (Magee p. 446)
> Volumetric measurements are commonly used to measure edema in the distal extremities. The measurement is typically performed by examining the amount of water displaced from a cylinder following immersion of an affected body part. It would be impractical to use this type of measurement in an area other than a distal extremity.
>
> 1. **A Colles' fracture refers to a fracture of the distal end of the radius. The injury would likely result in swelling in the wrist and hand which could be quantified with volumetric measurements.**
> 2. The location of the biceps tendon would require immersion of the upper extremity or the entire shoulder complex. The size of the upper extremity would make this unrealistic.
> 3. The location of the rotator cuff would require immersion of the entire shoulder complex which would also be unrealistic due to the size of the area.
> 4. Pulmonary edema refers to swelling or fluid accumulation in the lungs. This condition would be impossible to assess using volumetric measurements.
>
> System Specific: Cardiovascular/Pulmonary and Lymphatic Systems
> Content Outline: Physical Therapy Examination

## Exam One: Question 190

A three-year-old child throws frequent temper tantrums, usually contrived to gain attention. The physical therapist, recognizing the child's objective, refuses to acknowledge the action. This type of behavior therapy is BEST termed:

1. aversive conditioning
2. **extinction**
3. operant conditioning
4. rational emotive imagery

> **Correct Answer: 2** (Sadock p. 2502)
> By refusing to acknowledge the child's tantrums the physical therapist avoids reinforcing the behavior. As a result, the tantrums may decrease in frequency and eventually disappear.
>
> 1. Aversive conditioning is a behavioral therapy technique which reduces the appeal of a behavior by associating the behavior with physical or psychological discomfort. In aversive conditioning, the individual is exposed to an unpleasant stimulus while engaging in the targeted behavior. The goal would be to create an aversion to the targeted behavior.
> 2. **Extinction is the withholding of reinforcement for a previously reinforced behavior which decreases the future probability of that behavior. The goal of extinction is a reduction or a loss in the strength of a conditioned response when the unconditioned stimulus or reinforcement is withheld.**
> 3. Operant conditioning is learning that takes place when the learner recognizes the connection between the behavior and its consequences.
> 4. Rational emotive imagery is a form of intense mental practice for learning new emotional and physical habits. The behavioral technique focuses on uncovering irrational beliefs which may lead to unhealthy negative emotions and replacing them with more productive rational alternatives.
>
> System Specific: Neuromuscular and Nervous Systems
> Content Outline: Interventions

## Exam One: Question 191

A 61-year-old male referred to physical therapy complains of an excessive cough, sputum production, and shortness of breath. The patient indicates that he has been bothered by some combination of these symptoms for over 10 years. The patient's present condition is MOST indicative of:

1. idiopathic hypoventilation
2. chronic hypoxemia
3. Parkinson's disease
4. **chronic bronchitis**

**Correct Answer: 4** (Paz p. 70)

Excessive cough, sputum production, and shortness of breath are common symptoms of chronic obstructive pulmonary disease. Chronic bronchitis is defined as hypersecretion of mucus sufficient to cause a productive cough on most days for three months during two consecutive years.

1. Hypoventilation is a state in which a reduced amount of air enters the alveoli, resulting in decreased levels of oxygen and increased levels of carbon dioxide in the blood. It can be caused by shallow breathing, slow breathing or diminished lung function.

2. Chronic hypoxemia is a condition in which the arterial oxygenation is habitually below normal ($PaO_2$ of less than 80 mm Hg).

3. Parkinson's disease is a primary degenerative disorder of the nervous system characterized by a decrease in the production of dopamine in the basal ganglia.

4. **Chronic bronchitis is a form of obstructive pulmonary disease that is characterized by increased mucus secretions from the bronchioles and structural changes to the bronchi. Persistent cough, wheezing, shortness of breath, and cyanosis are common symptoms.**

System Specific: Cardiovascular/Pulmonary and Lymphatic Systems
Content Outline: Foundations for Evaluation, Differential Diagnosis, & Prognosis

## Exam One: Question 192

A patient appears to be somewhat anxious after learning her treatment will include soft tissue massage. The MOST appropriate massage stroke to begin treatment is:

1. **effleurage**
2. vibration
3. petrissage
4. tapotement

**Correct Answer: 1** (De Domenico p. 14)

Massage is a manual therapeutic modality that produces physiologic effects through different types of stroking, rubbing, and pressure. The specific massage technique to utilize depends on the established goals and the desired physiologic effects.

1. **Effleurage is a massage technique that is usually light in stroke and produces a reflexive response. The technique is often performed at the beginning and at the end of a massage to allow the patient to relax and should be directed towards the heart. Effleurage is also often used as a transitional stroke between different massage strokes.**

2. Vibration is a massage technique that places the therapist's hands or fingers firmly over an area and utilizes a rapid shaking motion that causes vibration to the treatment area. The therapist initiates this motion from the forearm while maintaining firm contact with the treatment area.

3. Petrissage is a massage technique described as kneading where the muscle is squeezed and rolled under the therapist's hands. Petrissage can be performed with two hands over larger muscle groups or with as few as two fingers over smaller muscles.

4. Tapotement is a massage technique that provides stimulation through rapid and alternating movements such as tapping, hacking, cupping, and slapping. The primary purpose of tapotement is to enhance circulation and stimulate peripheral nerve endings.

System Specific: Non-Systems
Content Outline: Equipment and Devices; Therapeutic Modalities

## Exam One: Question 193

A patient two days status post arthrotomy of the knee completes a quadriceps setting exercise while lying supine on a mat table. During the exercise the patient begins to experience severe pain. The MOST appropriate physical therapist action is:

1. have the patient perform the exercise in sidelying
2. have the patient flex the knee prior to initiating the exercise
3. place a pillow under the ankle
4. **discontinue the exercise**

**Correct Answer: 4** (Kisner p. 745)
A quadriceps setting exercise requires the patient to perform an isometric contraction of the quadriceps muscle. The resistive activity places minimal stress on the knee compared to many other resistive activities and as a result is often utilized early in a post-operative program.

1. Sidelying is often used to diminish the influence of gravity, however, in the described scenario the patient is performing an isometric activity with the lower extremity supported. As a result, it is possible that the patient would have more difficulty and associated pain completing the activity in sidelying.
2. Flexing the knee prior to initiating the exercise may decrease the patient's discomfort, however, the severity of the pain makes it critical that the exercise is discontinued.
3. Placing a pillow under the ankle would result in further extension of the knee. Given the patient's relative acuity secondary to their post-operative status, this position would likely increase the patient's pain.
4. **Severe pain in a patient rehabilitating from a surgical procedure is an acceptable reason to immediately discontinue an exercise. It is reasonable to attempt to modify an activity in the presence of pain, however, given the severity of the pain and the absence of information on the cause of the pain, discontinuing the exercise is a more desirable option.**

System Specific: Musculoskeletal System
Content Outline: Interventions

## Exam One: Question 194

A physical therapist enters a private treatment area and observes a patient collapsed on the floor. The patient appears to be moving slightly, however, seems to be in need of medical assistance. The MOST IMMEDIATE therapist action is:

1. **check for unresponsiveness**
2. monitor airway, breathing, and circulation
3. position the patient
4. phone emergency medical services

**Correct Answer: 1** (American Heart Association)
The first step in performing a primary survey is to determine responsiveness.

1. **To check for responsiveness, tap the victim on the shoulder and ask, "Are you all right?" If the patient is unresponsive (i.e., no movement or response to stimulation), the therapist should phone 911, get an automatic external defibrillator, provide cardiopulmonary resuscitation, and use the AED, if necessary.**
2. Monitoring airway, breathing, and circulation describes all of the elements of cardiopulmonary resuscitation. The current recommended sequence when performing CPR is compression, airway, and breathing.
3. Positioning the patient is only necessary if the patient is unresponsive and needs cardiopulmonary resuscitation. If an unresponsive victim is face down, the therapist should roll the victim to a face up position to open the airway.
4. The therapist should phone emergency medical services only after determining the patient is unresponsive.

System Specific: Non-Systems
Content Outline: Safety and Protection; Professional Responsibilities; Research

## Exam One: Question 195

A 48-year-old female rehabilitating from a fractured femur asks questions about her expected functional level following rehabilitation. Assuming an uncomplicated recovery, the MOST accurate prediction of functional level would be based on the patient's:

1. frequency of physical therapy visits
2. previous medical history
3. **previous functional level**
4. compliance with a home exercise program

**Correct Answer: 3** (Hertling p. 101)
A variety of factors can be useful when attempting to predict a patient's future functional level. Which variable is the most important is often determined by the unique characteristic of the patient's current disease or medical condition.

1. The frequency of physical therapy visits may be associated with the patient's rate of progress, however, it is not as strong of a predictor of functional level as the other options.

2. The previous medical history of a patient is often valuable information when predicting a patient's functional level, however, the option is more limited in scope than the patient's previous functional level. If the patient's previous medical history was significant there is a reasonable chance that it would already be reflected in the patient's previous functional level.

3. **A relatively young patient rehabilitating from a fractured femur should have a near complete recovery. As a result, the patient's previous functional level would serve as the best predictor of the patient's future functional level.**

4. A patient that is compliant with a home exercise program may have fewer complications than a patient who is less compliant, however, this variable alone remains a poor predictor of functional level.

System Specific: Musculoskeletal System
Content Outline: Foundations for Evaluation, Differential Diagnosis, & Prognosis

## Exam One: Question 196

A physical therapist attempts to strengthen the lumbricals on a patient with a low metatarsal arch. Which exercise would be the MOST appropriate?

1. resisted extension of the metatarsophalangeal joint
2. **resisted flexion of the metatarsophalangeal joint**
3. resisted abduction of the metatarsophalangeal joint
4. resisted adduction of the metatarsophalangeal joint

**Correct Answer: 2** (Kendall p. 404)
The lumbricals act to flex the metatarsophalangeal joints and assist in extending the interphalangeal joints of the second through fifth digits. The lumbricals are innervated by the tibial nerve.

1. The extensor digitorum longus extends the metatarsophalangeal joints of the second through fifth digits. The extensor digitorum brevis extends the metatarsophalangeal joints of the first through fourth digits.

2. **Resisted flexion of the metatarsophalangeal joint can be used to strengthen the lumbricals. This can be performed with manual resistance or by gathering a towel or another similar object placed on the floor.**

3. The dorsal interossei abduct the second through fourth digits from the axial line through the second digit and assist in flexion of the metatarsophalangeal joints.

4. The plantar interossei adduct the third, fourth, and fifth digits toward the axial line through the second digit and assist in flexion of the metatarsophalangeal joints.

System Specific: Musculoskeletal System
Content Outline: Interventions

## Exam One: Question 197

A 46-year-old male rehabilitating from a radial head fracture misses his third consecutive physical therapy treatment session. The therapist called the patient after the second missed appointment, but did not receive a return phone call. The MOST appropriate physical therapist action is:

1. contact the patient's insurance provider
2. design a home exercise program for the patient
3. schedule the patient with another physical therapist
4. **discharge the patient from physical therapy**

**Correct Answer: 4** (Shamus – Effective Documentation p. 219)

Patients receiving physical therapy services should demonstrate a commitment to attaining established goals. Failure to attend scheduled therapy sessions, particularly without providing advanced notice, is a strong indication that the patient is not currently exhibiting an appropriate level of commitment.

1. The situation should be formally addressed in the physical therapy clinic prior to contemplating the need to inform the insurance provider.

2. Designing a home exercise program for the patient could be a viable alternative, however, for this to be the correct response there would need to be evidence that suggests the patient has difficulty attending physical therapy sessions due to time constraints or other life activities.

3. The question does not provide any evidence to suggest that there is a conflict between the patient and the therapist or that the patient-therapist relationship is associated with the missed physical therapy sessions.

4. **Multiple missed appointments without a response to a phone call warrants discharging the patient from physical therapy. Failure to act in this manner limits the availability of physical therapy services for other patients.**

System Specific: Non-Systems
Content Outline: Safety and Protection; Professional Responsibilities; Research

## Exam One: Question 198

A physical therapist treats a patient with a decubitus ulcer using whirlpool. After treating the wound for 10 treatment sessions, the wound still shows little evidence of granulation. The MOST appropriate action is:

1. begin aggressive debridement
2. recommend a wound culture
3. apply aseptic ointment to the wound
4. **discontinue whirlpool treatments**

**Correct Answer: 4** (Sussman p. 224)

The *Criteria for Standards of Practice for Physical Therapy* published by the American Physical Therapy Association specifies the following: "The physical therapist re-examines the patient/client as necessary during an episode of care to evaluate progress or change in patient/client status and modifies the plan of care accordingly or discontinues physical therapy services."

1. Debridement is typically warranted when there is nonviable tissue present. Debridement can be selective debridement (e.g., sharp, enzymatic, and autolytic) or non-selective debridement (e.g., wet-to-dry dressings, wound irrigation, and hydrotherapy). The question indicates that the wound has not shown evidence of healing after hydrotherapy, however, it does not specify that the wound needs to be debrided.

2. A wound culture is a test in which microorganisms from a wound are grown in a special growth medium. It is performed to identify the microorganism causing an infection in a wound or an abscess. The described scenario does not offer direct evidence suggesting the need for a wound culture and in addition it would be a higher priority to discontinue the ineffective intervention.

3. Aseptic ointment is often used on contaminated or high risk wounds and can be applied to non-contaminated wounds that demonstrate early signs of infection. The question does not provide direct evidence to support aseptic ointment and in addition it would be a higher priority to discontinue the ineffective intervention.

4. **Physical therapists have an obligation to discontinue ineffective interventions. If the selected intervention was beneficial it is likely that 10 treatment sessions would have been adequate to generate supporting evidence such as signs of healing (e.g., presence of granulation tissue).**

System Specific: Other Systems
Content Outline: Interventions

## Exam One: Question 199

A physical therapist instructs a patient rehabilitating from a low back injury in a series of five pelvic stabilization exercises. The patient indicates he understands the exercises, however, frequently becomes confused and is unable to perform them correctly. The MOST appropriate therapist action is:

1. repeat the exercise instructions
2. **reduce the number of exercises in the series**
3. select a different treatment option
4. conclude the patient is not a candidate for physical therapy

**Correct Answer: 2** (Haggard p. 107)

A physical therapist should attempt to simplify the exercise session in order to reduce the patient's confusion.

1. Repeating the exercise instructions can be valuable, however, given that the patient "frequently becomes confused" this action is unlikely to resolve the patient's problem.

2. **Reducing the number of exercises in the series serves to simplify the program. Five pelvic stabilization exercises is a significant number for the patient to learn, and as a result, it is reasonable to hypothesize that the number of exercises may be the primary reason for the patient's difficulty.**

3. There is not enough evidence available to suggest that the patient is unable to learn the exercises or that the exercises, if performed appropriately, are not of value. As a result, selecting a different treatment option is not justified.

4. A therapist should attempt to alter the learning environment or the method of providing patient instruction prior to concluding that a patient is not a candidate for physical therapy.

System Specific: Musculoskeletal System
Content Outline: Interventions

## Exam One: Question 200

A physical therapist employed in a rehabilitation hospital prepares to perform a stand pivot transfer with a 42-year-old male rehabilitating from a motor vehicle accident. Prior to initiating the transfer, the therapist notices that the patient is wearing only a pair of hospital issued non-skid socks on his feet. The MOST appropriate therapist action is to:

1. ask another therapist for assistance and complete a dependent transfer
2. have the patient complete a sliding board transfer
3. perform the stand pivot transfer without socks
4. **perform the stand pivot transfer with the patient wearing the hospital-issued socks**

**Correct Answer: 4** (Pierson p. 172)

Physical therapists should not permit patients to perform transfer activities with standard socks since this action unnecessarily jeopardizes patient safety.

1. The physical therapist should have the patient actively participate in the transfer whenever possible. The use of non-skid socks is acceptable and would not impact the patient's ability to participate in the stand pivot transfer.

2. The question does not provide evidence to suggest that the stand pivot transfer is not appropriate for the patient. As a result, there is no reason to select an alternate type of transfer.

3. Patients should not complete transfers in bare feet. This action would create an unnecessary safety risk since the patient may slip if their feet are sweaty or if they fail to provide adequate traction. In addition, the patient increases their risk of acquiring or transmitting microorganisms.

4. **The hospital-issued socks are appropriate for transfers since the non-skid surface incorporates rubberized material that significantly improves traction when compared to traditional socks.**

System Specific: Musculoskeletal System
Content Outline: Interventions

# 12

## PHYSICAL THERAPY EXAM TWO

**Scott Giles**

794 Section One - Questions 1-50

819 Section Two - Questions 51-100

844 Section Three - Questions 101-150

869 Section Four - Questions 151-200

# PHYSICAL THERAPY
# EXAM TWO

# DIRECTION

**"If you don't know where you are going you could wind up some place else."**

— Yogi Berra

Candidates must be proactive throughout the study process and avoid relying on their past accomplishments.  Candidates that assess their progress throughout the study plan and make appropriate modifications often outperform candidates that prepare for the National Physical Therapy Examination in a more random fashion.

## Exam Two: Question 1

A note in a patient's medical record indicates a specific drug is taken through enteral administration. Which of the following is an example of enteral administration?

1. inhalation
2. injection
3. topical
4. **oral**

**Correct Answer: 4** (Ciccone p. 13)

Enteral administration of drugs involves the esophagus, stomach, and small and large intestines. The most common routes of enteral administration are oral, sublingual, and rectal.

1. Drugs that are in a gaseous or volatile state or that can be suspended as tiny droplets in an aerosol form can be administered through inhalation. Examples are general anesthetics and anti-asthmatic drugs.

2. Injection allows drugs to be introduced systemically or locally. Common types of injection include intravenous, intra-arterial, subcutaneous, intramuscular, and intrathecal. Examples are insulin and narcotic analgesics.

3. Topical administration refers to the application of drugs topically to the surface of the skin or mucous membranes. Topical administration is most often used to treat the outer layer of the skin and not other areas since most medications are absorbed poorly through the epidermis and into the systemic circulation.

4. **Oral administration is considered the easiest form of taking medication when self-medication is required and is relatively safe since drugs enter the system in a fairly controlled manner.**

System Specific: Other Systems
Content Outline: Foundations for Evaluation, Differential Diagnosis, and Prognosis

## Exam Two: Question 2

A patient is positioned in supine with the hips flexed to 90 degrees and the knees extended. As the patient slowly lowers her extended legs toward the horizontal, there is an increase in lordosis of the low back. This finding is indicative of weakness of the:

1. hip flexors
2. back extensors
3. hip extensors
4. **abdominals**

**Correct Answer: 4** (Kendall p. 212)

Muscle testing is often a standard component of a physical examination and can be useful in differential diagnosis and the treatment of musculoskeletal and neuromuscular conditions. Physical therapists should be aware of standard methods of assessing muscle strength and interpreting the results.

1. The strength of the hip flexors is assessed with the patient in short sitting. The patient is asked to raise their leg toward the ceiling. The physical therapist stabilizes the iliac crest of the test leg while placing a resistive downward force at the distal end of the femur. Weakness would be indicated by inability to maintain the leg off of the table or attempted substitution.

2. The strength of the back extensors is assessed with the patient in prone. The patient is asked to raise their trunk off of the surface of the table while clasping their hands behind the buttocks or behind the head. The physical therapist stabilizes by providing a downward force to the legs so that they remain firmly on the table. Resistance is provided by gravity. Weakness would be indicated by an inability to maintain the trunk off of the surface of the table or attempted substitution.

3. The strength of the hip extensors, as a group, is assessed in prone. The patient is asked to raise the leg off of the surface of the table, toward the ceiling. The physical therapist stabilizes the pelvis of the test leg while placing a resistive downward force at the distal end of the femur. Weakness would be indicated by an inability to maintain the leg off of the surface of the table.

4. **The supplied description of the resistive test in the question is a standard method to assess the strength of the lower abdominal muscles. Failure to maintain the low back flat on the surface of the table as the legs are lowered is indicative of muscle weakness.**

System Specific: Musculoskeletal System
Content Outline: Physical Therapy Examination

## Exam Two: Question 3

In a clinical trial, patient height is measured in centimeters and weight is measured in kilograms. What inference can the physical therapist make about the scale of measurement for height and weight?

1. **Height and weight are measurements on the ratio scale.**
2. Height and weight are measurements on the ordinal scale.
3. Height and weight are measurements on the nominal scale.
4. Height and weight are measurements on the interval scale.

**Correct Answer: 1** (Portney p. 71)

The four scales of measurement – nominal, ordinal, interval, and ratio – have different characteristics and a special set of rules for manipulating and interpreting numerical data.

1. **Measurements on the ratio scale have an absolute zero point**, meaning a score of 0 represents a total absence of the property being measured. Length in centimeters and mass in kilograms are examples of ratio scale measurements because the numbers represent the actual amount of the attributes being measured. All mathematical and statistical operations can be performed on ratio level measurements.

2. Measurements on an ordinal scale are rank-ordered according to an operationally defined characteristic or property. The measurements exhibit a greater than – less than relationship. Ordinal scale measurements are common in physical therapy. For example, scales of sensation (normal > impaired > absent), spasticity (none < minimal < moderate < severe), balance (good > fair > poor), and manual muscle test scores (trace < poor < fair < good < normal).

3. In the nominal scale or classification scale, elements are assigned to mutually exclusive categories according to some criterion. The categories may be coded by a name, number or symbol, which are used as labels for identification, but have no quantitative value. Gender, blood type, and diagnosis are examples of nominal variables. Counting the frequency or determining the percentages of elements within each category are the only permissible mathematical operations with nominal measurements.

4. The interval scale has the same rank-order characteristics as an ordinal scale, but also demonstrates known and equal distances or intervals between the units of measurement. Unlike the ratio scale, the interval scale has no true zero point. Temperature measured on the Celsius and Fahrenheit scales are examples of interval measurements.

System Specific: Non-Systems
Content Outline: Safety and Protection; Professional Responsibilities; Research

## Exam Two: Question 4 ✗

A physical therapist attempts to select an appropriate intervention to treat a patient with a 10 degree limitation in knee extension. Which of the following mobilization techniques would be indicated?

1. lateral glide of the patella
2. caudal glide of the patella
3. posterior glide of the tibia
4. **anterior glide of the tibia**

**Correct Answer: 4** (Kisner p. 696)

The patellofemoral articulation consists of a convex patella articulating with the concave femoral condyles. The tibiofemoral articulation consists of a concave tibial plateau articulating with the convex femoral condyles.

1. A lateral glide of the patella may be used to improve accessory motion of the patellofemoral joint, but would not be useful to improve knee extension.

2. A caudal glide refers to a downward glide (i.e., inferior) toward the feet. A caudal glide would not be useful to improve knee extension range of motion since the patella slides superiorly in knee extension.

3. A posterior glide of the tibia on the femur would be used to increase knee flexion range of motion.

4. **An anterior glide of the tibia on the femur would be used to increase knee extension range of motion.**

System Specific: Musculoskeletal System
Content Outline: Interventions

## Exam Two: Question 5 ✳

A patient with a right radial head fracture is examined in physical therapy. The patient's involved elbow range of motion begins at 15 degrees of flexion and ends at 90 degrees of flexion. The physical therapist should record the patient's elbow range of motion as:

1. 0 - 15 - 90
2. 15 - 0 - 90
3. **15 - 90**
4. 0 - 90

---

**Correct Answer: 3** (Norkin p. 31)
Physical therapists must accurately record the results of goniometric measurements in a manner that is easily interpreted by all health care providers. Any recording of range of motion must include the beginning of the range as well as the end of range.

1. This style of recording is not acceptable since it is not possible to have two distinct values to the right of the "0".

2. The use of "0" between the starting and ending value indicates the patient has 15 degrees of elbow hyperextension. The total available degrees of movement would be 105 degrees.

3. **The recording depicts a patient who begins in 15 degrees of elbow flexion and ends in 90 degrees of elbow flexion. The total available degrees of movement would be 75 degrees.**

4. The recording depicts a patient who is able to fully extend the elbow and flex the elbow to 90 degrees. The total available degrees of movement would be 90 degrees.

System Specific: Musculoskeletal System
Content Outline: Physical Therapy Examination

---

## Exam Two: Question 6

A physical therapist attempts to improve a patient's lower extremity strength. Which proprioceptive neuromuscular facilitation technique would be the MOST appropriate to achieve the therapist's goals?

1. contract-relax
2. **repeated contractions**
3. rhythmic stabilization
4. hold-relax

---

**Correct Answer: 2** (Sullivan p. 71)
There are a wide variety of proprioceptive neuromuscular facilitation techniques. Each technique is designed with a specific purpose and therapeutic objective. Repeated contractions is designed to initiate movement and promote strength while the other listed options are designed to increase range of motion or promote stability.

1. Contract-relax is a technique used to increase range of motion. As the extremity reaches the point of limitation the patient performs a maximal contraction of the antagonistic muscle group. The therapist resists the movement followed by relaxation and passive movement into newly gained range of motion.

2. **Repeated contractions are used to initiate movement and sustain a contraction through the range of motion. The therapist provides a quick stretch followed by isometric or isotonic contractions. Providing resistance at the point of weakness can enhance the effectiveness of repeated contractions.**

3. Rhythmic stabilization is a technique used to increase range of motion and coordinate isometric contractions. The technique requires isometric contractions of all muscles around a joint against progressive resistance.

4. Hold-relax uses isometric contractions to increase range of motion. The contractions are facilitated for all muscle groups at the limiting point within the range of motion. Relaxation occurs and the extremity moves through the newly acquired range to the next point of limitation.

System Specific: Neuromuscular & Nervous Systems
Content Outline: Interventions

## Exam Two: Question 7

A physical therapist performs an examination on a patient diagnosed with thoracic outlet syndrome. During the examination, the therapist initiates a special test as shown in the image. Which of the following would be considered a positive finding when performing the special test?

1. **inability to maintain the test position for three minutes**
2. subjective report of fatigue in the arms
3. absence of a radial pulse after one minute
4. failure of the hands to regain their normal color after 30 seconds

**Correct Answer: 1** (Magee p. 320)

Roos test is a commonly employed special test for patients with thoracic outlet syndrome. The test is performed with the patient positioned in sitting or standing with the arms positioned in 90 degrees of abduction, lateral rotation, and elbow flexion. The patient is asked to open and close their hands for three minutes.

1. **A positive Roos test is indicated by an inability to maintain the test position, weakness of the arms, sensory loss or ischemic pain.**

2. The act of opening and closing the hands for three minutes often produces a subjective report of fatigue in the arms. A subjective report of fatigue would also need to be accompanied by an inability to maintain the test position for three minutes to be considered a positive finding.

3. The absence of a radial pulse after one minute is not considered a positive test when performing Roos test. Unlike other tests for thoracic outlet syndrome (e.g., Adson's test, Halstead maneuver), Roos test does not require the radial pulse to be assessed during the testing procedure.

4. The color of the hands is not typically examined during Roos test. Other special tests such as Allen's test at the wrist or the capillary refill test would be more likely to assess this type of change in appearance.

System Specific: Musculoskeletal System
Content Outline: Physical Therapy Examination

## Exam Two: Question 8

A patient is limited in passive ankle dorsiflexion when the knee is extended, but is not limited when the knee is flexed. The MOST logical explanation is:

1. **the gastrocnemius is responsible for the limitation**
2. the soleus is responsible for the limitation
3. the popliteus is responsible for the limitation
4. the gastrocnemius and soleus are both responsible for the limitation

**Correct Answer: 1** (Kendall p. 375)

The gastrocnemius muscle consists of a medial and lateral head innervated by the tibial nerve. The medial head originates on the proximal and posterior part of the medial condyle and adjacent part of the femur and capsule of the knee joint. The lateral head originates on the lateral condyle and posterior surface of the femur, and capsule of the knee joint. The muscle inserts on the middle part of the posterior surface of the calcaneus.

1. **The gastrocnemius is a two-joint muscle that crosses both the knee and ankle joints. When the knee is flexed, the muscle is placed on slack which allows for normal ankle range of motion. A limitation in ankle range of motion when the knee is extended may indicate a restriction in the gastrocnemius and possibly the plantaris.**

2. The soleus is a one-joint muscle that plantar flexes the ankle joint and is innervated by the tibial nerve. The muscle's length would not be influenced by the position of the knee.

3. The popliteus muscle medially rotates the tibia on the femur and flexes the knee joint in non-weight bearing. The muscle acts to laterally rotate the femur on the tibia and flexes the knee joint in weight bearing. The popliteus muscle is also a one-joint muscle.

4. The gastrocnemius and soleus work together to plantar flex the ankle. The length of the gastrocnemius would be affected based on the position of the knee, however, the length of the soleus would not be affected since it is a one-joint muscle.

System Specific: Musculoskeletal System
Content Outline: Foundations for Evaluation, Differential Diagnosis, and Prognosis

## Exam Two: Question 9

A patient employed in a machine shop is referred to physical therapy with a diagnosis of carpal tunnel syndrome. The patient indicates that he is scheduled for a diagnostic test that may help to confirm the diagnosis. Which of the following electrodiagnostic tests would be the MOST appropriate?

1. electroencephalography
2. evoked potentials
3. **nerve conduction velocity**
4. electromyography

**Correct Answer: 3** (Tan p. 45)

Carpal tunnel syndrome results from repetitive compression of the median nerve where it passes through the carpal tunnel at the wrist. Nerve conduction velocity is commonly used to diagnose carpal tunnel syndrome. Less formal methods to assist in identifying carpal tunnel syndrome include Phalen's test and Tinel's sign.

1. Electroencephalography is the recording of the electrical activity of the brain. The electrical activity is collected by examining the difference between the electrical potential of two electrodes placed at different locations on the scalp. Electroencephalography is used to assess seizure activity, metabolic disorders, and cerebellar lesions.

2. An evoked potential refers to electrical activity recorded from the presentation of a stimulus. Signals can be recorded from the cerebral cortex, brain stem, spinal cord, and peripheral nerves. Evoked potentials can be used to determine how quickly and completely nerve signals reach the brain and can be used to assist with the diagnosis of several medical conditions including multiple sclerosis.

3. **Nerve conduction velocity refers to the speed by which an action potential travels down a peripheral nerve. The measure is recorded in meters per second. Nerve conduction velocity can be used to diagnose conditions such as carpal tunnel syndrome, peripheral neuropathy, and Guillain-Barre syndrome.**

4. Electromyography is the recording of the electrical activity of a selected muscle or muscle group at rest and during voluntary contraction. Electromyography is performed by inserting a needle electrode percutaneously into a muscle or through the use of surface electrodes. The test is commonly used to assess peripheral nerve injuries and to differentiate between various neuromuscular disorders.

System Specific: Neuromuscular & Nervous Systems
Content Outline: Foundations for Evaluation, Differential Diagnosis, & Prognosis

## Exam Two: Question 10 ✕

A physical therapist performs a goniometric measurement of the wrist on a patient diagnosed with carpal tunnel syndrome. Based on the presented image, which value would be MOST anticipated assuming the patient has normal wrist range of motion?

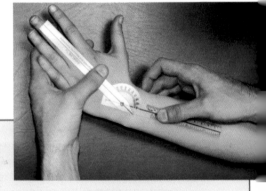

1. **0-20 degrees**
2. 0-30 degrees
3. 0-40 degrees
4. 0-70 degrees

**Correct Answer: 1** (Norkin p. 122)

The presented image depicts a physical therapist measuring radial deviation of the wrist. The measurement is performed with the axis of the goniometer aligned over the middle of the dorsal aspect of the wrist over the capitate. The stationary arm is aligned along the dorsal midline of the forearm using the lateral epicondyle of the humerus for reference. The moving arm is positioned over the dorsal midline of the third metacarpal.

1. **A measurement of 0-20 degrees is consistent with normal wrist radial deviation.**

2. A measurement of 0-30 degrees is consistent with normal wrist ulnar deviation.

3. A measurement of 0-40 degrees would be greater than the normal values of wrist radial or ulnar deviation.

4. A measurement of 0-70 degrees is consistent with normal wrist extension.

System Specific: Musculoskeletal System
Content Outline: Physical Therapy Examination

## Exam Two: Question 11

A physical therapist performs the talar tilt test on a 22-year-old female rehabilitating from an inversion ankle sprain. Which ligament does the talar tilt test examine?

1. anterior talotibial
2. **calcaneofibular**
3. deltoid
4. posterior talotibial

**Correct Answer: 2** (Magee p. 890)

The talar tilt test requires the patient to be positioned in supine or sidelying with the knee flexed to 90 degrees. The physical therapist stabilizes the distal tibia with one hand while grasping the talus with the other hand. The foot is maintained in a neutral position. The therapist tilts the talus into abduction and adduction. A positive test is indicated by excessive adduction and may be indicative of a calcaneofibular ligament sprain.

1. The anterior talotibial ligament extends from the tip of the medial malleolus to the anterior aspect of the medial surface of the talus. The ligament is extremely strong and resists abduction of the talus when it is in plantar flexion and eversion.

2. **The calcaneofibular ligament is a round cord that passes posteroinferiorly from the tip of the lateral malleolus to the lateral surface of the calcaneus. The integrity of the ligament can be assessed using the talar tilt test.**

3. The deltoid ligament refers to the collective medial ligaments of the ankle. The ligament as a whole attaches proximally to the medial aspect of the medial malleolus and fans out to the various distal attachments.

4. The posterior talotibial ligament extends from the medial malleolus to the medial side of the talus and the medial tuberosity of the talus. The ligament resists ankle dorsiflexion and lateral translation and external rotation of the talus.

System Specific: Musculoskeletal System
Content Outline: Physical Therapy Examination

## Exam Two: Question 12

A physical therapist completes a developmental assessment on a seven-month-old infant. Assuming normal development, which of the following reflexes would NOT be integrated?

1. asymmetrical tonic neck reflex
2. Moro reflex
3. **Landau reflex**
4. symmetrical tonic neck reflex

**Correct Answer: 3** (Ratliffe p. 30)

Integration of a reflex refers to the period of time when a reflex is no longer present despite an appropriate stimulus.

1. The asymmetrical tonic neck reflex is stimulated when the head is turned to one side. The response is a fencing posture (arm and leg on face side are extended, arm and leg on scalp side are flexed). The normal age of the response is from birth to 6 months.

2. The Moro reflex is stimulated when an infant's head is suddenly dropped into extension for a few inches. The response is that the arms abduct with fingers open, then cross the trunk into adduction; often followed immediately by crying. The normal age of the response is from 28 weeks of gestation to 5 months.

3. **The Landau reflex is an equilibrium response that occurs when a child responds to prone suspension by aligning their head and extremities in line with the plane of the body. Although the response begins around three months of age, it is not fully integrated until the child's second year.**

4. The symmetrical tonic neck reflex is stimulated by the head moving into flexion or extension. When the head is in flexion, the arms are flexed and the legs are extended. When the head is in extension, the arms are extended and the legs are flexed. The normal age of the response is from 6-8 months.

System Specific: Neuromuscular & Nervous Systems
Content Outline: Physical Therapy Examination

## Exam Two: Question 13

A physical therapist examines a patient with limited cervical range of motion. As part of the examination, the therapist attempts to screen the patient for possible vertebral artery involvement, but is unable to position the patient's head and neck in the recommended test position. The MOST appropriate action is to:

1. complete the vertebral artery test with the head and neck positioned in approximately 50 percent of the available cervical range of motion
2. **complete the vertebral artery test as far into the available cervical range of motion as tolerated**
3. avoid completing the vertebral artery test until the patient has full cervical range of motion
4. avoid all direct cervical treatment techniques until the vertebral artery test can be assessed at the limits of normal cervical range of motion

**Correct Answer: 2** (Dutton p. 1239)
The vertebral artery test is performed with the patient positioned in supine. The therapist places the patient's head in extension, lateral flexion, and rotation to the ipsilateral side. A positive test is indicated by dizziness, nystagmus, slurred speech or loss of consciousness and may be indicative of compression of the vertebral artery.

1. The vertebral artery test should be administered using the available cervical range of motion and as a result it would not make sense to utilize only a portion of the available range of motion.
2. **The physical therapist should perform the test and clear the patient's vertebral artery for their available range of motion. As the patient gains additional range of motion the test can be readministered.**
3. The vertebral artery test can be performed on patients that possess less than full cervical range of motion.
4. Direct cervical treatment techniques are often employed on patients with less than full cervical range of motion. In many cases it is still necessary to clear the vertebral artery using the patient's available cervical range of motion.

System Specific: Musculoskeletal System
Content Outline: Physical Therapy Examination

**Test Taking Tip:** In some cases two options express different ways of saying the exact same thing. When this happens the options mutually exclude each other since it would be impossible for one of the respective options to be correct and the other to be incorrect. In this particular question, option 3 and option 4 imply that the vertebral artery test, and therefore direct cervical treatment techniques, cannot be performed until the patient possesses full cervical range of motion. Regardless of a candidate's knowledge in this particular area it would be possible to eliminate options 3 and 4.

## Exam Two: Question 14

A 42-year-old female is admitted to a rehabilitation hospital after sustaining a stroke. During the examination the physical therapist identifies significant sensory deficits in the anterolateral spinothalamic system. Which sensation would be MOST affected?

1. barognosis
2. kinesthesia
3. graphesthesia
4. **temperature**

**Correct Answer: 4** (O'Sullivan p. 138)
Sensory information enters the spinal cord through the dorsal roots and is delivered to higher centers through the spinothalamic system or the dorsal columns. The spinothalamic system is involved with the transmission of nondiscriminative sensations which are activated by mechanoreceptors, thermoreceptors, and nociceptors.

1. Barognosis refers to the recognition of weight. Barognosis is tested by asking a patient to identify the comparative weight of similar sized objects presented in a series. This type of sensory information is transmitted through the dorsal columns.
2. Kinesthesia refers to the ability to identify the direction and extent of movement of a joint or body part. This type of sensory information is transmitted through the dorsal columns.
3. Graphesthesia refers to the ability to recognize symbols, letters or numbers traced on the skin. This type of sensory information is transmitted through the dorsal columns.
4. **Temperature information is transmitted through the spinothalamic system. The system consists of small diameter and relatively slow conducting afferent fibers. Conversely, the dorsal columns consist of large diameter, rapidly conducting afferent fibers.**

System Specific: Neuromuscular & Nervous Systems
Content Outline: Foundations for Evaluation, Differential Diagnosis, and Prognosis

## Exam Two: Question 15 ✳

A 13-year-old girl discusses the possibility of anterior cruciate ligament reconstruction with an orthopedic surgeon. The girl injured her knee while playing soccer and is concerned about the future impact of the injury on her athletic career. Which of the following factors would have the GREATEST influence on her candidacy for surgery?

1. anthropometric measurements
2. hamstrings/quadriceps strength ratio
3. **skeletal maturity**
4. somatotype

**Correct Answer: 3** (Hertling p. 518)
Physical therapists should possess a general idea of how specific factors such as normal growth and development influence a candidate's eligibility for selected medical and surgical procedures.

1. Common anthropometric measurements used for adults include height, weight, body mass index (BMI), waist-to-hip ratio, and percentage of body fat. These measures are then compared to reference standards to assess items such as weight status and the risk for various diseases.

2. Hamstrings/quadriceps strength ratio is a general measure of the relative strength of the hamstrings compared to the relative strength of the quadriceps. Strength is an important factor both prior to and post surgery, however, it is unlikely that this would influence candidacy for surgery.

3. **Due to the potential impact on future bone growth, lack of skeletal maturity can be a contraindication to anterior cruciate ligament reconstruction surgery.**

4. Somatotype is a term used to classify a system of body typing. The most common classifications of somatotype include endomorph, mesomorph, and ectomorph.

System Specific: Musculoskeletal System
Content Outline: Foundations for Evaluation, Differential Diagnosis, & Prognosis

## Exam Two: Question 16

A physical therapist identifies a bluish discoloration of the skin and nailbeds of a 55-year-old male referred to physical therapy for pulmonary rehabilitation. What does this objective finding indicate?

1. hyperoxemia
2. hyperoxia
3. hypokalemia
4. **hypoxemia**

**Correct Answer: 4** (Paz p. 70)
Individuals whose blood is deficient in oxygen tend to have a bluish discoloration of their skin called cyanosis. Cyanosis is most noticeable in mucous membranes and nailbeds.

1. Hyperoxemia refers to increased acidity of the blood.

2. Hyperoxia refers to increased oxygen in the blood.

3. Hypokalemia refers to severe potassium depletion in the circulating blood. The condition is commonly manifested by episodes of muscular weakness or paralysis and postural hypotension.

4. **Hypoxemia refers to a decreased oxygen concentration in the blood measured by arterial oxygen partial pressure ($PaO_2$) values. A $PaO_2$ less than 80 mm Hg constitutes hypoxemia.**

System Specific: Cardiovascular/Pulmonary and Lymphatic Systems
Content Outline: Physical Therapy Examination

## Exam Two: Question 17 ✳

A manager develops a policy on physical therapy utilization of continuing education resources. Which of the following would be the MOST appropriate action to enhance the quality of patient care?

1. offer continuing education resources to senior therapists in relation to their years of experience
2. divide the continuing education resources evenly among therapy staff
3. establish a committee to review requests for continuing education resources
4. **prioritize requests for continuing education resources based on established patient care standards**

---

**Correct Answer: 4** (Nosse p. 226)

Continuing education resources should be allocated in a manner that advances the established goals of the physical therapy department.

1. Providing resources to therapists based on experience would not specifically address the needs of all therapists. This type of continuing education strategy may be more effective as a method to retain experienced therapists.

2. Individual therapists have diverse interests that may or may not be compatible with the established goals of the physical therapy department. As a result, some form of oversight or prioritization would likely be necessary to ensure a meaningful impact on the quality of patient care.

3. Establishing a committee to review requests for continuing education resources provides necessary oversight and may be useful to enhance the quality of patient care, however, the strategy does not provide any specific insight as to how the established committee will enhance the quality of patient care.

4. **Prioritizing requests for continuing education resources based on established patient care standards is a specific strategy that will allocate resources directly toward educational opportunities which are consistent with established patient care standards. This type of allocation sends a strong message to all therapists about the priorities of the department and reinforces efforts to improve the quality of patient care.**

System Specific: Non-Systems
Content Outline: Safety and Protection; Professional Responsibilities; Research

---

## Exam Two: Question 18

A physical therapist uses the body mass index scale as a means of assessing a patient's total body composition. The therapist determines the body mass index by dividing the body weight in kilograms by height in meters squared. Which of the following values would be the MOST representative of a healthy male or female?

1. $14 \text{ kg/m}^2$
2. **$22 \text{ kg/m}^2$**
3. $28 \text{ kg/m}^2$
4. $37 \text{ kg/m}^2$

---

**Correct Answer: 2** (American College of Sports Medicine p. 267)

The body mass index (BMI) is used to assess weight relative to height and is calculated by dividing body weight (kilograms) by height (meters squared). A BMI of greater than 30 is associated with an increased risk of hypertension, hypercholesterolemia, coronary disease, and mortality. A BMI of less than 18.5 also increases the risk of cardiovascular disease.

1. A BMI of 14 is considered underweight since any value less than 18.5 is classified as underweight.

2. **A BMI from 18.5 – 24.9 is considered normal.**

3. A BMI of 28 is considered overweight since any value between 25.0 - 29.9 is classified as overweight.

4. A BMI of 37 is considered Obesity, Class II since any value between 35.0 - 39.9 is classified as obesity, Class II.

System Specific: Cardiovascular/Pulmonary and Lymphatic Systems
Content Outline: Physical Therapy Examination

---

## Exam Two: Question 19 ✳

A patient diagnosed with patellofemoral syndrome discusses his past medical history with a physical therapist. The patient reports having anterior cruciate ligament reconstruction surgery on his right knee two years ago, however, the therapist is not able to identify a scar over the anterior surface of the right knee. Assuming the surgeon utilized an autograft for the reconstruction, which of the following would be the MOST likely graft site?

1. semitendinosus and semimembranosus
2. **semitendinosus and gracilis**
3. semimembranosus and gracilis
4. semitendinosus and biceps femoris

**Correct Answer: 2** (Brotzman p. 214)
Anterior cruciate ligament (ACL) reconstruction refers to the use of a graft to replace a damaged anterior cruciate ligament. The graft is placed through drilled holes in the femoral and tibial tunnels and then anchored with a fixation device. The most common grafts used are the patellar tendon or the tendons of the semitendinosus and gracilis.

1. The semitendinosus and semimembranosus both function as medial hamstrings muscles. The muscles are innervated by the tibial branch of the sciatic nerve (L5-S1). The semimembranosus is not used as a graft for ACL reconstruction.
2. **The semitendinosus and gracilis tendons are commonly used together as a graft for anterior cruciate ligament reconstruction. The grafts result in a decreased incidence of post-operative patellofemoral knee pain, however, provide weaker initial fixation. The gracilis functions as a hip adductor and is innervated by the obturator nerve (L2-L4).**
3. The semimembranosus is not used as a graft for ACL reconstruction.
4. The semitendinosus and biceps femoris are hamstrings muscles. The semitendinosus is considered a medial hamstrings muscle and the biceps femoris is a lateral hamstrings muscle. The biceps femoris is not used as a graft for ACL reconstruction.

System Specific: Musculoskeletal System
Content Outline: Foundations for Evaluation, Differential Diagnosis, & Prognosis

## Exam Two: Question 20

A physical therapist assesses a one-month-old infant. During the treatment session the therapist strokes the cheek of the infant causing the infant to turn its mouth towards the stimulus. This action is utilized to assess the:

1. Moro reflex
2. **rooting reflex**
3. startle reflex
4. righting reflex

**Correct Answer: 2** (Ratliffe p. 26)
Primitive reflexes begin in utero and are typically integrated within the first year. Many of the primitive reflexes initially provide a useful purpose and the presence of the reflexes indicates normal functioning of the nervous system.

1. The Moro reflex is a primitive reflex that is normally present at 28 weeks gestation through five months of age. The reflex is stimulated by the head suddenly dropping into extension for a few inches. The response is abduction of the arms with the fingers open, followed by the arms crossing the trunk into adduction, and crying.
2. **The rooting reflex is a primitive reflex that is normally present from 28 weeks of gestation through three months of age. The reflex assists the mother when feeding an infant.**
3. The startle reflex is a primitive reflex that is normally present at 28 weeks gestation through five months of age. The reflex is stimulated by a loud, sudden noise. The response is similar to the Moro reflex, but the elbows remain flexed and the hands closed.
4. The righting reflex is a general term used to describe a group of reflexes that are responsible for the development of upright posture and smooth transitional movements. Equilibrium reactions occur in response to a change in body position or surface support to maintain body alignment.

System Specific: Neuromuscular & Nervous Systems
Content Outline: Physical Therapy Examination

## Exam Two: Question 21

A physical therapist elects to use mechanical lumbar traction for a patient rehabilitating from a back injury. The therapeutic goals of the session include decreasing the patient's muscle spasm. The MOST appropriate force based on the stated objective would be:

1. 10% of body weight
2. 15% of body weight
3. **25% of body weight**
4. 50% of body weight

> **Correct Answer: 3** (Cameron p. 301)
> The optimal amount of force when using traction depends on the patient's clinical presentation, the goals of the treatment, and the position selected. There are, however, some general guidelines that physical therapists can use. Guidelines are often expressed in percentages of total body weight instead of strictly an amount of force in pounds or kilograms since this method accommodates for patients of varying sizes.
>
> 1. Ten percent of the patient's body weight would be far less than the amount of force needed to accomplish the identified goal of decreasing the patient's muscle spasm.
> 2. Fifteen percent of the patient's body weight would be less than the amount of force needed, although it is possible that this amount of force could be used as a trial to determine how the patient will tolerate traction. Assuming the patient tolerates fifteen percent, the therapist could then move to twenty-five percent.
> 3. **Twenty-five percent of the patient's body weight is generally recommended when the goal of treatment is to decrease muscle spasm or stretch soft tissue in the lumbar spine.**
> 4. Fifty percent of the patient's body weight is required for mechanical separation of the lumbar spine, however, this amount of force would be excessive to diminish muscle spasm.
>
> System Specific: Non-Systems
> Content Outline: Equipment & Devices; Therapeutic Modalities

## Exam Two: Question 22

A physical therapist reviews a physician referral form that includes only the patient's name and the referring physician's signature. During the examination the patient indicates that she had knee surgery two weeks ago, however, is unable to provide more specific information. The therapist attempts to call the physician's office, but is unable to reach anyone. The MOST appropriate therapist action is:

1. initiate treatment based on the results of the examination
2. initiate treatment based on an established protocol following knee surgery
3. initiate treatment, however, avoid resistive exercises and high-level functional activities
4. **delay treatment until orders are received from the referring physician**

> **Correct Answer: 4** (Criteria for Standards of Practice)
> Physical therapists should not initiate treatment for patients following surgery until they have adequate medical information to develop an effective plan of care. Presently, the therapist only knows that the patient had knee surgery two weeks ago and was referred to physical therapy by their surgeon.
>
> 1. Initiating treatment without specific knowledge of the surgical procedure could be considered a negligent act and may unnecessarily jeopardize the integrity of the surgical procedure.
> 2. Initiating treatment based on an established protocol following knee surgery is too generic of an approach since there are a multitude of different protocols for each of the various types of commonly performed knee surgeries. It is critical that the physical therapist receives additional information on the surgical procedure directly from the referring physician or an appropriate intermediary (i.e., the referring physician's office).
> 3. Initiating treatment while avoiding resistive exercises and high-level functional activities limits the scope of the physical therapy session, however, it does not ensure that the chosen interventions are appropriate based on the patient's current status.
> 4. **Delaying treatment until orders are received from the referring physician ensures that the physical therapist has all of the relevant information prior to developing a plan of care. This action allows the therapist to be fully informed about relevant contraindications and precautions and allows the therapist to develop a plan of care based on the anticipated outcomes.**
>
> System Specific: Non-Systems
> Content Outline: Safety and Protection; Professional Responsibilities; Research

## Exam Two: Question 23

A physical therapist employed in an acute care hospital reviews the results of recent laboratory testing for one of his patients. A note in the medical record indicates that the patient was dehydrated at the time the blood sample was taken. Which finding would be MOST likely based on the patient's hydration status?

1. increased coagulation time
2. decreased hematocrit level
3. **increased blood urea nitrogen level**
4. decreased hemoglobin level

**Correct Answer: 3** (Goodman - Pathology p. 1640)

A blood urea nitrogen (BUN) test measures the amount of nitrogen in the blood that comes from the waste product urea. Urea is made when protein is broken down in the body.

1. Prothrombin time and partial thromboplastin time measure the coagulation of the blood. Increased coagulation time indicates an increased time to form a clot. Neither test is affected by hydration status.

2. Hematocrit measures the percentage of red blood cells in a volume of blood. Hematocrit may be increased when the body's water content is decreased from dehydration, diarrhea, vomiting, excessive sweating, severe burns, and the use of diuretics.

3. **A blood urea nitrogen test is performed to assess kidney function. An increased blood urea nitrogen level can be indicative of dehydration, renal failure or heart failure. Normal blood urea nitrogen levels for adults are 10-20 mg/dL.**

4. Hemoglobin is the iron-containing molecule of red blood cells that binds with oxygen. A low hemoglobin level is indicative of anemia and suggests the oxygen-carrying capacity of the blood is decreased. Hemoglobin may be increased when the body's water content is decreased from dehydration, diarrhea, vomiting, excessive sweating, severe burns, and the use of diuretics.

System Specific: Other Systems
Content Outline: Foundations for Evaluation, Differential Diagnosis, & Prognosis

## Exam Two: Question 24

A patient four days status post transtibial amputation is transported to physical therapy for a scheduled treatment session. Assuming an uncomplicated recovery, the MOST appropriate patient transfer to utilize from a wheelchair to a mat table is:

1. two-person lift
2. hydraulic lift
3. **stand pivot**
4. sliding board

**Correct Answer: 3** (Seymour p. 160)

Physical therapists should select transfers for patients based on their unique abilities and limitations. A patient status post transtibial amputation should be able to utilize their uninvolved lower extremity during the transfer and as a result, the therapist would not need to utilize a dependent transfer.

1. A two-person lift is used to transfer a patient between two surfaces of different heights or when transferring a patient to the floor.

2. A hydraulic lift is a device required for dependent transfers when a patient is obese, when there is only one therapist available to assist with the transfer or when the patient is totally dependent.

3. **A stand pivot transfer is used when a patient is able to stand and bear weight through one or both of the lower extremities. The patient must possess functional balance and the ability to pivot.**

4. A sliding board transfer is used for a patient who has sitting balance, some upper extremity strength, and can adequately follow directions.

System Specific: Musculoskeletal System
Content Outline: Interventions

## Exam Two: Question 25 ✳

A physical therapist positions a patient in supine prior to performing a manual muscle test of the supinator. To isolate the supinator and minimize the action of the biceps, the therapist should position the patient's elbow in:

1. 30 degrees of elbow flexion
2. 60 degrees of elbow flexion
3. 90 degrees of elbow flexion
4. **terminal elbow flexion**

**Correct Answer: 4** (Kendall p. 289)
The supinator is innervated by the radial nerve (C5, C6, C7) and acts to supinate the forearm. The biceps is innervated by the musculocutaneous nerve (C5-C6) and acts to flex the elbow and supinate the forearm. A therapist can isolate one muscle from another muscle with a similar action by placing the deemphasized muscle in a shortened position during the testing procedure. This finding is based on the length-tension relationship which specifies that a muscle can generate the greatest tension at its resting length.

1. The biceps is significantly lengthened in this position, however, 30 degree of elbow flexion allows the biceps to generate a reasonable amount of force.
2. The biceps is slightly lengthened in 60 degrees of elbow flexion, however, the muscle is able to generate a significant amount of force since the position is relatively close to the muscle's resting length.
3. The biceps is typically tested with the elbow in 90 degrees of flexion and therefore this is an undesirable position to minimize the action of the muscle.
4. **Placing the biceps in a maximally shortened position significantly limits the muscle's ability to function as a supinator. Physical therapists should avoid maximum pressure in this position since the shortened position of the biceps can result in significant cramping.**

System Specific: Musculoskeletal System
Content Outline: Physical Therapy Examination

## Exam Two: Question 26

During an examination a physical therapist attempts to determine a patient's general willingness to use an affected body part. What objective information would be the MOST useful for the therapist?

1. bony palpation
2. **active movement**
3. passive movement
4. sensory testing

**Correct Answer: 2** (Magee p. 28)
There are a multitude of tests and measures commonly utilized in physical therapy. Physical therapists must be familiar with these tests and measures and understand the relevance and type of information gathered.

1. Bony palpation is a passive technique that would not require the patient to actively participate.
2. **Active movement requires the patient to perform unassisted voluntary range of motion. The activity provides the therapist with information on the patient's willingness to use the affected body part, available range of motion, strength, and coordination.**
3. Passive movement refers to the arc of motion attained by a therapist without assistance from the patient. Passive range of motion is generally slightly greater than active range of motion. The activity provides the therapist with information on the integrity of the articular surfaces, extensibility of the joint capsule, ligaments, muscles, fascia, and skin.
4. Sensory testing is an umbrella term that includes the examination of superficial sensations, deep sensations, and combined cortical sensations. The vast majority of sensory tests would require the patient to verbalize and would not require the active use an affected body part.

System Specific: Musculoskeletal System
Content Outline: Physical Therapy Examination

## Exam Two: Question 27 ✳

A patient with right hemiplegia is observed during gait training. The patient performs sidestepping towards the hemiplegic side. The physical therapist may expect the patient to compensate for weakened abductors by:

1. hip hiking of the unaffected side
2. lateral trunk flexion towards the affected side
3. **lateral trunk flexion towards the unaffected side**
4. hip extension of the affected side

**Correct Answer: 3** (O'Sullivan p. 734)

Gait deviations result from many factors including potential weakness of the affected muscle groups, diminished proprioception, impaired trunk control, decreased awareness of the affected side, and contractures.

1. Hip hiking of the unaffected (left) side would not serve any purpose when side stepping to the right. The left lower extremity can step towards the right without the need to hip hike since motor function on the left is unaffected.

2. Lateral trunk flexion towards the affected (right) side while attempting to side step to the right will only further load the right lower extremity making it more difficult to step toward the right.

3. **Lateral trunk flexion towards the unaffected (left) side can compensate for weak hip abductors while sidestepping. This action unweights the right lower extremity and utilizes momentum along with the abductors to perform sidestepping.**

4. Hip extension of the affected (right) lower extremity would be important if the person was attempting to step backwards, but would not be a component of sidestepping.

System Specific: Neuromuscular & Nervous Systems
Content Outline: Interventions

## Exam Two: Question 28

A patient reports to a scheduled physical therapy session 25 minutes late. The patient has not been seen previously in physical therapy and was scheduled in a 45 minute block of time. The patient referral indicates the patient is 10 days status post arthroscopic medial meniscectomy. The MOST appropriate therapist action is:

1. **begin the examination**
2. design a home exercise program
3. consult with the patient's physician
4. ask the patient to reschedule

**Correct Answer: 1** (Criteria for Standards of Practice)

Physical therapists have to possess effective time management skills and adapt their schedule as necessary when warranted. It is important for therapists to attempt to accommodate patients when they happen to be early or late for scheduled appointments, however, they must also be careful that the accommodations do not disadvantage other patients.

1. **The physical therapist should have ample time (i.e., 20 minutes) to begin the examination. This may be particularly important in the described scenario because the patient is 10 days status post arthroscopic surgery.**

2. Although the patient may benefit from a home exercise program, it would be inappropriate to design a home exercise program without first completing a thorough examination.

3. The physician is responsible for the medical management of the patient, however, it is not necessary for a physical therapist to provide the physician with information related to timeliness.

4. Asking the patient to reschedule is a viable option, however, since there is still 20 minutes remaining in the session it is likely that the therapist can effectively use the time.

System Specific: Musculoskeletal System
Content Outline: Physical Therapy Examination

## Exam Two: Question 29

A physical therapist identifies that an infant is unable to roll from prone to supine. Which reflex could interfere with the infant's ability to roll?

1. **asymmetrical tonic neck reflex**
2. Moro reflex
3. positive support reflex
4. symmetrical tonic neck reflex

---

**Correct Answer: 1** (Ratliffe p. 25)

The asymmetrical tonic neck reflex interferes with rolling secondary to the tonal influence that is stimulated by turning of the head towards the side when preparing to roll.

1. **The onset of the asymmetrical tonic neck reflex is at birth. When the infant turns its head to one side, the upper and lower extremities on the face-side will extend while the upper and lower extremities on the skull-side flex. Without integration, the child will be unable to roll.**

2. The Moro reflex is stimulated by a sudden change in position of the head (i.e., when the head drops into extension). There is immediate abduction, extension, and splaying of the fingers followed by adduction of the upper extremities across the chest. This will normally cause an infant to cry.

3. The positive support reflex is stimulated as weight is placed on the balls of the feet when the infant is upright. This produces an extension response within the lower extremities and trunk.

4. The symmetrical tonic neck reflex is stimulated by movement of the head. With flexion, the upper extremities flex and lower extremities extend; with extension, the upper extremities extend and lower extremities flex.

System Specific: Neuromuscular & Nervous Systems
Content Outline: Interventions

---

## Exam Two: Question 30

A physical therapist reviews a laboratory report for a 41-year-old male diagnosed with chronic obstructive pulmonary disease. Which of the following would be considered a normal hemoglobin value?

1. 10 gm/dL
2. **15 gm/dL**
3. 20 gm/dL
4. 25 gm/dL

---

**Correct Answer: 2** (Paz p. 230)

Hemoglobin is the protein in red blood cells that carries oxygen. A blood test can determine how much hemoglobin is in the blood. The range of normal values for adult men is approximately 13.3-16.2 gm/dL.

1. 10 gm/dL is well below the normal range for adult men. Lower than normal hemoglobin levels can be due to anemia, acute blood loss, lead poisoning, nutritional deficiencies of iron, folate, and vitamins $B_{12}$ and $B_6$.

2. **Although the exact lower and upper values of normal may vary slightly depending on the source, 15 gm/dL is well within the range of normal.**

3. 20 gm/dL is well above the normal range for adult males. Higher than normal hemoglobin levels may be due to cor pulmonale, pulmonary fibrosis, and polycythemia vera (i.e., abnormal increase in blood cells).

4. 25 gm/dL is well above the normal range for adult males.

System Specific: Cardiovascular/Pulmonary and Lymphatic Systems
Content Outline: Foundations for Evaluation, Differential Diagnosis, & Prognosis

---

## Exam Two: Question 31

A patient diagnosed with an incomplete spinal cord lesion presents with muscle paralysis on the ipsilateral side of the lesion and a loss of pain, temperature, and sensitivity on the contralateral side of the lesion. This presentation BEST describes:

1. posterior cord syndrome
2. central cord syndrome
3. anterior cord syndrome
4. **Brown-Sequard's syndrome**

---

**Correct Answer: 4** (Umphred p. 607)

Brown-Sequard's syndrome is an incomplete spinal cord lesion resulting in hemisection of the spinal cord. There is paralysis and loss of vibration and position sense on the same side as the lesion (corticospinal tract and dorsal columns) and loss of pain and temperature sense on the opposite side of the lesion (lateral spinothalamic tract).

1. Posterior cord syndrome is a rare incomplete lesion that results from compression of the posterior spinal artery with subsequent loss of pain perception, stereognosis, proprioception, and two-point discrimination below the level of the lesion. Motor function remains intact.

2. Central cord syndrome is an incomplete lesion resulting from hyperextension. Damage to the spinothalamic tract, corticospinal tract, and dorsal columns produce greater upper extremity involvement than lower extremity; greater motor deficits exist as compared to sensory deficits.

3. Anterior cord syndrome is an incomplete lesion that results from compression to the anterior part of the spinal cord and anterior spinal artery. Presentation consists of a bilateral loss of motor function and pain and temperature sense below the level of the lesion (corticospinal and spinothalamic tracts).

4. **Brown-Sequard's syndrome most commonly occurs from a stab or bullet wound. True hemisection of the cord is rare; most injuries are irregular in nature with a mixture of symptoms.**

System Specific: Neuromuscular & Nervous Systems
Content Outline: Foundations for Evaluation, Differential Diagnosis, & Prognosis

## Exam Two: Question 32

A physical therapist reviews a physician's examination of a patient scheduled for physical therapy. The examination identifies excessive medial displacement of the elbow during ligamentous testing. Which ligament is typically involved with medial instability of the elbow?

1. annular
2. radial collateral
3. **ulnar collateral**
4. volar radioulnar

---

**Correct Answer: 3** (Hertling p. 360)

The medial collateral ligament, also termed the ulnar collateral ligament, is a fan shaped ligament that serves to restrict medial angulation of the ulna on the humerus.

1. The annular ligament is a strong, well-defined band that attaches to the anterior and posterior margins of the radial notch of the ulna. It acts as a restraining ligament preventing the downward displacement of the radial head.

2. The radial collateral ligament is a strong, triangular band attaching to a depression below the lateral epicondyle of the humerus and the lateral margin of the ulna. The ligament is assessed for potential instability by applying a varus force to the distal forearm.

3. **The ulnar collateral ligament extends from the medial epicondyle to the medial margin of the ulna's trochlear notch and is assessed for potential instability by applying valgus force to the distal forearm.**

4. The volar radioulnar ligament is located at the wrist joint and would not be implicated in an unstable elbow.

System Specific: Musculoskeletal System
Content Outline: Physical Therapy Examination

## Exam Two: Question 33

A patient is unable to take in an adequate supply of nutrients by mouth due to the side effects of radiation therapy. As a result, the patient's physician orders the implementation of tube feeding. What type of tube is MOST commonly used for short-term feeding?

1. endobronchial
2. **nasogastric**
3. endotracheal
4. tracheostomy

**Correct Answer: 2** (Pierson p. 281)

Patients in an acute care environment often utilize a variety of lines, tubes, and equipment. It is important for physical therapists to possess a basic understanding of these devices and be aware of signs and symptoms that may indicate the need for formal intervention.

1. An endobronchial tube, also called Carlen's catheter, is a flexible catheter for bronchospirometry and for isolation of a portion of the lung to control secretions into the remainder of the tracheobronchial tree during general anesthesia.

2. **A nasogastric tube is a plastic tube inserted through a nostril that extends into the stomach. The device is commonly used for liquid feeding, medication administration or to remove gas from the stomach. A gastric tube is inserted directly into the stomach for long-term feeding.**

3. An endotracheal tube is an airway catheter inserted in the trachea for endotracheal intubation.

4. A tracheostomy refers to an opening made in the trachea in order to insert a catheter or tube, most often to facilitate breathing.

System Specific: Other Systems
Content Outline: Foundations for Evaluation, Differential Diagnosis, and Prognosis

## Exam Two: Question 34

A physical therapist employed in an acute care hospital prepares to work on standing balance with a patient rehabilitating from abdominal surgery. The patient has been on extended bed rest following the surgical procedure and has only been out of bed a few times with the assistance of the nursing staff. The MOST important objective measure to assess after assisting the patient from supine to sitting is:

1. **systolic blood pressure**
2. diastolic blood pressure
3. perceived exertion
4. oxygen saturation rate

**Correct Answer: 1** (Pierson p. 339)

Orthostatic hypotension results from an inability to compensate quickly for changes in blood pressure. When a person stands up suddenly, gravity tends to cause blood to pool in the veins of the legs and lower body. As a result, the amount of blood returned to the heart is reduced and blood pressure falls. Dizziness or light-headedness is the most common symptom. Normally, the body quickly responds to a decrease in blood pressure, however, compensatory mechanisms may malfunction or function too slowly in patients who have been on extended bed rest.

1. **During bed rest, when the leg muscles are not used regularly, blood pools in the leg veins and is not pumped back to the heart. This results in diminished blood volume which serves to reduce blood pressure. Systolic blood pressure is the maximum arterial pressure during systole or contraction of the left ventricle. It is the most important measure to assess in a patient moving from supine to sitting after prolonged bed rest because of the risk of orthostatic hypotension. A decrease in systolic blood pressure of 20 mm Hg or greater is indicative of orthostatic hypotension.**

2. Diastolic blood pressure refers to the arterial pressure during diastole (between ventricular contractions), therefore, it is not as useful a measure to assess the patient's response to sitting up.

3. Rating of perceived exertion is a subjective measure of how hard the body is working. It is based on the sensations experienced during physical activity including increased heart rate, respiration rate, sweating, and muscle fatigue. It is not a useful measure to assess the patient's response to sitting up.

4. Oxygen saturation measures the percentage of hemoglobin binding sites in the blood bound to oxygen. It is not affected by changing positions.

System Specific: Other Systems
Content Outline: Interventions

## Exam Two: Question 35

A physical therapist inspects a burn obtained as a result of Iontophoresis. The therapist describes the burn as an acidic reaction. If the therapist is correct, the pH of the skin would MOST likely be:

1. **2**
2. 4
3. 6
4. 8

**Correct Answer: 1** (Prentice - Therapeutic Modalities p. 189)

Iontophoresis utilizes a continuous direct current which moves ions through the body's tissues. The direct current alters the normal pH of the skin and makes the patient susceptible to a chemical burn. The pH is a measure of the degree to which a solution is acidic or alkaline. Usually a pH of 7.0 indicates neutrality, a pH of less than 7.0 indicates acidity, and a pH of more than 7.0 indicates alkalinity. In this particular case, the acidic or alkaline reaction would be based on the relative change from the skin's normal pH of 3-4. Decreasing current density by increasing the size of the cathode relative to the anode can reduce the risk of a chemical burn.

1. **A pH of 2 would be considered an acidic reaction since it is below the typical pH of the skin.**
2. The normal pH of the skin is 3-4 and therefore a pH of 4 would fall at the upper limit of the normal range.
3. A pH of 6 would be considered an alkaline reaction since it is above the typical pH of the skin.
4. The pH of the skin would not typically reach a level approaching 8. This level exceeds the pH of the blood which is between 7.35-7.45.

System Specific: Other Systems
Content Outline: Interventions

## Exam Two: Question 36 ✳

A physical therapist attempts to palpate the lunate by moving his finger immediately distal to Lister's tubercle. Which wrist motion will allow the therapist to facilitate palpation of the lunate?

1. extension
2. **flexion**
3. radial deviation
4. ulnar deviation

**Correct Answer: 2** (Hoppenfeld p. 69)

The lunate is located in the center of the proximal row of carpals between the scaphoid and the triquetrum. The lunate is distinguished by its crescent-like outline and is just proximal to the capitate.

1. Extension and flexion of the wrist can be helpful to identify the lunate and capitate articulation, however, extension in isolation would not facilitate palpation of the lunate.
2. **The lunate is palpable just distal to the radial tubercle. Flexion of the wrist facilitates palpation of the lunate.**
3. Radial deviation would not be helpful to facilitate palpation of the lunate because the carpal bone is a midline structure.
4. Ulnar deviation would not be helpful to facilitate palpation of the lunate. Ulnar deviation can be used to facilitate palpation of the scaphoid since the motion causes the scaphoid to slide out from under the radial styloid process.

System Specific: Musculoskeletal System
Content Outline: Physical Therapy Examination

## Exam Two: Question 37 ✳

A physician indicates that a patient rehabilitating from a cerebrovascular accident has significant perceptual deficits. Which anatomical region would MOST likely be affected by the stroke?

1. primary motor cortex
2. **somatosensory cortex**
3. basal ganglia
4. cerebellum

**Correct Answer: 2** (DeMyer p. 54)

A lesion affecting the somatosensory cortex often results in numerous impairments including loss of sensation, perception, proprioception, and diminished motor control.

1. The primary motor cortex is located in the precentral gyrus within the frontal lobe and contains the largest concentration of corticospinal neurons. This area lies directly in front of the central sulcus and primarily controls contralateral voluntary movements.

2. The somatosensory cortex occupies the postcentral gyrus which is directly behind the central sulcus. The structure is responsible for complex processing of sensory information and damage can cause severely impaired perception. The somatosensory cortex receives information regarding touch, temperature, pain, and discriminative senses including stereognosis and position sense.

3. The basal ganglia are a group of nuclei (putamen, caudate nucleus, substantia nigra, subthalamis nuclei, globus pallidus) that are located at the base of the cerebral cortex. The basal ganglia influences movement and postural control.

4. The cerebellum regulates movement, muscle tone, and postural control. Symptoms of a cerebellar lesion include ataxia, tremor, hypotonia, and asthenia.

System Specific: Neuromuscular & Nervous Systems
Content Outline: Foundations for Evaluation, Differential Diagnosis, and Prognosis

## Exam Two: Question 38

A physical therapist treats a patient referred to physical therapy with incontinence. The patient describes her difficulty beginning after the birth of her son. After completing an examination the therapist concludes that the patient has extremely weak pelvic floor muscles. When instructing the patient in a pelvic floor muscle strengthening program, the MOST appropriate position to initiate treatment is:

1. sidelying
2. sitting
3. standing
4. **supine**

**Correct Answer: 4** (Hall p. 429)

A patient with weak pelvic floor muscles should be instructed in strengthening exercises in a position that minimizes the influence of gravity on the pelvic floor. As the patient's strength improves more challenging positions will be utilized for strengthening.

1. Although sidelying would be an acceptable position, it is more awkward than the supine position for most patients when initiating a pelvic floor muscle strengthening program.

2. Sitting requires the pelvic floor to contract against the resistance of gravity which would be too challenging for the initiation of pelvic floor exercises.

3. Standing requires the pelvic floor to contract against the resistance of gravity which would be too challenging for the initiation of pelvic floor exercises.

4. **Patients with extremely weak pelvic floor muscles should initiate strengthening exercises in a horizontal plane in order to avoid gravity exerting a downward force on the pelvic floor.**

System Specific: Other Systems
Content Outline: Interventions

## Exam Two: Question 39

A physical therapist prepares to administer the Berg Balance Scale to a patient rehabilitating from a cerebrovascular accident. Which of the following tools is considered a necessary piece of equipment when administering this outcome measure?

1. reflex hammer
2. goniometer
3. **stopwatch**
4. stethoscope

**Correct Answer: 3** (Physical Therapist's Clinical Companion p. 105)

The Berg Balance Scale is used for assessing a patient's risk of falling. The Berg consists of 14 tasks of everyday life that are scored according to a 0-4 scale. The maximum total score is 56, with a score of less than 45 indicating the patient is at an increased risk for falls. Observation and scoring should take approximately 15-20 minutes.

1. A reflex hammer may be used when examining a patient who has sustained a cerebrovascular accident, however, it is not a tool utilized for the Berg Balance Scale. A reflex hammer is most commonly used to assess deep tendon reflexes.
2. A goniometer may be used to quantify range of motion in a patient who has sustained a cerebrovascular accident, however, it is not a tool utilized for the Berg Balance Scale.
3. **Necessary equipment to administer the Berg includes a stopwatch, two chairs, a ruler, and a step stool.**
4. A stethoscope is used to assess respiratory rate, breath sounds, heart rate, and Korotkoff's (heart) sounds.

System Specific: Neuromuscular and Nervous Systems
Content Outline: Physical Therapy Examination

## Exam Two: Question 40

A physical therapist employed in a school setting observes a 10-year-old boy attempt to move from the floor to a standing position. During the activity, the boy has to push on his legs with his hands in order to attain an upright position. This type of finding is MOST commonly associated with:

1. cystic fibrosis
2. Down syndrome
3. **Duchenne muscular dystrophy**
4. spinal muscular atrophy

**Correct Answer: 3** (Campbell p. 500)

Duchenne muscular dystrophy is a sex-linked disorder characterized by progressive muscular weakness beginning between the ages of two and five. Life expectancy with Duchenne muscular dystrophy is late teens to early twenties due to respiratory or cardiac failure. The described method of standing upright is termed Gowers' sign.

1. Cystic fibrosis is a progressive autosomal recessive genetic disorder of the exocrine glands. The primary findings include pancreatic insufficiency, excessive pulmonary secretions within the lungs, and excessive electrolyte secretion of the sweat glands. Life expectancy has increased to 35 years of age.
2. Down syndrome (trisomy 21) is a chromosomal disorder that has an increased incidence in children of older parents. A moderate to severe decrease in cognition is typical, however, the mean life expectancy is 50-60 years of age.
3. **Gowers' sign is a descriptive term used to describe a specific method patients with muscular dystrophy often use to assume an upright position. The disease causes mechanical weakening and cell destruction. Pseudohypertrophy of the calf muscles is often the first observed finding, however, all muscles are eventually affected including respiratory and cardiac muscles.**
4. Spinal muscular atrophy is a progressive autosomal recessive genetic disorder characterized by anterior horn cell degeneration, paralysis, and intact cognition. Spinal muscular atrophy - Type 1 (Werdnig-Hoffman disease) has a life expectancy of less than three years while Type 2 has a slower progression and Type 3 (Kugelberg-Welander) has a normal life expectancy.

System Specific: Musculoskeletal System
Content Outline: Foundations for Evaluation, Differential Diagnosis, & Prognosis

## Exam Two: Question 41

A physical therapist uses repeated contractions to strengthen the quadriceps of a patient that fails to exhibit the desired muscular response throughout a portion of the range of motion. This proprioceptive neuromuscular facilitation technique should be applied:

1. with the extremity placed into a shortened range within the pattern
2. **at the point where the desired muscular response begins to diminish**
3. at the end of the available range of motion
4. with a maximal contraction of the antagonistic muscle group

**Correct Answer: 2** (Sullivan p. 71)
Repeated contractions should be applied at the point where the contraction begins to diminish. The technique utilizes an isometric contraction followed by subsequent manual stretching and resisted isotonic movement. Repeated contractions assist with enhancing motor neuron recruitment and strengthening of a muscle or group of muscles.

1. Hold-relax active movement is a technique to improve initiation of movement to muscles tested at 1/5 or less. An isometric contraction is performed once the extremity is passively placed into a shortened range within the pattern. Overflow and facilitation may be used to assist with the contraction. Upon relaxation, the extremity is moved into a lengthened position with a quick stretch. The patient then returns the extremity to the shortened position through an isotonic contraction.

2. **Repeated contractions, alternating isometrics, resisted progression, and timing for emphasis are all PNF techniques that are applied with the goal and purpose of increasing strength.**

3. Hold-relax is a technique that applies an isometric contraction at the end of available range to increase range of motion. The contraction is facilitated for all muscle groups at the limiting point in the range. Relaxation occurs and the extremity moves through the newly acquired range to the next point of limitation until there are no further gains in range of motion.

4. Contract-relax is a technique that applies a maximal contraction of the antagonistic muscle group as the extremity reaches the point of limitation. The therapist resists movement for eight to ten seconds with relaxation to follow. The technique is repeated until there are no further gains in range of motion.

System Specific: Neuromuscular & Nervous Systems
Content Outline: Interventions

## Exam Two: Question 42

A patient rehabilitating from extensive burns to the right upper extremity often complains of severe pain in the arm during physical therapy treatment sessions. The present plan of care emphasizes range of motion, stretching, and positioning. The MOST appropriate action to address the patient's complaint is to:

1. reduce the frequency and duration of the treatment sessions
2. **schedule treatment sessions when the patient's pain medication is most effective**
3. avoid treatment activities that are uncomfortable for the patient
4. request that the referring physician increase the dosage of the patient's pain medication

**Correct Answer: 2** (Paz p. 277)
Rehabilitation following a burn is extremely painful. Scheduling therapy to coincide with the maximum benefit from pain medication is a high priority. The reduction of pain level will allow for progression with the established plan of care.

1. Reducing the frequency and duration of treatment will not allow for adequate intervention and burn care. Patient participation may decrease as well secondary to pain if they are not treated in coordination with the pain medication schedule.

2. **A patient should receive the optimal benefit of pain medication during their scheduled therapy session. Greater tolerance may allow the patient to make more rapid progress in therapy.**

3. Patients with burns will likely have discomfort with all activities and treatments. Avoiding certain treatments (e.g., stretching) would be negligent.

4. The physician is responsible for prescribing the correct amount of medication. Increasing the dosage of the pain medication may not benefit the patient if physical therapy is not performed at an appropriate time.

System Specific: Other Systems
Content Outline: Interventions

# Exam Two: Question 43

A patient in the intensive care unit rehabilitating from a serious infection is connected to a series of lines and tubes. Which lower extremity intravenous infusion site would be the MOST appropriate to administer an intravenous line?

1. median cubital vein
2. basilic vein
3. cephalic vein
4. **saphenous vein**

**Correct Answer: 4** (Pierson p. 282)
The majority of intravenous insertions are made into superficial veins. Appropriate veins exist in the upper extremity, lower extremity, and scalp.

1. The median cubital vein is the communication between the basilic and cephalic veins in the cubital fossa.
2. The basilic vein is a large and superficial vein of the upper limb that assists with drainage of the hand and forearm.
3. The cephalic vein is located along the anterolateral surface of the biceps and is often visible through the skin.
4. **The saphenous vein is a superficial vein that extends from the foot to the saphenous opening. The vein is the only listed option that is located in the lower extremity.**

System Specific: Cardiovascular/Pulmonary and Lymphatic Systems
Content Outline: Foundations for Evaluation, Differential Diagnosis, & Prognosis

**Test Taking Tip:** On occasion, examination questions appear to be considerably more difficult than they actually are. In this particular item, candidates do not have to possess specific knowledge related to each of the options, rather they need to recognize that only one of the options is located in the lower extremity. Candidates must be sure they interpret each question correctly and attempt to make the question as simple as possible. Candidates who can do this consistently on the examination often score higher than other candidates with similar academic knowledge.

# Exam Two: Question 44

A physical therapist administers a neural tension test to a patient being treated in physical therapy with low back pain. Assuming the current testing procedure has been unable to reproduce the patient's symptoms, the MOST appropriate modification is to:

1. apply passive overpressure to cervical flexion
2. **apply passive overpressure to left ankle dorsiflexion**
3. passively extend the right knee
4. ask the patient to actively extend the right knee

**Correct answer: 2** (Dutton p. 429)
The slump test is a neural provocation test performed with the patient in sitting. The slump test is a series of progressive active and passive movements. At each portion of the test, the therapist asks the patient if they are experiencing symptoms (e.g., radicular pain, numbness, tingling). If symptoms are produced, the test would be considered positive. If symptoms are not produced, the therapist systematically increases the amount of dural stretch. The therapist initiates the test by asking the patient to flex the thoracic and lumbar spine. The patient is then asked to actively flex their cervical spine and the therapist applies overpressure. The therapist next asks the patient to actively extend their knee and then provides overpressure to ankle dorsiflexion.

1. The image already depicts the therapist applying passive overpressure to cervical flexion. As a result, there is no need for the therapist to apply additional pressure.
2. **Although the patient's left ankle appears to be dorsiflexed, applying passive overpressure to left ankle dorsiflexion would increase the amount of neural tension.**
3. The slump test requires the therapist to move through the described progression unilaterally prior to performing a bilateral assessment.
4. Actively extending the right knee would occur when assessing the right lower extremity. The right lower extremity would not be assessed until the described progression has been completed with the left lower extremity.

System Specific: Neuromuscular and Nervous Systems
Content Outline: Physical Therapy Examination

## Exam Two: Question 45

A physical therapist examines the foot of a 17-year-old female referred to physical therapy with lower leg pain. After placing the foot in subtalar neutral, the therapist determines that the medial border of the foot along the first metatarsal is higher than the lateral border of the foot along the fifth metatarsal. This position would MOST appropriately be documented as:

1. **forefoot varus**
2. forefoot valgus
3. rearfoot varus
4. rearfoot valgus

**Correct Answer: 1** (Magee p. 865)

Malalignment of the foot and ankle can alter the normal biomechanics of gait and distribute abnormal forces to other joints in the kinematic chain. Physical therapists must carefully assess the individual and collective functioning of the rearfoot, midfoot, and forefoot when assessing the foot and ankle.

1. **Forefoot varus refers to an inverted position of the forefoot in relationship to the rearfoot with the subtalar joint in a neutral position. Patients with low arches in weight bearing often exhibit forefoot varus with the subtalar joint in a neutral position.**

2. Forefoot valgus refers to an everted position of the forefoot in relation to the rearfoot with the subtalar joint in a neutral position. Forefoot valgus is often associated with high arches or cavus feet.

3. Rearfoot varus refers to the calcaneus assuming a position of inversion (calcaneus varus) with the subtalar joint in a neutral position. Three to four degrees of inversion is considered to be within normal limits.

4. Rearfoot valgus refers to the calcaneus assuming a position of eversion (calcaneus valgus) with the subtalar joint in a neutral position. Rearfoot valgus is often a result of compensation for forefoot varus.

System Specific: Musculoskeletal System
Content Outline: Physical Therapy Examination

## Exam Two: Question 46

A physical therapist reviews the medical record of a patient recently admitted to an inpatient rehabilitation hospital. The patient sustained a traumatic head injury in a motor vehicle accident five weeks ago. The medical record indicates that the patient is often disoriented and can frequently become agitated with little provocation. The MOST appropriate location for the therapist to make initial contact with the patient is:

1. **in the patient's room**
2. in the physical therapy gym
3. in a private treatment room
4. in the physical therapy waiting room

**Correct Answer: 1** (Umphred p. 550)

A patient with a head injury that is confused and can become agitated is likely functioning at level IV on the Rancho Los Amigos Scale.

1. **The patient's room is the most appropriate first meeting place since the patient will be familiar with the surroundings and may therefore be less distractible. The patient may tend to become agitated in the gym due to overstimulation from other patients and the overall level of activity.**

2. The physical therapy gym is a good option for the treatment of the general population, but becomes more difficult following brain injury due to the patient's decreased attention, lack of focus, and potential agitation.

3. A private treatment room may be too isolated if assistance is needed. Since the patient has a poor attention span, it will be helpful to use familiar surroundings, pictures, and personal effects.

4. The physical therapy waiting room is not an appropriate place to treat a patient. This patient would likely have a difficult time adjusting to the various distractions in the waiting room.

System Specific: Neuromuscular & Nervous Systems
Content Outline: Interventions

## Exam Two: Question 47

A physical therapist instructs a patient positioned in supine to bring her left leg toward her chest and maintain the position. Assuming the therapist observes the reaction shown in the picture, what muscle would MOST likely have insufficient length?

1. iliopsoas
2. quadratus lumborum
3. **rectus femoris**
4. sartorius

**Correct Answer: 3** (Magee p. 692)
The left hip and knee are flexed to the chest to flatten the lumbar spine and stabilize the pelvis. A hip flexion contracture would be denoted by the right leg rising off the table. The length of the rectus femoris can be assessed by examining the relative position of the knee (i.e., amount of knee flexion).

1. The iliopsoas acts to flex the hip. Tightness in the muscle could be identified using the Thomas test, however, the patient's right leg remains on the table which would be an indication of sufficient length in the one-joint hip flexors.

2. The quadratus lumborum originates on the iliolumbar ligament and the iliac crest. The muscle inserts on the inferior border of the last rib and the transverse processes of the upper four lumbar vertebrae. As a result, the muscle does not act on the hip.

3. **Extension of the right knee is an indication that the patient has tightness in the two-joint rectus femoris muscle. A patient without tightness in the rectus femoris would typically present with the knee in 90 degrees of flexion while maintaining the position.**

4. The sartorius is a two-joint muscle that crosses both the hip and knee. The muscle acts to flex, laterally rotate, and abduct the hip joint. The Thomas test is not specific enough to address tightness in the sartorius due to the diversity of the muscle's action. To specifically identify sartorius tightness the physical therapist would need to identify hip flexion, lateral rotation, and abduction of the hip during the Thomas Test.

System Specific: Musculoskeletal System
Content Outline: Physical Therapy Examination

## Exam Two: Question 48

A patient reports significant discomfort in the lower leg during ultrasound treatment. The therapist believes the discomfort is caused by periosteal pain from the ultrasound. Which scenario is most likely associated with the patient's subjective report of discomfort?

1. **an ultrasound unit with a high beam nonuniformity ratio**
2. an ultrasound unit with a low beam nonuniformity ratio
3. a transducer with a large effective radiating area
4. a transducer with a small effective radiating area

**Correct Answer: 1** (Prentice p. 370)
Beam nonuniformity ratio (BNR) is the ratio between the spatial peak intensity and spatial average intensity. The higher the quality of the crystal, the lower the BNR. The BNR is derived from the intrinsic factors and quality of the piezoelectric crystal.

1. **A high beam nonuniformity ratio produces a less uniform beam and therefore places the patient at greater risk for undesirable side effects such as periosteal pain or hot spots.**

2. A low beam nonuniformity ratio produces a more uniform beam and therefore allows for greater patient comfort and safety.

3. Large ultrasound transducers have relatively large effective radiating areas. Effective radiating area (ERA) refers to the area of the transducer that transmits ultrasound energy. The ERA is more relevant when considering the size of the transducer to utilize and the duration of treatment.

4. Small ultrasound transducers have small effective radiating areas. The ERA is always slightly smaller than the total size of the transducer head. A transducer with a small effective radiating area would be unlikely to produce the described discomfort without additional contributing variables.

System Specific: Non-Systems
Content Outline: Equipment and Devices; Therapeutic Modalities

## Exam Two: Question 49

A physical therapist attempts to obtain information on the ability of noncontractile tissue to allow motion at a specific joint. Which selective tissue tension assessment would provide the therapist with the MOST valuable information?

1. active range of motion
2. active-assistive range of motion
3. **passive range of motion**
4. resisted isometrics

**Correct Answer: 3** (Norkin p. 8)
Passive range of motion provides the physical therapist with information regarding the integrity of noncontractile tissues.

1. Active range of motion requires active contraction of muscles, which are composed of contractile tissue. Performing active range of motion will not allow an assessment of the noncontractile elements of a joint.

2. Active-assistive range of motion requires active contraction of muscles, which are composed of contractile tissue. While the therapist is assisting the patient in the movement, it is impossible to assess only the noncontractile elements of the joint since the musculature is actively contracting.

3. **Passive range of motion provides the therapist with information on the integrity of the articular surfaces and the extensibility of the joint capsule and associated ligaments. Passive range of motion is independent of a patient's strength.**

4. Resisted isometrics requires active contraction of the surrounding musculature. As a result, there is no ability to assess the noncontractile tissues of the joint.

System Specific: Musculoskeletal System
Content Outline: Physical Therapy Examination

## Exam Two: Question 50

A physical therapist attempts to transfer a dependent patient from a wheelchair to a bed. The therapist is concerned about the size of the patient, but is unable to secure another staff member to assist with the transfer. Which type of transfer would allow the therapist to move the patient with the GREATEST ease?

1. dependent standing pivot
2. **hydraulic lift**
3. sliding board
4. assisted standing pivot

**Correct Answer: 2** (Pierson p. 205)
The hydraulic lift can be used as a safe and efficient method to transfer large and/or dependent patients with little physical exertion. The transfer can be performed by one therapist under most circumstances.

1. A dependent standing pivot transfer would not be appropriate for a therapist that is concerned about the patient's size. This transfer requires the therapist to perform 100% of the activity.

2. **The hydraulic lift transfer allows the therapist to transfer the patient independently from the wheelchair to the bed without jeopardizing patient or staff safety.**

3. A sliding board transfer requires the patient to possess adequate sitting balance and actively participate in the transfer. This type of transfer would not be appropriate for a dependent patient.

4. An assisted standing pivot transfer requires the patient to stand and participate in the transfer.

System Specific: Non-Systems
Content Outline: Equipment & Devices; Therapeutic Modalities

## Exam Two: Question 51

A physical therapist reviews the surgical report of a patient that sustained extensive burns in a fire. The report indicates that at the time of primary excision, cadaver skin was utilized to close the wound. This type of graft is termed:

1. **allograft**
2. autograft
3. heterograft
4. xenograft

**Correct Answer: 1** (Paz p. 274)

Cadaver skin is removed from donors shortly after their deaths, then processed and distributed by skin and tissue banks. Cadaver skin is often used on patients with severe burns as a substitute until a graft of their own skin can be applied.

1. **An allograft is a temporary skin graft taken from another human, usually a cadaver, in order to cover a large burned area. A homograft is synonymous with the term allograft.**

2. An autograft is a permanent skin graft taken from a donor site on the patient's own body.

3. A heterograft is a temporary skin graft taken from another species.

4. A xenograft is synonymous with the term heterograft.

System Specific: Other Systems
Content Outline: Foundations for Evaluation, Differential Diagnosis, & Prognosis

## Exam Two: Question 52 ✳

A physician completes a physical examination on a 16-year-old male who injured his knee while playing in a soccer contest yesterday. The physician's preliminary diagnosis is a grade II anterior cruciate ligament injury. Which of the following diagnostic tools would be the MOST appropriate in the IMMEDIATE medical management of the patient?

1. bone scan
2. computed tomography
3. magnetic resonance imaging
4. **x-ray**

**Correct Answer: 4** (Magee p. 40)

A grade II anterior cruciate ligament injury most often presents with moderate pain and swelling, minimal instability of the joint, and decreased range of motion. The physician would make the diagnosis based on the patient's clinical presentation and the results of ligamentous testing such as the Lachman test, lateral pivot shift maneuver or anterior drawer test.

1. A bone scan is a diagnostic test that utilizes radioactive isotopes to identify areas of bone that are hypervascular or have an increased rate of bone mineral turnover. Bone scans are most commonly used to detect bone disease or stress fractures.

2. Computed tomography produces cross-sectional images based on x-ray attenuation. A computerized analysis of the changes in absorption produces a detailed reconstructed image. The test is commonly used to diagnose spinal lesions and in diagnostic studies of the brain.

3. Magnetic resonance imaging is a non-invasive diagnostic test that utilizes magnetic fields to produce an image of bone and soft tissue. The test is valuable in providing images of soft tissue structures such as muscles, menisci, ligaments, tumors, and internal organs. The test would be the most beneficial to confirm the presence of an anterior cruciate ligament injury, however, due to the cost of the diagnostic test and the availability of the testing units it is unlikely that the test would be used in the immediate medical management.

4. **X-ray is a radiographic photograph commonly used to assist with the diagnosis of musculoskeletal pathology such as fractures, dislocations, and bone loss. An x-ray is a relatively cost effective diagnostic test often utilized in the immediate medical management to rule out the possibility of an associated fracture.**

System Specific: Musculoskeletal System
Content Outline: Foundations for Evaluation, Differential Diagnosis, & Prognosis

## Exam Two: Question 53 ✳

A physical therapist performs goniometric measurements on a 38-year-old female rehabilitating from an acromioplasty. The therapist attempts to stabilize the scapula while measuring glenohumeral abduction. Failure to stabilize the scapula will lead to:

1. downward rotation and elevation of the scapula
2. downward rotation and depression of the scapula
3. **upward rotation and elevation of the scapula**
4. upward rotation and depression of the scapula

**Correct Answer: 3** (Norkin p. 70)

Normal glenohumeral abduction is 0-120 degrees. When measuring glenohumeral abduction, the axis of the goniometer should be placed over the anterior aspect of the acromial process. The stationary arm should be positioned parallel to the midline of the anterior aspect of the sternum and the moveable arm should be positioned on the medial midline of the humerus. Failure to stabilize the scapula will result in the obtained range of motion value being greater than the actual amount of glenohumeral abduction available.

1. Glenohumeral abduction requires upward rotation of the scapula and not downward rotation.
2. Glenohumeral abduction requires upward rotation and elevation of the scapula and not downward rotation and depression.
3. **Failure to stabilize the scapula when measuring glenohumeral abduction will result in upward rotation and elevation of the scapula. When measuring shoulder complex abduction, the thorax should be stabilized to prevent lateral flexion of the trunk.**
4. Glenohumeral abduction requires elevation of the scapula and not depression.

System Specific: Musculoskeletal System
Content Outline: Physical Therapy Examination

## Exam Two: Question 54

A physical therapist performs an examination on a 46-year-old male patient diagnosed with piriformis syndrome. The patient indicates he has experienced pain in his low back and buttock region for the last three weeks. Which motions would you expect to be weak and painful during muscle testing based on the patient's diagnosis?

1. **abduction and lateral rotation of the thigh**
2. abduction and medial rotation of the thigh
3. adduction and lateral rotation of the thigh
4. adduction and medial rotation of the thigh

**Correct Answer: 1** (Magee p. 696)

Piriformis syndrome refers to a condition in which the piriformis muscle irritates the sciatic nerve causing pain in the buttocks and referred pain along the course of the sciatic nerve. The piriformis muscle originates on the anterior surface of the sacrum and the sacrotuberous ligament and inserts on the greater trochanter of the femur. The muscle is innervated by the sacral plexus.

1. **The patient would likely present with pain and weakness with resisted abduction and lateral rotation of the thigh since the motions are consistent with the action of the piriformis muscle.**
2. The patient would likely present with pain and weakness with resisted abduction of the thigh, however, would not with resisted medial rotation.
3. The patient would not likely experience pain and weakness with resisted adduction, however, may with lateral rotation.
4. The patient would not likely experience pain and weakness with resisted adduction or medial rotation of the thigh since the motions are the exact opposite of the piriformis muscle's action.

System Specific: Other Systems
Content Outline: Physical Therapy Examination

## Exam Two: Question 55

A physical therapist examines a patient with a dorsal scapular nerve injury. Which muscles would you expect to be MOST affected by this condition?

1. serratus anterior, pectoralis minor
2. **levator scapulae, rhomboids**
3. latissimus dorsi, teres major
4. supraspinatus, infraspinatus

**Correct Answer: 2** (Kendall p. 348)
Damage to a peripheral nerve can significantly impair muscle function. The severity of the impact ranges from a mild disturbance to denervation.

1. The serratus anterior is innervated by the long thoracic nerve and the pectoralis minor is innervated by the medial pectoral nerve.
2. **The levator scapulae and rhomboids are innervated by the dorsal scapular nerve.**
3. The latissimus dorsi is innervated by the thoracodorsal nerve and the teres major is innervated by the lower subscapular nerve.
4. The supraspinatus and infraspinatus are innervated by the suprascapular nerve.

System Specific: Neuromuscular and Nervous Systems
Content Outline: Foundations for Evaluation, Differential Diagnosis, and Prognosis

**Test Taking Tip:** In some cases, a physical therapist may not have a full complement of academic information available to answer a given question, however, may still be able to identify the correct option or at least eliminate one or more of the incorrect options. For example, in option 1 the therapist may know that the serratus anterior is innervated by the long thoracic nerve, but may not know the innervation of the pectoralis minor. By recognizing that at least one of the muscles listed in option 1 is not associated with the dorsal scapular nerve, the therapist can safely eliminate this option. Candidates should not become anxious or unsettled when they identify information that they are not familiar with on the National Physical Therapy Examination and instead attempt to answer the question based on their existing academic knowledge. Candidates can use this strategy to enhance their examination score.

## Exam Two: Question 56

A 13-year-old female diagnosed with cerebral palsy is referred to physical therapy. The patient exhibits slow, involuntary, continuous writhing movements of the upper and lower extremities. This type of motor disturbance is MOST representative of:

1. spasticity
2. ataxia
3. hypotonia
4. **athetosis**

**Correct Answer: 4** (Tecklin p. 183)
Cerebral palsy is an umbrella term used to describe a group of non-progressive movement disorders that result from brain damage. Athetoid cerebral palsy involves damage to the cerebellum, cerebellar pathways or both.

1. Spasticity refers to an increased resistance to passive stretch. Spasticity is commonly observed with patients diagnosed with cerebral palsy due to upper motor neuron damage.
2. Ataxia is a generalized term used to describe motor impairments of cerebellar origin. It is characterized by the inability to perform coordinated movement and may affect gait, posture, and patterns of movements.
3. Hypotonia refers to decreased or absent tone where resistance to passive movement is decreased, stretch reflexes are diminished, and limbs are easily moved. Hypotonicity in children is often associated with motor delays.
4. **Athetosis refers to involuntary movements characterized as slow, irregular, and twisting. Peripheral movements occur without central stability. This type of motor disturbance makes it extremely difficult to maintain a static body position.**

System Specific: Neuromuscular & Nervous Systems
Content Outline: Foundations for Evaluation, Differential Diagnosis, and Prognosis

## Exam Two: Question 57 ✱

A physical therapist instructs a patient diagnosed with restricted shoulder mobility in a self-mobilization exercise. The therapist instructs the patient to attempt to lean in between their fixed arms (i.e., direct their upper thorax toward the mat surface). The primary objective of this activity is to improve:

1. glenohumeral abduction
2. **glenohumeral external rotation**
3. glenohumeral internal rotation
4. glenohumeral flexion

**Correct Answer: 2** (Kisner p. 491)
Self-mobilization exercises allow patients to improve joint capsule mobility. Physical therapists must offer explicit instructions for each exercise and observe the patient's ability to perform the technique correctly prior to formally including the exercises into the patient's home exercise program.

1. Glenohumeral abduction range of motion can be increased using a caudal glide of the humerus.
2. **The image depicts the recommended technique for administering a ventral glide of the humerus. A ventral glide of the humerus can be used to increase range of motion into glenohumeral external rotation, extension, and horizontal abduction.**
3. Glenohumeral internal rotation, flexion, and horizontal adduction range of motion can be increased using a dorsal glide of the humerus.
4. Glenohumeral internal rotation, flexion, and horizontal adduction range of motion can be increased using a dorsal glide of the humerus.

System Specific: Musculoskeletal System
Content Outline: Interventions

## Exam Two: Question 58

A physical therapist instructs a 55-year-old patient with significant bilateral lower extremity paresis to transfer from a wheelchair to a mat table. The patient has normal upper extremity strength and has no other known medical problems. The MOST appropriate transfer technique is a:

1. dependent squat pivot transfer
2. **sliding board transfer**
3. two-person lift
4. hydraulic lift

**Correct Answer: 2** (Pierson p. 189)
Physical therapists should select transfers for patients based on their unique abilities and limitations. Once a specific type of transfer is selected, the therapist should have the patient assist with the transfer to the greatest extent possible.

1. A dependent squat pivot transfer is used to transfer a patient who cannot stand independently, but can bear some weight through the trunk and lower extremities.
2. **A sliding board transfer is used for a patient who possesses sitting balance, good upper extremity strength, and can adequately follow directions. The use of the sliding board and the extent of upper extremity strength available make it possible for the patient to complete the transfer despite the presence of bilateral lower extremity paresis.**
3. A two-person lift is used to transfer a patient between two surfaces of different heights or when transferring a patient to the floor.
4. A hydraulic lift is a device required for dependent transfers when a patient is obese, when there is only one therapist available to assist with the transfer or when the patient is totally dependent.

System Specific: Non-Systems
Content Outline: Equipment & Devices; Therapeutic Modalities

## Exam Two: Question 59 ✳

A physical therapist instructs a patient to make a fist. The patient can make a fist, but is unable to flex the distal phalanx of the ring finger. This clinical finding can BEST be explained by:

1. a ruptured flexor carpi radialis tendon
2. a ruptured flexor digitorum superficialis tendon
3. **a ruptured flexor digitorum profundus tendon**
4. a ruptured extensor digitorum communis tendon

**Correct Answer: 3** (Hoppenfeld p. 101)

The flexor digitorum profundus muscle originates on the anterior and medial surfaces of the proximal portion of the ulna, interosseous membrane, and deep antebrachial fascia. The muscle inserts via four tendons into the anterior surface of the bases of the distal phalanges.

1. The flexor carpi radialis muscle acts to flex and abduct the wrist and may assist in pronation of the forearm and in flexion of the elbow.
2. The flexor digitorum superficialis muscle acts to flex the proximal interphalangeal joints of the second through fifth digits, and assists in flexion of the metacarpophalangeal joints and flexion of the wrist.
3. **The flexor digitorum profundus muscle acts to flex the distal interphalangeal joints of the index, middle, ring, and little finger, and assists in flexion of the proximal interphalangeal and metacarpophalangeal joints. A ruptured flexor digitorum profundus tendon would therefore make it impossible to flex the distal phalanx.**
4. The extensor digitorum communis muscle acts to extend the metacarpophalangeal joints and in conjunction with the lumbricals and interossei, extends the interphalangeal joints of the second through fifth digits. The muscle assists in abduction of the index, ring, and little finger and in extension and abduction of the wrist.

System Specific: Musculoskeletal System
Content Outline: Foundations for Evaluation, Differential Diagnosis, & Prognosis

**Test Taking Tip:** Candidates will often benefit from attempting to narrow down the possible options to a given examination question by eliminating options that they know are incorrect. In this particular question, a candidate should recognize that the answer cannot be option 4 since a rupture to an extensor tendon would result in an inability to extend and not to flex. Candidates who can use this type of pragmatic approach often achieve higher scores on the examination.

## Exam Two: Question 60 ✳

A physical therapist implements an aquatic program for a patient rehabilitating from a lower extremity injury. The program requires the patient to run in place using a flotation device while tethered to the side of the pool using an elastic cord. Which action would be the MOST appropriate to increase resistance?

1. increase the water temperature
2. **increase the speed of movement**
3. increase the depth of the water
4. remove the flotation device

**Correct Answer: 2** (Ruoti p. 20)

The therapeutic effects of immersion in water relate to the principles of hydrodynamics and thermodynamics. Some of the more relevant concepts associated with these principles include density, specific gravity, hydrostatic pressure, buoyancy, and viscosity.

1. Changes in the water temperature can influence variables such as oxygen uptake, but would not significantly influence resistance.
2. **The viscosity of water provides resistance to a body in motion. Viscosity refers to the thickness or resistance to the flow of a liquid. The faster the relative speed of the body, the greater the magnitude of resistance.**
3. Increasing the depth of the water would not result in a significant change in resistance since the patient is using a flotation device and therefore their level of immersion would remain relatively constant.
4. Removal of the flotation device would likely increase resistance since the patient may tend to move faster without the flotation device, however, it remains less desirable than simply continuing to use the belt and increasing the speed of movement.

System Specific: Other Systems
Content Outline: Interventions

## Exam Two: Question 61 ✳

A physical therapist measures passive forearm pronation and concludes that the results are within normal limits. Which measurement would be classified as within normal limits?

1. 60 degrees
2. **80 degrees**
3. 100 degrees
4. 120 degrees

---

**Correct Answer: 2** (Norkin p. 98)

Physical therapists should possess a thorough understanding of normal range of motion at different joints in the body. When measuring forearm pronation the axis of the goniometer is placed lateral to the ulnar styloid process. The proximal arm of the goniometer should be aligned parallel to the anterior midline of the humerus and the distal arm should be on the dorsal aspect of the forearm, just proximal to the styloid processes of the radius and ulna.

1. A value of 60 degrees of forearm pronation would be considered hypomobile.
2. **According to the American Academy of Orthopedic Surgeons and the American Medical Association normal forearm pronation is 0-80 degrees.**
3. A value of 100 degrees of forearm pronation would be considered hypermobile.
4. A value of 120 degrees of forearm pronation would be considered extremely hypermobile and would be unlikely given the joint structure of the superior and inferior radioulnar joints.

System Specific: Musculoskeletal System
Content Outline: Physical Therapy Examination

---

**Test Taking Tip:** There are sometimes small differences in reported ranges when using different academic sources. In the case of range of motion, acceptable academic sources may include groups such as the American Academy of Orthopedic Surgeons and the American Medical Association. Candidates must resist the urge to become too obsessive when reviewing this type of content and be confident that a scored examination question on the National Physical Therapy Examination would not require a candidate to differentiate between two acceptable sources.

## Exam Two: Question 62

A physical therapist discusses the importance of proper posture with a patient rehabilitating from back surgery at the L3-L4 spinal level. Which body position would place the MOST pressure on the lumbar spine?

1. standing in the anatomical position
2. standing with 45 degrees of hip flexion
3. **sitting in a chair slouching forward**
4. sitting in a chair with reduced lumbar lordosis

---

**Correct Answer: 3** (Hertling p. 880)

A study by Nachemson examined intradiskal pressures in the lumbar spine (L3 disc) as they relate to specific body positions. The order of body positions from the lowest total load to the greatest total load is as follows: lying in supine, sidelying, standing in the anatomical position, standing with 45 degrees of hip flexion, sitting in a chair with reduced lumbar lordosis, and sitting in a chair slouching forward.

1. Standing in the anatomical position resulted in the total load being greater than the load associated with lying in supine or sidelying.
2. Standing with 45 degrees of hip flexion resulted in the total load being greater than the load associated with lying in supine, sidelying, and standing in the anatomical position.
3. **Sitting in a chair slouching forward resulted in the total load being greater than any of the other five body positions measured.**
4. Sitting in a chair with reduced lumbar lordosis had the greatest total load of the positions measured with the only exception being sitting in a chair slouching forward.

System Specific: Musculoskeletal System
Content Outline: Interventions

## Exam Two: Question 63 ✷

A physical therapist works on transfer activities with a patient diagnosed with a complete C5 spinal cord injury. Which of the following muscles would the patient be able to utilize during the training session?

1.  brachioradialis
2.  pronator teres
3.  extensor carpi radialis brevis
4.  latissimus dorsi

**Correct Answer: 1** (Kendall p. 294)

A patient with C5 tetraplegia would be able to utilize muscles innervated at or above the C5 spinal level.

1.  **The brachioradialis is innervated by the radial nerve (C5-C6) and acts to flex the elbow joint and assists in pronating and supinating the forearm when these movements are resisted.**
2.  The pronator teres is innervated by the median nerve (C6-C7) and acts to pronate the forearm and assists in flexion of the elbow joint.
3.  The extensor carpi radialis brevis is innervated by the radial nerve (C6, C7, C8) and acts to extend the wrist and assists in wrist abduction.
4.  The latissimus dorsi is innervated by the thoracodorsal nerve (C6, C7, C8) and with the origin fixed acts to medially rotate, adduct, and extend the shoulder joint.

System Specific: Neuromuscular & Nervous Systems
Content Outline: Foundations for Evaluation, Differential Diagnosis, and Prognosis

## Exam Two: Question 64

A physical therapist treats a 32-year-old female diagnosed with thoracic outlet syndrome. While exercising the patient begins to complain of feeling lightheaded and dizzy. The therapist immediately ushers the patient to a nearby chair and begins to monitor her vital signs. The therapist measures the patient's respiration rate as 10 breaths per minute, pulse rate as 45 beats per minute, and blood pressure as 115/85 mm Hg. Which of the following statements is MOST accurate?

1.  pulse rate and respiration rate are below normal levels
2.  pulse rate and blood pressure are above normal levels
3.  blood pressure and respiration rate are above normal levels
4.  the patient's vital signs are within normal limits

**Correct Answer: 1** (Pierson p. 53)

Normal range for pulse rate is 60-100 beats per minute for an adult, while respiration rate is 12-20 breaths per minute. Normal blood pressures are 100-140 mm Hg systolic and 60-90 mm Hg diastolic.

1.  **A pulse of 45 beats per minute and a respiratory rate of 10 breaths per minute are below the normal range and can contribute to the patient's complaints.**
2.  A pulse of 45 beats per minute is below the normal range and a blood pressure of 115/85 mm Hg is within the normal range.
3.  A blood pressure of 115/85 mm Hg is within the normal range and a respiration rate of 10 breaths per minute is below the normal range.
4.  Blood pressure is the only vital sign that is within normal limits. Pulse rate and respiration rate are below normal.

System Specific: Cardiovascular/Pulmonary and Lymphatic Systems
Content Outline: Physical Therapy Examination

## Exam Two: Question 65

A physical therapist works with a patient diagnosed with anterior cruciate ligament insufficiency. The physician referral specifies closed kinematic chain rehabilitation. Which exercise would NOT be appropriate based on the physician order?

1. exercise on a stair machine
2. limited squats to 45 degrees
3. walking backwards on a treadmill
4. **isokinetic knee extension and flexion**

**Correct Answer: 4** (Dutton p. 956)

Closed-chain activities involve the body moving over a fixed distal segment. Closed-chain activities are often integrated into lower extremity strengthening programs. Open-chain activities involve the distal segment, usually the hand or foot, moving freely in space.

1. Exercising on a stair machine requires the patient to maintain contact with the stair mechanism with their feet which would maintain the lower extremity in a fixed position.

2. Limited squats to 45 degrees require the feet to stay in contact with the ground while the hips and knees are gradually flexed and the trunk remains erect.

3. Walking backwards on a treadmill, or retro-walking, requires the lower extremity to be in contact with the treadmill for the majority of the activity. As a result, the activity would be considered a form of closed-chain exercise.

4. **Isokinetic knee extension and flexion requires the distal segment to move freely in space, as a result the exercise is considered to be a form of open-chain exercise. Isokinetic contractions occur when a muscle is contracting at the same speed throughout the entire available range.**

System Specific: Musculoskeletal System
Content Outline: Interventions

## Exam Two: Question 66 ✕

A patient with complete paraplegia discusses accessibility issues with an employer in preparation for her return to work. The patient is concerned about her ability to navigate a wheelchair in certain areas of the building. What is the MINIMUM space required to turn 180 degrees in a standard wheelchair?

1. 32 inches
2. 48 inches
3. **60 inches**
4. 72 inches

**Correct Answer: 3** (Physical Therapist's Clinical Companion p. 330)

The Americans with Disabilities Act was designed to provide a clear and comprehensive national mandate for the elimination of discrimination. Title III provides information on public accommodations including minimum accessibility standards.

1. Thirty-two inches is the minimum required width of a doorway for wheelchair clearance, however, this space would not be adequate to turn 180 degrees in a standard wheelchair.

2. Forty-eight inches would be 12 inches less than the minimum required space to turn 180 degrees in a standard wheelchair.

3. **Sixty inches is the minimum required width to turn 180 degrees in a standard wheelchair according to the Americans with Disabilities Act.**

4. Seventy-two inches would be adequate to turn 180 degrees in a standard wheelchair, however, this value exceeds the minimum required space by 12 inches.

System Specific: Non-Systems
Content Outline: Safety and Protection; Professional Responsibilities; Research

## Exam Two: Question 67

A patient is referred to physical therapy following surgery to repair a torn rotator cuff. The physician referral does not include post-operative guidelines and also does not classify the extent or size of the tear. The physical therapist's MOST appropriate action is to:

1. consult various medical resources that discuss physical therapy management of rotator cuff repairs
2. consult various protocols of other surgeons in the area
3. **contact the referring physician and discuss the patient's care**
4. discuss the patient's care with other staff members who are more experienced in treating rotator cuff repairs

**Correct Answer: 3** (Criteria for Standards of Practice)
Physical therapists should consult with the referring physician when there is inadequate information available to direct the patient's plan of care. This is particularly important in surgical cases since there can be large variability in the post-operative management of even similar conditions.

1. Medical resources can serve to educate the therapist in regard to the specific injury and the typical management, however, would not offer specific insight on the patient's unique needs.

2. There are a variety of surgical approaches that can be used to repair a rotator cuff tear and in addition each tear is unique in terms of its location and magnitude. As a result, the protocols of other physicians may have little relevance to the rehabilitation needs of the patient.

3. **The physician would be the only individual who could provide the necessary level of specificity related to the surgical procedure and the associated rehabilitation parameters.**

4. Consulting with staff members may be helpful to draw on their expertise, however, does not provide the necessary clarification related to the patient's situation.

System Specific: Non-Systems
Content Outline: Safety and Protection; Professional Responsibilities; Research

## Exam Two: Question 68

A 52-year-old, self-referred male is examined in physical therapy. The patient states that over the last three months he has experienced increasing neck stiffness and pain at night. He also communicates that he recently had several episodes of dizziness. The patient has a family history of cancer and has smoked two packs of cigarettes a day for over twenty years. The date of his last medical examination was ten years ago. The physical therapist's MOST appropriate action is to:

1. treat the patient conservatively and document any changes in the patient's status
2. inform the patient that he is not a candidate for physical therapy
3. refer the patient to an oncologist
4. **refer the patient to his primary care physician**

**Correct Answer: 4** (Magee p. 2)
Physical therapists must carefully screen patients for any potential signs or symptoms (i.e., "red flags") that indicate the need for physician referral.

1. Failure to recognize the need to refer a patient to a physician despite the presence of "red flags" can jeopardize patient safety and may be considered professional negligence.

2. There is ample evidence provided that indicates the patient is not presently a candidate for physical therapy. Although this is important to convey to the patient, the need to refer the patient to a physician based on the presence of "red flags" is a greater priority since it addresses a potential underlying pathology.

3. The physical therapist should not attempt to make a medical diagnosis and would therefore be better served to refer the patient to the primary care physician. The physician would likely examine the patient and order a variety of laboratory and diagnostic testing and if necessary refer the patient to other medical personnel.

4. **The self-referred patient offers a medical history that reveals several significant issues including episodes of dizziness, neck stiffness with pain at night, and a family history of cancer. Based on the history and the date of the last medical examination, the patient should be referred to a physician.**

System Specific: Other Systems
Content Outline: Foundations for Evaluation, Differential Diagnosis, & Prognosis

## Exam Two: Question 69

A physical therapist wearing sterile protective clothing establishes a sterile field prior to changing a dressing on a wound. Which area of the protective clothing would NOT be considered sterile even before coming in contact with a non-sterile object?

1. gloves
2. sleeves of the gown
3. front of the gown above waist level
4. **front of the gown below waist level**

---

**Correct Answer: 4** (Pierson p. 38)

Once a sterile field has been established a physical therapist must be careful to maintain the sterile field and minimize any chance of contamination. The four rules of asepsis that a therapist should follow are: 1.) know which items are sterile, 2.) know which items are not sterile, 3.) separate sterile items from non-sterile items, 4.) if a sterile item becomes contaminated, the situation must be remedied immediately.

1. Gloves offer protection to the therapist's hands to reduce the likelihood of becoming infected with microorganisms and decrease the risk of the patient receiving microorganisms from the physical therapist. Sterile gloves are considered to be sterile after they are applied.

2. A gown is used to protect the therapist's clothing from being contaminated or soiled by a contaminant. The gown also reduces the probability of the physical therapist transmitting a microorganism from their clothing to the patient. The sleeves of a sterile gown are considered to be sterile after they are applied.

3. The front of the gown above the waist level is considered to be sterile after the gown is applied.

4. **The front of the gown below the waist level is not considered to be sterile after the gown is applied since there is an increased chance of incidental contact with a non-sterile object without the physical therapist's knowledge.**

System Specific: Non-Systems
Content Outline: Safety and Protection; Professional Responsibilities; Research

---

## Exam Two: Question 70

A physical therapist transports a patient with multiple sclerosis to the gym for her treatment session. The patient is wheelchair dependent and uses a urinary catheter. When transporting the patient, the MOST appropriate location to secure the collection bag is:

1. in the patient's lap
2. on the patient's lower abdomen
3. on the wheelchair armrest
4. **on the wheelchair cross brace beneath the seat**

---

**Correct Answer: 4** (Pierson p. 283)

Urine drains into a collection bag as a result of the effect of gravity; therefore the collection bag from a urinary catheter must be positioned below the level of the bladder.

1. Securing the collection bag in the patient's lap would result in the collection bag being at a similar level as the patient's bladder. The position would interfere with virtually any activity that required movement.

2. The lower abdomen is above the level of the bladder and would also interfere with any movement. Additionally, the patient may be embarrassed or bothered by having the collection bag in such a visible location.

3. The wheelchair armrest is above the level of the bladder and therefore would impede the flow of urine into the collection bag.

4. **Positioning the collection bag on the cross brace beneath the seat will allow it to be below the level of the bladder and will minimize the possibility that the bag or tubing will be pulled or snagged.**

System Specific: Other Systems
Content Outline: Foundations for Evaluation, Differential Diagnosis, and Prognosis

## Exam Two: Question 71

A physical therapist employed by a home health agency visits a patient status post total knee arthroplasty. The patient was discharged from the hospital yesterday and according to the medical record had an unremarkable recovery. The physician orders include the use of a continuous passive motion machine. The MOST appropriate rate of motion would be:

1. 2 cycles per minute
2. 4 cycles per minute
3. 6 cycles per minute
4. 8 cycles per minute

**Correct Answer: 1** (Kisner p. 61)

A continuous passive motion (CPM) machine is a mechanical device designed to provide continuous motion for a particular joint using a predetermined range and speed. The primary indication for CPM use is to improve range of motion that may have been impaired secondary to a surgical procedure. CPM can be used to prevent motion loss by inhibiting the formation of adhesions and contractures. CPM has been shown to accelerate healing, improve the orientation of collagen fibers, and inhibit edema formation. Any joint may be indicated for CPM use, however, the knee is the most common joint treated with CPM.

1. **A rate of two cycles per minute (one cycle = 30 seconds) typically allows the patient to tolerate the CPM without difficulty.**

2. A rate of four cycles per minute (one cycle = 15 seconds) represents a faster rate than is typically recommended. Faster rates are not usually tolerated as well primarily due to a patient's post-surgical status.

3. A rate of six cycles per minute (one cycle = 10 seconds) would not typically allow the patient to sufficiently relax and may result in protective muscle guarding.

4. A rate of eight cycles per minute (one cycle = 7.5 seconds) would be excessive and would likely result in the patient activating the stop button.

System Specific: Musculoskeletal System
Content Outline: Interventions

## Exam Two: Question 72

A physical therapist attempts to examine the extent of ataxia in a patient's upper extremities. The preferred method to examine and document ataxia is:

1. manual muscle test
2. sensory test for light touch
3. functional assessment of rolling in bed
4. **finger to nose**

**Correct Answer: 4** (DeMyer p. 380)

Ataxia refers to the inability to perform coordinated movements usually as a result of cerebellar pathology. Ataxia can affect gait, patterns of movement, and posture. The condition increases the incidence of errors in the rate, rhythm, and timing of responses.

1. Manual muscle tests are utilized to assess the strength of a muscle or muscle group. Ataxia is not necessarily due to weakness, rather the loss of muscular coordination.

2. A sensory test for light touch determines perception of tactile touch input. The test area is lightly touched or stroked using a brush, cotton ball or tissue. Sensory testing assesses the ascending pathways of the spinal cord.

3. Functional assessment of rolling in bed tests the overall mobility and strength of a patient, but is not a specific test for ataxia.

4. **A finger to nose test requires the patient to perform coordinated and controlled voluntary movement. A patient with ataxia may have difficulty completing the activity in an accurate and fluid manner.**

System Specific: Neuromuscular & Nervous Systems
Content Outline: Physical Therapy Examination

## Exam Two: Question 73 ✗

An eleven-month-old child with cerebral palsy attempts to maintain a quadruped position. Which reflex would interfere with this activity if it was NOT integrated?

1. Galant reflex
2. **symmetrical tonic neck reflex**
3. plantar grasp reflex
4. positive support reflex

**Correct Answer: 2** (Ratliffe p. 26)

Primitive reflexes are reflexes which begin in utero or in early infancy. Most of these reflexes become integrated as the infant ages. Integration denotes that the reflex is no longer present when the stimulus is provided. Failure to integrate primitive reflexes can lead to impaired movement.

1. The Galant reflex is stimulated by stroking lateral to the spine. The response is lateral sidebending to the same side as the side of the stimulus. An infant would typically be able to maintain the quadruped position if this reflex was stimulated.

2. **Head positioning is the stimulus for the symmetrical tonic neck reflex. When the head is flexed, the upper extremities flex and the lower extremities extend. When the head extends the upper extremities extend and the lower extremities flex. The reaction of the extremities would not allow the infant to maintain a quadruped position.**

3. The plantar grasp reflex is stimulated by placing pressure on the ball of the foot, generally in standing. The response is for the toes to curl or flex. The reflex will have no impact on an infant's ability to maintain quadruped since the balls of the feet are not in contact with the floor.

4. The positive support reflex is stimulated by bearing weight through the feet. The response is for the lower extremities to extend, thereby allowing the infant to bear weight through the lower extremities. The reflex will have no impact on an infant's ability to maintain quadruped since they are not bearing weight through the feet.

System Specific: Neuromuscular & Nervous Systems
Content Outline: Interventions

## Exam Two: Question 74

A physical therapist attempts to schedule a patient for an additional therapy session after completing the examination. The physician referral indicates the patient is to be seen two times a week. The therapist suggests several possible times to the patient, but the patient insists she can only come in on Wednesday at 4:30. The therapist would like to accommodate the patient, but already has two patients scheduled at that time. The MOST appropriate action is to:

1. schedule the patient on Wednesday at 4:30
2. attempt to move one of the patients scheduled on Wednesday at 4:30 to a different time
3. **schedule the patient with another physical therapist on Wednesday at 4:30**
4. inform the referring physician the patient will only be seen once this week in therapy

**Correct Answer: 3** (Guide for Professional Conduct)

The *Guide for Professional Conduct* published by the American Physical Therapy Association states that physical therapists shall respect the rights and dignity of all individuals. It is therefore necessary for the physical therapist to consider not only what is best for the patient in question, but also what is best for all of the patients being treated by the physical therapist.

1. Scheduling the patient on Wednesday at 4:30 will result in the physical therapist having three patients scheduled at the same time. It is unlikely that the physical therapist will be able to provide the requisite level of care for each patient given the number of patients.

2. Attempting to move a patient who is already scheduled to another appointment is not considerate of the patient's particular needs. It is the physical therapist's responsibility to ensure that each patient in their care is treated with the utmost respect.

3. **Scheduling with another physical therapist will allow the patient to be seen two times per week as indicated on the referral and will accommodate the patient's schedule.**

4. Informing the physician that the patient cannot be seen two times per week in physical therapy is not usually considered necessary information to communicate to the physician. When possible physical therapists should attempt to provide patients with the necessary frequency of physical therapy visits.

System Specific: Non-Systems
Content Outline: Safety and Protection; Professional Responsibilities; Research

## Exam Two: Question 75

While reading the Methods section of a research report, a physical therapist notes the investigators used a repeated measures design. This form of experimental design:

1. **controls for differences between subjects**
2. keeps the subjects "blind" to the identity of the treatment group
3. ensures that subjects with similar characteristics are assigned to different treatment groups
4. selects a homogenous group of subjects

**Correct Answer: 1** (Portney p. 172)

Researchers may employ a number of design strategies to manipulate and control variables and measurements to strengthen the validity of their experiment and demonstrate a cause-and-effect relationship between the independent and dependent variables.

1. **In a repeated measures design all subjects experience all levels of the independent variable. This provides an efficient method for controlling differences between subjects because characteristics that may affect the outcomes, such as gender, age, physical characteristics, remain constant for each subject. Differences in outcomes can be attributed to the treatment. Since each subject acts as his own control, a repeated measures design is also called a within-subjects design.**

2. In its most complete form, blinding involves hiding the identity of group assignments from the subjects, from those who provide treatment, from those who measure the outcome variables, and from those who analyze the data. A repeated measures design may or may not include "blinding."

3. The design strategy that ensures that subjects with similar characteristics are assigned to different treatment groups is called matching. A repeated measures design may or may not include matching.

4. By selecting subjects who are homogeneous with respect to a specific trait, the researcher eliminates these traits as variables that may interfere with the dependent variable. A repeated measures design may or may not use homogeneous subjects.

System Specific: Non-Systems
Content Outline: Safety and Protection; Professional Responsibilities; Research

## Exam Two: Question 76

A physical therapist reviews the parameters of several pain modulation theories using transcutaneous electrical nerve stimulation (TENS). When comparing sensory stimulation to motor stimulation, sensory stimulation requires:

1. greater phase duration
2. **greater frequency**
3. stronger amplitude
4. shorter treatment time

**Correct Answer: 2** (Cameron p. 218)

Motor stimulation requires sufficient phase charge to elicit a muscle contraction. This is accomplished by using a low frequency and long phase duration. Sensory stimulation, also called conventional TENS, requires a sufficient phase charge to achieve a sensory response, but is below the motor threshold. This is accomplished by using a high frequency and short phase duration.

1. Phase duration is shorter with sensory level stimulation compared to motor level stimulation.

2. **Frequency is significantly greater with sensory level stimulation compared to motor level stimulation.**

3. Sensory level stimulation requires lower amplitude than motor level stimulation.

4. Treatment time is highly variable with sensory and motor stimulation TENS.

System Specific: Non-Systems
Content Outline: Equipment & Devices; Therapeutic Modalities

## Exam Two: Question 77

A physical therapist performs an examination on a 27-year-old male diagnosed with iliotibial band syndrome. The patient is an avid distance runner who routinely ran between 45-60 miles per week before experiencing pain in his knee. Standing posture reveals a varus position at the knee and a cavus foot. When palpating the lateral portion of the lower extremity, which area would MOST likely exhibit marked tenderness?

1. **lateral femoral condyle**
2. lateral joint line
3. lateral tibial condyle
4. fibular head

**Correct Answer: 1** (Hertling p. 535)

Iliotibial band syndrome is characterized by localized pain approximately two centimeters above the knee joint line over the lateral femoral condyle. The syndrome can be caused by activities requiring frequent flexion of the knee such as running or cycling which produce an inflammatory reaction.

1. **The iliotibial band is a thickened strip of fascia that extends from the iliac crest to the tibial tubercle. In iliotibial band syndrome there is excessive contact between the iliotibial band and the lateral femoral condyle usually when the knee is in approximately 30 degrees of flexion.**

2. Tenderness along the lateral joint line is more commonly associated with a meniscal injury.

3. The lateral tibial condyle is not typically painful since the irritation tends to be superior in the area of the lateral femoral condyle.

4. The fibular head is located on the lateral side of the knee at the approximate level of the tibial tubercle. The bony structure serves as the insertion for the biceps femoris muscle, but would not typically be involved with iliotibial band syndrome.

System Specific: Musculoskeletal System
Content Outline: Foundations for Evaluation, Differential Diagnosis, & Prognosis

## Exam Two: Question 78

The measurement of blood pressure with an aneroid sphygmomanometer is said to have concurrent validity if the pressures measured by the sphygmomanometer are equal to the pressures measured at the same time by:

1. an electrocardiogram
2. **a pressure transducer inserted in the artery**
3. a physician using a mercury sphygmomanometer
4. a pulse oximeter

**Correct Answer: 2** (Portney p. 103)

Concurrent validity is demonstrated when the measurement to be validated and a "gold standard" are measured at relatively the same time so that they both reflect the same incident or behavior.

1. Since the electrocardiogram does not measure blood pressure, it could not provide evidence of the concurrent validity of a measurement of blood pressure.

2. **For blood pressure measured by an aneroid sphygmomanometer to have concurrent validity, the systolic and diastolic pressures would have to be similar to the pressures measured simultaneously by another instrument considered to be the "gold standard." A pressure transducer inserted in the patient's artery provides a direct and precise measurement of blood pressure.**

3. Like the aneroid sphygmomanometer, a mercury sphygmomanometer provides an indirect measure of blood pressure. The device would not be nearly as accurate as a pressure transducer inserted directly in the artery.

4. Since a pulse oximeter does not measure blood pressure, it could not provide evidence of the concurrent validity of a measurement of blood pressure.

System Specific: Cardiovascular/Pulmonary and Lymphatic Systems
Content Outline: Physical Therapy Examination

## Exam Two: Question 79

A physical therapist transfers a patient in a wheelchair down a curb with a forward approach. Which of the following actions would be the MOST appropriate?

1. have the patient lean forward
2. have the wheelchair brakes locked
3. **tilt the wheelchair backwards**
4. position yourself in front of the patient

**Correct Answer: 3** (Pierson p. 154)

When descending a curb using a forward approach, the wheelchair must remain tipped backward until the rear wheels are in contact with the surface below the curb.

1. The patient would likely fall forward out of the wheelchair if the patient leans forward as the wheelchair's front casters are lowered down a curb. The patient must keep their center of mass back so that the wheelchair can descend without forward momentum.

2. The wheelchair brakes need to remain off so that the wheelchair can roll down the curb under the direction of the physical therapist. If the brakes are locked, the wheelchair will not be able to move forward down the curb.

3. **The physical therapist must be competent in tilting the wheelchair back as it descends so that the activity does not create an unnecessary safety risk. The physical therapist must provide caregivers with consistent instructions on how to safely ascend and descend a curb.**

4. If the physical therapist is positioned in front of the patient then they will not be able to tilt the wheelchair backwards or effectively manage the wheelchair as it rolls down the curb. The patient may also come forward towards the therapist since the front casters will touch the ground first and allow for forward momentum.

System Specific: Non-Systems
Content Outline: Equipment & Devices; Therapeutic Modalities

## Exam Two: Question 80

A physical therapist working on an oncology unit reviews the medical chart of a male patient prior to initiating airway clearance techniques. The patient's cell counts are as follows: hematocrit 44%, white blood cells 8,500/mm³, platelets 30,000/µl, hemoglobin level 15 gm/dL. Which blood test value suggests that chest percussion for airway clearance is contraindicated?

1. hematocrit
2. white blood cells
3. **platelets**
4. hemoglobin

**Correct Answer: 3** (Paz p. 736)

Certain blood values may influence the physical therapist's choice of interventions and goals for the treatment session. The platelet value is significantly below the normal value and would therefore result in percussion being contraindicated.

1. The hematocrit is within the normal range for males (39-46%).

2. White blood cell count is within the normal range of 3.5-9.1 x 10³/mm³.

3. **The platelet count is well below the normal range of 165,000–415,000/µl. With a platelet count of 50,000/µl or less, the patient is thrombocytopenic and would be placed on thrombocytopenic precautions until the platelet count returns to normal. These precautions include restricting chest percussion due to the increased risk of bleeding. Alternative chest physical therapy techniques may include coughing, deep breathing exercises, and using an incentive spirometer.**

4. The hemoglobin is within the normal range for males (13.3-16.2 gm/dL).

System Specific: Cardiovascular/Pulmonary and Lymphatic Systems
Content Outline: Interventions

## Exam Two: Question 81

A physical therapist treats a patient with a fractured left hip. The patient is weight bearing as tolerated and uses a large base quad cane for gait activities. Correct use of the quad cane would include:

1. using the quad cane on the left with the longer legs positioned away from the patient
2. **using the quad cane on the right with the longer legs positioned away from the patient**
3. using the quad cane on the left with the longer legs positioned toward the patient
4. using the quad cane on the right with the longer legs positioned toward the patient

**Correct Answer: 2** (Minor p. 316)

A quad cane should be utilized in the upper extremity that is opposite from the affected lower extremity. The device is designed so that the longer legs are positioned away from the patient.

1. The quad cane should be used in the hand opposite the affected lower extremity.

2. **The quad cane, positioned in the right hand with the longer legs pointing away from the patient, will allow for proper distribution of the weight during gait and as a result, the patient will be less likely to trip over the longer legs of the cane.**

3. The quad cane should be used in the hand opposite the affected lower extremity with the longer legs of the quad cane positioned away from the patient.

4. The quad cane should be used with the longer legs positioned away from the patient so that the patient does not trip over them.

System Specific: Musculoskeletal System
Content Outline: Interventions

## Exam Two: Question 82

A 66-year-old female is referred to physical therapy with rheumatoid arthritis. During the examination the physical therapist notes increased flexion at the proximal interphalangeal joints and hyperextension at the metacarpophalangeal and distal interphalangeal joints. This deformity is MOST representative of:

1. **Boutonniere deformity**
2. mallet finger
3. swan neck deformity
4. ulnar drift

**Correct Answer: 1** (Magee p. 404)

There are a number of common hand and finger deformities that are often associated with specific medical diagnoses. Physical therapists should be familiar with the clinical presentation of these deformities. Boutonniere deformity, swan neck deformity, and ulnar drift are commonly observed in patients with rheumatoid arthritis.

1. **Boutonniere deformity is characterized by extension of the metacarpophalangeal and distal interphalangeal joints and flexion of the proximal interphalangeal joint. The deformity is caused by a rupture of the central tendinous slip of the extensor hood.**

2. Mallet finger is characterized by the distal phalanx of the finger resting in a flexed position. The deformity is caused by a rupture or avulsion of the extensor tendon.

3. Swan neck deformity is characterized by flexion at the distal interphalangeal joints and hyperextension of the proximal interphalangeal joints. The deformity is caused by a contraction of the intrinsic muscles or tearing of the volar plate.

4. Ulnar drift is characterized by ulnar deviation of the digits due to weakening of the capsuloligamentous structures of the metacarpophalangeal joints and the accompanying effect on the extensor communis tendons.

System Specific: Musculoskeletal System
Content Outline: Foundations for Evaluation, Differential Diagnosis, & Prognosis

## Exam Two: Question 83

A patient diagnosed with piriformis syndrome is referred to physical therapy for one visit for instruction in a home exercise program. After examining the patient, the physical therapist feels the patient's rehabilitation potential is excellent, but is concerned that one visit will not be sufficient to meet the patient's needs. The MOST appropriate action is to:

1. schedule the patient for treatment sessions as warranted by the results of the examination
2. explain to the patient that recent health care reforms have drastically reduced the frequency of physical therapy visits covered by third party payers
3. explain to the patient that she can continue with physical therapy beyond the initial session, but will be liable for all expenses not covered by her insurance
4. **contact the referring physician and request approval for additional physical therapy visits**

**Correct Answer: 4** (Criteria for Standards of Practice)
A physical therapist has an ethical and legal obligation to act in the patient's best interest.

1. Scheduling the patient for treatment sessions based on the results of the examination is appropriate, however, the physical therapist should contact the referring physician and attempt to have the visits approved.
2. Health care reforms have, in many cases, limited the frequency of physical therapy visits covered by third party payers, however, there is no indication that the patient would not have coverage for the additional visits.
3. Patients should understand that they may be responsible for the cost of unreimbursed physical therapy services, however, the physical therapist should take the necessary steps to insure that the services are both necessary and authorized by the referring physician.
4. **The physical therapist will need to seek physician approval for the additional visits in order to be working under a physician referral. Although this does not guarantee that the visits will be approved by the physician or that the visits will be covered by the third party payer, it provides the therapist with the opportunity to act in the patient's best interest.**

System Specific: Musculoskeletal System
Content Outline: Foundations for Evaluation, Differential Diagnosis, and Prognosis

## Exam Two: Question 84

A physical therapist completes lower extremity range of motion activities with a patient status post spinal cord injury. While performing passive range of motion, the therapist notices that the patient's urine is extremely dark and has a distinctive foul smelling odor. Which of the following is the MOST appropriate action?

1. verbally report the observation to the patient's physician
2. verbally report the observation to the patient's nurse
3. **document and verbally report the observation to the patient's nurse**
4. document and verbally report the observation to the director of rehabilitation

**Correct Answer: 3** (Pierson p. 283)
Physical therapists should report any abnormality in a patient's urine to the appropriate member of the health care team since this may indicate a change in the patient's medical status. Documentation of urine may include comments related to appearance (i.e., color, smell, quantity).

1. Verbally reporting the observation to a physician without also documenting the finding would be an incomplete response.
2. The nurse would be the most logical health care professional to initially receive this information, however, the option does not include documentation.
3. **The nurse is an appropriate member of the health care team to receive this information and it is necessary to document the findings.**
4. The director of rehabilitation is an administrative position within the health care organization and therefore would not typically be directly involved in the patient's care.

System Specific: Other Systems
Content Outline: Foundations for Evaluation, Differential Diagnosis, & Prognosis

## Exam Two: Question 85

A rehabilitation manager designs a system to monitor the productivity of the physical therapists. Which piece of data would be the LEAST beneficial to accomplish the manager's objective?

1. number of generated timed treatment units
2. **results of patient satisfaction survey data**
3. total hours of direct patient treatment time
4. number of regular payroll hours

**Correct Answer: 2** (Nosse p. 421)

Productivity is a term used to describe the efficiency of a given worker or group of workers. Productivity standards are used as performance targets to help direct management and staff. The established standards should be based on a measurable unit of output (e.g., billable units), objectively measured, understandable, and achievable.

1. The number of generated timed treatment units is most often expressed in 15 minute intervals and is necessary in order to determine the productivity of physical therapists.

2. **The results of patient satisfaction data would be considered a qualitative measure describing the general satisfaction of patients with selected aspects of the physical therapy services. Items commonly explored in this type of survey include direct patient care activities, staffing, environment, scheduling, hours of operation, and parking. Although measures of quality are often examined concurrently with productivity, they are not used to determine productivity.**

3. The total hours of direct patient treatment time is often compared to the number of generated timed treatment units.

4. The number of regular payroll hours is necessary to determine full-time equivalents. This measure is most often used to examine staffing patterns or staffing needs.

System Specific: Non-Systems
Content Outline: Safety and Protection; Professional Responsibilities; Research

## Exam Two: Question 86

A physical therapist observing a patient complete a leg curl exercise notices two prominent tendons visible on the posterior surface of the patient's left knee. The visible tendons are MOST likely associated with the:

1. semimembranosus and semitendinosus muscles
2. **semitendinosus and biceps femoris muscles**
3. popliteus and semitendinosus muscles
4. semimembranosus and biceps femoris muscles

**Correct Answer: 2** (Kendall p. 418)

The hamstrings muscles include the semitendinosus, semimembranosus, and biceps femoris. The muscles primary action is to flex the knee. As a result, the tendons of each of the hamstrings muscles become more prominent with resisted knee flexion.

1. The semimembranosus and semitendinosus are hamstrings muscles that act to flex the knee joint, however, they are both located on the medial aspect of the posterior knee joint. The image shows two tendons, one that is located on the medial aspect of the posterior surface of the knee joint and the other on the lateral aspect.

2. **The semitendinosus and biceps femoris are hamstrings muscles whose tendons become prominent when performing a leg curl. The biceps femoris is the lateral tendon, while the semitendinosus is the medial tendon.**

3. The popliteus muscle is located deep within the posterior surface of the knee joint and would not appear as a tendinous cord-like structure. The semitendinosus is a medial hamstrings muscle that would be prominent on the medial aspect of the posterior surface of the knee joint.

4. The semimembranosus muscle is a medial hamstrings muscle, however, the muscle's tendon is not nearly as prominent as the semitendinosus. The biceps femoris is a lateral hamstrings muscle that would be prominent on the lateral aspect of the posterior surface of the knee joint.

System Specific: Musculoskeletal System
Content Outline: Physical Therapy Examination

## Exam Two: Question 87

A physical therapist prepares to apply a hot pack to the low back of a patient diagnosed with degenerative disk disease. When examining the patient the therapist identifies several blisters on the patient's right side. The patient indicates they were caused by heat from a hot pack applied during the previous treatment session. The patient indicates he was hesitant to tell the therapist that the heat was too intense. The MOST appropriate therapist action is to:

1. **complete an incident report**
2. contact the referring physician
3. modify the documentation from the previous treatment session
4. avoid documenting the event since it occurred during the previous treatment session

**Correct Answer: 1** (Scott - Promoting Legal and Ethical Awareness p. 81)

An incident report is a factual written summary of an adverse event designed to memorialize specific details of the event and to limit future liability of the organization. Information obtained from the incident report is often used to guide risk management initiatives.

1. **The physical therapist must complete the incident report since they directly observed the blistered skin and heard the patient relate the cause of the burn to the hot pack.**

2. The referring physician may be informed of the event, however, the need to complete the incident report would be a higher priority given the described scenario.

3. Modifying documentation from a previous treatment session is not acceptable and would be considered a fraudulent act.

4. The patient's revelation to the therapist is important information to document despite the fact that the activity in question occurred during the previous treatment session. The therapist should document the objective findings (i.e., blisters) and the patient's claim that the blisters were caused by heat from the hot pack.

System Specific: Non-Systems
Content Outline: Safety and Protection; Professional Responsibilities; Research

## Exam Two: Question 88

A physical therapist attempts to calculate the target heart rate range for a 32-year-old female with no significant past medical history. The patient's resting heart rate is recorded as 60 beats per minute and the maximal heart rate is 180 beats per minute. Using the heart rate reserve method (Karvonen formula) and a range of 60-80% intensity, the patient's target heart rate range should be recorded as:

1. 96 - 120 beats per minute
2. **132 - 156 beats per minute**
3. 144 - 174 beats per minute
4. 164 - 185 beats per minute

**Correct Answer: 2** (American College of Sports Medicine p. 455)

There are a number of formulas used to prescribe exercise intensity based on heart rate. The heart rate (HR) reserve method, also known as the Karvonen method, uses resting heart rate subtracted from the maximal heart rate to obtain the heart rate reserve. Adding 60% and 80% of the heart rate reserve to resting heart rate results in the target heart rate range.

Target heart rate range = $[(HR_{max} - HR_{rest}) * 0.60$ and $0.80] + HR_{rest}$

1. 96 - 120 beats per minute is less than the target heart rate range calculated using the Karvonen formula and the patient's maximal and resting heart rates.

2. **Target heart rate range = [(180 – 60) * 0.60 and 0.80] + 60**
   **= [120*0.60 and 120*0.80] + 60**
   **= (72 + 60) and (96 + 60)**
   **= 132 - 156 beats per minute**

3. 144 - 174 beats per minute overlaps with a portion of the target heart rate range calculated from the Karvonen formula and the patient's maximal and resting heart rates, but is too high at the lower and upper ends.

4. 164 - 185 beats per minute is more than the target heart rate range calculated using the Karvonen formula and the patient's maximal and resting heart rates.

System Specific: Cardiovascular/Pulmonary and Lymphatic Systems
Content Outline: Interventions

## Exam Two: Question 89 ✕

A 47-year-old patient with a diagnosis of CVA with left hemiplegia is referred for orthotic examination. Significant results of manual muscle testing include: hip flexion 3+/5, hip extension 3/5, knee flexion 3+/5, knee extension 3+/5, ankle dorsiflexion 2/5, and ankle inversion and eversion 1/5. Sensation is intact and no abnormal tone is noted. The MOST appropriate orthosis for this patient is a:

1. knee-ankle-foot orthosis with a locked knee
2. **plastic articulating ankle-foot orthosis**
3. metal upright ankle-foot orthosis locked in neutral
4. prefabricated posterior leaf spring orthosis

**Correct Answer: 2** (Seymour p. 381)

The goal of an orthotic is to correct abnormal movement patterns and improve function using the least amount of intervention. A plastic ankle-foot orthosis (AFO) with an articulating ankle joint is the most appropriate orthotic based on the patient's strength, sensation and tone.

1. A knee-ankle-foot orthosis (KAFO) with a locked knee would be most appropriate for a patient that had no voluntary knee control. The locked knee ensures that the knee joint remains in an extended position and avoids genu recurvatum or collapsing of the knee during stance phase.

2. **The patient's strength at the hip and knee allows for an ankle-foot orthosis (AFO) to be used. A plastic AFO is appropriate since there is intact sensation and an articulating ankle joint is recommended to improve biomechanics during gait since there is an absence of tonal abnormalities.**

3. A metal upright AFO is normally prescribed for a patient that has fluctuating tone and/or a sensory deficit. An AFO may be locked in neutral at the ankle joint if an increase in tone exists or in the absence of voluntary motion.

4. A posterior leaf spring orthosis provides a dorsiflexion assist during gait. This type of AFO provides a spring-like dorsiflexion assist during terminal stance. Since the trim lines are posterior to the malleoli, dorsiflexion and plantar flexion can still occur during gait. The posterior leaf spring orthosis would not offer enough stability for the patient.

System Specific: Neuromuscular and Nervous Systems
Content Outline: Interventions

## Exam Two: Question 90

A 30-year-old female is seen in physical therapy secondary to benign paroxysmal positional vertigo. Which of the following physical therapy treatments would most benefit this patient?

1. Dix-Hallpike maneuver
2. **canalith repositioning maneuvers**
3. singular neurectomy
4. gaze stability exercises

**Correct Answer: 2** (Goodman - Pathology p. 1577)

Benign paroxysmal positional vertigo (BPPV) is an intense and intermittent vertigo that occurs in relation to rapid movement of the head in a particular direction and is believed to be a mechanical disorder of the labyrinths. Canaliths develop and float into the semicircular canals causing the brain to interpret their presence as an intense rotation of the head.

1. Dix-Hallpike maneuver is not a treatment for BPPV but rather a diagnostic tool. A patient that presents with BPPV will have torsional nystagmus when performing this maneuver. The patient moves from an upright posture to supine with the head hanging over the surface extended and rotated to 45 degrees. Nystagmus will occur in this position when the affected ear is toward the floor and should fatigue within 60 seconds.

2. **Canalith repositioning maneuvers are a highly effective treatment for BPPV and are designed to dislodge the provoking canaliths. This treatment technique attempts to move the canalith debris out of the affected semicircular canal and back to the otolith. Canalith repositioning maneuvers begin in the Dix-Hallpike position to provoke vertigo. Repeated head rolling utilizes gravity to assist with movement of the debris. Treatment continues until no further nystagmus is noted.**

3. A singular neurectomy is a surgical procedure that can assist with BPPV, but is rarely performed. This is not a physical therapy treatment but rather a selective surgical transection of the nerve supply to the posterior canal.

4. Gaze stability exercises are frequently used in the treatment of unilateral vestibular hypofunction with the goal of improving the vestibulo-ocular reflex and other systems that provide gaze stability while the head is in motion.

System Specific: Neuromuscular & Nervous Systems
Content Outline: Interventions

## Exam Two: Question 91

A physical therapist reviews the medical chart of a patient with a history of recurrent dysrhythmias. The therapist is concerned about the patient's past medical history and would like to monitor the patient during selected formal exercise activities. Which of the following monitoring devices would be the MOST beneficial?

1. pulmonary artery catheter
2. **electrocardiogram**
3. intracranial pressure monitor
4. pulse oximeter

**Correct Answer: 2** (Hillegass p. 331)

An electrocardiogram (ECG) is a recording of the electrical activity of the heart over time produced by an electrocardiograph, usually via skin electrodes. It is a common monitoring device for patients with known or suspected cardiac abnormalities.

1. A pulmonary artery catheter monitors cardiovascular pressures in the pulmonary artery.

2. **The electrocardiogram provides a graphic record of the electrical activity of the heart at rest or during exercise. Dysrhythmia is a general term used to denote disturbances in the heart's rhythm, which are best monitored by an electrocardiogram.**

3. An intracranial pressure monitor consists of a small plastic tube usually inserted in the left or right anterior portion of the brain. The monitor is often used to assess the pressure surrounding the brain of patients in the intensive care unit who have sustained head trauma, brain hemorrhage, brain surgery or conditions in which the brain may swell.

4. A pulse oximeter is an instrument that uses a light-emitting diode, a photodiode signal detector, and a microprocessor to determine the percentage of oxygen saturation of arterial blood.

System Specific: Cardiovascular/Pulmonary and Lymphatic Systems
Content Outline: Foundations for Evaluation, Differential Diagnosis, & Prognosis

## Exam Two: Question 92

A physical therapist observes a change in the muscle tone of an infant's extremities as a result of head rotation. Which developmental reflex would facilitate this type of response?

1. **asymmetrical tonic neck reflex**
2. symmetrical tonic neck reflex
3. symmetrical tonic labyrinthine reflex
4. crossed extension reflex

**Correct Answer: 1** (Ratliffe p. 26)

Primitive and tonic reflexes are normally present during infancy and gradually are integrated throughout early development by the central nervous system. Physical therapists should be familiar with the stimulus, response, and age of integration of common pediatric reflexes.

1. **The asymmetrical tonic neck reflex normally occurs in infants from birth to 6 months of age when the head is rotated to one side. This reflex causes extension of the extremity toward the side of rotation.**

2. The symmetrical tonic neck reflex normally occurs in infants from 6 to 8 months of age and is fully integrated by 8 to 12 months of age. It is stimulated by placing the head in either flexion or extension. When the head is in flexion, the upper extremities will flex while the lower extremities extend. When the head is extended, the upper extremities will extend while the lower extremities flex.

3. The symmetrical tonic labyrinthine reflex normally occurs at birth and is fully integrated by 6 months of age. It is stimulated by placing the infant in either prone or supine. When in the prone position, the body and extremities exhibit increased flexor tone and are held in flexion; in supine, the body and extremities exhibit increased extensor tone and are held in extension.

4. The crossed extension reflex normally occurs at 28 weeks gestation and is fully integrated by 1-2 months of age. The reflex is stimulated by a noxious stimulus to the ball of the foot, while the lower extremity is fixed in extension. This will elicit a response of the opposite lower extremity in which it will flex, then adduct and extend.

System Specific: Neuromuscular & Nervous Systems
Content Outline: Physical Therapy Examination

## Exam Two: Question 93 ✕

A physical therapy program designs a study that uses performance on the Scholastic Aptitude Test as a predictor of grade point average in a physical therapy academic program. The results of the study identify that the overall correlation between the variables is r =.87. Which statement is MOST accurate based on the results of the study?

1. A high grade point average in a physical therapy program is caused by a high score on the Scholastic Aptitude Test.
2. **Students in a physical therapy program with high scores on the Scholastic Aptitude Test tend to have high grade point averages.**
3. There is no relationship between grade point average in a physical therapy program and performance on the Scholastic Aptitude Test.
4. There is an inverse relationship between grade point average in a physical therapy program and performance on the Scholastic Aptitude Test.

**Correct Answer: 2** (Portney p. 525)
Correlation coefficients quantitatively describe the strength and magnitude of the relationship between two variables. The symbol "r" denotes the Pearson product-moment correlation coefficient, which is used to evaluate the strength and direction of the linear relationship between two continuous variables on the interval or ratio scales. The Pearson "r" can take values ranging from -1.00 (a perfect negative relationship) to 1.00 (a perfect positive relationship).

1. Correlation does not imply a causal relationship between two variables. A strong relationship between X and Y does not suggest that X causes Y or that Y causes X. Therefore, it cannot be said that the r = 0.87 suggests that a high score on the Scholastic Aptitude Test causes a high grade point average.
2. **A r = 0.87 indicates a good to excellent relationship between the Scholastic Aptitude Test (SAT) and grade point average (GPA). That is, low scores on the SAT tend to be associated with low GPAs and high scores on the SAT tend to be associated with high GPAs.**
3. No relationship between grade point average and performance on the Scholastic Aptitude Test would be indicated by an r = 0.0.
4. A r = 0.87 indicates a positive or direct relationship between grade point average in a physical therapy program and performance on the Scholastic Aptitude Test. A negative correlation coefficient would indicate an inverse relationship.

System Specific: Non-Systems
Content Outline: Safety and Protection; Professional Responsibilities; Research

## Exam Two: Question 94

A patient is referred to physical therapy with a C6 nerve root injury. Which of the following clinical findings would NOT be expected with this type of injury?

1. diminished sensation on the anterior arm and the index finger
2. weakness in the biceps and supinator
3. diminished brachioradialis reflex
4. **paresthesias of the long and ring fingers**

**Correct Answer: 4** (Magee p. 22)
Involvement of a specific nerve root often results in predictable impairments including diminished sensation, muscle weakness, impaired reflexes, and paresthesias.

1. Diminished sensation on the anterior arm and index finger is characteristic of a C6 nerve root injury and is assessed using light touch from a cotton ball.
2. Weakness in the biceps and supinator muscles is characteristic of a C6 nerve root injury and is assessed through resistive testing as part of an upper quarter screening examination and/or specific manual muscle testing.
3. A diminished brachioradialis reflex is characteristic of a C6 nerve root injury and is assessed by striking the blunt end of a reflex hammer at the distal end of the radius with the patient's elbow flexed to 90 degrees and the upper extremity supported by the therapist.
4. **Paresthesias of the long and ring fingers are commonly associated with the C7 nerve root. Other findings of a C7 nerve root injury include weakness of the triceps and wrist flexors, and a diminished triceps reflex.**

System Specific: Neuromuscular & Nervous Systems
Content Outline: Foundations for Evaluation, Differential Diagnosis, and Prognosis

## Exam Two: Question 95

A 22-year-old male status post traumatic brain injury receives physical therapy services in a rehabilitation hospital. The patient is presently functioning at Rancho Los Amigos level VI. The patient has progressed well in therapy, however, has been bothered by diplopia. Which treatment strategy would be the MOST appropriate to address diplopia?

1. provide non-verbal instructions within the patient's direct line of sight
2. **place a patch over one of the patient's eyes**
3. ask the patient to turn his head to one side when he experiences diplopia
4. instruct the patient to carefully focus on a single object

**Correct Answer: 2** (O'Sullivan p. 1159)
Diplopia refers to double vision resulting from defective function of the extraocular muscles that is typically caused by damage to the brain. A patient with diplopia is often instructed to wear a patch alternately over one of their eyes. Specific strengthening exercises of the extraocular muscles can serve to improve the patient's vision.

1. Verbal instruction is often more desirable than non-verbal instruction since double vision would tend to minimize the effectiveness of non-verbal instruction.
2. **A patient with diplopia will actually see two sets of the environment. If wearing the patch over the alternate eye does not resolve the problem, the patient may require prism glasses.**
3. The patient will not alleviate diplopia through positioning of the head. Double vision can result from damage to the brain and requires strengthening and the use of an eye patch.
4. A patient with diplopia can use the extraocular muscles of each eye, but they are not in focus. Verbal cueing to "focus" on a single object will not alleviate diplopia since strengthening is required.

System Specific: Neuromuscular & Nervous Systems
Content Outline: Interventions

## Exam Two: Question 96

A physical therapist completes an upper extremity manual muscle test on a patient diagnosed with rotator cuff tendonitis. Assuming the patient has the ability to move the upper extremities against gravity, which of the following muscles would NOT be tested with the patient in a supine position?

1. pronator teres
2. pectoralis major
3. biceps brachii
4. **middle trapezius**

**Correct Answer: 4** (Kendall p. 329)
The middle fibers of the trapezius originate on the spinous processes of the first through fifth thoracic vertebrae and insert on the medial margin of the acromion and superior lip of the spine of the scapula. The muscle is innervated by the spinal accessory nerve and ventral ramus C2, C3, C4.

1. The pronator teres is tested in a supine position. The test arm is positioned with forearm pronation and partial elbow flexion. The therapist provides pressure at the lower forearm in the direction of forearm supination.
2. The pectoralis major is tested with the patient in a supine position. The test arm is flexed to 90 degrees at the shoulder with slight medial rotation and elbow extension. Pressure is applied against the forearm in the direction of horizontal abduction.
3. The biceps brachii is tested with the patient in a supine position. The test arm is flexed at the elbow to 90 degrees with supination of the forearm. The therapist provides pressure at the distal end of the forearm in the direction of forearm pronation.
4. **The middle trapezius is tested with the patient in a prone position. The test arm is abducted at the shoulder to 90 degrees with lateral rotation and elbow extension. The therapist provides pressure against the forearm in a downward direction.**

System Specific: Musculoskeletal System
Content Outline: Physical Therapy Examination

## Exam Two: Question 97

A physical therapist prepares a patient education program for an individual with chronic venous insufficiency. Which of the following would NOT be appropriate to include in the patient education program?

1. wear shoes that accommodate to the size and shape of your feet
2. observe your skin daily for breakdown
3. **wear your compression stockings only at night**
4. keep your feet elevated as much as possible throughout the day

**Correct Answer: 3** (Kisner p. 833)

Chronic venous insufficiency is a common disorder of the lower extremity veins in which the veins do not work properly and blood pools in the lower extremities, leading to increased pressure within the veins. If uncontrolled, fluid may leak into the surrounding tissues in the ankles and feet and may eventually cause skin breakdown and ulceration.

1. Wearing shoes that accommodate to the size and shape of the foot is an important component of an education program for a patient with venous insufficiency. Successful implementation of the program reduces the risk of skin abrasions, ulcerations, and wound infections.

2. Swelling, cellulitis, and chronic lower extremity ulcers are common complications of venous insufficiency. Daily observation of the skin is a necessary component of an education program for a patient with venous insufficiency.

3. **Patients with chronic venous insufficiency often wear graduated compression stockings which attempt to improve circulation by preventing backward flow through the veins of the lower extremities. It is recommended that compression stockings are applied in the morning, since swelling is usually minimal in the morning and left on during the day for activity such as ambulation, to promote blood flow to the heart and avoid venous stasis.**

4. Elevating the feet throughout the day reduces pressure in the lower extremity veins and helps to improve blood flow. Positioning guidelines would be part of an education program for a patient with venous insufficiency.

System Specific: Cardiovascular/Pulmonary and Lymphatic Systems
Content Outline: Interventions

## Exam Two: Question 98

A physical therapist determines that a patient rehabilitating from ankle surgery has consistent difficulty with functional activities that emphasize the frontal plane. Which of the following would be the MOST difficult for the patient?

1. anterior lunge
2. **six-inch lateral step down**
3. six-inch posterior step up
4. eight-inch posterior step down

**Correct Answer: 2** (Norkin p. 5)

The frontal plane divides the body into front and back halves. Movements in the frontal plane occur as side to side movements such as abduction or adduction. Rotary motion in the frontal plane occurs around an anterior-posterior axis.

1. An anterior lunge would require the patient to perform hip flexion and extension (returning from the lunged position) which are sagittal plane motions.

2. **A lateral step-down would require the patient to perform hip abduction and adduction which are frontal plane motions.**

3. A posterior step up would require the patient to perform hip flexion and extension which are sagittal plane motions.

4. The posterior step down, regardless of the height of the step, would require the patient to perform hip flexion and extension which are sagittal plane motions.

System Specific: Musculoskeletal System
Content Outline: Interventions

## Exam Two: Question 99 ✕

A patient rehabilitating from a radial head fracture is examined in physical therapy. During the examination, the physical therapist notes that the patient appears to have an elbow flexion contracture. Which of the following would NOT serve as an appropriate <u>active exercise</u> technique to increase range of motion?

1. contract-relax
2. hold-relax
3. **maintained pressure**
4. rhythmic stabilization

**Correct Answer: 3** (Sullivan p. 64)
Maintained pressure is an effective technique that can be used to increase range of motion by facilitating local muscle relaxation, however, it is a passive technique.

1. Contract-relax is a technique used to increase range of motion. As the extremity reaches the point of limitation, the patient performs a maximal contraction of the antagonistic muscle group. The therapist resists movement for eight to ten seconds with relaxation to follow. The technique should be repeated until no further gains in range of motion are noted.

2. Hold-relax is an isometric contraction used to increase range of motion. The contraction is facilitated at the limiting point in the range of motion. Relaxation occurs and the extremity moves through the newly acquired range to the next point of limitation until no further increases in range of motion occur.

3. **Maintained pressure over the belly or tendon of a muscle can produce a calming effect and create relaxation of the musculotendinous unit. The effects of pressure are immediate, with little evidence of long-term effects.**

4. Rhythmic stabilization is a technique used to increase range of motion and coordinate isometric contractions. The technique requires isometric contractions of all muscles around a joint against progressive resistance. The patient should relax and move into the newly acquired range and repeat the technique.

System Specific: Musculoskeletal System
Content Outline: Interventions

## Exam Two: Question 100

A patient with a lengthy medical history of cardiac pathology is referred to a phase II cardiac rehabilitation program. During the first session the physical therapist prepares to measure the patient's blood pressure by inflating the cuff 20 mm Hg above the patient's estimated systolic value. Which of the following values describes the MOST appropriate rate to release the pressure when obtaining the blood pressure measurement?

1. **2-3 mm Hg per second**
2. 3-5 mm Hg per second
3. 5-7 mm Hg per second
4. 8-10 mm Hg per second

**Correct Answer: 1** (Pierson p. 60)
Deflating the cuff at a rate of 2-3 mm Hg per second is recommended to enable the physical therapist to identify normal Korotkoff's sounds and obtain a valid measure of the patient's blood pressure. Rates faster than 2-3 mm Hg will tend to increase the measurement error.

1. **After inflating the cuff to 20 mm Hg above the estimated systolic pressure, the therapist should carefully unscrew (open) the valve and deflate the bladder no more than 2-3 mm per second while listening for the Korotkoff sounds.**

2. 3-5 mm Hg per second is faster than the recommended rate of 2-3 mm Hg per second.

3. 5-7 mm Hg per second is more than twice as fast as the recommended rate of 2-3 mm Hg per second.

4. 8-10 mm Hg per second is more than three times as fast as the recommended rate of 2-3 mm Hg per second.

System Specific: Cardiovascular/Pulmonary and Lymphatic Systems
Content Outline: Physical Therapy Examination

## Exam Two: Question 101

A physically active 19-year-old male receives pre-operative instruction prior to anterior cruciate ligament reconstruction. The patient's past medical history includes a medial meniscectomy of the contralateral knee eight months ago. The MOST likely functional level of the patient following rehabilitation is:

1. able to participate in light recreational activities
2. able to participate in all recreational activities
3. able to return to recreational and competitive athletic activities with a derotation brace
4. **able to return to previous functional level**

**Correct Answer: 4** (Kisner p. 734)

Anterior cruciate ligament (ACL) reconstruction refers to the use of a graft to replace a damaged anterior cruciate ligament. The graft is placed through drilled holes in the femoral and tibial tunnels and then anchored with a fixation device.

1. The patient's anticipated functional level following anterior cruciate ligament reconstruction would allow the patient to participate in activities that are higher level than "light recreational activities."

2. "Recreational activities" would not typically include vigorous activities such as competitive sports. The patient should be able to return to his previous functional level which likely includes a combination of recreational activities and more physically challenging pursuits.

3. Derotation bracing can be an effective method to limit instability in patients with an anterior cruciate ligament deficient knee, however, research associated with the use of derotation bracing following anterior cruciate ligament reconstruction has shown little evidence to support enhanced knee function or reduced reinjury rates.

4. **A physically active, young patient should return to his previous functional level within 4-6 months following anterior cruciate ligament reconstruction.**

System Specific: Musculoskeletal System
Content Outline: Foundations for Evaluation, Differential Diagnosis, & Prognosis

## Exam Two: Question 102

A patient rehabilitating from an upper extremity injury uses a latissimus pull-down machine. The therapist specifically instructs the patient to pull the bar down behind his head. This action emphasizes strengthening of the:

1. **rhomboids and middle trapezius**
2. biceps brachii and pectoralis major
3. teres minor and middle trapezius
4. pectoralis major and rhomboids

**Correct Answer: 1** (Kendall p. 326)

Knowledge of functional anatomy allows physical therapists to analyze various resistive exercises and identify the primary muscles involved.

1. **The rhomboids and middle trapezius both function as strong adductors of the scapula. Adduction of the scapula (retraction) is required in order to complete the latissimus pull-down exercise with the bar positioned behind the patient's head. Physical therapists should use caution when using this exercise since without proper instruction, patients may have a tendency to significantly flex their neck.**

2. The biceps brachii acts to flex the elbow joint, supinate the forearm, and assists with shoulder flexion. The pectoralis major acts to adduct and medially rotate the humerus. The muscles primary actions are not consistent with the exercise.

3. The teres minor acts to laterally rotate the shoulder joint and stabilize the head of the humerus in the glenoid cavity. The middle trapezius acts to adduct the scapula. The teres minor would not be emphasized in the exercise.

4. The pectoralis major acts to adduct and medially rotate the humerus. The rhomboids act to adduct and elevate the scapula. The pectoralis major would not be emphasized in the exercise.

System Specific: Musculoskeletal System
Content Outline: Interventions

## Exam Two: Question 103

A physical therapist adjusts the on:off time on an electrical stimulation unit prior to beginning treatment. When using the unit for muscle re-education the MOST appropriate on:off ratio is:

1. 5:1
2. 15:1
3. **1:5**
4. 1:15

**Correct Answer: 3** (Prentice - Therapeutic Modalities p. 126)

The on:off ratio should be determined based on the established therapeutic objectives. The on:off ratio for muscle strengthening is most often expressed as 1:5 while a ratio of 1:1 may be more appropriate for a therapeutic objective such as relieving muscle spasm.

1. On time should be less than off time in order to prevent muscle fatigue. The ratio is expressed in the same order that the words appear in the ratio statement "on:off" and therefore a ratio of 5:1 would result in five times greater on time than off time.

2. A ratio of 15:1 would result in severe muscle fatigue due not only to the excessive period of on time, but also to the inadequate period of off time.

3. **The initial on:off ratio should be 1:5 in order to minimize muscle fatigue. As the patient gets stronger, the on:off ratio may be altered to 1:4 or 1:3.**

4. A ratio of 1:15 would provide excessive periods of rest following each contraction and would result in extremely long treatment sessions.

System Specific: Non-Systems
Content Outline: Equipment & Devices; Therapeutic Modalities

## Exam Two: Question 104

A physical therapist is scheduled to administer a whirlpool treatment to a patient that is HIV positive. The therapist is concerned about her ability to complete the treatment since she sustained a small paper cut on her fourth digit approximately three hours ago. The MOST appropriate therapist action is:

1. refuse to treat the patient and document the rationale in the medical record
2. **treat the patient using appropriate medical asepsis**
3. ask the patient to reschedule their appointment
4. select another appropriate treatment procedure

**Correct Answer: 2** (Pierson p. 28)

Standard precautions are designed for the care of all patients in hospitals regardless of the medical diagnosis. Health care professionals that follow established standard precautions do not place themselves or the patient at any significant risk for being contaminated or infected by pathogenic microorganisms.

1. A physical therapist cannot refuse to treat patients based on the presence of HIV or any other potentially infectious condition.

2. **A physical therapist should treat a patient that is HIV positive using established medical asepsis techniques to prevent the possible transmission of blood or body fluids.**

3. The physical therapist has an obligation to treat the patient despite their HIV status. Rescheduling the patient without adequate cause would be a violation of the patient's right to receive necessary health care services.

4. The question does not provide any evidence that the current treatment procedure is inappropriate for the patient. As a result, it would be unnecessary to select another treatment procedure.

System Specific: Other Systems
Content Outline: Interventions

## Exam Two: Question 105

A physical therapist examines a patient referred to physical therapy diagnosed with anterior compartment syndrome. The patient presents with an inability to dorsiflex the foot and a mild sensory disturbance between the first and second toes. The nerve MOST likely involved is the:

1. **deep peroneal nerve**
2. medial plantar nerve
3. tibial nerve
4. lateral plantar nerve

**Correct Answer: 1** (Magee p. 900)

Anterior compartment syndrome often affects the deep peroneal nerve as it passes under the extensor retinaculum. The result of nerve compression ranges from a mild sensory disturbance to an inability to dorsiflex the foot.

1. **The deep peroneal nerve innervates the tibialis anterior, extensor hallucis longus and brevis, lumbricals, interossei, extensor digitorum brevis, and peroneus tertius muscles.**

2. The medial plantar nerve is the larger of the two branches of the tibial nerve. The nerve supplies cutaneous branches to the medial three and a half digits, and motor branches to the abductor hallucis, flexor digitorum brevis, flexor hallucis brevis, and the most medial lumbrical muscles.

3. The tibial nerve innervates the tibialis posterior, abductor and adductor hallucis, flexor hallucis longus and brevis, flexor digitorum longus and brevis, quadratus plantae, soleus, gastrocnemius, plantaris, and popliteus muscles.

4. The lateral plantar nerve is the smaller of the two branches of the tibial nerve. The nerve supplies cutaneous branches to the lateral one and a half toes and motor branches to muscles of the sole of the foot that are not supplied by the medial plantar nerve.

System Specific: Neuromuscular & Nervous Systems
Content Outline: Physical Therapy Examination

## Exam Two: Question 106

A 35-year-old female is admitted to the hospital following a recent illness. Laboratory testing reveals a markedly high platelet count. This finding is typical with:

1. emphysema
2. metabolic acidosis
3. renal failure
4. **malignancy**

**Correct Answer: 4** (Goodman - Differential Diagnosis p. 487)

Thrombocytosis refers to an increased number of blood platelets. This condition is usually temporary and can occur as a compensatory measure after severe hemorrhage, surgery, iron deficiency, and as a manifestation of certain cancers.

1. Emphysema is defined as an abnormal permanent enlargement of air spaces distal to the terminal bronchioles. Blood values will include an increase in red blood cells to carry the oxygen and abnormal carbon dioxide and carbon monoxide. Pulmonary function tests will show an increase in total lung capacity, functional residual capacity, and residual volume. The vital capacity is decreased.

2. Metabolic acidosis is an acid-base disorder defined as an accumulation of acids or a deficit of bases within the blood. Causes may include renal failure, starvation, diabetic or alcoholic ketoacidosis. Blood values will show a decrease in serum pH due to a decrease in $HCO_3$ or an increase in H+ ions. An arterial pH < 7.35 in the absence of an elevated $PaCO_2$ is considered metabolic acidosis.

3. Renal failure is defined as an abrupt or rapid decline in renal filtration and function. There are three categories: prerenal, intrinsic, and post renal failure. Typical causes include hypovolemia, congestive heart failure, dehydration, sepsis, and autoimmune diseases. Blood values include hypocalcemia, hyperkalemia, elevated blood urea nitrogen, creatinine, magnesium, and uric acid.

4. Malignancy is defined as cells that have the ability to spread, invade, and destroy tissue. A tumor that is malignant may or may not respond to treatment or may return after removal. Blood values vary based on type, degree, and location of the malignancy, however, are often increased as a manifestation of an occult neoplasm such as lung cancer.

System Specific: Other Systems
Content Outline: Foundations for Evaluation, Differential Diagnosis, & Prognosis

## Exam Two: Question 107

A physical therapist interviews a patient referred to physical therapy with a diagnosis of chronic bronchitis. What finding obtained during the patient interview is MOST closely associated with the patient's medical diagnosis?

1. **patient is a smoker**
2. patient has a sedentary lifestyle
3. patient has numerous allergies
4. patient has severe scoliosis

**Correct Answer: 1** (Hillegass p. 216)
Smoking is a large risk factor for the development of chronic bronchitis. Over time, smokers will experience decreased alveolar ventilation and potentially hypoxia and acidosis. Persistent cough and sputum production create a cycle of impaired perfusion, oxygenation, and recurrent infection. Untreated, hypoxia can lead to cor pulmonale.

1. **Cigarette smoke irritates the bronchial lining and causes hypersecretion and hypertrophy of mucus producing cells of the larger bronchi. The excess secretion of mucus begins to obstruct the airways causing wheezing and coughing. The cilia begin to decrease in function and infection results from reduced clearance.**

2. A sedentary life style is a risk factor for cardiovascular disease. Regular, moderate physical activity helps prevent heart and blood vessel disease. Physical activity can assist in controlling cholesterol, diabetes, obesity, and blood pressure.

3. Allergies can enhance the effects of chronic bronchitis, but are not normally a causative factor in the development of the condition.

4. Scoliosis is classified as a restrictive lung disorder with more severe curves (>60 degrees) that produce reduced lung capacity and overall pulmonary insufficiency. Scoliosis, however, is not closely associated with the diagnosis of chronic bronchitis.

System Specific: Cardiovascular/Pulmonary and Lymphatic Systems
Content Outline: Foundations for Evaluation, Differential Diagnosis, & Prognosis

## Exam Two: Question 108

A physical therapist reviews the medical record of a 46-year-old female diagnosed with myasthenia gravis. A recent physician entry indicates that the patient is currently taking immunosuppressive medication. Which laboratory test should be the MOST frequently monitored based on the patient's medication?

1. hematocrit
2. hemoglobin
3. platelet count
4. **white blood cell count**

**Correct Answer: 4** (Ciccone p. 593)
Immunosuppressive medications are commonly used to prevent the rejection of organ transplant or to treat specific diseases caused by an autoimmune response. The medications lower a patient's resistance to infection.

1. Hematocrit measures the percentage of red blood cells in a volume of blood. Hematocrit may be decreased with anemia, nutritional deficiency, and leukemia. Hematocrit may be increased with dehydration, polycythemia, and burns.

2. Hemoglobin is the iron containing pigment in red blood cells that functions to carry oxygen in the blood. Low hemoglobin may indicate anemia or blood loss; elevated hemoglobin suggests polycythemia or dehydration.

3. Platelet count identifies the number of platelets present in whole blood. Platelets are small blood cells that are necessary for clotting. If the platelet level is high, it indicates increased risk of thrombosis and if the level is low, it indicates increased risk of bruising and bleeding.

4. **The majority of immunosuppressive medications act non-selectively and as a result the immune system is less able to resist infections and the spread of malignant cells. Leukopenia refers to a reduction in the number of leukocytes in the blood. The white blood cell count provides valuable information related to the degree of immunosuppression. It is essential for physical therapists to be aware of the patient's most recent white blood cell count prior to initiating treatment.**

System Specific: Other Systems
Content Outline: Foundations for Evaluation, Differential Diagnosis, & Prognosis

## Exam Two: Question 109

A physical therapist makes a conscious effort to demonstrate particular kinds of behavior that are significant and attainable for an eight-year-old patient. This type of behavior therapy is termed:

1. flooding
2. operant conditioning
3. role playing
4. **modeling**

**Correct Answer: 4** (Sadock p. 548)

Physical therapists often employ a number of strategies to influence patient behavior or to promote learning. Knowledge of a wide variety of techniques and their relative utility can assist therapists to achieve better outcomes with their patients.

1. Flooding is a technique to help patients heal their traumatic memories. The goal is to expose patients to their traumatic memories with the goal of reintegrating their repressed emotions with their current awareness. Flooding is commonly used to treat people to handle specific phobias.

2. Operant conditioning is a process where learning occurs when an individual engages in specific behaviors in order to receive certain consequences. Examples of specific operant conditioning techniques include positive reinforcement, negative reinforcement, extinction, and punishment.

3. Role playing requires participants to take the place of someone else by acting the part of that person in a particular situation. The rationale associated with the technique is that people can learn more from acting out a particular situation than from purely discussing it.

4. **Modeling refers to the process of learning by watching others. Learning often occurs through observation alone without any specific verbal direction from the therapist.**

System Specific: Neuromuscular and Nervous Systems
Content Outline: Interventions

## Exam Two: Question 110

A patient rehabilitating from knee surgery exhibits significant weakness in the involved extremity. During the most recent therapy session the patient was able to complete an independent straight leg raise as shown. What muscle is emphasized in the exercise?

1. vastus medialis
2. **rectus femoris**
3. vastus lateralis
4. sartorius

**Correct Answer: 2** (Kisner p. 745)

A straight leg raise is a commonly utilized lower extremity resistive exercise. The exercise requires dynamic hip flexion and an isometric contraction of the quadriceps. The resistance of gravity decreases gradually as the lower extremity is elevated.

1. A straight leg raise requires activation of muscles that cross both the hip and knee joints. The vastus medialis acts to extend the knee, but does not act on the hip. The muscle is innervated by the femoral nerve.

2. **The rectus femoris is the prime mover during a straight leg raise exercise. The muscle is a component of the quadriceps femoris muscle group and is innervated by the femoral nerve. The muscle is able to act on the hip as well as the knee due to the muscle originating on the anteroinferior iliac spine and the groove above the rim of the acetabulum.**

3. A straight leg raise requires activation of muscles that cross both the hip and knee joints. The vastus lateralis acts to extend the knee, but does not act on the hip. The muscle is innervated by the femoral nerve.

4. The sartorius is a two-joint muscle that crosses both the hip and knee. The muscle acts to flex, laterally rotate, and abduct the hip joint and is innervated by the femoral nerve. The muscle would likely be active during a straight leg raise, but would not be the prime mover.

System Specific: Musculoskeletal System
Content Outline: Interventions

## Exam Two: Question 111 ✳

A physical therapist reviews a laboratory report for a patient recently admitted to the hospital. The patient sustained burns over 25 percent of her body in a fire. Assuming the patient exhibits hypovolemia, which of the following laboratory values would be the MOST significantly affected?

1. **hematocrit**
2. erythrocyte sedimentation rate
3. oxygen saturation rate
4. prothrombin time

**Correct Answer: 1** (Paz p. 266)

Hypovolemia refers to a state of decreased blood volume, most often related to a decrease in blood plasma. The reduction of blood volume often occurs following a burn due to the shift in fluid to the interstitium, which reduces plasma and intravascular fluid volume. This results in a variety of hemodynamic and circulatory changes, however, hematocrit would likely be the laboratory value most affected.

1. **Hematocrit is the volume percentage of red blood cells in whole blood. The hematocrit rises immediately after a severe burn and gradually decreases with fluid replacement.**

2. Erythrocyte sedimentation rate is a non-specific test for inflammatory disorders often associated with conditions such as cancer, autoimmune diseases, and infection. The test is based on how quickly red blood cells sink to the bottom of a test solution containing anticoagulated blood.

3. Oxygen saturation indicates the saturation of hemoglobin with oxygen. Normal oxygen saturation is 95-98 percent. Oxygen saturation is not related to total blood volume.

4. Prothrombin time is most commonly used to monitor oral anticoagulant therapy or to screen for selected bleeding disorders.

System Specific: Other Systems
Content Outline: Foundations for Evaluation, Differential Diagnosis, & Prognosis

## Exam Two: Question 112

A physical therapist performs autolytic debridement in an attempt to remove nonviable tissue from a stage IV pressure ulcer. Autolytic debridement removes necrotic tissue by using:

1. a sharp instrument
2. an externally applied force
3. **the body's own mechanisms**
4. a commercially prepared enzyme

**Correct Answer: 3** (Sussman p. 445)

Autolytic debridement is typically performed using a moisture-retentive dressing. The dressing maintains a moist wound environment which promotes rehydration of viable tissue and allows the body's enzymes to digest necrotic tissue.

1. Sharp debridement requires the use of scalpel, scissors, and/or forceps to selectively remove nonviable tissue, foreign material or debris from a wound.

2. Wound irrigation removes nonviable tissue from the wound bed using pressurized fluid which serves as an externally applied force. Pulsatile lavage is an example of a specific wound irrigation technique.

3. **Autolytic debridement refers to using the body's own mechanisms to remove nonviable tissue. Common methods of autolytic debridement include transparent films, hydrocolloids, hydrogels, and alginates.**

4. Enzymatic debridement requires the application of a commercially prepared enzyme to the surface of nonviable tissue. The applied enzyme attempts to degrade the nonviable tissue through gradual digestion.

System Specific: Other Systems
Content Outline: Interventions

## Exam Two: Question 113

A physical therapist is responsible for supervising a physical therapist assistant at an off site location. Which of the following would not necessitate a supervisory visit by the physical therapist?

1. a change in the patient's medical status
2. a modification in the patient's plan of care
3. a request by the physical therapist assistant
4. **an alteration in the patient's level of motivation**

**Correct Answer: 4** (Guide to Physical Therapist Practice)
When a physical therapist delegates patient care responsibilities to physical therapist assistants or other supportive personnel, the physical therapist remains responsible for overseeing the physical therapy program.

1. A change in the patient's medical status requires reassessment and possibly a change in the established plan of care.

2. A physical therapist is solely responsible for modifying an established plan of care. A physical therapist assistant may be able to modify a parameter of an existing intervention within an established plan of care (i.e., changing the weight of a progressive resistive exercise).

3. The physical therapist is required to provide patient-related consultation at the request of another practitioner.

4. **Physical therapist assistants often deal with changes in patients' level of motivation. This observation in isolation would not warrant a supervisory visit by the physical therapist.**

System Specific: Non-Systems
Content Outline: Safety and Protection; Professional Responsibilities; Research

## Exam Two: Question 114

A physician instructs a 26-year-old male to utilize a knee derotation brace for all athletic activities. Which condition would MOST warrant the use of the derotation brace?

1. medial meniscus repair
2. anterior cruciate ligament reconstruction
3. **anterior cruciate ligament insufficiency**
4. posterior cruciate ligament reconstruction

**Correct Answer: 3** (Kisner p. 723)
Derotation braces are most effective in patients with ligamentous instability, usually involving the anterior and posterior cruciate ligaments. The literature is inconclusive on the efficacy of functional bracing following reconstruction.

1. A patient with a medial meniscus repair would not tend to experience functional instability unless there were other structures involved such as the anterior cruciate ligament. Meniscal repairs are most often performed when the lesion is in the vascular outer third of the medial or lateral meniscus.

2. Anterior cruciate ligament reconstruction is typically performed due to disabling instability or frequent episodes of the knee giving way. The purpose of the surgical procedure is to reduce functional instability. Full return to vigorous activities following ACL reconstruction often takes four to six months.

3. **A patient with anterior cruciate ligament insufficiency would be far more likely to experience functional instability than a patient who had anterior cruciate ligament reconstruction. As a result, the patient with the insufficiency would be a better candidate for the derotation brace.**

4. Posterior cruciate ligament reconstruction is considerably less common than anterior cruciate ligament reconstruction. The purpose of the surgical procedure is to reduce functional instability. Full return to vigorous activities following PCL reconstruction often takes nine months to one year.

System Specific: Musculoskeletal System
Content Outline: Foundations for Evaluation, Differential Diagnosis, & Prognosis

## Exam Two: Question 115

A physical therapist obtains a gross measurement of hamstrings length by passively extending the lower extremity of a patient in short sitting. The MOST common substitution to exaggerate hamstrings length is:

1. weight shift to the contralateral side
2. anterior rotation of the pelvis
3. **posterior rotation of the pelvis**
4. hiking of the contralateral hip

**Correct Answer: 3** (Magee p. 643)

The hamstrings muscles consist of the semitendinosus, semimembranosus, and biceps femoris. The semitendinosus and semimembranosus are considered the medial hamstrings since they insert on the medial surface of the tibia. The biceps femoris is considered the lateral hamstrings since the muscle inserts on the lateral surface of the tibia and the lateral surface of the head of the fibula.

1. Weight shifting to the contralateral side in short sitting without other compensatory movement would have minimal impact on measured hamstrings length.

2. Anterior rotation of the pelvis would tend to make the apparent hamstrings length shorter than the actual length due to the hamstrings origin on the tuberosity of the ischium.

3. **Posterior rotation of the pelvis would tend to make the apparent hamstrings length longer than the actual length due to the hamstrings origin on the tuberosity of the ischium. Patients often attempt to posteriorly rotate the pelvis in short sitting by leaning backwards.**

4. Hip hiking of the contralateral limb may cause the patient to weight shift toward the involved side. This adaptation would have minimal impact on measured hamstrings length.

System Specific: Musculoskeletal System
Content Outline: Physical Therapy Examination

## Exam Two: Question 116

A physical therapist conducts an upper quarter screening examination on a patient diagnosed with rotator cuff tendonitis. With the patient in sitting, the MOST appropriate action to facilitate palpation of the rotator cuff is:

1. passive abduction of the humerus
2. active medial and lateral rotation of the humerus
3. **passive extension of the humerus**
4. active extension and flexion of the elbow

**Correct Answer: 3** (Hoppenfeld p. 13)

The rotator cuff is composed of the supraspinatus, infraspinatus, teres minor, and subscapularis. The rotator cuff muscles are important in shoulder movement and in maintaining glenohumeral joint stability. Tenderness elicited during palpation may be due to localized inflammation, a tear or detachment of a tendon.

1. Passive abduction of the humerus would tend to keep the rotator cuff obscured beneath the acromion which would make palpation extremely difficult.

2. The therapist should make sure that the area being palpated is as relaxed as possible. As a result, active movement would be less desirable than passive movement. If the question had asked about palpating a specific contractile structure (e.g., tendon), active motion would likely be more desirable.

3. **The rotator cuff lies directly beneath the acromion and therefore must be rotated out from underneath the acromion before it can be palpated. Passive extension of the humerus makes it possible for a therapist to palpate a portion of the rotator cuff although the individual muscles cannot be easily distinguished from each other.**

4. The rotator cuff acts on the shoulder and not the elbow. As a result, elbow flexion and extension would not influence palpation of the rotator cuff.

System Specific: Musculoskeletal System
Content Outline: Physical Therapy Examination

## Exam Two: Question 117

A physical therapist prepares to formally assess the balance of a patient with a neurological disorder. The MOST appropriate method to assess the vestibular component of balance would be:

1. assess cutaneous sensation
2. **apply a perturbation to alter the body's center of gravity**
3. examine proprioception in a weight bearing posture
4. quantify visual acuity and depth perception

**Correct Answer: 2** (Goodman - Pathology p. 1566)

Balance requires complex integration of the vestibular, visual, and somatosensory systems. Each system is responsive to specific stimuli and therefore can be assessed individually or collectively.

1. Cutaneous sensation is commonly assessed as part of a neurological examination, however, would not be directly associated with the vestibular system. Cutaneous sensory receptors include free nerve endings, Ruffini endings, hair follicle endings, and Meissner's corpuscles.

2. **The vestibular system reports information to the brain regarding the position and movement of the head with respect to gravity and movement. Assessment of the vestibular system often includes perturbations that require the body to make automatic adjustments that restore normal alignment.**

3. The somatosensory system provides information about the relative orientation and movement of the body in relation to the support surface. Examining proprioception in a weight bearing posture would be a common method used for assessment of the somatosensory system.

4. The visual system allows individuals to perceive movement and detect the relative orientation of the body in space. Visual receptors allow for perceptual acuity regarding verticality, motion of objects and self, environmental orientation, postural sway, and movements of the head and neck. Visual acuity and depth perception contribute to the feedback gathered by the visual system.

System Specific: Neuromuscular & Nervous Systems
Content Outline: Physical Therapy Examination

## Exam Two: Question 118

A physical therapist inspects the skin of a child recently admitted to the hospital after sustaining a scald burn from hot water on his torso. The burn is moist and red with several areas of blister formation. The burn covers an area approximately four inches by three inches and blanches with direct pressure. The MOST likely burn classification is:

1. superficial
2. **superficial partial-thickness**
3. deep partial-thickness
4. full-thickness

**Correct Answer: 2** (Goodman - Pathology p. 436)

The extent and severity of a burn is dependent on a variety of factors including age, duration of burn, type of burn, and affected area. Burns are most appropriately classified according to the depth of tissue destruction.

1. A superficial burn involves only the outer epidermis. The involved area may be red with slight edema. Healing occurs without evidence of scarring.

2. **A superficial partial-thickness burn involves the epidermis and the upper portion of the dermis. The involved area may be extremely painful and exhibit blisters. Healing occurs with minimal to no scarring in approximately two weeks. A superficial partial-thickness burn is relatively common since many scalding water burns and intense sunburns fall into this category. The primary difference in appearance between superficial and superficial partial-thickness burns is the presence of blistering. This category of burn is the most painful since all nerve endings remain intact.**

3. A deep partial-thickness burn involves complete destruction of the epidermis and the majority of the dermis. The involved area may appear discolored with broken blisters and edema. Damage to nerve endings may result in only moderate levels of pain. Healing occurs with hypertrophic scars and keloids.

4. A full-thickness burn involves complete destruction of the epidermis and dermis along with partial damage of the subcutaneous fat layer. The involved area often presents with eschar formation and minimal pain. Patients with full-thickness burns require grafts and may be susceptible to infection.

System Specific: Other Systems
Content Outline: Foundations for Evaluation, Differential Diagnosis, & Prognosis

## Exam Two: Question 119

A physical therapist prepares to examine a patient's triceps using a reflex hammer. The MOST appropriate positioning of the patient's arm during the testing procedure is:

1. **shoulder extension and elbow flexion**
2. shoulder flexion and elbow extension
3. shoulder extension and elbow extension
4. shoulder flexion and elbow flexion

**Correct Answer: 1** (Bickley p. 698)

Deep tendon reflexes are performed to test the integrity of the spinal reflex. A physical therapist should assess a deep tendon reflex by placing the tendon on slight stretch. A reflex hammer is used to sharply tap over the tendon. Reflexes can be graded as normal, exaggerated (hyper) or depressed (hypo) or can be graded on a scale of 0-4.

1. **Shoulder extension and elbow flexion would be the most appropriate position to test the triceps reflex. The reflex is best elicited with the patient in sitting or standing with the arm supported by the physical therapist. The therapist strikes the triceps tendon with a reflex hammer where it crosses the olecranon fossa. Stimulation of the triceps reflex elicits involuntary contraction of the triceps. An acceptable alternate position to test the triceps reflex would be shoulder abduction and elbow flexion.**

2. Shoulder flexion and elbow extension would not place the triceps tendon on adequate stretch to elicit the triceps reflex.

3. Shoulder extension and elbow extension would result in an ineffective position to elicit the triceps reflex since the triceps is already in a maximally shortened position.

4. Shoulder flexion and elbow flexion place the triceps on total stretch secondary to the origin and insertion of the triceps muscle. A deep tendon reflex should be tested with the tendon on slight stretch.

System Specific: Neuromuscular & Nervous Systems
Content Outline: Physical Therapy Examination

## Exam Two: Question 120

If the forced expiratory volume in one second ($FEV_1$) test is negative for airway obstruction in 99% of individuals without lung disease, then the measurement of $FEV_1$ is:

1. sensitive
2. **specific**
3. reliable
4. valid

**Correct Answer: 2** (Portney p. 620)

The validity of a diagnostic test, such as the $FEV_1$ test, is evaluated by its accuracy in assessing the presence or absence of a target condition such as airway obstruction. A test is considered to be specific when the test is negative in persons who do not have the disease. A highly specific test will rarely be positive when a person does not have the disease.

1. Sensitivity is the probability of obtaining a positive test among individuals who have the disease. In this example, neither condition was met: the test result was negative for airway obstruction and the individuals tested did not have lung disease.

2. **Specificity is the probability of obtaining a negative test among individuals without the disease (who should test negative). Because 99 of 100 individuals without lung disease had a negative $FEV_1$ test for airway obstruction, the test is highly specific.**

3. Reliability refers to the extent to which a test or measurement is consistent or yields the same result on repeated trials. In this example, there is no indication that the $FEV_1$ was administered more than once, therefore no estimate of reliability is possible.

4. Validity refers to the degree to which a test or measurement accurately reflects or assesses the specific concept the clinician is attempting to measure. Validity is concerned with the success at measuring what was set out to be measured. In this example, the data does not provide useful information for assessing the extent to which $FEV_1$ is a valid way to identify airway obstruction.

System Specific: Cardiovascular/Pulmonary and Lymphatic Systems
Content Outline: Physical Therapy Examination

## Exam Two: Question 121

A physician examines a 36-year-old male with shoulder pain. As part of the examination the physician orders x-rays. Which medical condition could be confirmed using this type of diagnostic imaging?

1. bicipital tendonitis
2. **calcific tendonitis**
3. supraspinatus impingement
4. subacromial bursitis

**Correct Answer: 2** (Hertling p. 304)

The greater the density of the tissue, the more visible it will appear on x-ray. The majority of inflammatory conditions of the shoulder would be formally diagnosed using magnetic resonance imaging.

1. Bicipital tendonitis is an inflammatory process of the tendon of the long head of the biceps. The condition is characterized by subjective reports of a deep ache directly in front and on top of the shoulder made worse with overhead activities or lifting. Repeated full abduction and lateral rotation of the humeral head can lead to irritation that produces inflammation, edema, microscopic tears within the tendon, and degeneration of the tendon itself.

2. **Calcific tendonitis is often visible on x-ray due to the relative density of calcium. The greater the density of the tissue, the more visible it will appear on x-ray. The supraspinatus and infraspinatus tendons are common sites for calcific tendonitis.**

3. Supraspinatus impingement is caused by an inability of a weak supraspinatus muscle to adequately depress the head of the humerus in the glenoid fossa during elevation of the arm. The patient may experience a feeling of weakness and identify the presence of a painful arc of motion most commonly occurring between 60 and 120 degrees of active abduction.

4. Subacromial bursitis refers to inflammation of the subacromial bursa which lies between the deltoid muscle, supraspinatus tendon, and the fibrous capsule of the shoulder joint. The bursa facilitates movement of the deltoid muscle over the fibrous capsule of the shoulder joint and the supraspinatus tendon. The clinical presentation of the condition is very similar to the clinical presentation of supraspinatus impingement.

System Specific: Musculoskeletal System
Content Outline: Foundations for Evaluation, Differential Diagnosis, & Prognosis

## Exam Two: Question 122

A physical therapist designs a research study that will examine the effect of high voltage galvanic electrical stimulation on edema following arthroscopic knee surgery. The MOST appropriate method to collect data is:

1. anthropometric measurements
2. **circumferential measurements**
3. goniometric measurements
4. volumetric measurements

**Correct Answer: 2** (Hertling p. 501)

Physical therapists must utilize appropriate tests and measures to quantify the relative effectiveness of selected interventions. Therapists should carefully consider the reliability and validity of selected tests and measures when analyzing the collected data.

1. Common anthropometric measurements used for adults include height, weight, body mass index (BMI), waist-to-hip ratio, and percentage of body fat. These measures are then compared to reference standards to assess items such as weight status and the risk for various diseases.

2. **Circumferential measurements using a flexible tape measure allow physical therapists to obtain a gross estimate of edema in the knee. Pre-test and post-test measurements provide information on the effect of the electrical stimulation on the edema.**

3. Goniometric measurements are obtained with a goniometer and are designed to quantify available range of motion. If electrical stimulation is effective in reducing the edema, the patient may have improved range of motion, however, this would still not directly quantify the relative change in edema.

4. Volumetric measurements are often used to quantify the presence of edema in the wrist and hand by examining the amount of water displaced following immersion. Comparison with the uninvolved extremity provides a baseline measure. It would be impractical to attempt this type of measurement at the knee joint.

System Specific: Musculoskeletal System
Content Outline: Physical Therapy Examination

## Exam Two: Question 123

A physical therapist employed in an outpatient orthopedic clinic examines a patient diagnosed with cerebral palsy. The therapist has limited experience with cerebral palsy and is concerned about his ability to provide appropriate treatment. The MOST appropriate therapist action is:

1. inform the patient of your area of expertise
2. **co-treat the patient with another more experienced therapist**
3. treat the patient
4. refuse to treat the patient

**Correct Answer: 2** (Guide for Professional Conduct)
Physical therapists must make decisions that are consistent with their professional training. Since the therapist is concerned about his ability to provide appropriate treatment, he is in need of some form of external assistance.

1. Informing the patient of their area of expertise would likely make the patient question the therapist's competence.
2. **By co-treating the patient, the therapist receives external assistance and at the same time improves his skills with a particular patient population.**
3. The question states that the therapist is concerned about his ability to treat the patient. This type of admission makes it inappropriate to simply treat the patient without utilizing available resources.
4. Refusing to treat the patient would not be necessary since the therapist has available resources to offer assistance.

System Specific: Neuromuscular and Nervous Systems
Content Outline: Interventions

## Exam Two: Question 124

A patient status post Achilles tendon repair is examined in physical therapy. The physician referral includes a very specific post-operative protocol. If the therapist plans on deviating from the established protocol, the MOST appropriate action is to:

1. secure the patient's surgical report
2. complete a thorough examination
3. carefully document any modification
4. **contact the referring physician**

**Correct Answer: 4** (Guide for Professional Conduct)
A protocol traditionally outlines a detailed plan or sequence to be followed when treating a patient with a selected medical condition.

1. Familiarity with the surgical report would be helpful for the therapist, however, would not provide adequate justification for deviating from the established protocol.
2. A thorough examination must be completed regardless of whether the referral includes a very specific protocol or simply an order to "evaluate and treat."
3. When possible the therapist should contact the referring physician prior to making any modifications to a protocol, however, when a modification does occur it is necessary to document the change.
4. **Protocols are often established by physicians to ensure that health care providers progress patients in a predictable manner without jeopardizing the patients' post surgical status. As a result, it is necessary to contact the referring physician when deviating from the established protocol.**

System Specific: Musculoskeletal System
Content Outline: Interventions

## Exam Two: Question 125

A physical therapist examines the gait of a 62-year-old male with peripheral neuropathy. The therapist observes that the patient's right foot has a tendency to slap the ground during the loading response. The observation can BEST be explained by weakness of the:

1. iliopsoas
2. **tibialis anterior**
3. tibialis posterior
4. gastrocnemius

**Correct Answer: 2** (Kendall p. 410)

Peripheral neuropathy is a broad term that describes a lesion to a peripheral nerve. The condition can be caused by a multitude of factors including diabetes, compression, trauma or nutritional deficiencies. Patients with peripheral neuropathy may exhibit motor, sensory, and autonomic changes including extreme sensitivity to touch, loss of sensation, muscle weakness, and loss of vasomotor tone.

1. The iliopsoas is formed by the iliacus and psoas major muscles and acts to flex the hip and assists in lateral rotation and abduction. The iliacus is innervated by the femoral nerve and the psoas major is innervated by the lumbar plexus.

2. **The tibialis anterior acts to dorsiflex the ankle joint and assists in inversion of the foot. The muscle is innervated by the deep peroneal nerve. Injury to the deep peroneal nerve (L4, L5, S1) may produce dramatic weakness in dorsiflexion and resultant foot drop at initial foot contact. The patient will likely try to compensate for this by excessive hip and knee flexion in an attempt to avoid dragging the toe.**

3. The tibialis posterior acts to invert the foot and assists in plantar flexion of the ankle joint. The muscle is innervated by the tibial nerve.

4. The gastrocnemius acts to plantar flex the ankle joint and assists in flexion of the knee joint. The muscle is innervated by the tibial nerve.

System Specific: Neuromuscular & Nervous Systems
Content Outline: Physical Therapy Examination

## Exam Two: Question 126

A physical therapist compiles a table which identifies joint position at the hip, knee, ankle, and metatarsophalangeal joints for each subunit of the stance phase of gait. Which of the following is NOT accurate in describing normal joint position at the end of terminal stance?

1. 15 degrees of hip hyperextension
2. 0 degrees of knee extension
3. 0 degrees of ankle dorsiflexion
4. **10 degrees of metatarsophalangeal hyperextension**

**Correct Answer: 4** (Levangie p. 463)

Rancho Los Amigos stages of gait include initial contact, loading response, midstance, terminal stance, pre-swing, initial swing, midswing, and terminal swing. Each stage requires a specific amount of available range of motion at each of the lower extremity joints. Terminal stance begins when the stance limb's heel rises and ends when the other foot touches the ground.

1. The hip is in 10-20 degrees of hyperextension at the end of terminal stance.

2. The knee is in neutral (i.e., 0 degrees) at the end of terminal stance.

3. The ankle is in neutral (i.e., 0 degrees) at the end of terminal stance.

4. **The metatarsophalangeal joints are in 30 degrees of hyperextension at the end of terminal stance.**

System Specific: Musculoskeletal System
Content Outline: Physical Therapy Examination

## Exam Two: Question 127

A physical therapist positions a patient as shown in order to assess their claim of complete paresis of the right lower extremity. The therapist instructs the patient to perform a rapid straight leg raise with their left lower extremity. Which finding would BEST dispute the patient's claim?

1. The patient is unable to lift their left heel from the therapist's hand.
2. The patient experiences radiating pain into the right lower extremity.
3. **The patient exerts a downward force into the therapist's hand with their right heel.**
4. The patient reports severe pain while performing the straight leg raise.

**Correct Answer: 3** (Magee p. 577)
The Hoover test is often employed as a gross test for malingering. The physical therapist places one hand underneath each calcaneus with the patient lying in supine. The patient is then asked to perform a straight leg raise on the uninvolved extremity while the therapist simultaneously assesses motor output on the involved side.

1. The Hoover test relies on assessing the reaction of the contralateral limb rather than the quality of the straight leg raise.
2. The Hoover test is designed to provide insight on potential malingering rather than serving as a provocative test intended to create radiating pain or other signs or symptoms.
3. **A rapid straight leg raise of the left (uninvolved) lower extremity should result in the patient exerting a downward force into the therapist's hand with the right (involved) heel. This action would be considered a normal response due to the effort associated with performing the straight leg raise, therefore disputing the patient's claim of complete paresis of the right lower extremity.**
4. The Hoover test is not influenced by the presence or absence of pain.

System Specific: Neuromuscular & Nervous Systems
Content Outline: Physical Therapy Examination

## Exam Two: Question 128

A patient rehabilitating from a lower extremity injury has been non-weight bearing for three weeks. A recent physician entry in the medical record indicates the patient is cleared for weight bearing up to 25 pounds. The MOST appropriate device to use when instructing the patient on the new weight bearing status is:

1. an inclinometer
2. **a scale**
3. an anthropometer
4. a tape measure

**Correct Answer: 2** (Pierson p. 221)
There are a variety of surgical procedures and medical conditions that require patients to limit the amount of weight being borne through a lower extremity. Failure to comply with prescribed weight bearing restrictions can jeopardize or significantly delay a patient's recovery. It is therefore critical for therapists to educate patients on their prescribed weight bearing status.

1. Inclinometers, also termed gravity-dependent goniometers, use gravity's effect on pointers and fluid levels to measure joint position and motion.
2. **A scale can be a valuable tool for a patient to use to better understand what a selected amount of weight bearing feels like since it offers immediate feedback in the form of pounds.**
3. An anthropometer is a device used to gather data on the measurements and proportions of the human body. Common uses include measuring long bone length, skin folds or use in motion analysis studies.
4. Tape measures are designed to quantify distance. A common use in physical therapy would be to assess leg length or conduct girth measurements.

System Specific: Musculoskeletal System
Content Outline: Interventions

## Exam Two: Question 129

A physical therapist observes a patient complete hip abduction and adduction exercises in standing. Which axis of movement is utilized with these particular motions?

1. frontal
2. vertical
3. **anterior-posterior**
4. longitudinal

**Correct Answer: 3** (Levangie p. 7)

Motions are described as occurring around three cardinal planes of the body (frontal, sagittal, transverse). Movement in the cardinal planes occur around three corresponding axes (anterior-posterior, medial-lateral, vertical). The axis of any cardinal plane movement is always found perpendicular to its corresponding plane.

1. The frontal (coronal) plane divides the body into anterior and posterior sections. Motions in the frontal plane occur around an anterior-posterior axis. Although the described motions, hip abduction and adduction, occur in the frontal (coronal) plane, the question specifically asks about the axis of movement.

2. The term vertical or longitudinal axis of motion is used when the axis of motion passes through the length of a long bone. Motions in the transverse plane such as medial and lateral rotation occur around a vertical axis. The transverse plane divides the body into upper and lower sections.

3. **Motions in the frontal (coronal) plane such as abduction and adduction occur around an anterior-posterior axis. The frontal plane divides the body into anterior and posterior sections.**

4. The term longitudinal and vertical are synonyms and therefore respond to the same axis of movement.

System Specific: Musculoskeletal System
Content Outline: Physical Therapy Examination

## Exam Two: Question 130

A patient is treated using pulsed wave ultrasound at 1.2 W/cm$^2$ for seven minutes. The specific parameters of the pulsed wave are 2 msec on time and 8 msec off time for one pulse period. The duty cycle should be recorded as:

1. 10%
2. **20%**
3. 25%
4. 50%

**Correct Answer: 2** (Cameron p. 192)

Duty cycle is defined as the ratio of the on time to the total time. When ultrasound is used in a pulsed mode with a 20% or lower duty cycle, the heat produced during the on time of the cycle is dispersed during the off time and as a result, there is no measurable net increase in temperature. Ultrasound using a 20% or lower duty cycle would typically be used for nonthermal effects.

1. A 10% duty cycle would result if the parameters of the pulsed wave were 1 msec on time and 9 msec off time. Duty cycle = 1 msec / (1 msec + 9 msec) = .10 (100) = 10%.

2. **The question indicates that the parameters of the pulsed wave are 2 msec on time and 8 msec off time for one pulse period. As a result, duty cycle = 2 msec / (2 msec + 8 msec) = .20 (100) = 20%.**

3. This option may have been a common response for candidates who incorrectly answered the question since it is intuitive to take the on time and divide it by the off time. This calculation would be as follows: 2 msec / 8 msec = .25 (100) = 25%. Although the math is correct, the option remains incorrect since by definition duty cycle is defined as the ratio of the on time to the total time (not only the off time).

4. A 50% duty cycle would result any time the on time was the same as the off time. For example, if the parameters of the pulsed wave were 2 msec on time and 2 msec off time. Duty cycle = 2 msec / (2 msec + 2 msec) = .50 (100) = 50%.

System Specific: Non-Systems
Content Outline: Equipment & Devices; Therapeutic Modalities

# Exam Two: Question 131

A physical therapist examines the output from a single lead electrocardiogram of a patient with first degree atrioventricular heart block. The defining characteristic of this condition is:

1. inverted T wave
2. **prolonged PR interval**
3. bizarre QRS complex
4. ST segment depression

**Correct Answer: 2** (Brannon p. 212)

The PR interval is the time required to conduct the cardiac impulse from the sinoatrial node to the atrioventricular node. This is normally 0.12 to 0.20 seconds. Heart blocks, also known as conduction blocks, are characterized as 1st, 2nd or 3rd degree according to the severity of the disturbance in the conduction of the cardiac impulse through the electrical conduction system. A first-degree heart block is relatively benign. The defining feature is a prolonged PR interval (> 0.20 sec.).

1. A normal T wave is rounded, symmetric, and upright. An inverted T wave is commonly associated with myocardial ischemia.

2. **The normal duration of the PR interval is 0.12 to 0.20 second. A prolonged PR interval (> 0.20 sec) is the defining feature of first-degree atrioventricular block.**

3. A bizarre QRS complex refers to the characteristic shape and configuration of a premature ventricular contraction (PVC) arising from an ectopic focus in the ventricle that occurs before the expected time of normal ventricular depolarization.

4. ST segment depression is a classic sign of myocardial ischemia.

System Specific: Cardiovascular/Pulmonary and Lymphatic Systems
Content Outline: Foundations for Evaluation, Differential Diagnosis, & Prognosis

# Exam Two: Question 132

The first step a physical therapist should take to incorporate current best evidence into the practice of physical therapy is to:

1. **pose an answerable clinical question**
2. locate the most current best evidence from the literature
3. critically appraise the evidence for its validity, impact, and applicability
4. integrate the evidence into clinical decision making

**Correct Answer: 1** (Sackett p. 63)

The first step in evidence-based practice is to pose an answerable clinical question. This action is considered the starting point for searching the literature for information related to the question. A well built, answerable clinical question usually has four components: 1) patient/problem of interest; 2) intervention; 3) comparison intervention(s), if relevant; 4) clinical outcomes of interest. These components form the acronym P-I-C-O.

1. **The first step in evidence-based practice is to ask an answerable clinical question.**

2. The second step in evidence-based practice is to locate the best evidence to answer the question.

3. The third step in evidence-based practice is to critically appraise the evidence you find.

4. The fourth step in evidence-based practice is integrating the evidence, along with clinical experience and the patient's unique values and circumstances, to make clinical decisions.

System Specific: Non-Systems
Content Outline: Safety and Protection; Professional Responsibilities; Research

## Exam Two: Question 133

A patient diagnosed with ankylosing spondylitis exhibits a forward stooped posture. As part of the patient's care plan the physical therapist selects a number of active exercises that promote improved posture. Which proprioceptive neuromuscular facilitation pattern would be the MOST appropriate to achieve the therapist's objective?

1. D1 extension
2. D1 flexion
3. D2 extension
4. **D2 flexion**

**Correct Answer: 4** (Sullivan p. 300)

A proprioceptive neuromuscular facilitation approach utilizes methods that promote or hasten the response of the neuromuscular mechanism through stimulation of the proprioceptors. The two diagonal patterns are commonly referred to as D1 and D2 where "D" stands for diagonal and "1" and "2" refer to specific patterns of movement. To improve the patient's standing posture the therapist should use a pattern that requires the patient to move the arms upward and away from the body (D2 flexion).

1. The command for D1 extension would be to open your hand and push down and away from your body.

2. The command for D1 flexion would be to close your hand and pull up and across your body.

3. The command for D2 extension would be to close your hand and pull down and across your body.

4. **The command for D2 flexion would be to open your hand and pull up and away from your body. The pattern emphasizes shoulder flexion, abduction, and lateral rotation which would facilitate improved standing posture.**

System Specific: Neuromuscular & Nervous Systems
Content Outline: Interventions

## Exam Two: Question 134

A physical therapist completing a balance assessment positions a patient in standing prior to administering the Romberg test. When administering the Romberg test it would be MOST important for the therapist to determine:

1. the width of the base of support necessary in order to maintain standing
2. the amount of time the patient is able to maintain the test position
3. **the amount of sway present during the testing period**
4. the complexity of tasks the patient is able to perform with eyes open and eyes closed

**Correct Answer: 3** (Montgomery p. 191)

A positive Romberg test is indicative of a loss of proprioception often associated with a posterior column lesion in the spinal cord or a peripheral neuropathy.

1. The Romberg test is performed with the patient in standing with the feet together. The width of the base of support is not altered by the therapist during the test.

2. The Romberg test is most commonly administered during 30 second observational periods. The test does not attempt to quantify the amount of time a patient is able to maintain a static posture, rather the amount of sway present during the testing period.

3. **The amount of sway present during the testing period determines whether the Romberg test is positive or negative. A positive test is characterized by a patient being able to stand with no more than minimal sway with the eyes open, but presents with increased instability or falls with the eyes closed.**

4. The Romberg test is a static standing test where the variable being manipulated is whether the eyes are open or closed and not the complexity of the tasks.

System Specific: Neuromuscular & Nervous Systems
Content Outline: Physical Therapy Examination

## Exam Two: Question 135

A physical therapist reviews the medical record of a patient diagnosed with peripheral arterial disease prior to initiating treatment. Which objective finding would MOST severely limit the patient's ability to participate in an ambulation exercise program?

1. **signs of resting claudication**
2. decreased peripheral pulses
3. cool skin
4. blood pressure of 165/90 mm Hg

**Correct Answer: 1** (Kisner p. 830)

Peripheral arterial disease refers to a condition involving the arterial system that results in compromised circulation to the extremities. Resting claudication is typically considered a contraindication to active exercise in patients with peripheral arterial disease.

1. **Claudication pain is a symptom of ischemia of the lower extremity muscles caused by peripheral arterial disease. Resting claudication pain is typically considered a contraindication to exercise with peripheral arterial disease and may be an indication that the disease process is more advanced.**

2. Decreased peripheral pulses are a common sign associated with peripheral arterial disease, but would only severely limit ambulation if blood flow was markedly diminished or absent. Decreased peripheral pulses are a result of plaque buildup in the arteries which decreases blood flow and subsequently oxygen to the extremities.

3. Cool skin may be a sign of peripheral arterial disease, but would only severely limit ambulation if blood flow was markedly diminished or absent. Cool skin results from the diminished circulation, particularly in the extremities.

4. A blood pressure of 165/90 mm Hg is common during exercise and does not severely limit ambulation.

System Specific: Cardiovascular/Pulmonary and Lymphatic Systems
Content Outline: Interventions

## Exam Two: Question 136

A patient with limited elbow and forearm range of motion is referred to physical therapy. When mobilizing the humeroradial articulation, the treatment plane is considered to be:

1. in the concave radial head, parallel to the long axis of the radius
2. **in the concave radial head, perpendicular to the long axis of the radius**
3. in the convex radial head, parallel to the long axis of the radius
4. in the convex radial head, perpendicular to the long axis of the radius

**Correct Answer: 2** (Kisner p. 128)

The humeroradial joint is a uniaxial hinge joint between the capitulum of the humerus and the head of the radius. The humerus is convex and the radius is concave and therefore osteokinematic motion and arthrokinematic glide are in the same direction. The treatment plane is considered the plane perpendicular to a line running from the axis of rotation to the middle of the concave articular surface. The plane itself is located in the concave partner and is therefore determined by the position of the concave bone.

1. The radial head is the concave partner, however, the treatment plane is perpendicular and not parallel to the long axis of the radius.

2. **The radial head is the concave partner and the treatment plane is perpendicular to the long axis of the radius.**

3. The radial head is the concave partner and not the convex partner. The treatment plane is perpendicular and not parallel to the long axis of the radius.

4. The radial head is the concave partner and not the convex partner, however, the treatment plane is perpendicular to the long axis of the radius.

System Specific: Musculoskeletal System
Content Outline: Interventions

## Exam Two: Question 137

A physical therapist conducts an inservice on exercise guidelines for a group of senior citizens. As part of the inservice the therapist discusses the benefits of improving cardiovascular status through a low intensity activity such as a walking program. What frequency of exercise would be the MOST desirable to achieve the stated objective?

1. twice per day
2. one time per week
3. three times per week
4. **five times per week**

---

**Correct Answer: 4** (American College of Sports Medicine p. 452)

To minimize medical problems and promote long-term compliance with this population, exercise intensity should start low and progress gradually according to individual tolerance and preference. Exercise performed at a moderate intensity should be performed for 30 minutes on most days of the week. If exercise is at a vigorous level, it should be performed at least three times per week. Since the cited exercise is low intensity, five times per week is the most appropriate option.

1. The therapist can recommend that individuals who have difficulty sustaining exercise for 30 minutes continuously, or who prefer shorter bouts of exercise, should exercise for shorter periods (e.g., 10 minutes) several times each day. This is not the most desirable combination of exercise intensity and frequency, however, to improve cardiovascular status.

2. One time per week is an inadequate frequency to improve cardiovascular fitness when exercising at low intensity.

3. Three times per week is an appropriate frequency if the exercise is at a vigorous level. It would not be the most desirable frequency for low intensity exercise.

4. **Since walking is a low intensity activity, more frequent exercise sessions are needed to improve cardiovascular status. Five times per week is the most desirable option.**

System Specific: Cardiovascular/Pulmonary and Lymphatic Systems
Content Outline: Interventions

---

## Exam Two: Question 138

A physical therapist identifies the pisiform after palpating along the proximal row of carpals. Which carpal bone articulates with the pisiform?

1. trapezium
2. trapezoid
3. lunate
4. **triquetrum**

---

**Correct Answer: 4** (Hoppenfeld p. 70)

The proximal row of carpal bones from lateral to medial consists of the scaphoid, lunate, triquetrum, and pisiform. The distal row of carpal bones from lateral to medial consists of the trapezium, trapezoid, capitate, and hamate. The carpal bones articulate with each other at synovial joints and are connected via ligaments to form a compact mass.

1. The trapezium is located on the lateral side of the carpus between the scaphoid and the first metacarpal. It is distinguished by a deep groove on its palmar surface.

2. The trapezoid is the smallest carpal bone in the distal row and is noted for its wedge shaped form. The inferior surface of the bone articulates with the proximal end of the second metacarpal bone and the superior surface articulates with the scaphoid.

3. The lunate is located in the center of the proximal row between the scaphoid and the triquetrum. The lunate is distinguished by its crescent-like outline.

4. **The triquetrum is located on the medial side of the proximal row of carpals between the lunate and pisiform. The triquetrum is the third most often fractured carpal bone. The pisiform is located within the flexor carpi ulnaris tendon and lies immediately superior to the triquetrum.**

System Specific: Musculoskeletal System
Content Outline: Physical Therapy Examination

## Exam Two: Question 139

A physical therapist employed in an acute care hospital reviews the medical record of a patient diagnosed with congestive heart failure. The therapist would like to implement a formal exercise program, but is concerned about the patient's exercise tolerance. Which condition is MOST responsible for the patient's limited exercise tolerance?

1. diminished lung volumes
2. arterial oxygen desaturation
3. **insufficient stroke volume during ventricular systole**
4. excessive rise in blood pressure

**Correct Answer: 3** (Hillegass p. 94)

Congestive heart failure refers to the heart's inability to maintain a cardiac output that is adequate to meet the demands of the tissues due to an abnormality in the pumping ability of the heart muscle.

1. Diminished lung volumes are more commonly associated with obstructive or restrictive lung conditions and are not typically associated with congestive heart failure.

2. The level of arterial oxygenation is not significantly impacted with congestive heart failure, rather the primary issue is that a smaller volume of blood is pumped with each contraction of the ventricles.

3. **Congestive heart failure may be due to a diminished pumping ability of the ventricles due to muscle weakening (systolic dysfunction) or to stiffening of the heart muscle that impairs the ventricles' capacity to relax and fill (diastolic dysfunction). With systolic dysfunction, the weak heart pumps a smaller volume of blood for each contraction of the ventricles (stroke volume), reducing cardiac output. The resultant decrease in the delivery of oxygenated blood to the active tissues limits the patient's ability to exercise.**

4. Most patients with congestive heart failure take multiple medications including diuretics, vasodilators, ACE inhibitors, and beta blockers. The medications serve to reduce the hemodynamic response to exercise. An excessive increase in blood pressure is therefore unlikely.

System Specific: Cardiovascular/Pulmonary and Lymphatic Systems
Content Outline: Foundations for Evaluation, Differential Diagnosis, & Prognosis

## Exam Two: Question 140

A physical therapist measures a patient for a wheelchair. When measuring back height, which method is MOST accurate?

1. measure from the seat of the chair to the base of the axilla and subtract two inches
2. **measure from the seat of the chair to the base of the axilla and subtract four inches**
3. measure from the seat of the chair to the acromion process and subtract two inches
4. measure from the seat of the chair to the acromion process and subtract four inches

**Correct Answer: 2** (Pierson p. 136)

There are a variety of specific measurements that must be performed when fitting a patient for a wheelchair. Failure to obtain accurate measurements can result in a wheelchair that is not appropriately sized. Ramifications include increased difficulty with mobility and potential complications such as pressure sores or skin breakdown.

1. Measuring from the seat of the chair to the base of the axilla and subtracting two inches would result in the back height being at the mid-scapular level. This back height would be too high to allow for optimal mobility.

2. **Back height should be determined by measuring from the seat of the chair to the base of the axilla and subtracting four inches. This method will allow the back height to fall below the inferior angle of the scapula. The height of the seat cushion used, if applicable, must be added to the obtained measurement.**

3. Measuring from the seat of the chair to the acromion process and subtracting two inches would result in a back height that is excessive and would significantly restrict the patient's movement.

4. Measuring from the seat of the chair to the acromion process and subtracting four inches is more desirable than option 3, but would still not allow the back height to fall below the inferior angle of the scapula.

System Specific: Non-Systems
Content Outline: Equipment & Devices; Therapeutic Modalities

## Exam Two: Question 141

A patient diagnosed with infrapatellar tendonitis completes a series of functional activities. After completing the activities the physical therapist instructs the patient to use ice massage over the anterior surface of the knee. The MOST appropriate treatment time is:

1. 3-5 minutes
2. **5-10 minutes**
3. 10-15 minutes
4. 15-20 minutes

**Correct Answer: 2** (Cameron p. 145)

Ice massage is typically performed by freezing water in paper cups and applying the ice directly to the treatment area. Ice massage tends to create a more intense cooling since the ice is applied directly to a localized target area.

1. Sufficient cooling with ice massage would not occur with a 3-5 minute treatment time.
2. **Ice massage requires a treatment time of 5-10 minutes due to the intensity of the cooling.**
3. A treatment time of 10-15 minutes would be excessive with ice massage and could result in signs and symptoms of cold intolerance.
4. A treatment time of 15-20 minutes would be within the established range for an ice pack, but would not be acceptable for ice massage.

System Specific: Non-Systems
Content Outline: Equipment & Devices; Therapeutic Modalities

## Exam Two: Question 142

A physical therapist uses functional electrical stimulation as part of a treatment regimen designed to improve quadriceps strength. Which on:off time ratio would result in the MOST rapid onset of muscle fatigue?

1. 3:1
2. 1:4
3. **5:1**
4. 1:6

**Correct Answer: 3** (Prentice - Therapeutic Modalities p. 126)

The on:off time ratio is simply a method to show the relative duration of the on time versus the off time. The muscle contracts during the on time and relaxes during the off time. The greater the on time in relation to the off time, the more rapid the onset of muscle fatigue.

1. An on:off time ratio of 3:1 indicates that there is three seconds of on time for every one second of off time. This ratio would promote fatigue, however, it is not the best answer.
2. An on:off time ratio of 1:4 indicates that there is one second of on time for every four seconds of off time. This ratio has significantly greater rest periods and therefore fatigue would not tend to be a large factor.
3. **An on:off time ratio of 5:1 indicates that there is five seconds of on time for every one second of off time. This ratio would promote rapid fatigue given the extremely large on time in relation to the short off time.**
4. An on:off time ratio of 1:6 indicates that there is one second of on time for every six seconds of off time. This ratio has the greatest rest period and therefore fatigue would not tend to be a factor.

System Specific: Non-Systems
Content Outline: Equipment & Devices; Therapeutic Modalities

## Exam Two: Question 143

According to proponents of evidence-based medicine, the BEST source of information upon which to make clinical decisions about therapy for an individual patient is:

1. cohort study
2. randomized controlled trial
3. **systematic review**
4. case report

**Correct Answer: 3** (Sackett p. 98)
The hierarchy of evidence ranks the strength of the different types of clinical evidence, studies or clinical trials from those with the least amount of bias to those with the potential for the greatest amount of bias.

1. Cohort studies are observation studies in which subjects are classified according to the presence or absence of a particular risk factor or exposure and followed over time to determine disease outcomes. Cohort studies do not evaluate the effect of therapy.

2. In a randomized controlled trial, patients are randomized into an experimental and a control group. Both groups are followed up for the variables or outcomes of interest. Randomized-control trials provide strong evidence for or against a therapy, but are not considered to be the highest level of evidence.

3. **Systematic reviews are summaries of the medical literature that use explicit methods to perform a thorough literature search, a critical appraisal of individual studies, and statistical techniques to combine results. Systematic reviews are considered to provide the highest level of evidence for or against a therapy.**

4. A case report is an in-depth description of an interesting condition or response to treatment. A case report is the least rigorous form of research because of its inherent lack of control and limited generalizability.

System Specific: Non-Systems
Content Outline: Safety and Protection; Professional Responsibilities; Research

## Exam Two: Question 144

A physical therapist employed in an outpatient clinic observes a patient complete a series of exercises. During the treatment session the patient mentions to the therapist that he is experiencing angina. After resting for 20 minutes the patient's condition is unchanged, however, he insists it is something that he can work through. The MOST appropriate therapist action is:

1. allow the patient to resume exercise and continue to monitor the patient's condition
2. reduce the intensity of the exercise and continue to monitor the patient's condition
3. discontinue the treatment session and encourage the patient to make an appointment with his physician
4. **discontinue the treatment session and call an ambulance**

**Correct Answer: 4** (Hillegass p. 564)
Changes in anginal symptoms may reflect a change in coronary status. Any increase or change in anginal symptoms should be recorded and receive immediate medical attention.

1. Continued angina after 20 minutes of rest is cause for concern as it may indicate a serious change in the patients' coronary status. The patient should not be allowed to exercise, even if he says he can work through it.

2. Reducing the intensity of exercise does not negate the fact that the patient has continued angina after 20 minutes of rest.

3. Discontinuing the treatment session is necessary, however, encouraging the patient to make an appointment with his physician does not ensure that the patient will receive immediate medical attention.

4. **If anginal symptoms are not relieved by stopping exercise, or the use of three sublingual nitroglycerin tablets (one taken every five minutes), the patient should be transported to the nearest hospital emergency center.**

System Specific: Cardiovascular/Pulmonary and Lymphatic Systems
Content Outline: Interventions

## Exam Two: Question 145

A 55-year-old male status post myocardial infarction is referred to physical therapy. The patient has a history of cardiac disease and is moderately obese. The patient's age-predicted maximal heart rate should be recorded as:

1. 190
2. 185
3. **165**
4. 155

**Correct Answer: 3** (Brannon p. 254)
Heart rate is used as a guide to set exercise intensity because of the relatively linear relationship between heart rate and oxygen consumption. Although it is best to measure maximal heart rate during a progressive maximal exercise test, maximal heart rate is inversely related to age and may be estimated by the formula: 220 – age.

1. A patient with an age-predicted maximal heart of 190 would be 30 years old. $220 - 55 \neq 190$
2. A patient with an age-predicted maximal heart of 185 would be 35 years old. $220 - 55 \neq 185$
3. **A patient with an age-predicted maximal heart of 165 would be 55 years old. $220 - 55 = 165$**
4. A patient with an age-predicted maximal heart of 155 would be 65 years old. $220 - 55 \neq 155$

System Specific: Cardiovascular/Pulmonary and Lymphatic Systems
Content Outline: Interventions

## Exam Two: Question 146

A physical therapist transports a patient in a wheelchair to the parallel bars in preparation for ambulation activities. The patient is status post abdominal surgery and has not ambulated in over two weeks. The MOST appropriate action to facilitate ambulation is:

1. assist the patient to standing
2. monitor the patient's vital signs
3. **demonstrate ambulation in the parallel bars**
4. secure an additional staff member to offer assistance

**Correct Answer: 3** (Minor p. 306)
The physical therapist must provide clear and concise directions to the patient in order to minimize the risk associated with the activity. This may be particularly important in the described scenario since the patient has not ambulated in over two weeks and using the parallel bars is likely to be a novel activity.

1. Assisting the patient to standing will likely be necessary, however, this action without previously demonstrating the activity will place the patient at greater risk.
2. Monitoring a patient's vital signs (i.e., heart rate, blood pressure, respiration rate) may be necessary depending on the patient's response to the activity, however, it would not be considered the most appropriate action to facilitate ambulation.
3. **Demonstration allows the physical therapist to model the appropriate technique for the patient in a controlled learning environment.**
4. The stability provided by the parallel bars makes it unlikely the physical therapist would need to secure an additional staff member to offer assistance. Although this would be an acceptable option, it would not be as effective as demonstration.

System Specific: Other Systems
Content Outline: Interventions

## Exam Two: Question 147

A physical therapist prepares to transfer a patient from a wheelchair to a treatment table. The patient cannot stand independently, but is able to bear some weight through the lower extremities. The MOST appropriate transfer technique is:

1. sliding board transfer
2. hydraulic lift
3. **dependent squat pivot**
4. two-person lift

**Correct Answer: 3** (Minor p. 188)
Physical therapists should select transfers that allow patients to participate in the transfer to the greatest extent possible. Although the patient cannot stand independently, they can bear some weight through the lower extremities.

1. A sliding board transfer is used for a patient who has some sitting balance, some upper extremity strength, and can adequately follow directions.
2. A hydraulic lift is a device required for dependent transfers when a patient is obese, when there is only one therapist available to assist with the transfer or when the patient is totally dependent.
3. **A dependent squat pivot transfer is used when a patient can bear some weight through the lower extremities, however, cannot transfer independently.**
4. A two-person lift is used to transfer a patient between two surfaces of different heights or when transferring a patient to the floor.

System Specific: Non-Systems
Content Outline: Safety and Protection; Professional Responsibilities; Research

## Exam Two: Question 148

A risk management committee composed of various members of the rehabilitation team is charged with identifying methods to prevent employee exposure to blood and body fluids. The MOST appropriate INITIAL action is:

1. provide follow-up to employees if exposed to blood and body fluids
2. provide free hepatitis B immunizations to staff
3. **develop an infection control policy that conforms to Occupational Safety and Health Administration guidelines**
4. educate staff about the policies

**Correct Answer: 3** (Pierson p. 28)
The Occupational Safety and Health Administration (O.S.H.A.) requires that health care facilities provide employees with information and instruction in techniques to protect them from infectious diseases (e.g., blood borne diseases).

1. Health care facilities are required to provide follow up to employees exposed to blood and body fluids. This is an important action, however, the committee was charged with identifying methods to prevent employee exposure to blood and body fluids.
2. Health care facilities are required to offer the hepatitis B vaccine to employees who are at substantial risk of occupational exposure to hepatitis B. The vaccine does not have to be free, but usually is offered without charge or with a substantial discount.
3. **Health care facilities are required to have a formal infection control policy that is consistent with O.S.H.A. requirements. It is important for all health care facilities to establish a committee who develops an infection control policy and then closely monitors the policy to ensure that it remains consistent with current O.S.H.A. guidelines.**
4. Staff is required to be educated on established policies, however, the initial action needs to focus on developing a policy consistent with current O.S.H.A. guidelines.

System Specific: Non-Systems
Content Outline: Safety and Protection; Professional Responsibilities; Research

## Exam Two: Question 149

A physical therapist attempts to classify the amount of assistance a patient requires to complete a sit to stand transfer. After completing the transfer, the therapist estimates that he was required to exert approximately 20% of the physical work in order to ensure the transfer was completed safely. The MOST appropriate classification of the level of assistance would be:

1. independent
2. supervision
3. **minimal assistance**
4. moderate assistance

**Correct Answer: 3** (Pierson p. 170)
Classifying transfer status allows health care providers to communicate information regarding the level of assistance necessary during a transfer to other health care providers. Categories range from independent to maximum assistance.

1. Independent transfers require a patient to perform all aspects of the transfer, including the set-up, without assistance from others.
2. Supervision is used when it is necessary for a therapist to observe throughout the completion of the task.
3. **Minimal assistance is used for patients who can perform at least 75% of the activity.**
4. Moderate assistance is used for patients who can perform at least 50% of the activity.

System Specific: Non-Systems
Content Outline: Equipment and Devices; Therapeutic Modalities

**Test Taking Tip:** It is critical that candidates read each question carefully since even small lapses in concentration can lead to unnecessary test taking mistakes. In this particular question, it states clearly that the therapist estimates that he was required to exert approximately 20% of the physical work in order to ensure the transfer was completed safely. It would be very easy for a candidate to misinterpret this and believe that the patient was exerting 20% of the physical work instead of the physical therapist. Mistakes like this on the actual examination are particularly problematic since they result in candidates missing questions that they may have been academically prepared to answer correctly.

## Exam Two: Question 150

A patient explains to her therapist that she was instructed to bear up to five pounds of weight on her involved extremity. The patient's weight bearing status would be BEST described as:

1. non-weight bearing
2. toe touch weight bearing
3. **partial weight bearing**
4. weight bearing as tolerated

**Correct Answer: 3** (Pierson p. 221)
Physical therapists often classify a patient's weight bearing status using specific terminology ranging from non-weight bearing to full weight bearing. It is important for therapists to fully understand these terms since failure to follow the prescribed weight bearing status can jeopardize the safety of the patient and result in professional negligence.

1. Non-weight bearing occurs when a patient is unable to place any weight through the involved extremity and is not permitted to touch the ground or any surface.
2. Toe touch weight bearing occurs when a patient is unable to place any weight through the involved extremity, however, may place the toes on the ground to assist with balance.
3. **Partial weight bearing occurs when a patient is allowed to put a particular amount of weight through the involved extremity. The amount of weight bearing is expressed as allowable pounds of pressure or as a percentage of total weight. Partial weight bearing requires an assistive device.**
4. Weight bearing as tolerated occurs when a patient determines the proper amount of weight bearing based on comfort. The amount of weight bearing can range from minimal to full.

System Specific: Musculoskeletal System
Content Outline: Physical Therapy Examination

## Exam Two: Question 151

A physical therapist examines a patient who complains of occasional difficulty maintaining her balance when walking and frequent episodes of vertigo. The MOST likely cause of the patient's difficulty is a disorder of the:

1. visual system
2. somatosensory system
3. auditory system
4. **vestibular system**

**Correct Answer: 4** (Goodman - Pathology p. 1566)

Vestibular disorders are extremely common in clinical practice and it is estimated that up to five percent of the population in the United States experience some type of dizziness.

1. The visual system allows individuals to perceive movement and detect the relative orientation of the body in space.

2. The somatosensory system provides information about the relative orientation and movement of the body in relation to a supporting surface.

3. The auditory system is the sensory system associated with hearing. The auditory system is highly involved in vestibular functions and as a result, anything that disrupts auditory information can also affect vestibular functioning.

4. **The vestibular system reports information to the brain regarding the position and movement of the head with respect to gravity and inertia. Abnormalities of the vestibular system result in dizziness and impaired balance.**

System Specific: Neuromuscular & Nervous Systems
Content Outline: Foundations for Evaluation, Differential Diagnosis, and Prognosis

## Exam Two: Question 152

As a component of a cognitive assessment, a physical therapist asks a patient to count from one to twenty-five by increments of three. Which cognitive function does this task MOST accurately assess?

1. **attention**
2. constructional ability
3. abstract ability
4. orientation

**Correct Answer: 1** (O'Sullivan p. 230)

Attention is defined as the capacity of the brain to process information from the environment or from long-term memory. The complexity and familiarity of the task determines the degree of attention required to complete the task.

1. **Attention can be assessed by asking a patient to count from one to twenty-five by increments of three. The task should be relatively easy for most individuals, however, it requires the person to exert a sustained, consistent effort. Attention deficits are common with many neurological disorders including brain injury, stroke, and dementia.**

2. Constructional ability can be assessed by asking a person to copy figures consisting of varying sizes and shapes or to draw a known item such as a clock.

3. Abstract ability can be assessed by asking a person to interpret a common proverb or to describe similarities or differences between two objects.

4. Orientation can be assessed by asking a person to identify time (e.g., day, month, season), person (e.g., name), and place (e.g., city, state).

System Specific: Neuromuscular & Nervous Systems
Content Outline: Physical Therapy Examination

## Exam Two: Question 153

An 86-year-old female is partial weight bearing on the left lower extremity after a total hip arthroplasty. Her upper extremity strength is 3+/5 and she resides alone. Which assistive device would be the MOST appropriate for the patient?

1. Lofstrand crutches
2. axillary crutches
3. large base quad cane
4. **walker**

**Correct Answer: 4** (Pierson p. 217)

A physical therapist must select an assistive device based on the patient's weight bearing status and their abilities and limitations. The patient's post-operative status, age, and limited upper extremity strength make it important that the selected device offer adequate stability without relying too heavily on upper extremity strength.

1. Lofstrand crutches or forearm crutches allow altered levels of weight bearing. The patient, however, would not have the upper extremity strength and stability necessary to use the device.

2. Axillary crutches can be used with all levels of weight bearing, however, offer limited stability and require significantly more coordination than a walker.

3. A large base quad cane is a type of straight cane that has a broad base positioned on four short posts. The device provides a larger base of stability than a straight cane, however, does not allow for partial weight bearing.

4. **A walker provides the patient with the necessary stability without relying on significant upper extremity strength. The walker allows for varying degrees of weight bearing on the involved lower extremity.**

System Specific: Musculoskeletal System
Content Outline: Interventions

## Exam Two: Question 154

A patient with a suspected scaphoid fracture is referred to physical therapy. Which clinical sign is MOST indicative of a scaphoid fracture?

1. localized edema along the dorsum of the hand
2. crepitus with active range of motion
3. **localized bony tenderness in the anatomic snuff box**
4. pain with resisted wrist extension

**Correct Answer: 3** (Hertling p. 425)

The scaphoid links the proximal and distal carpal rows and helps provide stability to the wrist. A scaphoid fracture can occur as a result of a fall on an outstretched hand. This injury can be serious due to the potential for avascular necrosis. The fracture is usually treated with prolonged immobilization of the wrist and thumb.

1. Localized edema would be commonly associated with a scaphoid fracture, however, since edema is associated with a multitude of injuries to the wrist and hand it does not necessarily provide direct evidence of a scaphoid fracture. Small amounts of edema in this area may minimize the concavity of the anatomic snuffbox.

2. Crepitus refers to a grinding, crackling or popping noise often associated with cartilage loss or degeneration. Crepitus with active range of motion cannot easily be localized to a specific bony structure in the wrist and hand.

3. **The anatomic snuff box is located between the tendons of the extensor pollicis longus and extensor pollicis brevis. The scaphoid bone can be palpated inside the snuff box. Tenderness of the scaphoid bone upon palpation is often associated with a fracture.**

4. The primary muscles that extend the wrist do not insert on the scaphoid and as a result, pain with resisted wrist extension is not typically associated with a scaphoid fracture.

System Specific: Musculoskeletal System
Content Outline: Foundations for Evaluation, Differential Diagnosis, & Prognosis

## Exam Two: Question 155

A patient on prolonged bed rest attempts to get out of bed. Upon attaining a standing position the patient complains of lightheadedness and blurred vision. The MOST appropriate explanation is:

1. **decrease in blood pressure**
2. decrease in respiratory rate
3. increase in pulse rate
4. adverse reaction to medication

**Correct Answer: 1** (Pierson p. 339)

Lightheadedness and blurred vision are signs of decreased cerebral blood flow due to a drop in blood pressure. This often occurs when patients who have been on prolonged bed rest assume an upright position.

1. **Orthostatic hypotension refers to a decrease in blood pressure that often occurs in patients on prolonged bed rest when attempting to achieve an upright position.**

2. A decrease in respiratory rate is not associated with changes in position or symptoms of lightheadedness and blurred vision.

3. Although pulse rate may increase slightly when a patient on bed rest attempts to get out of bed, the relative magnitude of the change would not typically cause symptoms of lightheadedness and blurred vision.

4. There are a variety of medications that can cause lightheadedness or blurred vision, however, the described patient scenario (i.e., patient on extended bed rest, attaining a standing position) provides a more compelling case for the presented symptoms being caused by the decrease in blood pressure.

System Specific: Cardiovascular/Pulmonary and Lymphatic Systems
Content Outline: Interventions

## Exam Two: Question 156

A patient's job requires him to move boxes weighing 35 pounds from a transport cart to an elevated conveyor belt. The patient can complete the activity, however, is unable to prevent hyperextension of the spine. The MOST appropriate physical therapist action is:

1. implement a pelvic stabilization program
2. design an abdominal strengthening program
3. review proper body mechanics
4. **use an elevated platform when placing boxes on the belt**

**Correct Answer: 4** (Kisner p. 476)

Physical therapists often perform work site evaluations and make recommendations to modify existing work activities.

1. A pelvic stabilization program may be helpful to improve core stability, however, the question provides ample evidence that the problem is more likely related to the height of the elevated conveyor belt.

2. An abdominal strengthening program would also improve core stability, but would not accommodate for the height of the elevated conveyor belt.

3. Reviewing proper body mechanics may be desirable, however, the question states that the patient is unable to prevent hyperextension of the spine. Failure to prevent hyperextension of the spine is more likely to occur because of the height of the conveyor belt rather than lack of knowledge of proper body mechanics.

4. **In order to eliminate hyperextension of the spine it may be necessary to modify the workstation. The most reasonable modification would be to utilize an elevated platform in order to minimize the height of the conveyor belt. In many instances, it is possible to modify a work site without utilizing large amounts of resources (e.g., time, money).**

System Specific: Musculoskeletal System
Content Outline: Interventions

**SCORE**BUILDERS

## Exam Two: Question 157

A 21-year-old male patient informs a physical therapist that additional therapy visits will not be covered by his medical insurance provider. The patient is 12 weeks status post anterior cruciate ligament reconstruction and has had an unremarkable post-operative progression. The MOST appropriate therapist action is:

1. offer to treat the patient pro bono
2. devise an affordable payment plan
3. request additional visits from the third party payer
4. **discharge the patient with a home exercise program**

---

**Correct Answer: 4** (Kisner p. 734)

Physical therapists should discharge patients from physical therapy when the anticipated goals or expected outcomes have been achieved or the patient is no longer benefitting from physical therapy services.

1. Physical therapists are not permitted to offer pro bono services to selected patients based on factors such as reimbursement or the ability to pay. Therapists should strive to treat all patients equitably.

2. A payment plan permits a patient to pay for incurred physical therapy services in a gradual manner. This may be a more desirable option when a patient requires ongoing physical therapy services, but does not have adequate financial resources.

3. Requesting additional physical therapy visits from the third party payer is a possible option, however, based on the patient's diagnosis and post-operative progression additional visits may not be warranted.

4. **A patient 12 weeks status post anterior cruciate ligament reconstruction that has experienced an unremarkable recovery should be able to function independently using a well designed home exercise program. The program should incorporate activities such as jogging, strengthening, and agility drills.**

System Specific: Musculoskeletal System
Content Outline: Interventions

---

## Exam Two: Question 158

A physical therapist monitors the blood pressure response to exercise of a 52-year-old male on a stationary bicycle. The therapist notes a relatively linear increase in systolic blood pressure with increasing exercise intensity. The change in the patient's systolic blood pressure with exercise is BEST explained by:

1. **increased cardiac output**
2. decreased peripheral resistance
3. increased oxygen saturation
4. decreased myocardial oxygen consumption

---

**Correct Answer: 1** (Brannon p. 73)

Cardiac output is the volume of blood pumped into the systemic circulation per minute and is equal to the product of heart rate and stroke volume.

1. **The trend toward lower blood pressure during exercise brought about by a decrease in peripheral resistance is negated by an increase in cardiac output. The increased heart rate and force of contraction of the myocardium (stroke volume) has the net effect of increasing systolic blood pressure in a normal population.**

2. A decrease in peripheral resistance to blood flow tends to cause a decrease in blood pressure due to dilatation of blood vessels in the exercising muscles.

3. Oxygen saturation is not affected by exercise in individuals with healthy lungs. Oxygen saturation may decrease during exercise in patients with chronic lung disease.

4. An increase in heart rate while cycling will increase myocardial oxygen consumption as the heart muscle utilizes more oxygen. Cardiac output increases to supply oxygenated blood to the exercising muscles.

System Specific: Cardiovascular/Pulmonary and Lymphatic Systems
Content Outline: Foundations for Evaluation, Differential Diagnosis, and Prognosis

---

## Exam Two: Question 159

A 64-year-old female patient is admitted to the hospital with a stage III decubitus ulcer over her right ischial tuberosity. The patient's past medical history includes severe chronic obstructive pulmonary disease. The MOST appropriate position for the patient is:

1. supine with pillows under the knees
2. prone with pillows under the knees
3. **left sidelying with pillows between the knees**
4. right sidelying with pillows between the knees

**Correct Answer: 3** (Frownfelter p. 515)

Left sidelying would be the position of choice in order to relieve pressure on the ulcer and maximize the patient's respiration. Recognizing contraindications for chronic obstructive pulmonary disease as well as positioning for pressure relief will allow for safe and effective positioning to enhance recovery.

1. Although the supine position with pillows under the knees is a comfortable position that reduces lumbar lordosis and strain, there would be pressure directly over the right ischial tuberosity and this would hinder progress or worsen the decubitus ulcer.

2. A prone position would allow for pressure relief over the right ischial tuberosity, however, the patient has severe chronic obstructive pulmonary disease and should not lie in prone as breathing would be very difficult. Pillows are also not typically placed under the knees when a patient is in prone.

3. **Left sidelying does not compromise respiration and avoids placing stress on the right ischial tuberosity.**

4. A right sidelying position would assist the patient with breathing and would not compromise overall respiration, however, there would be significant pressure over the right ischial tuberosity.

System Specific: Other Systems
Content Outline: Interventions

## Exam Two: Question 160

A physical therapist performs a manual muscle test on a patient's shoulder medial rotators. Which muscle would NOT be involved in this specific test?

1. pectoralis major
2. teres major
3. latissimus dorsi
4. **teres minor**

**Correct Answer: 4** (Kendall p. 321)

The primary muscles being assessed while testing the shoulder medial rotators include the pectoralis major, latissimus dorsi, subscapularis, and teres major. The test is performed with the patient in supine and resistance is applied to the forearm in the direction of laterally rotating the humerus. The test can alternately be performed with the patient in prone.

1. The pectoralis major – upper fibers act to flex and medially rotate the shoulder joint, and horizontally adduct the humerus. The upper fibers are innervated by the lateral pectoral nerve. The pectoralis major – lower fibers act to depress the shoulder girdle and obliquely adduct the humerus. The lower fibers are innervated by the lateral and medial pectoral nerves.

2. The teres major acts to medially rotate, adduct, and extend the shoulder joint. The muscle is innervated by the lower subscapular nerve (C5, C6, C7).

3. The latissimus dorsi with the origin fixed acts to medially rotate, adduct, and extend the shoulder joint. The muscle is innervated by the thoracodorsal nerve (C6, C7, C8).

4. **The teres minor acts to laterally rotate the shoulder joint and stabilize the head of the humerus in the glenoid cavity. The muscle is innervated by the axillary nerve (C5, C6).**

System Specific: Musculoskeletal System
Content Outline: Physical Therapy Examination

## Exam Two: Question 161

A patient in an acute care hospital has a catheter inserted into the internal jugular vein. The catheter travels through the superior vena cava and into the right atrium. The device permits removal of blood samples, administration of medication, and monitoring of central venous pressure. The device is BEST termed:

1. arterial line
2. central venous pressure catheter
3. **Hickman catheter**
4. Swan-Ganz catheter

**Correct Answer: 3** (Pierson p. 278)

Patients in a medically compromised state often use a variety of lines, tubes, and special equipment. Physical therapists should be familiar with the handling and management of these devices and be aware of any precautions or contraindications.

1. An arterial line is a monitoring device consisting of a catheter that is inserted into an artery and attached to an electronic monitoring system. An arterial line is used to measure blood pressure or to obtain blood samples. The device is considered to be more accurate than traditional measures of blood pressure and does not require repeated needle punctures.

2. A central venous pressure catheter is a plastic intravenous tube used to measure pressure in the right atrium or the superior vena cava. Specifically, the device measures pressure associated with the filling of the right ventricle (i.e., diastolic pressure).

3. **A Hickman catheter (indwelling right atrial catheter) inserts into the right atrium of the heart. The catheter permits removal of blood samples, administration of medication, and monitoring of central venous pressure. Potential complications associated with the use of a Hickman catheter include sepsis and blood clots.**

4. A Swan-Ganz catheter is a soft, flexible catheter that is inserted through a vein and eventually into the pulmonary artery. The device is used to provide continuous measurements of pulmonary artery pressure. Patients must attempt to avoid activities that increase pressure on the catheter's insertion site.

System Specific: Cardiovascular/Pulmonary and Lymphatic Systems
Content Outline: Foundations for Evaluation, Differential Diagnosis, & Prognosis

## Exam Two: Question 162

A patient informs her physical therapist that she noticed a small lump on her right breast while dressing. The patient was referred to physical therapy with lateral epicondylitis and has no significant past medical history. The MOST appropriate therapist action is:

1. inspect the lump
2. **instruct the patient to make an immediate appointment with her physician**
3. inform the patient she may have cancer
4. document the patient's comment in the medical record

**Correct Answer: 2** (Goodman - Pathology p. 1022)

Ninety percent of breast cancer is discovered through self-identification. Research has demonstrated that in the United States one in nine women may be affected by breast cancer over the course of their life. As a result, it is imperative that the physical therapist impress upon the patient the importance of consulting with her physician.

1. Inspecting the lump would be inappropriate, especially when considering the patient's medical diagnosis. Physical therapists must refer patients to appropriate medical personnel when warranted based on the results of subjective and objective data.

2. **The patient's statement makes it imperative that the patient contact the physician. The physical therapist should be careful not to alarm the patient, however, must stress the importance of an appointment with the physician.**

3. It would be inappropriate for the physical therapist to suggest that the patient may have cancer. Physical therapists cannot medically diagnose and should avoid suggestive comments related to a given diagnosis.

4. It is acceptable to document the patient's comments in the medical record, however, the priority needs to be related to follow-up with the physician.

System Specific: Other Systems
Content Outline: Physical Therapy Examination

## Exam Two: Question 163

A physical therapist attempts to confirm the fit of a wheelchair for a patient recently admitted to a skilled nursing facility. After completing the assessment, the therapist determines the wheelchair has excessive seat width. Which adverse effect results from excessive seat width?

1. difficulty changing position within the wheelchair
2. insufficient trunk support
3. **difficulty propelling the wheelchair**
4. increased pressure to the distal posterior thighs

> **Correct Answer: 3** (O'Sullivan p. 1302)
>
> Seat width is determined by measuring the widest aspect of the user's buttocks, hips or thighs and adding approximately two inches. This provides space for bulky clothing, orthoses or clearance of the trochanters from the armrest side panel. The standard seat width for an adult wheelchair is 18 inches.
>
> 1. Difficulty changing position within the wheelchair may be due to a wheelchair that is too small and constricts movement. A seat with excess width would not prohibit the patient from moving within the wheelchair.
> 2. Insufficient trunk support may be due to a wheelchair that has less back support than is recommended. Back support is measured from the seat of the chair to the floor of the axilla with the patient's shoulder flexed to 90 degrees and then subtract approximately four inches. This will allow the back height to be below the inferior angles of the scapulae. The standard back height is 16 - 16.5 inches.
> 3. **Difficulty propelling a wheelchair may be due to excessive seat width. This will require the patient to stabilize at the shoulders and excessively abduct the upper extremities to reach the wheels. This produces a less functional push and increases the difficulty maneuvering through tight spaces.**
> 4. Increased pressure to the distal posterior thighs typically results from excessive seat depth. Seat depth is measured from the patient's posterior buttocks, along the lateral thigh to the popliteal fold; then subtract approximately two inches to avoid pressure from the front edge of the seat against the popliteal space. The standard seat depth for an adult wheelchair is 16 inches.
>
> System Specific: Non-Systems
> Content Outline: Equipment & Devices; Therapeutic Modalities

## Exam Two: Question 164

A patient uses a self-administered assessment tool as a method to record daily progress. What type of reliability would be the MOST essential using this tool?

1. reliability of parallel forms
2. internal consistency
3. **intratester**
4. intertester

> **Correct Answer: 3** (Portney p. 87)
>
> Since the assessment tool is used to record daily progress, it will be administered repeatedly. If changes in the scores are to be attributed to real progress made in physical therapy, and not to inconsistency or unreliable measurement, the tool should be evaluated for reliability.
>
> 1. Reliability of parallel forms refers to the consistency between results of two tests constructed in the same way from the same content domain. Parallel forms reliability is not an issue in this example because there is only one form of the assessment tool.
> 2. Internal consistency reliability refers to the consistency of results across items within a test. The reliability of the instrument is evaluated by estimating how well the different items within the test, which are supposed to reflect the same construct, do yield similar results. This is not of concern in the example.
> 3. **Intratester reliability refers to the extent to which scores on the tool obtained by the same tester are consistent. The tool should have intratester reliability so that any changes recorded can be attributed to progress in therapy and not to unreliable measurement.**
> 4. Intertester reliability refers to the extent of agreement of the scores recorded by two or more individuals. Interrater reliability addresses the consistency of the implementation of a rating system.
>
> System Specific: Non-Systems
> Content Outline: Safety and Protection; Professional Responsibilities; Research

## Exam Two: Question 165

A physical therapist administers the Mini-Mental State Examination to a patient recently admitted to an acute care medical facility. The MINIMUM patient score necessary in order to avoid being classified as possessing a cognitive impairment would be:

1. 18
2. **24**
3. 30
4. 34

**Correct Answer: 2** (Physical Therapist's Clinical Companion p. 113)

The Mini-Mental State Examination can be used to screen for cognitive dysfunction or dementia. The 11 question measure assesses five areas of cognitive function: orientation, registration, attention/calculation, recall, and language. The measure takes approximately 5-10 minutes to complete. Possible scores obtained on the Mini-Mental State Examination range from 0-30.

1. A score less than 20 may be associated with dementia, delirium, schizophrenia or an affective disorder.

2. **A score of 24 is the minimum score to avoid being classified as having a cognitive impairment.**

3. A score of 30 is a perfect score and would indicate that the patient is cognitively within normal limits.

4. A score of 34 exceeds the maximum score that can be attained on the Mini-Mental State Examination.

System Specific: Neuromuscular & Nervous Systems
Content Outline: Physical Therapy Examination

## Exam Two: Question 166

A physical therapist receives a referral to instruct a patient in stair training using axillary crutches. The patient is rehabilitating from a tibial fracture and is currently partial weight bearing on the involved extremity. The MOST important action prior to initiating the training session is:

1. apply a gait belt
2. maintain proper body mechanics
3. assess vital signs
4. **examine the patient's limitations and capabilities**

**Correct Answer: 4** (Pierson p. 214)

It is essential to determine the patient's limitations and capabilities prior to initiating an activity such as stair training. Failure of the physical therapist to accurately assess the patient's current status may unnecessarily jeopardize patient safety.

1. Applying a gait belt is a useful strategy to promote safety, however, therapists can effectively guard patients without the use of a gait belt. This fact makes it more important for the therapist to assess the patient's limitations and capabilities.

2. Maintaining proper body mechanics while guarding a patient is extremely important, however, the question asks specifically about the most important action prior to initiating the training session.

3. Vital signs should be assessed during the examination, however, given the patient's diagnosis and the proposed activity, it would not be as critical as some of the other presented options.

4. **Critical areas to assess prior to initiating the training session include uninvolved lower extremity strength, upper extremity strength, and ability to follow instructions.**

System Specific: Musculoskeletal System
Content Outline: Physical Therapy Examination

## Exam Two: Question 167

A physical therapist employed in an inpatient rehabilitation center works with a patient rehabilitating from a total knee arthroplasty. Which treatment activity would be the MOST appropriate to delegate to a physical therapy aide?

1. monitoring vital signs
2. measuring knee range of motion with a goniometer
3. **observing a patient complete a mat exercise program**
4. recording modality parameters in the medical record

**Correct Answer: 3** (Guide to Physical Therapist Practice)
The physical therapy aide is a non-licensed worker who is specifically trained under the direction and supervision of a physical therapist. Activities performed by the physical therapy aide are limited to those tasks that do not require clinical decision making by the physical therapist.

1. Monitoring vital signs is a skilled activity and therefore would be inappropriate for a physical therapy aide. Failure to accurately monitor vital signs can jeopardize patient safety.

2. Performing goniometric measurements is a skilled activity taught to physical therapists and physical therapist assistants as part of their academic training. A physical therapy aide would therefore not be permitted to perform this type of activity.

3. **Observing a patient complete a mat exercise program could be considered an unskilled activity and therefore appropriate for the physical therapy aide. It would be inappropriate for the physical therapy aide to expand their duties beyond an observational role (i.e., modify, interpret, progress) since this would require clinical decision making.**

4. Physical therapy aides should not make entries in the medical record. Recording parameters associated with a specific intervention should be completed by the physical therapist or in some cases the physical therapist assistant who performed the intervention.

System Specific: Non-Systems
Content Outline: Safety and Protection; Professional Responsibilities; Research

## Exam Two: Question 168

A physical therapist discusses common cognitive and behavioral changes associated with stroke with family members of a patient with right hemisphere damage and resultant left hemiplegia. Which term does NOT accurately describe the MOST typical patient presentation?

1. poor judgment
2. impulsive
3. quick
4. **overly cautious**

**Correct Answer: 4** (Umphred p. 870)
Physical therapists should be aware of commonly encountered behavioral differences in patients status post stroke with left hemisphere versus right hemisphere damage.

1. Patients with right hemisphere damage often have difficulty in grasping the whole idea of a task or activity and therefore may have difficulty with reasoning and judgment.

2. Patients with right hemisphere damage are often impulsive and tend to overestimate their abilities and underestimate their limitations. This combination makes the patient a greater safety risk compared to a patient with left hemisphere damage.

3. Patients with right hemisphere damage often are quick when performing mobility or tasks. Feedback must be given to encourage the patient to slow down and focus on each of the sequential steps of the activity.

4. **Patients with left hemisphere damage often are described as cautious, anxious, and disorganized. They often have difficulties communicating and in processing information in a sequential manner.**

System Specific: Neuromuscular & Nervous Systems
Content Outline: Foundations for Evaluation, Differential Diagnosis, & Prognosis

## Exam Two: Question 169

A physical therapist gathers a variety of equipment prior to administering a series of sensory tests. Which form of sensation would be examined by utilizing a tuning fork?

1. joint position
2. **vibration**
3. stereognosis
4. barognosis

**Correct Answer: 2** (Bickley p. 692)

A tuning fork is a small two pronged metal device that provides a fixed tone when struck. The base of the device is placed on a bony prominence after being struck and the patient attempts to perceive the vibratory stimulus. If vibration sense is intact, the patient will perceive the vibration. If there is impairment, the patient will be unable to distinguish between vibration and nonvibration.

1. Joint position sense and the awareness of joints at rest is termed proprioceptive awareness. This can be assessed by the therapist holding a joint in a static position followed by the patient verbally describing the position or duplicating the position with the contralateral extremity.

2. **Vibration sense can be assessed by placing a tuning fork vibrating at 128 Hz over a bony prominence. Vibration sense is often the first sensation to be compromised in the presence of a peripheral neuropathy.**

3. Stereognosis refers to the ability of a patient to identify objects placed in the hand without visual assistance. The objects are typically small and familiar such as a coin, key, comb, and pen.

4. Barognosis refers to the recognition of weight. The patient is asked to identify the comparative weights of similar sized objects presented in a series.

System Specific: Neuromuscular & Nervous Systems
Content Outline: Physical Therapy Examination

## Exam Two: Question 170

A physical therapist discusses the process of learning to drive an adapted van with a patient rehabilitating from a spinal cord injury. What is the highest spinal cord injury level where this activity would be a realistic independent functional outcome?

1. C4
2. **C6**
3. T1
4. T3

**Correct Answer: 2** (Umphred p. 632)

A patient with a spinal cord injury would need to have adequate upper extremity active movement to manipulate the hand controls. Prior to driving, an individual would have several unique tests that determine range of motion, strength, vision, and reaction time. The test is usually performed by a physical therapist, occupational therapist or a certified driving instructor.

1. A patient with a C4 spinal cord injury would not have adequate upper extremity movement to independently manipulate hand controls. The diaphragm and trapezius would be innervated.

2. **A patient with a C6 spinal cord injury would possess the requisite upper extremity movement to drive an adapted van with hand controls and use a lift to get the wheelchair in and out of the vehicle. The extensor carpi radialis, infraspinatus, latissimus dorsi, pectoralis major, pronator teres, serratus anterior, and teres minor would be innervated.**

3. A patient with a T1 spinal cord injury would be able to drive an adapted van. The patient would have full upper extremity innervation including a strong grasp. The option is not the correct response since the question asks the highest spinal cord injury level where driving is a realistic functional outcome.

4. A patient with a T3 spinal cord injury would also be able to drive an adapted van. The patient's clinical presentation would be consistent with the patient at the T1 level.

System Specific: Neuromuscular & Nervous Systems
Content Outline: Foundations for Evaluation, Differential Diagnosis, & Prognosis

## Exam Two: Question 171

A physical therapist searches the literature to find an appropriate cardiovascular screening test to identify individuals with known cardiovascular disease who should have a medical examination before starting an exercise program. The physical therapist should choose a screening test with:

1. **high positive predictive value**
2. low positive predictive value
3. high discriminant validity
4. high internal consistency

**Correct Answer: 1** (Portney p. 622)

To be clinically useful, a screening test should be efficient to use and yield accurate responses. The accuracy of the screening test is assessed by its predictive value.

1. **A positive predictive value estimates the probability that a person who tests positive on the screening test actually has the condition the screening test is intended to detect. A test with a high positive predictive value provides a strong estimate of the actual number of patients who have the condition.**

2. A screening test with a low positive predictive value would not be clinically useful as it would not accurately identify individuals with the condition or disease.

3. Discriminant validity is a way to assess the construct validity of a measurement. When measurements that are believed to assess different characteristics are shown to be different, or have a low correlation, then one measurement is said to have discriminant validity with respect to the second measurement. This is not the most important attribute for a screening test.

4. Internal consistency is a form of reliability of a measurement, assessing the degree to which a set of items in an instrument all measure the same trait. This is not the most important attribute for a screening test.

System Specific: Cardiovascular/Pulmonary and Lymphatic Systems
Content Outline: Physical Therapy Examination

## Exam Two: Question 172

A patient classifies the intensity of exercise as a 16 using Borg's (20-point) Rating of Perceived Exertion Scale. This classification BEST corresponds to:

1. 40 percent of the maximum heart rate range
2. 60 percent of the maximum heart rate range
3. 70 percent of the maximum heart rate range
4. **85 percent of the maximum heart rate range**

**Correct Answer: 4** (Brannon p. 316)

Borg's Rating of Perceived Exertion Scale (RPE) may be used as an alternative means to monitor the intensity of exercise once the patient becomes familiar with the feeling of exertion associated with exercise at the appropriate target level. The 20-point RPE scale ranges from a minimum value of 6 to a maximum value of 20.

1. A rating of 16 is relatively close to the maximum value and would therefore not correspond to a heart rate percent that is less than 50% of heart rate range.

2. 60% of the heart rate range corresponds to an RPE of 12 to 13 (somewhat hard).

3. 70% of the heart rate range corresponds to an RPE of 14 or 15 (between somewhat hard and hard).

4. **A rating of 16 (hard+) on the 20-point RPE scale corresponds to 85% of the heart rate range.**

System Specific: Cardiovascular/Pulmonary and Lymphatic Systems
Content Outline: Interventions

## Exam Two: Question 173

A male patient rehabilitating from a lower extremity injury is referred to physical therapy for gait analysis. The physical therapist begins the session by observing the patient at free speed walking. The normal degree of toe-out at this speed is:

1. 3 degrees
2. **7 degrees**
3. 14 degrees
4. 21 degrees

---

**Correct Answer: 2** (Levangie p. 528)

The degree of toe-out is measured by determining the angle formed by each foot's line of progression and a line intersecting the center of the heel and the second toe.

1. A measurement of 3 degrees of toe-out may be associated with walking at a relative fast rate of speed since the normal degree of toe-out decreases as the speed of walking increases.
2. **The degree of toe-out during free speed walking is approximately 7 degrees.**
3. A measurement of 14 degrees is greater than normal and may be associated with a wide range of orthopedic or neurologic abnormalities.
4. A measurement of 21 degrees is excessive and may be associated with more severe orthopedic or neurologic abnormalities.

System Specific: Musculoskeletal System
Content Outline: Physical Therapy Examination

---

## Exam Two: Question 174

A patient with Alzheimer's disease is referred to physical therapy for instruction in an exercise program. The MOST appropriate INITIAL step is:

1. provide verbal and written instructions
2. frequently repeat multiple step directions
3. **assess the patient's cognitive status**
4. avoid using medical terminology

---

**Correct Answer: 3** (Bickley p. 151)

Physical therapists should attempt to provide exercise instructions that are consistent with the abilities and limitations of the target audience. This is particularly important with Alzheimer's disease since cognitive status can vary greatly from patient to patient.

1. Providing verbal and written instructions is an effective method to improve patient understanding and can be particularly important in the case of a home exercise program. The breadth and depth of the instructions would be heavily influenced by the patient's cognitive status.
2. Repetition is an effective technique to enhance learning and memory. The appropriate amount of repetition will be dictated in part by the patient's cognitive status.
3. **It is essential for the physical therapist to determine the patient's cognitive status prior to providing formal exercise instruction. The patient's cognitive status will have a significant impact on a variety of factors including the ability to interpret instructions, the ability to perform exercises correctly, and the ability to recall elements of the exercise program.**
4. Physical therapists should avoid using medical terminology whenever possible. Although this is good advice, it would not be as important as assessing the patient's cognitive status.

System Specific: Neuromuscular & Nervous Systems
Content Outline: Physical Therapy Examination

---

## Exam Two: Question 175

A physician provides a group of physical therapists with an overview of diagnostic imaging techniques commonly used in clinical practice. Which imaging technique would NOT be considered invasive?

1. arthrography
2. myelography
3. discography
4. **computed tomography**

**Correct Answer: 4** (Magee p. 62)

Diagnostic imaging techniques are often used to confirm a clinical opinion. Familiarity with these techniques will allow the physical therapist to play a more active role in the medical management of their patients and assist them to comprehend and perhaps interpret the results of diagnostic imaging.

1. Arthrography is an invasive test utilizing a contrast medium to provide visualization of joint structures through radiographs. Soft tissue disruption can be identified by leakage from the joint cavity and capsule. The test is commonly used at peripheral joints such as the hip, knee, ankle, elbow, and wrist.

2. Myelography is an invasive test that combines fluoroscopy and radiography to evaluate the spinal subarachnoid space. The test utilizes a contrast medium that is injected into the epidural space by spinal puncture. Myelography is used to identify bone displacement, disk herniation, spinal cord compression or tumors.

3. Discography is an invasive test that involves injecting a radiopaque dye into the nucleus pulposus of an intervertebral disc using radiographic guidance. The technique can be used to identify disruptions of the nucleus pulposus or the annulus fibrosus.

4. **Computed tomography is a non-invasive imaging technique that uses cross-sectional images based on x-ray attenuation. Computer enhancement allows the imaging to have significantly better contrast resolution when compared to conventional x-rays.**

System Specific: Musculoskeletal System
Content Outline: Foundations for Evaluation, Differential Diagnosis, & Prognosis

## Exam Two: Question 176

A physical therapist completing a lower quarter screening examination attempts to palpate the tendon of the tibialis anterior. The MOST appropriate therapist action to facilitate palpation is:

1. ask the patient to actively move the foot into dorsiflexion and eversion
2. **ask the patient to actively move the foot into dorsiflexion and inversion**
3. passively move the patient's foot into dorsiflexion and eversion
4. passively move the patient's foot into dorsiflexion and inversion

**Correct Answer: 2** (Kendall p. 410)

The tibialis anterior acts to dorsiflex the ankle joint and assists in inversion of the foot. The muscle is innervated by the deep peroneal nerve.

1. Active movement would be helpful to facilitate palpation of the tendon, however, the tibialis anterior assists to invert the foot and not evert.

2. **The action of the tibialis anterior is to dorsiflex the ankle and invert the foot. To facilitate palpation of the tendon the patient must actively move in the direction of the muscle's action.**

3. Passive movement would not be as useful as active movement to assist with facilitation of a contractile structure.

4. Dorsiflexion of the ankle and inversion of the foot is consistent with the action of the tibialis anterior, however, passive movement would not be as desirable as active movement to facilitate palpation of the tendon.

System Specific: Musculoskeletal System
Content Outline: Physical Therapy Examination

## Exam Two: Question 177

A physical therapist transports a patient with a brain injury to the physical therapy gym. Each day after arriving in the gym, the patient asks the therapist, "Where am I?" Recognizing the patient has short-term memory loss, the therapist's MOST appropriate response should be:

1. You know where you are.
2. You are in the same place you were yesterday at this time.
3. **You are in the physical therapy gym for your treatment session.**
4. You are in the hospital because of your injury.

**Correct Answer: 3** (O'Sullivan p. 914)

A patient's question should be answered in a direct and forthcoming manner whenever possible.

1. The statement implies that the patient knows where they are and is simply withholding information. The more likely reality is that the patient's short-term memory loss is responsible for the difficulty with orientation.
2. The statement provides information for the patient by informing them that they were in the same location that they were yesterday, however, because of the short-term memory loss this may still be of little value.
3. **The statement provides a specific and informative response to the question asked by the patient. Frequent repetition is a component of any treatment plan for patients with short-term memory loss.**
4. The statement provides some useful information for the patient, but lacks the specificity of option 3 given that the patient has been transported to the physical therapy gym.

System Specific: Neuromuscular & Nervous Systems
Content Outline: Interventions

## Exam Two: Question 178

A physical therapist completes a balance assessment on a patient recently admitted to a skilled nursing facility. The therapist concludes that the patient is able to maintain their balance without support in standing, however, cannot maintain balance during weight shifting or with any form of external perturbation. The MOST appropriate balance grade would be:

1. normal
2. good
3. **fair**
4. poor

**Correct Answer: 3** (O'Sullivan p. 254)

The patient's ability to maintain balance in standing and inability to maintain balance with weight shifting or outside challenges is typical of a patient with fair standing balance.

1. A balance grade of normal indicates that the patient would weight shift in all directions and accept maximal perturbation while maintaining their balance.
2. A balance grade of good indicates that the patient would maintain balance without support and accept moderate perturbation while maintaining their balance.
3. **A balance grade of fair indicates that the patient would maintain balance without support, but cannot weight shift without losing their balance.**
4. A balance grade of poor indicates that the patient would require some assistance in order to maintain balance in standing and cannot weight shift or accept any perturbation.

System Specific: Neuromuscular & Nervous Systems
Content Outline: Physical Therapy Examination

## Exam Two: Question 179

A physical therapist completes a respiratory assessment on a patient with T2 paraplegia. As a component of the assessment, the therapist measures the amount of chest excursion during inspiration. The MOST appropriate patient position to conduct the measurement is:

1. sitting
2. **supine**
3. prone
4. sidelying

**Correct Answer: 2** (Umphred p. 626)

The primary muscles of inspiration are the diaphragm and external intercostals. The primary muscles of expiration are the abdominals and internal intercostals. Normal mechanics of inspiration allow for an increase in the diameter of the thorax. Normal mechanics of resting expiration is through recoil of the lungs, however, the abdominals and intercostals contribute in several ways. The loss of these muscles significantly decreases the overall respiratory efficiency. Supine is the most appropriate position to assess chest excursion and initially strengthen.

1. The sitting position is a higher level activity for patients with any form of respiratory weakness and compromise. Patients should be assessed and initiate strengthening in the supine position with the goal of progressing to a sitting position. Abdominal binders assist the patient with respiration in sitting by maintaining pressure that is normally lost in patients with lesions at T12 or above.

2. **The supine position creates support and resistance to the diaphragm. There is a direct correlation between the amount of chest expansion and intercostal strength.**

3. The prone position would not be recommended for a patient with a spinal cord injury due to the patient's body weight and force of gravity upon the weakened muscles of respiration.

4. The sidelying position would not be indicated for measurement of chest excursion during inspiration since one portion of the thorax would be supported by the surface that the patient is sidelying on.

System Specific: Cardiovascular/Pulmonary and Lymphatic Systems
Content Outline: Physical Therapy Examination

## Exam Two: Question 180

A physical therapist working in an outpatient physical therapy clinic guards a patient descending a step with axillary crutches. Based on the photograph, the MOST likely patient scenario is:

1. **partial weight bearing secondary to a left lateral ankle sprain**
2. partial weight bearing secondary to a right lateral ankle sprain
3. toe touch weight bearing secondary to a left lateral ankle sprain
4. toe touch weight bearing secondary to a right lateral ankle sprain

**Correct Answer: 1** (Pierson p. 251)

When descending a step with axillary crutches the involved lower extremity and crutches are moved from the step to the ground, while the upper extremities and the uninvolved lower extremity are used to slowly lower the body.

1. **The patient should use the upper extremities and the uninvolved lower extremity to slowly lower the body when descending a step. As a result, the patient's left ankle would be the involved ankle. Partial weight bearing occurs when a patient is allowed to put a particular amount of weight through the involved extremity.**

2. If the right ankle was the involved ankle, the patient would use the upper extremities and the left lower extremity to slowly lower the body when descending a step.

3. The patient's left ankle is the involved ankle, however, the picture does not depict toe touch weight bearing. Toe touch weight bearing occurs when a patient is unable to place any weight through the involved extremity, however, can place the toes on the ground to assist with balance.

4. The right ankle is not the involved ankle and the depicted weight bearing status is better described as partial weight bearing.

System Specific: Musculoskeletal System
Content Outline: Interventions

## Exam Two: Question 181

A physical therapist prepares a patient recovering from a total hip arthroplasty using a posterolateral surgical approach for discharge from the hospital. The patient is a 65-year-old and resides alone. Assuming an uncomplicated recovery, which of the following pieces of adaptive equipment would NOT be necessary for home use?

1. long handled shoehorn
2. raised toilet seat
3. **sliding board**
4. tub bench

**Correct Answer: 3** (Kisner p. 657)

Contraindications following total hip arthroplasty using a posterolateral surgical approach include hip flexion greater than 90 degrees, adduction, and medial rotation beyond neutral. Adaptive equipment allows the patient to perform necessary activities of daily living without compromising the integrity of the total hip arthroplasty.

1. A long handled shoehorn allows the patient to put on shoes without flexing the affected hip greater than 90 degrees.
2. A raised toilet seat allows the patient to use the toilet without flexing the hips greater than 90 degrees. A normal toilet seat requires greater than 90 degrees of hip flexion.
3. **A patient scheduled for discharge from the hospital following total hip arthroplasty surgery should be able to perform transfers independently without using a sliding board.**
4. A tub bench provides a stable base for the patient to use when showering. The stability offered by the tub bench allows the patient to safely shower without concerns or fear of falling.

System Specific: Musculoskeletal System
Content Outline: Interventions

## Exam Two: Question 182

A physical therapist records the end-feel associated with forearm supination as firm in the medical record. Which of the following is NOT consistent with an end-feel categorized as firm?

1. muscular stretch
2. capsular stretch
3. **soft tissue approximation**
4. ligamentous stretch

**Correct Answer: 3** (Norkin p. 9)

Supination occurs in the transverse plane around a longitudinal axis with the patient in the anatomical position. Normal supination is 0-80 degrees. The end-feel is typically classified as firm due to tension in the palmar radioulnar ligament of the inferior radioulnar joint, interosseous membrane, pronator teres, and pronator quadratus muscles.

1. Muscular stretch is a type of firm end-feel described as a "rubbery" feel resembling what would be felt at the extremes of a straight leg raise due to tension in the hamstrings muscles.
2. Capsular stretch is a type of firm end-feel with a "leathery" feeling with slight creep. An example is extension of the metacarpophalangeal joints of the fingers resulting from tension in the anterior capsule.
3. **Soft tissue approximation is a type of soft end-feel. This type of end-feel could occur with knee flexion resulting from contact between the soft tissue of the posterior leg and the posterior thigh.**
4. Ligamentous stretch is a type of firm end-feel with no give or creep. This type of end-feel could occur with forearm supination resulting from tension in the palmar radioulnar ligament of the inferior radioulnar joint and interosseous membrane.

System Specific: Musculoskeletal System
Content Outline: Physical Therapy Examination

## Exam Two: Question 183

A physical therapist examines several superficial reflexes on a patient diagnosed with an upper motor neuron lesion. When assessing the cremasteric reflex the MOST appropriate stimulus is:

1. stroke the skin beneath the costal margins and above the inguinal ligament
2. **stroke the skin of the superior and medial thigh**
3. prick the skin of the perianal region
4. prick the skin of the glans penis

**Correct Answer: 2** (DeMyer p. 333)

The physical therapist should stroke the skin in the area of the superior and medial thigh in order to elicit the cremasteric reflex. The anticipated response is elevation of the testicle on the same side as the stimulus.

1. Stroking the skin beneath the costal margins and above the inguinal ligament assesses the abdominal reflex. A normal response will produce a contraction of the abdominal muscles in the stimulated quadrant.

2. **Stroking of the skin of the superior and medial thigh will elicit the cremasteric reflex. Upper and lower motor neuron disorders as well as a spinal injury at the L1-L2 level can cause the reflex to be absent.**

3. Pricking the skin of the perianal region assesses the superficial anal reflex. A normal response will produce a contraction of the rectal sphincter.

4. Pricking the skin of the glans penis assesses the bulbocavernosus reflex. A normal response will produce a contraction of the bulbous urethra.

System Specific: Neuromuscular & Nervous Systems
Content Outline: Physical Therapy Examination

## Exam Two: Question 184

A 35-year-old male diagnosed with ankylosing spondylitis is referred to physical therapy for instruction in a home exercise program. Which general treatment objective would be the MOST beneficial for the patient?

1. strengthening of the rectus abdominus
2. strengthening of the internal and external obliques
3. strengthening of the quadratus lumborum
4. **strengthening of the back extensors**

**Correct Answer: 4** (Dutton p. 276)

Ankylosing spondylitis is a form of systemic rheumatic arthritis that results in inflammation of the axial skeleton with subsequent back pain. The condition is associated with an increase in thoracic kyphosis and loss of the lumbar curve. The patient often develops a forward stooped posture observed in standing.

1. Strengthening of the rectus abdominus will produce a flexion moment in the trunk. This will further accentuate the thoracic kyphosis and decrease the lumbar lordosis.

2. Strengthening of the internal and external obliques when contracting bilaterally will produce a flexion moment of the trunk and when contracting unilaterally will produce a rotary moment of the trunk. General core strengthening is desirable, however, the emphasis would be on strengthening the back extensors.

3. Strengthening of the quadratus lumborum will produce a lateral bending of the trunk when performed in a closed-chain activity and a hip hiking movement when performed in an open-chain activity. These motions would not be the emphasis of a strengthening program for a patient with ankylosing spondylitis. The quadratus lumborum also assists with extension, however, the muscle is just one of many muscles that serve this function.

4. **Extension exercises are often an important component of a comprehensive plan of care to assist patients with ankylosing spondylitis to maintain the normal curves of the spine while at the same time limiting the forward bending nature of the disease.**

System Specific: Musculoskeletal System
Content Outline: Interventions

## Exam Two: Question 185

A 73-year-old male patient receiving outpatient physical therapy begins to experience acute angina. The patient indicates he uses nitroglycerin to alleviate the angina. The MOST appropriate mode of administration is:

1. oral
2. buccal
3. **sublingual**
4. topical

**Correct Answer: 3** (Ciccone p. 309)

Drugs can be administered through the alimentary canal or through nonalimentary routes. Each route has distinct advantages and disadvantages.

1. Oral administration is the most common method of administration. It is considered the easiest form of taking medication when self-medication is required and is relatively safe since drugs enter the system in a fairly controlled manner.

2. Buccal administration occurs when the drug is placed between the cheeks and gums. Drugs administered in this manner are absorbed through the oral mucosa.

3. **Sublingual administration occurs when placing drugs under the tongue. Sublingual administration of nitroglycerin is the most appropriate mode of administration with acute angina due to the rapid absorption into the systemic circulation.**

4. Topical administration refers to the application of drugs topically to the surface of the skin or mucous membranes. Topical administration is used most often to treat the outer layer of the skin and not other areas since most medications are absorbed poorly through the epidermis and into the systemic circulation.

System Specific: Cardiovascular/Pulmonary and Lymphatic Systems
Content Outline: Foundations for Evaluation, Differential Diagnosis, and Prognosis

## Exam Two: Question 186

A physical therapist prepares to conduct a manual muscle test of the hip flexors. Assuming a grade of poor, the MOST appropriate testing position is:

1. prone
2. **sidelying**
3. supine
4. standing

**Correct Answer: 2** (Kendall p. 422)

A grade of poor indicates that the hip flexors can produce movement with gravity-eliminated, but cannot function against gravity. Muscles acting to flex the hip include the iliopsoas, sartorius, rectus femoris, and pectineus.

1. A prone position would place the hip flexors in an elongated position and make it impossible for the therapist to offer resistance in a direction opposite of the muscle's action.

2. **The hip flexors would need to be tested in sidelying due to the grade of "poor." If the hip flexors were given a grade of "good" or "normal" the recommended testing position would be sitting upright with the knees bent over the side of the table.**

3. A supine position would not be considered gravity-eliminated and therefore would not be appropriate given the muscle's current grade. A supine position is sometimes employed as a substitute for sitting upright, most often in situations where the muscle's strength is "good" or "normal."

4. Testing the hip flexors in standing would be problematic since the muscles would need to work against gravity and it would be impossible to adequately stabilize the patient during the testing.

System Specific: Musculoskeletal System
Content Outline: Physical Therapy Examination

## Exam Two: Question 187 ✳

A physical therapist administers the Functional Reach Test to a patient rehabilitating from a neurological disorder. Which bony landmark would be the MOST appropriate to utilize when formally measuring the distance the patient reached during each trial?

1. distal tip of the third digit
2. **third metacarpal**
3. radial styloid process
4. ulnar styloid process

---

**Correct Answer: 2** (Montgomery p. 192)

The Functional Reach Test was developed to assess standing balance and the risk for falls. The test is reliable, however, the standard error of measurement may be relatively high and the test measures sway only in a forward direction. A person is required to stand upright against a wall with a static base of support. The patient is then asked to make a fist and raise the arm nearest the wall to 90 degrees of shoulder flexion. The therapist records the beginning position on a yardstick. The patient is then asked to lean forward as far as possible and the ending position is recorded. The beginning position is then subtracted from the ending position to obtain the final value.

1. The distal tip of the third digit is in the midline of the hand, but is not the identified landmark used on the Functional Reach Test.

2. **The Functional Reach Test requires the therapist to measure the position of the patient's third metacarpal on the yardstick after making a fist.**

3. The radial styloid process is located on the lateral side of the distal radius with the hand in the anatomic position. The most prominent part of the radial styloid process is just proximal to the carpal joint.

4. The ulnar styloid process is located on the medial side of the ulna with the hand in the anatomic position. The ulna articulates with the distal radius, but does not articulate with the carpals.

System Specific: Neuromuscular and Nervous Systems
Content Outline: Physical Therapy Examination

---

## Exam Two: Question 188

A physical therapist measures elbow flexion while a patient grasps the handgrip of a walker in standing. The therapist records elbow flexion as 35 degrees. Which statement BEST describes the height of the walker?

1. the walker height is too low for the patient
2. **the walker height is too high for the patient**
3. the walker height is appropriate for the patient
4. not enough information is given to assess walker height

---

**Correct Answer: 2** (Pierson p. 219)

A patient using a properly fitting walker should exhibit 20–25 degrees of elbow flexion. This position of the elbow would allow the patient to most effectively use the upper extremities during ambulation. A walker can be used with all levels of weight bearing and offers a large base of support which promotes stability.

1. A walker height that is too low for the patient would result in elbow flexion less than the recommended 20-25 degrees. Any deviation from the recommended fit would decrease the efficiency of using the walker and increase the potential safety risk.

2. **A walker height that is too high for the patient would result in elbow flexion greater than the recommended 20-25 degrees.**

3. Elbow flexion of 35 degrees exceeds the upper limit of the acceptable range of elbow flexion (i.e., 20-25 degrees) when using a walker. As the height of the walker increases, the amount of elbow flexion will also increase.

4. The amount of elbow flexion is the primary indicator of the relative height of the walker. As a result, there is ample information provided to assess the height of the walker.

System Specific: Non-Systems
Content Outline: Equipment & Devices; Therapeutic Modalities

## Exam Two: Question 189

A physical therapist often makes errors when completing daily documentation. Which of the following statements would be the MOST appropriate advice to the therapist when an error occurs?

1. use correction fluid as needed on your documentation
2. **place a single line through the error, write "error", date, and initial it**
3. use pencil when completing your documentation
4. use erasable ink when completing your documentation

**Correct Answer: 2** (Shamus - Effective Documentation p. 12)

Physical therapists often make mistakes when writing entries in the medical record. It is critical that when this occurs, therapists correct the mistake in a manner that makes the medical record accurate and also makes it clear how the record was altered.

1. Correction fluid provides a mechanism to correct mistakes, however, obscures the original entry.

2. **Place a single line through the error, write "error", date, and initial it provides the physical therapist with a valid method to correct the mistake while preserving the integrity of the original entry.**

3. Pencil is not acceptable to utilize when completing documentation since it is not permanent.

4. Erasable ink is not acceptable since by virtue of being "erasable" it lacks permanence.

System Specific: Non-Systems
Content Outline: Safety and Protection; Professional Responsibilities; Research

## Exam Two: Question 190

A 22-year-old male rehabilitating from a motor vehicle accident is referred to physical therapy for gait training. The patient sustained multiple injuries including a fractured tibia and a traction injury to the brachial plexus. The patient is partial weight bearing and has good upper extremity strength. The MOST appropriate assistive device is:

1. axillary crutches
2. **Lofstrand crutches**
3. walker with platform attachment
4. cane

**Correct Answer: 2** (Pierson p. 217)

Physical therapists often have to consider a variety of factors when determining an appropriate assistive device for a patient. In this particular question, the therapist has to consider the patient's brachial plexus injury and the present weight bearing status.

1. Axillary crutches would accommodate the patient's weight bearing status, however, have the potential to transmit pressure through the axillary region which could exacerbate the brachial plexus injury.

2. **Lofstrand or forearm crutches avoid transmitting pressure to the brachial plexus area and accommodate for the weight bearing status of the involved lower extremity. The patient's age and upper extremity strength make Lofstrand crutches the most appropriate device.**

3. A walker with a platform attachment would be an appropriate option for the patient, however, given the patient's age and upper extremity strength, the device may offer more stability than the patient requires.

4. A cane or bilateral canes do not permit partial weight bearing and instead are used to promote balance.

System Specific: Neuromuscular and Nervous Systems
Content Outline: Interventions

## Exam Two: Question 191

A 29-year-old female status post Colles' fracture is referred to physical therapy. The patient has moderate edema in her fingers and the dorsum of her hand and complains of pain during active range of motion. The MOST appropriate method to quantify the patient's edema is:

1. **volumetric measurements**
2. circumferential measurements
3. girth measurements
4. anthropometric measurements

**Correct Answer: 1** (Magee p. 446)
Volumetric measurements are often used to quantify the presence of edema in the wrist and hand by examining the amount of water displaced following immersion.

1. **A patient with moderate edema in the fingers and dorsum of the hand would displace more water than the contralateral extremity due to the involved limb's increased volume. Although the contralateral extremity serves as an effective baseline measure, it is important to recognize that there may normally be a small difference between the dominant and non-dominant hand.**
2. Circumferential measurements using a flexible tape measure are most commonly used to obtain a gross estimate of edema or muscle atrophy. The test would not commonly be used for the hand due to the difficulty associated with obtaining an accurate measurement because of the relative nonuniformity of the hand.
3. Girth measurements are synonymous with circumferential measurements.
4. Common anthropometric measurements used for adults include height, weight, body mass index (BMI), waist-to-hip ratio, and percentage of body fat. These measures are then compared to reference standards to assess items such as weight status and the risk for various diseases.

System Specific: Musculoskeletal System
Content Outline: Physical Therapy Examination

## Exam Two: Question 192

The MOST important contribution case reports make to evidence-based practice in physical therapy is:

1. A case report demonstrates a causal relationship between treatment and outcome in a single patient.
2. **A case report provides information that can be used to generate inductive hypotheses for future studies.**
3. A case report provides data on the natural history of disease states.
4. A case report uses triangulation to test a hypothesis with more than one source of data.

**Correct Answer: 2** (Portney p. 316)
Describing interesting, new and unique cases is one means of building a foundation for clinical science. The case report is a practical approach to research in the clinical sciences because it is directly applicable to patient care, but it is also the least rigorous because of its lack of control and limited generalizability.

1. Due to the lack of control and the number of different interventions the patient may receive (medical, surgical, nursing, social, recreational, etc.), it is not reasonable to try to suggest a direct causal relationship between one treatment and the outcome in a single patient.
2. **Case reports are important for generating and testing theory and for providing information that may be used to generate inductive hypotheses that can be tested by exploratory or experimental methods.**
3. Longitudinal studies of many patients followed for a long period of time are the preferred means of studying the natural history of a disease.
4. Case reports do not triangulate data from multiple sources to test hypotheses. In most case reports, the data comes from a single patient.

System Specific: Non-Systems
Content Outline: Safety and Protection; Professional Responsibilities; Research

## Exam Two: Question 193

A physical therapist treats an infant diagnosed with torticollis with marked lateral flexion of the neck to the right. As part of the infant's plan of care the therapist performs passive stretching activities to improve the patient's range of motion. The MOST appropriate stretch for the patient is:

1. lateral flexion to the right and rotation to the right
2. lateral flexion to the left and rotation to the left
3. lateral flexion to the right and rotation to the left
4. **lateral flexion to the left and rotation to the right**

**Correct Answer: 4** (Long p. 190)
Torticollis is characterized by lateral flexion of the head toward the affected side and rotation toward the unaffected side. The condition is caused by a contracture of the sternocleidomastoid muscle.

1. Stretching in lateral flexion to the right would be inappropriate since the question indicates that the patient presents with marked lateral flexion of the neck to the right. The direction of the stretch for the rotation component is accurate.

2. Stretching in lateral flexion to the left would be beneficial, however, patients with torticollis present with rotation to the opposite side. As a result, the rotation component should be stretched to the right and not the left.

3. This option more accurately characterizes the clinical presentation of the patient than it does the necessary stretch. The question indicates that the patient presents with marked lateral flexion of the neck to the right and therefore it would not make sense to stretch to the right. The direction of stretch for the rotation component is also inaccurate.

4. **Stretching the patient in lateral flexion to the left and rotation to the right is the correct answer since it is opposite of the patient's current contracture (i.e., marked lateral flexion of the neck to the right and rotation to the left).**

System Specific: Musculoskeletal System
Content Outline: Interventions

**Test Taking Tip:** It is possible for a candidate to eliminate two of the presented options without having any specific knowledge related to torticollis. The question indicates that the patient presents with marked lateral flexion of the neck to the right. Based on the that particular clinical finding it becomes apparent that the stretch would need to be in the opposite direction (i.e., to the left). Often when presented with information that is unfamiliar, candidates fail to recognize that they can still narrow down the presented options. It is critically important for candidates to use this valuable skill since it can significantly increase the probability of identifying the correct response.

## Exam Two: Question 194

A physical therapist instructs a patient to close her eyes and hold out her hand. The therapist places a series of different weights in the patient's hand one at a time. The patient is then asked to identify the comparative weight of the objects. This method of sensory testing is used to examine:

1. **barognosis**
2. graphesthesia
3. recognition of texture
4. stereognosis

**Correct Answer: 1** (O'Sullivan p. 147)
Barognosis, graphesthesia, recognition of texture, and stereognosis are considered combined cortical sensations.

1. **Barognosis refers to the ability of a patient to identify the comparative weight of objects in a series. This can be done by placing a series of different weights in the same hand or by placing different weights in each hand simultaneously.**

2. Graphesthesia refers to the ability of a patient to verbally identify letters or numbers traced on the palm of the hand typically with a fingertip or the eraser of a pencil.

3. Recognition of texture refers to the ability to differentiate among various textures such as cotton, wool or silk. Items may be identified by name or texture such as rough or smooth.

4. Stereognosis refers to the ability to identify an object without sight. Objects used are typically easily obtainable and familiar objects such as a coin, key or comb. Patients are asked to verbally identify the object by name.

System Specific: Neuromuscular & Nervous Systems
Content Outline: Physical Therapy Examination

## Exam Two: Question 195

A physical therapist assesses the pulse rate of a patient exercising on a treadmill. The therapist notes that the rhythm of the pulse is often irregular. The MOST appropriate action to ensure an accurate measurement of pulse rate is:

1. select a different pulse site
2. **measure the pulse rate for 60 seconds**
3. use a different stethoscope
4. document the irregular pulse rate in the patient's medical record

**Correct Answer: 2** (Pierson p. 54)

An irregular pulse rate is characterized by beats occurring at varying intervals. The lack of predictability will increase measurement error particularly when the time used to assess the pulse is relatively small (e.g., 15 seconds).

1. Pulse site will not have an impact on the regularity or irregularity of the pulse.

2. **The longer the duration of the measurement, the closer the obtained measure will be to the patient's actual pulse rate. Although 60 seconds may seem excessive to assess the pulse in a patient with a regular heart rhythm, it is often necessary in the presence of an irregular rhythm in order to ensure a valid measure of pulse rate.**

3. The question does not provide any evidence to suggest that the stethoscope used is defective. In addition, the type of stethoscope used would primarily influence the quality of audible sound and not other items such as rhythm.

4. Documenting the irregular rhythm is necessary, however, the question specifically asks for the most appropriate method to ensure an accurate measurement of pulse rate.

System Specific: Cardiovascular/Pulmonary and Lymphatic Systems
Content Outline: Physical Therapy Examination

## Exam Two: Question 196

A physical therapist participates in a community fitness program by conducting anthropometric measurements designed to determine percent body fat. Which site is NOT typically utilized when measuring skinfolds?

1. suprailiac
2. subscapular
3. triceps
4. **lateral calf**

**Correct Answer: 4** (American College of Sports Medicine p. 269)

Measuring body composition by determining skinfold measurements is based on the principle that the amount of subcutaneous fat is proportional to the total amount of body fat. The technique provides a better estimate of body fat than height, weight, and circumference; however, is not as accurate as hydrostatic weighing.

1. The suprailiac site is taken by obtaining a diagonal fold; in line with the natural angle of the iliac crest taken in the anterior axillary line immediately superior to the iliac crest.

2. The subscapular site is taken by obtaining a diagonal fold; 1-2 cm below the inferior angle of the scapula.

3. The triceps site is taken by obtaining a vertical fold; on the posterior midline of the upper arm, halfway between the acromion and olecranon process, with the arm held freely to the side of the body.

4. **The lateral calf is not a site used for obtaining skinfold measurements, rather the medial calf is used. The medial calf site is taken by obtaining a vertical fold; at the maximum circumference of the calf on the midline of its medial border.**

System Specific: Musculoskeletal System
Content Outline: Physical Therapy Examination

## Exam Two: Question 197

A physical therapist prepares to administer ultrasound to a patient with lateral epicondylitis. When applying ultrasound the amount of heat absorbed is LEAST dependent upon:

1. the intensity
2. the duration of exposure
3. **the choice of the coupling agent**
4. the size of the area sonated

**Correct Answer: 3** (Prentice – Therapeutic Modalities p. 378)

A number of factors play a significant role in determining the amount of heat absorbed using ultrasound. Physical therapists must ensure that the selected parameters are consistent with the desired physiologic effect.

1. Intensity refers to the power per unit area of the sound head, most often expressed in $W/cm^2$. The amount of heat absorbed will increase as the intensity increases assuming that other parameters remain constant.

2. The amount of heat absorbed will increase as the duration of exposure increases assuming that the other parameters remain constant. The duration of exposure is measured in minutes.

3. **A coupling agent is used to transmit ultrasound energy between the transducer and the target area since ultrasound waves do not travel well through air. Examples of coupling agents include gels, lotions, bladders or water. The choice of coupling agent has a relatively small impact when compared to the other presented options.**

4. The amount of heat absorbed will increase as the size of the area sonated decreases assuming that other parameters remain constant. Surface area is most often measured in $cm^2$. Surface area two to three times the size of the transducer typically requires a duration of five minutes of treatment.

System Specific: Non-Systems
Content Outline: Equipment & Devices; Therapeutic Modalities

## Exam Two: Question 198

A physical therapist employed in a rehabilitation hospital utilizes the services of a physical therapy aide. Which variable BEST determines the extent to which physical therapy aides are involved in patient care activities?

1. the number of years of experience
2. the scope of formal training
3. **the discretion of the physical therapist**
4. the quantity of continuing education courses

**Correct Answer: 3** (Guide to Physical Therapist Practice)

The physical therapy aide is a non-licensed worker who is specifically trained under the direction and supervision of a physical therapist. Activities performed by the aide are limited to those tasks that do not require clinical decision making by the physical therapist.

1. Regardless of the number of years of training the aide remains a non-licensed health care provider.

2. The scope of the formal training of the physical therapy aide may influence how the aide is utilized, however, to what extent this factor is considered will depend on the judgment of the physical therapist.

3. **The determination of what tasks are appropriately directed to the aide must be made by the physical therapist or, where allowable by law or regulations, the physical therapist assistant.**

4. The quantity of continuing education courses may provide the physical therapy aide with specialized knowledge in selected areas of clinical practice, however, how this influences the aides' role in patient care activities remains the responsibility of the physical therapist.

System Specific: Non-Systems
Content Outline: Safety and Protection; Professional Responsibilities; Research

## Exam Two: Question 199

A physical therapist prepares to treat a patient with cystic fibrosis using postural drainage. The MOST appropriate patient position when treating the superior segments of the lower lobes is:

1. sitting, leaning back at a 30-40 degree angle
2. head down on left side, 1/4 turn backward
3. supine with two pillows under the knees
4. **prone with two pillows under the hips**

**Correct Answer: 4** (Rothstein p. 445)

Postural drainage for the superior segments of the lower lobes requires the physical therapist to clap over the middle of the back at the tip of the scapula on either side of the spine.

1. Sitting, leaning back 30-40 degrees describes the postural drainage position for the apical segments of the right and left upper lobes.

2. Head down on left side, 1/4 turn backward describes the postural drainage position for the right middle lobe.

3. Supine with two pillows under the knees describes the postural drainage position for the anterior segments of the left and right upper lobes.

4. **Prone with two pillows under the hips describes the postural drainage position for the superior segments of the left and right lower lobes.**

System Specific: Cardiovascular/Pulmonary and Lymphatic Systems
Content Outline: Interventions

## Exam Two: Question 200

A patient rehabilitating from a knee injury completes an isokinetic examination. The patient produces 88 ft/lbs of torque with the hamstrings at 120 degrees per second. Assuming normal quadriceps/hamstrings ratio, which of the following MOST accurately reflects the predicted quadriceps value?

1. 67 ft/lbs
2. 109 ft/lbs
3. **136 ft/lbs**
4. 183 ft/lbs

**Correct Answer: 3** (Hamill p. 236)

The most commonly accepted ratio of quadriceps to hamstrings strength is 3:2. As the speed of movement increases above 200 degrees per second the ratio approaches 1:1.

1. A quadriceps value of 67 ft/lbs would indicate that the quadriceps are not as strong as the recorded hamstrings value (i.e., 0.8:1.0).

2. A quadriceps value of 109 ft/lbs would result in a quadriceps/hamstrings ratio of slightly greater than 1:1 (i.e., 1.2:1.0).

3. **A quadriceps value of 136 ft/lbs would result in a quadriceps/hamstrings ratio of approximately 3:2 (i.e., 1.5:1.0).**

4. A quadriceps value of 183 ft/lbs would result in a quadriceps/hamstrings ratio of over 2:1 (i.e., 2.1:1.0).

System Specific: Musculoskeletal System
Content Outline: Physical Therapy Examination

# 13

## PHYSICAL THERAPY EXAM THREE

Scott Giles

896  Section One - Questions 1-50

921  Section Two - Questions 51-100

946  Section Three - Questions 101-150

971  Section Four - Questions 151-200

# PHYSICAL THERAPY
# EXAM THREE

# EXCELLENCE

**"Aiming for perfection is always a goal in progress."**

— Thomas J. Watson Jr.

Candidates do not have to be perfect to pass the National Physical Therapy
Examination, however, should attempt to strive for perfection. The relative
importance of the examination makes it imperative that candidates become
intolerant of any risk of failure.

## Exam Three: Question 1

A physical therapist would like to minimize the likelihood of a burn when using iontophoresis. Which action would be the MOST consistent with the therapist's objective?

1. **increase the size of the cathode relative to the anode**
2. decrease the space between the electrodes
3. increase the current intensity
4. decrease the moisture of the electrodes

**Correct Answer: 1** (Prentice - Therapeutic Modalities p. 180)

Current density (mA/cm²) is calculated by taking the current amplitude (mA) and dividing by the surface area (cm²). Greater current density will result in an increased risk of an electrochemical burn.

1. **Increasing the size of the cathode relative to the anode serves to decrease current density and therefore reduces the probability of a burn when using iontophoresis. The cathode refers to the negatively charged electrode in a direct current system and the anode refers to the positively charged electrode. The accumulation of positively charged ions in a small area creates an alkaline reaction that is more likely to create tissue damage. As a result, it is desirable to increase the size of the cathode.**

2. Decreasing the space between the electrodes decreases the surface area and therefore increases current density resulting in an increased risk of an electrochemical burn.

3. Increasing the current intensity will increase the force and speed of propulsion of the ions and increase ion uptake. The result of this is increased current density and an increased risk of an electrochemical burn.

4. Commercially produced electrodes most commonly used with iontophoresis have a small chamber covered by a semipermeable membrane which houses the ionized solution. This type of electrode eliminates the need to soak a more traditional electrode in water or saline and instead, is simply self-adherent.

System Specific: Non-Systems
Content Outline: Equipment & Devices; Therapeutic Modalities

## Exam Three: Question 2

A physical therapist reviews a patient coverage form that lists the parameters used during a recent ultrasound treatment to the right anterior shoulder: 1.5 W/cm², pulsed 20%, 1 MHz, 6 minutes. Assuming the objective of the ultrasound was to increase tissue temperature, which parameter would be the MOST critical for the therapist to alter?

1. time
2. **duty cycle**
3. frequency
4. intensity

**Correct Answer: 2** (Cameron p. 192)

Physical therapists must select specific parameters when using ultrasound based on the desired physiological effect. Failure to select the correct parameters will minimize the effectiveness of the session and could potentially jeopardize patient safety in extreme cases.

1. The duration of the ultrasound is an important parameter, however, it is typically determined based on the size of the area to be treated and not by the desired increase in tissue temperature.

2. **Duty cycle is defined as the ratio of the on time to the total time. When ultrasound is used in a pulsed mode with a 20% or lower duty cycle, the heat produced during the on time of the cycle is dispersed during the off time and as a result there is no measurable net increase in temperature. To increase tissue temperature it would be necessary to significantly increase the duty cycle or use a continuous mode.**

3. The frequency of ultrasound selected primarily determines the depth of penetration. A frequency setting of 1 MHz is used for heating of deeper tissues (up to five centimeters). A frequency setting of 3 MHz produces a more rapid heating with a depth of penetration of less than two centimeters.

4. Intensity for continuous ultrasound is normally set between .5 to 2.0 W/cm² for thermal effects. Pulsed ultrasound is normally set between .5 to .75 W/cm² with a 20% duty cycle for nonthermal effects.

System Specific: Non-Systems
Content Outline: Equipment & Devices; Therapeutic Modalities

## Exam Three: Question 3

A physical therapist examines a patient with a C6 spinal cord injury. Which muscle would NOT be innervated based on the patient's level of injury?

1. biceps
2. deltoid
3. **triceps**
4. diaphragm

**Correct Answer: 3** (Magee p. 22)

A patient with a C6 spinal cord injury would not possess motor, sensory or reflex function below the C6 level. As a result, any muscle or structure innervated below this level would not be active.

1. The biceps muscle is innervated by the musculocutaneous nerve (C5-C6).

2. The deltoid muscle is innervated by the axillary nerve (C5-C6).

3. **The triceps muscle is innervated by the radial nerve (C7-C8).**

4. The diaphragm is innervated by the phrenic nerve (C3, C4, C5).

System Specific: Neuromuscular & Nervous Systems
Content Outline: Physical Therapy Examination

## Exam Three: Question 4

A physical therapist attempts to assess the integrity of the vestibulocochlear nerve by administering the Rinne test on a patient with a suspected upper motor neuron lesion. After striking the tine of the tuning fork to begin vibration, which bony prominence should the therapist utilize to position the stem of the tuning fork?

1. midline of the skull
2. occipital protuberance
3. inion
4. **mastoid process**

**Correct Answer: 4** (Magee p. 115)

The Rinne test is designed to compare bone conduction hearing with air conduction hearing. A therapist uses a vibrating tuning fork placed on the mastoid process and then placed next to the ear. Air conducted sound should be approximately twice as long as bone conducted sound.

1. The Weber test is another commonly used hearing test that requires placing a tuning fork on the midline of the skull on the patient's forehead.

2. The occipital protuberance refers to a prominence on the outer surface of the occipital bone.

3. The inion refers to the most prominent projecting point of the occipital bone at the midline of the base of the skull. The inion marks the center of the superior nuchal line.

4. **The mastoid process refers to a protruding bony area in the lower part of the skull situated behind the ear.**

System Specific: Neuromuscular & Nervous Systems
Content Outline: Physical Therapy Examination

## Exam Three: Question 5

A physical therapist prepares to apply a topical antibiotic to a small portion of the upper arm of a patient with a deep partial-thickness burn. When applying the topical antibiotic, the therapist should utilize which form of medical asepsis?

1. gloves
2. **sterile gloves**
3. sterile gloves, gown
4. sterile gloves, gown, mask

**Correct Answer: 2** (Paz p. 290)

Topical antibiotics are often utilized in the treatment of burns. They serve to reduce bacterial count, provide a covering for the wound, reduce stiffness, and reduce evaporative loss. Since topical antibiotics are applied directly to the affected area, sterile gloves should be worn.

1. Gloves offer protection to the physical therapist's hands to reduce the likelihood of becoming infected with microorganisms from a patient and reduce the risk of the patient receiving microorganisms from the physical therapist. Non-sterile gloves are typically used with intact skin.

2. **Topical antibiotics are applied directly to the burn and therefore require the use of sterile gloves. Failure to use sterile technique increases the probability of contamination.**

3. A gown is used to protect the physical therapist's clothing from being contaminated or soiled by a contaminant. The gown also reduces the probability of the physical therapist transmitting a microorganism from their clothing to the patient. The size and the location of the burn make it unnecessary to use a gown.

4. A mask is designed to reduce the spread of microorganisms that are transmitted through the air. The mask protects the physical therapist from inhalation of particles or droplets that may contain pathogens and also reduces the transmission of pathogens from the physical therapist to the patient. The mask would not be necessary since there is minimal risk of microorganisms being transmitted through the air in the described scenario.

System Specific: Other Systems
Content Outline: Interventions

## Exam Three: Question 6

A patient involved in a motor vehicle accident sustains a proximal fibula fracture. The fracture damaged the motor component of the common peroneal nerve. Ankle dorsiflexion and eversion are tested as 2/5. The MOST appropriate intervention to assist the patient with activities of daily living would be:

1. electrical stimulation
2. **orthosis**
3. exercise program
4. aquatic program

**Correct Answer: 2** (Seymour p. 31)

There are a variety of interventions that can assist patients to perform activities of daily living following a peripheral nerve injury. Physical therapists must select the most appropriate interventions to accomplish each of the established goals. In this particular question, the candidate is asked to identify the most appropriate intervention to assist the patient with activities of daily living.

1. Electrical stimulation can be used to facilitate motor activity within the affected muscle, however, the effectiveness of this intervention may be limited depending on the severity of the damage to the nerve. In addition, the intervention would not immediately assist the patient with activities of daily living.

2. **The use of an orthosis would ensure adequate foot clearance and stability during activities of daily living. This form of intervention would have an immediate impact on the patient's ability to perform activities of daily living.**

3. An exercise program would be beneficial for the patient for a variety of reasons. The patient will need to perform selected movements in a different manner since the lower extremity musculature has been affected. Exercise will also be necessary to strengthen the surrounding musculature to provide additional stability. Despite the stated benefits, the intervention would not provide the same magnitude of benefit as the orthosis when performing activities of daily living.

4. An aquatic program allows the patient to exercise in a decreased weight bearing environment, however, the intervention is unlikely to have an immediate impact on the patient's ability to perform activities of daily living.

System Specific: Other Systems
Content Outline: Interventions

## Exam Three: Question 7

A physical therapist discusses the importance of a proper diet with a patient diagnosed with congestive heart failure. Which of the following substances would MOST likely be restricted in the patient's diet?

1. high-density lipoproteins
2. low-density lipoproteins
3. **sodium**
4. triglycerides

**Correct Answer: 3** (Goodman - Pathology p. 572)

Patients with congestive heart failure tend to have excessive fluid retention in the pulmonary and systemic circulation. As a result, a diet high in potassium is prescribed, while items high in sodium are restricted.

1. High-density lipoproteins (HDL) are the smallest particles in the classes of lipoproteins. They are composed of proteins, cholesterol, and a small amount of triglyceride. HDL plays an important role in lipid metabolism by transporting cholesterol back to the liver from the cells. High levels of HDL reduce the incidence of coronary artery disease. There is no association between HDL and congestive heart failure.

2. Low-density lipoproteins (LDL) are the major carriers of cholesterol in plasma. Elevated LDL is a cause of coronary artery disease. There is no association between LDL and congestive heart failure.

3. **Due to poor cardiac output in congestive heart failure, renal and extrarenal sensors initiate a process to retain fluid to increase arterial blood flow. Retention of sodium is part of that process. By controlling sodium intake and water retention, congestive heart failure can be more effectively controlled.**

4. Triglycerides are combinations of glycerol and fatty acids. Elevated triglycerides are not independently predictive of coronary artery disease, but are associated with known risk factors for atherosclerosis, including low HDL cholesterol level and uncontrolled diabetes. There is no association between triglycerides and congestive heart failure.

System Specific: Cardiovascular/Pulmonary and Lymphatic Systems
Content Outline: Interventions

## Exam Three: Question 8

A physical therapist instructs a patient with a pulmonary disease in energy conservation techniques. Which of the following techniques would be the MOST effective when assisting a patient to complete a selected activity without dyspnea?

1. diaphragmatic breathing
2. **pacing**
3. pursed-lip breathing
4. ventilatory muscle training

**Correct Answer: 2** (Kisner p. 865)

Pacing is a technique that can allow patients to complete functional activities without shortness of breath or dyspnea.

1. Diaphragmatic breathing is a breathing technique that can decrease the work of breathing by lowering respiratory rate, increasing tidal volume, and decreasing the use of accessory muscles of respiration by facilitating use of the diaphragm. Diaphragmatic breathing can be used with pacing when necessary.

2. **Pacing is an integral component of energy-saving techniques used by patients who present with dyspnea during activity. Pacing refers to dividing an activity into component parts so that the patient does not exceed the limits of their breathing capacity throughout each portion of the task. For example, climbing up stairs is performed only on exhalation and by taking only one or two steps at a time.**

3. Pursed-lip breathing is a breathing technique performed by inhaling through the nose and exhaling through pursed lips. Patients with chronic obstructive pulmonary disease have been shown to benefit from pursed lip breathing by decreasing respiratory rate, increasing tidal volume, and decreasing the sense of dyspnea. When used in isolation the technique would not be as effective as pacing to assist the patient to complete the activity without dyspnea.

4. Ventilatory muscle training is accomplished by devices called inspiratory muscle trainers, which strengthen the inspiratory muscles by providing resistance to inspiration.

System Specific: Cardiovascular/Pulmonary and Lymphatic Systems
Content Outline: Interventions

## Exam Three: Question 9

A physical therapist reviews the medical record of a patient 24 hours status post total hip arthroplasty. A recent entry in the medical record indicates that the patient was placed on anticoagulant medication. Which of the following laboratory values would be MOST affected based on the patient's current medication?

1. hematocrit
2. hemoglobin
3. **prothrombin time**
4. white blood cell count

---

**Correct Answer: 3** (Physical Therapist's Clinical Companion p. 145)

Anticoagulant drugs are often prescribed post-operatively for patients at risk for acquiring deep vein thrombosis.

1. Hematocrit is used in the identification of abnormal states of hydration, polycythemia, and anemia. A low hematocrit may result in a feeling of weakness, chills or dyspnea. A high hematocrit may result in an increased risk of thrombus.

2. Hemoglobin is used to assess blood loss, anemia, and bone marrow suppression. Low hemoglobin may indicate anemia or recent hemorrhage, while elevated hemoglobin suggests hemoconcentration caused by polycythemia or dehydration.

3. **Prothrombin time is often used as a screening procedure to examine extrinsic coagulation factors (V, VII, X, prothrombin, and fibrinogen) and to determine the effectiveness of oral anticoagulant therapy. An abnormal prothrombin time is most often caused by liver disease, injury or by treatment with blood thinners. Abnormal values can place patients at risk for side effects ranging from a high likelihood of bleeding to a high likelihood of developing a clot.**

4. White blood cell count is commonly used to identify the presence of infection, allergens, bone marrow integrity or the degree of immunosuppression. An increase in white blood cell count can occur after hemorrhage, surgery, coronary occlusion or malignant growth.

System Specific: Cardiovascular/Pulmonary and Lymphatic Systems
Content Outline: Foundations for Evaluation, Differential Diagnosis, & Prognosis

---

## Exam Three: Question 10

A physical therapist discusses the plan of care for a 61-year-old male diagnosed with spinal stenosis with the referring physician. During the discussion the physician shows the therapist a picture of the patient's spine obtained through computed tomography. What color would vertebrae appear when using this imaging technique?

1. black
2. light gray
3. dark gray
4. **white**

---

**Correct Answer: 4** (Magee p. 62)

Computed tomography produces cross-sectional images based on x-ray attenuation. The test is commonly used to diagnose spinal lesions and in diagnostic studies of the brain. The relative color of each item using computed tomography is dependent on the relative density. The greater the density, the less penetration of x-rays and the whiter the image will appear. Specific structures listed in descending degree of density are metal, bone, soft tissue, water, fat, and air.

1. Cerebrospinal fluid would appear as black using computed tomography since it is radiolucent.

2. Soft tissue structures would appear as various shades of gray depending on their relative density.

3. A structure that is darker gray has less relative density than a structure that appears as a lighter shade of gray.

4. **Vertebrae are composed of extremely dense bone and therefore appear to be white.**

System Specific: Musculoskeletal Systems
Content Outline: Foundations for Evaluation, Differential Diagnosis, & Prognosis

---

## Exam Three: Question 11

A physical therapist identifies a number of substances that influence circulation. Which of the following substances is stimulated by decreased arterial pressure and acts as a vasoconstrictor?

1. **angiotensin**
2. histamine
3. epinephrine
4. norepinephrine

**Correct Answer: 1** (Ciccone p. 297)

Physical therapists should possess a general sense of the role of different substances and their influence on normal body processes such as circulation.

1. **Angiotensin is a polypeptide in the blood that causes vasoconstriction, increased blood pressure, and the release of aldosterone from the adrenal cortex. Release of angiotensin is stimulated by decreased arterial pressure.**

2. Histamine is an endogenous chemical that is involved in the normal regulation of a variety of physiologic functions such as gastric secretion as well as various hypersensitivity or allergic reactions.

3. Epinephrine is a naturally occurring hormone released by the adrenal glands. The hormone is released in the fight or flight response. The hormone boosts the supply of oxygen and glucose to the brain and muscles while suppressing other non-emergency body processes such as digestion.

4. Norepinephrine serves dual roles as a hormone and neurotransmitter. Norepinephrine affects parts of the brain where attention and responding actions are controlled and in conjunction with epinephrine underlies the fight or flight response by increasing heart rate, releasing glucose from energy stores, and increasing blood flow to skeletal muscles.

System Specific: Cardiovascular/Pulmonary and Lymphatic Systems
Content Outline: Foundations for Evaluation, Differential Diagnosis, and Prognosis

## Exam Three: Question 12

A patient diagnosed with C5 tetraplegia receives physical therapy services in a rehabilitation hospital. The patient has made good progress in therapy and is scheduled for discharge in one week. During a treatment session, the patient informs the physical therapist that one day in the future he will walk again. The MOST appropriate therapist response is:

1. Your level of injury makes walking unrealistic.
2. **Future advances in spinal cord research may make your goal a reality.**
3. You can have a rewarding life even if confined to a wheelchair.
4. Completing your exercises on a regular basis will help you to walk.

**Correct Answer: 2** (Umphred p. 639)

Physical therapists should encourage patients to reach for their goals even in cases where presently it may be unrealistic. In this scenario, the patient is not asking the therapist directly about their future functional level, rather the patient is simply sharing their optimism about the possibility of one day being able to walk. It would, therefore, be inappropriate for the therapist to do anything to diminish this optimism.

1. The response is accurate, however, it would serve to significantly dampen the patient's current enthusiasm and is not warranted given the described scenario.

2. **Responding in this manner leaves open the possibility that the patient may one day walk, without providing the patient with a sense of false hope.**

3. The response would likely be construed as negative given the patient's proclamation and is made worse by the terminology selected (i.e., "confined to a wheelchair").

4. The response implies that compliance with an exercise program can facilitate walking. This is not accurate based on the patient's level of injury and therefore may provide the patient with a sense of false hope.

System Specific: Neuromuscular & Nervous Systems
Content Outline: Foundations for Evaluation, Differential Diagnosis, & Prognosis

## Exam Three: Question 13

A physical therapist performs several surface palpations on a patient diagnosed with an acromioclavicular injury. Which anatomical landmark is MOST consistent with the location of the therapist's finger?

1. manubrium
2. sternoclavicular joint
3. **suprasternal notch**
4. xiphoid process

**Correct Answer: 3** (Hoppenfeld p. 6)
Physical therapists must possess knowledge of surface anatomy and be able to identify anatomical structures through observation or palpation. It is often important to inspect the integrity of selected structures within a reasonable proximity of the primary injury.

1. The manubrium refers to the broad upper portion of the sternum. The manubrium has a quadrangular shape and articulates with the clavicles and the first two ribs.
2. The sternoclavicular joint consists of the clavicle articulating with the manubrium of the sternum.
3. **The anatomical landmark consistent with the therapist's finger is the suprasternal notch. The suprasternal notch refers to the "V" shaped notch at the top of the sternum.**
4. The xiphoid process refers to the small extension of the lower portion of the sternum. The xiphoid process is cartilaginous at birth and usually ossifies and unites with the body of the sternum by 40 years of age.

System Specific: Musculoskeletal System
Content Outline: Physical Therapy Examination

## Exam Three: Question 14

A physical therapist discusses the plan of care for a patient rehabilitating from total hip arthroplasty surgery (posterolateral approach) with the patient's surgeon. During the discussion the surgeon indicates that he would like the patient to continue to wear a knee immobilizer in order to help prevent hip dislocation. The PRIMARY rationale for this action is:

1. The knee immobilizer serves as a constant reminder to the patient that the hip is susceptible to injury.
2. **The knee immobilizer reduces hip flexion by maintaining knee extension.**
3. The knee immobilizer facilitates quadriceps contraction during weight bearing activities.
4. The knee immobilizer limits post-operative edema and as a result, promotes lower extremity stability.

**Correct Answer: 2** (Paz p. 105)
Hip flexion greater than 90 degrees is often considered a contraindication following total hip arthroplasty surgery using a posterolateral surgical approach. Other contraindications in the early post-operative phase include restricting adduction and medial rotation beyond neutral.

1. A knee immobilizer can serve as an external feedback mechanism to remind the patient that the hip is vulnerable to injury, however, this would not be the primary rationale to use the device.
2. **A knee immobilizer limits hip flexion by maintaining the knee in an extended position. The immobilizer can be particularly helpful in patients who are unable to maintain posterior hip precautions independently.**
3. A knee immobilizer is commonly used following knee surgery to provide stability to the lower extremity. The immobilizer is most often prescribed in the presence of quadriceps weakness to prevent "buckling" or "giving way" of the knee. The knee immobilizer would, however, offer limited stability to a patient following total hip arthroplasty surgery.
4. The knee immobilizer offers some compression to the knee, however, would have little impact on the patient's post-operative edema particularly since the surgery involved the hip. In addition, limiting post-operative edema would play a relatively minor role in promoting lower extremity stability.

System Specific: Musculoskeletal System
Content Outline: Interventions

## Exam Three: Question 15

A physical therapist administers a submaximal exercise test to a patient in a cardiac rehabilitation program. The protocol requires the patient to ride a cycle ergometer for a predetermined amount of time using progressive workloads. In order to predict the patient's maximum oxygen uptake it is necessary to determine the relationship between:

1. heart rate and rate of perceived exertion
2. **heart rate and workload**
3. blood pressure and rate of perceived exertion
4. blood pressure and workload

**Correct Answer: 2** (American College of Sports Medicine p. 308)

Because maximal exercise testing is not always feasible, practitioners often rely on submaximal exercise tests to assess cardiorespiratory fitness. In addition to the heart rate response, it is recommended that the individual's functional response to exercise is examined.

1. Rate of perceived exertion (RPE) is one of the indices commonly measured as a response to exercise. However, oxygen uptake cannot be determined from heart rate and RPE.
2. **The physical therapist can use the heart rate response to one or more submaximal workloads to predict maximum oxygen uptake.**
3. Rate of perceived exertion (RPE) and blood pressure are commonly measured as a response to exercise. However, oxygen uptake cannot be determined from blood pressure and RPE.
4. Blood pressure is one of the indices commonly measured as a response to exercise. However, oxygen uptake cannot be determined from blood pressure and workload.

System Specific: Cardiovascular/Pulmonary and Lymphatic Systems
Content Outline: Interventions

## Exam Three: Question 16

A physical therapist employed in a large medical center reviews the chart of a 63-year-old male referred to physical therapy for pulmonary rehabilitation. The chart indicates the patient has smoked one to two packs of cigarettes a day since the age of 25. The admitting physician documented that the patient's thorax was enlarged with flaring of the costal margins and widening of the costochondral angle. Which pulmonary disease does the chart MOST accurately describe?

1. asthma
2. bronchiectasis
3. chronic bronchitis
4. **emphysema**

**Correct Answer: 4** (Hillegass p. 214)

Due to the pathologic changes in alveoli, patients with emphysema often have increased total lung capacity from "air trapping." Over time, many patients develop a barrel-shaped configuration of the thorax. The anteroposterior diameter enlarges to approximate the transverse diameter. The diaphragm is depressed and the sternum pushed forward with the ribs attached in a horizontal, not angular, fashion. As a result, the chest appears continuously in the inspiratory position.

1. Asthma is a chronic inflammatory disease of the airways. Clinical features include cough, dyspnea, and wheezing, but not an enlarged thorax.
2. Bronchiectasis is a permanent, abnormal dilatation of one or more bronchi caused by destruction of the elastic and muscular components of the bronchial walls. Common clinical features include recurrent pulmonary infections with cough and copious mucopurulent sputum, but not an enlarged thorax.
3. Chronic bronchitis is defined as hypersecretion of mucus sufficient to cause a productive cough on most days for three months during two consecutive years, but not an enlarged thorax.
4. **Emphysema is an obstructive pulmonary disease characterized by destruction of alveoli leading to hyperinflation of the lungs. A barrel-shaped configuration of the thorax is a common clinical feature of the disease.**

System Specific: Cardiovascular/Pulmonary and Lymphatic Systems
Content Outline: Foundations for Evaluation, Differential Diagnosis, & Prognosis

## Exam Three: Question 17

A physical therapist reviews the results of pulmonary function testing on a 44-year-old female diagnosed with emphysema. Assuming the patient's testing was classified as unremarkable, which of the following lung volumes would MOST likely approximate 10% of the patient's total lung capacity?

1. **tidal volume**
2. inspiratory reserve volume
3. residual volume
4. functional residual capacity

**Correct Answer: 1** (Hillegass p. 28)

Tidal volume is the total volume of air inhaled or exhaled during quiet breathing. Total lung capacity is the maximum volume of air to which the lungs can be expanded. Normal tidal volume is approximately 10% of total lung capacity.

1. **While there is wide variability in tidal volume in the normal population, the average for a healthy adult is around 500 mL (± 100 mL). Total lung capacity is the maximum volume of air to which the lungs can be expanded, typically 4,000 – 6,000 mL. Thus, normal tidal volume is approximately 10% of total lung capacity.**

2. Inspiratory reserve volume is the additional volume of air that can be inhaled beyond the normal tidal inhalation. The inspiratory reserve volume varies, however, should represent approximately 55% to 60% of the total lung capacity.

3. Residual volume is the volume of air remaining in the lungs after a forced expiratory effort. This volume is usually 1,000 mL, and approximates 25% of total lung capacity.

4. Functional residual capacity is the amount of air remaining in the lungs at the end of a normal tidal exhalation. This volume approximates 40% of total lung capacity.

System Specific: Cardiovascular/Pulmonary and Lymphatic Systems
Content Outline: Physical Therapy Examination

## Exam Three: Question 18

A physical therapist measures a patient's shoulder complex medial rotation with the patient positioned in supine, the glenohumeral joint in 90 degrees of abduction, and the elbow in 90 degrees of flexion. The therapist records the patient's shoulder medial rotation as 0 - 70 degrees and classifies the end-feel as firm. Which portion of the joint capsule is primarily responsible for the firm end-feel?

1. anterior joint capsule
2. **posterior joint capsule**
3. inferior joint capsule
4. superior joint capsule

**Correct Answer: 2** (Norkin p. 76)

The glenohumeral joint is a synovial ball and socket joint, in which the round head of the humerus (convex) articulates with the shallow glenoid cavity (concave) of the scapula. The glenohumeral joint has three degrees of freedom. The capsule of the glenohumeral joint is reinforced by the superior glenohumeral ligament, middle glenohumeral ligament, inferior glenohumeral ligament, and the coracohumeral ligament.

1. A firm end-feel caused by the anterior joint capsule would most often be associated with lateral rotation of the glenohumeral joint as the humeral head slides anteriorly on the glenoid fossa.

2. **A firm end-feel caused by the posterior joint capsule would most often be associated with medial rotation of the glenohumeral joint as the humeral head slides posteriorly on the glenoid fossa.**

3. A firm end-feel caused by the inferior joint capsule would most often be associated with flexion and abduction of the glenohumeral joint. In flexion, the humeral head moves posteriorly and inferiorly, and in abduction the humeral head moves inferiorly.

4. A firm end-feel caused by the superior joint capsule would most often be associated with extension and adduction of the glenohumeral joint. In extension, the humeral head moves anteriorly and superiorly, and in adduction the humeral head moves superiorly.

System Specific: Musculoskeletal System
Content Outline: Physical Therapy Examination

## Exam Three: Question 19 ✗

A physician suspects a stress fracture in a 16-year-old distance runner after completing an examination. Assuming the physician's preliminary diagnosis is correct, which of the following diagnostic tests would be the MOST appropriate to identify the stress fracture?

1. **bone scan**
2. magnetic resonance imaging
3. telethermography
4. ultrasound scan

**Correct Answer: 1** (Magee p. 63)

Physical therapists should be familiar with commonly employed diagnostic tests since the results of these tests are frequently encountered in the medical record. Awareness of the purpose of the diagnostic tests may also assist the physical therapist to make specific recommendations to the referring physician when appropriate.

1. **A bone scan is a diagnostic test that utilizes radioactive isotopes to identify areas of bone that are hypervascular or have an increased rate of bone mineral turnover.** Bone scans can demonstrate bone disease or stress fractures with as little as 4-7% bone loss.

2. Magnetic resonance imaging is a non-invasive diagnostic test that utilizes magnetic fields to produce an image of bone and soft tissue. The test is valuable in providing images of soft tissue structures such as muscles, menisci, ligaments, tumors, and internal organs.

3. Telethermography is a diagnostic test that demonstrates thermal alterations in the body. For example, a hyperthermic image may be observed in the presence of an inflammatory reaction or a hypothermic image may be observed in the presence of compression or a degenerative process.

4. Ultrasound can be used as a diagnostic test by administering high frequency sound waves into the tissues. The depth of each structure is determined based on the amount of time it takes for an echo to return to the transducer. Ultrasound provides good image detail and cross-sectional multi-planar images.

System Specific: Musculoskeletal System
Content Outline: Foundations for Evaluation, Differential Diagnosis, & Prognosis

## Exam Three: Question 20

A physical therapist positions a patient in prone to measure passive knee flexion. Range of motion may be limited in this position due to:

1. active insufficiency of the knee extensors
2. active insufficiency of the knee flexors
3. **passive insufficiency of the knee extensors**
4. passive insufficiency of the knee flexors

**Correct Answer: 3** (Kisner p. 44)

Passive insufficiency occurs when a two-joint muscle is passively stretched across two joints at the same time resulting in an inability to permit normal elongation simultaneously over both joints. When the muscle is in a lengthened position, the actin filaments are pulled away from the myosin heads so that they cannot create as many cross-bridges. Active insufficiency occurs when a two-joint muscle is incapable of shortening to the extent necessary to produce full range of motion at all joints crossed simultaneously. When the muscle is in a shortened position the overlap of actin and myosin reduces the number of sites available for cross-bridge formation.

1. Active insufficiency occurs with active movement and not passive movement. The question specifically asks about passive knee flexion.

2. Active insufficiency occurs with active movement and not passive movement.

3. **Passive insufficiency refers to a lack of muscle length. When performing passive knee flexion the two-joint knee extensors are placed on stretch and therefore in the presence of insufficient length, may contribute to a limitation in knee flexion.**

4. When performing passive knee flexion, the knee flexors would shorten and therefore would not limit knee flexion range of motion.

System Specific: Musculoskeletal System
Content Outline: Physical Therapy Examination

## Exam Three: Question 21

A physical therapist incorporates electrical stimulation as part of the plan of care for a patient rehabilitating from a lower extremity injury. Which of the following recommendations would be LEAST effective to minimize electrode resistance?

1. keep the sponge interface well moistened
2. **use small electrodes**
3. maintain even, firm contact with the skin
4. remove hair from the skin

---

**Correct Answer: 2** (Prentice - Therapeutic Modalities p. 112)
Resistance refers to the opposition to electron flow in a conducting material.

1. Water serves as a conductive substance that reduces electrode resistance.

2. **Small electrodes increase electrode resistance, while large electrodes decrease electrode resistance.**

3. Uneven or inadequate contact or pressure from the electrodes increases electrode resistance and can severely limit the effectiveness of electrotherapy.

4. Hair can cause nonuniform conduction at the skin-electrode interface and therefore it is important that the skin be appropriately prepared by cleaning and potentially clipping if necessary.

System Specific: Non-Systems
Content Outline: Equipment & Devices; Therapeutic Modalities

---

## Exam Three: Question 22

A physical therapist reviews the results of a pulmonary function test. Assuming normal values, which of the following measurements would you expect to be the GREATEST?

1. **vital capacity**
2. tidal volume
3. residual volume
4. inspiratory reserve volume

---

**Correct Answer: 1** (Brannon p. 48)
Vital capacity is defined as the amount of air that can be exhaled following a maximal inspiratory effort.

1. **Vital capacity is comprised of inspiratory reserve volume (IRV), tidal volume (TV), and expiratory reserve volume (ERV). Vital capacity is approximately 4,000 - 5,000 mL, but varies directly with height and indirectly with age.**

2. Tidal volume is the amount of air inspired and expired during normal resting ventilation. This volume is approximately 500 mL.

3. The lungs are not emptied of air even after maximal exhalation. The residual volume is the amount of air remaining in the lungs after the expiratory reserve volume has been exhaled. This volume is approximately 900 - 1,200 mL.

4. Inspiratory reserve volume is the volume that can be inhaled in excess of tidal breathing. This volume is approximately 2,300 - 3,000 mL.

System Specific: Cardiovascular/Pulmonary and Lymphatic Systems
Content Outline: Physical Therapy Examination

---

## Exam Three: Question 23

A patient involved in a motor vehicle accident sustains an injury to the posterior cord of the brachial plexus. Which muscle would NOT be affected by the injury?

   1. **infraspinatus**
   2. subscapularis
   3. latissimus dorsi
   4. teres major

> **Correct Answer: 1** (Kendall p. 248)
> The brachial plexus extends from the neck to the axilla and arises from the ventral rami of the fifth through eighth cervical nerves and most of the first thoracic nerve. The brachial plexus innervates the entire upper extremity as well as the muscles of the scapula. Knowledge of its components is critical to proper identification and treatment of upper extremity impairments.
>
>   1. **The infraspinatus muscle is innervated by the suprascapular nerve (C4, C5, C6) that extends from the superior trunk of the brachial plexus.**
>
>   2. The subscapularis is innervated by the upper (C5, C6) and lower subscapular nerve (C5, C6, C7) which extends from the all three trunks of the brachial plexus, via the posterior cord.
>
>   3. The latissimus dorsi is innervated by the thoracodorsal nerve (C6, C7, C8) which extends from all three trunks of the brachial plexus, via the posterior cord.
>
>   4. The teres major is innervated by the lower subscapular nerve (C5, C6, C7) which extends from all three trunks of the brachial plexus, via the posterior cord.
>
> System Specific: Neuromuscular & Nervous Systems
> Content Outline: Physical Therapy Examination

## Exam Three: Question 24

A physical therapist designs a training program for a patient without cardiovascular pathology. The therapist calculates the patient's age-predicted maximal heart rate as 175 beats per minute. Which of the following would be an acceptable target heart rate for the patient during cardiovascular exercise?

   1. 93 beats per minute
   2. **135 beats per minute**
   3. 169 beats per minute
   4. 195 beats per minute

> **Correct Answer: 2** (American College of Sports Medicine p. 455)
> The target heart rate for exercise can be approximated using a percentage of the maximum heart rate, which can be estimated as 220 – age. With this approach, 70-85% of maximum heart rate or 50-70% of maximum oxygen uptake ($VO_{2max}$) is the recommended exercise intensity according to the American College of Sports Medicine. If the maximal heart rate is 175 beats per minute, the target heart rate range is (70% x 175) to (85% x 175), or 123 to 149 beats per minute. Some sources recommend a more broadly defined target heart rate range of 60-90%. In either case, the correct answer would be option 2.
>
>   1. 93 beats per minute is below the recommended range for exercise intensity. 93 beats per minute corresponds to 53% of the maximum heart rate.
>
>   2. **135 beats per minute is within the recommended range for exercise intensity. 135 beats per minute corresponds to 77% of the maximum heart rate.**
>
>   3. 169 beats per minute is above the recommended range for exercise intensity. 169 beats per minute corresponds to 97% of the maximum heart rate.
>
>   4. 195 beats per minute is above the recommended range for exercise intensity. 195 beats per minute corresponds to 111% of the maximum heart rate.
>
> System Specific: Cardiovascular/Pulmonary and Lymphatic Systems
> Content Outline: Interventions

## Exam Three: Question 25

A patient with complete C5 tetraplegia works on a forward raise for pressure relief. The patient utilizes loops that are attached to the back of the wheelchair to assist with the forward raise. Which muscles need to be particularly strong in order for the patient to be successful with the forward raise?

1. brachioradialis, brachialis
2. rhomboids, levator scapulae
3. **biceps, deltoids**
4. triceps, flexor digitorum profundus

**Correct Answer: 3** (Rothstein p. 404)

A patient with C5 tetraplegia would not have muscles innervated below the C5 level. Primary innervations and actions for each of the muscles are listed.

1. The brachioradialis (C5-C6) and brachialis (C5-C6) would both be innervated. The primary action of the brachioradialis and brachialis is to flex the elbow.
2. The rhomboids (C4-C5) and levator scapulae (C3-C5) would both be innervated. The rhomboids adduct and rotate the scapula downward. The levator scapulae elevate and rotate the scapula downward.
3. **The biceps (C5-C6) and deltoids (C5-C6) would both be innervated. The deltoids (anterior, middle, posterior) assist with all shoulder motions with the exception of adduction. The biceps act to flex the shoulder, flex the elbow, and supinate the forearm.**
4. The triceps (C7-C8) and flexor digitorum profundus (C8-T1) would not be innervated in a patient with C5 tetraplegia.

System Specific: Neuromuscular & Nervous Systems
Content Outline: Interventions

## Exam Three: Question 26

A patient sustained a fracture of the acetabulum that was treated with open reduction and internal fixation. The injury occurred in a motor vehicle accident approximately seven weeks ago. Which objective measure would be the MOST influential variable when determining the patient's weight bearing status?

1. visual analogue pain scale rating
2. **radiographic confirmation of bone healing**
3. lower extremity manual muscle testing
4. balance and coordination assessment

**Correct Answer: 2** (Magee p. 57)

The primary determinant of weight bearing status following a fracture is based on the relative stability of the fracture. The amount of time since the injury (i.e., seven weeks) should allow for bone healing to be visible using diagnostic imaging.

1. The pain level following a fracture is not directly correlated with the relative stability of the acetabulum.
2. **An x-ray is a radiographic photograph commonly used to assist with the diagnosis of musculoskeletal problems such as fractures, dislocations, and bone loss. The diagnostic tool provides the physician with the best indicator of the relative stability of the fracture and therefore would be the most influential variable when determining weight bearing status.**
3. A manual muscle test would assess the relative strength of selected muscles, but would not provide information on the relative stability of the fracture.
4. A balance and coordination assessment may be useful when determining an appropriate assistive device or the level of assistance needed, however, this is not directly related to the relative stability of the fracture.

System Specific: Musculoskeletal System
Content Outline: Foundations for Evaluation, Differential Diagnosis, & Prognosis

## Exam Three: Question 27

A patient two weeks status post transtibial amputation is instructed by his physician to remain at rest for two days after contracting bronchitis. The MOST appropriate position for the patient in bed is:

1. supine with a pillow under the patient's knees
2. supine with a pillow under the patient's thighs and knees
3. **supine with the legs extended**
4. sidelying in the fetal position

**Correct Answer: 3** (Seymour p. 145)

It is important for a patient with a transtibial amputation to keep the knee extended in order to prevent shortening of the hamstrings muscles and avoid developing a flexion contracture at the knee.

1. Lying in supine with a pillow under the knees is a comfortable position for the patient after transtibial amputation. However, placing a pillow under the knee puts the knee in a partially flexed position. This promotes the development of hamstrings muscle tightness, which may lead to a flexion contracture at the knee.

2. Lying in supine with a pillow under the thighs puts the hip and knee in a flexed position. This promotes the development of hip flexor and hamstrings muscle tightness, which may lead to flexion contractures at the hip or knee.

3. **The supine position with the legs extended is the most appropriate position since it promotes lengthening of the hip flexors and hamstrings muscles and prevents the development of flexion contractures.**

4. Sidelying in the fetal position places the hips and knees in a flexed position. This promotes the development of hip flexor and hamstrings muscle tightness, which may lead to flexion contractures at the hip or knee.

System Specific: Other Systems
Content Outline: Interventions

## Exam Three: Question 28

A patient with T10 paraplegia is working with a therapist on how to react in the event of a backward fall. The patient is instructed to place one hand behind the head and the other across their lap as seen in the image. This directive will protect the head and:

1. allow the patient to remain within the chair upon landing
2. allow the patient to hold onto one armrest to stabilize the wheelchair
3. **prevent the lower extremities from hitting the patient's face**
4. allow the patient to secure the brake to slow the fall

**Correct Answer: 3** (Pierson p. 167)

Patients that use wheelchairs as their primary mode of mobility should be proficient with all aspects of wheelchair mobility, including a backward fall. Patients with tetraplegia and paraplegia must stabilize their lower extremities during a backward fall to avoid injury secondary to the backward momentum. Patients can also learn how to return the wheelchair to an upright position, however, this is unrealistic for the majority of patients with a complete spinal cord injury.

1. The patient will likely not remain completely within the chair after a backward fall secondary to limited trunk control and lower extremity paralysis.

2. Holding the armrest is a preventative measure to decrease the movement of the lower extremities, not to stabilize the wheelchair.

3. **The primary goal of placing one arm across the lap is to limit the movement of the lower extremities with the forearm so that they do not fall into the patient's face during the backward fall.**

4. Even if the patient is able to reach the brake with the hand placed across the lap, this would not slow the progression of the fall and is not the primary purpose of placing one arm across the lap.

System Specific: Non-Systems
Content Outline: Equipment and Devices; Therapeutic Modalities

## Exam Three: Question 29

A 27-year-old female diagnosed with anterior compartment syndrome reports to an outpatient clinic for physical therapy services. While reviewing the physician referral supplied by the patient, the physical therapist identifies that the referral form is over 90 days old. The MOST appropriate therapist action is:

1. continue with the session since the existing referral is acceptable
2. **attempt to contact the physician's office by telephone to receive verbal orders**
3. send the physician written correspondence requesting an updated referral
4. discontinue the session until the patient secures an updated referral

**Correct Answer: 2** (Nosse p. 217)

Physical therapists should attempt to ensure that physician referrals are as current as possible. This action is a risk management strategy that increases the probability of patients being appropriate candidates for physical therapy services.

1. Ninety days is a significant amount of time and it is possible that the patient's health status or another relevant variable has changed during this period.

2. **Contacting the physician's office by telephone provides the fastest, most direct method to update the referral without further delaying treatment. Relying on a verbal order would not be problematic in this case since the physical therapist already has the original referral.**

3. Sending the physician written correspondence requesting an updated referral would unnecessarily delay physical therapy services.

4. Discontinuing the session until the patient secures an updated referral would delay physical therapy services. The option places the burden for retrieving the referral on the patient and although this is acceptable, the task could likely be handled without difficulty by the physical therapist or the office staff.

System Specific: Non-Systems
Content Outline: Safety and Protection; Professional Responsibilities; Research

## Exam Three: Question 30

A physical therapist assesses the deep tendon reflexes of a patient as part of a lower quarter screening examination. The therapist determines that the right and left patellar tendon reflex and the left Achilles tendon reflex are 2+, while the right Achilles tendon reflex is absent. The clinical condition that could BEST explain this finding is:

1. cerebral palsy
2. multiple sclerosis
3. **peripheral neuropathy**
4. intermittent claudication

**Correct Answer: 3** (Goodman – Differential Diagnosis p. 649)

A reflex is a motor response to a sensory stimulation that can be used to assess the integrity of the nervous system. Deep tendon reflexes (DTR) elicit a muscle contraction when the muscle's tendon is stimulated. A grade of 2+ would be considered a normal response.

1. Cerebral palsy is a neuromuscular disorder of posture and controlled movement, however, the clinical presentation is highly variable based on the area and extent of central nervous system damage. It is unlikely that a reflex would be absent in an upper motor neuron disorder like cerebral palsy.

2. Multiple sclerosis is a chronic autoimmune inflammatory disease of the central nervous system characterized by demyelination of the myelin sheaths that surround nerves within the brain and spinal cord. Symptoms can include visual problems, paresthesias and sensory changes, clumsiness, weakness, ataxia, balance dysfunction, and fatigue. Deep tendon reflexes would not typically be absent with multiple sclerosis since it is an upper motor neuron disorder.

3. **Peripheral neuropathy is a broad term that describes a lesion to a peripheral nerve. Patients with peripheral neuropathy may exhibit motor, sensory, and autonomic changes including extreme sensitivity to touch, loss of sensation, muscle weakness, and loss of vasomotor tone. Deep tendon reflexes may be asymmetrical based on the location of the involved peripheral nerve and usually present as diminished or absent.**

4. Intermittent claudication occurs as a result of insufficient blood supply and ischemia in active muscles. Symptoms most commonly include pain and cramping in muscles distal to the occluded vessel. Deep tendon reflexes would not typically be affected.

System Specific: Neuromuscular & Nervous Systems
Content Outline: Foundations for Evaluation, Differential Diagnosis, & Prognosis

## Exam Three: Question 31

An employee with a disclosed disability informs her employer that she is unable to perform an essential function of her job unless her workstation is modified. Which of the following would provide the employer with a legitimate reason for NOT granting the employee's request?

1. the accommodation would cost hundreds of dollars
2. the accommodation would require an expansion of the employee's present workstation
3. **the accommodation would fundamentally alter the operation of the business**
4. the accommodation would not address the needs of other employees

**Correct Answer: 3** (Pierson p. 348)

The Americans with Disabilities Act was designed to provide a clear and comprehensive national mandate for the elimination of discrimination. Employers are required to make reasonable accommodations for qualified individuals with a disability who satisfy the job-related requirements of a position held or desired.

1. An accommodation that costs hundreds of dollars does not necessarily indicate that the accommodation is unreasonable or creates an "undue hardship" for the employer.

2. Workstation modifications are common and are most often designed to allow a qualified employee or applicant to perform an essential job function.

3. **An accommodation that fundamentally alters the operation of a business would be considered an "undue hardship."**

4. The Americans with Disabilities Act applies primarily, but not exclusively, to "disabled" individuals. It is not necessary to ensure that an accommodation made for a qualified individual addresses the needs of other employees.

System Specific: Non-Systems
Content Outline: Safety and Protection; Professional Responsibilities; Research

## Exam Three: Question 32

A patient is directed to reach for an object beyond their arm's length during therapeutic activities emphasizing core training and balance activities as depicted in the image. The desired response with this activity would be:

1. left trunk elongation, left weight shift, right hip hiking
2. right trunk elongation, right weight shift, right hip hiking
3. left trunk elongation, left weight shift, left hip hiking
4. **right trunk elongation, right weight shift, left hip hiking**

**Correct Answer: 4** (Gillen p. 171)

When treating patients, therapists must be cognizant of the goals of specific activities and use therapeutic interventions that relate to the goal. For example, reaching above shoulder level will produce trunk elongation and weight shift ipsilaterally and reaching towards the floor will produce trunk elongation and weight shift contralaterally.

1. A patient that presents with left trunk elongation, left weight shift, and right hip hiking is likely reaching for an object just beyond their reach at shoulder height or higher on their left side.

2. A patient that presents with right trunk elongation and right weight shift would typically be reaching for an object beyond arm's length at shoulder level or higher on their right side. They would, however, present with left hip hiking, not right hip hiking.

3. A patient that presents with left trunk elongation and left weight shift would typically be reaching for an object beyond arm's length at shoulder level or higher on their left side. They would, however, present with right hip hiking, not left hip hiking.

4. **A patient that presents with right trunk elongation, right weight shift, and left hip hiking is likely reaching for an object just beyond reach at shoulder height or higher on their right side.**

System Specific: Neuromuscular and Nervous Systems
Content Outline: Interventions

## Exam Three: Question 33

A physical therapist attempts to palpate the tibialis posterior tendon. To facilitate palpation of this structure the therapist should:

1. **ask the patient to invert and plantar flex the foot**
2. ask the patient to evert and dorsifex the foot
3. ask the patient to invert and dorsiflex the foot
4. passively evert and plantar flex the foot

**Correct Answer: 1** (Kendall p. 411)

A tendon is a band of dense fibrous tissue forming the termination of a muscle which attaches the muscle to a bone. A tendon becomes more prominent when the associated muscle is active. The tendon of the tibialis posterior can be palpated posterior and inferior to the medial malleolus.

1. **The tibialis posterior originates on the interosseous membrane, lateral portion of the posterior surface of the tibia, and proximal two thirds of the medial surface of the fibula. The muscle acts to invert the foot and assists with plantar flexion of the ankle joint. As a result, the tendon is more prominent with active inversion and plantar flexion.**

2. Eversion and dorsiflexion are opposite of the action of the tibialis posterior. As a result, the active movement would not facilitate palpation of the muscle's tendon.

3. The tibialis anterior acts to dorsiflex the ankle joint and assists with inversion of the foot. As a result, the tendon is more prominent with active dorsiflexion and inversion. The tendon of the muscle is easily palpated where it crosses the ankle joint to its insertion on the medial aspect of the base of the first metatarsal and the medial cuneiform bone.

4. Passive movement would not be as desirable as active movement to facilitate palpation of the tendon since muscular activity is necessary to make the tendon prominent. In addition, the tibialis posterior inverts the foot and assists with plantar flexion of the ankle joint.

System Specific: Musculoskeletal System
Content Outline: Physical Therapy Examination

## Exam Three: Question 34

A physical therapist participating in a research project uses a simple random sample to draw a sample from the population. By selecting this type of sample, the therapist ensures:

1. the data collected from the sample will be normally distributed
2. the sample size will be large
3. the sample will have proportional representation from all parts of the population
4. **that every member of the population has an equal opportunity of being chosen**

**Correct Answer: 4** (Portney p. 148)

Probability samples are created through a process of random selection. Each selection is independent and every member of the population has an equal chance of being selected for the sample.

1. Simple random sampling does not ensure that the data collected will be normally distributed. The shape of the distribution of the data collected from the sample is independent of the type of sample.

2. Simple random sampling does not determine the size of the sample.

3. To ensure that the sample will have proportional representation from all parts of the population, the therapist would create a proportional stratified sample.

4. **A simple random sample is unbiased; each member of the population has an equal chance of being chosen.**

System Specific: Non-Systems
Content Outline: Safety and Protection; Professional Responsibilities; Research

## Exam Three: Question 35

The goals for a patient status post total knee arthroplasty include general conditioning and independent household mobility. Which component of the patient's treatment would be the MOST appropriate to delegate to a physical therapy aide?

1. stair training
2. progressive gait training with a straight cane
3. patient education regarding the surgical procedure
4. **ambulation with a walker for endurance**

**Correct Answer: 4** (Guide to Physical Therapist Practice)
A physical therapy aide is a non-licensed worker, trained under the direction of a physical therapist, who requires continuous on-site supervision. A physical therapist is required, before delegating any component of a treatment plan, to have an understanding of the physical therapy aide's level of training as well as the patient's current abilities.

1. Stair training is a skilled activity that requires the constant supervision of a licensed physical therapist. The term "training" implies that the patient is being taught a new skill. Delegating this type of skilled activity to a physical therapy aide is inappropriate and would potentially jeopardize patient safety.

2. Progressive gait training implies that there will be some progression within the activity based on the patient's performance. The decision to progress a patient during an activity is the responsibility of the physical therapist and would be inappropriate for a physical therapy aide.

3. Patient education regarding the surgical procedure requires an individual to possess specific knowledge of the actual surgical procedure performed by the surgeon. A physical therapy aide does not possess the educational background to provide the patient with this information.

4. **A physical therapist, and in some jurisdictions a physical therapist assistant, may delegate ambulation activities to an aide if the physical therapist feels the aide's training is adequate to complete the activity. This decision would be heavily influenced by the patient's current status and competence with ambulation. Ambulation for endurance implies that the patient already possesses basic competence with the activity.**

System Specific: Musculoskeletal System
Content Outline: Interventions

## Exam Three: Question 36

A physical therapist examines the heart sounds of a 48-year-old female status post coronary artery bypass graft. When auscultating, the therapist identifies the heart sound associated with closing of the mitral and tricuspid valves. This heart sound BEST describes:

1. **S1**
2. S2
3. S3
4. S4

**Correct Answer: 1** (Hillegass p. 105)
The heart sounds are the noises generated by the beating heart and the resultant flow of blood through it. The therapist uses a stethoscope to listen for these sounds, which provide important information about the condition of the heart.

1. **The first heart sound, S1 (the lub of the lub-dub), is associated with the closing of the mitral and tricuspid valves, corresponding to the onset of ventricular systole.**

2. The second heart sound, S2, (the dub of the lub-dub), is associated with the closing of the aortic and pulmonary valves, corresponding to the onset of ventricular diastole.

3. A third heart sound, S3, occurs early in diastole while the ventricle is rapidly filling. The sound occurs immediately after S2 (lub-dub-dub). The S3 sound may occur in healthy children and young adults, and is referred to as a physiologic third heart sound. It also indicates a loss of ventricular compliance in the presence of heart disease or heart failure. In this case, it is called a ventricular gallop.

4. A fourth heart sound, S4, occurs late in diastole just before S1 (la-lub-dub) and is associated with atrial contraction and an increased resistance to ventricular filling. The heart sound is referred to as an atrial gallop. The sound is common in patients with hypertension, a history of myocardial infarction or coronary bypass surgery.

System Specific: Cardiovascular/Pulmonary and Lymphatic Systems
Content Outline: Physical Therapy Examination

## Exam Three: Question 37

During a balance assessment of a patient with left hemiplegia, it is noted that in sitting the patient requires minimal assistance to maintain the position and cannot accept any additional challenge. The physical therapist would appropriately document the patient's sitting balance as:

1. normal
2. good
3. fair
4. **poor**

> **Correct Answer: 4** (O'Sullivan p. 254)
> Sitting balance can be graded in an objective manner by using a scale that ranges from poor to normal. A patient that requires assistance to maintain a sitting position would be graded as having poor sitting balance.
>
> 1. A grade of normal is indicative of a person that is able to sit unsupported, move in and out of the base of support, and accept maximal challenge without loss of balance.
> 2. A grade of good is indicative of a person that is able to sit unsupported, move in and out of the base of support, and accept some challenge without loss of balance.
> 3. A grade of fair is indicative of a person that is able to maintain their balance in sitting unsupported, but cannot accept any challenge or go outside of their base of support without loss of balance.
> 4. A grade of poor is indicative of a person that is unable to maintain their balance in sitting without external support or assistance.
>
> System Specific: Neuromuscular & Nervous Systems
> Content Outline: Physical Therapy Examination

## Exam Three: Question 38

A physical therapist is treating a patient with a head injury who begins to perseverate. In order to refocus the patient and achieve the desired therapeutic outcome, the therapist should:

1. focus on the topic of perseveration for a short period of time in order to appease the patient
2. **guide the patient into an interesting new activity and reward successful completion of the task**
3. take the patient back to his room for quiet time and attempt to resume therapy once he has stopped perseverating
4. continue with repetitive verbal cues to cease perseveration

> **Correct Answer: 2** (O'Sullivan p. 723)
> Perseveration is the continued repetition of a word, phrase or movement. Initiating a new activity during therapy may allow the patient to redirect attention and subsequently receive positive reinforcement for attending to the selected task.
>
> 1. It is not necessary to attempt to appease the patient since the patient cannot independently move beyond whatever they are perseverating on. Staying with the topic will not assist in moving forward.
> 2. **Patients with a lesion in the premotor or prefrontal cortex often exhibit perseveration. Since the patient typically continues the repetition of a word, phrase or movement after the cessation of the original stimulus, the best intervention would be to redirect the patient away from the current activity.**
> 3. The patient will not benefit from "quiet time" since the patient is not perseverating due to a behavioral issue. Redirecting the patient may successfully allow the patient to move forward and continue with therapy without interruption.
> 4. Verbal cueing is not an effective technique to cease perseveration. The patient typically requires a redirection of their attention to another activity or environment.
>
> System Specific: Neuromuscular & Nervous Systems
> Content Outline: Interventions

## Exam Three: Question 39

A patient rehabilitating from congestive heart failure is examined in physical therapy. During the examination the patient begins to complain of pain. The MOST IMMEDIATE physical therapist action is to:

1. notify the nursing staff to administer pain medication
2. contact the referring physician
3. discontinue the treatment session
4. **ask the patient to describe the location and severity of the pain**

> **Correct Answer: 4** (Magee p. 5)
> Congestive heart failure is characterized by the inability of the heart to maintain adequate cardiac output. Before the physical therapist can adequately respond to the patient's report of pain, it is essential to gather additional information.
>
> 1. Administering pain medication is premature until more information is known about the pain. Once additional information is collected, the nursing staff will be able to make a more informed decision.
>
> 2. Contacting the physician is premature until more information is known about the location and severity of the pain. This type of detailed information is necessary to provide the physician with a better sense of what the patient is currently experiencing.
>
> 3. Discontinuing the treatment session based on a subjective report of pain is a viable option particularly given the patient's diagnosis, however, the physical therapist would need to gather additional information about the pain prior to making a definitive decision.
>
> 4. **Having the patient describe the location and severity of the pain is the most immediate action the physical therapist should take. The information can be collected in a timely manner and may be useful to determine the relative seriousness of the patient's subjective report of pain.**
>
> System Specific: Cardiovascular/Pulmonary and Lymphatic Systems
> Content Outline: Physical Therapy Examination

## Exam Three: Question 40

A physical therapist reviews the medical record of a patient diagnosed with chronic obstructive pulmonary disease. The medical record indicates that the patient's current condition is consistent with chronic respiratory acidosis. Which testing procedure was likely used to identify this condition?

1. **arterial blood gas analysis**
2. pulmonary function testing
3. graded exercise testing
4. pulse oximetry

> **Correct Answer: 1** (Paz p. 60)
> Arterial blood gas analysis (ABG) provides information on the functioning of the lungs (i.e., oxygenation and elimination of carbon dioxide). Respiratory acidosis is characterized by elevated $PaCO_2$ and below normal pH due to hypoventilation.
>
> 1. **Abnormal acid-base balance will result in respiratory alkalosis, respiratory acidosis, metabolic alkalosis or metabolic acidosis depending on the cause. These conditions can become life threatening without intervention to normalize the pH within the body, which is typically 7.35-7.45. ABG analysis provides values for $PaCO_2$, $PaO_2$, $O_2$ saturation, and $CO_2$.**
>
> 2. Pulmonary function testing is a series of measurements that measure and evaluate how well the lungs take in and release air and how well they move oxygen into and remove carbon dioxide from the blood. There are reference values based on height, weight, sex, and age and results are considered abnormal if they are not within 80% of these reference values for a given test.
>
> 3. Graded exercise testing is used to measure the response of the heart to a graded increase in oxygen demand. Exercise occurs using a systematic protocol that can assess other variables such as evaluation of arrhythmias, functional capacity, and significance of coronary artery disease.
>
> 4. An oximeter is a photoelectric device used to determine the oxygen saturation of blood. The device is most commonly applied to the finger or the ear. Oximetry is often used by therapists to assess activity tolerance.
>
> System Specific: Cardiovascular/Pulmonary and Lymphatic Systems
> Content Outline: Foundations for Evaluation, Differential Diagnosis, & Prognosis

## Exam Three: Question 41 ✗

A physical therapist employed in a work hardening program performs an examination on a patient diagnosed with fibromyalgia. During the examination the therapist identifies an inconsistency between the measured lumbar range of motion and the amount of lumbar range of motion observed while lifting a milk crate from the floor to a table. The MOST appropriate therapist action is:

1. **avoid discussing the identified inconsistency with the patient**
2. confront the patient with the identified inconsistency
3. discuss the identified inconsistency with the referring physician
4. discharge the patient from physical therapy

**Correct Answer: 1** (O'Sullivan p. 1127)

Symptom magnification is best identified by inconsistencies in the presentation of function. Physical therapists should be extremely cautious to avoid labeling patients as "symptom magnifiers" or "malingerers" without adequate evidence to support their hypothesis.

1. **There is not enough information presented to form a definitive conclusion and therefore the physical therapist should not address the observation with the patient. The therapist would be better served by continuing the examination and gathering additional information during future treatment sessions.**
2. The physical therapist has identified a given inconsistency, however, it would be inappropriate to immediately confront the patient based on a single observation.
3. There are a variety of legitimate reasons why a physical therapist could observe an inconsistency such as the described scenario. As a result, the finding does not warrant consultation with the physician.
4. There is not any presented information that would suggest the patient is not a candidate for physical therapy.

System Specific: Neuromuscular and Nervous Systems
Content Outline: Physical Therapy Examination

## Exam Three: Question 42

A former patient calls to ask for advice after injuring his low back in a work related accident. The patient explains that he cannot bend down and touch his toes without severe pain and has muscle spasms throughout the entire low back. The physical therapist works in a state without direct access, but would like to help the former patient. The MOST appropriate response would be:

1. explain to the patient that you would be happy to treat him, however, since you have not completed a formal examination it would be unfair to prescribe treatment
2. arrange a time for the patient to come into your clinic for immediate treatment
3. prescribe flexion exercises and ice every three hours
4. **refer the patient to a qualified physician**

**Correct Answer: 4** (Guide for Professional Conduct)

The *Guide for Professional Conduct* published by the American Physical Therapy Association states: "A physical therapist shall make professional judgments that are in the patient/client's best interests."

1. The physical therapist correctly recognizes that the patient cannot be treated without a formal examination, however, needs to also consider that the patient was hurt in a work related accident and works in a state without direct access.
2. Arranging a time for treatment without first completing an examination is inappropriate.
3. Prescribing exercises of any type without adequate clinical justification can be considered a negligent act.
4. **Referring the patient to a physician will allow the patient to receive a thorough examination, and if indicated, a referral to physical therapy.**

System Specific: Musculoskeletal System
Content Outline: Foundations for Evaluation, Differential Diagnosis, and Prognosis

## Exam Three: Question 43

A physical therapist treats a patient with superficial partial-thickness burns to the anterior surface of his lower legs. In an attempt to assist the patient to control the pain associated with the burns, the therapist rewards the patient with a lengthy rest period after successfully completing an exercise sequence. This type of psychological approach is MOST representative of:

1. distraction
2. extinction
3. classical conditioning
4. **operant conditioning**

**Correct Answer: 4** (Richard p. 486)

Physical therapists often use specific teaching and learning strategies to influence or shape patient behavior. Many of the most common strategies employed are derived from the field of educational psychology. Physical therapists should be familiar with commonly used teaching and learning strategies and recognize opportunities to integrate them into patient care activities.

1. Distraction is a general term that refers to something that diverts attention.

2. Extinction refers to removing selected variables that reinforce a specific behavior. It can also refer to the lack of any consequence following a behavior. The theory is that when a behavior is inconsequential, producing neither favorable nor unfavorable consequences, it will occur with less frequency.

3. Classical conditioning is a process where learning occurs when an unconditioned stimulus is repeatedly preceded by a neutral stimulus. The neutral stimulus serves as a conditioned stimulus and the learned reaction that results is termed the conditioned response.

4. **Operant conditioning is learning that takes place when the learner recognizes the connection between the behavior (completing an exercise progression) and its consequences (lengthy rest period).**

System Specific: Other Systems
Content Outline: Interventions

## Exam Three: Question 44

A physical therapist reviews a research study that examines knee flexion range of motion two weeks following arthroscopic surgery. Assuming knee flexion range of motion two weeks after arthroscopic surgery is a normally distributed variable, what percentage of patients in the population would achieve a goniometric measurement value between the mean and one standard deviation above the mean?

1. 14%
2. **34%**
3. 48%
4. 68%

**Correct Answer: 2** (Portney p. 399)

Because of the standard properties of the normal distribution, it is possible to determine the proportional areas under the curve represented by the standard deviation. 34.13% of the area under the curve of a normal distribution is bounded by the mean and 1 standard deviation above or below the mean.

1. 14% is the approximate area under the normal curve between 1 and 2 standard deviations above or below the mean.

2. **34% is the approximate area under the normal curve bounded by 1 standard deviation above or below the mean.**

3. 48% is the approximate area under the normal curve bounded by 2 standard deviations above or below the mean.

4. 68% is the approximate area under the normal curve bounded by 1 standard deviation below the mean and 1 standard deviation above the mean.

System Specific: Non-Systems
Content Outline: Safety and Protection; Professional Responsibilities; Research

## Exam Three: Question 45

A physical therapist uses intermittent compression to treat a patient with an acute ankle sprain. The patient is positioned in supine with the leg elevated on a 40 degree wedge. The therapist uses an inflation pressure of 50 mm Hg with an on:off time of 40 seconds on and 20 seconds off. The treatment time is scheduled for 20 minutes. After five minutes of treatment the patient reports some discomfort in the ankle. The MOST appropriate modification to the current treatment parameters would be:

1. increase the inflation pressure
2. **increase the off time**
3. increase the total treatment time
4. increase the elevation of the leg

**Correct Answer: 2** (Prentice - Therapeutic Modalities p. 530)
Intermittent compression is often used in combination with elevation to limit edema following an acute ankle sprain. The physical therapist should modify the parameters of the intervention based on relevant subjective data such as a report of discomfort.

1. Increasing the inflation pressure would likely serve to exacerbate the patient's pain level.

2. **Increasing the off time greater than the current 20 second interval would provide the patient with a greater rest period and may therefore decrease the patient's discomfort.**

3. Increasing the total treatment time without modifying other parameters (e.g., on:off time, inflation pressure) would likely result in the level of discomfort remaining the same or worsening as the session continues.

4. Increasing the elevation of the leg beyond 40 degrees would not likely decrease the patient's discomfort without concurrently decreasing another treatment parameter.

System Specific: Non-Systems
Content Outline: Equipment & Devices; Therapeutic Modalities

## Exam Three: Question 46

A physical therapist examines the electrocardiogram of a patient during exercise. What change in the electrocardiogram would be most indicative of myocardial ischemia?

1. P wave changes
2. PR interval changes
3. QRS complex changes
4. **ST segment changes**

**Correct Answer: 4** (Brannon p. 183)
ST segment depression is the most common manifestation of exercise-induced myocardial ischemia.

1. The P wave is normally the first wave of the ECG tracing and represents depolarization of the atria. Normally, the P wave is upright, rounded, and symmetric with only one P wave for each QRS complex. Abnormal configuration of P waves occurs in various conditions including wandering atrial pacemaker, premature atrial complexes, atrial tachycardia, atrial fibrillation, atrial flutter, and nodal or junctional arrhythmias.

2. The PR interval represents the time (in seconds) from the beginning of the P wave (onset of atrial depolarization) to the beginning of the QRS complex (onset of ventricular depolarization). The normal PR interval duration range is from 0.12 seconds - 0.20 seconds, measured from the initial deflection of the P wave to the initial deflection of the QRS complex. A prolonged PR interval can correspond to impaired AV node conduction and results in various types of heart block.

3. The QRS complex represents depolarization of the ventricles. Abnormal configuration of the QRS complex occurs in various conditions including premature ventricular contractions, ventricular tachycardia, and ventricular fibrillation.

4. **The ST segment is the portion of the ECG tracing from the end of the S wave to the beginning of the T wave. It represents the initiating of ventricular repolarization and is a sensitive indicator of ischemia of the ventricles. The standard criterion for a positive exercise test is greater than or equal to 1 mm of horizontal or downsloping ST segment depression.**

System Specific: Cardiovascular/Pulmonary and Lymphatic Systems
Content Outline: Foundations for Evaluation, Differential Diagnosis, & Prognosis

## Exam Three: Question 47

A physical therapist treats a patient diagnosed with chronic arterial disease. The patient exhibits cool skin, decreased sensitivity to temperature changes, and intermittent claudication with activity. The primary treatment goal is to increase the patient's ambulation distance. The MOST appropriate ambulation parameters to facilitate achievement of the goal are:

1. **short duration, frequent intervals**
2. short duration, infrequent intervals
3. long duration, frequent intervals
4. long duration, infrequent intervals

**Correct Answer: 1** (Kisner p. 830)

Intermittent claudication occurs as a result of insufficient blood supply and ischemia in active muscles. The condition occurs with activity, subsides during periods of rest, and as a result can limit the duration of exercise activities. Symptoms most commonly include pain and cramping in muscles distal to the occluded vessel.

1. **Treadmill and track walking are the most effective modes of exercise to reduce claudication. The initial workloads are set to elicit claudication symptoms within three to five minutes. This is followed by a period of standing or sitting to allow symptoms to resolve. The exercise-rest-exercise pattern is repeated throughout the exercise session. Because of the short duration of each bout of exercise before the onset of symptoms, more frequent exercise bouts are indicated.**

2. Because the patient can only exercise for shorter durations before the onset of symptoms, exercising at infrequent intervals would not allow the patient to progress toward the goal of increasing ambulation distance.

3. Patients who experience claudication from chronic arterial disease usually can only walk for short periods before the onset of pain limits their ability to continue exercise. Therefore, long duration of exercise with frequent intervals is not a realistic plan to progress toward the goal of increasing ambulation distance.

4. Although the infrequent intervals may provide the patient with less total activity, the long duration of the exercise remains problematic.

System Specific: Other Systems
Content Outline: Interventions

## Exam Three: Question 48

A patient rehabilitating from a bone marrow transplant is referred to physical therapy for instruction in an exercise program. The physical therapist plans to use oxygen saturation measurements to gain additional objective data related to the patient's exercise tolerance. Assuming the patient's oxygen saturation was measured as 95% at rest, which of the following guidelines would be the MOST appropriate?

1. discontinue exercise when the patient's oxygen saturation is below 95%
2. **discontinue exercise when the patient's oxygen saturation is below 90%**
3. discontinue exercise when the patient's oxygen saturation is below 85%
4. discontinue exercise when the patient's oxygen saturation is below 80%

**Correct Answer: 2** (Paz p. 441)

An oxygen saturation at rest greater than 95% is considered to be within normal limits. A rate of 90% or less is often used as a guideline to discontinue exercise activities. Supplemental oxygen may be indicated if oxygen saturation is 90% or less.

1. An oxygen saturation of 95% is within normal limits.

2. **When oxygen saturation falls below 90% exercise should be discontinued and the patient should rest. This corresponds to a partial pressure of oxygen ($PaO_2$) of approximately 60 mm Hg, which represents a state of arterial hypoxemia. This is the most common indication for supplemental oxygen therapy.**

3. A patient with an oxygen saturation of 85% is in a state of hypoxemia. Exercise should have been terminated before this level of hypoxemia was reached.

4. A patient with an oxygen saturation of 80% is in a severe hypoxemic state. Exercise should have been terminated before this level of hypoxemia was reached.

System Specific: Other Systems
Content Outline: Interventions

## Exam Three: Question 49

A physical therapist reviews a patient's medical history prior to administering intermittent compression. Which of the following conditions would be considered a contraindication to the use of this mechanical device?

1. venous stasis ulcer
2. **acute pulmonary edema**
3. intermittent claudication
4. lymphedema

**Correct Answer: 2** (Prentice - Therapeutic Modalities p. 537)
Intermittent compression is effective in controlling edema since it increases the extravascular hydrostatic pressure and circulation. Intermittent compression is most commonly used to control edema due to venous insufficiency or lymphatic dysfunction.

1. Venous stasis ulcers occur secondary to inadequate functioning of the venous system resulting in inadequate circulation and eventual tissue damage and ulceration. Intermittent compression improves venous circulation and facilitates the healing of previously formed ulcers.
2. **Acute pulmonary edema should not be treated with intermittent compression since the shift of fluid from the peripheral to the central circulation may significantly increase stress on the heart.**
3. Intermittent claudication occurs when blood flow is not adequate to meet the demand of the peripheral tissue, most often during activity. The result is ischemia which produces symptoms such as muscle pain, numbness, tingling, and fatigue. Intermittent claudication would not be a contraindication for intermittent compression.
4. Lymphedema refers to an abnormal accumulation of tissue fluid in the interstitial spaces. Stagnation of the tissue fluid promotes the inflammatory response and increases the probability of infection. Intermittent compression is commonly used to treat lymphedema.

System Specific: Non-Systems
Content Outline: Equipment & Devices; Therapeutic Modalities

## Exam Three: Question 50

A 62-year-old female is restricted from physical therapy for two days following surgical insertion of a urinary catheter. This type of procedure is MOST commonly performed with a:

1. condom catheter
2. Foley catheter
3. **suprapubic catheter**
4. Swan-Ganz catheter

**Correct Answer: 3** (Pierson p. 284)
An internal or indwelling catheter is inserted through the urethra and into the bladder. Females can utilize internal catheters, while males can use internal or external catheters.

1. An external catheter is applied over the shaft of the penis and is held in place by a padded strap or adhesive tape. The catheter has no practical application for females.
2. A Foley catheter is an indwelling urinary tract catheter that has a balloon attachment at one end. The balloon, which is filled with air or sterile water, must be deflated before the catheter can be removed. The catheter does not require surgical insertion.
3. **A suprapubic catheter is an indwelling urinary catheter that is surgically inserted directly into the patient's bladder. Insertion of a suprapubic catheter is performed under general anesthesia.**
4. A Swan-Ganz catheter is a soft, flexible catheter that is inserted through a vein into the pulmonary artery. The device is used to provide continuous measurements of pulmonary artery pressure.

System Specific: Other Systems
Content Outline: Foundations for Evaluation, Differential Diagnosis, & Prognosis

## Exam Three: Question 51 ✗

A physical therapist instructs a patient in residual limb wrapping. Which bandage would be the MOST appropriate to utilize for a patient with a transfemoral amputation?

1. two-inch
2. four-inch
3. **six-inch**
4. eight-inch

**Correct Answer: 3** (Seymour p. 132)
A six-inch bandage is used to wrap the residual limb of a patient with a transfemoral amputation. The bandage should be applied in a figure-eight pattern using angular turns. The bandage provides a pressure gradient that is greatest distally with decreasing pressure proximally. The bandage should be applied well into the groin area to avoid an adductor roll and should be rewrapped approximately every four hours in order to maintain proper pressure and fit.

1. A two-inch bandage would not be appropriate for wrapping the residual limb of a patient following transfemoral amputation due to the large surface area. The limited width of the bandage may have a tendency to cause a tourniquet effect.

2. A four-inch bandage would be appropriate when wrapping the residual limb of a patient following a transtibial amputation, however, would not be the most appropriate for a transfemoral amputation.

3. **A patient with a transfemoral amputation should wrap the residual limb with two to three six-inch bandages and include a hip spica to assist with securing the bandage. The six-inch bandage is appropriately sized to cover the necessary surface area of the thigh and waist.**

4. An eight-inch bandage is too wide for use on a typical residual limb. The patient would be at an increased risk for multiple wrinkles and folds since the residual limb would not possess the necessary surface area to accommodate the eight-inch bandage.

System Specific: Other Systems
Content Outline: Interventions

## Exam Three: Question 52

A physical therapist measures body composition using skinfold measurements prior to initiating an exercise program. When measuring the abdominal skinfold the MOST appropriate method is:

1. **utilize a vertical fold approximately 2 cm to the right of the umbilicus**
2. utilize a horizontal fold approximately 2 cm to the right of the umbilicus
3. utilize a vertical fold approximately 2 cm to the left of the umbilicus
4. utilize a horizontal fold approximately 2 cm to the left of the umbilicus

**Correct Answer: 1** (American College of Sports Medicine p. 269)
Anthropometry studies body dimensions and includes the use of skinfold measurements. The theory associated with skinfold measurements is that the amount of subcutaneous fat is proportional to the total amount of body fat. The exact proportion of subcutaneous to total fat varies with gender, age, and ethnicity. Acceptable skinfold sites include the biceps, triceps, abdominal, suprailiac, thigh, chest, midaxillary, medial calf, and subscapular areas. Each site has specific guidelines for attaining measurements in order to maximize consistency and decrease measurement error. A healthy range of body fat is 12-18% for males and 18-23% for females.

1. **The abdominal skinfold site utilizes a vertical fold approximately 2 cm to the right of the umbilicus.**

2. The abdominal skinfold requires the use of a vertical fold and not a horizontal fold.

3. All skinfold measurements are made using the right side of the body.

4. The abdominal skinfold requires the use of a vertical fold using the right side of the body.

System Specific: Musculoskeletal System
Content Outline: Physical Therapy Examination

## Exam Three: Question 53

A physical therapist observes that a patient has an exaggerated heel strike on the left during ambulation activities. Which term is MOST consistent with heel strike using Rancho Los Amigos nomenclature?

1. terminal swing
2. loading response
3. **initial contact**
4. midstance

**Correct Answer: 3** (Levangie p. 526)

The phases of gait are classified based on either points in time (traditional terminology) or periods of time (Rancho Los Amigos terminology). It is important for physical therapists to be familiar with both sets of terminology. Standard terminology includes heel strike, foot flat, midstance, heel off, toe off, acceleration, midswing, and deceleration. Rancho Los Amigos terminology includes initial contact, loading response, midstance, terminal stance, pre-swing, initial swing, midswing, and terminal swing.

1. Terminal swing begins when the tibia is perpendicular to the floor and ends when the foot touches the ground.

2. Loading response corresponds to the amount of time between initial contact and the beginning of the swing phase for the other leg.

3. **Initial contact refers to the beginning of the stance phase when the foot touches the ground.**

4. Midstance corresponds to the point in stance phase when the other foot is off the floor until the body is directly over the stance limb.

System Specific: Musculoskeletal System
Content Outline: Physical Therapy Examination

## Exam Three: Question 54

A physical therapist obtains the past medical history of a patient recently referred to physical therapy after being diagnosed with adhesive capsulitis. Which medical condition is associated with an increased incidence of adhesive capsulitis?

1. **diabetes mellitus**
2. hemophilia
3. peripheral vascular disease
4. osteomalacia

**Correct Answer: 1** (Goodman – Pathology p. 494)

Adhesive capsulitis refers to an inflammation and adherence of the articular capsule resulting in limited joint play and restricted active and passive movement. The condition is more common in women than in men and tends to appear in the fourth, fifth, and sixth decades of life.

1. **Diabetes mellitus is a group of metabolic diseases characterized by high blood sugar levels that result from defects in insulin secretion, the actions of insulin, or both. Patients with diabetes mellitus have an increased incidence of adhesive capsulitis and often experience a longer duration of symptoms and greater limitation of motion.**

2. Hemophilia is a bleeding disorder of genetic etiology. It is a sex-linked autosomal recessive trait. Patients with hemophilia are prone to hemarthrosis, intramuscular hemorrhage, and secondary complications from hematomas. The condition is not associated with an increased incidence of adhesive capsulitis.

3. Peripheral vascular disease refers to any disease or pathology of the circulatory system outside of the brain and heart. The disease is characterized by narrowing of the arteries, and reduced blood flow to the legs, arms, brain and other organs. The cause, in most cases, is atherosclerosis. The condition is not associated with an increased incidence of adhesive capsulitis.

4. Osteomalacia refers to softening of the bone without loss of bone matrix. There is insufficient mineralization of the bone matrix normally caused by insufficient calcium absorption and increased renal phosphorus losses. Symptoms include bone pain, aching, fatigue, and periarticular tenderness. The condition is not associated with an increased incidence of adhesive capsulitis.

System Specific: Other Systems
Content Outline: Foundations for Evaluation, Differential Diagnosis, & Prognosis

## Exam Three: Question 55

A physical therapist notices that a patient with a transfemoral amputation consistently takes a longer step with the prosthetic limb than the contralateral limb. The MOST likely cause of the deviation is:

1. weak abdominal muscles
2. **hip flexion contracture**
3. weak residual limb
4. fear and insecurity

**Correct Answer: 2** (Seymour p. 232)
A hip flexion contracture on the prosthetic side can result in an uneven step length. Hip flexion contractures are the most common type of contracture following a transfemoral amputation. Activities such as prone lying can decrease the incidence of developing the contracture.

1. A patient with weak abdominal muscles may have difficulty maintaining standard step length secondary to weakness of the trunk and inadequate stability. The physical therapist would not tend to observe an increased step length secondary to weakened abdominals.
2. **A hip flexion contracture would cause decreased hip extension during late stance on the prosthetic side allowing for a shorter step on the uninvolved side and a longer step with the prosthetic limb.**
3. A patient with a weak residual limb would not typically take a longer step with the prosthetic limb since the hip flexors would be weak and unable to create the necessary force. A weak limb would typically result in a shorter step on the prosthetic side or the use of compensatory techniques (vaulting or circumduction) to advance the prosthesis.
4. A patient that exhibits fear and insecurity would typically demonstrate an overall shorter step length bilaterally. The patient may exhibit a shuffling gait in order to minimize single stance phase on either lower extremity.

System Specific: Musculoskeletal System
Content Outline: Physical Therapy Examination

## Exam Three: Question 56

A physical therapist designs a research study that examines body composition as a function of aerobic exercise and diet. Which method of data collection would provide the therapist with the MOST valid measurement of body composition?

1. anthropometric measurements
2. bioelectrical impedance
3. **hydrostatic weighing**
4. skinfold measurements

**Correct Answer: 3** (American College of Sports Medicine p. 268)
Body composition is defined as the relative percentage of body weight that is comprised of fat and fat-free tissue. There are multiple methods for testing the percentage of body fat including hydrostatic weighing, skinfold measurements, plethysmography, body mass index (BMI), and bioelectrical impedance analysis.

1. Common anthropometric measurements used for adults include height, weight, BMI, waist-to-hip ratio, and percentage of body fat. These measures are then compared to reference standards to assess items such as weight status and the risk for various diseases.
2. Bioelectric impedance measures body composition by using electrical current to determine the resistance or opposition to current flow. The technique is based on the principle that resistance to electrical current is inversely related to the composition of water within the body. Limitations include the requisite hydration status of the patient and the ability of the examiner to follow the established testing protocol.
3. **Hydrostatic weighing calculates the density of the body by immersing a person in water and measuring the amount of water that becomes displaced. The percentage of body fat is then determined by calculating the measured amount of water displaced in an equation based on Archimedes' principle. This measurement technique is considered the criterion or gold standard for determining body composition. Limitations include the relative availability and expense of the necessary equipment and the amount of time needed to administer the technique.**
4. Skinfold measurements can be used to determine the overall percentage of body fat through the measurement of nine standardized sites. The theory associated with skinfold measurements is that the amount of subcutaneous fat is proportional to the total amount of body fat. Limitations of this method include the availability of an experienced examiner as well as variance from the standards based on gender, age, and ethnicity.

System Specific: Other Systems
Content Outline: Physical Therapy Examination

## Exam Three: Question 57

A physical therapist examines a patient diagnosed with post-polio syndrome. Which of the following areas is the LEAST likely to be affected based on the patient's diagnosis?

1. strength
2. **sensation**
3. endurance
4. functional mobility

**Correct Answer: 2** (Goodman - Pathology p. 1624)

Post-polio syndrome is a term used to describe symptoms that occur years after the onset of poliomyelitis. The condition is characterized by a weakening of the muscles that were originally affected by polio. Symptoms include progressive muscle weakness, fatigue, and muscle atrophy.

1. Patients with post-polio syndrome experience a decrease in strength. This finding may be related to the degeneration of individual nerve terminals in the motor units that remain after the initial illness.

2. **The polio virus attacks specific neurons in the brainstem and anterior horn cells of the spinal cord. As a result, sensation is not typically affected.**

3. Endurance is compromised in patients with post-polio syndrome secondary to the loss of strength, vasomotor abnormalities, joint pain, and myalgias.

4. Functional mobility will decrease as a result of the patient's loss of strength and endurance. Pain will also often increase with physical activity which may result in the patient becoming less active.

System Specific: Neuromuscular & Nervous Systems
Content Outline: Foundations for Evaluation, Differential Diagnosis, & Prognosis

## Exam Three: Question 58

A physical therapist prepares to perform manual vibration as a means of airway clearance with a patient diagnosed with chronic obstructive pulmonary disease. When performing vibration the MOST appropriate form of manual contact over the affected lung segment is:

1. contact with a cupped hand
2. **contact with the entire palmar surface of the hand**
3. contact with the ulnar border of the hand
4. contact with the distal phalanx of the middle finger

**Correct Answer: 2** (Hillegass p. 573)

Vibration is administered by contracting the muscles of the upper extremities and intentionally causing a vibration to the chest wall with the hands. Vibration should produce a gentle, high frequency force and is a viable alternative to percussion in acutely ill patients with chest wall discomfort or pain.

1. Contact with a cupped hand would be indicated when performing percussion. Percussion refers to a rhythmical clapping applied over an affected lung segment. Percussion is used to loosen retained secretions.

2. **Vibration requires the palmar aspect of the physical therapist's hands to be in full contact with the affected lung segment. The therapist may elect to partially or fully overlap the hands during manual vibration. Vibration is applied at the end of a deep inspiration and is maintained through the end of expiration.**

3. Contact with the ulnar border of the hand can be used as a method to assess tactile fremitus. Tactile fremitus refers to the vibration of spoken words felt through the chest wall. The palmar surface of one or both hands can also be used. Tactile fremitus provides information about the density of the lungs and the thoracic cavity.

4. Mediate percussion is used to evaluate changes in lung density. The technique requires the physical therapist to place the middle finger of one hand flat on the chest wall along the intercostal space between two ribs while the other fingers are lifted off of the chest wall. The opposing hand acts as a fulcrum using the middle finger to strike the middle finger of the opposite hand positioned on the chest wall. The quality of the generated sound provides the therapist with information on lung density.

System Specific: Cardiovascular/Pulmonary and Lymphatic Systems
Content Outline: Interventions

## Exam Three: Question 59

A physical therapist completes an upper quarter screening examination on a patient with a suspected cervical spine lesion. Which objective finding is NOT consistent with C5 involvement?

1. **muscle weakness in the supinator and wrist extensors**
2. diminished sensation in the deltoid area
3. muscle weakness in the deltoid and biceps
4. diminished biceps and brachioradialis reflexes

**Correct Answer: 1** (Magee p. 22)
Involvement of a specific nerve root often results in predictable impairments including diminished sensation, muscle weakness, impaired reflexes, and paresthesias.

1. **Muscle weakness of the supinator (C5, C6, C7) and the extensor digitorum (C6, C7, C8) is associated with C6 involvement.**

2. Diminished sensation in the deltoid area and the anterior aspect of the entire arm to the base of the thumb is associated with the C5 dermatome.

3. Muscle weakness of the deltoid (C5, C6) and the biceps (C5, C6) is associated with the C5 myotome.

4. Diminished biceps (C5, C6) and brachioradialis (C5, C6) reflexes are associated with C5 involvement.

System Specific: Neuromuscular & Nervous Systems
Content Outline: Foundations for Evaluation, Differential Diagnosis, & Prognosis

## Exam Three: Question 60

A physical therapist employed in a rehabilitation hospital reviews the medical record of a 26-year-old patient recently admitted to the facility. The medical record indicates that the patient sustained a spinal cord injury four weeks ago in a diving accident. Which medical diagnosis would result in the patient being MOST susceptible to autonomic dysreflexia?

1. **T4 paraplegia**
2. T12 paraplegia
3. cauda equina injury
4. posterior cord syndrome

**Correct Answer: 1** (O'Sullivan p. 943)
Autonomic dysreflexia is caused when a noxious stimulus below the level of the lesion triggers the autonomic nervous system causing a sudden elevation in blood pressure. Symptoms include profuse sweating, bradycardia, goose bumps, headache, and vasodilation (flushing) above the level of the injury. This condition should be treated as a medical emergency.

1. **Autonomic dysreflexia is common in patients with spinal cord lesions above the T6 level. The condition should be treated as a medical emergency. Immediate medical management includes assisting the patient to a sitting position in an attempt to reduce blood pressure and examining the urinary drainage system since this often serves as the noxious stimulus that triggers the autonomic response.**

2. A patient with T12 paraplegia would not typically be at risk for autonomic dysreflexia since the level of the lesion is below T6.

3. Cauda equina injury occurs below the L1 spinal level where the long nerve roots transcend. Characteristics include flaccidity, areflexia, and impairment of bowel and bladder function. Full recovery is not typical due to the distance needed for axonal regeneration.

4. Posterior cord syndrome refers to a relatively rare incomplete lesion caused by compression of the posterior spinal artery and is characterized by loss of pain perception, proprioception, two-point discrimination, and stereognosis. Motor function is preserved.

System Specific: Neuromuscular & Nervous Systems
Content Outline: Foundations for Evaluation, Differential Diagnosis, & Prognosis

## Exam Three: Question 61

A physical therapist utilizes neuromuscular electrical stimulation by attaching an electrode over the motor point of the peroneus longus. The MOST appropriate location to attach the electrode is:

1. along the lateral border of the popliteal fossa
2. **on the anterolateral surface of the lower leg**
3. proximal to the first metatarsophalangeal joint
4. immediately inferior to the lateral malleolus

**Correct Answer: 2** (Kendall p. 365)

A motor point refers to a point on the skin where the application of an electrical stimulus via an electrode will cause the contraction of an underlying muscle. A physical therapist can attempt to identify a motor point based on their knowledge of a muscle's origin and insertion.

1. The popliteal fossa refers to an area or shallow depression located on the posterior surface of the knee. The area is significantly superior to the origin and insertion of the peroneus longus and therefore could not serve as a motor point for the muscle.

2. **The peroneus longus originates on the head and upper two-thirds of the lateral surface of the fibula and inserts on the lateral side of the base of the first metatarsal and the medial cuneiform. The muscle acts to evert the foot and assists in plantar flexion of the ankle joint. The anterolateral surface of the lower leg is consistent with the muscle's motor point.**

3. A motor point proximal to the first metatarsophalangeal joint would likely be associated with one of the intrinsic muscles of the foot.

4. While the location immediately inferior to the lateral malleolus would correspond to an area that the peroneus longus passes over, by the time the muscle reaches this distal point, it is mostly tendon and therefore an electrical stimulus would not produce the desired motor response.

System Specific: Musculoskeletal System
Content Outline: Interventions

## Exam Three: Question 62 ✗

A patient diagnosed with shoulder pain of unknown etiology is referred by his physician for magnetic resonance imaging. Results of the test reveal a partial tear of the infraspinatus muscle. Which muscle group would be the MOST seriously affected by the injury?

1. **shoulder lateral rotators**
2. shoulder medial rotators
3. shoulder abductors
4. shoulder adductors

**Correct Answer: 1** (Kendall p. 321)

The infraspinatus muscle originates on the medial two-thirds of the infraspinous fossa of the scapula and inserts on the greater tubercle of the humerus. The muscle is innervated by the suprascapular nerve.

1. **The primary action of the infraspinatus is lateral rotation of the shoulder joint. The muscle also plays an important role in stabilizing the head of the humerus in the glenoid cavity. Other muscles that function as shoulder lateral rotators include the teres minor and posterior deltoid.**

2. The shoulder medial rotators include the subscapularis, teres major, pectoralis major, latissimus dorsi, and anterior deltoid muscles.

3. The shoulder abductors include the middle deltoid and supraspinatus muscles.

4. The shoulder adductors include the pectoralis major, latissimus dorsi, and teres major muscles.

System Specific: Musculoskeletal System
Content Outline: Physical Therapy Examination

## Exam Three: Question 63

A physical therapist reads in the medical record that a wound located near a patient's ischial tuberosity was classified as "Black" using the Red-Yellow-Black system. The MOST relevant finding associated with a "Black" classification would be the presence of:

1. granulation tissue
2. exudate
3. slough
4. **eschar**

**Correct Answer: 4** (Sussman p. 83)
The Red-Yellow-Black system uses a wound's surface color to direct treatment. A red wound is the most desirable, followed by yellow, and then black.

1. Granulation tissue is produced during the proliferative phase of wound healing and is rich with macrophages, fibroblasts, collagen, and blood vessels. Granulation tissue is classified as "Red" using the Red-Yellow-Black system.

2. Exudate is a fluid rich in protein and cellular debris that has escaped from blood vessels due to inflammation. The characteristics of exudate from a given wound assist physical therapists to diagnose wound infection, evaluate the effectiveness of selected interventions, and monitor wound healing. Exudate is not part of the Red-Yellow-Black system.

3. Slough is a form of necrotic tissue that is usually moist, stringy, and viscous and is most often yellow in color. Slough is classified as "Yellow" using the Red-Yellow-Black system.

4. **Eschar describes a particular type of necrosis, usually presenting as brown or black with a hard or soft appearance. Eschar is indicative of full-thickness tissue destruction. Eschar is classified as "Black" using the Red-Yellow-Black system.**

System Specific: Other Systems
Content Outline: Foundations for Evaluation, Differential Diagnosis, & Prognosis

## Exam Three: Question 64

A physical therapist instructs a patient with a unilateral amputation to ascend and descend stairs. Which amputation level would you expect to have the MOST difficulty performing the described task?

1. transmetatarsal
2. transtibial
3. **transfemoral**
4. Syme's

**Correct Answer: 3** (Tan p. 245)
As the level of amputation increases, the necessary energy expenditure, balance, and coordination required to complete functional activities also increases.

1. A transmetatarsal amputation will have very little effect on a patient's ability to ascend and descend stairs. A transmetatarsal amputation is an amputation that occurs through the midsection of the metatarsals.

2. A transtibial amputation will result in an increased energy expenditure of approximately twenty-five percent with mobility compared to a person with two healthy lower extremities. The amount is significantly less than the increased energy expenditure associated with a transfemoral amputation.

3. **A transfemoral amputation will have the largest impact on energy expenditure during functional activities. A patient ambulating with a transfemoral prosthesis has an increased energy expenditure of approximately two times that of a person with two healthy lower extremities. As a result, ascending and descending stairs will be the most difficult for a patient with a transfemoral amputation.**

4. A Syme's amputation occurs when the ankle is disarticulated and the heel pad is attached to the distal tibia. The amputation causes an increased energy expenditure during mobility, but due to the long length of the lever arm and distal point of amputation, the increase in energy expenditure is minimal.

System Specific: Musculoskeletal System
Content Outline: Foundations for Evaluation, Differential Diagnosis, & Prognosis

## Exam Three: Question 65

A physical therapist receives a referral for a 48-year-old female diagnosed with lung cancer. The patient reports smoking three packs of cigarettes a day for the last 25 years. Assuming the patient was diagnosed with cancer two months ago, which of the following pieces of data would provide the therapist with the MOST valuable information when establishing the plan of care and the associated goals?

1. premorbid lifestyle
2. **staging of cancer**
3. past medical history
4. motivation level

**Correct Answer: 2** (Goodman – Pathology p. 350)

Lung cancer is the most frequent form of cancer in the United States and refers to a malignancy of the epithelium of the respiratory tract. The majority of lung cancers are detected on routine chest x-ray in patients presenting with an unrelated medical condition. The staging of the cancer is used to estimate prognosis and to determine appropriate intervention strategies.

1. The patient's premorbid lifestyle is relevant, however, would not be the primary factor when establishing the plan of care and associated goals.

2. **The TNM Classification System (T=tumor, N=node, M=metastasis) is a commonly used cancer classification system that describes the extent of a particular malignant tumor. "T" refers to the extent of the primary tumor, "N" refers to the absence or presence and extent of regional lymph node metastasis, and "M" refers to the absence or presence of distant metastasis. This type of staging offers guidance to health care professionals when determining treatment options, life expectancy, and prognosis for complete resolution.**

3. Past medical history provides a basic snapshot of a patient's overall health status. This information would be considered when establishing the plan of care and associated goals, but it would not be as critical as other pieces of information (i.e., cancer staging).

4. Motivation level is particularly important once a plan of care is established, however, the patient's motivation level would be of only modest value when establishing the plan of care and associated goals.

System Specific: Other Systems
Content Outline: Foundations for Evaluation, Differential Diagnosis, & Prognosis

## Exam Three: Question 66

A physical therapist treats a 54-year-old male rehabilitating from a tibial plateau fracture. While completing a resistive exercise, the patient indicates that lifting weights often causes him to void small amounts of urine. The MOST appropriate therapist action is:

1. refer the patient to a support group
2. instruct the patient in pelvic floor muscle strengthening exercises
3. discontinue resistive exercises as part of the established plan of care
4. **educate the patient about incontinence**

**Correct Answer: 4** (Kisner p. 581)

Incontinence refers to an inability to control the release of urine, feces or gas and is a common occurrence for many men and women. The causes of incontinence may include weak pelvic floor muscles or medical conditions such as an enlarged prostate, prostatitis, cancer, neurological disorders or obstruction. Proper diagnosis is necessary in order to effectively treat this condition.

1. The use of a support group would be a potential adjunct activity for the patient, however, at this time, education is the appropriate action.

2. It would be inappropriate to begin pelvic floor exercises without a referral from a physician since the cause of the incontinence is unknown.

3. The physical therapist should not discontinue resistive exercises since strengthening is a necessary component of a rehabilitation program for a patient following a tibial plateau fracture. This action also does not directly address the current issue of uncontrolled voiding of urine.

4. **The patient may significantly benefit from formal education about incontinence. The action would provide the patient with necessary information and make the patient more likely to see a physician about this issue. A vast majority of patients with incontinence can be successfully treated with non-invasive measures such as pelvic floor exercises.**

System Specific: Other Systems
Content Outline: Interventions

# Exam Three: Question 67

A patient two days status post transfemoral amputation demonstrates decreased strength and generalized deconditioning. Which of the following positions should be utilized when instructing the patient to wrap their residual limb?

1. sidelying
2. standing
3. **supine**
4. prone

**Correct Answer: 3** (Seymour p. 124)

A physical therapist should instruct a patient to wrap their residual limb in a manner that allows full access to the residual limb and provides a secure and stable environment that does not jeopardize patient safety.

1. A sidelying position would make it difficult for the patient to utilize the upper extremities to manipulate the bandage. Viewing the residual limb in sidelying would also be more difficult than in supine.

2. Standing on the uninvolved lower extremity would not provide an adequate base of support for wrapping the residual limb. Wrapping the residual limb in standing requires high levels of coordination and balance.

3. **A supine position would provide the patient with adequate access to the residual limb and provide a secure and stable environment to complete the wrapping.**

4. A prone position would make it extremely challenging for the patient to wrap the residual limb and would make it impossible for the patient to inspect the wrapping. A prone position may be contraindicated for patients with particular cardiac or respiratory pathologies.

System Specific: Other Systems
Content Outline: Interventions

# Exam Three: Question 68

A physical therapist employed in an outpatient private practice receives a referral for a patient diagnosed with spondylolisthesis. Which of the following scenarios would be MOST consistent with the medical diagnosis?

1. **a 13-year-old female gymnast with no significant medical history**
2. a 17-year-old female tennis player with a 15 degree lateral curvature of the spine
3. a 28-year-old male machinist with a history of recurrent low back pain
4. a 67-year-old male with a previous diagnosis of ankylosing spondylitis

**Correct Answer: 1** (Brotzman p. 532)

Spondylolisthesis refers to a condition where one vertebra slips forward on the one below it due to a bilateral fracture of the pars interarticularis. This condition most commonly occurs at L4-L5 or L5-S1.

1. **Children ages 10-15 who are involved in activities such as gymnastics, weight lifting, volleyball, and pole vaulting are particularly susceptible to spondylolisthesis.**

2. Lateral curvature of the spine is indicative of scoliosis and not spondylolisthesis. Scoliosis has many causes including changes in bony structure of the spine (i.e., wedging of a vertebral body), neuromuscular disorders (i.e., cerebral palsy, muscular dystrophy) or an impairment of an extremity (i.e., leg length discrepancy). Scoliosis can also have idiopathic etiology.

3. This patient's age and occupation are not typically consistent with the incidence of spondylolisthesis. The recurrence of the patient's low back pain is more suggestive of a muscular strain than a fracture.

4. Ankylosing spondylitis is a systemic condition that is characterized by inflammation of the spine and larger peripheral joints. The chronic inflammation causes destruction of the ligamentous-osseous junction with subsequent fibrosis and ossification of the area. Men are at a two to three time greater risk than women and onset is typically seen between twenty and forty years of age.

System Specific: Musculoskeletal System
Content Outline: Foundations for Evaluation, Differential Diagnosis, & Prognosis

## Exam Three: Question 69

A patient diagnosed with Cushing's syndrome is referred to physical therapy. Which of the following signs and symptoms is NOT consistent with this syndrome?

1. distension of the abdomen
2. swelling in the facial area
3. **adrenal hypoplasia**
4. cardiac hypertrophy

**Correct Answer: 3** (Goodman - Pathology p. 481)

Cushing's syndrome is produced by an excess of free circulating cortisol from the adrenal cortex. Physical therapists may be more likely to treat patients who have developed medication-induced Cushing's syndrome, usually after receiving large doses of cortisol or cortisol derivatives.

1. Distention of the abdomen and subsequent central obesity is consistent with Cushing's syndrome. Weakening of the muscles and elastic tissue in combination with abnormal fat distribution results in distention of the abdomen. Thinning of the skin with striae on the breasts, axillary areas, and abdomen are often observed.

2. Swelling in the facial area is a common characteristic of Cushing's syndrome. This condition is often referred to as "moon-shaped face."

3. **Cushing's syndrome is a condition characterized by hyperfunction of the adrenal cortex. Addison's disease is a condition characterized by hypoplasia of the adrenal cortex.**

4. Physiological manifestations of Cushing's syndrome include hypertension caused by potassium depletion, and sodium and water retention. Hypertension can result in left ventricular hypertrophy and increased risk of congestive heart failure or CVA.

System Specific: Other Systems
Content Outline: Foundations for Evaluation, Differential Diagnosis, & Prognosis

## Exam Three: Question 70

A physical therapist completes an examination on a patient diagnosed with complete C7 tetraplegia. The patient problem list includes inability to complete an independent bed to wheelchair transfer, decreased passive lower extremity range of motion, tissue breakdown over the ischial tuberosities, and decreased upper extremity strength. Which of the following treatment activities should be given the highest priority?

1. **pressure relief activities**
2. transfer training using a sliding board
3. self-range of motion activities
4. upper extremity strengthening exercises

**Correct Answer: 1** (O'Sullivan p. 465)

A physical therapist should give the highest priority to educating the patient on appropriate skin care including pressure relief activities. A patient with C7 tetraplegia can perform lateral and forward weight shifting in the wheelchair to assist with pressure relief.

1. **Education and instruction in pressure relief activities is the highest priority for a patient that has compromised sensation. The patient can perform independent relief through weight shifting each two-hour period to avoid further skin breakdown and infection.**

2. Transfer training using a sliding board will be a component of the treatment plan, but would not be the highest priority. Weight shifting is a precursor to performing a sliding board transfer.

3. Self-range of motion will be a component of the treatment plan. Patients must maintain an expected length in each muscle group in order to function at maximum potential. Pressure relief must be given the highest priority, however, so that the patient can progress through rehabilitation without skin breakdown.

4. Upper extremity strengthening will be a component of the treatment plan and focuses on maximizing strength in the available muscles. Although strengthening is desirable, failure to prevent tissue breakdown will place the patient at considerable risk for serious medical complications.

System Specific: Neuromuscular & Nervous Systems
Content Outline: Interventions

## Exam Three: Question 71

A physical therapist treats a 56-year-old male status post transfemoral amputation with a hip flexion contracture. As part of the treatment regimen the therapist performs passive stretching exercises to the involved hip. The MOST appropriate form of passive stretching is:

1. **moderate tension over a prolonged period of time**
2. moderate tension over a brief period of time
3. maximal tension over a prolonged period of time
4. maximal tension over a brief period of time

**Correct Answer: 1** (Kisner p. 79)
The effectiveness of a stretching program is influenced by a multitude of variables including intensity, duration, speed, frequency, and mode of stretch. Physical therapists must carefully select the parameters of a stretching program based on the established therapeutic goals.

1. **Moderate tension over a prolonged period of time would be the most appropriate form of stretching for the hip flexors. Moderate tension will minimize muscle guarding and the duration of the stretch will promote gradual gains in muscle length.**

2. Moderate tension over a brief period of time is an appropriate option, however, the time period would be less effective than a prolonged period of time to increase muscle length.

3. Maximal tension over a prolonged period of time would not likely be tolerated by the patient. The amount of tension would result in significant muscle guarding that would limit the effectiveness of the stretching activity.

4. Maximal tension over a brief period of time may be a slightly better option than the prolonged period of time, however, the intensity of the stretch would still likely result in muscle guarding that would limit the effectiveness of the stretching activity.

System Specific: Musculoskeletal System
Content Outline: Interventions

## Exam Three: Question 72

A physical therapist treats a patient diagnosed with Parkinson's disease. When working on controlled mobility, which of the following would BEST describe the physical therapist's objective?

1. facilitate postural muscle control
2. **promote weight shifting and rotational trunk control**
3. emphasize reciprocal extremity movement
4. facilitate tone and rigidity

**Correct Answer: 2** (Sullivan p. 77)
Controlled mobility refers to the ability to move within a weight bearing position or rotate around a long axis. Controlled mobility is one component of the Stages of Motor Control (mobility, stability, controlled mobility, and skill).

1. Stability refers to the ability to maintain a position or posture through cocontraction and tonic holding around a joint. Unsupported sitting with midline control is an example of stability.

2. **Controlled mobility activities should emphasize weight shifting and trunk control with rotation. This type of activity may serve to decrease rigidity and improve the fluidity of gait in a patient with Parkinson's disease.**

3. A patient must possess prerequisite stability and dynamic postural control in order to perform reciprocal extremity movement. Coordination training often focuses on reciprocal extremity movement.

4. Facilitation techniques are used to increase tone in patients with hypotonia. These techniques are not often used to treat Parkinson's disease since patients with this condition typically exhibit hypertonia or in more severe cases, rigidity.

System Specific: Neuromuscular & Nervous Systems
Content Outline: Interventions

## Exam Three: Question 73

A physical therapist assesses the strength of selected lower extremity muscles on a patient rehabilitating from a knee injury. The pictured test would be MOST effective to examine the strength of the:

1. hip abductors
2. hip adductors
3. hip medial rotators
4. **hip lateral rotators**

**Correct Answer: 4** (Kendall p. 430)

The hip lateral rotators include the gluteus maximus, obturator internus, obturator externus, piriformis, gemelli, and sartorius. Weakness of the lateral rotators usually results in medial rotation of the femur accompanied by pronation of the foot and a tendency toward a valgus position at the knee.

1. The strength of the hip abductors is assessed with the patient in sidelying with the test leg raised. The physical therapist should apply pressure to the distal aspect of the femur, pushing the leg downward in an attempt to adduct the thigh. The hip abductors include the gluteus minimus, gluteus medius, piriformis, and obturator internus.

2. The strength of the hip adductors is assessed with the patient in sidelying with the test leg closest to the surface adducted. The physical therapist should apply pressure to the distal aspect of the femur, pushing the leg downward in an attempt to abduct the thigh. The hip adductors include the adductor longus, adductor brevis, adductor magnus, and gracilis.

3. The strength of the hip medial rotators is assessed with the patient in sitting. The physical therapist should apply pressure to the lateral side of the leg above the ankle, pushing the leg inward in an attempt to rotate the thigh laterally. The hip medial rotators include the pectineus, adductor longus, tensor fasciae latae, gluteus minimus, and gluteus medius.

4. **The strength of the hip lateral rotators is assessed with the patient in sitting. The physical therapist should apply pressure to the medial side of the leg above the ankle, pushing the leg outward in an attempt to rotate the thigh medially.**

System Specific: Musculoskeletal System
Content Outline: Physical Therapy Examination

## Exam Three: Question 74

A physical therapist employed in a rehabilitation hospital treats a patient status post traumatic brain injury. During the treatment session the therapist notices that the patient's toes are discolored below a bivalved lower extremity cast. The cast was applied approximately five hours ago in an attempt to reduce a plantar flexion contracture. The MOST appropriate therapist action is to:

1. discontinue the use of the anterior portion of the cast
2. contact the staff nurse and request that the cast is removed
3. refer the patient to an orthotist
4. **remove the cast**

**Correct Answer: 4** (Tan p. 501)

Discoloration of the patient's toes is an indication that the cast is too tight and is likely impeding the patient's circulation. This objective finding would make it necessary to remove the bivalved cast for further inspection.

1. The anterior and posterior portions of the bivalved cast would need to be removed in order to assess the patient's skin integrity and circulation. Removal of only the anterior portion of the cast would not be adequate to fully inspect the lower extremity.

2. The physical therapist would be able to remove the bivalved cast by simply unfastening the Velcro straps which secure the anterior and posterior portions. As a result, the physical therapist would not need to rely on the nurse.

3. Referral to an orthotist is not necessary since a bivalved cast is easily removed and the observed finding requires immediate attention.

4. **A physical therapist possesses the requisite skills and training to remove the bivalved cast.**

System Specific: Other Systems
Content Outline: Interventions

**SCORE**BUILDERS

## Exam Three: Question 75

A physical therapist treats a patient rehabilitating from a traumatic brain injury by applying approximation to the pelvis to increase bilateral lower extremity weight bearing. The patient exhibits significant hypertonicity and the presence of the positive support reflex. The therapist is MOST likely using the therapeutic ball to:

1. **avoid a mass extensor pattern in standing**
2. encourage active assistive range of motion
3. allow the patient partial weight bearing through the ball
4. limit range of motion at the shoulder

**Correct Answer: 1** (Umphred p. 672)

The positive support reflex is an abnormal reflex that occurs with weight bearing through the ball of the foot. The response produces an increase in extensor tone through the lower extremities and trunk. The use of trunk flexion with lower extremity weight bearing activities using the therapeutic ball assists the patient to avoid a mass extensor pattern in standing. A therapeutic ball can be utilized for facilitation, inhibition, and range of motion.

1. **In this particular scenario, the patient uses the therapeutic ball to allow for supported trunk flexion when standing. This avoids a mass extensor response and allows for weight bearing and weight shifting through the lower extremities.**

2. The therapeutic ball can be used to promote active assistive range of motion, however, the use of the therapeutic ball in this scenario is more related to supported standing with the trunk flexed to avoid a mass extensor pattern.

3. The therapeutic ball can be used for weight bearing through the upper extremities, however, the use of the therapeutic ball in this scenario is more related to supported standing with the trunk flexed to avoid a mass extensor pattern.

4. The therapeutic ball may be used for increasing range of motion of a given joint, however, it is rarely used to limit range of motion. Decreasing upper extremity range of motion would not be beneficial to limit the mass extensor pattern.

System Specific: Neuromuscular and Nervous Systems
Content Outline: Interventions

## Exam Three: Question 76

A physical therapist asks a patient who has been inconsistent with his attendance in physical therapy, why he is having difficulty keeping scheduled appointments. The patient responds that it is difficult to understand the scheduling card that lists the appointments. The therapist's MOST appropriate action would be to:

1. contact the referring physician to discuss the patient's poor attendance in therapy
2. make sure the patient is given a scheduling card at the conclusion of each session
3. **write down the patient's appointments on a piece of paper in a manner that the patient can understand**
4. discharge the patient from physical therapy

**Correct Answer: 3** (Falvo p. 19)

In order to determine if the patient's poor attendance in therapy is due to difficulty understanding the scheduling card, the information must be presented in a manner the patient can understand.

1. Contacting the referring physician may eventually be warranted, however, the initial focus should be directed toward improving the patient's understanding of his scheduled appointments.

2. Since the patient has expressed that he has difficulty reading the scheduling card, it would not be helpful to provide the same card at more frequent intervals.

3. **The physical therapist can improve the patient's understanding of the scheduling card by writing the appointments in a more understandable format.**

4. A patient should not be discharged from physical therapy unless the physical therapist has already taken steps to improve the patient's compliance with scheduled appointments.

System Specific: Non-Systems
Content Outline: Safety and Protection; Professional Responsibilities; Research

## Exam Three: Question 77

A physical therapist treats a patient status post right cerebrovascular accident with resultant left hemiplegia for a colleague on vacation. A note left by the primary therapist indicates that the patient exhibits "pusher syndrome." When examining the patient's sitting posture, which of the following findings would be MOST likely?

1. **sitting with increased lean to the left along with increased weight bearing through the left buttocks**
2. sitting with increased lean to the right along with increased weight bearing through the right buttocks
3. sitting with increased weight bearing through the right buttocks and the head rotated to the right; unresponsive to stimuli on the left
4. sitting with unequal weight bearing and the head rotated to the left; unresponsive to stimuli on the right

---

**Correct Answer: 1** (O'Sullivan p. 750)

Pusher syndrome is characterized by a significant lateral deviation toward the hemiplegic side. Pusher syndrome more commonly occurs in patients that have sustained a right CVA. Therapeutic intervention for a patient that exhibits pusher syndrome may include the use of a mirror, a small wedge placed under the left lateral thigh, weight shifting across midline, and facilitation techniques for trunk control.

1. **A patient with right CVA (left hemiplegia) with pusher syndrome would typically exhibit a lateral lean to the left in sitting with increased weight bearing on the left buttocks.**
2. A patient with right CVA (left hemiplegia) without pusher syndrome would typically exhibit less weight bearing through the left side due to the existing sensory and motor deficits. Intervention would include midline orientation and weight shifting in sitting.
3. A patient with right CVA (left hemiplegia) who demonstrates the inability to interpret stimuli on the left side of the body is exhibiting unilateral neglect. Neglect is most often associated with a lesion of the right frontal lobe of the brain.
4. A patient with right CVA (left hemiplegia) would not typically rotate the head towards the affected (left) side, but rather away from it secondary to neglect. The patient would be more responsive to stimuli on the right.

System Specific: Neuromuscular & Nervous Systems
Content Outline: Foundations for Evaluation, Differential Diagnosis, & Prognosis

---

## Exam Three: Question 78

A physical therapist working in a school system develops long-term goals as part of an Individualized Educational Plan for a child with Down syndrome. The MOST appropriate time frame to attain these goals is:

1. one month
2. four months
3. six months
4. **one year**

---

**Correct Answer: 4** (Tecklin p. 659)

An Individualized Educational Plan (IEP) is designed for any school-aged child that requires therapy services. Long-term goals are based on a one-year plan. These services are provided through federal legislation through the Individuals with Disabilities Education Act (IDEA).

1. A goal with a one-month time frame is designed for a patient that requires therapeutic intervention for an injury or condition that will steadily progress and improve. This time frame is not within the framework of the IEP.
2. A four-month time frame may be an appropriate interval to informally reassess the child and quantify the actual progress towards the established goals, however, it is typically an insufficient amount of time to expect the established goals to be accomplished.
3. A six-month time frame may be an appropriate interval for review of established goals for the IEP since it is a midpoint in the year. This time frame, however, is not typically sufficient to accomplish the long-term goals.
4. **Federal legislation mandates the review of an IEP on a one-year basis. Goals relate to improving a child's educational experience. IDEA also provides for children 0-5 years of age through early intervention programs.**

System Specific: Non-Systems
Content Outline: Safety and Protection; Professional Responsibilities; Research

# Exam Three: Question 79

A two-year-old with T10 spina bifida receives physical therapy for gait training. Initially, the preferred method to teach a child how to maintain standing is with the use of:

1. bilateral hip-knee-ankle-foot orthoses (HKAFO) and forearm crutches
2. **parapodium and the parallel bars**
3. bilateral knee-ankle-foot orthoses (KAFO) and the parallel bars
4. bilateral ankle-foot orthoses (AFO) and the parallel bars

**Correct Answer: 2** (Tecklin p. 254)

The parapodium provides the necessary amount of support and is optimal to assist with standing activities for children with thoracic and high level lumbar lesions. The parallel bars are the most stable assistive device to initiate standing and gait training.

1. HKAFOs would require a swing-through or reciprocal gait pattern. Using HKAFOs with forearm crutches requires a high level of balance and energy expenditure and is not appropriate for initial standing activities.
2. **The parapodium is a HKAFO with a thoracolumbar orthosis that supports the trunk and lower extremities. It has a large base of support and is used with or without an assistive device. This would be ideal for a patient with T10 spina bifida to initiate standing within the parallel bars.**
3. A patient with T10 spina bifida would not initially use KAFOs in the parallel bars when working on standing activities due to the deficits in strength and sensation below the T10 level.
4. A patient with T10 spina bifida would not possess the necessary motor function to use bilateral AFOs.

System Specific: Neuromuscular & Nervous Systems
Content Outline: Interventions

# Exam Three: Question 80

A physical therapist notices a small area of skin irritation under the chin of a patient wearing a Philadelphia collar. The patient expresses that the area is not painful, but is becoming increasingly itchy. The MOST appropriate therapist action is:

1. instruct the patient to apply 1% hydrocortisone cream to the area twice daily
2. apply powder to the area and instruct the patient to avoid scratching
3. **provide the patient with a liner to use as a barrier between the skin and the orthosis**
4. discontinue use of the orthosis until the skin has become less irritated

**Correct Answer: 3** (Physical Therapist's Clinical Companion p. 316)

Patients can experience itching or skin irritation when using a cervical orthosis. Since an orthosis is applied directly over the skin, it is imperative to utilize a liner that maximizes comfort, promotes cleanliness, limits moisture, and reduces skin irritation. Failure to select an appropriate liner may result in skin breakdown.

1. Hydrocortisone may be used to treat an existing area of irritation, however, it does not address the primary cause of irritation.
2. Powder may assist to temporarily reduce friction over a particular area, but it does not address the primary cause of irritation.
3. **Liners made from lambs' wool are commonly utilized and prevent chafing and irritation of the patient's skin. This liner is easily donned and provides an adequate barrier between the skin and orthosis.**
4. Discontinuing the use of the cervical orthosis would be undesirable since it is prescribed based on medical necessity.

System Specific: Other Systems
Content Outline: Interventions

## Exam Three: Question 81

A patient with muscle weakness and compromised balance uses a four-point gait pattern with two canes. The physical therapist would like to instruct the patient to ascend and descend the stairs according to the normal flow of traffic. When ascending stairs the MOST practical method is to:

1. **use the handrail with the right hand and place the two canes in the left hand**
2. use the handrail with the left hand and place the two canes in the right hand
3. place one cane in each hand and avoid using the handrail
4. place the two canes in the left hand and avoid using the handrail

**Correct Answer: 1** (Minor p. 428)
Since the normal flow of traffic assumes ascending on the right and descending on the left, the patient should grasp the railing with the right hand and use the two canes in the left hand when ascending and descending the stairs.

1. **Since the patient does not have unilateral weakness, it is most appropriate to ascend the stairs on the right in order to utilize the handrail and remain consistent with the normal flow of traffic.**

2. Since the normal flow of traffic assumes ascending on the right and descending on the left, the patient would be going against the normal flow of traffic by grasping the handrail with the left hand and using the two canes in the right hand.

3. The patient should use a handrail when available in order to improve stability and balance.

4. Failure to use the handrail would significantly increase the patient's relative risk of falling.

System Specific: Non-Systems
Content Outline: Equipment & Devices; Therapeutic Modalities

## Exam Three: Question 82

A patient rehabilitating from a total hip arthroplasty receives home physical therapy services. The patient is currently full weight bearing and is able to ascend and descend stairs independently. The patient expresses that her goal following rehabilitation is to walk one mile each day. The MOST appropriate plan to accomplish the patient's goal is to:

1. continue home physical therapy services until the patient's goal is attained
2. refer the patient to an outpatient orthopedic physical therapy clinic
3. **design a home exercise program that emphasizes progressive ambulation**
4. admit the patient to a rehabilitation hospital

**Correct Answer: 3** (Guide for Professional Conduct)
The patient's goal of walking one mile each day does not warrant continued physical therapy services. The physical therapist should assist the patient to achieve their individual goals by implementing a home exercise program that includes progressive ambulation.

1. Home physical therapy is warranted for patients that are "homebound." This patient would not qualify for home physical therapy services secondary to her current functional status.

2. The patient's current functional status does not appear to warrant continued physical therapy services regardless of practice setting. Since the patient is now independent in the home and her goal includes ambulating one mile each day, the outpatient orthopedic clinic is not an appropriate setting. The patient can meet her goal independently by following a home program.

3. **The physical therapist can assist the patient with her long-term goal by designing a home exercise program that incorporates ongoing exercise and progressive ambulation activities. This patient would not typically qualify for further physical therapy services.**

4. A rehabilitation hospital is appropriate for patients with functional deficits and acute rehabilitation needs. The patient's current functional status makes the intensity of rehabilitation offered in this setting unnecessary.

System Specific: Musculoskeletal System
Content Outline: Interventions

## Exam Three: Question 83

A physical therapist completes a work site analysis for a patient with T3 paraplegia. The patient is employed in the marketing department of an advertising agency and relies on a wheelchair for daily locomotion. Which of the following is likely to be the MOST significant architectural barrier for the patient?

1. hardwood floors
2. **an entrance ramp (one inch of vertical rise for every six inches of ramp length)**
3. one-quarter inch thresholds at each door
4. pedestal type sinks

**Correct Answer: 2** (O'Sullivan p. 409)

An entrance ramp that has one inch of vertical rise for every six inches of ramp length would not satisfy the 1:12 (rise:run) minimum ratio identified in the Americans with Disabilities Act (ADA).

1. Hardwood floors allow for easier propulsion, turning, and function with the wheelchair. Floor surfaces must be firm, stable, and slip resistant. A patient would expect increased difficulty using a wheelchair on carpet or outside terrain.

2. **An entrance ramp designed with one inch of vertical rise for every six inches of ramp length would be twice as steep as the 1:12 (rise:run) minimum ratio. The 1:12 ratio allows for a maximum ramp grade of 8.3 percent.**

3. A threshold of one-quarter inch is an acceptable height as a transition surface. Thresholds with beveled edges up to one-half inch are permissible.

4. Pedestal type sinks would not serve as an architectural barrier since the underside of the sink is open and allows for close wheelchair access. A sink encased with a vanity style cabinet would be more restrictive.

System Specific: Non-Systems
Content Outline: Safety and Protection; Professional Responsibilities; Research

## Exam Three: Question 84

A patient requires inpatient physical therapy after sustaining brain damage in a motor vehicle accident. Upon entering the patient's room, the physical therapist finds the patient as shown in the image. The patient's MOST likely perceptual deficit is:

1. diplopia
2. apraxia
3. **somatoagnosia**
4. anosognosia

**Correct Answer: 3** (O'Sullivan p. 1173)

Perception is the integration of sensory impressions into information that is meaningful and that can be interpreted. Perception allows individuals to have awareness of things and experiences in a constantly changing environment. Damage to the central nervous system can produce many forms of perceptual deficits that can significantly influence patient outcomes.

1. Diplopia (i.e., double vision) is a visual deficit where an individual sees two images of the same object. The duplicate image can be seen vertically, horizontally or diagonally in relation to the other image.

2. Apraxia is the inability to perform purposeful learned movements or activities despite the absence of a motor or sensory impairment that would hinder completion of the task.

3. **Somatoagnosia is an impairment of body schema where there is a lack of awareness of a body structure and its relationship to other body parts, to oneself or to others. This patient is attempting to brush their hair, however, does not realize that the mirror image is not the true body part.**

4. Anasognosia is a severe denial or awareness of the presence or severity of one's neurologic defect or illness in general, especially paralysis. Patient's may deny that a paretic extremity belongs to them or lie as to the reasons for why an extremity doesn't move as it should.

System Specific: Neuromuscular and Nervous Systems
Content Outline: Foundations for Evaluation, Differential Diagnosis, and Prognosis

## Exam Three: Question 85

A physical therapist observes that a number of aides appear to be unfamiliar with appropriate guarding techniques. The MOST appropriate remedial strategy to improve their performance is to:

1. offer assistance to the aides when the inappropriate behavior is observed
2. refer the aides to textbooks that explain proper guarding techniques
3. **develop a mandatory inservice on guarding techniques for the aides**
4. inform the director of rehabilitation that the aides are incompetent

**Correct Answer: 3** (Nosse p. 217)

A mandatory inservice would allow the physical therapist to provide formal education for the aides to ensure consistent use of appropriate guarding techniques.

1. Aides must be competent with all guarding, transfers, and other duties within their job description. Offering assistance to an aide when they are guarding a patient incorrectly may assist with an isolated incident, however, does not fully address the issue of competency.

2. A textbook may be able to educate an aide on general guarding techniques, however, a textbook cannot take the place of an inservice or other forms of experiential training.

3. **An aide should receive mandatory inservicing for all expected job related duties. Each aide should be able to demonstrate proficiency during the inservice in order to ensure patient safety across the spectrum of activities.**

4. Informing the director that the aides are incompetent does not assist the department to improve the competency of the aides.

System Specific: Non-Systems
Content Outline: Safety and Protection; Professional Responsibilities; Research

## Exam Three: Question 86

A physical therapist attends an inservice entitled "Principles of Exercise for the Obstetric Patient." During the session, the speaker identifies several conditions that are considered to result in high risk pregnancies. Which of the following conditions would NOT be considered high risk?

1. **diastasis recti**
2. incompetent cervix
3. pre-eclampsia
4. multiple gestation

**Correct Answer: 1** (Kisner p. 804)

Diastasis recti refers to a separation of the two halves of the rectus abdominus muscle at the linea alba. This condition is often associated with pregnancy during the second and third trimesters, however, does not place a pregnancy at high risk.

1. **The etiology of diastasis recti is unknown with separation greater than two centimeters considered significant. This condition is not considered high risk for pregnancy, however, can produce low back pain due to a limited ability of the abdominal muscles to stabilize the pelvis and lumbar spine.**

2. The increase in pressure associated with pregnancy may cause the cervix to open prematurely. Incompetent cervix may lead to miscarriage or premature delivery and results in a high risk pregnancy. Causative factors include previous cervical surgeries, damage during a previous birth, malformed cervix or DES exposure.

3. Pre-eclampsia is a rapidly progressive condition characterized by high blood pressure and protein in the urine. Swelling, sudden weight gain, headaches, and changes in vision are common symptoms. The condition is considered a medical emergency with high risk to both the mother and baby.

4. Multiple gestation pregnancies are considered high risk since the fetal mortality rate for twins is four times that of single births. Twins have increased frequency of congenital anomalies, placenta previa, abruptio placenta, pre-eclampsia, cord accidents, and malpresentations.

System Specific: Other Systems
Content Outline: Foundations for Evaluation, Differential Diagnosis, & Prognosis

## Exam Three: Question 87

A physical therapist reviews the medical record of a patient with a spinal cord injury. A note recently entered by the physician indicates that the patient contracted a respiratory infection. Which patient would be MOST susceptible to this condition?

1. **a patient with complete C4 tetraplegia**
2. a patient with a cauda equina lesion
3. a patient with Brown-Sequard's syndrome
4. a patient with posterior cord syndrome

**Correct Answer: 1** (Umphred p. 626)

A patient with complete C4 tetraplegia will present with a loss of motor and sensory function secondary to damage to the spinal cord. Since the primary muscle of respiration, the diaphragm, is impaired the patient will be unable to voluntarily or effectively ventilate.

1. **A patient with complete C4 tetraplegia will have a reduced ventilatory capacity due to muscle paralysis. The patient will exhibit limited ability to clear secretions, impaired chest mobility, and alveolar hypoventilation.**

2. A cauda equina lesion is an injury that occurs below the L1 spinal level where the long nerve roots transcend. Cauda equina injuries are frequently incomplete due to the large number of nerve roots in the area and as a result are often considered to be peripheral nerve injuries. Characteristics include flaccidity, areflexia, and impairment of bowel and bladder function.

3. Brown-Sequard's syndrome is an incomplete lesion usually caused by a stab wound, which produces hemisection of the spinal cord. There is paralysis and loss of vibratory and position sense on the same side as the lesion due to the damage to the corticospinal tract and dorsal columns. There is a loss of pain and temperature sense on the opposite side of the lesion from damage to the lateral spinothalamic tract.

4. Posterior cord syndrome is an extremely rare condition that presents with a loss of proprioception, two-point discrimination, graphesthesia, and stereognosis below the level of the lesion. Patients typically present with a wide-based steppage gait.

System Specific: Other Systems
Content Outline: Foundations for Evaluation, Differential Diagnosis, & Prognosis

## Exam Three: Question 88

A patient with a T3 spinal cord injury exercising on a treatment table in supine begins to exhibit signs and symptoms of autonomic dysreflexia including a dramatic increase in blood pressure. The MOST IMMEDIATE action to address the patient's blood pressure response is to:

1. elevate the patient's legs
2. call for assistance
3. **sit the patient upright**
4. check the urinary drainage system

**Correct Answer: 3** (Pierson p. 343)

The physical therapist should immediately position the patient in sitting to address the autonomic nervous system response and reduce the patient's elevated blood pressure. After the patient has been positioned in sitting, the urinary drainage system should be checked since a blocked catheter is a common noxious stimulus that triggers the sympathetic response.

1. Elevation of the patient's legs would be contraindicated since the position would serve to increase the return of circulation and further increase blood pressure.

2. Calling for assistance is an acceptable option given the seriousness of autonomic dysreflexia, however, the action would not be the most immediate action to address the patient's blood pressure response.

3. **Autonomic dysreflexia is caused by a noxious stimulus below the level of the lesion that triggers the autonomic nervous system causing a sudden elevation in blood pressure. If untreated, this condition can lead to convulsions, hemorrhage, and death.**

4. The common causes of autonomic dysreflexia include distended or full bladder, kink or blockage in the catheter, bladder infections, pressure ulcers, extreme temperature changes, tight clothing or an ingrown toenail. A physical therapist should check the urinary drainage system immediately after moving the patient into a sitting position.

System Specific: Neuromuscular and Nervous Systems
Content Outline: Interventions

## Exam Three: Question 89

A physical therapist treats a patient following a lower extremity amputation. The patient is currently one week post amputation and has a post-operative rigid dressing. Which of the following is NOT a benefit of the rigid dressing?

1. limits the development of post-operative edema in the residual limb
2. allows for earlier ambulation with the attachment of a pylon and foot
3. allows for earlier fitting of a definitive prosthesis
4. **allows for daily wound inspection and dressing changes**

**Correct Answer: 4** (Seymour p. 126)

A rigid dressing, usually made from plaster of Paris or fiberglass, does not allow for wound inspection or dressing changes. The rigid dressing is applied in the operating room and remains on the residual limb approximately 7-14 days until the sutures are removed and proper shaping occurs.

1. The rigid dressing limits the development of post-operative edema by maintaining total contact with the surface of the residual limb.

2. The rigid dressing allows for earlier ambulation since the rigid construction of the cast allows for pylon attachment and weight bearing.

3. The rigid dressing allows for earlier fitting of a definitive prosthesis since healing occurs more rapidly. The limb also receives better protection and is less likely to develop a flexion contracture since the rigid dressing limits knee motion.

4. **A rigid dressing does not allow for wound inspection and dressing changes since the rigid dressing remains on the residual limb for an extended period of time. An elastic bandage or a shrinker would be examples of soft dressings that allow for frequent wound inspection and dressing changes.**

System Specific: Other Systems
Content Outline: Foundations for Evaluation, Differential Diagnosis, & Prognosis

## Exam Three: Question 90

A patient rehabilitating from a traumatic head injury is lethargic since being placed on Phenobarbital. The PRIMARY purpose of the medication is to:

1. decrease agitation
2. **prevent seizures**
3. reduce spasticity
4. limit arrhythmias

**Correct Answer: 2** (Ciccone p. 107)

Physical therapists must possess an awareness of commonly used pharmacological agents, their indications, and potential side effects. Failure to recognize anticipated side effects from a medication may significantly jeopardize patient safety.

1. The most common side effect of Phenobarbital is sedation. As a result, agitation is typically diminished, however, the primary purpose of the medication is to prevent seizures.

2. **Phenobarbital is classified as a barbiturate and is prescribed most often to prevent adult seizures. Side effects include sedation, vitamin deficiencies, nystagmus, and ataxia.**

3. There are many medications that treat spasticity, but the most common include Baclofen, Diazepam, and Dantrolene sodium.

4. Antiarrhythmic drugs are typically classified into four groups: sodium channel blockers, beta-blockers, drugs that prolong repolarization, and calcium channel blockers.

System Specific: Neuromuscular & Nervous Systems
Content Outline: Foundations for Evaluation, Differential Diagnosis, and Prognosis

## Exam Three: Question 91

A patient with a transtibial amputation ambulates in the physical therapy gym. The patient exhibits an extended knee throughout early stance phase on the prosthetic side. The MOST appropriate action to resolve the patient's difficulty is:

1. plantar flex the foot
2. soften the heel wedge
3. move the foot anteriorly
4. **dorsiflex the foot**

**Correct Answer: 4** (Rothstein p. 724)

The prosthesis requires slight ankle dorsiflexion to allow for subsequent knee flexion during early stance. A prosthesis with excessive plantar flexion will promote full knee extension during early stance.

1. A prosthetic foot that is plantar flexed will present with an increased extension moment and impede sufficient knee flexion during early stance. The prosthesis must be set into neutral or slight dorsiflexion to allow for knee flexion during stance phase.
2. Softening the heel wedge of a transtibial prosthesis will create an increased extension moment and impede sufficient knee flexion during stance phase.
3. Moving the foot of a transtibial prosthesis anteriorly will create an increased extension moment and impede sufficient knee flexion during stance phase.
4. **A prosthetic foot that is set in slight dorsiflexion will present with an increased flexion moment and assist with knee flexion during stance and when advancing the prosthesis.**

System Specific: Musculoskeletal System
Content Outline: Interventions

## Exam Three: Question 92

A physical therapist examines a patient diagnosed with carpal tunnel syndrome. As part of the examination the therapist assesses end-feel. The therapist classifies the end-feel associated with wrist extension as firm. The MOST logical explanation is:

1. tension in the dorsal radiocarpal ligament and the dorsal joint capsule
2. contact between the ulna and the carpal bones
3. contact between the radius and the carpal bones
4. **tension in the palmar radiocarpal ligament and the palmar joint capsule**

**Correct Answer: 4** (Norkin p. 120)

End-feel is the type of resistance that is felt when passively moving a joint through the end range of motion. Certain tissues and joints have a consistent end-feel and are described as firm, hard or soft. Pathology can be identified through noting the type of abnormal end-feel within a particular joint.

1. A firm end-feel with wrist flexion can result from tension in the dorsal radiocarpal ligament and the dorsal joint capsule.
2. The ulna articulates with the radius at the distal radioulnar joint, however, does not articulate with the carpal bones.
3. Contact between the radius and the carpal bones would result in a hard end-feel and not a firm end-feel.
4. **A firm end-feel with wrist extension can result from tension in the palmar radiocarpal ligament and the palmar joint capsule. Tension in the ulnocarpal ligament can also contribute to the firm end-feel.**

System Specific: Musculoskeletal System
Content Outline: Physical Therapy Examination

## Exam Three: Question 93

A physical therapist examines a patient diagnosed with patellofemoral syndrome. As part of the examination the therapist elects to measure the patient's Q angle. Which three bony landmarks are used to measure the Q angle?

1. anterior superior iliac spine, superior border of the patella, tibial tubercle
2. **anterior superior iliac spine, midpoint of the patella, tibial tubercle**
3. anterior superior iliac spine, inferior border of the patella, midpoint of the patella tendon
4. greater trochanter, midpoint of the patella, tibial tubercle

**Correct Answer: 2** (Hertling p. 499)

The Q angle refers to the angle between the quadriceps muscles and the patella tendon. The angle represents the angle of quadriceps muscle force. Normal Q angle values are 13 degrees for males and 18 degrees for females. An increased Q angle above 18 degrees may be associated with patellar tracking dysfunction, subluxing patella, increased femoral anteversion or increased lateral tibial torsion.

1. The anterior superior iliac spine and tibial tubercle are landmarks used when measuring Q angle, however, the midpoint of the patella should be used as the axis instead of the superior border of the patella.
2. **The most accurate measure of quadriceps muscle force (i.e., Q angle) utilizes the origin and insertion of the quadriceps muscle and the midpoint of the patella.**
3. The inferior border of the patella is located too far distally to use as the axis when measuring Q angle. The midpoint of the patella tendon is relatively close to the axis and may be difficult to accurately locate compared to a bony landmark such as the tibial tubercle.
4. The greater trochanter is not associated with the origin of the quadriceps muscle and is located too far laterally to use as a landmark when measuring Q angle.

System Specific: Musculoskeletal System
Content Outline: Physical Therapy Examination

## Exam Three: Question 94

A patient in a rehabilitation hospital begins to verbalize about the uselessness of life and the possibility of committing suicide. The MOST appropriate physical therapist action is:

1. suggest the patient be placed on a locked unit
2. ask nursing to check on the patient every 15 minutes
3. **discuss the situation with the patient's case manager**
4. review the patient's past medical history for signs and symptoms of mental illness

**Correct Answer: 3** (Bailey p. 317)

Any formal or informal indication that a patient may be suicidal should be taken seriously. The case manager communicates with all of the members of the rehabilitation team and is therefore an appropriate individual for the physical therapist to contact.

1. The physical therapist is not trained or qualified to determine a course of action for a patient that is potentially suicidal.
2. A nurse can frequently check on a patient, however, this action does not ensure the patient's safety given their tenuous mental state.
3. **The case manager would likely contact the attending physician or appropriate mental health provider for direct intervention.**
4. The patient's past medical history may or may not have any bearing on the patient's current status. In addition, the action does not address the patient's expressed suicidal intent.

System Specific: Non-Systems
Content Outline: Safety and Protection; Professional Responsibilities; Research

## Exam Three: Question 95

A physical therapist positions a patient as shown prior to testing for clonus. The MOST appropriate action to complete the test is:

1. **provide a quick stretch to the plantar flexors**
2. provide a quick stretch to the dorsiflexors
3. provide a quick stretch to the plantar flexors while extending the knee
4. provide a quick stretch to the dorsiflexors while extending the knee

**Correct Answer: 1** (DeMyer p. 311)
Clonus refers to rhythmic oscillation of a body part resulting from a quick stretch. The test is ideally performed by providing a stretch to the plantar flexors with the gastrocnemius in a relaxed position.

1. **Clonus is evaluated by supporting the knee in a partially flexed position, encouraging the patient to relax, and passively moving the foot. The therapist provides a quick stretch into dorsiflexion and observes any rhythmic oscillations between plantar flexion and dorsiflexion.**

2. When assessing clonus, the therapist provides a quick stretch to the plantar flexor muscle group, not the dorsiflexor muscle group.

3. When assessing clonus, the therapist provides a quick stretch to the plantar flexor muscle group, however, the knee should be partially flexed rather than extended in order to successfully place the gastrocnemius on slack and elicit the response.

4. When assessing clonus, the therapist should provide a quick stretch to the plantar flexor muscle group and maintain the knee in slight flexion. This option is completely opposite (i.e., quick stretch to the dorsiflexors while extending the knee).

System Specific: Neuromuscular & Nervous Systems
Content Outline: Physical Therapy Examination

## Exam Three: Question 96

A 29-year-old male diagnosed with ankylosing spondylitis reports progressive stiffening of the spine and associated pain for more than five years. The patient's MOST typical standing posture demonstrates:

1. posterior thoracic rib hump
2. **flattened lumbar curve, exaggerated thoracic curve**
3. excessive lumbar curve, flattened thoracic curve
4. lateral curvature of the spine with fixed rotation of the vertebrae

**Correct Answer: 2** (Goodman – Differential Diagnosis p. 471)
Ankylosing spondylitis is a form of systemic rheumatic arthritis that is associated with an increase in thoracic kyphosis and loss of the lumbar curve. Ankylosing spondylitis occurs three times more often in males than females with a typical age of onset of 20-40 years.

1. A posterior thoracic rib hump is characteristic of scoliosis. The rotated vertebrae cause a rotation in the corresponding rib segments and result in posterior displacement of the rib cage.

2. **The clinical presentation of ankylosing spondylitis initially includes recurrent and insidious onset of back pain, morning stiffness, and impaired spinal extension. Chronic inflammation causes destruction of the ligamentous-osseous junction with subsequent fibrosis and ossification. The patient may exhibit flexion at the hips, spinal kyphosis, fatigue, weight loss, and peripheral joint involvement. If the costovertebral joints are affected there may be impaired chest mobility, compromised breathing, and decreased vital capacity.**

3. Excessive lumbar curve with a flattened thoracic curve is opposite from the typical clinical presentation of ankylosing spondylitis.

4. Lateral curvature of the spine with fixed rotation of the vertebrae is descriptive of scoliosis.

System Specific: Musculoskeletal System
Content Outline: Foundations for Evaluation, Differential Diagnosis, & Prognosis

## Exam Three: Question 97

A physical therapist completes a developmental assessment on an infant. Which pediatric reflex would the therapist expect to be integrated at the youngest age?

1. plantar grasp reflex
2. Moro reflex
3. Landau reflex
4. **Galant reflex**

**Correct Answer: 4** (Ratliffe p. 26)

Integration of a reflex refers to the period of time when a reflex is no longer present despite an appropriate stimulus.

1. The plantar grasp reflex is stimulated by placing pressure on the ball of the foot, generally in standing. The response is flexion and curling of the toes. The normal age of the response is from 28 weeks of gestation to nine months.

2. The Moro reflex is stimulated when an infant's head is suddenly allowed to fall into extension. The action causes a "startled look" followed by upper extremity abduction with the fingers open, then crossing the trunk into adduction. The normal age of the response is from 28 weeks of gestation to five months.

3. The Landau reflex is an equilibrium response that occurs when a child responds to prone suspension by aligning their head and extremities in line with the plane of the body. Although the response begins around three months of age, it is not fully integrated until the child's second year.

4. **The Galant reflex is stimulated by touching the skin along the spine from the shoulder to the hip. The response is lateral flexion of the trunk to the side of the stimulus. The normal age of the response is from 30 weeks of gestation to two months.**

System Specific: Neuromuscular & Nervous Systems
Content Outline: Physical Therapy Examination

## Exam Three: Question 98

A physical therapist examines a patient with a limited straight leg raise of 40 degrees due to inadequate hamstrings length. Which proprioceptive neuromuscular facilitation technique would be the MOST appropriate to increase the patient's hamstrings length?

1. **contract-relax**
2. rhythmic initiation
3. rhythmic stabilization
4. rhythmic rotation

**Correct Answer: 1** (Sullivan p. 66)

Contract-relax is a proprioceptive neuromuscular facilitation (PNF) technique utilized to increase range of motion on one side of a joint. This technique utilizes isometric as well as isotonic contractions.

1. **Contract-relax is used to improve range of motion. As the extremity reaches the point of limitation, the patient performs a maximal contraction of the antagonistic muscle group. The therapist resists movement for eight to ten seconds followed by a period of relaxation. The technique is repeated until no further gains in range of motion are noted.**

2. Rhythmic initiation is used to initiate movement when hypertonia exists. Movement progresses from passive ("let me move you"), to active assistive ("help me move"), to slightly resistive ("move against resistance"). Movements are slow and rhythmical to reduce tone and allow for full range of motion.

3. Rhythmic stabilization is used to increase range of motion and coordinate isometric contractions. The technique requires isometric contractions of all muscles around a joint against progressive resistance. The patient should attempt to relax and move into the newly acquired range of motion.

4. Rhythmic rotation is a passive technique used to decrease hypertonia by slowly rotating an extremity around the longitudinal axis. Relaxation of the extremity promotes an increase in available range of motion.

System Specific: Neuromuscular & Nervous Systems
Content Outline: Interventions

## Exam Three: Question 99

A physical therapist examines a patient following a transtibial amputation. The patient resides in a retirement community and describes herself as socially active. She is presently using a temporary prosthesis consisting of a plastic socket, a pylon, and a solid ankle cushion heel (SACH) foot. The patient expresses concern that the permanent prosthesis will look awful and will be obvious to everyone. Which type of prosthesis would be the MOST appropriate for the patient?

1. endoskeletal shank and single-axis articulated foot-ankle assembly
2. **endoskeletal shank and solid ankle cushion heel (SACH) foot**
3. exoskeletal shank and single-axis articulated foot-ankle assembly
4. exoskeletal shank and solid ankle cushion heel (SACH) foot

**Correct Answer: 2** (Tan p. 247)
An endoskeleton or modular shank is designed to incorporate a synthetic foam cover shaped like the opposite leg. As a result, the device is more cosmetically attractive and would likely make the patient more socially comfortable. A SACH foot is the most frequently prescribed foot-ankle assembly. It is considered to be a nonarticulated foot since it does not incorporate a mechanical joint at the ankle.

1. An endoskeletal shank would be an appropriate choice given the patient's concerns, however, a single-axis articulated foot-ankle assembly would be heavier and requires more maintenance than the SACH foot. Since the patient is of retirement age and does not plan on heavy activity, this type of foot would not be appropriate.

2. **Since the patient is of retirement age and expects low impact on the prosthesis, the endoskeletal shank and SACH foot will provide the patient with durability, low maintenance, and cosmesis.**

3. An exoskeletal shank would not be appropriate for the patient since it less cosmetically desirable and heavier with the hard, thermoplastic resin shell. The single-axis articulated foot-ankle assembly would be heavier and require more maintenance than the SACH foot.

4. An exoskeletal shank would not be as desirable for the patient as the endoskeletal shank. The SACH foot is appropriate for the patient.

System Specific: Musculoskeletal System
Content Outline: Interventions

## Exam Three: Question 100

A physical therapist observes a patient during gait training. The patient has normal strength and equal leg length. As the patient passes midstance he slightly vaults and exhibits early toe off. The MOST likely cause of this deviation is:

1. weakness of the dorsiflexors
2. weakness of the hip abductors
3. limited plantar flexion
4. **limited dorsiflexion**

**Correct Answer: 4** (Magee p. 964)
A patient with limited dorsiflexion may compensate with a vault or bounce through mid to late stance. Approximately ten degrees of dorsiflexion is required for late stance through toe off.

1. Weakness of the dorsiflexors will typically create a "steppage gait pattern." The patient will present with foot slap at initial contact and compensate by lifting the knee higher than normal to clear the foot and avoid dragging the toe.

2. Weakness of the hip abductors (gluteus medius and minimus) will typically create a contralateral dip of the pelvis during the stance phase of the weak side, also known as a Trendelenburg gait pattern. The observed contralateral dip of the pelvis results from the inability of the weak hip abductors to stabilize the pelvis during contralateral swing phase.

3. Limited plantar flexion would not result in a vaulting gait pattern. The patient would require plantar flexion to vault (ascend onto the toes) during gait. Plantar flexion of 0-20 degrees is required for normal gait biomechanics with approximately 15 degrees during the loading response and 20 degrees during the pre-swing phase.

4. **Limited dorsiflexion will typically result in premature elevation of the heel during midstance. The patient will appear to have a bounce during gait secondary to the gastroc-soleus tightness.**

System Specific: Musculoskeletal System
Content Outline: Foundations for Evaluation, Differential Diagnosis, & Prognosis

## Exam Three: Question 101

A physical therapist attempts to auscultate over the aortic valve. Which of the following areas is the MOST appropriate to isolate the desired valve?

1. second left intercostal space at the left sternal border
2. **second right intercostal space at the right sternal border**
3. fourth left intercostal space along the lower left sternal border
4. fifth left intercostal space at the midclavicular line

**Correct Answer: 2** (Rothstein p. 504)
Auscultation of the heart requires selective listening for each component of the cardiac cycle over the main topographic areas for auscultation.

1. The second left intercostal space at the left sternal border denotes the pulmonary area and is best for auscultating the pulmonic valve.
2. **The second right intercostal space at the right sternal border denotes the aortic area and is best for auscultating the aortic valve.**
3. The fourth left intercostal space along the lower left sternal border denotes the tricuspid area and is best for auscultating the tricuspid valve.
4. The fifth left intercostal space at the midclavicular line denotes the mitral area or apex of the heart and is best for auscultating the mitral valve.

System Specific: Cardiovascular/Pulmonary and Lymphatic Systems
Content Outline: Physical Therapy Examination

## Exam Three: Question 102

A physical therapist attempts to estimate the energy expenditure in calories for a patient performing a selected activity for 15 minutes. Assuming the therapist has a metabolic equivalent value for the activity, what other variables are necessary in order to obtain an estimate of the patient's energy expenditure?

1. patient's height
2. **patient's body weight**
3. patient's stroke volume
4. patient's residual volume

**Correct Answer: 2** (Rothstein p. 540)
To estimate the energy expended (calories) of an activity, it is necessary to know the patient's body weight (kg) and the metabolic equivalent (MET) value of the activity.

1. Height is not needed to estimate the energy expenditure of an activity. Height and weight are needed to calculate body mass index.
2. **A metabolic equivalent (MET) is a measure of oxygen consumption, 1 MET = 3.5 mL $O_2$ per kg of body weight per minute. Therefore, the caloric expenditure of any activity can be estimated using the number of METs for the activity, the body weight (kg), and the duration of the activity.**
3. Stroke volume is the volume of blood ejected from the ventricles with each contraction. Stroke volume is not needed to estimate the energy expenditure of an activity. Stroke volume and heart rate are needed to calculate cardiac output.
4. Residual volume is the volume of air that remains in the lungs after a maximum forced exhalation. Residual volume is not needed to estimate the energy expenditure of an activity.

System Specific: Cardiovascular/Pulmonary and Lymphatic Systems
Content Outline: Interventions

## Exam Three: Question 103

A patient in a work hardening program completes a training program consisting of ten different exercises requiring upper and lower extremity strength and endurance. The patient indicates that he is frustrated since he has been unable to increase the weight on a selected carrying activity in over two weeks. The MOST appropriate physical therapist action is:

1. provide the patient with verbal encouragement
2. attempt to substitute a different exercise for the carrying activity
3. **vary the order of the exercises**
4. decrease the number of repetitions

**Correct Answer: 3** (Prentice – Techniques p. 379)
Physical therapists must be able to modify existing training programs based on the rate of patient progress and the stated therapeutic objectives.

1. Verbal encouragement is desirable, however, given the two week time frame it is likely that an attempt to modify the program would be more appropriate.

2. The described scenario does not provide enough evidence to indicate that the carrying activity should be discontinued. The question states only that the patient is frustrated since he has been unable to increase the weight. It would therefore be more valuable to modify the program in a manner that allows the patient to progress with the originally selected activity.

3. **Varying the order of the exercises in the program is a strategy often employed when a patient experiences a plateau. For example, by encountering the activity earlier in the program the patient may be less fatigued and able to progress.**

4. The question discusses the patient's inability to increase the weight on the carrying activity, however, it does not discuss the number of repetitions. If the therapist decreases the number of repetitions from the present level it may deemphasize the focus on endurance.

System Specific: Musculoskeletal System
Content Outline: Interventions

## Exam Three: Question 104

A patient prepares for discharge from a rehabilitation hospital after completing three months of therapy. The patient has made significant progress in his rehabilitation, however, expresses concern that his previous employer may not want him to return to work due to his injury. The MOST appropriate action is to:

1. explain to the patient that to return to work after a serious injury is very difficult
2. **inform the patient of his rights according to the Americans with Disabilities Act**
3. request that the patient consider vocational retraining
4. refer the patient to a psychologist to assist with the transition back to work

**Correct Answer: 2** (Minor p. 1)
The Americans with Disabilities Act (ADA) is federal legislation designed to eliminate discrimination against individuals with disabilities. Physical therapists have an ethical obligation to make patients aware of their rights according to the ADA.

1. A physical therapist should be empathetic and supportive about the patient's return to work, however, it is more critical to make the patient aware of their rights according to the ADA.

2. **The patient may have some of their expressed concern eliminated by learning that they have certain rights according to the ADA.**

3. The question does not provide any evidence to suggest that the patient is unable to complete their previous role at work. As a result, it would be premature to suggest vocational retraining.

4. The patient is worried that the employer may not want him to return to work, however, the question does not imply that the patient's concern has a psychological origin.

System Specific: Non-Systems
Content Outline: Safety and Protection; Professional Responsibilities; Research

## Exam Three: Question 105

A physical therapist employed in an acute care hospital attempts to identify a standardized instrument that measures level of consciousness. The MOST appropriate standardized instrument is the:

1. **Glasgow Coma Scale**
2. Modified Rankin Scale
3. Barthel Index
4. Sickness Impact Profile

**Correct Answer: 1** (Rothstein p. 360)

The Glasgow Coma Scale provides a practical method for assessing the degree of conscious impairment in the critically ill patient. The scale utilizes eye opening, verbal responses, and motor responses to determine the level of consciousness and degree of dysfunction.

1. **The Glasgow Coma Scale is a neurological assessment tool used initially after injury to determine arousal and cerebral cortex function. A score of eight or less correlates to a severe brain injury, a score of 9 to 12 indicates a moderate brain injury, and a score of 13 to 15 indicates a mild brain injury.**

2. The Modified Rankin Scale measures independence rather than the performance of specific tasks. The scale is a measure of disability or dependence in activities of daily living and is frequently used with patients with CVA.

3. The Barthel Index measures the patient's performance in 10 activities of daily living. It is considered a reliable disability scale for patients with CVA. Scored items relate to self-care (feeding, grooming, bathing, dressing, bowel and bladder care, and toileting) and mobility (ambulation, transfers, and stair climbing).

4. The Sickness Impact Profile is a generic measure used to evaluate the impact of disease on both physical and emotional functioning. Patients are asked to respond to the items based on their current status.

System Specific: Neuromuscular & Nervous Systems
Content Outline: Physical Therapy Examination

## Exam Three: Question 106

A physical therapist critically analyzes the methodology used in a published research study. Which type of sampling procedure would result in the GREATEST degree of sampling error?

1. simple random sample
2. systematic sample
3. **cluster sample**
4. stratified random sample

**Correct Answer: 3** (Portney p. 152)

Cluster sampling involves successive random sampling of a series of units in the population. Cluster sampling is often utilized when a researcher is unable to know all elements in the population in advance.

1. A simple random sample is a type of probability sample where every element of the population has an equal chance of being selected for the sample.

2. A systematic sample is a type of probability sample where elements are chosen from lists of population members using specified intervals, such as every 4th element.

3. **A cluster sample is a probability sample in which large subgroups (clusters) are randomly selected first, and then smaller units are selected from the clusters. Because the technique requires two or more samples to be drawn, each sample is subject to sampling error, potentially compounding the accuracy of the final sample.**

4. A stratified random sample is a type of probability sample in which elements of the population are chosen at random from homogenous groups based on some characteristic. Organizing elements into homogenous groups before selection decreases the sampling error.

System Specific: Non-Systems
Content Outline: Safety and Protection; Professional Responsibilities; Research

## Exam Three: Question 107

A physical therapist attempts to identify an appropriately sized wheelchair for a patient recently referred to a rehabilitation hospital. The physical therapist determines that the patient's hip width in sitting and the measurement from the back of the buttocks to the popliteal space are each 16 inches. Given these measurements, which of the following wheelchair specifications would BEST fit this patient?

1. seat width 16 inches, seat depth 14 inches
2. seat width 18 inches, seat depth 18 inches
3. seat width 16 inches, seat depth 18 inches
4. **seat width 18 inches, seat depth 14 inches**

> **Correct Answer: 4** (Pierson p. 136)
> Seat width is determined by measuring the widest aspect of the user's buttocks, hips or thighs and adding two inches. Seat depth is measured from the user's posterior buttock, along the lateral thigh to the popliteal fold; then subtracting two inches. In the described scenario, seat width and depth should be calculated as follows: seat width = hip width (16 inches) + 2 inches = 18 inches; seat depth = posterior buttock to the popliteal space (16 inches) - 2 inches = 14 inches.
>
> 1. The described wheelchair would have inadequate seat width, however, the seat depth would be appropriate. Inadequate seat width could result in the development of a pressure sore.
> 2. The described wheelchair would have appropriate seat width, however, the seat depth would be excessive. Excessive seat depth could result in increased pressure in the popliteal area leading to discomfort or circulatory compromise.
> 3. The described wheelchair would have inadequate seat width and the seat depth would be excessive.
> 4. **A seat width of 18 inches and a seat depth of 14 inches are consistent with the presented formula based on the obtained measurements.**
>
> System Specific: Non-Systems
> Content Outline: Equipment & Devices; Therapeutic Modalities

## Exam Three: Question 108

A physical therapist employed in an acute care hospital conducts an initial interview with a patient referred to physical therapy. During the interview, the therapist asks the patient if he feels dependent on coffee, tea or soft drinks. Which clinical scenario would MOST appropriately warrant this type of question?

1. a 27-year-old female status post arthroscopic medial meniscectomy
2. **a 42-year-old male with premature ventricular contractions**
3. a 37-year-old female with restrictive pulmonary disease
4. a 57-year-old male with respiratory alkalosis

> **Correct Answer: 2** (Brannon p. 206)
> Premature ventricular contractions (PVCs) are premature beats arising from an ectopic focus in one of the ventricles of the heart. Coffee, tea, and soft drinks may contain caffeine, a stimulant that may precipitate premature ventricular contractions. Other causes of PVCs are nicotine, stress, alcohol, and certain electrolyte imbalances.
>
> 1. It would not be important to know if a patient who is post arthroscopic medial meniscectomy has a dependence on coffee, tea, and soft drinks, since these drinks would have no affect on their condition or course of physical therapy.
> 2. **It would be important to know if a patient known to have PVCs has a dependence on coffee, tea, and soft drinks since these drinks may contain caffeine, a stimulant that can precipitate PVCs. The physical therapist should inform the patient about the possible connection between these drinks and the occurrence of PVCs.**
> 3. It would not be important to know if a patient who has restrictive pulmonary disease has a dependence on coffee, tea, and soft drinks, since these drinks have no known affect on their condition or course of physical therapy.
> 4. It would not be important to know if a patient with respiratory alkalosis has a dependence on coffee, tea, and soft drinks, since these drinks would have no affect on their condition or course of physical therapy.
>
> System Specific: Cardiovascular/Pulmonary and Lymphatic Systems
> Content Outline: Foundations for Evaluation, Differential Diagnosis, & Prognosis

## Exam Three: Question 109

A physical therapist assigns a manual muscle test grade of 4 to patient A and a grade of 2 to patient B. Which of the following is the BEST interpretation of the strength of the patients?

1. patients A and B have equal strength
2. **patient A is stronger than patient B**
3. patient A is twice as strong as patient B
4. patient B is twice as strong as patient A

**Correct Answer: 2** (Portney p. 68)

Manual muscle test grades are examples of ordinal measurements, which in essence represent labels specifying relative rank or position. Ordinal measurements are rank-ordered into categories that have a "greater than – less than" relationship. The intervals between ranks on an ordinal scale may not be consistent and may not be known.

1. The numerical scale used in manual muscle testing ranks the strength by strongest (equivalent to the grade of 5) and weakest (equivalent to the grade of 0). In this situation, the grades are not equal, 4 does not equal 2 therefore they cannot have equal strength.

2. **Based on the traditional 0 – 5 manual muscle grading scale, a grade of 4 represents more muscle strength than a grade of 2.**

3. The numerical scale does not provide an "absolute" value, therefore, it is impossible to say that a grade of 4 is two times stronger than a grade of 2. Furthermore, the testing positions of these grades are not the same and as a result they cannot be compared in this manner.

4. The numerical order of the manual muscle testing scale indicates that a grade of 5 is the strongest and a grade of 0 is the weakest. Therefore, a grade of 2 cannot indicate greater strength than a grade of 4.

System Specific: Musculoskeletal System
Content Outline: Physical Therapy Examination

## Exam Three: Question 110

A physical therapist inspects a patient's wound prior to applying a dressing. When documenting the findings in the medical record the therapist classifies the exudate from the wound as serous. Based on the documentation, the MOST likely color of the exudate is:

1. **clear**
2. pink
3. red
4. yellow

**Correct Answer: 1** (Sussman p. 458)

It is normal during the stages of healing to observe exudate from a wound. The physical therapist should inspect the various types of exudate and determine whether it is a normal response to healing or an abnormal response that needs to be reported.

1. **Serous exudate is described as clear or light color fluid with a thin, watery consistency. This particular type of exudate is normal during the inflammatory and proliferative phases of healing.**

2. Serosanguinous (pink) exudate can be a normal exudate in a healthy healing wound.

3. Sanguinous (red) exudate indicates a bloody discharge which may be indicative of either new blood vessel growth (normal healing tissue) or a disruption of blood vessels (abnormal).

4. Purulent (yellow) exudate is generally indicative of infection.

System Specific: Other Systems
Content Outline: Physical Therapy Examination

## Exam Three: Question 111

A patient coverage form indicates selective debridement is to be performed on a patient rehabilitating from a lower extremity burn. Based on the coverage form, the MOST likely intervention would be:

1. whirlpool
2. wet-to-dry dressings
3. **enzymatic debridement**
4. wound irrigation

**Correct Answer: 3** (Sussman p. 442)
Selective debridement involves removing only nonviable tissues from a wound. Non-selective debridement involves removing both viable and nonviable tissues from a wound.

1. Whirlpool uses a turbine to produce agitation and aeration which creates movement of the water in the tank. The movement of the water results in the softening and loosening of adherent necrotic tissue. The inability to isolate necrotic tissue using whirlpool makes the intervention a form of non-selective debridement.

2. Wet-to-dry dressings refer to the application of a moistened gauze dressing placed in an area of necrotic tissue. The dressing is then allowed to dry completely and is later removed along with the necrotic tissue that has adhered to the gauze. This type of debridement should be used sparingly on wounds with both necrotic tissue and viable tissue since granulation tissue will be traumatized in the process. As a result, a wet-to-dry dressing is a form of non-selective debridement.

3. **Enzymatic debridement is considered to be selective since the topical preparation of the enzymes used (collagenolytic, proteolytic) will greatly influence the treatment outcome.**

4. Wound irrigation removes necrotic tissue from the wound bed using pressurized fluid. Most devices permit varying pressure settings and provide suction for removal of the exudate and debris. Wound irrigation is a form of non-selective debridement.

System Specific: Other Systems
Content Outline: Interventions

## Exam Three: Question 112

A physical therapist participates in a community-based screening program designed to identify individuals with osteoporosis. Which group would have the highest risk for developing osteoporosis?

1. **Caucasian females over the age of 60**
2. African American females over the age of 60
3. Caucasian females under the age of 40
4. African American females under the age of 40

**Correct Answer: 1** (Goodman - Differential Diagnosis p. 439)
Osteoporosis is a metabolic bone disease characterized by increased bone resorption resulting in a reduction in bone mass. Osteoporosis is more prevalent in females than in males, in older than younger individuals, and in Caucasians than African Americans.

1. **Caucasian females experience an increased incidence of osteoporosis compared to African American females. The relative risk of osteoporosis increases with age since there is decreased production of estrogen and a greater loss of bone density following menopause.**

2. African American females have an increased risk of osteoporosis with increasing age, however, this group is at less risk than Caucasian females because bone mass has a positive correlation to the color and pigmentation of the skin. Therefore, African American females generally have greater bone mass than the statistically equivalent Caucasian females.

3. Caucasian females under the age of 40 are typically not at high risk for osteoporosis. Bone mass will normally peak between 25 and 35 years of age, followed by a progressive increase in bone resorption compared to bone formation that may result, decades later, in osteopenia and osteoporosis.

4. African Americans under the age of 40 are typically not at high risk for osteoporosis. Bone mass will normally peak between 25 and 35 years of age. Bone resorption and bone formation occur in a similar manner as described in option 3.

System Specific: Other Systems
Content Outline: Foundations for Evaluation, Differential Diagnosis, & Prognosis

## Exam Three: Question 113

A physical therapist positions a patient in sidelying in preparation for postural drainage activities. Which lung segment would be indicated based on the patient's position?

1. posterior basal segment of the lower lobes
2. anterior apical segment of the upper lobes
3. **lateral basal segment of the lower lobes**
4. anterior segment of the upper lobes

**Correct Answer: 3** (Frownfelter p. 314)

When performing postural drainage, the physical therapist should position the patient so that the bronchus of the involved lung segment is perpendicular to the ground. Specific positioning for each lung segment allows gravity to assist in the drainage of the secretions.

1. Posterior basal segment of the lower lobes would require positioning in prone with a pillow under the hips with the foot of the bed elevated 18 inches from the floor.
2. The anterior apical segment of the upper lobes would require a seated position where the patient is leaning back at a 30 degree angle against the therapist.
3. **The lateral basal segment of the lower lobes requires positioning in sidelying with an inclination of 18 inches of the foot of the bed.**
4. The anterior segment of the upper lobes would require a supine position with a pillow under the knees.

System Specific: Cardiovascular/Pulmonary and Lymphatic Systems
Content Outline: Interventions

## Exam Three: Question 114

A patient with acute back pain is given a transcutaneous electrical nerve stimulation unit to use at home. The physical therapist provides detailed instructions on the care and use of the unit. Which of the following activities is NOT the responsibility of the patient?

1. modulate the current intensity
2. application of new electrodes
3. change the battery
4. **alter the pulse rate and width**

**Correct Answer: 4** (Cameron p. 214)

Physical therapists routinely educate patients on how to use various portable electrical devices such as a transcutaneous electrical nerve stimulation (TENS) unit at home. Therapists must be sure that patients understand which parameters they are able to modify and which parameters should be modified by the patient.

1. Patients need to adjust the current intensity of the TENS with each use. Current intensity refers to the movement of charged particles and is most often measured in amperes.
2. Electrodes often need to be replaced during the course of treatment since they may no longer adequately adhere to the skin.
3. Changing the battery of a TENS unit is a relatively easy task that does not require changing any of the specified treatment parameters.
4. **Specific pulse rates and widths are selected by the therapist based on the TENS technique selected. Common techniques include conventional TENS, acupuncture-like TENS, brief-intense TENS, and noxious-TENS. Pulse rate and width should not be altered by the patient throughout the duration of treatment, unless specified by the therapist.**

System Specific: Non-Systems
Content Outline: Equipment & Devices; Therapeutic Modalities

## Exam Three: Question 115

A patient with chronic pulmonary dysfunction is placed on a corticosteroid medication to reduce mucosal edema and inflammation. The MOST common cardiovascular side effect of corticosteroids is:

1. palpitations
2. arrhythmias
3. **increased blood pressure**
4. tachycardia

**Correct Answer: 3** (Ciccone p. 378)

Increased blood pressure or hypertension is a side effect that is associated with heavy or prolonged use of corticosteroids (also known as glucocorticoids). Other side effects include osteoporosis, muscle wasting, skin breakdown, cataracts, adrenocorticosuppression, and hyperglycemia.

1. A palpitation is a sensation in which a person is aware of an irregular, hard or fast heartbeat that may skip or beat irregularly. The word palpitation is sometimes used synonymously with arrhythmia, however, a palpitation may or may not be caused by an arrhythmia. Many palpitations are benign, but the underlying cause is important to diagnose.

2. An arrhythmia is defined as a significant deviation from normal sinus rhythm. Many medications have potential side effects of arrhythmias including other cardiac medications, tricyclic antidepressants, and minerals such as calcium.

3. **Corticosteroid use can increase blood pressure secondary to the sodium and water retention properties of the corticosteroid. Long-term use of corticosteroids must be closely monitored due to the stated adverse effects.**

4. Tachycardia refers to a heart rate in excess of 100 beats per minute in an adult. It may occur normally in response to fever, exercise or excitement.  Many substances have potential side effects of tachycardia including alcohol, caffeine, nicotine, and certain anti-anxiety and cardiac medications.

System Specific: Cardiovascular/Pulmonary and Lymphatic Systems
Content Outline: Foundations for Evaluation, Differential Diagnosis, and Prognosis

## Exam Three: Question 116

A physical therapist inspects a wound that has large quantities of exudate which requires frequent dressing changes. If the therapist applies a dressing that cannot handle the quantity of exudate present, the MOST likely outcome is:

1. **maceration**
2. granulation
3. epithelialization
4. infection

**Correct Answer: 1** (Sussman p. 376)

Transparent film is an example of a type of dressing that would be unable to handle a significant amount of exudate. Conversely, an alginate dressing would be a better choice for a wound with a significant amount of exudate since the dressing is highly permeable and would therefore tend to absorb the exudate.

1. **Maceration refers to a softening of connective tissue fibers due to excessive moisture. The result is a loss of pigmentation and a wound that is highly susceptible to breakdown or enlargement.**

2. Granulation refers to perfused, fibrous connective tissue that replaces a fibrin clot in a healing wound. The tissue is highly vascular and fills the defects of full-thickness wounds.

3. Epithelialization refers to the process of epidermal resurfacing and appears as pink or red skin.

4. Signs and symptoms of infection include the production of pus, redness, pain, and swelling. More generalized symptoms of infection may include fever, chills, and an increased pulse rate. Laboratory values associated with infection include an increased erythrocyte sedimentation rate and white blood cell count.

System Specific: Other Systems
Content Outline: Interventions

## Exam Three: Question 117

A patient refuses physical therapy services after being transported to the gym. The physical therapist explains the potential consequences of refusing treatment, however, the patient does not reconsider. The MOST appropriate INITIAL therapist action is:

1. treat the patient
2. convince the patient to have therapy
3. contact the referring physician
4. **document the incident in the medical record**

**Correct Answer: 4** (Scott - Promoting Legal and Ethical Awareness p. 231)
The Guide for Professional Conduct published by the American Physical Therapy Association states that "A physical therapist shall respect the patient's/client's right to make decisions regarding the recommended plan of care, including consent, modification or refusal."

1. A therapist does not have the right to treat a patient against their wishes.
2. The therapist is obligated to inform the patient of the potential consequences of refusing treatment, however, the purpose of this action is to allow the patient to make an informed decision and not to "convince" them to have therapy.
3. Contacting the referring physician when a patient refuses treatment is appropriate and necessary, however, it would not be the "initial" therapist action.
4. **The therapist must document that the patient refused treatment and was informed of the potential consequences associated with this decision. Failure to document this important information in a timely manner could place the therapist at unnecessary legal risk.**

System Specific: Non-Systems
Content Outline: Safety and Protection; Professional Responsibilities; Research

## Exam Three: Question 118

A physical therapist completes an examination on a 36-year-old female diagnosed with multiple sclerosis. After completing the examination, the therapist should FIRST:

1. develop long-term goals
2. develop short-term goals
3. **develop a problem list**
4. justify the need for physical therapy services

**Correct Answer: 3** (Quinn p. 34)
A physical therapist should generate a problem list after completing an examination. The problem list will assist the physical therapist to determine the patient's need for physical therapy services, the frequency of therapy sessions, and the short and long-term goals.

1. The development of long-term goals is vital to the plan of care. The physical therapist will generate long-term goals based on current patient status, typical expected outcome based on diagnosis, patient goals, and the expected time frame of physical therapy services.
2. Short-term goals are developed to assist in attaining a long-term goal in a step by step manner. The physical therapist will generate short-term goals with a predetermined time frame based on current patient status and the established long-term goal.
3. **Once an examination has been completed, the physical therapist reviews all of the data and generates a problem list. The problem list assists the therapist to determine if physical therapy services are warranted and to develop an effective and individualized plan of care.**
4. A physical therapist must justify the need for physical therapy services based on the results of the examination, however, the problem list would be developed first to assist the therapist to make an informed decision.

System Specific: Non-Systems
Content Outline: Safety and Protection; Professional Responsibilities; Research

## Exam Three: Question 119

An electrical equipment safety committee develops a policy to limit electrical hazards arising from ground faults. Which action would be the MOST appropriate to meet the committee's objective?

1. report all equipment defects or failures
2. **manually test each ground fault circuit interrupter on a monthly basis**
3. follow manufacturer recommendations for electrical equipment care and service
4. mandate an introductory inservice on all new electrical equipment

**Correct Answer: 2** (Prentice - Therapeutic Modalities p. 150)

Policies are used to guide or in some instances, standardize certain behaviors within an organization. It is important to recognize that the question asks specifically about a policy related to electrical hazards arising from ground faults.

1. The identification of defects or failures is essential for corrective action to be taken, however, the action is reactive rather than proactive.
2. **Ground fault circuit interrupters are designed to identify the presence of ground faults and quickly switch off power to that circuit. The automatic device provides personal protection from electrical shock. Manually testing each ground fault circuit interrupter on a fixed interval allows for proactive monitoring.**
3. Manufacturers' recommendations for electrical equipment care and service should be followed. This action, although desirable, does not specifically address the goal of limiting electrical hazards arising from ground faults.
4. Physical therapists should be oriented to all new electrical equipment and possess a thorough understanding of how to operate the equipment prior to clinical use. This action in isolation does not specifically address the prevention of ground faults.

System Specific: Non-Systems
Content Outline: Safety and Protection; Professional Responsibilities; Research

## Exam Three: Question 120

A 21-year-old female is examined in physical therapy after sustaining a grade I ankle sprain two days ago in a marching band competition. The patient's description of the mechanism of injury is consistent with inversion and plantar flexion. Which of the following ligaments would MOST likely be affected?

1. **anterior talofibular ligament**
2. calcaneofibular ligament
3. anterior tibiofibular ligament
4. deltoid ligament

**Correct Answer: 1** (Magee p. 859)

A grade I ankle sprain is a minor injury that involves stretching of the ligament or perhaps a small partial tear of the ligament. Treatment consists of rest, ice, compression, and elevation.

1. **The anterior talofibular ligament is a thickening of the anterior joint capsule that extends from the anterior surface of the lateral malleolus to the lateral facet of the talus and the lateral surface of the talar neck. The ligament functions to resist ankle inversion with the foot in plantar flexion. Regardless of the position of the foot, the anterior talofibular ligament is the most likely ligament torn with an inversion injury.**
2. The calcaneofibular ligament is a round cord that passes posteroinferiorly from the tip of the lateral malleolus to the lateral surface of the calcaneus. The ligament functions to resist ankle inversion and dorsiflexion.
3. The anterior tibiofibular ligament provides support to the distal tibiofibular joint. The ligament resists distal and posterior glide of the fibula.
4. The deltoid ligament refers to the collective medial ligaments of the ankle. The ligament as a whole attaches proximally to the medial aspect of the medial malleolus and fans out to the various distal attachments.

System Specific: Musculoskeletal System
Content Outline: Physical Therapy Examination

## Exam Three: Question 121

A physical therapist prepares to administer iontophoresis over the anterior surface of a patient's knee. The therapist would like to keep the current density low in order to avoid skin irritation. Which of the listed parameters would BEST accomplish the therapist's objective?

1. **current amplitude of 4 mA; electrode with an area of 12 cm²**
2. current amplitude of 4 mA; electrode with an area of 4 cm²
3. current amplitude of 3 mA; electrode with an area of 6 cm²
4. current amplitude of 3 mA; electrode with an area of 4 cm²

**Correct Answer: 1** (Cameron p. 223)
The current density may be altered either by increasing or decreasing current intensity or by changing the size of the electrode. Current density with iontophoresis equals current amplitude (mA) divided by electrode size (cm²). Failure to select appropriate treatment or failure to monitor the patient's response to treatment creates an unnecessary safety risk.

1. **Current density = 4 mA / 12 cm² = .33 mA/cm²**
2. Current density = 4 mA / 4 cm² = 1.0 mA/cm²
3. Current density = 3 mA / 6 cm² = .50 mA/cm²
4. Current density = 3 mA / 4 cm² = .75 mA/cm²

System Specific: Non-Systems
Content Outline: Equipment & Devices; Therapeutic Modalities

## Exam Three: Question 122

To practice physical therapy according to the tenets of evidence-based medicine, a physical therapist must:

1. use tests and measurements with known reliability and validity
2. use systematic reviews and randomized controlled trials as sources of research evidence
3. **integrate the best research evidence, clinical expertise, and patient values in clinical decision-making**
4. respect the rights and dignity of patients

**Correct Answer: 3** (Sackett p. 1)
Evidence-based medicine is the integration of the best research evidence with clinical expertise and patient values. Best research evidence refers to clinically relevant research, especially patient-centered clinical research. Clinical expertise refers to the clinician's clinical skills and past experiences, but also may refer to published clinical practice guidelines. Patient values refer to the unique preferences, concerns, and expectations each patient brings to the clinical encounter.

1. Using tests and measurements with known reliability and validity is important to the practice of physical therapy, but is not specific to evidence-based practice.
2. Using systematic reviews and randomized controlled trials as sources of research evidence is important to the practice of physical therapy, but is not specific to evidence-based practice.
3. **Evidence-based medicine is the integration of the best research evidence with clinical expertise and patient values.**
4. Respecting the rights and dignity of patients is important to the practice of physical therapy, but is not specific to evidence-based practice.

System Specific: Non-Systems
Content Outline: Safety and Protection; Professional Responsibilities; Research

## Exam Three: Question 123

A physical therapist completes a coordination assessment on a 67-year-old patient with central nervous system involvement. After reviewing the results of the assessment, the therapist concludes the clinical findings are indicative of cerebellar dysfunction. Which finding is NOT associated with cerebellar dysfunction?

1. dysmetria
2. **hypertonia**
3. ataxia
4. nystagmus

---

**Correct Answer: 2** (O'Sullivan p. 198)

Cerebellar pathology is often characterized by incoordinated movement. Specific motor impairments associated with cerebellar pathology include ataxia, hypotonicity, dysmetria, dysdiadochokinesia, nystagmus, tremor, and scanning speech.

1. Dysmetria refers to the inability to control the range of a movement and the force of muscular activity. The result of this is often overshooting or undershooting.

2. **Cerebellar dysfunction would typically be associated with hypotonia and not hypertonia. Hypotonia causes the patient to have difficulty fixating the limb, leading to incoordination with movement.**

3. Ataxia refers to the inability to perform coordinated movements. Ataxia can affect gait, patterns of movement, and posture. The condition increases the incidence of errors in the rate, rhythm, and timing of responses.

4. Nystagmus refers to abnormal eye movement that entails nonvolitional, rhythmic oscillation of the eyes. The speed of movement is typically faster in one direction than the other direction.

System Specific: Neuromuscular & Nervous Systems
Content Outline: Foundations for Evaluation, Differential Diagnosis, & Prognosis

---

## Exam Three: Question 124

A patient status post open knee meniscectomy is referred to physical therapy for neuromuscular electrical stimulation. The MOST beneficial frequency of treatment to promote strengthening is:

1. two times per day
2. one time per week
3. **three times per week**
4. once every two weeks

---

**Correct Answer: 3** (Prentice - Therapeutic Modalities p. 130)

The question indicates that the focus of the intervention is to increase strength and therefore it is necessary for the intervention to be performed multiple times each week. Frequency is also influenced by variables such as intensity, repetitions, and sets.

1. Two times per day would be excessive since the intensity of the strengthening activity would require more recovery time. Failure to have sufficient recovery time may lead to delayed-onset muscle soreness, excessive microtrauma, and possible injury.

2. One time per week is insufficient based on the stated goal of promoting muscle strength. This frequency may be more appropriate for a maintenance program.

3. **Three times per week is a general guideline for strengthening activities. The frequency allows for adequate intensity and sufficient rest time to minimize microtrauma and avoid delayed onset muscle soreness.**

4. Once every two weeks is insufficient for virtually any therapeutic purpose, most notably strengthening.

System Specific: Musculoskeletal System
Content Outline: Interventions

## Exam Three: Question 125

A 67-year-old male with longstanding cardiac pathology is referred to physical therapy. The medical record indicates the patient is taking Nitrostat. The PRIMARY indication for this medication is:

1. to strengthen the heart's pumping force
2. **to produce a general vasodilation of vascular structures**
3. to increase excretion of sodium and water
4. to decrease electrical conduction

> **Correct Answer: 2** (Ciccone p. 309)
> Nitrates are commonly used to treat angina pectoris. Potential adverse reactions when using nitrates includes headache, hypotension, dizziness, vertigo, weakness, and flushing. Nitrostat and NitroQuick are commonly used brand names of nitrates.
>
> 1. Cardiac glycosides are a category of drugs that increase the myocardial contraction force. Cardiac glycosides increase myocardial contractility by elevating intracellular calcium levels and facilitating actin-myosin interaction in cardiac cells.
> 2. **Nitrates are administered to produce a general vasodilation throughout the body. Nitrates decrease the amount of blood returning to the heart as well as the amount of work the heart must perform which decreases myocardial oxygen demand.**
> 3. Diuretics decrease the volume of water within the vascular system by increasing the renal excretion of sodium and water.
> 4. Antiarrythmics such as sodium channel blockers normalize the rate of sodium entry into cardiac tissues and thereby help control cardiac excitation and conduction.
>
> System Specific: Cardiovascular/Pulmonary and Lymphatic Systems
> Content Outline: Foundations for Evaluation, Differential Diagnosis, and Prognosis

## Exam Three: Question 126

A physical therapist interviews a patient recently involved in a motor vehicle accident. The patient sustained multiple lower extremity injuries as a result of the accident and appears to be very depressed. In an attempt to encourage active dialogue the therapist asks open-ended questions. Which of the following would NOT be considered an open-ended question?

1. How does your knee feel today?
2. What are your goals for physical therapy?
3. **Do you have trouble sleeping at night?**
4. Tell me about your present condition?

> **Correct Answer: 3** (Goodman - Differential Diagnosis p. 36)
> Open-ended questions allow patients to answer with a myriad of responses, while closed-ended questions can often be answered with a yes or no response.
>
> 1. The question "How does your knee feel today?" provides the patient with a variety of potential answers and will likely result in the patient elaborating about the pain level today in relation to the baseline pain level.
> 2. The question "What are your goals for physical therapy?" provides the patient with the opportunity to elaborate on what they hope to achieve in physical therapy and is often extremely helpful for the therapist when designing an individualized program for the patient.
> 3. **The question "Do you have trouble sleeping at night?" would likely be answered by a simple "yes" or "no" and therefore is considered to be a closed-ended question.**
> 4. The question "Tell me about your present condition?" requires the patient to provide the therapist with a variety of information related to the history of their medical condition and current status.
>
> System Specific: Non-Systems
> Content Outline: Safety and Protection; Professional Responsibilities; Research

## Exam Three: Question 127 ✗

A group of physical therapists employed in an acute care hospital is responsible for developing departmental guidelines for electrical equipment care and safety. What is the MINIMUM required testing interval for electrical equipment?

1. 3 months
2. 6 months
3. **12 months**
4. 24 months

**Correct Answer: 3** (Belanger p. 237)
Electrical equipment should be inspected according to the specified intervals outlined by the manufacturer. The regular schedule, once established, can be modified based on variables such as increased frequency of use or reports of faulty performance.

1. Three months would be a reasonable testing interval for devices that are used more frequently or devices that tend to have greater difficulty remaining properly calibrated.

2. Six months would be a reasonable testing interval for some equipment, although the question asks for the minimum required testing interval.

3. **Testing intervals may often be more frequent than every twelve months, however, it is unacceptable for any electrical equipment to be uninspected for more than a twelve-month period.**

4. Twenty-four months would typically exceed all manufacturer's recommendations for equipment testing.

System Specific: Non-Systems
Content Outline: Equipment & Devices; Therapeutic Modalities

**Test Taking Tip:** Candidates must pay close attention to specific qualifiers used within the question. The question asks for "the MINIMUM required testing interval." In some cases, candidates fail to identify this type of qualifier and as a result select another option. In this particular question a candidate could easily select a three month or six month interval based on the premise that more frequent inspection would lead to better functioning electrical equipment with less risk to the patient. Although this is correct, the question is specifically asking the candidate to identify "the MINIMUM required testing interval."

## Exam Three: Question 128

A physical therapist participates in a research study to determine the effect of noise level on the ability to perform a physical skill. In the study, noise is the:

1. **independent variable**
2. dependent variable
3. criterion variable
4. extraneous variable

**Correct Answer: 1** (Portney p. 129)
The independent variable is also known as the experimental or predictor variable. It is the condition, intervention or characteristic that will predict or cause an outcome in an experimental study.

1. **Noise level is the independent variable because it is the condition or characteristic that the researcher will manipulate to see how it changes physical skill.**

2. The dependent variable is also known as the outcome variable, which is the response or effect that is presumed to vary with the independent variable. Physical skill is the dependent variable because it is presumed to vary depending on noise level.

3. The term criterion variable is a synonym for dependent variable.

4. An extraneous variable is also known as a nuisance or intervening variable. An extraneous variable is any factor that is not related to the purpose of the study, but that may affect the dependent variable.

System Specific: Non-Systems
Content Outline: Safety and Protection; Professional Responsibilities; Research

## Exam Three: Question 129

A patient with a C6 spinal cord injury is examined in physical therapy. Which objective finding would be the strongest indication the spinal cord injury is NOT complete?

1. intact sensation on the lateral portion of the shoulder
2. absent triceps reflex
3. **diminished sensation over the hypothenar eminence**
4. weakness of the biceps muscle

> **Correct Answer: 3** (Goodman - Pathology p. 1502)
> A patient with a complete C6 spinal cord injury would not possess motor, sensory or reflex function below the C6 level. As a result, any identified finding below this level could provide evidence that the injury is not complete.
>
> 1. The dermatome associated with the lateral portion of the shoulder is C5 and therefore sensation in this area would typically be intact in a complete spinal cord injury at the C6 level.
>
> 2. The triceps reflex is associated with the C7-C8 nerve root and therefore the reflex would be absent in a complete spinal cord injury at the C6 level.
>
> 3. **The dermatome that corresponds to the hypothenar eminence is at the C8 level. As a result, the finding of diminished sensation (not absent) at a level below the level of injury (i.e., C6) indicates that the injury is incomplete.**
>
> 4. The biceps muscle is innervated by C5-C6 and therefore weakness is often associated with a spinal cord injury at this level.
>
> System Specific: Neuromuscular & Nervous Systems
> Content Outline: Foundations for Evaluation, Differential Diagnosis, & Prognosis

## Exam Three: Question 130

When is it considered acceptable for a clinical trial to include a non-treatment control group as a basis for comparison with a new experimental therapy?

1. **when there is no known effective form of therapy to treat the patient's condition**
2. when the experimental therapy has shown positive results in animal studies
3. when the study is reviewed by the facility's Institutional Review Board (IRB)
4. when subjects are randomly assigned to a group

> **Correct Answer: 1** (Portney p. 49)
> According to the current Declaration of Helsinki, in research with human beings, a placebo control may be used in clinical conditions for which no treatments have been effective or when the purpose of the research is to determine if a particular treatment is not effective. In all cases, the researcher is obliged to inform the potential human subjects when the study includes a control group.
>
> 1. **A non-treatment control group may be used in clinical conditions for which no treatments have been effective.**
>
> 2. Positive results in animal studies do not make the use of a non-treatment control group acceptable in research on humans.
>
> 3. Federal regulations in the United States require that an Institutional Review Board (IRB) research proposals using human subjects prior to implementation to ensure that the rights of the subjects are protected. However, review by the IRB does not make the use of a non-treatment control group acceptable.
>
> 4. Random assignment to groups is the best way to control for confounding variables that could affect the outcomes of the study. However, it does not make the use of a non-treatment control group acceptable.
>
> System Specific: Non-Systems
> Content Outline: Safety and Protection; Professional Responsibilities; Research

## Exam Three: Question 131

A physical therapist treats a patient diagnosed with spinal stenosis. As part of the treatment program the patient lies prone on a treatment plinth with a hot pack draped over the low back. The MOST effective method to monitor the patient while using the hot pack is:

1. check on the patient at least every ten minutes
2. **supply the patient with a bell to ring if the hot pack becomes too hot**
3. instruct the patient to remove the hot pack if it becomes too hot
4. select an alternate superficial heating modality

**Correct Answer: 2** (Michlovitz p. 68)

A hot pack consists of a canvas or nylon covered pack filled with a hydrophilic silicate gel that provides a moist heat. A hot pack must be stored in hot water between 158 to 167 degrees Fahrenheit (70 to 75 degrees Celsius). Application requires six to eight layers of towels around the hot pack. Given the potential for burns, formal measures must be adopted to ensure safe use throughout the treatment session.

1. Checking on a patient on a frequent basis is desirable, however, 10 minutes is not frequent enough particularly when considering that the duration of treatment with a hot pack may only be 15-20 minutes.

2. **Supplying the patient with a bell to ring if the hot pack becomes too intense provides a form of instant communication with the therapist.**

3. It may be challenging for the patient to independently remove the hot pack based on the selected positioning. In addition, this option places the burden solely on the patient to make a definitive decision on whether or not to continue using the hot pack. This decision should be made by the therapist with feedback from the patient.

4. There is no need to discontinue a selected intervention in the absence of data to support this decision. Hot packs can be a safe and effective form of superficial heat when applied with the necessary precautions.

System Specific: Non-Systems
Content Outline: Equipment & Devices; Therapeutic Modalities

## Exam Three: Question 132

A physical therapist asks a patient to complete a pain questionnaire. The questionnaire utilizes an ascending numeric scale ranging from "0" equaling no pain to "10" equaling excruciating pain. This type of measurement scale is BEST described as:

1. nominal
2. **ordinal**
3. interval
4. ratio

**Correct Answer: 2** (Portney p. 68)

Four scales of measurement have been identified – nominal, ordinal, interval, ratio – each with its own set of rules for manipulating and interpreting numerical data.

1. The nominal scale of measurement is also known as the classificatory scale. Objects or things are classified in categories according to some criterion, e.g., name, letter, or symbol, which do not have any quantitative value. The nominal scale is the lowest scale of measurement.

2. **The ordinal scale of measurement requires that the categories be ranked or ordered according to some defined characteristic or property, so that the numbers on the scale have a greater than – less than relationship. The intervals between ranks need not be equal, and may not be known, as is the case with measurement of pain on a 0 to 10 scale. While an "8" indicates greater pain than a "4" it cannot be said to represent twice as much pain because the magnitude of pain associated with each number is unknown and may vary among patients. Also, the difference between an 8 and 4 does not indicate the same difference in pain as the difference between a 6 and 2.**

3. The interval scale has the rank-order characteristics of an ordinal scale, but also demonstrates known and equal distances or intervals between the units of measurement. This latter property permits relative difference and equivalence to be determined. Measures of temperature on the Fahrenheit and Celsius scales are at the interval level.

4. The ratio scale is the highest level of measurement because, in addition to the known and equal distances or intervals, the scale has an absolute zero point representing a total absence of the property being measured. Range of motion, height, weight, and force are examples of clinical measurements on the ratio scale.

System Specific: Non-Systems
Content Outline: Safety and Protection; Professional Responsibilities; Research

## Exam Three: Question 133

An attorney contacts you by phone and requests specific information on a patient he claims to represent. Questions asked include the extent of the patient's disability and his willingness to return to work. The MOST appropriate response is:

1.  answer the questions asked by the attorney
2.  **request the attorney provide a completed release of patient medical information form**
3.  tell the attorney not to bother you at work
4.  send the attorney a copy of the patient's medical records

**Correct Answer: 2** (Scott - Promoting Legal and Ethical Awareness p. 78)

Physical therapists have an ethical and legal obligation to appropriately secure protected health information. Releasing this type of information without written patient consent would be considered a negligent act.

1.  Answering questions asked by the attorney without the appropriate release forms would violate the rights of the patient.
2.  **The attorney should be reminded of the appropriate procedure to obtain medical records.**
3.  It is inappropriate to be rude to the attorney despite the fact that the attorney should be aware of the appropriate procedure to obtain medical records.
4.  Sending the attorney a copy of the patient's medical records violates the patient's rights since there is no indication that the attorney has followed the appropriate procedure to have the records released.

System Specific: Non-Systems
Content Outline: Safety and Protection; Professional Responsibilities; Research

## Exam Three: Question 134

A patient four weeks status post anterior cruciate ligament reconstruction questions a physical therapist as to why he is still partial weight bearing. An acceptable rationale is:

1.  **the patient does not have full active knee extension**
2.  the patient has good quadriceps strength
3.  the patient has fair hamstrings strength
4.  the patient has diminished superficial cutaneous sensation

**Correct Answer: 1** (Kisner p. 733)

The physician is responsible for determining a patient's weight bearing status following surgery. Physical therapists should possess an understanding of relevant factors associated with the prescribed weight bearing status and understand what is necessary for the patient to progress to full weight bearing.

1.  **A patient status post anterior cruciate ligament reconstruction surgery may continue to use an assistive device for weight bearing if they do not possess full active knee extension. Ambulation on a flexed knee can result in excessive irritation of the patellofemoral joint.**
2.  The quadriceps control the amount of knee flexion during initial contact (loading response) and then extend the knee toward midstance. The quadriceps also control the amount of knee flexion during pre-swing (heel off to toe off) and prevent excessive heel rise during initial swing. Good quadriceps strength would be adequate for full weight bearing on the involved lower extremity assuming the absence of other relevant clinical findings. A grade of good indicates that the patient completes range of motion against gravity with moderate resistance.
3.  The hamstrings are responsible for controlling the forward swing of the leg during terminal swing. The hamstrings provide posterior support to the knee capsule when the knee is extended during stance. Fair hamstrings strength would be adequate for full weight bearing on the involved lower extremity assuming the absence of other relevant clinical findings. A grade of fair indicates that the patient completes range of motion against gravity without manual resistance.
4.  Diminished superficial cutaneous sensation is common following surgery particularly in close proximity to an incision. The presence of diminished superficial cutaneous sensation would not influence a patient's weight bearing status.

System Specific: Musculoskeletal System
Content Outline: Interventions

## Exam Three: Question 135 ✕

A physical therapist palpates medially along the spine of the scapula. Which spinous process is at the same level as the vertebral end of the spine?

1. T2
2. **T3**
3. T4
4. T5

**Correct Answer: 2** (Hoppenfeld p. 11)

Physical therapists often use selected bony prominences to assist them to identify a specific vertebral level. For example, in the lumbar spine the top of the iliac crest is at the same level as the L4-L5 interspace and in the sacral spine the posterior superior iliac spine is at the same level as S2.

1. The scapula's medial border extends from the level of spinous processes T2-T7.

2. **The vertebral end of the spine of the scapula is at the same level as the spinous process of T3.**

3. The spinous process of T4 is slightly below the level of the vertebral end of the spine of the scapula. Like all thoracic vertebrae, T4 articulates with the ribs and possesses a spinous process that is easily identifiable, particularly when the spine is flexed.

4. The spinous process of T5 is significantly inferior to the level of the vertebral end of the spine of the scapula. The body of the middle four vertebrae in the thoracic spine (T5-T8) when viewed from the superior aspect are heart shaped and their vertebral foramina are circular.

System Specific: Musculoskeletal System
Content Outline: Physical Therapy Examination

## Exam Three: Question 136

A physical therapist observes a patient status post transfemoral amputation lying in supine with a pillow positioned under the residual limb. This position results in the patient being MOST susceptible to a:

1. knee extension contracture
2. knee flexion contracture
3. **hip flexion contracture**
4. hip extension contracture

**Correct Answer: 3** (Seymour p. 145)

Proper positioning is required to avoid a contracture of the residual limb. A patient with a transfemoral amputation is particularly susceptible to a hip flexion contracture.

1. A patient with a transfemoral amputation would not possess a knee joint on the affected side. As a result, a contracture involving the affected lower extremity would only involve the hip.

2. A patient with a transtibial amputation lying in supine with a pillow under the residual limb would be more likely to develop a knee flexion contracture.

3. **A hip flexion contracture can occur if the patient lies supine with a pillow under the residual limb. The positioning into hip flexion along with the relative strength of the hip flexors places the patient at high risk for contracture. Intermittent prone lying is often a recommended activity following a transfemoral amputation.**

4. Lying in supine would not make the patient susceptible to a hip extension contracture since the hip remains in a neutral or a flexed position when in supine.

System Specific: Musculoskeletal System
Content Outline: Interventions

**Test Taking Tip:** This question demonstrates how easy it can be to make a test taking mistake on the National Physical Therapy Examination. Some candidates may have selected option 2 knee flexion contracture after reading key words such as supine and pillow under the residual limb. If they selected option 2 it is likely that they were thinking about a transtibial amputation despite the fact that the question clearly indicates transfemoral amputation. Candidates must be careful to identify key words within the question and possess a clear understanding of what the question is asking prior to identifying the correct answer. Test taking mistakes result in a candidate's score not representing their true ability and as a result, make them more at risk for failing the National Physical Therapy Examination. Increased awareness of individual tendencies is one proactive approach to reduce the frequency of test taking mistakes.

## Exam Three: Question 137

A physical therapist conducts an examination on a patient diagnosed with Parkinson's disease. Which of the following clinical findings would the therapist expect to identify?

1. aphasia
2. ballistic movements
3. severe muscle atrophy
4. **cogwheel rigidity**

---

**Correct Answer: 4** (O'Sullivan p. 200)

Parkinson's disease is a degenerative disorder characterized by a decrease in production of dopamine (neurotransmitter) within the corpus striatum portion of the basal ganglia. Clinical presentation may include hypokinesia, difficulty initiating and stopping movement, festinating and shuffling gait, bradykinesia, poor posture, and "cogwheel" or "lead pipe" rigidity.

1. Aphasia is an acquired neurological communication impairment caused by damage to the brain. The condition is most commonly associated with brain injury, head trauma, CVA, tumor or infection.

2. Ballistic movements refer to large amplitude involuntary movements affecting the proximal limb musculature, manifested in jerking, flinging movements of the extremity. Ballismus usually results from a lesion in the subthalamic nucleus. Often only one side of the body is involved, resulting in hemiballismus.

3. Severe muscle atrophy is an expected clinical finding in diseases that affect the nerves that control muscles (e.g., poliomyelitis, amyotrophic lateral sclerosis, Guillain-Barre syndrome) and diseases affecting the muscles directly (e.g., muscular dystrophy, myotonia congenita).

4. **Cogwheel rigidity refers to a jerky, rachet-like resistance to passive movement as muscles sequentially tense and relax. The condition is most often associated with Parkinson's disease.**

System Specific: Neuromuscular & Nervous Systems
Content Outline: Foundations for Evaluation, Differential Diagnosis, & Prognosis

---

## Exam Three: Question 138

A patient rehabilitating from a CVA requires an orthosis due to occasional dragging of the toe during swing phase. The patient presents with weakness of the dorsiflexors and has good medial/lateral stability at the ankle. The MOST appropriate option for the patient is:

1. solid ankle-foot orthosis
2. tone reducing foot orthosis
3. **posterior leaf spring orthosis**
4. custom articulating ankle-foot orthosis with anterior trim lines

---

**Correct Answer: 3** (Seymour p. 383)

A posterior leaf spring (PLS) orthosis is a type of ankle-foot orthosis that provides a dorsiflexion assist during swing phase. The trim line is posterior to the malleoli and as a result the device offers minimal medial or lateral ankle support.

1. A solid ankle-foot orthosis (AFO) is typically indicated for diminished strength of the dorsiflexors, plantar flexors, evertors or invertors. The solid AFO will control the ankle and influence the knee joint during gait. The solid AFO maintains the ankle in a static position, however, may assist with tonal influence and lower extremity weakness. The AFO provides more stability than the patient requires.

2. A tone reducing foot orthosis is typically indicated to decrease hypertonicity and normalize tone. The foot orthosis provides total contact under the foot allowing for areas of pressure that function to decrease tone.

3. **The PLS orthosis is designed with flexibility so that both dorsiflexion and plantar flexion can occur during the gait cycle. The PLS allows for improved biomechanics during gait secondary to its flexibility and therefore would be the most appropriate type of orthosis for the patient given their level of medial/lateral stability.**

4. A custom articulating ankle-foot orthosis (AFO) with anterior trim lines typically provides total contact and a significant amount of stability. The articulating joint promotes improved biomechanics allowing the tibia to advance over the foot during stance phase. The patient, however, would not require the level of stability offered by this type of AFO.

System Specific: Neuromuscular and Nervous Systems
Content Outline: Interventions

## Exam Three: Question 139

A physical therapist prescribes a wheelchair for a 34-year-old patient with bilateral lower extremity amputations. The MOST important feature of a wheelchair designed for the patient should be:

1. friction surface handrims
2. **the drive wheels are set behind the vertical back supports**
3. reclining back with elevating legrests
4. removable armrests

**Correct Answer: 2** (Seymour p. 160)

A patient with bilateral lower extremity amputations requires offset rear wheels to accommodate for the change in the center of gravity. An anti-tipping device may also be used to prevent the wheelchair and patient from falling backwards.

1. Friction surface handrims are used when patients do not have a functional grip or strength to adequately propel a wheelchair. Patients with C6-C7 tetraplegia commonly rely on this feature.

2. **A wheelchair with offset rear wheels is an adaptation that moves the axis posterior to the center support and provides greater stability during propulsion over varying surfaces. An active patient will use all available options to enhance the stability of the chair.**

3. A wheelchair with a reclining back and elevating legrests would be appropriate for a patient that does not tolerate an upright posture or possess postural control. This would not be appropriate for a patient with bilateral amputations since it would move the center of gravity in a posterior direction as the chair reclines.

4. Removable armrests are appropriate for many patients including those with bilateral amputations to improve safety and ease of transfers, however, the most important adaptation should be the offset rear wheels to ensure safety within the wheelchair.

System Specific: Non-Systems
Content Outline: Equipment & Devices; Therapeutic Modalities

## Exam Three: Question 140

A physical therapist assesses a patient's heart rate by measuring the time necessary for 30 beats. Assuming the therapist measures this value as 22 seconds, the patient's heart rate should be recorded as:

1. **82 beats per minute**
2. 86 beats per minute
3. 90 beats per minute
4. 95 beats per minute

**Correct Answer: 1** (Pierson p. 56)

To determine the beats per minute, calculate the number of beats in one second, then multiply the obtained value by 60 seconds per minute.

1. **The number of beats in one second = 1.36 (30 beats / 22 seconds = 1.36 beats per second). Multiplying 1.36 beats per second by 60 seconds per minute yields heart rate in beats per minute: 1.36 beats per second x 60 seconds per minute = 81.6 beats per minute (rounded up to 82).**

2. 1.36 beats per second x 60 seconds per minute ≠86

3. 1.36 beats per second x 60 seconds per minute ≠90

4. 1.36 beats per second x 60 seconds per minute ≠95

System Specific: Cardiovascular/Pulmonary and Lymphatic Systems
Content Outline: Physical Therapy Examination

## Exam Three: Question 141

A patient diagnosed with Guillain-Barre syndrome works on weight shifting activities while standing in the parallel bars. The PRIMARY objective of this activity is to improve:

1. mobility
2. stability
3. **controlled mobility**
4. skill

**Correct Answer: 3** (Sullivan p. 77)

Functional training uses postures and activities to improve motor control. Physical therapists select activities for patients that are designed to progressively increase the effects of gravity and body weight.

1. Mobility, the first stage of motor control, refers to the ability to initiate movement through a functional range of motion.
2. Stability, the second stage of motor control, refers to the ability to maintain a position or posture through cocontraction and tonic holding around a joint.
3. **Controlled mobility, the third stage of motor control, refers to the ability to move within a weight bearing position or rotate around a long axis.**
4. Skill, the fourth stage of motor control, refers to the ability to consistently perform functional tasks and manipulate the environment with normal postural reflex mechanisms and balance reactions. Skill activities include ADLs and community locomotion.

System Specific: Neuromuscular & Nervous Systems
Content Outline: Interventions

## Exam Three: Question 142

A physical therapist asks a physical therapist assistant to complete a lower extremity isokinetic test on a patient. The physical therapist assistant is willing to complete the test, however, indicates it has been quite some time since they have set up the isokinetic device. The MOST appropriate physical therapist action is:

1. provide verbal cueing for the physical therapist assistant prior to beginning the set up
2. instruct the physical therapist assistant to refer to the owner's manual
3. **observe the physical therapist assistant complete the set up**
4. ask another physical therapist assistant to complete the set up

**Correct Answer: 3** (Nosse p. 217)

A physical therapist should establish and maintain an ongoing professional relationship with a physical therapist assistant. The physical therapist should delegate appropriate patient care duties to the physical therapist assistant that are within their established scope of practice. The physical therapist assistant must clearly communicate their needs to the physical therapist and work in a collaborative manner.

1. Verbal cueing allows the physical therapist to assist the physical therapist assistant to set up the isokinetic device through verbal input, however, it does not ensure that the device is set up correctly.
2. Referring the physical therapist assistant to the owner's manual provides the physical therapist assistant with a general reference to guide them through the set up, but like the previous option does not ensure that the device is set up correctly.
3. **Observing the physical therapist assistant complete the set up allows the physical therapist to assist the physical therapist assistant as needed and at the same time ensures the device is set up correctly. Direct involvement of the physical therapist is collaborative and may assist the physical therapist assistant to complete the set up independently in the future.**
4. The physical therapist assistant is capable of completing the set up with assistance. As a result, it is not necessary to secure another physical therapist assistant to complete the set up. In addition, the question does not provide direct evidence that another physical therapist assistant is available who possesses the requisite knowledge to complete the activity.

System Specific: Musculoskeletal System
Content Outline: Physical Therapy Examination

## Exam Three: Question 143

A physical therapist administers ultrasound over a patient's anterior thigh. After one minute of treatment, the patient reports feeling a slight burning sensation under the soundhead. The therapist's MOST appropriate action is to:

1. explain to the patient that what she feels is not out of the ordinary when using ultrasound
2. **temporarily discontinue treatment and examine the amount of coupling agent utilized**
3. discontinue treatment and contact the referring physician
4. continue with treatment utilizing the current parameters

**Correct Answer: 2** (Michlovitz p. 102)

A patient report of a slight burning sensation under the soundhead can be due to inadequate coupling, loosening of the crystal or hot spots due to a high beam nonuniformity ratio.

1. A complaint of a slight burning sensation would be an abnormal response when using ultrasound. As a result, it would be inappropriate to inform the patient that what she feels is "not out of the ordinary." It may be normal to feel a dull warming, however, a slight burning sensation would require an immediate response.

2. **The complaint of a slight burning sensation may indicate improper coupling. By temporarily discontinuing the treatment and examining the amount of coupling agent used, the physical therapist may be able to continue with treatment. If the physical therapist adds coupling agent and the patient reports a similar sensation the intervention should be discontinued and the ultrasound unit should be formally inspected by a qualified technician.**

3. Discontinuing treatment would be an acceptable option, however, there is not presently a need to contact the referring physician. A physical therapist may elect to contact the physician in situations where the patient has been injured by a physical therapy intervention or if there has been a change in the patient's medical status.

4. Continuing with treatment utilizing the current parameters is not appropriate since the patient has already reported a slight burning sensation. Failure to respond specifically to the patient's subjective report creates an unnecessary safety risk.

System Specific: Non-Systems
Content Outline: Equipment & Devices; Therapeutic Modalities

## Exam Three: Question 144

A patient ambulating in the physical therapy gym suddenly grabs the physical therapist's arm and indicates that he feels faint. The MOST appropriate IMMEDIATE action is:

1. assess the patient's pulse rate
2. ask the patient if he has ever previously fainted
3. loosen tight clothing
4. **assist the patient to a sitting position**

**Correct Answer: 4** (Code of Ethics)

The physical therapist must take immediate action to ensure patient safety. By assisting the patient to a chair, the therapist can adequately assess the patient without compromising patient safety.

1. Assessing the patient's pulse rate may provide the physical therapist with additional information on the patient's current medical status, however, the more immediate concern would be to assist the patient to a stable and secure position to minimize the risk of a fall.

2. Gathering additional information on the patient's past medical history will eventually be warranted, however, the action does not specifically address the immediate safety concern.

3. Loosening tight clothing may assist the patient to be more comfortable, however, this action would not be appropriate until the patient is in a secure position.

4. **The physical therapist's primary responsibility is to preserve patient safety. Assisting the patient to a sitting position takes the patient out of immediate danger. Each of the remaining options is viable, however, only after patient safety has been preserved.**

System Specific: Cardiovascular/Pulmonary and Lymphatic Systems
Content Outline: Interventions

## Exam Three: Question 145

A physical therapist uses a manual wheelchair during a training session with a patient with C5 quadriplegia. Which wheelchair would be the most appropriate based on the patient's level of injury?

1. manual wheelchair with sip and puff controls
2. **manual wheelchair with handrim projections**
3. manual wheelchair with friction surface handrims
4. manual wheelchair with standard handrims

**Correct Answer: 2** (O'Sullivan p. 962)

A patient with C5 tetraplegia would typically be able to utilize a manual wheelchair with handrim projections to assist with propulsion. The projections are typically angled at 30 degrees and may have friction surfaces for greater ease of movement.

1. Sip and puff controls are used only on power wheelchairs. These types of controls are most often used on patients with C4 tetraplegia. Innervation at the C4 level includes the diaphragm, trapezius, face, and neck muscles.

2. **A manual wheelchair with handrim projections would be appropriate to use during a training session for a patient with C5 quadriplegia, however, may not be used as the primary mode of mobility due to the limited upper extremity muscle innervation and the associated endurance issues.**

3. A manual wheelchair with friction surface handrims would be more appropriate for a patient with C6-C7 tetraplegia secondary to the motor innervation at the C6 and C7 levels.

4. A patient with paraplegia (full upper extremity innervation) can propel a wheelchair without adaptation of the wheelrims. Standard handrims are used for patients with injury at the C8 level and below.

System Specific: Neuromuscular and Nervous Systems
Content Outline: Interventions

## Exam Three: Question 146

A physical therapist employed in a rehabilitation hospital creates a professional development plan as part of his annual performance appraisal. Which of the following would be the MOST appropriate plan to facilitate the therapist's development in his present practice setting?

1. attend continuing education courses approved by the Federation of State Boards of Physical Therapy
2. attend continuing education courses featuring nationally recognized experts
3. attend a minimum of two continuing education courses annually
4. **attend continuing education courses related to primary patient care responsibilities**

**Correct Answer: 4** (Guide for Professional Conduct)

Facilitating the physical therapist's development in his present practice setting requires the physical therapist to attend continuing education courses related to his primary care responsibilities. Continuing education courses allow the physical therapist to refine existing skills and learn new skills. By taking courses related to primary patient care responsibilities the therapist will be able to immediately integrate selected skills into their daily practice.

1. The Federation of State Boards of Physical Therapy does not approve continuing education courses.

2. Attending continuing education courses featuring nationally recognized experts does not ensure that the courses will be more beneficial to the therapist than courses taught by less known speakers. The physical therapist should evaluate each course based on its relevant merit and the direct relevance to their patient care duties.

3. The quality of the continuing education courses a physical therapist attends is a more important variable to consider than the actual number of courses attended. For example, a physical therapist could attend several courses with little direct relevance to their present patient care duties and as a result receive little practical benefit.

4. **The physical therapist should attend continuing education courses that directly relate to their primary patient care responsibilities. Developing this particular skill set will allow the physical therapist to improve the quality of patient care within their current practice setting.**

System Specific: Non-Systems
Content Outline: Safety and Protection; Professional Responsibilities; Research

## Exam Three: Question 147

A male physical therapist examines a female diagnosed with subacromial bursitis. After taking a thorough history, the therapist asks the patient to change into a gown. The patient seems very uneasy about this suggestion, but finally agrees to use the gown. The MOST appropriate course of action would be to:

1. continue with treatment as planned
2. attempt to treat the patient without using the gown
3. **bring a female staff member into the treatment room and continue with treatment**
4. offer to transfer the patient to a female physical therapist

**Correct Answer: 3** (Nosse p. 217)
The physical therapist should be sensitive to the patient's apparent discomfort with the situation, however, must also take appropriate steps to manage their relative risk. Physical therapists must be willing to modify their approach with each patient encounter based on the unique presented circumstances.

1. The patient's original reluctance to wear the gown makes it prudent to have a witness present during treatment. The decision to continue with treatment without any formal action places the physical therapist at unnecessary risk.

2. Failure to wear the gown may make it more difficult for the physical therapist to treat the patient or depending on the chosen intervention could risk damaging or soiling the patient's clothes.

3. **The male physical therapist should bring a female staff member into the treatment room. The presence of a witness is a form of risk management that protects the physical therapist in the event of any alleged misconduct and may make the patient more comfortable.**

4. It would be impractical to transfer a patient to another physical therapist simply because the patient seemed to be uncomfortable when asked to change into the gown.

System Specific: Musculoskeletal Systems
Content Outline: Physical Therapy Examination

## Exam Three: Question 148 ✗

A physical therapist treats a patient status post CVA. Which action would be MOST likely to facilitate elbow extension in a patient with hemiplegia?

1. **turn the head to the affected side**
2. turn the head to the unaffected side
3. extend the lower extremities
4. flex the lower extremities

**Correct Answer: 1** (Sullivan p. 19)
Patients status post CVA are likely to exhibit abnormal tonic reflexes. Eliciting the reflexes will produce sustained posturing and abnormal movement patterns.

1. **The asymmetrical tonic neck reflex produces extension of the affected upper extremity when the patient's head is turned toward the affected side. The upper extremity on the skull side will flex.**

2. If the patient's head is turned toward the unaffected side, the unaffected upper extremity will extend and the affected upper extremity will flex due to the influence of the asymmetrical tonic neck reflex (ATNR).

3. The symmetrical tonic labyrinthine reflex (STLR) promotes a tendency for extension when a patient is in supine and reduced extensor influence when the patient is in prone. STLR would not facilitate elbow extension in isolation as noted with ATNR.

4. Flexion of the lower extremities does not have a direct influence on upper extremity flexion or extension.

System Specific: Neuromuscular & Nervous Systems
Content Outline: Interventions

## Exam Three: Question 149

A physical therapist examines a patient three days following shoulder surgery. The patient complains of general malaise and reports a slightly elevated body temperature during the last twenty-four hours. Physical examination reveals an edematous shoulder that is warm to the touch. A small amount of yellow fluid is observed seeping from the incision. The MOST appropriate therapist action is:

1. send the patient to the emergency room
2. **communicate the information to the referring physician**
3. document the findings in the medical record
4. ask the patient to make an appointment with the referring physician

**Correct Answer: 2** (Anemaet p. 547)
Physical therapists must be aware of any signs or symptoms of infection, particularly in patients following surgery. Common signs of infection include elevated body temperature, purulent exudate, swelling, edema, and redness.

1. The patient's presentation requires the physical therapist to take formal action, but would not be indicative of an emergent condition that requires the patient to be seen in the emergency room.

2. **The possibility of infection in a patient three days status post surgery warrants immediate consultation with the referring physician.**

3. The subjective and objective information gathered by the physical therapist should be documented in the medical record, however, this action would not address the primary issue which is the possibility of an infection.

4. Asking the patient to make an appointment with the physician is not an appropriate action since it places the burden solely on the patient. The physical therapist is responsible for communicating any potential change in a patient's medical status to the physician in a timely manner.

System Specific: Other Systems
Content Outline: Interventions

## Exam Three: Question 150

A physical therapist instructs a patient how to fall safely to the floor when using axillary crutches. Which of the following should be the FIRST to occur in the case of a forward fall?

1. reach towards the floor
2. turn your face towards one side
3. **release the crutches**
4. flex the trunk and head

**Correct Answer: 3** (Pierson p. 261)
Physical therapists are responsible for instructing patients how to properly use various assistive devices. The instructions typically include training in fall prevention and strategies to minimize injury in the event of a fall.

1. Reaching forward toward the floor would be a desirable action in the event of a forward fall, however, the question specifically asks for the "first" action.

2. Turning the face towards one side would be a desirable action in the event of a forward fall to minimize the relative trauma to the face, however, this would not be the "first" action.

3. **A patient should release the crutches in the event of a forward fall in order to utilize the upper extremities to minimize the impact of the fall.**

4. Flexing the trunk and head are instructions that are necessary when teaching a patient to properly fall backward. The coupled motions are used to facilitate the patient to fall on their buttocks instead of directly landing on their head.

System Specific: Musculoskeletal System
Content Outline: Interventions

## Exam Three: Question 151 ✕

A patient with an acute burn is referred to physical therapy less than 24 hours after being admitted to the hospital. The patient's burns range from superficial partial-thickness to deep partial-thickness and encompass approximately 35 percent of the patient's total body surface area. Which of the following findings would be MOST predictable based on the patient's injury?

1. **increased oxygen consumption**
2. hypernatremia
3. increased intravascular fluid
4. decreased core temperature

**Correct Answer: 1** (Paz p. 266)
An acute burn produces hypermetabolism that results in increased oxygen consumption, increased minute ventilation, and an increased core temperature. Intravascular, interstitial, and intracellular fluids are all diminished.

1. **Pulmonary function is affected by the presence of a burn injury. In addition to increased oxygen consumption, the patient can also experience increased minute ventilation up to five times the normal value.**

2. Hyponatremia or low sodium concentration, initially occurs (within the first 36 hours) secondary to extracellular changes from the increased cellular permeability. In patients that sustain burns above 20% of the total body surface area, fluid and electrolyte replacement is a component of immediate medical management in order to control the hypermetabolic cycle that results from the burn.

3. Intravascular fluid will decrease due to the increased vascular permeability and overall hematologic changes. Cardiac output can decrease secondary to a combination of an increase in blood viscosity, decrease in intravascular fluid, and an overall increase in peripheral resistance.

4. A patient with a significant burn injury is at risk for an increased core temperature due to the increased metabolic and catabolic activity. The one to two degree increase occurs secondary to the "recalibrating" of the hypothalamic temperature centers in the brain. Patients that have sustained extensive burns require a warmer ambient temperature in order to reduce their metabolic rate. Average room temperature will create continued heat loss and perpetuate the hypermetabolic state.

System Specific: Other Systems
Content Outline: Foundations for Evaluation, Differential Diagnosis, & Prognosis

## Exam Three: Question 152

A patient sustains a deep partial-thickness burn to the anterior surface of the right upper extremity and a superficial partial-thickness burn to the anterior surface of the trunk. According to the "rule of nines", the patient has burns over:

1. 13.5 percent of the body
2. **22.5 percent of the body**
3. 27 percent of the body
4. 36 percent of the body

**Correct Answer: 2** (Rothstein p. 963)
The "rule of nines" is commonly utilized to assess the percentage of the body surface affected by a burn. Each area of the body has a specific percentage allotted to it in order to approximate the total percentage of the body surface affected. The values are as follows: head (9%), each upper extremity (9%), the trunk (36%), each lower extremity (18%), and the genital area (1%).

1. A value of 13.5% is less than the percentage of body surface affected. A candidate may have generated an answer of 13.5% by allocating only 9% for the anterior trunk instead of 18% and then adding 4.5% for the anterior surface of the upper extremity.

2. **The anterior surface of the right upper extremity equals 4.5% and the anterior surface of the trunk equals 18% (4.5%+18%=22.5%).**

3. A value of 27% is greater than the percentage of body surface affected in the described scenario. A candidate may have generated an answer of 27% by incorrectly allocating 9% for the anterior surface of the right upper extremity and then adding 18% for the anterior surface of the trunk.

4. The entire trunk is valued at 36% of the body using the "rule of nines."

System Specific: Other Systems
Content Outline: Physical Therapy Examination

## Exam Three: Question 153

The treatment plan for a patient with hemiplegia is based on the theory of reinforcing normal movement through key points of control and avoiding all reflex movement patterns and associated reactions. This approach MOST closely resembles:

1. **Bobath**
2. Kabat
3. Rood
4. Brunnstrom

**Correct Answer: 1** (Scott - Foundations p. 156)

The Bobath approach for neurological rehabilitation is often termed Neurodevelopmental Treatment (NDT). The patient learns to control movement through functional activities that promote normal movement patterns that integrate function.

1. **The Bobath approach recognizes that interference of normal brain function caused by central nervous system damage leads to a slowing down or cessation of motor development and the inhibition of righting reactions, equilibrium reactions, and automatic movements. Emphasis on normal movement and rotational patterns are key components of this therapeutic model.**

2. The Kabat, Knott, and Voss approach is based on the premise that stronger parts of the body are utilized to stimulate and strengthen weaker parts. Normal movement and posture is based on a balance between control of antagonist and agonist muscle groups. Movement patterns follow diagonals or spirals that each possess a flexion, extension, and rotatory component and are directed toward or away from midline.

3. The Rood approach is based on Sherrington and the reflex stimulus model. Rood believed that all motor output was the result of both past and present sensory input. Rood introduced the use of sensory stimulation to facilitate or inhibit responses, such as icing and brushing, in order to elicit desired reflex motor responses.

4. The Brunnstrom approach created and defined the term synergy and initially encouraged the use of synergy patterns during rehabilitation. The patient was encouraged to immediately practice synergy patterns and subsequently develop combinations of movement patterns outside of the synergy.

System Specific: Neuromuscular & Nervous Systems
Content Outline: Interventions

## Exam Three: Question 154 X

A patient with several motor and sensory abnormalities exhibits signs of autonomic nervous system dysfunction. Which of the following is NOT an indicator of increased sympathetic involvement?

1. anxiety, distractibility
2. mottled, cold, shiny skin
3. **constriction of the pupils**
4. rapid, shallow breathing

**Correct Answer: 3** (Sullivan p. 60)

The autonomic nervous system (sympathetic and parasympathetic divisions) function together to maintain homeostasis. The sympathetic division prepares the body for stressful situations using the "fight or flight" response. The parasympathetic division ("rest and digest") controls body processes during ordinary situations.

1. Anxiety and distractibility are characteristics seen with an increase in sympathetic activity. Increased sweating, abnormal circulation, a lowered pain threshold, and heightened reflex activity are additional characteristics of a sympathetic response.

2. Skin that appears mottled and shiny is indicative of an increase in sympathetic activity. Other characteristics include hypersensitivity to touch, a rapid heart rate, dilation of the lungs, and increased muscle tension and strength.

3. **Constriction of the pupils is characteristic of a parasympathetic response. The parasympathetic division will also decrease heart rate, stimulate digestion, constrict the lungs, and stimulate other internal organs.**

4. Rapid and shallow breathing is a characteristic of increased sympathetic activity. Treatment techniques to decrease sympathetic stimulation include maintained touch, massage, rocking, deep breathing, generalized warmth, and midline pressure.

System Specific: Other Systems
Content Outline: Foundations for Evaluation, Differential Diagnosis, & Prognosis

## Exam Three: Question 155 ✗

A 55-year-old patient, six months status post CVA with right hemiparesis, attends physical therapy on an outpatient basis. As the patient lies supine on the mat, the physical therapist applies resistance to right elbow flexion. The therapist notes mass flexion of the right lower extremity as the resistance is applied. The therapist should document this as:

1. Raimiste's phenomenon
2. Souques' phenomenon
3. coordination synkinesis
4. **homolateral synkinesis**

**Correct Answer: 4** (Sullivan p. 25)
Homolateral synkinesis is an associated reaction that can occur after neurological damage. Resistance to flexion of the involved upper extremity will cause flexion in the involved lower extremity.

1. Raimiste's phenomenon occurs when the involved lower extremity abducts or adducts with applied resistance to the uninvolved lower extremity in the same direction.

2. Souques' phenomenon is observed when a patient raises the involved upper extremity above 100 degrees with the elbow extended. This action produces extension and abduction of the involved fingers.

3. Coordination synkinesis refers to voluntary contraction of certain muscle groups on the involved side that, in turn, gives rise to involuntary contractions of synergistic muscles.

4. **Homolateral synkinesis is a condition often associated with hemiplegia where there is mutual dependency between the involved upper and lower extremities. Certain theories of neurological rehabilitation avoid utilizing associated reactions while other theories utilize them to increase movement.**

System Specific: Neuromuscular & Nervous Systems
Content Outline: Interventions

## Exam Three: Question 156

A physical therapist orders a wheelchair for a patient with C4 tetraplegia. Which wheelchair would be the MOST appropriate for the patient?

1. manual wheelchair with friction surface handrims
2. manual wheelchair with handrim projections
3. **power wheelchair with sip and puff controls**
4. power wheelchair with joystick controls

**Correct Answer: 3** (O'Sullivan p. 961)
A patient with C4 tetraplegia would require a power wheelchair with a sip and puff, head, mouth or chin controls. The wheelchair would also require a tilt-in-space frame to allow for pressure relief.

1. Friction surface handrims are used when patients do not have a functional grip or the strength necessary to adequately propel a wheelchair. Patients with C6-C7 tetraplegia commonly rely on this feature.

2. Handrim projections add depth to the wheel and allow the patient to more easily propel the wheelchair. This is indicated at C5 where the lowest innervation includes the biceps, brachialis, brachioradialis, deltoids, rhomboids, and supinator. Although a patient with C5 tetraplegia may utilize handrim projections, the necessary energy expenditure may necessitate the use of a power wheelchair for mobility.

3. **A patient with C4 tetraplegia will have innervation of the face and neck, diaphragm, and trapezius muscles. The patient should be able to verbally direct all aspects of wheelchair management and would be a candidate for a power wheelchair with head or mouth controls.**

4. A patient with C5 tetraplegia is appropriate for a power wheelchair with joystick control. Patients utilize a power wheelchair for community mobility secondary to the high energy expenditure of using a manual wheelchair with handrim projections.

System Specific: Neuromuscular and Nervous Systems
Content Outline: Interventions

## Exam Three: Question 157

A child with a unilateral hip disarticulation works on advanced gait training activities. Which of the following activities would be the MOST difficult for the patient?

1. rising from a wheelchair
2. ascending stairs with a handrail
3. descending stairs with a handrail
4. **ascending a curb**

**Correct Answer: 4** (Seymour p. 256)

Patients with amputations experience greater energy use when completing functional skills. The higher the level of amputation, the greater the metabolic demand will be for a given activity. A hip disarticulation refers to the surgical removal of the lower extremity from the pelvis.

1. Rising from a wheelchair is performed with double leg support allowing for use of the arm rests to provide assistance with upward movement during the transfer. This requires less energy expenditure than ascending a curb.
2. Ascending stairs with a handrail is a challenging activity for a patient with a hip disarticulation, however, the presence of a handrail likely provides the patient with the necessary balance and stability to complete the activity.
3. Descending stairs with a handrail is typically slightly less difficult for a patient with a hip disarticulation compared to ascending stairs since the patient does not need to overcome the force of gravity.
4. **A child with a hip disarticulation would have the greatest difficulty ascending a curb during prosthetic training since there are no external supports (handrails) to assist with the activity.**

System Specific: Musculoskeletal System
Content Outline: Foundations for Evaluation, Differential Diagnosis, & Prognosis

## Exam Three: Question 158

A physical therapist examines the gait of a patient with a transtibial amputation. The patient exhibits delayed and limited knee flexion after heel strike on the prosthetic side. The MOST likely cause of the deviation is:

1. foot positioned in dorsiflexion
2. **heel wedge is too soft**
3. foot positioned too far posteriorly
4. socket is too large

**Correct Answer: 2** (Seymour p. 203)

A physical therapist must be able to analyze the gait of a patient following amputation and identify any deviation from normal. Once identified, therapists should attempt to determine the likely cause of the deviation and if necessary make an adjustment or refer the patient to the prosthetist.

1. If the foot of the prosthesis is positioned in dorsiflexion the knee will move anteriorly in relation to the center of gravity and cause a greater flexion moment during heel strike and stance. The knee will subsequently exhibit excessive knee flexion during stance.
2. **If the heel wedge is too soft, it will create an extension moment at the knee. The prosthesis will not advance over the foot to allow for flexion that normally occurs after initial contact. The heel cushion should only compress approximately 3/8 inch.**
3. If the foot of the prosthesis is positioned too far posteriorly, it will cause a greater flexion moment and result in excessive flexion upon initial contact and stance. Conversely, a foot positioned too far anteriorly may delay and limit knee flexion due to the increased extension moment.
4. If the socket of the prosthesis is too large, it may cause a greater flexion moment due to diminished support between the socket and the residual limb. The residual limb will flex in an attempt to maintain the fit of the prosthesis causing premature knee flexion during initial contact and stance.

System Specific: Musculoskeletal System
Content Outline: Foundations for Evaluation, Differential Diagnosis, & Prognosis

## Exam Three: Question 159

A physical therapist consults with an orthotist regarding the need for an ankle-foot orthosis for a patient status post CVA. The patient has difficulty moving from sitting to standing when wearing a prefabricated plastic ankle-foot orthosis (AFO). The therapist indicates the patient has poor strength at the ankle, intact sensation, and does not have any edema or tonal influence. The MOST appropriate type of AFO for the patient would incorporate:

1. **an articulation at the ankle joint**
2. tone reducing features
3. metal uprights
4. dorsiflexion assist

**Correct Answer: 1** (Seymour p. 382)

A plastic AFO with an articulating ankle joint is more cosmetic and lighter than a metal upright AFO. The orthosis provides total contact and therefore should not be used on patients with fluctuating edema or significant sensory deficits.

1. **An articulation at the ankle joint would allow the tibia to advance forward over the fixed foot. This would assist the patient with weight shifting during the sit to stand transfer as well as during ambulation.**

2. This patient would not require an AFO with tone reducing features since they do not present with tonal influence. A total contact footplate can be used to normalize tonal abnormalities and improve function and gait in patients that present with increased tone.

3. A metal AFO consists of two metal uprights connected proximally to a calf band and distally to a mechanical ankle joint and shoe. The ankle joint can be locked or set to have limited anterior/posterior capability. Since this design does not provide total contact it does not pose a risk to patients with fluctuating edema or significant sensory deficits.

4. A posterior leaf spring (PLS) is a plastic AFO with a trim line posterior to the malleoli. The primary purpose of the orthosis is to provide a dorsiflexion assist to prevent foot drop. The patient's lack of strength at the ankle (i.e., poor) makes it unlikely that they would possess the necessary medial/lateral stability to use this orthotic.

System Specific: Neuromuscular and Nervous Systems
Content Outline: Interventions

## Exam Three: Question 160

A physical therapist measures a patient for a straight cane prior to beginning ambulation activities. Which gross measurement method would provide the BEST estimate of cane length?

1. measuring from the head of the fibula straight to the floor and multiplying by two
2. measuring from the iliac crest straight to the floor
3. **measuring from the greater trochanter straight to the floor**
4. dividing the patient's height by two and adding three inches

**Correct Answer: 3** (Pierson p. 220)

The straight cane can be used with a variety of gait patterns, but does not permit partial weight bearing. The patient should have 20-25 degrees of elbow flexion while grasping the handgrip. A straight cane provides minimal support and is used primarily for assisting with balance.

1. Measuring from the head of the fibula and multiplying by two would not be an accurate method to determine the appropriate length of a straight cane. The formula doesn't take into account the differences that may exist in sizing of a patient's long bones or overall body type.

2. Measuring from the iliac crest to the floor would be in excess of the required height for proper fit of a straight cane. If the straight cane is too long, the angle of elbow flexion will increase beyond 20-25 degrees and the cane will be less effective.

3. **The handgrip of a cane that is properly fit should be at the approximate level of the greater trochanter.**

4. Dividing the patient's height by two and adding three inches is not an accurate formula to fit a straight cane. The formula doesn't take into account where the greater trochanter lies in relation to height from the floor or the patient's body type.

System Specific: Non-Systems
Content Outline: Equipment & Devices; Therapeutic Modalities

## Exam Three: Question 161

A physical therapist recommends a wheelchair for a patient rehabilitating from a CVA with the goal of independent mobility. The left upper and lower extremities are flaccid and present with edema. There is normal strength on the right, however, the patient's trunk is hypotonic. The patient is cognitively intact. The MOST appropriate wheelchair for the patient is:

1. solid seat, solid back, elevating legrests, and anti-tippers
2. sling seat, sling back, arm board, and elevating legrests
3. **light weight, solid seat, solid back, arm board, and elevating legrests**
4. light weight, solid seat, solid back, arm board, and standard footrests

**Correct Answer: 3** (Pierson p. 140)

A physical therapist must carefully select a wheelchair for a patient that possesses the necessary adaptations to meet the patient's unique needs. Failure to select an adequately equipped wheelchair can significantly compromise the patient's progress in rehabilitation.

1. The flaccid upper extremity would need to be supported using an arm board. Anti-tippers would not typically be necessary for this patient.
2. A sling seat and sling back promote poor positioning and would not provide the necessary stability the patient requires.
3. **Independent propulsion is facilitated by the use of a lightweight wheelchair, while a solid seating system assists with posture and activities. An arm board allows the flaccid upper extremity to be supported and an elevating legrest will assist to decrease dependent edema.**
4. The wheelchair is appropriate for the patient, however, the presence of lower extremity edema makes it desirable to incorporate elevating legrests.

System Specific: Neuromuscular and Nervous Systems
Content Outline: Interventions

## Exam Three: Question 162

A patient is scheduled to undergo a transtibial amputation secondary to gangrene of his left foot. In addition, the patient is one month status post right total knee arthroplasty due to osteoarthritis. Given the patient's past and current medical history, the physical therapist can expect which of the following tasks to be the MOST difficult for the patient following his amputation?

1. rolling from supine to sidelying
2. moving from sitting to supine
3. **moving from sitting to standing**
4. ambulating in the parallel bars

**Correct Answer: 3** (O'Sullivan p. 1045)

All of the listed tasks are reasonable expectations for the patient, however, moving from sitting to standing would be the most difficult due to the required lower extremity strength and the necessary balance required to complete the activity.

1. Rolling from supine to sidelying should be a relatively easy task for the patient since they can utilize upper extremity strength to initiate the movement.
2. Transferring from sitting to supine should be a relatively easy task for the patient since it is a non-weight bearing activity. The patient's sitting balance should not be impaired and the patient should be able to transfer to sitting using upper extremity support.
3. **Transferring from sitting to standing would be the most difficult for the patient since the activity requires adequate strength and dynamic balance. The patient's strength will be decreased in the right lower extremity secondary to the recent total knee arthroplasty and balance will be altered due to the left transtibial amputation.**
4. Ambulating in the parallel bars requires greater strength and balance than performing bed mobility, however, the patient is able to use the parallel bars to provide a stable base of support. The patient can use upper extremity strength to decrease some of the demand on the right lower extremity and to maintain balance during the activity.

System Specific: Musculoskeletal System
Content Outline: Foundations for Evaluation, Differential Diagnosis, & Prognosis

## Exam Three: Question 163 ✗

A patient diagnosed with T5 paraplegia is discharged from a rehabilitation hospital following 16 weeks of therapy. Assuming a normal recovery, which of the following MOST accurately describes the status of the patient's bathroom transfers?

1. independent with the presence of an attendant
2. independent with a sliding board
3. **independent with bathroom adaptations**
4. independent

**Correct Answer: 3** (Umphred p. 619)
A patient with T5 paraplegia should be able to complete bathroom transfers with selected adaptations. The patient would possess full upper extremity innervation and limited trunk control.

1. An attendant would not be necessary based on the patient's upper extremity innervation and the availability of bathroom adaptations.
2. Use of a sliding board when transferring to or from a toilet or tub bench could create an unnecessary safety risk for the patient due to the inherent space limitations in the bathroom and the relative stability of the sliding board on different surfaces.
3. **A patient with T5 paraplegia should be independent for all transfers using bathroom adaptations such as a grab bar, tub bench or commode seat.**
4. A patient with any form of complete spinal cord lesion will require various adaptations in order to attain independence.

System Specific: Neuromuscular & Nervous Systems
Content Outline: Foundations for Evaluation, Differential Diagnosis, & Prognosis

## Exam Three: Question 164

A physical therapist educates a patient status post transfemoral amputation on the importance of frequent skin checks. The MOST appropriate resource for the patient to utilize when inspecting the posterior aspect of the residual limb is:

1. **hand mirror**
2. video camera
3. nurse
4. prosthetist

**Correct Answer: 1** (Seymour p. 138)
The use of a mirror during skin inspection of the residual limb will enable the patient to view the entire limb without being dependent on another person.

1. **A patient should regularly inspect all areas of the residual limb using a mirror in order to maintain healthy skin. Proper skin care is important for all patients following amputation.**
2. A video camera would not be the most appropriate resource to inspect the residual limb since it can be cumbersome to use and may not be readily available for all patients.
3. A nurse is capable of viewing areas of the residual limb that the patient cannot see, however, a mirror will enable the patient to inspect their skin independently.
4. A prosthetist, like the nurse, could inspect the skin, however, this option would result in the patient being dependent on another person.

System Specific: Other Systems
Content Outline: Interventions

## Exam Three: Question 165

A physical therapist examines a 26-year-old female whose subjective complaints include morning stiffness of her hands and visible swelling. The patient indicates that the stiffness seems to diminish with activity. This description BEST describes:

1. carpal tunnel syndrome
2. osteoporosis
3. **rheumatoid arthritis**
4. osteoarthritis

**Correct Answer: 3** (Paz p. 375)

Rheumatoid arthritis is a chronic systemic autoimmune disorder of unknown etiology characterized by inflammatory changes in joints and related structures. The disease is two to three times more common in women than men.

1. Carpal tunnel syndrome is a medical condition caused by compression of the median nerve resulting in paresthesias, numbness, and muscle weakness in the hand. Symptoms include night pain, muscle atrophy, decreased grip strength, and decreased wrist mobility.

2. Osteoporosis is a metabolic condition that presents with a decrease in bone mass resulting in a greater risk of fracture. Symptoms include compression and other fractures, low thoracic or lumbar pain, loss of lumbar lordosis, kyphosis, decrease in height, Dowager's hump, and postural changes.

3. **Symptoms of rheumatoid arthritis include morning stiffness, limited range of motion, effusion, pain with movement, and low grade fever. Smaller peripheral joints are initially affected, however symptoms may progress to larger synovial joints.**

4. Osteoarthritis is a chronic disease that is characterized by degeneration of articular cartilage typically in weight bearing joints. Subsequent deformity and thickening of subchondral bone results in impaired functional status. The most commonly affected sites include the hands, hips, spine, and knees.

System Specific: Other Systems
Content Outline: Foundations for Evaluation, Differential Diagnosis, & Prognosis

## Exam Three: Question 166

A physical therapist provides pre-operative instructions to a patient scheduled for lower extremity amputation. Which of the following is the MOST common cause of lower extremity amputation?

1. tumor
2. trauma
3. **peripheral vascular disease**
4. cardiac disease

**Correct Answer: 3** (Seymour p. 10)

Peripheral vascular disease refers to diseases of blood vessels outside the heart and brain. The condition is often caused by narrowing of vessels that carry blood to the legs, arms, stomach or kidneys.

1. Certain tumors will require extremity amputation, however, this is not the most common causative factor for lower extremity amputation. Sarcomas are the most common type of malignant tumor that require amputation.

2. Trauma may result in the need for amputation, however, this is not the most common causative factor for lower extremity amputation. Trauma remains the most common cause of upper extremity amputation.

3. **Peripheral vascular disease is caused by atherosclerotic or inflammatory processes causing lumen narrowing (stenosis), embolism, vasospasm, trauma or thrombus formation. Initially, symptoms may include intermittent claudication and in severe cases, the condition can progress to amputation. The relative risk of limb amputation is largely dependent on the number and severity of cardiovascular risk factors (i.e., smoking, hypertension, diabetes).**

4. Cardiac disease itself is not a common causative factor for lower extremity amputation.

System Specific: Other Systems
Content Outline: Foundations for Evaluation, Differential Diagnosis, & Prognosis

## Exam Three: Question 167

A physical therapist instructs a patient diagnosed with C6 tetraplegia in functional activities. Which of the following activities would be LEAST appropriate?

1. independent raises for skin protection
2. manual wheelchair propulsion
3. assisted to independent transfers with a sliding board
4. **independent self-range of motion of the lower extremities**

**Correct Answer: 4** (Umphred p. 617)

A patient with C6 tetraplegia does not have sufficient motor innervation to consistently perform independent self-range of motion of the lower extremities. The lowest motor innervation at the C6 level includes extensor carpi radialis, infraspinatus, latissimus dorsi, pectoralis major, teres minor, pronator teres, and serratus anterior.

1. A patient with C6 tetraplegia can provide pressure relief using a wheelchair with push handles or loops attached.

2. A patient with C6 tetraplegia can perform manual wheelchair propulsion with friction surface handrims or rim projections.

3. A patient with C6 tetraplegia can perform assisted to independent transfers using a sliding board. A patient with C7 tetraplegia is typically independent with transfers with or without a sliding board.

4. **A patient with C6 tetraplegia cannot typically perform self-range of motion of the lower extremities. The activity is more appropriate for a patient with C7 tetraplegia.**

System Specific: Neuromuscular & Nervous Systems
Content Outline: Interventions

## Exam Three: Question 168

A physical therapist examines the residual limb of a patient following ambulation activities with a patellar tendon bearing prosthesis. The therapist identifies excessive redness over the patella. The MOST likely cause is:

1. **settling due to limb shrinkage**
2. socket not properly aligned
3. excessive withdrawal in sitting
4. excessive number of residual limb socks

**Correct Answer: 1** (O'Sullivan p. 1048)

Redness over the patella most often occurs when a patient's residual limb sits too low in the prosthesis. This is most often caused by shrinking of the residual limb or an inadequate number of residual limb socks.

1. **A physical therapist may elect to add additional one-ply socks to the residual limb of a patient with excessive redness over the patella in order to more normally distribute weight bearing forces.**

2. If the socket was improperly aligned, it would be unlikely that the residual limb would only receive excess pressure directly over the patella.

3. If the patient's residual limb experienced excessive withdrawal during sitting, the patella would come further out of the socket as opposed to sitting lower within the socket. This would not cause excessive redness over the patella.

4. An excessive number of residual limb socks would elevate the patella tendon above the patella tendon bearing surface of the prosthesis. This would cause the patella to move further out of the socket and therefore would be unlikely to cause redness over the patella.

System Specific: Musculoskeletal System
Content Outline: Interventions

## Exam Three: Question 169

A patient with increased sympathetic output is examined in physical therapy. Which treatment technique would NOT be beneficial in decreasing the level of sympathetic activity?

1. connective tissue massage
2. rotating the lower trunk in hooklying
3. **slow reversal hold of the quadriceps and hamstrings**
4. gentle manual pressure to the abdomen

**Correct Answer: 3** (Sullivan p. 60)

The sympathetic division of the autonomic nervous system prepares the body for stressful situations using the "fight or flight" response. It increases heart rate, dilates the airways, and allows the body to release stored energy. This division also causes the palms to sweat, pupils to dilate, and hair to stand on end.

1. Connective tissue massage is a technique that can be used to decrease sympathetic activity. Massage can influence muscle tension via the circulatory and autonomic systems with noted changes in vital signs and muscle tone.

2. Passive rotation of the lower trunk while in a hooklying position is an example of rhythmical movement which produces reflexive autonomic changes and an overall calming effect.

3. **Slow reversal hold is a proprioceptive neuromuscular facilitation technique used primarily to improve stability surrounding a joint. The technique uses slow and resisted concentric contractions of agonists and antagonists around a joint with an isometric contraction that is performed at the end of each movement. Slow reversal hold would not decrease sympathetic activity.**

4. Maintained touch is used to promote a parasympathetic response and produce a generalized calming effect due to the stimulation of tonic sensory receptors. Gentle manual pressure to the abdomen is an example of maintained touch.

System Specific: Neuromuscular & Nervous Systems
Content Outline: Interventions

## Exam Three: Question 170

A patient who sustained a CVA four weeks ago is beginning to show the ability to produce movement patterns outside of limb synergies. According to Brunnstrom, this patient is in which stage of recovery?

1. two
2. three
3. **four**
4. six

**Correct Answer: 3** (Brunnstrom p. 45)

Brunnstrom separates neurological recovery into separate stages based on progression through abnormal tone and spasticity. The stages range from stage one "flaccidity" to stage seven "normal coordinated movement." The stages of recovery describe tone, reflex activity, and volitional movement.

1. Stage two is characterized by the appearance of basic limb synergies and the beginning of spasticity.

2. Stage three is characterized by voluntary movement within synergies and increased spasticity.

3. **Stage four is characterized by movement patterns beginning outside of synergy patterns with diminished spasticity.**

4. Stage six is characterized by isolated coordinated joint movements with the disappearance of spasticity.

System Specific: Neuromuscular & Nervous Systems
Content Outline: Physical Therapy Examination

## Exam Three: Question 171

A recent entry in the medical record indicates a patient exhibits dysdiadochokinesia. Based on the patient's documented deficit, which activity would be the MOST difficult for the patient?

1. **alternate supination and pronation of the forearms**
2. perform a standing squat
3. march in place
4. walk along a straight line

**Correct Answer: 1** (Umphred p. 842)

Dysdiadochokinesia refers to the inability to perform rapid, alternating movements. This condition results in inappropriate timing of muscle firing and difficulty with cessation of ongoing movement.

1. **When the patient attempts pronation and supination of the forearms, the movement is slow and will lose range and rhythm quickly. The presence of dysdiadochokinesia is commonly associated with a cerebellar lesion.**

2. Performing a standing squat is not a velocity-based activity requiring alternating movement and therefore does not assess dysdiadochokinesia. The activity requires concentric and eccentric muscle control of the trunk and lower extremities.

3. Marching in place to a specific cadence is sometimes used to test for a cerebellar movement disorder. A positive test occurs when a patient is unable to follow the rhythm of the cadence.

4. Walking along a straight line is often used to identify signs of cerebellar pathology such as ataxia. Characteristics of an ataxic gait include uneven step length, increased base of support, inability to walk a straight line without lurching, impaired rhythm, and a high stepping pattern.

System Specific: Neuromuscular & Nervous Systems
Content Outline: Interventions

## Exam Three: Question 172

A physical therapist recognizes that a child has significant difficulty flexing the neck while in a supine position. Failure to integrate which reflex could explain the child's difficulty?

1. **symmetrical tonic labyrinthine reflex**
2. Moro reflex
3. asymmetrical tonic neck reflex
4. symmetrical tonic neck reflex

**Correct Answer: 1** (Ratliffe p. 26)

The symmetrical tonic labyrinthine reflex promotes a tendency for extension when a patient is in supine and reduced extensor influence when the patient is in prone. The persistence of a primitive reflex is generally seen with a neurological insult.

1. **The symmetrical tonic labyrinthine reflex serves to limit the child's ability to flex the neck when in a supine position. The child should lie in sidelying or in supine with hip flexion and/or knee flexion in order to decrease the influence of the reflex.**

2. The Moro reflex is elicited by a sudden change in the position of the head, usually having the head drop backwards. The typical response is crying along with extension and abduction of the upper extremities followed by flexion and adduction across the chest.

3. The asymmetrical tonic neck reflex is elicited through rotation of the neck. If the patient's head is turned, the upper and lower extremities on the face side extend and the upper and lower extremities on the skull side flex. The asymmetrical tonic neck reflex does not influence the child's ability to flex the neck while in a supine position.

4. The symmetrical tonic neck reflex is elicited by flexion or extension of the neck. When the head is flexed, upper extremities flex and lower extremities extend. When the head is extended, upper extremities extend and lower extremities flex. The symmetrical tonic neck reflex does not influence the child's ability to flex the neck while in a supine position.

System Specific: Neuromuscular & Nervous Systems
Content Outline: Physical Therapy Examination

## Exam Three: Question 173

A physical therapist discusses the importance of a well-balanced diet with a patient diagnosed with type 2 diabetes mellitus. The MOST appropriate action to emphasize the importance of diet is:

1. provide a handout from the American Diabetes Association which outlines an appropriate diet
2. ask other patients that have made dietary changes to speak to the patient
3. **arrange for a consultation with a dietician**
4. provide copies of recent research articles which cite the benefit of a well-balanced diet

**Correct Answer: 3** (Goodman - Pathology p. 490)

Type 2 diabetes mellitus (DM) is the most common form of diabetes. In type 2 DM, there is a combination of cellular resistance to insulin and an inadequate compensatory insulin secretory response. In most cases, this form of DM can be controlled with proper diet, exercise, weight control, and oral insulin supplementation.

1. A handout from the American Diabetes Association may serve as a helpful resource, however, type 2 diabetes mellitus is a condition where appropriate diet is critical to the management of the condition. As a result, a more proactive and formal action would be warranted.

2. Requesting that a patient with type 2 diabetes mellitus speak to other patients who have made dietary changes would qualify as a form of peer support, but would not provide the patient with enough information to make necessary dietary changes.

3. **Consultation with a dietician will provide the patient with education and a dietary program that typically includes a personal menu and recommendations for lifestyle modifications.**

4. Research articles on the benefits of a well-balanced diet may be of interest to some patients, however, the action would not be an appropriate substitute for a consultation with a dietician.

System Specific: Other Systems
Content Outline: Interventions

## Exam Three: Question 174

A physical therapist instructs a patient in an exercise designed to increase pelvic floor awareness and strength. The exercise requires the patient to tighten the pelvic floor as if attempting to stop the flow of urine. The patient is instructed to hold the isometric contraction for five seconds and complete ten repetitions. The MOST appropriate INITIAL position for the exercise is:

1. **supine**
2. sitting
3. tall kneeling
4. standing

**Correct Answer: 1** (Kisner p. 814)

The pelvic floor muscles follow the same general strengthening principles as other muscles of the body. As a result, the initial position for the pelvic floor exercise should remove or minimize the influence of gravity. As the patient demonstrates mastery of the initial position, the physical therapist can select positions that will provide the patient with a greater challenge.

1. **Kegel exercises or isometric contractions of the pelvic floor, are often utilized as part of a treatment program for incontinence. Supine and sidelying are the typical gravity-eliminated positions to initiate strengthening. A patient may also use a gravity-assisted position where the hips are above the level of the heart such as supported bridging or on elbows and knees in order to have gravity assist the contraction.**

2. A patient would progress to sitting once there is adequate strength and awareness of the pelvic floor muscles. Sitting requires exercise against gravity and therefore would not be the most appropriate initial position.

3. A patient would progress to tall kneeling once there is adequate strength and awareness of the pelvic floor in a sitting position. Tall kneeling requires proximal control and balance to maintain the position.

4. Standing is the highest level in the general progression of pelvic floor strengthening. The normal sequence is supine or sidelying followed by quadruped, sitting, tall kneeling, and standing.

System Specific: Other Systems
Content Outline: Interventions

## Exam Three: Question 175 ✗

A physical therapist attempts to assess the dynamic balance of an elderly patient. Which screening tool would be the MOST helpful to test balance and gait?

1. Functional Independence Measure
2. **Tinetti Performance Oriented Mobility Assessment**
3. Fugl-Meyer Assessment
4. Barthel Index

**Correct Answer: 2** (Physical Therapists Clinical Companion p. 123)

The Tinetti Performance Oriented Mobility Assessment is an outcome measurement tool used to identify if there is an increased risk for falling. The tool measures balance and gait using a two to three point ordinal scale and takes 5-15 minutes to administer. The risk of falling increases as the total score decreases.

1. The FIM is a tool used in rehabilitation hospitals to determine a patient's level of disability and burden of care. A seven-point scale is utilized to examine 18 areas including self-care, sphincter control, transfers, locomotion, communication, and social cognitive activities. This tool is used as a predictor of disability.

2. **The Tinetti Performance Oriented Mobility Assessment has two sections. The first section assesses balance through sit to stand and within the standing position. The second section assesses gait at normal and rapid speeds. There is a total maximum score of 28 with patients scoring less than 19 considered to be at high risk for falling.**

3. The Fugl-Meyer Assessment is an ordinal scale used to measure recovery post CVA. The framework is based on Brunnstrom's sequence of recovery. The five areas of assessment are joint movement and pain, balance, upper extremity motor function, sensation, and lower extremity motor function. The maximum combined score for upper and lower extremity motor function is 100 and can be interpreted as a percentage of motor recovery. For example, a score of 63 indicates approximately 63% return of motor function.

4. The Barthel Index is designed to measure the amount of assistance needed to perform ten different ADL and mobility activities with a total maximum score of 100. The index does not account for cognitive or safety issues and is not sensitive to higher level patients regarding their level of disability.

System Specific: Neuromuscular and Nervous Systems
Content Outline: Physical Therapy Examination

## Exam Three: Question 176

A physical therapist monitors the blood pressure of a 28-year-old male during increasing levels of physical exertion. Assuming a normal physiologic response, which of the following BEST describes the patient's blood pressure response to dynamic exercise?

1. systolic pressure decreases, diastolic pressure increases
2. systolic pressure remains the same, diastolic pressure increases
3. systolic pressure and diastolic pressure remain the same
4. **systolic pressure increases, diastolic pressure remains the same**

**Correct Answer: 4** (Pierson p. 62)

The normal response to dynamic exercise is a progressive increase in systolic blood pressure, and no change or a slight decrease in diastolic pressure. The magnitude of increase in systolic blood pressure is approximately 5-10 mm Hg per metabolic equivalent.

1. A decrease in systolic blood pressure and an increase in diastolic blood pressure are both abnormal responses.

2. No change in systolic blood pressure and an increase in diastolic blood pressure are both abnormal responses. An increase in diastolic blood pressure of more than 10 mm Hg may be indicative of exertional ischemia.

3. No change in either systolic or diastolic blood pressure is an abnormal response.

4. **An increase in systolic blood pressure while diastolic blood pressure remains the same is a normal response to dynamic exercise.**

System Specific: Cardiovascular/Pulmonary and Lymphatic Systems
Content Outline: Interventions

## Exam Three: Question 177

A physical therapist examines the reflex status of a patient. The therapist should use which technique to assess the patient's superficial reflexes?

1. brushing the skin with a light, feathery object
2. passive joint range of motion
3. **stroking the skin with a non-cutting, but pointed object**
4. tapping over a muscle tendon

**Correct Answer: 3** (O'Sullivan p. 238)

Superficial cutaneous reflexes are elicited with a light stroke of the skin. The anticipated response is a small or brief contraction of the muscles innervated by a given spinal segment that received the light stroking.

1. Light touch sensation is assessed by brushing the skin with a light, feathery object.
2. Passive joint range of motion is performed to assess the influence of noncontractile structures on range of motion or tone (hypertonicity or hypotonicity).
3. **The plantar reflex (S1, S2) is an example of a superficial reflex. The reflex is elicited by stroking the lateral aspect of the foot from the heel to the ball of the foot with a blunt object. A normal response is indicated by flexion of the great toe, while an abnormal response is indicated by extension of the great toe with fanning of the four other toes (Babinski sign). The Babinski sign is often associated with upper motor neuron damage.**
4. Deep tendon reflexes are performed to test the integrity of the spinal reflex and are elicited by tapping over a muscle tendon. A physical therapist should strike the tendon with a reflex hammer after placing the tendon on slight stretch.

System Specific: Neuromuscular & Nervous Systems
Content Outline: Physical Therapy Examination

## Exam Three: Question 178

A patient returns to an outpatient physical therapy clinic two hours after a physical therapy session complaining of increased back pain. The patient has been in physical therapy for three previous visits and has had little difficulty with a program consisting of palliative modalities and pelvic stabilization exercises. The patient was referred to physical therapy after injuring his back two weeks ago. The MOST appropriate physical therapist action is:

1. contact the referring physician to discuss the patient's care plan
2. **instruct the patient to discontinue the pelvic stabilization exercises and re-examine the patient at his next visit**
3. refer the patient to the emergency room of a local hospital
4. instruct the patient to cancel existing physical therapy visits and schedule an appointment with the physician

**Correct Answer: 2** (Criteria for Standards of Practice)

Physical therapists must carefully assess a patient's response to physical therapy interventions. The severity of the patient's signs and symptoms combined with the therapist's knowledge of their medical condition assists the therapist to make an informed decision regarding an appropriate course of action.

1. The patient's current complaints do not suggest the need for immediate consultation with the referring physician.
2. **The physical therapist should have the patient discontinue any activities that increase their pain. The therapist can re-examine the patient at the next scheduled visit and determine an appropriate course of action based on the findings.**
3. The patient's current complaints are not severe enough to warrant referral to an emergency room.
4. Physical therapists most often refer patients back to the referring physician due to a change in medical status or failure to make anticipated progress in physical therapy. The patient's recent increase in symptoms does not suggest that the patient is not a candidate for physical therapy.

System Specific: Musculoskeletal System
Content Outline: Interventions

## Exam Three: Question 179

A physical therapist reviews the medical record of a patient rehabilitating from a stroke. The patient exhibits paralysis and numbness on the side of the body contralateral to the vascular accident. Which descending pathway is MOST likely damaged based on the patient's clinical presentation?

1. **corticospinal tract**
2. vestibulospinal tract
3. tectospinal tract
4. rubrospinal tract

**Correct Answer: 1** (O'Sullivan p.195)
The corticospinal tract is the largest descending pathway where 80% of the fibers decussate and descend on the opposite side; 20% continue to descend ipsilaterally. The corticospinal tract carries information from the motor cortex directly to the spinal cord.

1. **The corticospinal tract is concerned with skilled fine motor control primarily of the distal limbs.**
2. The vestibulospinal tract is responsible for gross postural adjustments subsequent to head movements and acceleration.
3. The tectospinal tract is responsible for visual information related to spatial awareness. The tract ends at the cervical spine and controls the musculature of the neck as well as head position.
4. The rubrospinal tract communicates with the thalamus and cerebellum and plays an important role in the coordination of movement.

System Specific: Neuromuscular & Nervous Systems
Content Outline: Physical Therapy Examination

## Exam Three: Question 180

A patient exhibits pain and sensory loss in the posterior thigh, lateral calf, and dorsal foot. Extension of the hallux is poor, however, the Achilles reflex is normal. What spinal level would you expect to be involved?

1. L4
2. **L5**
3. S1
4. S2

**Correct Answer: 2** (Magee p. 16)
Involvement of a specific spinal level often results in predictable impairments including diminished sensation, muscle weakness, impaired reflexes, and paresthesias.

1. L4 nerve root:
   Dermatome - medial buttock, lateral thigh, medial leg, dorsum of foot, great toe
   Myotome - tibialis anterior, extensor hallucis
   Reflexes - patellar

2. **L5 nerve root:**
   **Dermatome - buttock, posterior and lateral thigh, lateral aspect of leg, dorsum of foot, medial half of sole, first, second, and third toes**
   **Myotome - extensor hallucis, peroneals, gluteus medius, dorsiflexors, hamstrings, plantar flexors**
   **Reflexes - medial hamstrings, posterior tibial**

3. S1 nerve root:
   Dermatome - lateral and plantar aspect of foot
   Myotome - hamstrings, peroneals, plantar flexors
   Reflexes - Achilles

4. S2 nerve root:
   Dermatome - buttock, thigh, posterior leg
   Myotome - hamstrings, plantar flexors
   Reflexes - Achilles

System Specific: Neuromuscular & Nervous Systems
Content Outline: Physical Therapy Examination

## Exam Three: Question 181

A physical therapist performs goniometric measurements for elbow flexion with a patient in supine. In order to isolate elbow flexion the therapist should stabilize the:

1. **distal end of the humerus**
2. proximal end of the humerus
3. distal end of the ulna
4. proximal end of the radius

**Correct Answer: 1** (Norkin p. 96)

When measuring elbow flexion the physical therapist should align the fulcrum of the goniometer over the lateral epicondyle of the humerus. The stationary arm should be aligned with the lateral midline of the humerus using the center of the acromial process as a reference. The moveable arm should be aligned with the lateral midline of the radius using the radial head and radial styloid process as references. Normal elbow flexion is 0-150 degrees.

1. **The distal end of the humerus should be stabilized when measuring elbow flexion to prevent flexion of the shoulder. The therapist should place a pad (i.e., folded towel) between the table and the distal humerus to prevent extension of the shoulder.**

2. Stabilization of the proximal end of the humerus is too far away from the elbow to adequately stabilize the joint during elbow flexion.

3. The distal end of the radius and ulna would be stabilized when measuring wrist flexion and extension or wrist radial and ulnar deviation.

4. Any attempt to stabilize the proximal end of the radius would interfere with elbow flexion range of motion.

System Specific: Musculoskeletal System
Content Outline: Physical Therapy Examination

## Exam Three: Question 182

A patient rehabilitating from a radial head fracture performs progressive resistive exercises designed to strengthen the forearm supinators. Which muscle would be of particular importance to achieve the desired outcome?

1. brachialis
2. brachioradialis
3. **biceps brachii**
4. anconeus

**Correct Answer: 3** (Kendall p. 268)

A physical therapist should have a strong understanding of anatomy including primary and secondary actions of muscles and their innervations.

1. The brachialis muscle flexes the elbow joint. The muscle is innervated by the musculocutaneous nerve.

2. The brachioradialis muscle flexes the elbow joint and assists in supination and pronation when the movements are resisted. Although the muscle plays a role in supination of the forearm, the biceps brachii is a much more powerful supinator. The muscle is innervated by the radial nerve.

3. **The biceps brachii muscle flexes the elbow joint and supinates the forearm. The muscle is innervated by the musculocutaneous nerve.**

4. The anconeus muscle extends the elbow joint and assists to stabilize the ulna during supination and pronation. The muscle is innervated by the radial nerve.

System Specific: Musculoskeletal System
Content Outline: Interventions

## Exam Three: Question 183

A physical therapist examines a patient with a suspected injury to the thoracodorsal nerve. Which objective finding would be consistent with this injury?

1. shoulder medial rotation weakness
2. **shoulder extension weakness**
3. paralysis of the rhomboids
4. paralysis of the diaphragm

**Correct Answer: 2** (Kendall p. 279)
The thoracodorsal nerve (C6, C7, C8) is a branch of the posterior cord of the brachial plexus. The nerve follows the course of the subscapular artery along the posterior wall of the axilla to the latissimus dorsi.

1. The medial rotators of the shoulder include the subscapularis, teres major, pectoralis major, latissimus dorsi, and anterior deltoid. The latissimus dorsi would be affected by an injury to the thoracodorsal nerve, however, the presence of a number of other muscles which act to medially rotate the humerus would be adequate to compensate for any impairment in the latissimus dorsi.

2. **The latissimus dorsi is innervated by the thoracodorsal nerve (C6, C7, C8). Weakness in this prime mover for shoulder extension would produce impaired strength during shoulder extension resistive testing despite the fact that several other muscles also function to extend the shoulder. These muscles include the posterior deltoid and teres major.**

3. The rhomboids are innervated by the dorsal scapular nerve (C4, C5).

4. The diaphragm is innervated by the phrenic nerve (C3, C4, C5).

System Specific: Neuromuscular & Nervous Systems
Content Outline: Physical Therapy Examination

## Exam Three: Question 184

A physical therapist works with a patient using a flotation device positioned vertically in the deep end of a pool. Which area of the patient's body would experience the GREATEST amount of hydrostatic pressure?

1. shoulders
2. torso
3. hips
4. **feet**

**Correct Answer: 4** (Cameron p. 247)
Hydrostatic pressure refers to the pressure exerted by a fluid on a body immersed in the fluid. Hydrostatic pressure increases as the depth of immersion increases.

1. When positioned vertically, the shoulders would be only partially immersed since the patient is using a flotation device. The hydrostatic pressure on the shoulders would be negligible.

2. When positioned vertically, the torso will likely be partially or perhaps fully immersed. The hydrostatic pressure on the torso will be greater than the hydrostatic pressure on the shoulders, but less than the hydrostatic pressure on the hips or feet.

3. When positioned vertically, the hips will be fully immersed. The hydrostatic pressure on the hips will be less than the hydrostatic pressure on the feet since the feet are immersed to a greater depth.

4. **When positioned vertically, the feet would experience the greatest amount of hydrostatic pressure since they are the deepest immersed body part.**

System Specific: Other Systems
Content Outline: Interventions

## Exam Three: Question 185

A physical therapist elects to begin a trial of mechanical lumbar traction on a 165 pound male diagnosed with suspected nerve root impingement. The MOST appropriate amount of force to initiate the session is:

1. 15 lbs.
2. **30 lbs.**
3. 60 lbs.
4. 80 lbs.

**Correct Answer: 2** (Cameron p. 302)

Mechanical traction refers to the application of forces to the body using a machine to separate joint surfaces and stretch periarticular structures. Traction is indicated for many diagnoses and allows for variation and adjustment of the established protocol based on individual patient needs. Traction affects many of the body's systems and requires ongoing monitoring and reassessment of treatment parameters.

1. 15 lbs. is an insufficient amount of force to use when initiating a trial of mechanical traction due to the relative weight of the patient's body.

2. **A traction force of 25-50 lbs. is recommended when initiating mechanical lumbar traction. The amount of force is low enough to reduce the risk of protective muscle guarding and spasm, but is sufficient to determine if traction is likely to aggravate the patient's symptoms.**

3. 60 lbs. is greater than the recommended range of 25-50 lbs. for initial treatment. This amount of force may cause muscle guarding secondary to patient fear, anxiety or pain.

4. 80 lbs. is almost 50% of the patient's body weight and corresponds to the approximate amount of force (i.e., 50%) necessary to cause mechanical separation in the lumbar spine. This amount of force may be appropriate depending on the established treatment objectives, however, would not be appropriate for the initial session.

System Specific: Non-Systems
Content Outline: Equipment & Devices; Therapeutic Modalities

## Exam Three: Question 186

A physical therapist completes an examination on a patient diagnosed with Parkinson's disease. Results of the examination include 4/5 strength in the lower extremities, 10 degree flexion contracture at the hips, and exaggerated forward standing posture. The patient has difficulty initiating movement and requires manual assistance for gait on level surfaces. The MOST appropriate activity to incorporate into a home program is:

1. **prone lying**
2. progressive relaxation exercises
3. lower extremity resistive exercises with ankle weights
4. postural awareness exercises in standing

**Correct Answer: 1** (Umphred p. 787)

Prone lying is a commonly employed positional technique designed to stretch the hip flexors in patients with Parkinson's disease. Increased flexibility of the hip muscles will improve standing posture and enable the body's center of gravity to remain within the base of support. Although some of the other options are appropriate, they would not provide the same degree of benefit for the patient based on the described clinical presentation.

1. **Prone lying is a static positioning activity designed to stretch the hip flexors. If the patient was unable to tolerate prone lying, the physical therapist could place one or more pillows under the patient's hips and gradually remove pillows over time as the patient improves their flexibility.**

2. Progressive relaxation exercises can be incorporated using gentle rocking or segmental trunk rotation, however, the patient needs to have adequate range of motion in the hip flexors to optimize their functional status.

3. Strengthening is a restorative intervention used with patients with Parkinson's disease, however, the patient's strength in the lower extremities is already good (i.e., 4/5) and therefore would not be an immediate treatment priority.

4. Postural awareness exercises in standing are an appropriate intervention, however, the relative benefit of the activity is limited without adequate muscle length. By improving the patient's hip flexibility, the patient would be able to exhibit improved standing posture.

System Specific: Neuromuscular and Nervous Systems
Content Outline: Interventions

## Exam Three: Question 187

A patient four days status post right total hip arthroplasty loses his balance and falls to the ground during a physical therapy session. The patient is visibly shaken by the fall, but insists that he is uninjured. The physical therapist examines the right hip and although active motion elicits pain, all other findings are inconclusive. The therapist should:

1. continue with the current treatment so the patient does not focus on the incident
2. notify the supervisor about the incident
3. **document the incident and contact a physician to examine the patient before resuming treatment**
4. document the incident and gradually resume prior treatment

**Correct Answer: 3** (Scott - Promoting Legal and Ethical Awareness p. 81)

If a patient has fallen or has been injured during physical therapy, the physical therapist must inform the patient's physician of the incident and request medical clearance prior to continuing with treatment. Failure to inform the physician would be considered a form of negligence.

1. A physical therapist must place the patient's well-being above any other present concern. An attempt to manipulate the patient for fear of personal liability is never an appropriate course of action.

2. A physical therapist may choose to notify their supervisor about the incident, however, the primary therapist action must be directed toward making sure the patient is unharmed and ensuring the integrity of the hip arthroplasty.

3. **The described incident combined with the patient's post-operative status provides adequate justification for physician involvement and documentation. In addition to traditional documentation, the physical therapist will need to complete an incident report.**

4. The incident must be documented, however, it would be inappropriate to resume treatment without first having the patient examined by a physician.

System Specific: Musculoskeletal System
Content Outline: Interventions

## Exam Three: Question 188

The medical record indicates a patient has been diagnosed with chronic respiratory alkalosis. The MOST consistent laboratory finding with this condition is:

1. **elevated arterial blood pH, low $PaCO_2$**
2. low arterial blood pH, elevated $PaCO_2$
3. elevated arterial blood pH, elevated $PaCO_2$
4. low arterial blood pH, low $PaCO_2$

**Correct Answer: 1** (Rothstein p. 440)

Analysis of arterial blood gases provides information about acid-base balance, ventilation, and oxygenation.

1. **Elevated arterial blood pH and low $PaCO_2$ are consistent with respiratory alkalosis. This condition can be caused by alveolar hyperventilation due to dizziness or syncope.**

2. Low arterial blood pH and elevated $PaCO_2$ are consistent with respiratory acidosis. This condition can be caused by alveolar hypoventilation due to anxiety, confusion, and coma.

3. Elevated arterial blood pH and elevated $PaCO_2$ are consistent with a partially compensated metabolic alkalosis. Causes of metabolic alkalosis include bicarbonate ingestion, vomiting, diuretics, steroids, and adrenal disease.

4. Low arterial blood pH and low $PaCO_2$ are consistent with a partially compensated metabolic acidosis. Causes of metabolic acidosis include metabolic diseases or disturbances such as diabetes, lactic acid, uremic acidosis, and chronic diarrhea.

System Specific: Cardiovascular/Pulmonary and Lymphatic Systems
Content Outline: Foundations for Evaluation, Differential Diagnosis, & Prognosis

## Exam Three: Question 189

A patient with a transtibial amputation is observed ambulating with excessive knee flexion from heel strike through midstance on the prosthetic side. A possible cause for this deviation is:

1. the foot is set in neutral
2. the socket is set posterior in relation to the foot
3. the prosthesis is too short
4. **the socket is aligned in excessive flexion**

**Correct Answer: 4** (Seymour p. 204)

If the socket of a transtibial prosthesis is aligned in excessive flexion, there will be excessive flexion during stance causing instability of the prosthetic limb. Anatomical contributing factors include a knee flexion contracture, knee extensor weakness or a hip flexion contracture.

1. A neutral foot setting would not cause excessive knee flexion from heel strike to midstance.

2. A transtibial socket that is set posteriorly to the foot will create an increased extension moment at the knee and result in insufficient knee flexion during early stance.

3. A prosthesis that is too short would typically create an increased extension moment at the knee and result in insufficient knee flexion during early stance. A prosthesis that is too long may cause excessive flexion during heel strike through midstance.

4. **A socket that is aligned in excessive flexion will create an increased flexion moment at the knee which will result in excessive flexion from heel strike through stance phase.**

System Specific: Musculoskeletal Systems
Content Outline: Physical Therapy Examination

## Exam Three: Question 190

A physical therapist monitors a patient's vital signs while completing 20 minutes of jogging at 5 mph on a treadmill. As the session approaches its conclusion, the therapist incorporates a cool down period. The anticipated response during the post-exercise period is:

1. a progressive increase in systolic blood pressure
2. **a progressive decrease in systolic blood pressure**
3. a progressive increase in diastolic blood pressure
4. a progressive increase in rate pressure product

**Correct Answer: 2** (American College of Sports Medicine p. 55)

Incorporating a cool down period provides a gradual recovery and a return of the heart rate and blood pressure to near resting values. Additional benefits of cool down include enhanced venous return, increased dissipation of body heat, increased removal of lactic acid, and reduced likelihood of ventricular arrhythmias.

1. A progressive increase in systolic blood pressure is the normal response to an increase in workload and therefore would not be associated with the post-exercise period.

2. **A progressive decrease in systolic blood pressure is the normal post-exercise response.**

3. A progressive increase in diastolic blood pressure would be considered an abnormal response since it should not occur during an increase in work or during the post-exercise period.

4. Rate pressure product or double-product, is the product of heart rate and systolic blood pressure. Both heart rate and systolic blood pressure are expected to decrease during the post-exercise period. Rate pressure product is an indicator of myocardial oxygen consumption.

System Specific: Cardiovascular/Pulmonary and Lymphatic Systems
Content Outline: Physical Therapy Examination

# Exam Three: Question 191

A patient status post stroke ambulates with a large base quad cane. The patient presents with left neglect and diminished proprioception. The MOST appropriate method to ensure patient safety is:

1. provide continuous verbal cues
2. utilize visual cues and demonstration
3. **offer manual assistance on the left side**
4. offer manual assistance on the right side

**Correct Answer: 3** (O'Sullivan p. 1169)

A physical therapist must carefully consider a patient's current limitations and identify remedial strategies to assist the patient to achieve established goals. The presence of left neglect and diminished proprioception requires the therapist to take formal action to avoid jeopardizing patient safety.

1. Verbal cues may be beneficial for the patient, however, without concurrent manual assistance the patient would likely still have increased difficulty with ambulation and may be at increased risk for a fall.

2. Demonstration prior to practice is important, however, this type of educational strategy would not directly address the left neglect and diminished proprioception.

3. **The physical therapist should offer manual assistance on the patient's left side during ambulation activities. The manual assistance can facilitate motor activity and weight bearing, as well as proprioception on the affected side. Manual contact significantly reduces the risk for fall or injury.**

4. The patient presents with left neglect and as a result manual assistance would not typically be necessary on the right side of the body.

System Specific: Neuromuscular and Nervous Systems
Content Outline: Interventions

# Exam Three: Question 192 X

A patient elevated on a tilt table to 60 degrees suddenly begins to demonstrate signs and symptoms of orthostatic hypotension. The MOST appropriate physical therapist action is to:

1. lower the tilt table 10 degrees and monitor the patient's vital signs
2. lower the tilt table 20 degrees and monitor the patient's vital signs
3. lower the tilt table 40 degrees and monitor the patient's vital signs
4. **lower the tilt table completely and monitor the patient's vital signs**

**Correct Answer: 4** (Pierson p. 339)

Signs and symptoms of orthostatic hypotension include a 20 mm Hg or greater decrease in systolic blood pressure, dizziness, and nausea. The signs and symptoms are caused by reduced venous return from the lower extremities which is often precipitated by vertical positioning. The reduced venous return results in decreased filling of the left ventricle and diminished cardiac output and cerebral perfusion.

1. Lowering the tilt table 10 degrees would not likely be sufficient to adequately resolve the patient's current signs and symptoms of orthostatic hypotension.

2. Lowering the tilt table 20 degrees would serve as a relatively modest change in the degree of vertical positioning and would therefore be more appropriate if the patient had experienced only mild dizziness or another isolated sign or symptom of orthostatic hypotension.

3. Lowering the tilt table 40 degrees would be a viable option, however, the sudden onset of signs and symptoms of orthostatic hypotension make it more appropriate to lower the tilt table to a horizontal position.

4. **The magnitude of the positional change (i.e., 60 degrees to horizontal) would likely be adequate to reduce the patient's signs and symptoms of orthostatic hypotension. The patient's vital signs should be checked to ensure that the patient's blood pressure is within normal limits.**

System Specific: Cardiovascular/Pulmonary and Lymphatic Systems
Content Outline: Interventions

## Exam Three: Question 193

A physical therapist and a physical therapist assistant work as a team in an orthopedic private practice. Which activity would be inappropriate for the physical therapist assistant?

1. application of a superficial modality
2. **completing a discharge summary**
3. leading a group exercise program
4. performing an isokinetic test

**Correct Answer: 2** (Guide to Physical Therapist Practice)

The physical therapist assistant is a technically educated health care provider who assists the physical therapist in the provision of physical therapy services. The physical therapist of record is directly responsible for the actions of the physical therapist assistant and should therefore possess a comprehensive understanding of the physical therapist assistant's scope of practice.

1. Physical therapist assistants routinely perform interventions such as the application of superficial modalities as part of an established plan of care.
2. **The physical therapist is solely responsible for the establishment of the discharge summary and the associated documentation.**
3. Physical therapist assistants often instruct individual patients and groups of patients in exercise programs. The activity would be within the physical therapist assistant's scope of practice.
4. An isokinetic test is a resistive test designed to collect data regarding a patient's strength. Physical therapist assistants perform tests and measures as part of their daily practice.

System Specific: Non-Systems
Content Outline: Safety and Protection; Professional Responsibilities; Research

## Exam Three: Question 194

A physical therapist obtains a complete medical history prior to administering cryotherapy. Which condition would NOT be considered a contraindication to cryotherapy?

1. Raynaud's disease
2. cryoglobulinemia
3. **cancer**
4. cold urticaria

**Correct Answer: 3** (Cameron p. 140)

Commonly used cryotherapeutic agents include cold whirlpool, ice packs, ice massage, cold sprays, and contrast baths. Physical therapists should be aware of indications and contraindications for all superficial agents.

1. Raynaud's disease is a condition that causes arteries supplying blood to the skin to narrow resulting in diminished circulation. Symptoms include pallor, rubor, cyanosis, and numbness and tingling in the digits and hand. Raynaud's disease is considered a contraindication for cryotherapy.
2. Cryoglobulinemia is a condition where abnormal blood protein transforms to gel when exposed to cold temperatures. The gel-like state can lead to ischemia and gangrene if prolonged exposure exists. Cryoglobulinemia is considered a contraindication for cryotherapy.
3. **Cryotherapy is not contraindicated for patient's with cancer, however, secondary impairments such as diminished sensation can make cryotherapy an unacceptable treatment option.**
4. Cold urticaria refers to an allergic-like response producing hives or large welts on the skin following exposure to cold. In more severe cases, the patient may experience a significant decrease in blood pressure, an increase in heart rate, and syncope. Cold urticaria is considered a contraindication for cryotherapy.

System Specific: Non-Systems
Content Outline: Equipment & Devices; Therapeutic Modalities

## Exam Three: Question 195

A patient with T10 paraplegia is discharged from a rehabilitation hospital following 12 weeks of intense rehabilitation. Which of the following pieces of equipment would be the MOST essential to assist the patient with functional mobility?

1. ambulation with Lofstrand crutches
2. ambulation with Lofstrand crutches and ankle-foot orthoses
3. ambulation with Lofstrand crutches and knee-ankle-foot orthoses
4. **wheelchair**

**Correct Answer: 4** (Rothstein p. 408)

A patient with a lesion above T12 would not be a functional ambulator due to the extreme energy demands and therefore would utilize a wheelchair as their primary mode of mobility.

1. A patient with an incomplete lesion may ambulate without an orthotic using Lofstrand crutches, however, this would not be an option for a complete spinal cord lesion.

2. A patient with a complete lesion at L4 or L5 would typically ambulate with crutches or canes and bilateral AFOs. The extensor digitorum, medial hamstrings, posterior tibialis, quadriceps, tibialis anterior, and low back muscles would be the lowest innervated muscles.

3. A patient with a complete lesion at L2 or L3 would typically ambulate with crutches and bilateral KAFOs. Patients at this level of injury may also use a manual wheelchair for energy conservation and convenience. The gracilis, iliopsoas, quadratus lumborum, rectus femoris, and sartorius would be the lowest innervated muscles.

4. **A patient with T10 paraplegia will require a wheelchair for community ambulation due to the increased energy expenditure associated with ambulation. The lower abdominals and intercostals would be the lowest innervated muscles.**

System Specific: Neuromuscular and Nervous Systems
Content Outline: Interventions

## Exam Three: Question 196

A physical therapist instructs a patient's spouse to remove and reapply a bandage. Which of the following instructional methods would be the MOST appropriate to ensure the task is performed appropriately?

1. have the patient instruct the spouse how to remove and reapply the bandage
2. provide written instructions on how to remove and reapply the bandage
3. **instruct the spouse to remove and reapply the bandage and observe her performance**
4. instruct the spouse to contact the physical therapy department if she has specific questions on how to remove or reapply the bandage

**Correct Answer: 3** (Hall p. 40)

The physical therapist should observe the removal and reapplication of the bandage in order to determine if the spouse is capable of performing the task. Although this will not ensure the task is done appropriately in the future, it will provide the patient with the opportunity for feedback based on their current performance.

1. If the patient instructs the spouse how to remove and reapply the bandage, the therapist can conclude that the patient can explain the task, but this does not ensure that the spouse can independently perform the task.

2. Written instructions are helpful for the patient and spouse as a resource, but will not ensure independence. Demonstration is the best instructional method to ensure proper technique and independence.

3. **Patient and family education is a critical component of a comprehensive plan of care following amputation. Direct observation of the spouse's performance is the best method to increase the probability that the activity will be performed correctly.**

4. The physical therapist would be exercising poor judgment if they requested the patient to call the department with questions on bandaging without providing additional instruction. The therapist must provide instruction and observe the family members' performance to ensure competence.

System Specific: Other Systems
Content Outline: Interventions

## Exam Three: Question 197 ✗

A physical therapist instructs a patient in an upper extremity proprioceptive neuromuscular facilitation pattern by telling the patient to begin by grasping an imaginary sword positioned in a scabbard on their left hip using their right hand. This type of command would be MOST appropriate to initiate:

1. D1 extension
2. D1 flexion
3. D2 extension
4. **D2 flexion**

**Correct Answer: 4** (Kisner p. 196)

Proprioceptive neuromuscular facilitation (PNF) patterns are upper and lower extremity movement patterns that are designed to improve stability and strengthen the extremities, trunk, and neck. The patterns are performed unilaterally or bilaterally, symmetrically or asymmetrically. Resistance using tubing, weights or manual resistance can increase the level of difficulty.

1. The D1 extension pattern begins with the patient positioned in shoulder flexion, adduction, and lateral rotation. The patient follows the directive of "open your hand and push down and away from your body" to complete the diagonal pattern.

2. The D1 flexion pattern begins with the patient positioned in shoulder extension, abduction, and medial rotation. The patient follows the directive of "close your hand and pull up and across your body" to complete the diagonal pattern.

3. The D2 extension pattern begins with the patient positioned in shoulder flexion, abduction, and lateral rotation. The patient follows the directive of "close your hand and pull down and across your body" to complete the diagonal pattern.

4. **The D2 flexion pattern begins with the patient positioned in shoulder extension, adduction, and medial rotation. The patient follows the directive of "open your hand and pull up and away from your body" to complete the diagonal pattern.**

System Specific: Neuromuscular & Nervous Systems
Content Outline: Interventions

## Exam Three: Question 198

A physical therapist develops a plan of care for a patient status post unilateral transtibial amputation that has been approved for inpatient rehabilitation. Assuming an uncomplicated recovery, what is the MOST appropriate amount of time for prosthetic training?

1. 1-2 days
2. **1-2 weeks**
3. 4-6 weeks
4. 6-8 weeks

**Correct Answer: 2** (Lusardi p. 716)

A patient with a unilateral transtibial amputation would typically require one to two weeks for prosthetic training. Training includes donning and doffing, prosthetic management, transfers, ambulation, and stair training.

1. Prosthetic training requires careful observation of prosthetic fit and mastering all functional activities including gait, stairs, community training, transferring to and from the floor, and total care of the prosthesis. This cannot be accomplished in a one or two day period.

2. **A patient with a unilateral transtibial amputation would typically enter inpatient rehabilitation for one to two weeks for prosthetic training. This period permits sufficient time for the majority of patients to develop adequate proficiency in functional training activities.**

3. A patient with a unilateral transtibial amputation would not typically require four to six weeks of inpatient rehabilitation for prosthetic training. The patient should be able to master all aspects of prosthetic training within a one to two week time frame.

4. A patient with a unilateral transtibial amputation would not typically require six to eight weeks of inpatient rehabilitation for prosthetic training. A time frame of six to eight weeks would be more indicative of a patient with a complete spinal cord injury resulting in paraplegia.

System Specific: Musculoskeletal System
Content Outline: Foundations for Evaluation, Differential Diagnosis, & Prognosis

## Exam Three: Question 199

After observing a patient during an exercise session, a physical therapist concludes that the patient commonly uses the Valsalva maneuver. Which activity would have the GREATEST probability of producing the Valsalva maneuver?

1. **lifting a 40 lb. package from the floor to a counter at waist level**
2. walking at 4 mph on a treadmill
3. stationary cycling at 80 revolutions per minute
4. using an upper extremity ergometer at 40 revolutions per minute

**Correct Answer: 1** (Kisner p. 392)

The Valsalva maneuver refers to a contraction of the muscles of the abdomen, chest wall, and diaphragm in a forced expiratory effort against a closed glottis. This action produces an increase in intrathoracic and intra-abdominal pressures that lead to decreased venous blood flow to the heart.

1. **Patients commonly use the Valsalva maneuver during heavy resistance exercise. Forty pounds would be a sufficiently heavy load that would result in most patients straining and holding their breath while lifting the package from the floor.**

2. Walking at 4 mph on a treadmill is a rhythmical form of exercise that would not require the patient to hold their breath in a Valsalva maneuver. Patients typically establish a steady breathing pattern when walking at a constant speed on a treadmill.

3. Stationary cycling at 80 revolutions per minute is a rhythmical form of exercise. The continuous nature of the activity combined with the high revolutions per minute would not require the patient to hold their breath in a Valsalva maneuver.

4. Using an upper extremity ergometer at 40 revolutions per minute is a rhythmical form of exercise that requires continuous motion of the upper extremities. The Valsalva maneuver is more commonly observed in strenuous, shorter duration activities.

System Specific: Cardiovascular/Pulmonary and Lymphatic Systems
Content Outline: Interventions

## Exam Three: Question 200

A physical therapist receives a referral to instruct a patient in pelvic floor muscle strengthening exercises. Which of the following explanations would be the MOST effective to assist the patient to perform a pelvic floor contraction?

1. tighten your muscles like you were trying to expel a large amount of urine in a very short amount of time
2. **pull your muscles upward and inward as if attempting to stop the flow of urine**
3. tighten your abdominal muscles and anteriorly rotate your pelvis
4. gently push out as if you had to pass gas

**Correct Answer: 2** (Hall p. 429)

The pelvic floor muscles support the pelvic organs against intra-abdominal pressure, provide closure of the urethra and rectum for continence, and support sexual function. Pelvic floor exercises, also known as Kegel exercises, assist to maintain the strength and function of the pelvic floor muscles.

1. Placing a downward pressure on the pelvic floor serves to increase intra-abdominal pressure and encourage protrusion or prolapse of the pelvic organs.

2. **The correct technique for pelvic floor exercises includes pulling the pelvic floor muscles up and in. Isometric contractions should be held for five to ten seconds with complete relaxation after each contraction. Five to ten contractions should be performed in a series and three to four series should be performed each day.**

3. Tightening the abdominal muscles will trigger reflexive contraction of the pelvic floor, however, anteriorly rotating the pelvis will lengthen the abdominal muscles. Performing both actions simultaneously will reduce the strength of any pelvic floor contraction.

4. The act of "pushing out as if you had to pass gas" places a downward pressure on the pelvic floor muscles. This action is opposite of the necessary action for pelvic floor strengthening.

System Specific: Other Systems
Content Outline: Interventions

# EXAM REFERENCES, EXAM & ACADEMIC REVIEW INDEXES, MOTIVATIONAL MOMENTS, AND RESOURCES

997 Exams Scoring Summary

998 Computer-Based Exam References

1000 Computer-Based Exam Index

1006 Academic Review Index

1023 PTEXAM: The Complete Study Guide

1024 Motivational Moment One

1025 Online Advantage

1026 Online Advantage Research Abstract

1027 PT Content Master - Flash Card

1028 Motivational Moment Two

1029 On-Campus Review Course

1030 Motivational Moment Three

1031 Applications

1032 Motivational Moment Four

1033 CD Installtion Instructions

SCOREBUILDERS

# Computer-Based Exams Scoring Summary

|  | Available Questions | Correct Questions | % Correct |
|---|---|---|---|
| Exam One | 200 |  |  |
| Exam Two | 200 |  |  |
| Exam Three | 200 |  |  |

# Computer-Based Exam References

American Heart Association, www.americanheart.org, 2011

American College of Sports Medicine. *ACSM's Resource Manual for Guidelines for Exercise Testing and Prescription.* Eighth Edition. Lippincott Williams & Wilkins. 2010.

Anemaet W, Moffa-Trotter M. *Home Rehabilitation: Guide to Clinical Practice.* Mosby Inc. 2000.

Bailey D, Robinson D. *Therapeutic Approaches in Mental Health/Psychiatric Nursing.* Fourth Edition. F.A. Davis Company. 1997.

Belanger AY. *Evidence-Based Guide to Therapeutic Physical Agents.* Lippincott Williams & Wilkins. 2003.

Bickley L, Szilagyi P. Bates' *Guide to Physical Examination and History Taking.* Tenth Edition. Lippincott Williams & Wilkins. 2009.

Brannon F, Foley M, Starr J, Saul L. *Cardiopulmonary Rehabilitation: Basic Theory and Application.* Third Edition. F.A. Davis Company.1998.

Brotzman SB, Manske RC. *Clinical Orthopedic Rehabilitation.* Third Edition. Mosby Inc. 2011.

Brunnstrom S. *Movement Therapy in Hemiplegia.* Harper and Row Publishers Inc. 1992.

Cameron M. *Physical Agents in Rehabilitation: From Research to Practice.* Third Edition. WB Saunders Company. 2008.

Cameron M, Monroe L. *Physical Rehabilitation: Evidence Based Examination. Evaluation, and Intervention.* Saunders. 2007.

Campbell S. *Physical Therapy for Children.* Fourth Edition. W.B. Saunders Company. 2011.

Ciccone C. *Pharmacology for Rehabilitation.* Fourth Edition. F.A. Davis Company. 2007.

*Code of Ethics.* American Physical Therapy Association. HOD S06-00-12-23.

*Criteria for Standards of Practice for Physical Therapy.* American Physical Therapy Association. BOD S03-06-16-38.

Davis C. *Patient Practitioner Interaction.* Fourth Edition. Slack Inc. 2006.

De Domenico G, Wood E. *Beard's Massage.* Fifth Edition. WB Saunders Company. 2007.

DeMyer W. *Technique of the Neurologic Examination.* McGraw-Hill Companies. 2004.

Dutton M. *Orthopaedic Examination, Evaluation, and Intervention.* Second Edition. McGraw-Hill Inc. 2008.

Falvo DR. *Effective Patient Education.* Fourth Edition. Jones and Bartlett Publishers. 2010.

Frownfelter D, Dean E. *Cardiovascular and Pulmonary Physical Therapy: Evidence and Practice.* Fifth Edition. Mosby-Year Book Inc. 2012.

Goodman CC, Fuller KS. *Pathology: Implications for the Physical Therapist.* Third Edition. Saunders Elsevier. 2009.

Goodman C, Snyder T. *Differential Diagnosis for Physical Therapists.* Fifth Edition. W.B. Saunders Company. 2013.

*Guide for Conduct of the Physical Therapist Assistant.* American Physical Therapy Association.

*Guide to Physical Therapist Practice.* 2nd ed. Phys Ther. 2001; 81:583.

Haggard A. *Handbook of Patient Education.* Aspen Publishers. 1989.

Hall C, Brody L. *Therapeutic Exercise: Moving Toward Function.* Third Edition. Lippincott Williams & Wilkins. 2011.

Hamill J, Knutzen K. *Biomechanical Basis of Human Movement.* Third Edition. Lippincott Williams & Wilkins. 2008.

Hertling D, Kessler R. *Management of Common Musculoskeletal Disorders.* Fourth Edition. Lippincott Williams & Wilkins. 2005.

Hillegass E, Sadowsky S. *Essentials of Cardiopulmonary Physical Therapy.* Third Edition. W.B. Saunders Company. 2011.

Hoppenfeld S. *Physical Examination of the Spine and Extremities.* Appleton-Century-Crofts. 1982.

Kendall F, McCreary E. Provance P. *Muscle Testing and Function.* Fifth Edition. Lippincott Williams & Wilkins. 2005.

Kisner C, Colby L. *Therapeutic Exercise Foundations and Techniques.* Fifth Edition. F.A. Davis Company. 2007.

Levangie P, Norkin C. *Joint Structure and Function: A Comprehensive Analysis.* Fifth Edition. F.A. Davis Company. 2011.

Long T, Toscano K. *Handbook of Pediatric Physical Therapy.* Second Edition. Lippincott Williams & Wilkins. 2002.

Lusardi M, Nielsen C. *Orthotics and Prosthetics in Rehabilitation.* Elsevier Inc. 2007.

Magee D. *Orthopedic Physical Assessment.* Fifth Edition. W.B. Saunders Company. 2007.

# Computer-Based Exam References

Michlovitz S, Bellew J, Nolan T. *Modalities for Therapeutic Intervention.* Fifth Edition. F.A. Davis Company. 2012.

Minor M, Minor S. *Patient Care Skills.* Sixth Edition. Prentice Hall. 2009.

Montgomery PC, Connolly BH. *Clinical Applications for Motor Control.* Slack Inc. 2003.

Myers D. *Psychology*. Ninth Edition. Worth Publishers. 2009.

Norkin C, White D. *Measurement of Joint Motion: A Guide to Goniometry.* Fourth Edition. F.A. Davis Company. 2009.

Nosse L, Friberg D. *Managerial and Supervisory Principles for Physical Therapists.* Third Edition. Lippincott Williams & Wilkins. 2010.

O'Sullivan S, Schmitz T. *Physical Rehabilitation: Assessment and Treatment.* Fifth Edition. F.A. Davis Company. 2007.

Paz J, West MP. *Acute Care Handbook for Physical Therapists.* Third Edition. Saunders. 2008.

*Physical Therapist's Clinical Companion.* Springhouse Corporation. 2000.

Pierson F, Fairchild S. *Principles and Techniques of Patient Care.* Fifth Edition. WB Saunders Company. 2013.

Portney LG, Watkins MP. *Foundations of Clinical Research: Applications to Practice.* Third Edition. Upper Saddle River. NJ; Prentice Hall. 2009.

Prentice W, Voight M. *Techniques in Musculoskeletal Rehabilitation.* McGraw-Hill Inc. 2008.

Prentice W. *Therapeutic Modalities in Rehabilitation.* Fourth Edition. McGraw-Hill Inc. 2011.

Purtilo R, Haddad A. *Health Professional and Patient Interaction.* Seventh Edition. WB Saunders Company. 2007.

Quinn L, Gordon J. *Functional Outcomes: Documentation for Rehabilitation*. Elsevier Science. 2003.

Ratliffe KT. *Clinical Pediatric Physical Therapy: A Guide for the Physical Therapy Team.* Mosby Inc. 1998.

Richard R, Staley M. *Burn Care and Rehabilitation*: *Principles and Practice*. F.A. Davis Company. 1994.

Rothstein JM, Echternach JL. *Primer on Measurement: An Introductory Guide to Measurement Issues.* American Physical Therapy Association. 1993.

Rothstein J, Roy S, Wolf S. *The Rehabilitation Specialist's Handbook.* Third Edition. F.A. Davis Company. 2005.

Ruoti RG, Morris DM. *Aquatic Rehabilitation.* Lippincott Williams & Wilkins. 1997.

Sackett DL, Straus SE, Richardson WS, Rosenburg W, Haynes RB. *Evidence-Based Medicine. How to Practice and Teach EBM.* Fourth Edition. Churchill Livingstone. 2011.

Sadock B, Sadock V. *Kaplan & Sadock's Comprehensive Textbook of Psychiatry*. Ninth Edition. Lippincott Williams & Wilkins. 2009.

Scott R. *Foundations of Physical Therapy: A 21st Century-Focused View of the Profession*. McGraw-Hill Inc. 2002.

Scott R. *Promoting Legal and Ethical Awareness*. Mosby Inc. 2009.

Seymour R. *Prosthetics and Orthotics: Lower Limb and Spinal*. Lippincott Williams & Wilkins. 2002.

Shamus E, Stern D. *Effective Documentation for the Physical Therapy Professional.* Second Edition. McGraw-Hill Inc. 2011.

Sullivan P, Markos P. *Clinical Decision Making in Therapeutic Exercise*. Appleton & Lange. 1995.

Sussman C, Bates-Jensen B. *Wound Care: A Collaborative Practice Manual for Health Professionals.* Fourth Edition. Philadelphia, Pennsylvania; Wolters Kluwer Health/Lippincott Williams & Wilkins. 2012.

Tan JC. *Practical Manual of Physical Medicine and Rehabilitation.* Second Edition. Mosby Inc. 2005.

Tecklin J. *Pediatric Physical Therapy.* Fourth Edition. Lippincott Williams & Wilkins. 2007.

Umphred D. *Neurological Rehabilitation.* Fifth Edition. Mosby Inc. 2006.

Van Deusen J. *Assessment in Occupational and Physical Therapy*. WB Saunders Company. 1997.

# Computer-Based Exam Index

## Directions for Using the Computer-Based Exams Index

The Computer-Based Exams Index allows candidates to identify specific academic content in each of the three sample examinations. For example, consider the following entry: **Breathing exercises 1:** 52, 196; **3:** 108. The bold numbers represent the exam number and the non-bold numbers that follow represent the question number within the respective exam. Therefore, questions pertaining to breathing exercises are located in Exam One: Question 52, 196 and in Exam Three: Question 108. The index provides candidates with an efficient and effective method to review selected academic content after completing each of the sample examinations.

**Accessibility**
  **1:** 127, 131; **2:** 66; **3:** 83
**Active/passive insufficiency**
  **2:** 8; **3:** 20
**Adhesive capsulitis**
  **3:** 54
**Administration**
  **1:** 143, 146; **2:** 17, 22, 85, 157; **3:** 29, 127, 133, 146
**Advanced directives**
  **1:** 146
**Airway clearance**
  **1:** 103, 162; **3:** 58
**Alzheimer's disease**
  **2:** 174
**Americans with Disabilities Act (ADA)**
  **1:** 127, 131; **2:** 66; **3:** 31, 83, 104
**Amputation**
  **1:** 35; **2:** 24; **3:** 27, 51, 55, 64, 67, 89, 91, 99, 136, 139, 157, 158, 162, 164, 166, 168, 189, 198
**Anatomic snuff box**
  **2:** 154
**Anatomy**
  **1:** 5, 55, 87, 117, 119, 153, 171, 178, 179; **2:** 11, 32, 59, 77, 86, 96, 182; **3:** 13, 18, 61, 92, 101, 120, 135
**Anemia**
  **1:** 4, 14, 144
**Angina**
  **2:** 144, 185
**Ankylosing spondylitis**
  **2:** 133, 184; **3:** 96
**Anterior compartment syndrome**
  **2:** 105
**Anterior cruciate ligament**
  **1:** 22, 45, 174; **2:** 15, 19, 52, 101, 114, 157; **3:** 134
**Anthropometry**
  **1:** 17; **2:** 18, 196; **3:** 52
**Aquatic therapy**
  **2:** 60
**Arrhythmias**
  **1:** 128; **3:** 108
**Arterial blood gas analysis**
  **3:** 40

**Arterial line**
  **1:** 75, 109
**Assistive/adaptive devices**
  **1:** 44, 135; **2:** 81, 153, 166, 180, 181, 188, 190; **3:** 81, 150, 160
**Ataxia**
  **2:** 72
**Athetosis**
  **1:** 88; **2:** 56
**Auscultation**
  **1:** 76; **3:** 101
**Autonomic dysreflexia**
  **1:** 97; **3:** 60, 88
**Autonomic nervous system**
  **3:** 154, 169
**Axes of motion**
  **2:** 129
**Balance**
  **1:** 74; **2:** 117, 134, 151, 178; **3:** 32, 37, 175
**Bandaging**
  **3:** 51, 67, 196
**Barthel Index**
  **1:** 23
**Berg Balance Scale**
  **2:** 39
**Biomechanics**
  **1:** 25; **2:** 62
**Blood pressure**
  **1:** 17, 97, 99; **2:** 34, 100, 155; **3:** 176, 190, 192
**Body composition**
  **1:** 93; **2:** 18, 196; **3:** 52, 56
**Body mass index**
  **2:** 18
**Borg's Rating of Perceived Exertion Scale**
  **2:** 172
**Brachial plexus**
  **3:** 23
**Bracing/splinting**
  **2:** 114
**Breath sounds**
  **1:** 76, 139, 182

# Computer-Based Exam Index

**Breathing exercises**
  **1:** 96, 152; **3:** 8
**Bronchial drainage**
  **1:** 145; **3:** 113
**Brown-Sequard's syndrome**
  **2:** 31
**Brunnstrom's Stages of Recovery**
  **1:** 158; **3:** 170
**Burns**
  **1:** 13, 60, 64; **2:** 42, 51, 111, 118; **3:** 5, 111, 151, 152
**Calcific tendonitis**
  **2:** 121
**Cardiac rehabilitation**
  **1:** 30, 141; **3:** 15
**Cardiopulmonary resuscitation (CPR)**
  **1:** 136, 194
**Cardiovascular fitness**
  **2:** 137
**Carpal tunnel syndrome**
  **2:** 9
**Carpals**
  **1:** 153; **2:** 36, 138, 154
**Cerebral palsy**
  **2:** 56
**Chest excursion**
  **1:** 12, 37; **2:** 179
**Chest physical therapy**
  **2:** 80, 199; **3:** 58
**Chronic arterial disease**
  **3:** 47
**Chronic bronchitis**
  **1:** 76, 191; **2:** 107
**Chronic venous insufficiency**
  **2:** 97
**Circulation**
  **2:** 16, 43, 135; **3:** 11, 74
**Circumferential measurements**
  **1:** 27
**Closed-chain activities**
  **2:** 65
**Cognition**
  **1:** 42, 156; **2:** 152, 165, 174, 177
**Cold immersion bath**
  **1:** 53
**Communication**
  **1:** 47; **3:** 12, 39, 41, 126
**Computed tomography (CT) scan**
  **2:** 175; **3:** 10
**Congestive heart failure**
  **1:** 123; **2:** 139; **3:** 7, 39
**Consultation**
  **1:** 3, 39, 84, 85, 155, 157; **2:** 22, 67, 68, 83, 84, 123, 124; **3:** 29, 42, 94, 149, 173, 187
**Continuous passive motion machine (CPM)**
  **1:** 166; **2:** 71

**Coordination**
  **2:** 72; **3:** 123
**Coronary artery bypass graft (CABG)**
  **3:** 36
**Coronary artery disease**
  **1:** 36
**Correlation**
  **2:** 93
**Coughing**
  **1:** 103, 162
**Cranial nerves**
  **1:** 173; **3:** 4
**Cryotherapy**
  **1:** 53, 120; **2:** 141; **3:** 194
**Cushing's syndrome**
  **3:** 69
**Cystic fibrosis**
  **1:** 12
**Data collection**
  **1:** 177; **2:** 122
**Debridement**
  **2:** 112; **3:** 111
**Deep tendon reflexes**
  **1:** 83, 137; **2:** 119; **3:** 30
**Deep vein thrombosis**
  **1:** 147, 163; **3:** 9
**Delegation**
  **2:** 167, 198; **3:** 35, 193
**Diabetes mellitus**
  **1:** 185; **3:** 54, 173
**Diagnostic imaging/testing**
  **1:** 69, 108; **2:** 9, 23, 52, 121, 175; **3:** 10, 19, 26
**Diplopia**
  **2:** 95
**Discriminative sensations**
  **1:** 90; **2:** 194
**Documentation**
  **1:** 16, 31, 143; **2:** 5, 84, 189; **3:** 78, 117, 133, 187
**Dressings**
  **1:** 50; **3:** 89, 116
**Duchenne muscular dystrophy**
  **1:** 9; **2:** 40
**Dysdiadochokinesia**
  **3:** 171
**Dysmetria**
  **1:** 46
**Edema**
  **1:** 66, 189; **2:** 122, 191
**Electrical stimulation**
  **1:** 1, 140; **2:** 76, 103, 122, 142; **3:** 21, 61, 114, 124
**Electrocardiogram**
  **1:** 8, 49, 124; **2:** 91, 131; **3:** 46
**Electromyography**
  **1:** 69

# Computer-Based Exam Index

**Emergent conditions**
1: 97, 185, 194; 2: 144; 3: 88

**Emphysema**
1: 54; 3: 16

**End-feel**
1: 15, 107, 171; 2: 182; 3: 18, 92

**Endurance**
1: 7, 63

**Energy conservation**
3: 8

**Energy expenditure**
3: 64, 102, 157

**Ergonomics**
2: 156; 3: 31, 199

**Eschar**
3: 63

**Ethics**
1: 41, 91; 3: 104, 117, 130, 133

**Evidence-based practice**
1: 183; 2: 132, 143; 3: 122

**Exercise prescription**
1: 18, 160, 174; 2: 65, 88, 137, 139, 145, 158, 184; 3: 24, 47, 103, 174

**Exercise testing**
1: 63, 67; 3: 15

**Exercise tolerance**
1: 14, 95; 3: 48, 176, 190

**Extension lag**
1: 57

**Exudate**
3: 110

**Foot and ankle alignment**
1: 25; 2: 45

**Fractures**
1: 195; 3: 26

**Froment's sign**
1: 149

**Functional Reach Test**
2: 187

**Functional Independence Measure (FIM)**
1: 112

**Gait**
1: 33, 70, 87, 98, 116; 2: 27, 125, 126, 173; 3: 53, 55, 64, 81, 91, 100, 157, 158, 189, 191

**Glasgow Coma Scale**
1: 169; 3: 105

**Goniometry**
1: 26, 57, 122; 2: 5, 10, 53; 3: 181

**Gower's sign**
2: 40

**Growth and development**
1: 92; 2: 12, 15; 3: 97

**Hand washing**
1: 125

**Heart block**
2: 131

**Heart rate**
1: 21, 49, 67, 86, 124; 2: 88, 145, 172, 195; 3: 15, 24, 140

**Heart sounds**
3: 36, 101

**Heat disorders**
1: 93

**Heimlich maneuver**
1: 136

**Heterotopic ossification**
1: 15

**Hierarchy of evidence**
2: 143

**Hoover test**
2: 127

**Hot packs**
1: 159; 3: 131

**Human immunodeficiency virus (HIV)**
2: 104

**Hydrostatic weighing**
3: 56

**Hydrotherapy**
1: 24, 38, 180; 3: 184

**Hypertension**
1: 113; 3: 115

**Hyperthermia**
1: 38

**Hypoxemia**
2: 16

**Iliotibial band syndrome**
2: 77

**Incentive spirometry**
1: 152

**Incontinence**
2: 38; 3: 66, 200

**Independent variable**
3: 128

**Individual Educational Plan (IEP)**
3: 78

**Informed consent**
1: 41, 105

**Innervation**
1: 83, 173, 186, 187; 2: 55, 63, 94, 105, 170; 3: 3, 23, 25, 59, 87, 129, 145, 156, 167, 180, 183, 195

**Inspection and maintenance**
1: 134, 142

**Institutional Review Board (IRB)**
1: 61

**Intermittent claudication**
3: 47

**Intermittent compression**
3: 45, 49

# Computer-Based Exam Index

**Intravenous line (IV)**
1: 115
**Iontophoresis**
1: 72, 77, 80; 2: 35; 3: 1, 121
**Ischemia**
3: 46
**Laboratory values**
1: 36; 2: 23, 30, 80, 106, 108, 111; 3: 9, 40
**Levels of measurement**
2: 3; 3: 109, 132
**Levels of weight bearing**
2: 128, 150, 180
**Ligamentous testing**
2: 32
**Lines, tubes, and devices**
1: 32, 75, 109, 115, 155; 2: 33, 43, 70, 161; 3: 50
**Malingering**
2: 127; 3: 41
**Manual muscle testing**
1: 106; 2: 2, 25, 96, 186; 3: 73, 109
**Massage**
1: 192
**Mechanical device parameters**
1: 81, 166; 2: 21, 71; 3: 45, 49, 185
**Mechanical traction**
1: 81; 2: 21; 3: 185
**Medical equipment**
1: 66; 2: 50, 91; 3: 119
**Metabolic equivalents (METs)**
1: 141; 3: 102
**Mini-Mental State Examination**
2: 165
**Mobilization**
1: 79, 181; 2: 4, 57, 136
**Modality parameters**
1: 40, 72, 117, 126, 129, 140, 151, 172; 2: 76, 103, 130, 141, 142, 197; 3: 1, 2, 21, 114, 121, 124, 143
**Motor control**
1: 19; 3: 72, 141
**Muscle action**
1: 2, 52, 55, 59, 94, 196; 2: 2, 25, 26, 59, 102, 110, 125, 160, 176; 3: 25, 33, 62, 73, 182, 183
**Muscle length**
1: 59; 2: 47, 115; 3: 20, 71, 98, 100, 136
**Myocardial infarction**
1: 128
**Neuroanatomy**
1: 88, 173, 186, 187; 2: 37, 94, 105, 168; 3: 123, 154, 179
**Neurodevelopmental Treatment (NDT)**
3: 153
**Normal distribution**
3: 44

**Nutrition**
3: 7
**Obstetrics**
3: 86
**Oncology**
1: 111; 2: 106, 162; 3: 65
**Orthostatic hypotension**
1: 99; 2: 34, 155; 3: 192
**Orthotics**
1: 68, 161; 2: 89; 3: 6, 79, 80, 138, 159
**Osteogenesis imperfecta**
1: 6
**Osteokinematic and arthrokinematic motions**
2: 136
**Osteoporosis**
1: 71; 3: 112
**Outcome measurement tools**
1: 7, 23, 112; 2: 39, 165, 187; 3: 175
**Outcomes**
1: 195; 2: 101
**Oxygen saturation**
1: 82, 95; 3: 48
**Pain**
1: 148, 170, 193; 2: 42; 3: 39, 132
**Palpation**
2: 36, 77, 116, 138, 176; 3: 13, 33, 135
**Parkinson's disease**
1: 33; 3: 72, 137, 186
**Patient management**
1: 20, 41, 47, 73, 84, 85, 121, 132, 133, 157, 160, 164, 167, 188, 190, 197, 198; 2: 28, 74; 3: 76, 94, 117, 118, 144, 147, 178
**Patient rights**
1: 146
**Pelvic floor exercises**
2: 38; 3: 174, 200
**Perceptual deficits**
2: 37; 3: 84
**Peripheral nerve injury**
1: 186; 2: 55, 105; 3: 6
**Peripheral neuropathy**
2: 125; 3: 30
**Peripheral vascular disease**
2: 135; 3: 166
**Perseveration**
3: 38
**pH**
2: 35; 3: 188
**Pharmacology**
1: 8, 13, 21, 77, 85, 147; 2: 1, 108, 185; 3: 9, 90, 115, 125
**Phonophoresis**
1: 172
**Physical therapist assistant role**
2: 113; 3: 142, 193

# Computer-Based Exam Index

**Physical therapy aide role**
1: 175; 2: 167, 198; 3: 35, 85

**Piriformis syndrome**
2: 54

**Plan of care**
1: 6; 2: 157; 3: 70, 82, 118, 198

**Planes of motion**
1: 58; 2: 98, 129

**Pleural effusion**
1: 139

**Positioning**
1: 6, 104, 113, 162; 2: 159; 3: 27, 88, 113, 136

**Post-polio syndrome**
3: 57

**Postural strategies**
1: 74

**Posture**
2: 62, 133; 3: 77, 96, 186

**Pressure garments**
1: 66

**Pressure relief**
1: 104; 2: 159; 3: 25, 70

**Pressure ulcers**
1: 51; 2: 159

**Primitive reflexes**
1: 11, 78; 2: 12, 20, 29, 73, 92; 3: 75, 97, 148, 172

**Professional development**
2: 17

**Properties of water**
2: 60; 3: 184

**Proprioceptive neuromuscular facilitation**
2: 6, 41, 99, 133; 3: 98, 169, 197

**Prosthetics**
3: 99, 158, 168, 189, 198

**Pulmonary function testing**
1: 28, 54; 3: 17, 22

**Pusher syndrome**
3: 77

**Q-angle**
3: 93

**Rancho Los Amigos Levels of Cognitive Functioning Scale**
1: 121; 2: 46

**Range of motion**
1: 59; 2: 8, 10, 49, 61, 115; 3: 20

**Red-Yellow-Black System**
3: 63

**Reliability**
1: 165, 184; 2: 164

**Rescue breathing**
1: 114

**Research**
1: 29, 61, 62, 65, 100, 165, 177, 183, 184; 2: 75, 78, 93, 120, 132, 164, 171, 192; 3: 34, 44, 106, 109, 122, 128, 130, 132

**Residual limb care**
1: 35; 3: 51, 67, 89, 164, 168

**Respiration**
1: 52; 2: 64, 159, 179; 3: 8, 87

**Respiratory acidosis/alkalosis**
3: 40, 188

**Reverse Trendelenburg**
1: 113

**Rheumatoid arthritis**
2: 82; 3: 165

**Rinne test**
3: 4

**Risk factors**
1: 10, 36; 2: 107; 3: 7, 16, 54, 68, 86, 87, 108, 112, 149, 166

**Risk management**
2: 87, 148; 3: 127, 147

**Romberg test**
2: 134

**Rotator cuff**
1: 48, 55; 2: 116; 3: 62

**Rule of Nines**
3: 152

**Safety**
1: 35, 72, 73, 134, 135, 138, 142, 166, 200; 2: 146, 166; 3: 28, 85, 114, 127, 130, 131, 143, 144, 187, 191

**Sampling**
1: 29; 3: 34, 106

**Scaphoid fracture**
2: 154

**Scoliosis**
1: 39

**Scope of practice**
1: 3, 110, 155, 175; 2: 22, 67, 68, 83, 113, 123, 124, 162; 3: 42, 74, 142, 173, 187, 193

**Screening**
1: 39, 71; 2: 171; 3: 59, 112

**Segmental breathing**
1: 96

**Sensitivity**
1: 62

**Sensory testing**
1: 90, 154; 2: 14, 169, 194

**Serial/inhibitive casting**
3: 74

**Six-Minute Walk Test**
1: 7

**Skin graft**
2: 51

**Slump test**
2: 44

**Spasticity**
1: 102

# Computer-Based Exam Index

**Special tests**
1: 45, 149; 2: 7, 11, 13, 44, 47, 127, 134
**Specificity**
2: 120
**Spina bifida**
1: 68, 161; 3: 79
**Spinal cord injury**
1: 43, 98, 101, 103; 2: 31, 63, 170, 179; 3: 3, 12, 25, 28, 60, 70, 79, 83, 88, 129, 145, 156, 163, 167, 195
**Spinal tracts**
2: 14
**Spondylolisthesis**
1: 10; 3: 68
**Sprains/strains**
1: 22, 53, 117, 178; 2: 11; 3: 120
**Stability**
1: 19; 3: 72, 197
**Stabilization**
2: 53
**Standard precautions**
1: 50, 114, 115, 125, 168, 176; 2: 69, 104, 148; 3: 5
**Sterile technique**
2: 69
**Strengthening**
1: 55, 58, 94, 193, 196, 199; 2: 6, 41, 102, 110, 200; 3: 103, 124, 182, 197
**Stretching**
1: 5; 2: 193; 3: 71, 98, 186
**Stroke**
1: 158; 2: 27, 89, 168; 3: 77, 138, 148, 155, 159, 161, 170, 179, 191
**Substitution**
2: 115
**Superficial heat**
1: 40, 129
**Superficial reflexes**
2: 183; 3: 177
**Surgical management**
1: 22, 48, 111, 163, 174, 193; 2: 19; 3: 14, 36, 50, 134
**Target heart rate**
1: 86; 3: 24
**Teaching and learning**
1: 20, 34, 56, 110, 132, 160, 163, 164, 167, 190, 199; 2: 97, 109, 128, 146; 3: 28, 38, 43, 66, 76, 82, 85, 104, 142, 146, 150, 196
**Thomas test**
2: 47
**Thoracic outlet syndrome**
2: 7
**Tilt table**
3: 192
**Tinetti POMA**
3: 175

**TNM cancer classification system**
3: 65
**Torticollis**
2: 193
**Total hip arthroplasty**
2: 181; 3: 14
**Transfers**
1: 34, 101, 118, 138, 200; 2: 24, 50, 58, 147, 149; 3: 162, 163
**Traumatic brain injury**
1: 15, 44, 121, 169; 2: 46, 95, 177; 3: 38, 75, 84
**Trendelenburg gait**
1: 87
**Trendelenburg position**
1: 145
**Triceps reflex**
2: 119
**Trochanteric bursitis**
1: 89
**Ultrasound**
1: 117, 126, 134, 142, 151; 2: 48, 130, 197; 3: 2, 143
**Upper motor neuron lesion**
2: 183; 3: 95
**Validity**
1: 100; 2: 78
**Valsalva maneuver**
3: 199
**Vertebral artery test**
2: 13
**Vestibular system**
2: 90, 117, 151
**Vibration**
3: 58
**Visual Analogue Scale**
1: 150, 170
**Vital signs**
1: 30; 2: 64, 100
**Volumetric measurements**
1: 189, 2: 191
**Wheelchairs**
1: 43, 102, 130, 131, 138; 2: 66, 79, 140, 163; 3: 28, 107, 139, 145, 156, 161, 195
**Whirlpool**
1: 24, 38, 180, 198
**Wound care**
1: 50, 77, 111, 168, 198; 2: 112, 159; 3: 63, 70, 110, 111, 116, 149
**X-ray**
1: 10, 108; 2: 52, 121; 3: 26

# Academic Review Index

Abnormal gait patterns  80
Abrasion  315
Accessibility
    Accessibility requirements  491
    Americans with Disabilities Act  490
    Ramps  490
Achilles tendon rupture
    Template  559, 568-569
Achilles tendonitis  104
Acid base metabolic disorders
    Metabolic acidosis  334
    Metabolic alkalosis  334
Acromioclavicular joint
    Arthro/osteokinematics  50, 101
    Capsular pattern  50, 72
    Close/open packed position  50, 71
Active cycle of breathing  280
Acute respiratory distress syndrome  249
Adaptive equipment  415
Addison's disease  341
Adenosine triphosphate (ATP)  45, 335
Adhesive capsulitis  104-105
    Template  559, 570-571
Administration of services  507-508
Adrenal glands  337, 339, 341
Adson maneuver  93
Adventitious breath sounds  266
Aerobic exercise prescription  279-280
Aerobic metabolism  45, 335
Affective disorders  374
Agnosia  196
Agraphesthesia  196
Airborne precautions  488
Airway adjuncts  262
Airway clearance techniques  280-284
Airway suctioning  262
Akinesia  165
Alexia  196
Allen test (thoracic outlet syndrome)  93
Allen test (vascular insufficiency)  95
Alzheimer's disease  176
    Template  559, 572-573
Ambulation
    Assistive devices  416-417, 419
    Gait patterns  418
    Guarding  417-418
    Levels of weight bearing  417
    Stair training  419-420
Americans with Disabilities Act  490
Amputations and prosthetics
    Complications  118
    Gait deviations  119
    Lower extremity amputations  115
    Lower extremity prosthesis  116

Post-operative dressings  116
Prosthetic training  117
Upper extremity amputations  115
Wrapping guidelines  118
Amyotrophic lateral sclerosis  176
    Template  559, 574-575
Anabolism  335
Anaerobic metabolism  45, 335
Anatomical position  45, 46
Aneurysm  243
Angina pain scales  263
Angina pectoris  243-244, 290
Angiography  256
Ankle-brachial index (ABI)  263
Ankle-foot orthotics  113-114
Ankle and foot joints
    Arthro/osteokinematics  57, 102
    Articulations  57
    Balance strategy  167
    Goniometric technique  87-88
    Muscle action  49, 57
    Orthotics  113-114
    Primary structures  57-58
    Range of motion norms  82
    Special tests  100
Ankylosing spondylitis
    Template  559, 576-577
Anosognosia  196
Antalgic gait pattern  80
Anterior cord syndrome  197
Anterior cruciate ligament sprain  105
    Template  559, 578-579
Anterior drawer test (ankle)  100
Anterior drawer test (knee)  98
Anterograde memory impairments  207
Anthropometry
    Skinfold measurement  67
Antisocial behavior  375
Anuria  363
Anxiety disorder  374
Aphasia  172-173, 196
Apley's compression test  99
Apprehension tests for shoulder dislocation  92
Apraxia  173, 196
Arterial blood gas test  253, 254
Arterial blood pressure  263-264
Arterial insufficiency ulcers  315, 317
Arteriography  422
Arthritis
    Juvenile rheumatoid arthritis (JRA)  106, 562, 620-621
    Osteoarthritis (OA)  107, 563, 632-633
    Rheumatoid arthritis (RA)  108, 565, 652-653
Arthrography  422
Arthrogryposis multiplex congenita (AMC)  214

# Academic Review Index

**Arthrokinematic motions**　101-103
**Asepsis**　489
**ASIA impairment scale**　197-198
**Assistive devices**
　Axillary crutches　416, 419
　Cane　417, 419
　Lofstrand crutches　417
　Parallel bars　416
　Walkers　416, 419
**Astereognosis**　196
**Asthenia**　165
**Asthma**　249-250
**Astrocytoma**　369
**Asymmetrical tonic neck reflex**　208
**Ataxia**　165, 177
**Ataxic gait pattern**　80
**Atelectasis**　250
**Atherectomy**　260
**Atherosclerosis**　244
**Athetosis**　165
**Atlantoaxial joint**　60
**Atlanto-occipital joint**　60
**Atrial fibrillation**　270
**Atrial septal defect (ASD)**　245
**Atrioventricular conduction blocks**　270-271
**Auscultation**
　Heart sounds　264-265
　Lung sounds　265-267
**Autolytic debridement**　321
**Automatic implantable cardioverter-defibrillator**　260
**Autonomic dysreflexia**　42, 199, 319
**Autonomic nervous system**　136, 137
**Avulsion wound**　315
**Avulsion fracture**　111
**Axillary crutches**　416, 419
**Axonotmesis**　163
**Balance**
　Postural strategies　167
　Reflexes　167
　Somatosensory input　166
　Tests and measures　170-171
　Visual input　167
　Vestibular input　167
　Vertigo　168-169
**Balloon angioplasty**　260
**Balloon valvuoplasty**　260
**Bariatrics**
　Diagnostic tools　379
　Interventions　379-380
　Pharmacological management　380
　Risk factors　378
**Barlow's test**　97
**Baroreceptor reflex**　238
**Bed mobility**　405

**Behavioral therapy**　379
**Bell's palsy**　176-177
**Benign neoplasm**　373
**Benign paroxysmal positional vertigo (BPPV)**　168
**Benign prostatic hypertrophy**　363
**Berg Balance Scale**　170
**Bicipital tendonitis**
　Template　559, 580-581
**Biofeedback**　458-459
**Biopsy**　366
**Biotherapy**　371
**Bipolar disorder**　374
**Bladder**　355, 358-359
**Blood components**　239
**Body composition**
　Anthropometry　67
　Body mass index　267
　Densitometry　66
　Other techniques　67
**Body mechanics**　485
**Body schema**　196
**Bone scan**　366, 422
**Bounce home test**　99
**Brachial plexus**　152
**Bradykinesia**　165
**Brain**
　Anatomy　138-141
　Blood supply　141-143
　Cancer　367
　Hemispheric specialization　138-139
　Supporting systems　143-144
**Breast cancer**　367
　Template　560, 582-583
**Breathing exercises**　284-287
**Broca's aphasia**　173
**Bronchial carcinoma**　250
**Bronchiectasis**　250
**Bronchitis**　250
**Bronchophony**　267
**Brown-Sequard's syndrome**　146, 197
**Brush test**　99
**Bunnel-Littler test**　95
**Burns**
　Anticipated deformities　328
　Classification　327
　Rule of nine　328
　Scar management　329
　Topical agents　330
　Types　327
**Bursae**
　Knee　56
　Subacromial　51
　Subscapular　51
**Bursitis**　113

# Academic Review Index

Cane  417, 419
Capillary refill time  267
Cancer (see Oncology)
Cardiac ablation  260
Cardiac catheterization  256
Cardiac pacemaker  260
Cardiomyopathy  244
Cardiopulmonary system
  Diagnostic testing  256-257
  Interventions  279-294
  Laboratory tests  253-256
  Metabolic equivalents (METS)  289-291
  Reference values  255
  Tests and measures  263-278
Cardiovascular system
  Anatomy and physiology  235-238
  Cardiac cycle  238-239
  Conduction system  238
  Medical procedures  260-261
  Neural reflexes  238
  Pathology  243-249
  Pharmacological management  258-259
  Rehabilitation  287-293
  Tests and measures  263-278
Cardioversion  260
Carotid ultrasound  256
Carpal tunnel syndrome  177
  Template  560, 584-585
Carpometacarpal joint
  Goniometric technique  85
  Range of motion norms  82
Cartilaginous joints (amphiarthroses)
  Symphysis  47
  Synchrondrosis  46-47
Catabolism  336
Cauda equina injuries  197, 203
Cellulitis  331
Central cord syndrome  197
  Template  560, 586-587
Central nervous system
  Anatomy and physiology  135, 138-146
Cerebellar disorder  177
Cerebellar gait pattern  80
Cerebral angiogram
  Neurological dysfunction  173
Cerebral palsy (CP)  214
  Template  560, 588-589
Cerebrovascular accident
  Characteristics  181-183
  Classification  181-182
  Synergy patterns  183
  Template  560, 590-591
  Tests and measures  183
Cervical cancer  367

Cervical spine
  Articulations  60
  Capsular pattern  60, 72
  Close/open packed position  60, 72
  Goniometric technique  88-89
  Muscle action  48, 60
  Orthoses  114
  Osteokinematic motions  60
  Primary structures  60
  Range of motion norms  82
  Special tests  100-101
Chemoreceptor reflex  238
Chemotherapy  370-371
Chest radiograph  256
Chest tube  422
Cholecystitis  351-352
Cholelithiasis  351-352
Cholesterol test  253
Chorea  165
Chronic obstructive pulmonary disease (COPD)  250-251
Chronic venous insufficiency  244
Circumduction gait pattern  80
Circumferences for limb edema  268
Cirrhosis of the liver  351
Clarke's sign  100
Clasp knife response  165
Classical conditioning (Pavlov)  514
Claudication test  268
Clonus  165
Closed chain activities  63
Closed fracture  111
Coarctation of the aorta  245
Coccydynia  360
Cogwheel rigidity  165
Colonization  315
Colorectal cancer  368
Coma  205
Comminuted fracture  111
Communication disorders
  Broca's aphasia  173
  Conduction aphasia  172
  Dysarthria  173
  Fluent aphasia  172
  Global aphasia  173
  Non-fluent aphasia  172, 173
  Verbal apraxia  173
  Wernicke's aphasia  172
Complete blood count  253
Completed stroke  181
Compound fracture  111
Compression
  Compression garments  329, 447
  Intermittent compression  447
  Static compression  446-447
Computed tomography (CT scan)

# Academic Review Index

Cardiopulmonary testing  256
Diagnostic testing  422, 423
Neurological dysfunction  173
Oncology  366
**Concentric muscle contraction**  62
**Concussion**  205
**Congenital heart defects**
Atrial septal defect (ASD)  245
Coarctation of the aorta  245
Patent ductus arteriosus  245
Tetralogy of Fallot  245-246
Ventricular septal defect (VSD)  245
**Congenital hip dysplasia**  105
**Congenital limb deficiencies**  105
**Congenital torticollis**  105
Template  560, 592-593
**Congestive heart failure (CHF)**  246-247
Template  560, 594-595
**Consciousness**  205
**Constipation**  349
**Constructional apraxia**  196
**Contact dermatitis**  331
**Contact precautions**  488
**Contamination**  315, 489
**Continuous passive motion machine**  448
**Contusion**  113, 326
**Conversion disorder**  375
**Cor pulmonale**  246
**Coronary arteries**  235-237
**Coronary artery bypass graft surgery (CABG)**  260
**Coronary artery disease**  246
**Coronary veins**  238
**Corset**  114
**Corticospinal tract (anterior)**  145
**Corticospinal tract (lateral)**  145
**Costoclavicular syndrome test**  93
**Cozen's test**  94
**Crackles (formerly rales)**  266
**Craig-Scott knee-ankle-foot orthosis**  114
**Craig's test**  98
**Cranial nerves and testing**  149-151
**Cushing's syndrome**  341
**Cyrotherapy**
Cold bath  428, 429
Cold pack  427, 429
Controlled cold compression unit  428, 429
Cyro Cuff  428, 429
Ice massage  426-427, 429
Vapocoolant spray  429, 430
**Cystic fibrosis**  251
Template  561, 596-597
**Cystocele**  363
**Data and measurements**  523-524
**Decerebrate rigidity**  196

**Decorticate rigidity**  196
**Deep vein thrombosis (DVT)**  118, 198, 246
**Degenerative spondylolisthesis**
Template  561, 598-599
**Dehiscence**  326
**Delegation and supervision**
Physical therapist assistant  503-504, 505
Health care professionals  504-506
**Delirium**  205
**Densitometry**
Hydrostatic weighing  66
Plethysmography  66
**Deoxyribonucleic acid (DNA)**  336
**Depression**  374
**Dermatomes**  65, 147-148, 203
**Dermis**  326
**Desiccated**  326
**Desquamation**  326
**Developmental concepts**  208
**Diabetes mellitus**  344-345, 351
Template  561, 600-601
**Diabetic neuropathy**  177
**Diaphragmatic breathing**  284-285
**Diarrhea**  349
**Diastasis recti**  360
**Dietary modification**  380
**Diplopia**  196
**Directed cough and huffing**  280-281
**Discography**  174
**Dissociative disorders**  374-375
**Diverticulitis**  350
**Dix-Hallpike test**  168
**Documentation**
Diagnosis  493, 497
Discharge summary  492, 493, 497, 509
Evaluation  493, 497
Examination  493, 494-496
Guidelines  492-494, 509-510
Measurements  499
Military time  499
Plan of care  493, 497
Prognosis  493, 497
Progress note  492
Reexamination  493, 497
S.O.A.P. note  492
Symbols  498
Therapeutic modalities  433
Types  492
Wounds  320
**Doppler ultrasonography**  422
**Double step gait pattern**  80
**Down syndrome**  214
Template  561, 602-603
**Draping**  405

# Academic Review Index

**Drop arm test**  92
**Droplet precautions**  488
**Duchenne muscular dystrophy**  214
   Template  561, 604-605
**Dysarthria**  173, 196
**Dysdiadochokinesia**  165
**Dysmetria**  165
**Dysphagia**  196
**Dysplasia**  374
**Dyspnea**
   Dyspnea scales  268
   Positions to relieve  287
**Dysprosody**  196
**Dystonia**  165
**Eating disorders**  381
**Eccentric muscle contraction**  62
**Ecchymosis**  326
**Echocardiography**  257
**Ectopic bone**  199
**Eczema**  331
**Edema**  113, 268
**Education**
   Patient education  515-518
   Team models  518
**Effect size**  526
**Egophony**  267
**Elbow joint**
   Arthro/osteokinematics  51, 101
   Articulations  51
   Capsular pattern  51, 72
   Close/open packed position  51, 71
   Goniometric technique  84
   Muscle action  49, 51
   Primary structures  51-52
   Range of motion norms  82
   Special tests  94-95
**Electrocardiogram (ECG)**  256, 268-272, 423
**Electroencephalography (EEG)**
   Diagnostic testing  423
   Neurological dysfunction  174
**Electromyography (EMG)**
   Diagnostic testing  423
   Neurological dysfunction  174
   Therapeutic modality  457-458
**Electrophysiologic testing**  257
**Electrotherapy**
   Biofeedback  458-459
   Electrodes  451
   Electromyography  457-458
   Inferential current  454-455
   Iontophoresis  455-457
   Muscle and nerve cell excitation  449
   Neuromuscular electrical stimulation (NMES)  452-453
   Parameters  451-452

**Principles of electricity**  449
   Therapeutic currents  449-450
   Transcutaneous electrical stimulation (TENS)  453-454
   Waveforms  450
**Ely's test**  96
**Embolism**  42, 181-182, 252
**Emotional lability**  196
**Emphysema**  251
   Template  561, 606-607
**End-feel**  72
**Endocarditis**  246
**Endocrine system**
   Functions  337
   Glands  337-340
   Hormones  338-340
   Pathology  340-345
   Pharmacological management  345-346
**Endometriosis**  356
**Endoscopy**  366
**Endotracheal tube**  262
**Enhanced extracorporeal counterpulsation**  260
**Enzymatic debridement**  321
**Epidemiology**  532
**Epidermis**  326
**Epidural hematoma**  205
**Epilepsy**  177-178
   Antiepileptic agents  175
**Equine gait pattern**  80
**Erb's palsy**
   Template  561, 608-609
**Erectile dysfunction**  357
**Ergonomic guidelines**  485
**Erythema**  326
**Eschar**  320
**Esophagus**  346, 348
**Ethics**
   Code of ethics  510-512
   Malpractice  500
   Research  522, 532
   Standards of practice  507
   Terminology  500
   Theories and issues  500
**Evidence based practice**  519-520
**Exercise**
   Aerobic exercise prescription  279-280
   Bariatric  379-380
   Cancer  369
   Cardiac rehabilitation  288-293
   DeLorme protocol  64
   Environmental considerations  292
   Isokinetic exercise  63
   Isometric exercise  63
   Isotonic exercise  63
   Oxford technique protocol  64

# Academic Review Index

Pelvic floor exercises 361-362
PNF 193-194
Pregnancy and exercise 361-363
Pulmonary rehabilitation 293-294
**Experimental controls** 525-526
**Experimental designs** 524-525
**Exudate classification** 319
**Fasciculation** 165
**Fasciculus cuneatus** 145
**Fasciculus gracilis** 145
**Feedback** 185
**Feeding devices**
Gastric tube 420
Intravenous system 420-421
Jejunostomy tube 420
Nasogastric tube 420
**Festinating gait pattern** 80
**Fibromyalgia**
Template 562, 610-611
**Fibrous joints**
Suture 46
Syndesmosis 46
Gomphosis 46
**Finkelstein test** 96
**Fluent aphasia** 172, 196
**Fluoroscopy** 257, 423
**Foot orthotics** 113
**Foraminal compression test** 100
**Forearm**
Arthro/osteokinematics 101-102
Goniometric technique 84
Range of motion norms 82
**Forefoot joints**
Arthro/osteokinematics 102
Articulation 57
**Fractures** 111
**Friable** 326
**Froment's sign** 95-96
**Fugl-Meyer assessment** 170, 183
**Full-thickness burn** 327
Template 562, 612-613
**Full-thickness wound** 317
**Functional Independence Measure (FIM)** 183
**Functional reach test** 170
**Gait**
Abnormal gait patterns 80
Normal gait 78-79
Patterns 418
Peak muscle activity 79
Rancho Los Amigos terminology 77
Range of motion requirements for normal gait 79
Stair training 419-420
Standard terminology 77
Terminology 77, 80

**Gait deviations**
Amputations and prosthetics 119
Ankle and foot 81
Knee 81
Hip 81
**Galant reflex** 208
**Gallbladder** 347, 351-352
**Gangrene (dry)** 331-332
**Gangrene (wet)** 332
**Gangrene tissue** 320
**Gastritis** 348
**Gastroesophageal reflux** 348
**Gastrointestinal system**
Functions 346-347
Pathology 347-352, 353
Pharmacological management 352-353
**Gene** 336
**Genetic disorders**
Down syndrome 214, 561, 602-603
Duchenne muscular dystrophy 214, 561, 604-605
Osteogenesis imperfecta 107, 563, 634-635
Paget's disease 335
Phenylketonuria 333
Prader Willi syndrome 215
Spinal muscular atrophy 215
Tay-Sachs disease 333
Wilms' tumor 370
Wilson's disease 333-334
**Genitourinary system**
Functions 354-356
Obstetrics 360-363
Pathology 356-360
Pharmacological management 363, 364
Terminology 363-364
**Genu valgum** 113
**Genu varum** 113
**Glasgow coma scale** 206
**Glenohumeral instability** 105-106
**Glenohumeral joint (see Shoulder joint)**
**Glenoid labrum tear test** 93
**Gomphosis** 46
**Goniometric technique**
Ankle 87-88
Carpometacarpal 85
Cervical spine 88-87
Distal interphalangeal 86
Documentation 90
Elbow 84
Forearm 84
Hip 86-87
Knee 87
Metacarpophalangeal 85-86
Proximal interphalangeal 86
Shoulder 83-84

# Academic Review Index

Subtalar  88
Thoracolumbar  89-90
Wrist  84-85
**Graphs**  527-528
**Graves' disease**  342
**Greenstick fracture**  111
**Grind test**  96
**Gross and fine motor skill development**  210-212
**Growth factors for wound healing**  322
**Guarding**  417-418
**Guillain-Barre syndrome**  178
Template  562, 614-615
**Halo vest orthosis**  114
**Hand washing**  487, 489
**Handheld dynamometry**  76
**Hawkins-Kennedy impingement test**  93
**Head-hips relationship**  203
**Healing by intention**
Primary intention  314
Secondary intention  314
Tertiary intention  314
**Health behavior models**
Health belief model  514
Social cognitive (learning) theory  514-515
Trans-theoretical model  515
**Health insurance**
Reimbursement coding  513-514
Types  512-513
**Heart**
Anatomy and physiology  235-238
Innervation  238
**Heart failure**  246-247
**Heart murmur**  247, 265
**Heart transplant**  260
**Hematocrit test**  253, 255
**Hematoma**  205, 326
**Hematuria**  364
**Hemiballism**  165
**Hemiparesis**  196
**Hemiplegia**  196
**Hemiplegic gait pattern**  80
**Hemodialysis**  358
**Hemorrhage**  182
**Hepatitis**  350-351
**Hip-knee-ankle-foot orthosis (HKAFO)**  114
**Hip joint**
Arthro/osteokinematics  55, 102
Articulations  55
Balance strategy  167
Capsular pattern  55, 72
Close/open packed position  55, 71
Goniometric technique  86-87
Muscle action  49, 55
Orthoses  114

Primary structures  55
Range of motion norms  82
Special tests  96-98
**Homan's sign**  273
**Homonymous hemianopsia**  196
**Hughston's plica test**  100
**Human immunodeficiency virus (HIV)**
Template  562, 616-617
**Huntington's disease**  179
Template  562, 618-619
**Hydrocephalus**  144
**Hydrostatic weighing**  66
**Hydrotherapy**  321, 440
Contrast bath  443
Pool therapy  442
Properties of water  441
Safety  443
Types of tanks  442
Whirlpool  442
**Hyperbaric oxygen**  322
**Hypergranulation**  326
**Hyperkeratosis tissue**  320
**Hyperpigmentation**  326
**Hyperplasia**  374
**Hypertension**  247
**Hypertrophic scar**  326
**Hypochondriasis disorder**  375
**Hypothalamus**  140, 337, 338, 340
**Hypothesis testing**  526-527
**Hypovolemic shock**  42
**Ideational apraxia**  196
**Ideomotor apraxia**  196
**Iliofemoral joint (see Hip joint)**
**Impingement syndrome**  106
**Incentive spirometry**  287
**Incisional wound**  315
**Incontinence**  325, 358-359
Urinary stress incontinence template  567, 686-687
**Infection**  315
**Infection control**
Infectious disease  487
Nosocomial infections  488-489
Personal protective equipment  489
Standard precautions  487-488
Sterile field guidelines  489
Terminology  489
Transmission-based precautions  488
**Inflammatory phase**  313
**Inherited metabolic disorders**
Mitochondrial disorders  333
Phenylketonuria  333
Tay-Sachs disease  333
Wilson's disease  333-334
**Inspiratory muscle training**  285

# Academic Review Index

**Insulin** 338, 340
**Integumentary system**
  Burns 327-330
  Functions 313
  Pathology 331-332
  Skin graft 331
  Terminology 326
  Wound assessment 317-320
  Wound healing phases 313
  Wound interventions 321-326
  Wound types 315-317
**Interdisciplinary team** 518
**International Classification of Functioning, Disability and Health (ICF) Model** 502
**Interosseous membrane**
  Tibiofibular 58
  Wrist 52
**Interphalangeal joints**
  Arthro/osteokinematics 102
  Goniometric technique 86
  Range of motion norms 82
**Intervertebral disks** 60, 61
**Intervertebral joints**
  Cervical spine 60
  Thoracolumbar spine 61
**Intestines** 346-347, 349-350
**Intraaortic balloon counterpulsation** 260
**Invasive hemodynamic monitoring** 257
**Involuntary movement disorders** 165
**Iontophoresis** 327, 455-457
**Irritable bowel syndrome** 349-350
**Ischemic attack** 181-182
**Isokinetic dynamometry** 76
**Isokinetic muscle contraction** 62
**Isometric dynamometry** 76
**Isometric muscle contraction** 62
**Isotonic muscle contraction** 62
**Joint classification**
  Cartilaginous joints 46-47
  Fibrous joints 46
  Synovial joints 47
**Joint mobilization**
  Convex-concave rule 103
  Mobilization technique 103
**Joint positions**
  Close packed positions 71
  Common capsular patterns 72
  Descriptions of specific positions 71
  Loose packed positions 71
**Joint receptors**
  Free nerve endings 47
  Golgi ligament endings 47
  Golgi-Mazzoni corpuscles 47
  Pacinian corpuscles 47
  Ruffini endings 47

**Juvenile rheumatoid arthritis** 106
  Template 562, 620-621
**Keloid** 326
**Kidneys** 355, 357-358
**Kinesthesia** 159, 165
**Knee-ankle-foot orthosis** 114
**Knee joint**
  Arthro/osteokinematics 55, 102
  Articulations 55-56
  Goniometric technique 87
  Muscle action 49, 56
  Orthoses 114
  Primary structures 56-57
  Range of motion norms 82
  Special tests 98-100
**Kyphosis** 113
**Laceration** 315
**Lachman test** 98
**Lateral epicondylitis** 106
  Template 562, 622-623
**Lateral epicondylitis test** 94
**Lateral pivot shift test** 98-99
**Lead pipe rigidity** 165
**Legal matters** 503
**Legg-Calve-Perthes disease** 106
**Legislation acts and amendments for the education of children with disabilities** 216
**Leukemia** 369
**Levels of consciousness**
  Coma 205
  Consciousness 205
  Delirium 205
  Obtundity 205
  Stupor 205
**Levels of evidence** 520
**Lever classification** 46
**Lifting guidelines** 485-486
**Limbic system** 137
**Liver** 347, 350-351
**Lobectomy** 262
**Lofstrand crutches** 417
**Lordosis** 113
**Lower motor neuron disease** 164
**Ludington's test** 92
**Lumbar plexus** 61
**Lung cancer** 368
**Lung sounds**
  Abnormal breath sounds 266-267
  Auscultation 265-267
  Normal breath sounds 265-266
  Voice sounds 267
**Lung transplant** 262
**Lung volumes and capacities** 242-243
**Lymphedema** 247, 268, 367
  Template 563, 624-625

# Academic Review Index

Lymphoma  368
Maceration  326
Magnetic resonance imaging (MRI)
    Cardiopulmonary testing  257
    Diagnostic testing  423
    Neurological dysfunction  174
Malignant neoplasm  374
Mammography  366
Management  501
Mania  374
Manual muscle testing
    Dynamometry  76
    Manual muscle testing grades  73
    Muscle insufficiency  76
    Positioning for muscle testing  73-75
Massage  459-461
Maturation phase  313
McGill pain questionnaire  63
McMurray test  99
Measurements  499, 523-524
Mechanical ventilation  41, 262, 422
Medial collateral ligament sprain  106-107
    Template  563, 626-627
Medial epicondylitis test  94
Medical equipment
    Diagnostic tests  422-424
    Feeding devices  420-421
    Miscellaneous  422
    Monitoring devices  421
    Oxygen therapy  421
    Skeletal traction  421-422
    Urinary catheters  422
Memory impairments
    Anterograde memory  207
    Post-traumatic amnesia  207
    Retrograde amnesia  207
Meniscus tear  107
Metabolic acidosis  254, 334
Metabolic alkalosis  254, 334
Metabolic bone disease
    Osteomalacia  334-335
    Osteoporosis  335
    Paget's disease  335
Metabolic equivalents (METS)  290-291
Metabolic system
    Functions  333
    Pathology  333-336
    Terminology  335-336
Metabolism  336
Metacarpophalangeal joints
    Arthro/osteokinematics  102
    Capsular pattern  72
    Close/open packed position  71
    Goniometric technique  85-86
    Range of motion norms  82

Metaplasia  374
Midcarpal joints  52
Midtarsal joints
    Arthro/osteokinematics  57, 102
    Articulations  57
    Capsular pattern  57, 72
    Close/open packed position  57, 71
Military time  499
Mill's test  95
Milwaukee orthosis  114
Minerals  383-384
Minimal detectable difference  527
Minimally clinically important difference  527
Mitochrondria  336
Mitochondrial disorders  333-334
Mobility
    Ambulation  416-420
    Bed mobility  405
    Draping  405
    Preparation  405
    Transfers  405-407
    Wheelchairs  408-414
Models of disability
    Nagi model  501
    International classification of functioning, disability and health (ICF) model  502
Modified Ashworth scale  166
Moisture and occlusion  325-326
Monitoring devices
    Arterial line  421
    Central venous pressure catheter  421
    Indwelling right atrial catheter  421
    Intracranial pressure monitor  421
    Oximeter  421
    Pulmonary artery catheter  421
Moro reflex  209
Motor control  184-186
Motor learning  184-186
Movement disorders
    Athetosis  165
    Chorea  165
    Dystonia  165
    Tics  165
    Tremors  165
Multidisciplinary team  518
Multiple personality disorder  375
Multiple sclerosis  179
    Template  563, 628-629
Murphy sign  96
Muscle action
    Ankle joint  49, 57
    Cervical intervertebral joints  48, 60
    Elbow joint  49, 51
    Hip joint  49, 55

# Academic Review Index

Knee joint   49, 56
Radioulnar joint   49
Scapula   48
Shoulder joint   48, 50
Temporomandibular joint   48
Thoracic and lumbar intervertebral joints   48, 61
Wrist joint   49, 52
Muscle contraction types   62
Muscle physiology
 Classification of muscle fibers   62
 Functional characteristics of muscle fibers   62
Muscle receptors
 Golgi tendon organs   62
 Muscle spindles   62
Musculoskeletal system
 Amputations   114-119
 Anatomy and physiology   46-62
 Arthro/osteokinematics   101-103
 Capsular pattern   72
 Close/open packed positions   71
 End-feel   72
 Examination   64-66
 Fractures   111
 Gait   77-81
 Goniometric technique   83-90
 Joint mobilization   103-104
 Muscle action   48-49
 Muscle testing   73-76
 Orthotics   113-114
 Pathology   104-110
 Pharmacological management   112
 Posture   68-70
 Prosthetics   113-119
 Range of motion norms   82
 Special tests   90-101
 Terminology   113
Myasthenia gravis   179, 180
Myelography
 Diagnostic testing   423
 Neurological dysfunction   174
Myelotomy   203
Myocardial infarction   247-248, 271
 Template   563, 630-631
Myocardial perfusion imaging   257
Myocarditis   248
Myotomes   147-148, 203
Nagi model   501
Necrotic tissue types   320
Neer impingement test   93
Negative pressure wound therapy   322
Neglect   196
Neoadjuvant   374
Neologism   196
Nephrolithiasis   364

Nerve conduction velocity (NCV) testing   174
Nerve roots   147-148
Neurapraxia   162
Neurectomy   203
Neuroblastoma   369-370
Neurogenic bladder   203, 358
Neurologic level   203
Neurological rehabilitation
 Bobath: neuromuscular developmental treatment   187-189
 Brunnstrom: movement therapy   189-190
 Carr and Shepherd: motor relearning   186-187
 Kabat, Knott, and Voss: PNF   190-194
 Levels of motor control   193
 Motor control   184-186
 PNF – lower extremity patterns   192
 PNF – therapeutic exercise   194
 PNF – upper extremity patterns   192
 Rood   195
Neuromuscular electrical stimulation (NMES)   452-453
Neuromuscular system
 Anatomy and physiology   135-148, 152-153
 Balance   166-172
 Cerebrovascular accident   181-183
 Communication disorders   172-173
 Developmental concepts   208-212
 Diagnostic tests   173-174
 Pathology   162-166, 176-181
 Pediatric pathology   214-215
 Pharmacological management   175
 Rehabilitation   184-195
 Spinal cord injury   197-204
 Terminology   196
 Tests and measures   147-162, 170-171, 197-198, 208-209
 Traumatic brain injury   205-207
Neuropathic ulcers   316, 317
Neuroses disorders   374
Neurotmesis   163
Noble compression test   100
Nocturia   364
Non-fluent aphasia   172, 173
Nonreflexive bladder   203
Non-selective debridement
 Hydrotherapy   321
 Wet-to-dry dressings   321
 Wound irrigation   321
Nonunion fracture   111
Normotrophic scar   326
Nosocomial infections   488-489
Numerical rating scale   63
Nutrition   381-384
Nystagmus   169
Ober's test   96
Obesity (see Bariatrics)

# Academic Review Index

**Obsessive compulsive disorder**  374
**Obstetrics**
  Pathology  360-361
  Pelvic floor exercises  361-362
  Pregnancy  361-363
**Obtundity**  205
**Oliguria**  364
**Onychomycosis**  332
**Oncology**
  Diagnostic tools  366
  Pathology  367-369
  Pediatric pathology  369-370
  Pharmacological management  372-373
  Prevention  365
  Signs and symptoms  365
  Staging  366
  Terminology  373-374
  Tissue and tumor classification  365
  Treatment options  370-372
**Open chain activities**  63
**Operant conditioning (B.F. Skinner)**  514
**Orthostatic hypotension**  199
**Orthotics**  113-114
**Ortolani's test**  97
**Osgood Schlatter disease**  107
**Osteoarthritis**  107
  Template  563, 632-633
**Osteogenesis imperfecta**  107
  Template  563, 634-635
**Osteogenic sarcoma**  370, 680-681
**Osteokinematic motions**  102-103
**Osteomalacia**  334-335
**Osteopenia**  336
**Osteopetrosis**  336
**Osteoporosis**  335, 336
  Template  564, 636-637
**Ovaries**  338, 339, 345, 354
**Oxygen therapy**  263, 421
**Paced breathing**  285-286
**Paget's disease**  335
**Pain assessment**  63
**Palliative care**  371-372
**Palmar grasp reflex**  209
**Pancreas**  338, 340, 344-345, 347, 351
**Pancreatic cancer**  368
**Paradoxical breathing**  203, 278
**Parallel bars**  416
**Paraplegia**  203
**Parapodiums**  114
**Parathyroid gland**  337, 340, 343
**Paresthetic areas**  147-148
**Parkinson's disease**  179-180
  Template  564, 638-639
**Parkinsonian gait pattern**  80

**Partial-thickness wound**  317
**Patellar apprehension test**  100
**Patellar tap test**  99
**Patellofemoral joint**
  Arthro/osteokinematics  102
  Articulations  56
  Pathology  107-108
**Patellofemoral syndrome**  107-108
  Template  564, 640-641
**Patent ductus arteriosus**  245
**Pathology**
  Cardiovascular system  243-249
  Endocrine system  340-345
  Gastrointestinal system  347-352
  Genitourinary system  356-360
  Integumentary system  331-332
  Metabolic system  333-325
  Musculoskeletal system  104-110
  Neuromuscular system  176-181
  Obstetric  360-361
  Oncology  367-370
  Pediatric neuromuscular system  214-215
  Psychological disorders  374-375
  Pulmonary system  249-253
**Patient education**
  Cultural influences  516-517
  Domains of learning  515-516
  Guidelines  515, 516, 517-518
  Learning styles  516
  Materials  517
  Patient communication  516
  Principles of motivation  516
  Stages of dying  518
  Teaching methods  516
**Patient/client management**  506, 508-510
**Patrick's test**  98
**Pediatrics**
  Childhood obesity  379
  Concepts of development  208
  Gross and fine motor skills  210-212
  Legislation acts and amendments for education of children with disabilities  216
  Pathology  214-215
  Reflexes  208-209
  Special tests  97
  Therapeutic positioning  213
**Penetrating wound**  315
**Penis**  355, 357
**Peptic ulcer disease**  348-349
**Percussion**  273-274, 281-284
**Pericarditis**  248
**Peripheral arterial disease**  248-249
**Peripheral nerve lesions**
  Axonotmesis  163

# Academic Review Index

Lower motor neuron disease  164
Neurapraxia  162
Neurotmesis  163
Peripheral neuropathy  162
Polyneuropathy  162
Upper motor neuron disease  164
**Peripheral nerve classification**  147
**Peripheral nervous system**
Anatomy and physiology  136, 146-149
Brachial plexus  152
Cranial nerves and testing  149-151
Dermatomes  147-148
Lower extremity innervation  153
Myotomes  147-148
Nerve roots  147-148
Paresthetic areas  147-148
Reflexes  147-148, 154-157
Sensation testing  158-162
Terminology  146-147
**Peripheral neuropathy**  157, 162, 164, 316
**Peripheral pulses**  274-275
**Peripheral vascular disease**
Template  564, 642-643
**Perseveration**  196
**Personal protective equipment**  489
**Personality disorders**  375
**pH**  254, 327, 336
**Phalen's test**  96
**Pharmacology**
Bariatrics  380
Cardiovascular system  258-259
Endocrine system  345-346
Gastrointestinal system  352-353
Genitourinary system  363
Integumentary system  330
Musculoskeletal system  112
Neuromuscular system  175
Oncology  372-373
Psychological disorders  375-378
Pulmonary system  261-262
**Phenylketonuria**  333
**Phobia disorder**  374
**Phonocardiography**  257
**Physical therapist assistant**  503-504, 505
**Physical therapy practice**
Administration of services  507-508
Code of ethics  510-512
Ethics  500, 507
Patient/client management  506, 508-510
Standards of practice  507
**Piriformis syndrome**  361
**Piriformis test**  97
**Pituitary gland**  337, 339, 340-341
**Plaque psoriasis**  332

**Planes of the body**
Frontal (coronal) plane  45
Sagittal plane  45
Transverse plane  45
**Plantar fasciitis**  108
Template  564, 644-645
**Plantar grasp reflex**  209
**Pleuroscopy**  257
**Plethysmography**  66
**Pneumonia**  251
**Polyneuropathy**  162
**Polyuria**  364
**Positron emission tomography (PET)**
Cardiopulmonary testing  257
Neurological dysfunction  174
**Post-polio syndrome**  180-181
**Post-traumatic amnesia**  207
**Posterior cord syndrome**  197
**Posterior cruciate ligament sprain**  108
**Posterior drawer test (knee)**  99
**Posterior sag sign**  99
**Positive support reflex**  209
**Postural drainage**  281-283
**Postural strategies**
Ankle  167
Hip  167
Stepping  167
Suspensory  167
**Posture**
Good and faulty posture, summary chart  68-69
Ideal plumb line alignment  70
Kyphosis  113
Lordosis  113
Workstation  485
**Practice**  185
**Prader-Willi syndrome**  215
**Pregnancy**  361-363
**Pressure ulcers**  199-200, 316, 319
Staging  318
Template  564, 646-647
**Proliferative phase**  313
**Proprioception**  158, 159
**Proprioceptive neuromuscular facilitation (PNF)**
Lower extremity patterns  192
Techniques  193-194
Upper extremity patterns  192
**Prostate**  355, 357, 368
**Prosthetics**
Gait deviations  119
Lower extremity prosthesis  116
Prosthetic training  117
Upper extremity prosthesis  115
**Prothrombin time (PT)**  256
**Psychogenic amnesia**  374

# Academic Review Index

**Psychological disorders**
Affective disorders  374
Dissociative disorders  374-375
Neuroses disorders  374
Personality disorders  375
Pharmacological management  375-378
Schizophrenia disorders  375
Somatoform disorders  375
**Pulmonary edema**  252
**Pulmonary embolism**  42, 252
**Pulmonary fibrosis**  252
**Pulmonary function testing**  275-276
**Pulmonary system**
Anatomy and physiology  240-243
Circulation  242
Control of breathing  242
Innervation of lungs  242
Lung volumes and capacities  242-243
Oxygen and carbon dioxide transport  243
Pathology  249-253
Pharmacological management  261-262
Rehabilitation  293-294
Tests and measures  262-278
**Pulse oximetry**  276
**Puncture**  315
**Pursed-lip breathing (PLB)**  286
**Purulent exudate**  319
**Pushing or pulling an object**  486
**Q angle**  113
**Quadrant scouring test**  98
**Radiation**  370
**Radical mastectomy**  364
**Radiocarpal joint**
Arthro/osteokinematics  52, 102
Articulations  52
Capsular pattern  52, 72
Close/open packed position  52, 71
**Radiohumeral joint**
Arthro/osteokinematics  51, 101
Articulations  51
Capsular pattern  51, 72
Close/open packed position  51, 71
**Radioulnar joint**
Arthro/osteokinematics  51, 101-102
Articulations  51
Capsular pattern  51, 72
Close/open packed position  51, 71
**Ramps**  490
**Rancho Los Amigos gait terminology**  77
**Rancho Los Amigos Levels of Cognitive Functioning**  205-206
**Range of motion norms**  82
**Rating of perceived exertion**  276-277
**Reciprocating gait orthosis**  114

**Rectocele**  364
**Red-Yellow-Black system**  321
**Referred pain**  353
**Reflex sympathetic dystrophy**
Template  565, 648-649
**Reflexes**
Adult  147-148, 154-157
Grading  155
Pediatric  208-209
**Reimbursement coding**  513-514
**Reliability**  523
**Renal failure**  357-358
**Research**
Data and measurements  523-524
Descriptive statistics  529-530
Epidemiology  532
Ethics  522
Evaluating studies  519
Evidence based practice  519-520
Experimental controls  525-526
Experimental designs  524-525
Graphs  527-528
Hypothesis testing  526-527
Inferential statistics  530-532
Levels of evidence  520
Practice guidelines  519-520
Statistical measures of validity  532
Subjects and sampling  524
Types of research  521
**Respiratory rate/rhythm/pattern**  277-278
**Respiratory system (see Pulmonary system)**
**Restrictive lung dysfunction**  252-253
Template  565, 650-651
**Reticulospinal tract**  145
**Retrograde amnesia**  207
**Rheumatic fever**  249
**Rheumatoid arthritis**  108
Template  565, 652-653
**Rhizotomy**  203
**Rhonchi**  267
**Rigidity**  165
**Romberg test**  171
**Roos test**  93
**Rooting reflex**  209
**Rotator cuff tear**  108-109
**Rotator cuff tendonitis**
Template  565, 654-655
**Rubrospinal tract**  145
**Rule of nines**  328
**Sacral plexus**  61
**Sacral sparing**  203
**Sacroiliac joint stress test**  101
**Sacrum**  62
**Safety and protection**
Body mechanics  485

# Academic Review Index

Ergonomic guidelines  485
Lifting guidelines  485-486
Pushing or pulling an object  486
Workstation posture  485
**Sampling**  524
**Sanguineous exudate**  319
**Scapulothoracic joint**  50
**Scar management**  329
**Schizophrenia disorders**  375
**Sciatica**
Template  565, 656-657
**Scissor gait pattern**  80
**Scoliosis**  109
Template  565, 658-659
**Segmental breathing**  286
**Selective debridement**
Autolytic debridement  321
Enzymatic debridement  321
Sharp debridement  321
**Sensory testing**  158-162, 316
**Serous exudate**  319
**Serosanguineous exudate**  319
**Seropurulent exudate**  319
**Sharp debridement**  321
**Shoulder joint**
Arthro/osteokinematics  50, 101
Articulations  50
Capsular pattern  50, 72
Close/open packed position  50, 71
Goniometric technique  83-84
Muscle action  48, 50
Primary structures  51
Range of motion norms  82
Special tests  92-94
**Sitting flexion test**  101
**Six-minute walk test (6MWT)**  278
**Skin cancer**  368-369
**Skin care products**  326
**Skin grafts**
Types  331
**Skin tear**  315
**Skinfold measurement**  67
**Slocum test**  99
**Slough**  320
**Somatic nervous system**  137
**Somatization disorder**  375
**Somatoform disorders**  375
**Spastic gait pattern**  80
**Spasticity**
Antispasticity agents  175
Modified Ashworth scale  166
Spinal cord injury complications  200
**Special tests**
Ankle  91, 100

Cervical spine  92, 100-101
Elbow  91, 94-95
Hip  91, 96-98
Knee  91, 98-100
Lumbosacral  92, 101
Shoulder  90, 92-94
Wrist and hand  91, 95-96
**Speed's test**  92
**Spina bifida**  215
Template  566, 660-661
**Spinal cord**
Ascending tracts  145
Descending tracts  145
Supporting systems  143-144
**Spinal cord injury**
Functional outcomes  200-202
Potential complications  198-200
Template (C7)  566, 662-663
Template (L3)  566, 664-665
Terminology  203
Tests and measures  197
Types  197
**Spinal muscular atrophy (SMA)**  215
**Spinal puncture (lumbar)**
Neurological dysfunction  174
**Spinal shock**  203
**Spinocerebellar tract (dorsal)**  145
**Spinocerebellar tract (ventral)**  145
**Spino-olivary tract**  145
**Spinoreticular tract**  145
**Spinotectal tract**  145
**Spinothalamic tract (anterior)**  145
**Spinothalamic tract (lateral)**  145
**Spiral fracture**  111
**Spondylolithesis**
Template  566, 666-667
**Sprain**  113
**Stages of dying**  518
**Standard gait terminology**  77
**Standard precautions**  487-488
**Standards of practice**  507-512
**Standing flexion test**  101
**Startle reflex**  209
**Statistics**  529-532
**Steppage gait pattern**  80
**Stepping strategy**  167
**Sterile field**  489
**Sternoclavicular joint**
Arthro/osteokinematics  50, 101
Articulations  50
Capsular pattern  50, 72
Close/open packed position  50, 71
**Stomach**  346, 348-349
**Strain**  113

# Academic Review Index

Stress fracture   111
Stress test
  Exercise   272-273
  Pharmacological   257
Stridor   267
Stroke (see Cerebrovascular accident)
Stroke in evolution   181
Stupor   205
Subdural hematoma   205
Subtalar joint
  Arthro/osteokinematics   57, 102
  Articulations   57
  Capsular pattern   57, 72
  Close/open packed position   57, 71
  Goniometric technique   88
  Range of motion norms   82
Subcutaneous wound   317
Supraspinatus test   93
Surgery
  Bariatrics   380
  Oncology   370
Suspensory strategy   167
Superficial wound   317
Suture joint   46
Symmetrical tonic neck reflex   208
Symphysis   47
Synchondrosis   46-47
Syndesmosis   46
Synergy
  Definition   196
  Patterns   183
Synovial joints (diarthroses)
  Uniaxial joints   47
  Biaxial joints   47
  Multi-axial joints   47
Systemic circulation   239
Systemic lupus erthematosus
  Template   566, 668-669
Tabetic gait pattern   80
Talar tilt test   100
Talipes equinovarus   109
Talocrural joint
  Arthro/osteokinematics   57, 102
  Articulations   57
  Capsular pattern   57, 70
  Close/open packed position   57, 71
Tay-Sachs disease   333
Taylor brace   114
Teaching and learning
  Maslow's hierarchy of needs   514
  Classical conditioning (Pavlov)   514
  Operant conditioning (B.F. Skinner)   514
Team Models   518
Tectospinal tract   145

Temporomandibular joint
  Arthro/osteokinematics   103
  Muscle action   48
  Template   566, 670-671
Tendodesis   203
Tendonitis   113
Tenotomy   203
Testes   338, 340, 345, 355
Tetraplegia   203
Tetrology of Fallot   245-246
Therapeutic modalities
  Compression   446-447
  Continuous passive motion machine   448
  Cyrotherapy   426-430
  Deep thermotherapy   434-439
  Electrotherapy   448-459
  Hydrotherapy   440-443
  Massage   459-461
  Principles of heat transfer   425-426
  Superficial thermotherapy   430-433
  Traction   444-446
  Ultraviolet light   439-440
Therapeutic positioning in pediatrics   213
Thermotherapy
  Diathermy   437-439
  Fluidotherapy   431-432, 438
  Hot packs   430-431, 438
  Infrared lamp   432, 438
  Paraffin   432-433, 438
  Ultrasound   434-437, 438
  Ultraviolet light   439-443
Thomas test   97
Thompson test   100
Thoracentesis   257
Thoracic outlet syndrome
  Special tests   93
  Template   566, 672-673
Thoracolumbar spine
  Articulations   61
  Capsular pattern   61, 72
  Close/open packed position   61, 71
  Goniometric technique   89-90
  Muscle action   48, 61
  Orthoses   114
  Osteokinematic motions   61
  Primary structures   61-62
  Range of motion norms   82
  Special tests   92, 101
Thoracolumbosacral orthosis   114
Thrombolytic agents   259
Thrombus   182
Thyroid gland   337, 340, 341-343
Tibial torsion test   100

# Academic Review Index

**Tibiofemoral joint**
Arthro/osteokinematics  55, 102
Articulations  55
Capsular pattern  55, 72
Close/open packed position  55, 71
Muscle action  49, 56
**Tibiofibular joint**
Arthro/osteokinematics  102
Capsular pattern  72
Distal tibiofibular joint  57
**Tics**  165
**Tight retinacular ligament test**  95
**Timed get up and go test**  171
**Tinea pedis**  332
**Tinel's sign (elbow)**  95
**Tinel's sign (wrist)**  96
**Tinetti performance oriented mobility assessment**  171
**Tissue and tumor classification**  365
**Tonic labyrinthine reflex**  208
**Total hip arthroplasty**  109-110
Template  567, 674-675
**Total knee arthroplasty**  110
Template  567, 676-677
**Total shoulder arthroplasty**
Template  567, 678-679
**Tracheostomy**  263
**Tracheostomy tube**  262
**Traction**
Mechanical cervical traction  445-446
Mechanical lumbar traction  444-445
Skeletal traction  421-422
**Transdisciplinary team**  518
**Transcutaneous electrical stimulation (TENS)**  453-454
**Transfemoral amputation**  115
Template  567, 680-681
**Transfers**
Communication  405
Guidelines  405-406
Levels of physical assistance  405
Types  406-408
**Transient ischemic attack (TIA)**  181
**Transtibial amputation**  115
Template  567, 682-683
**Traumatic brain injury**
Glasgow coma scale  206
Levels of consciousness  205
Rancho Los Amigos Levels of Cognitive Functioning  205-206
Template  567, 684-685
Types  205
**Tremor**  165
**Trendelenburg gait pattern**  80
**Trendelenburg test**  98
**Tripod sign**  97

**True leg length discrepancy test**  100
**Tumor**  374
**Turgor**  326
**Ulcers**  315-319, 326
**Ulnohumeral joint**
Arthro/osteokinematics  51, 101
Articulations  51
Capsular pattern  51, 72
Close/open packed position  51, 71
**Ultrasound**  434-438
**Unilateral neglect**  196
**Upper limb tension test**  93-94
**Upper motor neuron disease**  164
**Urinary catheters**  422
**Urinary incontinence (see Incontinence)**
**Urinary stress incontinence**
Template  567, 686-687
**Urinary tract infection**  359
**Uterus**  354, 356
**Uterine prolapse**  356
**Valgus stress test (elbow)**  94
**Valgus stress test (knee)**  99
**Validity**  523-524, 526, 532
**Valsalva maneuver**  238
**Valve replacement**  260
**Valvular heart disease**  249
**Vapocoolant spray**  429-430
**Varus stress test (elbow)**  94
**Varus stress test (knee)**  99
**Vaulting gait pattern**  80
**Venography**  257, 423
**Venous insufficiency ulcers**  316-317
**Ventilation-perfusion scan**  257
**Ventricular arrhythmias**  271
**Ventricular assist devices**  261
**Ventricular septal defect (VSD)**  245
**Vertebral artery test**  101
**Vestibular rehabilitation**  171-172
**Vestibuloocular reflex (VOR)**  167
**Vestibulospinal reflex (VSR)**  167
**Vestibulospinal tract**  145
**Vertigo**
Benign paroxysmal positional vertigo (BPPV)  168
Dix-Hallpike test  168
Etiologies  168
Nystagmus  169
**Vibration**  281-284
**Visual analogue scale**  63
**Vitamins**  381-383
**Voice sounds**
Bronchophony  267
Egophony  267
Whispered pectoriloquy  267

# Academic Review Index

**Wagner ulcer grade classification system**  318
**Waist circumference**  278
**Walker**  416, 419
**Walking (stepping) reflex**  209
**Weight bearing**
  Full weight bearing (FWB)  417
  Non-weight bearing (NWB)  417
  Partial weight bearing (PWB)  417
  Toe touch weight bearing (TTWB)  417
  Weight bearing as tolerated (WBAT)  417
**Wernicke's aphasia**  172
**Wet-to-dry dressings**  321
**Wheelchair**
  Accessibility requirements  491
  Measurements  408-409
  Mobility  414
  Prescription  410-413
**Wheeze**  267
**Whispered pectoriloquy**  267
**Wilms' tumor**  370
**Wilson's disease**  333-334
**Wounds**
  Assessment  316, 317-321
  Classification by depth  317
  Debridement  321
  Dressings  323-325
  Exudate classification  319
  Modalities and physical agents  322-323
  Necrotic tissue types  320
  Pressure ulcer staging  318
  Red-Yellow-Black system  321
  Skin care  325-326
  Types  315-317
  Wagner ulcer grade classification system  318
**Wound healing**
  Phases  313
  Healing by intention  314
  Factors that influence  314-315
**Wound irrigation**  321
**Wright test**  93
**Wrist joint**
  Arthro/osteokinematics  52, 102
  Articulations  52
  Capsular pattern  52, 72
  Close/open packed positions  52, 71
  Goniometric technique  84-85
  Muscle action  49, 52
  Primary structures  52
  Range of motion norms  82
  Special tests  95-96
**X-ray**  424
**Yergason's test**  92

**Zone of injury**
  Zone of coagulation  327
  Zone of hyperemia  327
  Zone of stasis  327
**Zone of preservation**  203
**Zygapophyseal joints**
  Cervical spine  60
  Thoracolumbar spine  61

# PTEXAM: The Complete Study Guide

The new edition is the most comprehensive resource available for the NPTE. The resource is a virtual visual delight with full color and hundreds of images. The detailed academic review section includes chapter essentials and proficiency exercises to ensure student mastery of critical NPTE content.

**PTEXAM: The Complete Study Guide** includes 600 clinically-oriented questions with expansive explanations of the correct and incorrect answers. Students routinely comment that our multiple-choice questions are extremely realistic and the most consistent with the difficulty level of the actual NPTE.

**Author:** Scott Giles PT, DPT, MBA
**ISBN:** 978-1-890989-32-3
**Price:** $85.00

# SCOREBUILDERS

Your Ticket to Success

www.scorebuilders.com

# Motivational Moment

*Imagine the impact you will make on the lives of your patients during a long and distinguished physical therapy career!*

# Online Advantage

Candidates utilize **Online Advantage** by purchasing an access code that permits entry to a full-length examination for a 30 day period. The elaborate performance analysis summary classifies candidate performance using a Mastery Meter in five content outline and five system specific areas.

**Online Advantage** consists of two distinctly separate offerings:

**Student version** – The student version provides candidates with an ideal opportunity to assess their current examination performance relative to the performance of other licensing examination candidates. Comprehensive summary reports identify both areas of strength and weakness as well as offer specific suggestions for remedial activities.

**Academic version** – The academic version is designed to provide academic programs with the opportunity to administer a comprehensive examination to their graduating students. A detailed performance analysis section generates individual and group data and therefore is an ideal tool for individual and program assessment.

Visit our web site **www.scorebuilders.com** to learn additional information on this innovative product and to view **Online Advantage** research.

# SCOREBUILDERS

Your Ticket to Success

SCOREBUILDERS

# Online Advantage Research Abstract

## TITLE

An evaluation of the usefulness of a comprehensive examination as a predictor of score on the national physical therapy examination

## AUTHORS

Giles, Scott M.[1]; Wetherbee, Ellen[2]

## INSTITUTIONS

1. Department of Physical Therapy, University of New England, Portland, ME, USA.

2. Department of Physical Therapy, University of Hartford, West Hartford, CT, USA

## ABSTRACT

Purpose/Hypothesis: Academic programs use a variety of methods to assist students with their preparation for the National Physical Therapy Examination (NPTE) including comprehensive examinations (CE). Previous research has suggested that CE scores can be used to predict NPTE scores, however, the studies have utilized data from only a single academic program and have used CEs developed by the program's academic faculty. The purpose of the study is to determine if there is a relationship between scores on a commercially available CE (PTEXAM: Online Advantage) and scores on the NPTE.

Number of Subjects: Academic programs using a CE product, PTEXAM: Online Advantage, in 2005-2006 were invited to participate in the research study.

Materials/Methods: Program chairs completed a survey describing how they administered the CE. Additionally, chairs provided data which anonymously compared students' CE scores and their associated scale scores on the NPTE. Descriptive statistics were used to analyze how the CE was administered. Regression analysis was used to identify a correlation coefficient between scores on the CE and scores on the NPTE; and to determine an individual's minimum CE score in order to obtain a NPTE scale score of 600 (i.e., minimum passing score) or greater with 95% confidence. The research study was approved by the University of New England Institutional Review Board.

Results: A geographically diverse sample of 12 physical therapist academic programs representing 332 students participated in the study. Ten (83.3%) of the academic programs offered the CE between 0-3 months before graduation and 11 (91.7%) administered the CE in a computer classroom. Nine (75%) of the academic programs encouraged students to prepare in advance and 8 (66.7%) established a minimum score for the CE. Minimum scores were established based on a variety of methods. A correlation coefficient of .674 was computed when comparing individual CE scores to individual NPTE scores. Linear regression was used to determine that a student who scores 144 (72.0%) on the CE has a 95% chance to score 600 or greater on the NPTE. There were no significant differences in the CE scores of students who were encouraged to prepare in advance or those whose academic programs required a minimum score.

Conclusions: Score on the CE using PTEXAM: Online Advantage was strongly correlated with score on the NPTE. The strength of the correlation suggests predictive validity of the CE and supports the use of CEs in physical therapist academic programs.

Clinical Relevance: A CE that is positively correlated with results on the NPTE may assist educators in identifying physical therapy students at risk for performing poorly on the NPTE. Early identification of "at risk" students has the potential to improve outcomes for academic programs and allow graduates to make more informed decisions on their readiness to take the actual examination.

Keywords: National Physical Therapist Examination, Comprehensive Examination.

*Abstract submitted and accepted for 2008 APTA Combined Sections Meeting in Nashville, Tennessee

# PT Content Master - Flash Cards

Make reviewing essential academic content enjoyable! **Physical Therapy Content Master** is designed to assist physical therapists to possess full command of core academic content using flash cards. Vibrant colors and visually pleasing layouts make the flash cards a perfect learning resource to review academic content.

## Features

• 200 double-sided flash cards covering only the most essential academic content from our entire physical therapy product line.

• The flash cards provide users with the opportunity to frequently review academic content and in the process, commit the information to long-term memory.

**Author:** Scott Giles PT, DPT, MBA

**ISBN:** 978-1-890989-30-9

**Price:** $45.00

# SCOREBUILDERS

Your Ticket to Success

www.scorebuilders.com

SCOREBUILDERS

# Motivational Moment

*Studying for the NPTE is hard work, but you are only months away from experiencing something that you have not experienced in a very long time . . . Positive Cash Flow!*

# On-Campus Review Course

Our review course provides students with the most personal, effective, and efficient method to maximize performance on the NPTE. The course introduces students to challenging multiple-choice questions, recent examination trends, a myriad of study tools, and resources designed to increase mastery of essential exam content. Our goal is to maximize the efficiency of a student's study plan by focusing on critical exam content at an appropriate level of breadth and depth.

**Scorebuilders** offers over 160 review courses annually at academic institutions and is the largest provider of PT and PTA review courses in the United States. Our expert instructors are experienced educators who are superior teachers.

**Participants attending our on-campus review course will:**

- Improve decision making skills when answering challenging multiple-choice questions.

- Develop a comprehensive study plan to maximize efficiency and performance.

- Identify indicators to determine readiness to take the examination.

All participants attending the course receive a detailed course manual that includes sample questions, assessment activities, study tools, and other valuable resources including an application to assist students to select appropriate remedial strategies and determine readiness to take the NPTE.

# SCOREBUILDERS

## Your Ticket to Success

## www.scorebuilders.com

SCOREBUILDERS

# Motivational Moment

*Picture yourself lounging in this hammock in a tropical oasis. Make a list of other possible celebration activities after you pass the NPTE!*

# Applications

## Physical Therapy Content Master*

Physical therapists have the option of utilizing flash cards with an app. The app consists of a content review mode covering the same academic content as the traditional flash cards plus an additional 750 multiple-choice questions designed to assess a candidate's knowledge of the

information within the content review mode. The questions are unique to the app and are not utilized in any other Scorebuilders' product.

**Price: $29.99**

## Physical Therapy Question of the Day**

Question of the Day provides users with a unique daily opportunity to assess their mastery of essential physical therapy content through multiple-choice questions. A complete explanation of both correct and incorrect options is offered for all questions. The app provides users with a method to track their individual performance over time and to compare their results to the relative performance of other physical therapists.

**Price: $9.99 for six-month subscription**

\* Available through the iTunes and Android App Stores
** Available only through the iTunes App Store

# SCOREBUILDERS

## Your Ticket to Success

## www.scorebuilders.com

# Motivational Moment

*If it was easy, everyone would be a physical therapist. Recognize that you still have some work left to do, but are incredibly close to achieving your goal of being a physical therapist.*

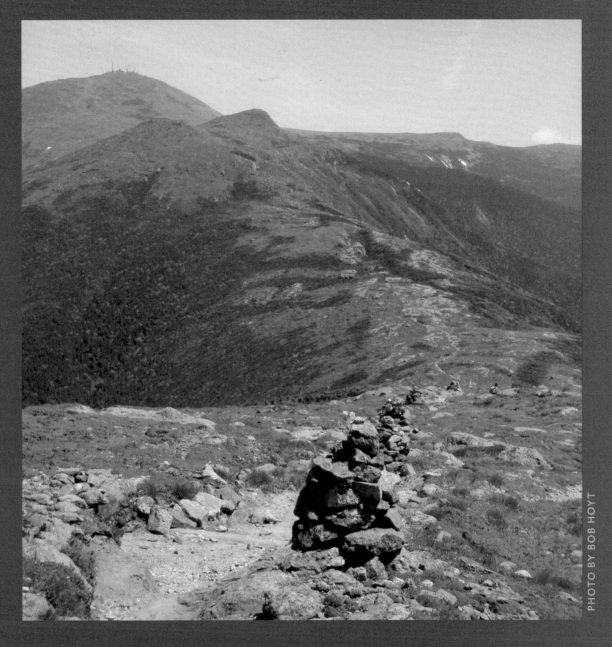

PHOTO BY BOB HOYT

# PTEXAM: The Complete Study Guide Companion CD
## CD Installation Instructions

### System Requirements: Windows

- Intel® Pentium® III processor (Pentium 4 recommended)
- Microsoft® Windows® XP Home, Professional, or Tablet PC Edition with Service Pack 2 or 3, Windows Server® 2003, Windows Vista® Home Premium, Business, Ultimate, or Enterprise (including 64-bit editions) with Service Pack 1, Windows 7 or Windows 8
- 512MB of RAM (1GB recommended)

### System Requirements: Macintosh

- Intel Core™ Duo or faster processor
- Mac OS X v10.4 (Tiger), v10.5 (Leopard), v10.6 (Snow Leopard), v10.7 (Lion) or v10.8 (Mountain Lion)
- 512MB of RAM (1GB recommended)

This application is optimized for higher resolution displays. A minimum of a 1280 x 1024 resolution is recommended.

# Installation Instructions: Companion CD for Windows

### Microsoft Windows 7 and Vista

1. Insert the Scorebuilders–The Complete Study Guide (PT) CD into your computer's CD drive. When the AutoPlay dialog box appears, select the "Run Scorebuilders_Windows_Installer.exe" option.
2. You will be prompted to ensure that you wish to proceed with the installation. If you wish to proceed, select the Install button.
3. You will be prompted to configure advanced installation preferences. No interaction is required to proceed with the default settings. Select the continue button and choose to proceed to step 4.

*If you do not have Adobe Air version 2.0.3 or higher installed on your computer, you will be required to install it at this time. The prerequisite installation files for Adobe Air 2.0.3 are included on this CD and will be installed by default as part of this installation.*

4. Next you will be prompted to review the Adobe Air license agreement. Upon completion of this review, indicate your acceptance by selecting the I Agree button and proceed with the installation.
5. Windows 7 or Vista will now prompt you to ensure your approval of Adobe Air installation on this computer. Select the Install button to proceed. The application is now installed on this computer.

*More detailed installation instructions with associated screen shots are available in the Help section of our web site* **www.scorebuilders.com/help**

### Microsoft Windows XP

1. Insert the Scorebuilders–The Complete Study Guide (PT) CD into your computer's CD drive. When the AutoPlay dialog box appears, it will momentarily prepare for installation.
2. You will be prompted to ensure that you wish to proceed with the installation. If you wish to proceed, select the Install button.
3. You will be prompted to configure advanced installation preferences. No interaction is required to proceed with the default settings. Select the continue button and proceed to step 4.

*If you do not have Adobe Air version 2.0.3 installed on your computer, you will be required to install it at this time. The prerequisite installation files for Adobe Air 2.0.3 are included on this CD and will be installed by default as part of this installation.*

4. Next you will be prompted to review the Adobe Air license agreement. Upon completion of this review, indicate your acceptance by selecting the I Agree button and proceed with the installation. The application is now installed on this computer.

*More detailed installation instructions with associated screen shots are available in the Help section of our web site* *www.scorebuilders.com/help*

## Installation Instructions: Companion CD for Macintosh

**Macintosh OSX v10.4 and higher**

1. Insert the Scorebuilders–The Complete Study Guide (PT) CD into your computer's CD drive. Navigate to the contents of the CD drive by either selecting the desktop icon or opening a finder window and selecting Scorebuilders–The Complete Study Guide (PT) from the list of mounted devices.
2. Initiate installation by selecting the Scorebuilders_Mac_Installer via double click.
3. You will be prompted to ensure that you wish to proceed with the installation. If you wish to proceed, select the Install button.
4. You will be prompted to configure advanced installation preferences. No interaction is required to proceed with the default settings. Select the Continue button and proceed to step 5.

*If you do not have Adobe Air version 2.0.3 or higher installed on your computer, you will be required to install it at this time. The prerequisite installation files for Adobe Air 2.0.3 are included on this CD and will be installed by default as part of this installation.*

5. Next you will be prompted to review the Adobe Air license agreement. Upon completion of this review, indicate your acceptance by selecting the I Agree button and proceed with the installation.
6. OSX will now require you to authenticate with your account Name and Password to proceed with installation. Upon successful authentication, installation will commence.
7. If you selected the default option to start the application after installation, you will see the screen with the Scorebuilders name and logo appear. The application is now installed on this computer.
8. To locate this application post-installation, navigate to your Applications folder, select the SCOREBUILDERS-PTEXAM folder and double-click the Scorebuilders-PTEXAM.air.app.

QUICK TIP - Once the application is running you may opt to keep it in your dock by clicking and holding down the mouse button on the Scorebuilders logo. An additional options menu will appear. Select Options, Keep in Dock for quick dock access to this application.

More detailed installation instructions with associated screen shots are available in the Help section of our web site *www.scorebuilders.com/help*

**SCOREBUILDERS**

Your Ticket to Success

www.scorebuilders.com